OXFORD MEDICAL PUBLICATIONS

Oxford Handbook of
General Practice

Oxford Handbook of
General
Practice

Second Edition

Chantal Simon
University of Southampton

Hazel Everitt
University of Southampton

Tony Kendrick
University of Southampton

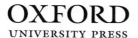

OXFORD
UNIVERSITY PRESS

OXFORD
UNIVERSITY PRESS

Great Clarendon Street, Oxford OX2 6DP

Oxford University Press is a department of the University of Oxford.
It furthers the University's objective of excellence in research, scholarship,
and education by publishing worldwide in

Oxford New York

Auckland Cape Town Dar es Salaam Hong Kong Karachi
Kuala Lumpur Madrid Melbourne Mexico City Nairobi
New Delhi Shanghai Taipei Toronto

With offices in

Argentina Austria Brazil Chile Czech Republic France Greece
Guatemala Hungary Italy Japan Poland Portugal Singapore
South Korea Switzerland Thailand Turkey Ukraine Vietnam

Oxford is a registered trade mark of Oxford University Press
in the UK and in certain other countries

Published in the United States
by Oxford University Press, Inc., New York

© Oxford University Press, 2005

A catalogue record for this title is available from the British Library

Library of Congress Cataloging in Publication Data
Simon, Chantal.

Oxford handbook of general practice / Chantal Simon, Hazel Everitt, Tony Kendrick.—2nd ed.
Includes bibliographical references and index.

1. Physicians (General practice)–Handbooks, manuals, etc. 2. Primary care (Medicine)–
Practice–Handbooks, manuals, etc. 3. Family medicine–Practice–Handbooks, manuals, etc.
[DNLM: 1. Family Practice–Handbooks. 2. Evidence-Based Medicine–Handbooks. 3. Primary
Health Care–Handbooks. WB 39 S593o 2005] I. Everitt, Hazel. II. Kendrick, Tony. III. Title.
R729.5.G4O95 2005   616–dc22   2005015604

Typeset by Newgen Imaging Systems (P) Ltd., Chennai, India
Printed in Italy
on acid-free paper by LegoPrint S.p.A

ISBN 0–19–856581–X (flexicover: alk. paper)
     978–0–19–856581–9 (flexicover: alk. paper)

10 9 8 7 6 5 4 3 2 1

Preface

This is the second edition of the *Oxford Handbook of General Practice*—so what's changed? When we wrote the first edition, we spent many long hours debating what to include and what to exclude. It wasn't an easy task, as general practice has no boundaries and, inevitably, we excluded topics we should have included and vice versa.

In this edition, we have updated the first edition material: we have completely rewritten the general practice section to include the new GP contract and updated clinical topics in line with new national and international guidelines. As a result of feedback from readers, we have tried to make the text clearer and more evidence-based. We have also included several new topics such as complementary medicine, elderly care, and chronic disease management, as well as expanding some of the pre-existing sections.

We have lost two of our authors. Jon Birtwistle has moved to a new post and no longer works in general practice. Brian Stevenson has retired and is enjoying life to the full travelling the world. In their place, we have gained Tony Kendrick, Professor of Primary Care at Southampton University, as a guest author for this edition. He has a special interest in mental health problems in primary care and has considerably updated that section in this edition, as well as providing invaluable feedback on many other sections.

Having 'test driven' this edition for several months in our own surgeries, we think it is a big improvement on the last but, as always, any feedback is welcomed. A 'comments card' is provided for this purpose or you can contact us via the OUP website:
http://www.oup.co.uk/isbn/0-19-856581-X

July 2005

CS
HE
AK

Acknowledgements

We would like to give special thanks to all the staff in the Department of Primary Care at Southampton University for their patience and tolerance whilst we worked on this edition of the *Oxford Handbook of General Practice*. We would also like to thank all the staff at the Orchard Surgery in Christchurch, Dorset, who have (I think without exception) been asked to comment on sections of this book.

Thanks also go to many others who have read chapters, provided feedback on the first edition, or otherwise contributed (in no particular order): Liz Oliver, Dr. R. Oliver, Dr. D. Rogers, Rita Rogers, Dr. J. White, Dr. I. Wright, Dr. S. Kumar, Dr. A. Wilson, Dr. H. Brown, David Gough, Dr. H. Roberts, Dr. R. Davies, Dr. W. Scott Jupp, Mr. S. Darke, Dr.G. Lewith, Prof. P. Little, Dr. P. Brooke, Prof. P. Durrington, Dr. P. Sawney, Dr. C. Saddler, Dr. E. Kingston, Dr. D.A. Orlans, Mr. M. Uglow, Dr. N. Jones, Dr. F. van Dorp, Deborah Morris, Dr. M. O'Riordan, Dr. K.C.L. Leung.

If there are any omissions from this list, we apologize—please tell us and we will add you to the list at the first opportunity.

Lastly, we would like to thank the many unnamed reviewers, asked for feedback by Oxford University Press, for their criticisms and helpful hints—many of which were very constructive. You will all see some of your ideas incorporated into this edition.

Contents

Detailed contents

18 Neurology

Abbreviations and symbols

Evidence-based superscripts

N   NICE guideline
CE Clinical evidence
G   Guideline from a major guideline-producing body
S   Systematic review or meta-analysis published in a major peer-reviewed journal
C   Cochrane review
R   Randomized controlled trial published in a major peer-reviewed journal
ND Notifiable disease

Referral times

E   Emergency admission
U   Urgent referral
S   Soon referral
R   Routine referral

Handbook symbols

❶   Note
⚠   Warning
📖 OHGP cross reference
🖳 Weblink
☎   Telephone number
♀   Female
♂   Male
🕭 Controversy
1°   Primary
2°   Secondary
↑   Increased/increasing
↓   Decreased/decreasing
→   Leading to/resulting in
~   Approximately
≈   Approximately equal
±   With or without

Standard abbreviations

µg/mcg	Micrograms
AA	Attendance allowance
AAA	Abdominal aortic aneurysm
ACE	Angiotensin converting enzyme
ACTH	Adrenocorticotrophic hormone
ADH	Antidiuretic hormone
AF	Atrial fibrillation
AFP/αFP	Alpha fetoprotein
AIDS	Acquired immune deficiency syndrome
Alk phos	Alkaline phosphatase
ALT	Alanine aminotransferase
ANF	Antinuclear factor
APH	Antepartum haemorrhage
ASD	Atrial septal defect
ASO	Antistreptolysin O
AST	Aspartate aminotransferase
AV	Arterio-venous
AXR	Abdominal X-ray
bd	Twice daily
BMA	British Medical Association
BMJ	British Medical Journal
BNF	British National Formulary
BP	Blood pressure
bpm	Beats per minute
Ca^{2+}	Calcium
CABG	Coronary artery bypass graft
CCF	Congestive cardiac failure
CHD	Coronary heart disease
CNS	Central nervous system
COC	Combined oral contraceptive
COPD	Chronic obstructive airways disease
Cr	Creatinine
CRP	C-reactive protein
CT	Computerized tomography
CVA	Cerebrovascular accident
CVD	Cardiovascular disease
CVS	Cardiovascular system
CXR	Chest X-ray
d.	Days
DIP	Distal interphalangeal

DLA	Disability living allowance
DM	Diabetes mellitus
DN	District nurse
DoH	Department of Health
DRE	Digital rectal examination
DTB	Drugs and Therapeutics Bulletin
DVLA	Driver and Vehicle Licensing Authority
DVT	Deep vein thrombosis
EBV	Epstein-Barr virus
ECG	Electrocardiogram
Echo	Echocardiogram
EEG	Electroencephalogram
ENT	Ear, nose, and throat
ESR	Erythrocyte sedimentation rate
ESRF	End-stage renal failure
FBC	Full blood count
FH	Family history
FSH	Follicle stimulating hormone
g	Grams
GA	General anaesthetic
GGT/γGT	Gamma glutamyl transferase
GI	Gastrointestinal
GMC	General Medical Council
GP	General practitioner
GPC	General Practitioner Committee
GTT	Glucose tolerance test
GU	Genito-urinary
GUM	Genito-urinary medicine
h.	Hours
Hb	Haemoglobin
HBsAg	Hepatitis B surface antigen
HDL	High density lipoprotein
HIV	Human immunodeficiency virus
HRT	Hormone replacement therapy
HSV	Herpes simplex virus
HV	Health visitor
HVS	High vaginal swab
ICP	Intracranial pressure
Ig	Immunoglobulins
IHD	Ischaemic heart disease
Im/IM	Intramuscular
INR	International normalized ratio

IUCD	Intrauterine contraceptive device
iv/IV	Intravenous
IVP	Intravenous pyelogram
JVP	Jugular venous pressure
K^+	Potassium
kg	Kilograms
KUB	X-ray of kidneys, ureters, and bladder
l	Litres
LA	Local anaesthetic
LBBB	Left bundle branch block
LFT	Liver function tests
LH	Luteinizing hormone
LIF	Left iliac fossa
LMP	Last menstrual period
LRTI	Lower respiratory tract infection
LUQ	Left upper quadrant
LVF	Left ventricular failure
LVH	Left ventricular hypertrophy
M,C&S	Microscopy, culture, and sensitivity
m.	Metres
mane	In the morning
MAOI	Monoamine oxidase inhibitor
MCP	Metacarpophalangeal
MCV	Mean cell volume
mg	Milligrams
MI	Myocardial infarct
min.	Minutes
mL	Millilitres
mmHg	Millimetres of mercury
MMR	Measles, mumps, and rubella
MND	Motor neurone disease
mo.	Months
MRI	Magnetic resonance imaging
MS	Multiple sclerosis
MSU	Midstream urine
Na^+	Sodium
NHS	National Health Service
NICE	National Institute of Clinical Excellence
nocte	At night
NSAID	Non-steroidal anti-inflammatory drug

OA	Osteoarthritis
od	Once daily
PAN	Polyarteritis nodosa
PCO	Primary care organization
PCT	Primary care trust
PD	Parkinson's disease
PE	Pulmonary embolus
PEFR	Peak expiratory flow rate
PET	Pre-eclamptic toxaemia
PHCT	Primary healthcare team
PMH	Past medical history
PN	Practice nurse
po	Oral
POP	Progesterone only pill
PPH	Postpartum haemorrhage
PR	Per rectum
prn	As needed
qds	Four times daily
RA	Rheumatoid arthritis
RBBB	Right bundle branch block
RCGP	Royal College of GeneralPractitioners
RhD	Rhesus factor
RIF	Right iliac fossa
RTA	Road traffic accident
RUQ	Right upper quadrant
sc/s/cut	Subcutaneous
sec	Seconds
SLE	Systemic lupus erythematosis
SOL	Space occupying lesion
SSRI	Selective serotonin reuptake inhibitor
stat	Immediately
STD	Sexually transmitted disease
TB	Tuberculosis
TCA	Tricyclic antidepressant
tds	Three times daily
TFT	Thyroid function tests
TIA	Transient ischaemic attack
u	Units
U&E	Urea and electrolytes
URTI	Upper respiratory tract infection

US(S)	Ultrasound scan
UTI	Urinary tract infection
VF	Ventricular fibrillation
VSD	Ventriculoseptal defect
VT	Ventricular tachycardia
WCC	White cell count
wk.	Weeks
y.	Years

❶ *All other abbreviations are defined in the text on the page in which they appear.*

General practice

What is general practice?

In the early 19th century, when apothecaries, physicians, and surgeons provided medical care, the term 'general practitioner' was applied to apothecaries taking the Membership Examination of the Royal College of Surgeons of England.

Over the past 50y., general practice has established itself as the cornerstone of most national healthcare systems. In so doing, GPs or family physicians have shown the intellectual framework within which they operate is different from, complementary to, but no less demanding than that of specialists.

GPs diagnose illness, treat minor illness within the community, promote better health, prevent disease, certify disease, monitor chronic disease, and refer patients requiring specialist services. General practice is the primary point of access to healthcare services.

Although 80% of patients have seen their GP within the past year, only 13% are referred for hospital care. Everything else is dealt with in the primary care, general practice setting. In order to do this, GPs must:
- Have a working knowledge of the whole breadth of medicine.
- Maintain on-going relationships with their patients—they are the only doctors to remain with their patients through sickness and health.
- Focus on patients' response to illness rather than the illness itself taking into account personality, family patterns, and the effect of these on the presentation of symptoms.
- Be interested in ecology of health and illness within communities and in the cultural determinants of health beliefs.
- Be able to draw on a far wider range of resources than are taught in medical school, including intuition, knowledge of medicine, communication skills, business skills, and our own humanity.

Is general practice a specialty? In English 'generalist' and 'specialist' are opposites. GPs do not have in-depth knowledge about a specific biomedical topic unique to general practice. General practice is, however, an academic discipline with its own curriculum, research base, and peer reviewed journals. Is it therefore a specialty? In many countries, GPs have needed to claim specialist status to achieve recognition for their level of training and to be deemed a separate discipline. In the UK, this recognition has been accomplished through showing expertise of the generalist is complementary to that of the specialist. To achieve equal standing and status as their hospital-based colleagues, GPs must claim to be specialists—but specialists in general and holistic care of their patients.

Defining general practice: The aim of a definition of general practice is to state the core content and function of the discipline. The breadth and comprehensiveness of general practice makes that difficult—so why define it? Potential reasons include:
- To allow doctors performing broadly similar roles to communicate and work together across healthcare systems and national boundaries;
- To set clinical and administrative boundaries if needed;
- To provide a framework for teaching, training, and research.

The definition should be universal and independent of country-specific systems, settings, or working methods but there is no ideal definition as yet.

Commonly used definitions

Leeuwenhorst 1974: 'The GP is a licensed medical graduate who gives personal, primary and continuing care to individuals, families and a practice population irrespective of age, sex and illness. It is the synthesis of these functions which is unique.'

McWhinney 1997: 9 principles of family medicine. Family physicians:
1. Are committed to the person rather than to a particular body of knowledge, group of diseases, or special technique
2. Seek to understand the context of the illness
3. See every contact with their patient as an opportunity for prevention or health education
4. View the patients in their practice as a population at risk
5. See themselves as part of a community-wide network of supportive and healthcare agencies
6. Should ideally share the same habitat as their patients
7. See patients in their homes
8. Attach importance to the subjective aspects of medicine
9. Manage resources

Olesen 2000: 'The GP is a specialist trained to work in the front line of a healthcare system and to take the initial steps to provide care for any health problem(s) that patients may have. The GP takes care of individuals in a society, irrespective of the patient's type of disease or other personal and social characteristics, and organizes the resources available in the healthcare system to the best advantage of the patients. The GP engages with autonomous individuals across the fields of prevention, diagnosis, cure, care, and palliation, using and integrating the sciences of biomedicine, medical psychology, and medical sociology.'

Further information

Olesen et al. (2000) BMJ **320**: 354–7
Heath et al. (2000) BMJ **320**: 326–7
McWhinney (1997) A textbook of family medicine, OUP

General practice in the UK

Today, along with opticians, dentists, and pharmacists, GPs form the 'front line' of the NHS, providing primary medical care and acting as 'gatekeepers' to the secondary care system.

Workload: ~97% of the British population is registered with a GP. Patients register with a practice of their choice in their area—whole families are often registered with the same practice. Once registered, patients stay with that practice for an average 12y. GPs carry out ~300 million consultations/y.—80% at the surgery and 10% at the patient's home. 70% of the GP's total workload is spent with a patient, while >20% is currently spent on administration.

Working hours: 8 a.m.–6.30 p.m. on normal working weekdays. Practices may opt to provide out-of-hours cover too (☐ p.52) or provide services outside those times as an enhanced service (☐ p.35) or as part of routine services. How workload is distributed between individual doctors and other primary healthcare team staff is a matter for each practice to decide.

Primary care provider: New term used to designate any practice providing NHS primary care services.

Partnerships: Traditionally groups of independent contractor GPs working together for mutual benefit. Under terms of the new GP contract, a partnership can become a provider as long as ≥1 partner is a GP. Practices can now include practice managers, nurses, allied health professionals, and pharmacists within their partnership. As the new GMS contract is with a provider not an individual GP, individual doctors within a practice can retire or leave without affecting the contractual obligations of that practice to the PCO (unless the partnership splits). This imparts a new flexibility for practices as they can adapt both the size and constituents of their workforce according to need without it affecting their global income. There is no longer an obligation to obtain permission from the PCO to create a new GP post or to alter GP hours.

Health service bodies: A practice can opt to become a health service body. This means that the GMS/PMS contract becomes an NHS contract (or in Northern Ireland, a Health and Social Services contract). The major difference this makes is that contract disputes are resolved formally in accordance with Dispute Resolution Regulations.

Primary care performer list: List of all doctors deemed competent to provide primary medical care.

GP contract: Currently there are 2 forms of contract which GP practices may have with their local PCOs—General Medical Services (☐ p.34) or Personal Medical Services (☐ p.42). The contract defines the services they will provide, standards to achieve, and payment they will receive.

Organizations important to British general practice: ☐ p.18–21

Independent contractor status: ¾ GPs work as independent contractors under contract to provide core primary healthcare services and additional services as negotiated within the GP contract (see opposite). As such, these GPs are self-employed, running small businesses or practices. They have management responsibilities for staff, premises, and equipment. Since most GPs receive a profit share, the amount each GP is paid depends not only on income to the practice, but also expenditure.

Income

- *Private work:* Sources of private fees include: private appointments (e.g. clinical assistant, industrial appointments); insurance examinations and reports; private medial examinations and certificates (e.g. HGV licence applications).
- *Income from the NHS:* GMS (📖 p.36)/PMS (📖 p.42) contract work.

Expenditure

- *Running costs of the practice:* Staff salaries; cost of the premises (rent, rates, repairs, maintenance, and insurance); service costs (heating, water, electricity, gas and telephone bills, stationery, and postage); training costs; etc..
- *Capital expenses:* Purchase of new medical and office equipment.

Salaried GP: A GP employed by a PCO/practice. PCOs and GMS practices are bound by a nationally agreed model contract, with a salary within a range set by the Review Body. PMS practices can make their own arrangements but are unlikely to be able to recruit GPs if they offer less favourable terms and conditions.

Salaried posts have advantages for those who do not want to commit themselves to long-term working within 1 practice or who do not want to become involved with managerial tasks. Pay tends to be less than that of independent contractors.

GP with special interest (GpwSI): 📖 p.32

GP retainer: Provides an opportunity for doctors with other commitments to maintain medical skills before returning to full- or part-time employment at a later date (usually within 5y.). Practices approved for the retainer scheme must provide adequate education, supervision, and support. Members of the scheme must:
- Have 'right to practice' (📖 p.25) and maintain their GMC registration.
- Work ≥ 12, but ≤ 208 paid service sessions a year (one session = 3.5h.). Most work 2–4 sessions/wk..
- Undertake ≥ 28h. of educational sessions/y. and take a professional journal.

Freelance GP or locum: Works for practices or PCOs by a regular or intermittent arrangement or by providing medical cover on a one-off basis. Tends to be self-employed and charge on a sessional basis. Long-term locums should make their own pension provision or apply to join the NHS scheme.

GP registrar: 📖 p.24

Registration and practice leaflets

The registration process: Patients can apply to join a practice list by handing in their medical card at the practice or completing an application form. For children, a parent or a guardian can make the application.

- **Open lists:** Practices with open lists must consider all applications to join their list. They can only refuse if they have reasonable grounds for doing so which do not relate to the applicant's race, gender, social class, age, religion, sexual orientation, appearance, disability, or medical condition. Reasonable grounds include living outside the practice area. When an application is refused, the practice must inform the applicant in writing of the reasons for refusal.
- **Closed lists:** Practices with closed lists can only consider applications from immediate family members of patients already registered.

Once the practice has accepted the application, it must then inform the PCO. The PCO confirms the application has been accepted in writing to practice and patient.

Newly registered patients: When a patient has been accepted onto a practice list, or assigned to a practice list by a PCO, the practice must offer the patient a consultation for a routine health check (the 'new patient check') within 6mo. of registration.

Routine health checks for other groups: Practices must offer a consultation for a routine health check to all:

- Patients aged 16–75y. who have not been seen by a healthcare professional within the practice in the past 3y.
- Patients aged >75y. who have not been seen by a healthcare professional within the past year.

Temporary residents: Patients may register with a practice on a short-term basis for treatment or advice if they are living temporarily (for >24h. but <3mo.) in the practice area.

Emergency and immediately necessary treatment: A practice must provide services required in core hours for the immediately necessary treatment of:

- Anyone injured or acutely unwell as a result of an accident or medical emergency at any place in its practice area.
- Anyone whose application for inclusion in the practice list (as a permanent or temporary resident) has been refused and who is not registered with another provider in the area.
- Anyone who is in the practice area for <24h.

Removing patients from the practice list: 📖 p.64

List closure: Practices wishing to close their lists to new registrations must inform the PCO in writing. The PCO must then enter into discussion with the practice to provide support to keep the list open. If that is not possible, the list will be closed for a specified period of time. Often closure is requested due to high list size. In that instance, a list size can be set so that the list re-opens when it falls below that limit.

Assignments: PCOs may assign patients to any open practice list if the patient has problems registering with a practice. PCOs can only assign patients to closed lists if all other local practice lists are also closed and an assessment panel has approved the placement.

Practice leaflets: Each practice is required to produce a practice leaflet to distribute to patients. In Wales, the practice leaflet must be in Welsh and English. The practice leaflet aims to inform patients about the practice, the services provided, and how to access them. In addition, it informs patients of their rights and responsibilities. Most practices also take the opportunity to include general health information and information about self-management of minor illness.

The practice leaflet *must* be updated annually *and* include details of:
- The name of the practice (and if the contract is with a partnership, names of partners and status within the partnership; if the contract is with a company, names of directors, company secretary, shareholders, and the address of the company's registered office).
- Names and professional qualifications of those providing medical care.
- Whether the practice teaches or trains healthcare professionals.
- Practice area including reference to a map, plan, or postcode.
- Addresses of all practice premises, telephone and fax numbers, and website address (if any).
- Services available including details of routine health checks for patients aged >75y. not seen in the past year or aged 16–75y. and not seen in the previous 3y.
- Access for disabled patients and, if not, alternative arrangements for providing them with services.
- Registration process.
- Opening hours and methods of accessing services (including home visits) within those hours.
- Out-of-hours arrangements (including who is responsible for their provision) and how to access them.
- Arrangements for dispensing drugs (if applicable) and repeat prescriptions.
- Name and address of any local walk-in centre and telephone number of NHS Direct and details of NHS Direct online.
- Complaints procedure.
- Rights and responsibilities—including the right of patients to express a preference of practitioner (and the way they can express that); responsibility to keep appointments.
- Action that will be taken if a patient is aggressive or abusive.
- Access to patient information and the patient's rights of confidentiality.
- Name, address, and telephone number of the responsible PCO.

Practice in other countries

It is beyond the scope of this book to discuss different systems of healthcare and practice regulations outside the UK. However, in most countries there is a registration body (usually termed the 'medical council') which ensures doctors are qualified and fit to practice; an organization representing the interests of the medical profession generally (often termed the 'medical association'); and separate specialist bodies representing the interests of family practitioners. Details can be obtained from the following websites:

International Directory of Medical Regulatory Authorities:
Lists worldwide medical regulatory bodies and contact details.
🖥 http://www.iamra.com

World Organization of Family Doctors (WONCA): Includes a list of member organizations and contact details.
🖥 http://www.globalfamilydoctor.com

European Union of Family Doctors: Gives overview of different healthcare systems in member states and contacts for member organizations. 🖥 http://www.uemo.org

Medical Association of South East Asian Nations (MASEAN):
Contains contact details for medical associations in Brunei, Cambodia, Indonesia, Laos, Malaysia, Myanmar (Burma), Philippines, Singapore, Thailand, and Vietnam. 🖥 http://www.masean.org

Specific country information

Australia
- Australian Medical Council: 🖥 http://www.amc.org.au
- Australian Medical Association: 🖥 http://www.ama.com.au
- Royal Australian College of General Practitioners:
  🖥 http://www.racgp.org.au

Canada
- Medical Council of Canada: 🖥 http://www.mcc.ca
- Canadian Medical Association: 🖥 http://www.cma.ca
- College of Family Physicians of Canada: 🖥 http://www.cfpc.ca

Hong Kong
- Medical Council of Hong Kong: 🖥 http://www.mchk.org.hk
- Hong Kong Medical Association: 🖥 http://www.hkma.org
- Hong Kong College of Family Physicians: 🖥 http://www.hkcfp.org.hk

India
- Medical Council of India: 🖥 http://mciindia.org
- Indian Medical Association (and IMA College of GPs):
  🖥 http://www.imanational.com

Ireland (Eire)
- Irish Medical Council: 🖳 *http://www.medicalcouncil.ie*
- Irish Medical Organization: 🖳 *http://www.health.ie*
- The Irish College of General Practitioners: 🖳 *http://www.icgp.ie*

New Zealand
- Medical Council of New Zealand: 🖳 *http://www.mcnz.org.nz*
- New Zealand Medical Association: 🖳 *http://www.nzma.org.nz*
- Royal New Zealand College of General Practitioners:
  🖳 *http://www.rnzcgp.org.nz*

Pakistan
- Pakistan Medical and Dental Council: 🖳 *http://www.pmdc.org.pk*
- Pakistan Medical Association: 🖳 *http://www.pma.org.pk*

Singapore
- Singapore Medical Council: 🖳 *http://www.smc.gov.sg*
- Singapore Medical Association: 🖳 *http://www.sma.org.sg*
- College of Family Physicians Singapore: 🖳 *http://www.cfps.org.sg*

South Africa
- Health Professions Council of South Africa: 🖳 *http://www.hpcsa.co.za*
- South African Medical Association: 🖳 *http://www.samedical.org*
- South African College of Family Practice/Primary Care:
  🖳 *http://www.fam-med.org*

USA
- Educational Commission for Foreign Medical Graduates (ECFMG)
  🖳 *http://www.ecfmg.org*
- American Medical Association (AMA): 🖳 *http://www.ama-assn.org*
- Federation of State Medical Boards: 🖳 *http://www.fsmb.org*
- American Board of Family Practice: 🖳 *http://www.abfp.org*
- American Academy of Family Physicians: 🖳 *http://www.aafp.org*

Good medical practice for GPs

'All patients are entitled to good standards of practice and care from their doctors.'
GMC: 'Good medical practice for GPs'

GMC duties of a doctor*

- Make the care of your patient your first concern
- Treat every patient politely and considerately
- Respect patients' dignity and privacy
- Listen to patients and respect their views
- Give patients information in a way they can understand
- Respect the right of patients to be fully involved in decisions about their care
- Keep your professional knowledge and skills up to date
- Recognize the limits of your professional competence
- Be honest and trustworthy
- Respect and protect confidential information
- Make sure your personal beliefs do not prejudice your patient's care
- Act quickly to protect patients from risk if you have good reason to believe you or a colleague may not be fit to practise
- Avoid abusing your position as a doctor
- Work with colleagues in the ways that best serve patients' interests.

In all these matters you must never discriminate unfairly against your patients or colleagues and you must always be prepared to justify your actions to them.

Good medical practice for GPs**

- *Good clinical care:* Provide the best possible clinical care for patients.
- *Maintaining good medical practice:* Monitor, review, and continuously strive to improve the performance of yourself and your practice.
- *Relationships with patients:* Communicate with and listen to views and opinions of your patients; use terms/information they can understand; respect their privacy and dignity at all times.
- *Working with colleagues:* Ensure effective communication channels within and outside the practice; ensure environment for personal and professional development for everyone working within the practice.
- *Teaching and training, appraising and assessing:* 📖 p.28
- *Probity:* Behave in a proper fashion ensuring honesty and openness in all matters. Avoid conflicts between personal and professional roles. Research—📖 p.92.
- *Health and performance of other doctors:* 📖 p.80

---

* Reproduced with permission of the GMC
** Summarized from 'Good medical practice for GPs': 🖥 http://www.rcgp.org.uk

Continuity of care: A patient seeing the same healthcare worker over time. In the UK this has been the norm but continuity of care is becoming less available.

Reasons for continuity of care: A practitioner's sense of responsibility toward his/her patients ↑ with duration of relationship and number of contacts. Continuity builds trust, creates a context for healing, and ↑ practitioner and patient knowledge of each other.

Evidence: ↑ patient and doctor satisfaction, ↑ compliance, ↑ uptake of, preventive care, and better use of resources (time spent in the consultation, discriminatory use of laboratory tests, and admission to hospitals).

Patients' desire for personal care depends on the reason for the encounter. Most find it important to see their own GP for serious medical conditions and emotional problems.

Reasons why continuity of care is becoming less available
Problems balancing accessibility, flexibility, and continuity of care:
• *Doctor factors:* Flexible careers, special interests, and managerial responsibilities all limit the availability of GPs to their patients.
• *Patient factors:* 24-h. society in which patients want to be seen at their convenience rather than when their GP is available makes it impossible to maintain continuous care. For minor problems and emergencies, patients do not mind who they see—as long as they see someone who can deal with their problem quickly.
• *System factors:* Changing roles—nurse practitioners and other healthcare professionals commonly take on tasks which used to be done by GPs; clinical governance structures mean that patients with particular conditions are managed in clinics specifically for those conditions within the practice; other primary healthcare providers e.g. NHS Direct, walk-in clinics, and separate out-of-hours cover arrangements further fragment care.

Rationing: A full discussion on rationing healthcare is beyond the scope of this handbook but with continued innovation, rising demand, and limited resources it will become an increasingly important factor in medicine worldwide. To some extent there is already rationing by default—patients in different areas of the country have access to different services (the so-called 'postcode lottery') and medicines and certain treatments are not provided on the NHS or have very long waiting lists. Government bodies such as NICE are trying to evaluate services and develop guidelines for healthcare professionals about medicines and services which are both clinically and cost-effective. Inevitably this will mean that some groups will feel they are being deprived of the treatment they require. It will remain a contentious issue.

Essential reading
Appraisal and revalidation: 📖 p.30
GMC/RCGP: Good medical practice for GPs 🖥 *http://www.rcgp.org.uk*
GMC: Duties of a doctor 🖥 *http://www.gmc-uk.org*
Hjortdahl (2001) *BJGP* **51**(470): 699–700

The NHS in England

In 1911, the National Insurance Act was passed, ensuring free GP care for all working men. In 1948, the National Health Service (NHS) was formed, giving free comprehensive healthcare for the entire population of the UK, paid for by the taxpayer.

The NHS Plan: Will determine changes in the NHS until 2010. It promises:
- more power and information for patients;
- more hospitals and beds;
- more doctors and nurses;
- much shorter waiting times for hospital and doctor appointments;
- cleaner wards, better food and facilities in hospitals;
- improved care for older people;
- tougher standards for NHS organizations and better rewards for the best.

To achieve these aims, priority areas have been targeted—changes most urgently needed to improve people's health and well-being and diseases that are the biggest killers e.g. cancer and heart disease.

Modernisation Board: Leading the changes. Headed by the Health Secretary, the board has an advisory role and comprises figures from healthcare institutions (e.g. Royal Colleges), clinical staff, managers from within the NHS, and patient representatives.

Task forces: 10 task forces drive forward strategies outlined in The NHS Plan:
- 6 focus on service provision—CHD; cancer; mental health; older people; children; waiting time and access to services.
- 4 focus on how improvements can be made—the NHS workforce; quality; reducing inequalities and promoting public health; investment in facilities and information technology.

Modernisation Agency: Ensures commitments in the plan are translated into reality. The agency helps local NHS staff and NHS organizations, such as hospital trusts and PCOs, improve services for patients. The Modernisation Agency is due to be incorporated into a new agency—the *Institute for Learning, Skills, and Innovation*—in July 2005.

The structure of the NHS: Varies from country to country within the UK. The structure of the NHS in England is described opposite. The structure of the NHS in Northern Ireland, Scotland, and Wales is described on the following 2 pages.

Further information

- *http://www.modernnhs.nhs.uk*
- *http://www.dh.gov.uk*
- *http://www.nhs.uk/England*

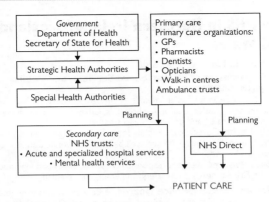

Figure 1.1 Structure of the NHS in England

Structure of the NHS in England: Figure 1.1

- *Secretary of State for Health:* Head of the National Health Service. Accountable to Parliament.
- *Department of Health (DoH):* Sets overall health policy in England, is the headquarters for the NHS, and is responsible for developing and putting policy into practice. It also sets targets for the NHS and monitors performance through its 4 Directors of Health and Social Care.
- *Strategic Health Authorities (StHA):* Key link between DoH and NHS. Responsible for developing strategies for local health services, ensuring high-quality performance, and ensuring national priorities are integrated into local plans.
- *Special Health Authorities:* Provide health services to the whole population of England, not just to a local community e.g. National Blood Authority, NICE.
- *NHS Trusts:* Provide hospital and specialist community services. Services are commissioned by PCTs (see below). Accountable to PCOs. Since April 2004, high-performing Trusts have been eligible to become Foundation Trusts—these Trusts will have greater freedom to control their budgets and provide services tailored to local needs.
- *Primary Care Trusts (PCTs):* Cornerstone of the new NHS—303 PCTs are responsible for planning, providing, and commissioning health services from service providers (□ p.16), and improving the health of the local population. In addition, they are responsible for integrating health and social care. They control 75% of the NHS budget.

The NHS in Northern Ireland, Scotland, and Wales

The NHS in Northern Ireland

The Department of Health, Social Services, and Public Safety (DHSSPS)

- *Health and Personal Social Services:* An integrated service which includes policy and legislation for hospitals, family practitioner services, community health, and personal social services.
- *Public Health:* Covers responsibility for policy and legislation to promote and protect the health and well-being of the population of Northern Ireland.
- *Public Safety:* Encompasses responsibility for the policy and legislation for the Fire Authority, food safety, and emergency planning.

Health and Social Service Boards: 4 Boards cover the whole of Northern Ireland (Eastern, Northern, Southern, and Western). They are agents of the DHSSPS in planning, commissioning, and purchasing services for the residents in their areas, including primary care services.

Health and Social Service Trusts: 18 Trusts provide health and social services.

Future reforms in Northern Ireland: Following recommendations of the Hayes Report (2001), the Northern Ireland Assembly has proposed a radical shake-up of healthcare in Northern Ireland. It proposes reducing the number of acute hospitals and setting up additional local hospitals to deal with non-acute work; removing all 4 health and social service boards; and merging or replacing some of the 18 current health trusts.

Further information: 🖳 *http://www.n-i.nhs.uk*

The NHS in Scotland

Minister of Health and Community Care: Responsible to the Scottish Parliament for all matters relating to the NHS in Scotland.

Scottish Executive Health Department (SEHD): Responsible for health policy and the administration of the National Health Service in Scotland; for social work policy and, in particular, community care and voluntary issues.

Health boards: 15 health boards have responsibility for planning health services for people in their area with responsibilities for: health protection; health improvement (including Health Improvement Plans—HIPs) and health promotion; needs assessment; service development; resource allocation and utilization; and performance management of trusts.

Special NHS Boards: 6 Special NHS Boards have national responsibilities:

- *NHS Quality Improvement Scotland:* Sets and monitors clinical standards.

- *NHS Health Scotland:* Aims to improve health education and public health
- *NHS24:* 24-h telephone advice and information service—📖 p.53
- *NHS Education for Scotland:* Professional postgraduate education.
- *State Hospitals Board for Scotland:* High-security forensic psychiatric care.
- *Common Services Agency:* Specialized services with a nationwide remit e.g. blood transfusion, tissue and bone banking; legal advice; fraud investigation; national statistic and health surveillance.

Trusts: In each health board area (except the Islands and West Lothian health boards) there are 2 types of Trust:
- *Acute Hospital Trusts (AHT):* For acute hospital services.
- *Primary Care Trusts (PCT):* For primary, community, and mental health services and community hospitals. Role includes providing support to GPs; contributing to the Health Improvement Programmes and implementing local healthcare strategies; and delivering and continuing to improve quality and standards of care through clinical governance.
- In addition, there is 1 Scotland-wide Ambulance Trust.

Further information: 🖥 *http://www.show.scot.nhs.uk*

The NHS in Wales: Wales' largest employer (7% workforce)

The Welsh Assembly Government is responsible for policy direction and for allocating funds to the NHS in Wales.

Local Health Boards (LHBs): Replaced Health Authorities in Wales from 2003. 22 boards receive ~¾ of the Welsh NHS budget to plan and pay for health services for people living in their areas. Each board covers the same area as the 22 local authorities and they have a statutory duty to work together to produce strategies for improving health and social care for the people living in their area. LHBs are also responsible for commissioning GP services directly from practices, and community and secondary care services from NHS Trusts.

The Health Commission Wales (Specialized Services): Provides specialist services, operating across the whole of Wales e.g. blood transfusion.

The National Public Health Service: Provides advice and guidance to LHBs on a range of issues e.g. disease protection and control; child protection.

NHS Trusts: 14 Trusts manage hospitals and community health services across Wales; 1 Trust manages an all-Wales ambulance service.

Further information: 🖥 *http://www.wales.nhs.uk*

Commissioning

Commissioning represents a collaborative/cross-organizational boundary process, informed by patients and the public. It includes, at the outset, an assessment of health and social care needs for the local population. Commissioning allows GPs, other health professionals, and members of the public, combining at a local level, to plan primary care health services appropriate for their area.

The role of PCOs: PCOs are responsible for deciding exactly which health services the local population needs and ensuring the continual provision of these services. They do this by providing some services themselves, and commissioning others from other service providers.

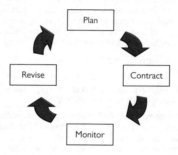

Figure 1.2 The commissioning cycle

Planning: An assessment is made of available resources, together with capacity to meet need. Where identified needs do not have matching resources, stakeholders work together to identify, attract, or develop the necessary resource or capacity to meet that need.

Contracting: Once resource and need are matched, contracts are made to define service within agreed parameters. These parameters include quality, standards, access targets, volumes, prices, and other issues.

Monitoring: Agreed measures are put in place to monitor delivery, and controls are built in to ensure that delivery is kept on track. Funding passes from the PCO to the provider under the terms of the contract.

Revision: If delivery is not on track, agreements are reviewed and revised and plans are adjusted.

Key steps in the commissioning process

Health needs assessment: Long-term forecast, looking 10y. ahead at the health needs of the communities served by a PCO. Helps determine—and justify—commissioning objectives.

Health equity audit: The purpose of a health equity audit is to inform the planning and commissioning process on health inequalities in a local area, to support PCOs in taking decisions about service organization designed to narrow health inequalities and to measure the impact of change.

National targets: The NHS Plan sets the objectives for service improvement to 2005 and 2008. These are the minimum standards that the NHS must reach.

Current pattern of services: A summary of the current services by care group (acute, primary care, mental health, elderly, maternity, children, learning disability, ambulance, etc.). This baseline should include:
• activity information
• access rates per 1000 population
• the recurring cost of services
• a brief description of the current style of service delivery.

Capacity planning: Forecast of demand and capacity in the light of the needs assessment and the current pattern of services. Should be used to test different assumptions e.g. outcome if access rates change; impact of a new provider.

Comparative performance: Both within the PCO and between PCOs. Aims to ensure community is receiving enough services and value for money. Should include:
• relative access rates for services
• comparative cost of services
• the relative spending levels on different care areas.

Local delivery plan: Draws together all the information gathered above to create a clear 3y. plan with intermediate milestones of achievement to be delivered within the available resources.

Service level agreements: Detailed agreements with providers giving effect to the volumes, quality, and costs of care agreed in the local delivery plan.

Practice based commissioning: 📖 p.43

Further information

DoH: The NHS contractors' companion. Part 1: commissioning and contracting
  🖥 http://www.dh.gov.uk
NatPact: The Commissioning friend for PCOs
  🖥 http://www.natpact.nhs.uk

Organizations important to British general practice (A-K)

British Medical Association (BMA): Voluntary professional association and independent trade union of doctors. >80% of practising UK doctors are members. Also runs a publishing house producing books and journals (including the *BMJ*); negotiates doctors' pay and terms of service; provides advice about matters related to work practice; provides educational and research facilities, accommodation, dining facilities, and financial services. The General Practitioners Committee (GPC) is a sub-group of the BMA (see opposite page).

Further information
☎020 7387 4499. ▣ http://www.bma.org.uk

Commission for Healthcare Audit and Inspection (CHAI)/ Healthcare Commission: Acts as an independent inspectorate aiming to provide an integrated approach to assessing the quality of care provided to patients, wherever they are treated, and to assessing the capacity of the organizations delivering healthcare and public health to deliver services of high quality.

• Assesses arrangements in place to promote public health.
• Reviews local healthcare organizations in the NHS every 3–4y.
• Ensures standards set by the Government, through health policies, NSF, and clinical guidance, are met.
• Carries out/assists in investigations and enquiries into serious service failures.
• Carries out independent review of patient complaints (2nd stage in the NHS complaints procedure—▣ p.58).
• Helps NHS organizations draw up action plans to tackle problems or areas of weakness.
• Carries out/publishes studies of the efficiency, effectiveness, and economy of healthcare.

Eventually it is expected that CHAI will also take over the role of the Mental Health Act Commission.

Further information
▣ http://www.chai.org.uk

Commission for Patient and Public Involvement in Health: Partly replaces role of Community Health Councils in England (still exist in Scotland and Wales). It is an independent, non-departmental public body, sponsored by the DoH. Its remit is to ensure that the public is involved in decision making about health and health services by:

• Providing advice and training material to patients' fora (▣ p.21) and setting standards for them.
• Ensuring local people have a say in decisions made about their health service.
• Reporting to Government on how the system of patient and public involvement in the NHS is working.
• Setting quality standards for the ICAS (opposite).

Further information
▣ http://www.cppih.org

General Medical Council (GMC): Licenses doctors to practice medicine in the UK. They investigate complaints against doctors, and have the authority to revoke a doctor's licence if appropriate. They also monitor standards of undergraduate, postgraduate, and continuing medical education and provide information about good medical practice.

Further information: 🖳 http://www.gmc-uk.org

General Practitioners Committee (GPC): BMA committee with authority to deal with all matters affecting NHS GPs, representing all doctors in general practice, whether or not they are a member of the BMA. The committee is recognized as the sole negotiating body for general practice by the DoH.

Further information: 🖳 http://www.bma.org.uk

Independent Complaints Advocacy Services (ICAS): In process of being set up in every NHS Trust and PCO. ICAS will focus on helping individuals to pursue complaints about the NHS through advice and/or advocacy. It will aim to ensure complainants have access to the support they need to articulate their concerns and navigate the complaints system.

Joint Committee on Postgraduate Training for General Practice (JCPTGP)

• Issues certificates to doctors who have successfully completed vocational training for general practice in the UK.
• Issues certificates of acquired rights and equivalent experience (📖 p.25).
• Is responsible for the approval of all general practice training posts in hospitals and GP surgeries.

The NHS National Plan announced the merger of the JCPTGP with the Specialist Training Authority to form a new body, the Medical Education Standards Board, but, at the time of going to press, the JCPTGP is still performing its current functions.

Further information: ☎020 7930 7228. 🖳 http://www.jcptgp.org.uk

Organizations important to British general practice (L-Z)

Local Medical Committee (LMC): Committee of GPs representative of GPs in their area. Since 1999, all GPs (including locums and non-principals) are represented by LMCs. Functions:

- *Statutory:* Consultation regarding administration of the GMS and PMS contracts; involvement with disciplinary and professional conduct committees; representation of GPs as a whole.
- *Non-statutory:* Advice on all matters concerning GPs; communication between GPs; links with other bodies; helping individual GPs.

Further information: 🖥 http://www.bma.org.uk

National Association of Sessional GPs (NASGP): Acts as a voice and resource for all NHS GPs who work independently of the traditional 'GP principal' model. Usually includes GP locums, retainers, salaried GPs, and GP assistants.

Further information: 🖥 http://www.nasgp.org.uk

National Clinical Assessment Authority (NCAA): Special health authority aiming to provide support services to health authorities, PCOs, and hospital and community trusts faced with concerns over the performance of an individual doctor or dentist.

Further information: 🖥 http://www.ncaa.nhs.uk

National Institute for Health and Clinical Excellence (NICE): Special health authority which aims to provide the NHS (patients, health professionals and the public) in England and Wales with authoritative guidance on 'best practice' and thus improve the quality and consistency of health services across the country. It evaluates health technologies and reviews management of specific conditions.

Further information: 🖥 http://www.nice.org.uk

National Patient Safety Agency (NPSA): Special health authority created to co-ordinate the efforts across the UK to report and learn from mistakes and problems that affect patient safety.

Further information: 🖥 http://www.npsa.nhs.uk

NHS Health Scotland: Aims to improve health education and public health in Scotland.

Further information: 🖥 http://www.healthscotland.com

NHS Quality Improvement Scotland: Sets standards and monitors performance; provides advice, guidance, and support to NHS Scotland on effective clinical practice and service improvements.

Further information: 🖳 http://www.nhshealthquality.org

Patients' forum: Set up in every NHS trust and PCO. Made up of local people, the forum's main role is to provide input from patients on how local NHS services are run and could be improved. Each patient's forum has a representative on the trust board.

Patient Advice and Liaison Service (PALS): Provided by all trusts running hospitals, GP, or community health services. Aims to:
● Advise and support patients, their families, and carers;
● Provide information on NHS services;
● Listen to and record concerns, suggestions, or queries; PALS can liaise directly with NHS staff and managers regarding patients' concerns;
● Help sort out problems quickly;
● Direct NHS users to sources of independent advice and support e.g. Independent Complaints Advocacy Services (ICAS) (📖 p.19).

Prescription Pricing Authority (PPA): 📖 p.123

Royal College of General Practitioners (RCGP): Founded to 'encourage, foster and maintain high standards within general practice and to act as the voice of GPs on issues concerned with education, training, research and standards'. Services include: library and educational publications (including *British Journal of General Practice*); representation on committees; research support. 3 grades of membership:
● *Members:* Are entitled to speak and vote at meetings and to use the designation, MRCGP—📖 p.26
● *Fellows:* Highest grade of membership—📖 p.27
● *Associates:* For doctors still in training or those who have not sat the MRCGP examination. Associates can participate in College activities but cannot vote or use the designation, MRCGP.

Further information: 🖳 http://www.rcgp.org.uk

International perspective

Comité Permanent des Médecins Européens/Standing Committee of EU Doctors (🖳 http://www.cpme.be): Non-profit-making international organization made up of European national medical associations. Its objectives are:
- study and promotion of medical training, medical practice, and health-care within the EU
- representation of the medical profession

Commonwealth Medical Trust
(🖳 http://www.commat.org): Non-governmental organization of Commonwealth nations. Main objective is to assist and strengthen capacities of Commonwealth countries to improve health and well-being of their communities, particularly vulnerable members of their populations. Important current concerns include: HIV/AIDS; reproductive and sexual health services; medical ethics; medical migration and recruitment of health workers; and, human rights.

European Union (EU) (🖳 http://europa.eu.int/comm/health): Works to protect and promote the health of European people through its public health programme. Areas covered include: monitoring health indicators across the EU; communicable diseases; rare diseases; injury prevention; bio-terrorism; smoking; nutrition; environmental health; and blood, tissue, and organ donation.

International Committee of the Red Cross (🖳 http://www.icrc.org): Works around the world, on a strictly neutral and impartial basis, to protect and assist people affected by armed conflicts and internal disturbances.

United Nations (UN) (🖳 http://www.un.org): Brings all nations of the world together to work for peace and development, based on principles of justice, human dignity, and well-being of all people. Organizations include:
- World Health Organization (WHO)—see below
- UN Programme on Ageing (🖳 http://www.un.org/esa/socdev/ageing)
- UN Disability Programme (🖳 http://www.un.org/esa/socdev/enable)
- UN Drug Control Programme and Commission on Narcotic Drugs (🖳 http://www.unodc.org)
- Joint UN Programme on HIV/AIDS (🖳 http://www.unaids.org)
- UN Refugee Agency (🖳 http://www.unhcr.ch)
- UN Childrens' Fund (UNICEF) (🖳 http://www.unicef.org)
- World Food Programme (🖳 http://wfp.org)

World Health Organization (WHO) (🖳 http://who.int): Specialized agency of the UN with 191 member states. WHO promotes technical cooperation for health among nations, carries out programmes to control and eradicate disease, and strives to improve the quality of human life.

World Medical Association (WMA) (🖫 *http://www.wma.net*): International organization representing doctors from ~70 countries. Created to ensure independence of physicians, and to work towards highest standards of ethical behaviour and care.

Becoming a GP in the UK

Prospective GPs must normally undertake 3y. vocational training once they have achieved full GMC registration—2y. in hospital posts and 1y. (often as 2 × 6mo. periods) in an approved GP surgery as a GP Registrar (GPR). Part-time training is possible but must be completed within 7y. Options:

- **Formal scheme:** Package of pre-determined posts over a 3y. period including 1y. in a designated training practice as a GPR, and the remaining time in hospital training posts as a Senior House Officer. Hospital posts must cover ≥2 specialties relevant to general practice e.g. paediatrics, general medicine, geriatrics, obstetrics, psychiatry, or A&E.
- **Self-constructed:** The doctor designs his/her own training scheme by applying for individual posts in hospitals and training practices. The training must still consist of 3y. divided between approved hospital posts and a training practice, but there is greater freedom to decide which posts to undertake. Ensure each post is educationally approved.[*]

❶ In the Armed Services, 18mo. are spent in general practice and 18mo. in hospital posts.

Summative assessment: Legal requirement for GP registrars completing vocational training in the UK. Tests:
1. If factual medical knowledge is sufficient to perform a GP's duties.
2. Ability to apply factual knowledge to management of problems in general practice.
3. Effective communication, both orally and in writing.
4. Ability to consult with general practice patients.
5. Ability to review and critically analyse own working practices and manage any necessary changes.
6. Clinical skills.
7. Ability to synthesize all these skills and apply them appropriately in a general practice setting.

There are 4 components of summative assessment
- Trainer's report
- Multiple choice questionnaire (MCQ)
- Assessment of consultation skills, using video
- Written submission of practical work (usually clinical audit)

[*] Educational approval of training posts: For more information, see *Recommendations on the selection and re-selection of hospital posts for GP training*, published by the JCTGP in 1998.

Extended training: Is offered to:

- Doctors who fail summative assessment: Usually offered 6mo. more training.
- GPRs who are not making sufficient progress: If a GPR is unlikely to pass summative assessment in the allotted time, extra training can be applied for through the JCTGP.
- Higher Professional Training Fellows (Scotland only): 2y. period after vocational training is completed, working 4 sessions/wk. in practice while undertaking further training in a specific area e.g. education.
- GPRs with special interests: There are limited opportunities for GPRs to spend longer in their registrar posts, as long as there is a specific objective in doing this (e.g. research) and funding can be secured.

Prescribed or equivalent experience

'Prescribed experience': Training received as a GPR/SHO. Doctors must ensure they obtain a form confirming satisfactory completion of each part of their training—VTR1 forms for GPR posts, VTR2 forms for hospital posts. Forms are available via the JCPTGP website (below). At the end of training, forms are submitted to the Joint Committee on Postgraduate Training for General Practice (JCPTGP—📖 p.19). If satisfied, the JCPTGP issues a 'certificate of prescribed experience'.

'Equivalent experience': Some doctors may have other medical experience (e.g. locum or overseas work) that may count towards their accreditation. The JCPTGP then issues a certificate of 'equivalent experience'.

'Acquired right': Doctors trained in other EEC countries may practise in the UK without undergoing further medical training. They must apply to the JCTGP for a 'certificate of acquired right'.

At present, all certificates issued by JCPTGP are valid indefinitely.

Returning GPs scheme: Intended for qualified GPs who have taken a career break from general practice. Training will usually consist of a mixture of taught courses and supervised practice under the mentorship of a GP trainer. Amount and type of training is tailored to the individual and determined by the local director of GP education. Contact local PCO for more details.

Additional qualifications: There are a number of additional qualifications offered by medical Royal Colleges and faculties that can be obtained. All these qualifications are gained through examinations and include the Membership of the Royal College of General Practitioners (📖 p.26), the Diploma in Child Health (DCH) (📖 p.814), and Diploma in Obstetrics and Gynaecology (DRCOG) (🖥 http://www.rcog.org.uk).

Further information

Royal College of General Practitioners. ☎0207 581 3232. E-mail: info@rcgp.org.uk.
🖥 http://www.rcgp.org.uk
Joint Committee on Postgraduate Training for General Practice (JCPTGP). ☎020 7930 7228
🖥 http://www.jcptgp.org.uk
National Office for Summative Assessment 🖥 http://www.nosa.org.uk

Membership of the Royal College of General Practitioners

Membership of the Royal College of General Practitioners (MRCGP) can be obtained through examination or assessment of performance (MAP).

Eligibility to sit the examination: Anyone eligible to be an independent practitioner of general practice (family medicine), or undergoing vocational training with this in view.

Applying to sit the examination: Application form is available from the RCGP (by mail/internet). Candidates must then apply and pay a fee (currently ~£260) to sit each of the 4 modules of the examination. Covers all aspects of general practice (see Table 1.1). Average pass rate ≈80%.

Modules

Paper 1: 2 sittings each year (May and October) and a choice of venues. 3½ h. written paper consisting of ~12 questions requiring short note answers. Designed to test knowledge and interpretation of general practice literature; ability to evaluate and interpret written material; and ability to integrate and apply theoretical knowledge and professional values within the setting of primary healthcare in the UK.

Paper 2: Can be sat 2x/y.—either separately or together with paper 1. Multiple-choice paper containing questions on: medicine (65%); administration and management (15%), and research, epidemiology, and statistics (20%). A pass in this module exempts the candidate from the multiple-choice component of summative assessment (📖 p.24).

Consulting skills: Assessed by one of 2 methods:
- *Video recordings* of the candidate consulting with patients (who have given their consent to be recorded). Instructions about how to make a video are available from the RCGP. A pass in this module exempts the candidate from the video recording component of summative assessment (📖 p.24).
- *'Simulated surgery'*: The candidate consults with a series of standardized patients who are portrayed by role players. Only available for candidates who can convince the examiners they are unable to make a video recording.

Oral examination: Held 2x/y. in London and Edinburgh. Attendance is conditional on passing the written examinations (paper 1 and 2). Assesses decision making, and the professional values underpinning it, in the contexts of: care of patients; working with colleagues; social role of general practice; and the doctor's personal responsibilities.

CPR certificate: Evidence of proficiency in cardio-pulmonary resuscitation (CPR). Must be submitted before completing the examination. Blank certificates are available from the RCGP.

Membership by Assessment of Performance (MAP): Equivalent to membership by examination and allows experienced GPs (>5y. post registrar practice and working >3 sessions/wk. for >1y.), who can show evidence of good-quality practice, to become members of the College without sitting the membership examination. 3 elements:
• Video assessment or simulated surgery
• A portfolio of written evidence
• A practice visit
Further details can be obtained from the RCGP.

Fellowship of the RCGP

Fellowship by nomination: Awarded to members of the College of >5y. continuous standing following recommendation by existing Fellows and the faculty's provost.

Fellowship by assessment: Any member of the RCGP can apply for fellowship through this route as long as they have been in practice for >5y., including 2y. in the present practice. Candidates must demonstrate they consistently meet high standards in all aspects of general practice. Contact the RCGP for further details.

Further information

Royal College of General Practitioners. ☎ 0207 581 3232. E-mail: *info@rcgp.org.uk.*
🖳 *http://www.rcgp.org.uk.*

Table 1.1 Domains of competence required by a GP

• *Factual knowledge*	• *Verbal communication:* the consultation process
• *Evolving knowledge:* uncertainty, 'hot topics', qualitative research	• *Practice context:* 'team' issues, practice management, business skills
• *Evidence base of practice:* knowledge of literature, quantitative research	• *Regulatory framework of practice*
• *Critical appraisal skills:* interpretation of literature, principles of statistics	• *Wider context:* medico-political, legal, and societal issues
• *Application of knowledge:* justification, prioritizing, audit	• *Ethnic and transcultural issues*
• *Problem-solving:* general, case-specific, and clinical	• *Values and attitudes:* ethics, integrity, consistency, caritas
• *Personal care:* matching principles to individual patients	• *Self-awareness:* insight, reflective learning, 'the doctor as a person'
• *Written communication*	• *Commitment to maintaining standards:* personal and professional growth, continuing medical education

Continuing professional development

The aim of continuing professional development (CPD) is to sustain the professional development of general practitioners and help them to provide high quality patient care throughout their careers.

Doctors need to demonstrate that they have up-to-date knowledge across the spectrum of general practice to become a registered GP, and then need to show they are continuing to update and expand their knowledge to meet requirements of appraisal and revalidation (🕮 p.30). Teaching and training for general practice should:

- Be based on evidence;
- Train the doctor to be part of an integrated and comprehensive healthcare system;
- Have a balanced agenda across clinical topics (prevention, diagnosis, cure, care, and palliation), practice organization and management, team working, audit, and research.

Learning styles: Different people have different learning styles. Depending on a person's preferred learning style, the starting point for an educational initiative will be different:

- *'Why'* (concrete, reflective) learners learn best when they know why something is relevant and how it will apply to their work.
- *'What'* (abstract, reflective) learners learn best when given plenty of time to think about things and link different concepts in their mind.
- *'How'* (abstract, active) learners like to work actively on well-defined tasks and learn by trial and error.
- *'What if'* (concrete, active) learners learn best by applying course material in new situations and solving problems they create for themselves.
- *Serialist* learners like to see the 'big picture' first.
- *Holist learners* like to take learning bit by bit, in small chunks.
- *Individual learners* prefer to learn on their own.
- *Group learners* prefer to learn with others.

Principles of self-directed and adult learning: The learner takes responsibility for defining learning needs; setting goals; identifying resources; implementing appropriate activities; and evaluating outcomes. Adults are motivated by education that:

- Is based on mutual trust and respect
- Allows them to take responsibility for their own learning
- Actively involves them
- Is perceived as relevant
- Is based on, and builds on, previous experience
- Is focused on problems
- Can be immediately applied in practice
- Involves cycles of action and reflection

Personal development plans (PDPs): Outline areas of knowledge in need of update and ways in which these needs can be met. PDPs are an integral part of the appraisal process (📖 p.30). Ask:
* *What* you need to learn—specific, measurable objectives
* *Why* you need to learn it
* *How* you plan to learn it
* *How* you will know *whether* you have learnt it
* How your intentions link to *past* and *future* learning
* The *timescale* for your learning

'SMART' criteria: Learning objectives should be:
Specific
Measurable
Achievable
Realistic
Timed (i.e. there should be a deadline for achieving them)

Methods of identifying learning needs: Numerous—include:
* Gap analysis
* Significant event audit (📖 p.91)
* Objective tests of knowledge and skill (e.g. phased evaluation project (PEP)—see below)
* Self-assessment through diary, log book, or weekly review
* Video assessment of performance
* Criterion-based audit (📖 p.90)
* Patient satisfaction surveys (📖 p.88)
* Risk assessment (📖 p.73)
* Peer assessment

Teaching in general practice: Most GPs are involved in teaching to some extent. This may involve: teaching medical students or GP registrars within the practice; helping to train new practice staff; arranging your own and/or your colleagues' continuing education programme. Teaching can be very rewarding but also brings stresses (e.g. preparation of material). Payments are available to GPs who take medical students into their surgeries for teaching and there are a few teaching posts within UK universities for GPs. Medical students are taught in general practice as:
* *Early patient contact* is helpful to enable students to relate theoretical concepts to the reality of medical practice. General practice settings are especially good for teaching concepts of health and illness behaviour and the effect of family and social settings on illness.
* *Clinical skills* can be taught successfully in general practice and the one-to-one teaching that can be undertaken within GP surgeries is an excellent teaching resource.

As a teacher it is your responsibility to ensure you are competent to fulfil the task. Take steps to acquire proficiency in teaching skills. Local medical schools often run courses for prospective teachers.

Further information

Phased evaluation project (PEP) 🖥 http://www.rcgp.org.uk
Grant J (2000) *BMJ* **354**: 156–9

Appraisal and revalidation

Appraisal: Requires all doctors wishing to practice medicine in the UK to undergo a formal review on a yearly basis. It aims to:

- Set out personal and professional development needs, career paths and goals, and agree plans for them to be met;
- Review the doctor's performance and consider the doctor's contribution to quality and improvement of local healthcare services;
- Optimize the use of skills and resources in achieving the delivery of high-quality care;
- Offer an opportunity for doctors to discuss and seek support for their participation in activities;
- Identify the need for adequate resources to enable service objectives to be met.

Based on the GMC's document *Good Medical Practice* (GMC, 2001), the appraisal will be divided into the following sections:

- Good clinical care
- Maintaining good medical practice
- Teaching and training
- Relationships with patients
- Working with colleagues
- Probity
- Health

The appraiser: Chief Executives of NHS organizations are accountable for ensuring appraisal takes place, and that appraisers are properly trained to carry out this role and are in a position to undertake appraisal of a doctor's whole practice, including clinical performance, and where appropriate, specialist aspects of performance e.g. research, service delivery, or management issues. In general, appraisers for GPs will be other GPs.

The appraisal process

- *Before the interview:* Doctors must prepare an appraisal folder containing information and supporting evidence about their practice and personal needs. Folders should be submitted to the appraiser ≥ 2wk. prior to appraisal interviews to allow adequate time for preparation. An electronic 'toolkit' and further information is available at 🖳 www.appraisals.nhs.uk
- *At the interview:* Doctor and appraiser agree a summary of achievement in the past year, objectives for the next year, key elements of a personal development plan, and actions expected of the organization.
- *After the interview:* A summary document is produced (usually by the doctor being appraised) and a joint declaration signed that the appraisal has been carried out properly.

Further information

🖳 http://www.appraisals.nhs.uk

⚠ **Concerns about performance:** In the first instance, any GP with concerns about their own or a colleague's performance should discuss the matter confidentially with the secretary of their LMC, with the clinical governance lead/performance information manager of their PCO, or with the GMC.

Revalidation:

The regular demonstration by doctors that they remain fit to practise.

Revalidation was due to start in April 2005 but has been delayed to allow routes of revalidation to be reassessed. Every doctor practising in the UK will need to revalidate their GMC licence to practice medicine every 5y.

Routes to revalidation: Doctors will need to be able to show the GMC that they have followed the standards within *Good Medical Practice* relevant to their specialty and practice. It is the doctor's responsibility, not that of anyone else. 2 routes:
• *The appraisal route:* The doctor must show that, during the revalidation period, he or she has worked in a managed environment and has participated in an annual appraisal system (see above). For doctors within managed organizations, 5 sets of completed annual appraisal forms can be submitted to the GMC as evidence to support revalidation. Alternatively, the evidence gathered for the appraisal process could also be submitted to the GMC as evidence to support revalidation. Following the report of the Shipman Enquiry, it is likely that the appraisal process will be made more stringent in the near future.
• *The independent route:* The doctor must show he or she is adopting the standards of *Good Medical Practice* within professional practice and undertaking appropriate continuing medical education or professional development.

Outcomes of revalidation
• *Revalidation:* Licence to practise will remain valid.
• *Insufficient information:* The GMC cannot revalidate the doctor because he or she has not given it enough information. It will ask the doctor to send additional information, and then reconsider the case.
• *Inadequate information:* The GMC is not persuaded by the information the doctor has provided, including any additional information that was asked for, that he or she should be revalidated.

Withdrawing a licence to practise: The GMC will withdraw a licence if:
• The doctor tells them they no longer want it.
• The doctor does not pay the appropriate fee.
• The doctor does not take part in the revalidation process when asked to
• A Fitness to Practise panel directs that the doctor's registration should be suspended or erased.
A doctor has a right of appeal against any decision to withdraw, or refuse to restore, their licence to practise.

Further information
GMC: 🖥 *http://www.gmc-uk.org*

Career options for GPs

Times are changing in general practice. Doctors considering a life as a GP want a more flexible and varied career than in the past. The new GP GMS contract encourages GPs to develop additional clinical and non-clinical interests.

Career options within the NHS

Clinical assistant or hospital practitioner: The GP works within a hospital setting on the wards or in out-patients providing a specialist service under direct supervision of a hospital consultant. Posts usually advertised in medical/GP press ± locally. Generally poorly paid.

GP with special clinical interests (GpwSI): GPs who, in addition to their normal GP duties, provide a specialist service to meet the needs of their local PCO. They might deliver a specialist clinical service beyond the scope of normal general practice, undertake advanced procedures, or develop services. The main difference between a GPwSI and clinical assistant is that the GPwSI receives referrals from other GPs and will decide on the appropriate treatment independently and not under direct supervision of a consultant, but with the support of secondary care. In order to be classed as having a special interest, GPs must:
- Have undertaken particular training in the specialty, or have a proven track record of expertise in the specialty
- Regularly update knowledge through attendance at courses, conferences, or meetings and through reading
- Look after a specific group of patients with the condition
- Audit practice in the specialty area, thereby demonstrating quality of care.
Apply to local PCO. More information: 🖳 http://www.natpact.nhs.uk

Medical adviser or consultant in primary care: Medical advisers or directors in ambulance trusts, NHS Direct sites, etc. Some national NHS agencies have GP advisers or directors too e.g. National Clinical Assessment Authority and National Clinical Governance Support Team. Posts are either advertised or obtained by direct approach.

Providing GMS/PMS ± enhanced medical services—📖 p.34

Providing postgraduate medical education: e.g. GP tutor, GP trainer (1:8 GPs are GP trainers), course organizer. Approach local director or dean of postgraduate medical education.

Working for a local PCO: e.g. serving on a committee, clinical tutor, GP appraiser, etc. Contact local PCO.

Opportunities outside the NHS

Academic posts: A GP may be employed solely by a university or jointly by a university and the NHS. Posts include undergraduate teachers, lecturers, and research posts. Contact local university departments of general practice or look for posts advertised in the medical/GP press.

Clinical sessions for commercial companies and charities e.g. school doctor for a private school.

Complementary medicine: Seek specialist training. Contact representative bodies of the specialty chosen—📖 p.141–156.

Forensic work e.g. police surgeon (🖳 *http://www.apsweb.org.uk*), coroner (☎020 8979 6805), expert witness (🖳 *http://www.ewi.org.uk*).

Media work/medical author: Some sort of professional journalism qualification is useful. The *BMJ* offers a 1y. registrar post for doctors with 3–5y. experience. Courses are also available through the BMA and Medical Journalists Association (🖳 *http://www.mja-uk.org*). If you have an idea for a book, contact the medical commissioning editor of a reputable publisher to discuss your ideas.

Medical adviser posts within GP and other medical organizations: e.g. RCGP, MDU, GMC. Posts may be advertised or appointments made through election or direct approach. Contact the relevant organization.

Medicals for benefits: Nestor Disability Analysis (🖳 *http://www.nda.uk.com*) recruits and administers payments to doctors carrying out disability assessments on behalf of the Department for Work and Pensions (DWP). Applications can be made on-line.

Medical politics: GPs serve on local medical committees (LMCs) on an elected basis. Contact local LMC and ask about standing for election.

Work for government agencies e.g. armed forces as a civilian medical practitioner or the territorial army. Usually civilian posts are advertised in the medical/GP press. For commissioned posts contact service recruitment offices.

Occupational medicine: Contact—Faculty for Occupational Medicine (🖳 *http://www.facoccmed.ac.uk*)

Prison doctor: Posts are usually advertised in the medical/GP press.

Sports medicine: e.g. for professional sportsmen; in private clinics. Doctors are required to have a knowledge of sports injuries, their treatment, rehabilitation, and prevention. They also need to know about other aspects of sport e.g. drugs in sport, nutrition, travel problems. Contact: British Association of Sport and Exercise Medicine (🖳 *http://www.basem.co.uk*), National Sports Medicine Institute (🖳 *http://www.nsmi.org.uk*) or United Kingdom Association of Doctors in Sport (🖳 *http://www.ukadis.org*)

Work abroad: Contact: RCGP International Department (☎0207 581 3232); International Health Exchange (🖳 *http://www.ihe.org.uk*); Voluntary Service Overseas (🖳 *http://www.vso.org.uk*). Overseas posts are also advertised in the medical press.

The General Medical Services (GMS) contract

Although there may be some differences in process in each of the four countries of the UK, the principles of the GMS contract apply to all.

The contract: Made between an individual practice and a PCO. All the partners of the practice, at least one of whom must be a GP, have to sign the contract. It includes:
- National terms applicable to all practices (the 'practice contract')
- Which services will be provided by that practice i.e.
  - essential (see below)
  - additional, if not opted out (see below)
  - out-of-hours, if not opted out (🕮 p.52)
  - enhanced, if opted in (see opposite)
- Level of quality of essential and additional services that the practice 'aspires' to (🕮 p.36)
- Support arrangements e.g. IT, premises
- Total financial resources i.e. global sum (including MPIG if necessary—🕮 p.36) + quality payments (🕮 p.40) + enhanced services payments (see opposite) + premises (🕮 p.70) + IT (🕮 p.76) + dispensing (🕮 p.37)

Essential services: All practices must undertake these services which include:
- ***Day-to-day medical care of the practice population:*** Health promotion, management of minor and self-limiting illness, and referral to secondary care services and other agencies as appropriate
- ***General management of patients who are terminally ill***
- ***Chronic disease management:*** 🕮 p.165–79

Additional services: Services the practice will usually undertake but may 'opt out' of. If the practice opts out, the PCO takes responsibility for providing the service instead. The practice then receives a ↓ global sum payment (🕮 p.36). Services included:
- Cervical screening—opting out → 1.1% ↓ in global sum
- Contraceptive services—opting out → 2.4% ↓ in global sum
- Vaccinations and immunizations—opting out → 2% ↓ in global sum; opting out of childhood immunizations → 1% ↓ in global sum
- Child health surveillance (excluding the neonatal check)—opting out → 0.7% ↓ in global sum
- Maternity services, excluding intra-partum care (which will be an enhanced service)—opting out → 2.1% ↓ in global sum
- Certain minor surgical procedures: curettage, cautery, cryocautery of warts/verrucae and other skin lesions—opting out → 0.6% ↓ in global sum

Out-of-hours: 🕮 p.52

Enhanced services: Commissioned by the PCO and paid for *in addition* to the global sum payment (📖 p.36). 3 types:
- Directed enhanced services: See below.
- National enhanced services: Services with national minimum standards and benchmark pricing but not directed (i.e. PCOs do not have to provide these services) e.g. anticoagulation monitoring; treatment of drug/alcohol abuse; minor injury services.
- Services developed locally to meet local needs (local enhanced services) e.g. enhanced care of the homeless.

Directed enhanced services: Enhanced services under national direction with national specifications and benchmark pricing which all PCOs must commission to cover their relevant population. Include:
- *Access to general medical services:* Meeting national access targets— patients can see a primary care professional in <24h. and a GP in <48h. (does not include weekends or bank holidays and does not have to be GP/primary care professional of the patient's choice).
- *Childhood immunizations:* Routine immunizations for children ≤ 2y. and routine pre-school boosters for children ≤ 5y. Practices must meet a 70% target to claim the lower payment and 90% target to claim the higher payment.
- *Influenza immunizations:* For all patients ≥ 65y. and those in at-risk groups—chronic lung, heart, or renal disease; DM; immunosuppression; patients living in long-term care.
- *Minor surgery:* Injections of muscles, tendons or joints; injection of piles or varicose veins; invasive procedures including incisions/excisions.
- *Access for violent patients:* Providing GMS services for patients removed from a practice list due to violent or aggressive behaviour.
- *Quality information preparation:* Time-limited payment for producing accurate summaries of patient notes—not available from 1.4.2005.

Further detail: Other parts of the GMS contract covered in greater detail in this book include:
- Carr–Hill formula 📖 p.38
- Dispensing 📖 p.37
- GP pay 📖 p.36
- IT 📖 p.76
- Minimum practice income guarante 📖 p.36
- Practices, providers, and partnerships 📖 p.4
- Premises 📖 p.70
- Quality framework 📖 p.40
- Recruitment/retention payments 📖 p.37
- Seniority 📖 p.37

Further information
DoH: The GMS contract. 🖥 http://www.dh.gov.uk
BMA: The 'Blue book' and supporting documents 🖥 http://www.bma.org.uk

GP pay under the GMS contract

A total sum for GMS services is given to each PCO as part of a bigger unified budget allocation. PCOs are responsible for managing the GMS budget locally.

Total financial resources = global sum (including MPIG) + quality payments (📖 p.40) + enhanced services payments (📖 p.35) + premises (📖 p.70) + IT (📖 p.76) + dispensing

The global sum: Major part of the money paid to practices. Paid monthly and intended to cover practice running costs. Includes provision for: delivery of essential services and additional/OOH services, if not opted out; staff costs; career development; locum reimbursement (e.g. for appraisal, career development, and protected time).

Carr–Hill allocation formula: GMS resource allocation formula for allocating funds for the global sum and quality payments. The formula takes the practice population and then makes a series of adjustments based on the profile of the local community, taking account of determinants of relative practice workload and costs—📖 p.38.

Preparation payments: Available for the first 3y. of the new contract (i.e. until 2005/6). Helps practices collect initial data to find out where they are in the quality framework (📖 p.40) and what their aspirations should be. Lump sum allocated on the basis of the Carr–Hill formula to each practice annually.

Aspiration payments: Advance payments to allow practices to develop services to achieve higher quality standards. Practices agree their aspirations for quality points for the following year with their PCO. Aspiration payments are made monthly, alongside global sum payments, and amount to 1/3 of the points total the practice is aspiring to (e.g. if a practice currently has 300 points and aspires to 600 points the following year, as long as there is a realistic chance of achieving that level, it will receive 200 points in aspiration payments that year).

Achievement payments: Payments made for the practice's achieved number of points in the quality and outcomes framework as measured at the start of the following year. Aspiration payments already received are deducted from the total i.e. payment for actual points less aspiration pay.

Minimum practice income guarantee (MPIG): Protects those practices that lost out under the redistribution effect of the new resource allocation formula. Calculated from the difference between the global sum allocation (GSA) under the new GMS contract (see above) and the global sum equivalent (GSE)—the amount the practice would have earned for providing the same service under the old GMS contract ('The Red Book')—see Table 1.2. If GSA < GSE, a correction factor (CF), will be applied, as long as necessary, so that GSA + CF = GSE.

Payment for extra services: Paid to practices that provide directed enhanced services, national enhanced services, and/or local enhanced services to meet local needs (📖 p.34).

Seniority payments: Payment system based on years of NHS service. Superannuable income is used as a measure of that service. Salaried GPs will have seniority reflected in their salary scales.

Dispensing GPs: Any GP, in an area classified as rural, may apply to dispense to any of his patients living >1 mile from the local pharmacist, as long as this would not render the pharmacist's business unviable. A series of fees are paid for providing this service, in a similar way to that in which community pharmacists are funded and in addition to the GMS global sum.

Recruitment and retention packages

Golden hello: lump sum payment to GPs taking up their first eligible post in general practice since qualifying as a GP, leaving the retainer scheme, or returning to general practice after a break. Different arrangements apply in Scotland, Wales, and NI.

Delayed retirement: annual lump sum payment for each year a GP delays retirement after 60y. (i.e. GPs aged 61–64y. are eligible). Different arrangements apply in Scotland, Wales and NI.

Flexible working scheme (FWS): Any GP wishing to undertake a salaried post less < ½ time is eligible. 2 components:
- Payment to employers of flexible career scheme GPs to cover the costs of employing a FWS GP. Level of subsidy ↓ with time.
- Payments to FWS GPs to cover professional expenses.

OOH: 📖 p.52   **IT:** 📖 p.76   **Premises:** 📖 p.70

Table 1.2 'Red Book' payments subsumed by global allocation

• Basic practice allowance	• Minor surgery fees (part)	• Practice staff reimbursements
• Capitation fees	• Child health surveillance fees	• Telephone fees
• Health promotion payments (excluding chronic disease management)	• Emergency treatment fees	• Vaccination and immunization payments (except target payments)
• Night visit fees	• Immediately necessary treatment	• Cervical cytology payments (part)
• Night allowance	• Anaesthetic administration fees	• Primary care work-force review (part)
• Contraceptive service fees (except IUD fees)	• Arrest of dental haemorrhage fees	• Postgraduate education allowance
• Maternity medical service fees (excluding intrapartum care)	• Rural practice payments	• Appraisal and other protected time
• Temporary resident fees	• Chapter 10.5 payments	• Employers' and practitioners' superannuation
• Deprivation payments	• Inducement payments	
• Registration fees		

The Carr–Hill allocation formula

Geographical and social factors result in differing workloads for GPs—see Table 1.4. The Carr–Hill formula allocates payment to practices on the basis of the practice population, weighted for factors that influence relative needs and costs in order to reflect the differences in workload these factors generate.

Age–sex adjustments: Older people and children <5y. require the most GP care. The Carr–Hill formula uses an age–sex curve to adjust payments to practices based on the age and gender of their registered populations.

Table 1.3 Age–sex workload index (using males aged 5–14 = 1)

Age →	0–4	5–14	15–44	45–64	65–74	75–84	85+
Male	3.97	1	1.02	2.15	4.19	5.18	6.27
Female	3.64	1.04	2.19	3.36	4.9	6.56	6.72

❶ A different age–sex curve is used for Scotland

Nursing and residential homes: Patients in nursing and residential homes generate more workload through ↑ travelling time. The workload factor applied is 1.43.

List turnover: Areas with high list turnover often have higher workloads, as patients tend to have more consultations in their first year of registration with a practice. A factor of 1.46 is applied to all new registrations.

Additional needs: In the UK (apart from Scotland), Standardized Limited Long-Standing Illness (SLLI) and the Standardized Mortality Ratio for those <65y. (SMR < 65) are best at explaining variations in workload over and above age and sex. They are related to workload by a complex formula used to make the payment adjustment.

Scotland: SMR<65 together with unemployment rate, elderly people (>65y.) on income support, and households with ≥2 indicators of deprivation are used in the adjustment formula.

Staff market forces factor (MFF): Reflects geographical variation in staff costs.

Rurality: Rural practices have ↑ practice costs. Adjustment is made to payments based on a complex formula using average distance patients live from the practice and population density. An additional adjustment is made for a few small practices in Scotland to allow for economies of scale (small practices incur disproportionately high costs as many expenses—particularly relating to premises—must be met, regardless of practice size).

Table 1.4 Comparison of inner city and rural practice

	Inner city practice	Rural practice
Deprivation	Above average unemployment; workers on low pay; ↑ single parents; ↑ sick and disabled.	1:4 rural households live in poverty. Deprivation is more covert.
Access to care	Highly mobile populations → fragmented care. Non-English speakers (e.g. refugees) have limited access to care. Cultural issues can restrict care.	Public transport is often poor; costs of private transport are increasingly making it impossible for some patients to attend the surgery or hospital. Home visiting rates are ↑ and visiting arranged by geography rather than urgency.
Patterns of illness	Social class gradients are found for many different causes of morbidity and mortality.	Certain conditions are rarely seen in the town e.g. poisoning with organo-phosphate insecticides.
Workload	Social deprivation → ↑ consultation rates, ↓ consultation times, multiple problems, and heavy workload. ↑ land costs, elderly buildings, and ↑ crime rates → poor premises and ↓ patient, GP, and staff morale.	GPs in rural areas take longer to do home visits etc. and may need to travel further to attend meetings or educational events.
Recruitment	Potential recruits are dissuaded from applying due to heavy workload, environment, and high property costs.	Difficulty recruiting due to ↑ working hours, ↓ income, lack of out-of-hours cover (still the case in some rural Scottish practices), and difficulties covering time off for educational activities.

Further information

DoH: The GMS contract—annex D. 🖳 http://www.dh.gov.uk

The GMS quality and outcomes framework

Emphasis is now on rewards for quality as well as quantity of practice. The quality and outcomes framework was developed specifically for the new GMS contract but similar arrangements are in place for those GPs working within PMS contracts (□ p.42). Financial incentives are used to encourage high-quality care.

The domains: The GMS quality framework is divided into 4 domains:
- Clinical
- Organizational
- Additional services
- Patient experience

See Table 1.5

Indicators: Every domain has a set of 'indicators' which relate to quality standards or guidelines that can be achieved within that domain. The indicators were developed by an expert group based on the best available evidence at the time and will be updated regularly. All data should be obtainable from practice clinical systems, and new read codes (□ p.76) are being developed to make this easier. Indicators are split into 3 different types:
- *Structure:* e.g. is a disease register in place?
- *Process:* e.g. is a particular measure being recorded? Is action being taken where appropriate?
- *Outcome:* e.g. how well is the condition being controlled?

Quality points: All achievement against quality indicators converts to points. Each point has a monetary value. A maximum 1050 points is available.
- *Yes/no indicators:* All the points are allocated if the result is +ve and none if it is –ve.
- *Range of attainment:* For most of clinical indicators it is not possible to attain 100% results (even if allowed exceptions are applied), so a range of satisfactory attainment is specified. Minimum standard is 25%. Points are allocated in a linear fashion based on comparison with attainment of the practice against the maximum standard e.g. if the maximum % for an indicator is 85% and the minimum 25%, and the practice achieves 65%, the practice will receive 40/60 (i.e. 2/3) of the available points.

Reporting on quality: Every year each practice must complete a standard return form recording level of achievement and the evidence for that. In addition, there is an annual quality review visit by the PCO. Based on these, the PCO confirms level of achievement funding attained and discusses points the practice will 'aspire' to the following year (□ p.36). The process is confirmed in writing by the PCO and signed off by the practice. The Commission for healthcare audit and inspection (or equivalents in Scotland/NI) checks PCO-wide quality against other PCOs countrywide.

Payment: □ p.36

Table 1.5 Calculation of points for quality framework payments

Components of total points score	Points	Way in which points are calculated
Clinical indicators	550	Achieving pre-set standards in management of: • CHD (including left ventricular dysfunction) • Stroke and TIA • Hypertension • Hypothyroidism • DM • Mental health • COPD • Asthma • Epilepsy • Cancer
Organizational	184	Achieving pre-set standards in: • Records and information about patients • Information for patients • Education and training • Medicines management • Practice management
Additional services	36	Achieving pre-set standards in: • Cervical screening • Child health surveillance • Maternity services • Contraceptive services
Patient experience	100	Achieving pre-set standards in: • Patient survey • Consultation length
Holistic care	100	Reflects range of achievement across clinical indicators—calculated by ranking clinical indicators in terms of proportion of points gained (1–10). Proportion of the points gained by the 3rd lowest indicator (i.e. indicator ranked 7) is the proportion of the holistic care points obtained.
Quality practice	30	Reflects achievement across organizational, additional services and patient experience domains. Calculated in much the same way as holistic care points.
Access	50	For maintaining improved access
Total possible	**1050**	

In 2005/6, the average value of 1 point = £124.60.

Further information

DoH: The GMS contract 🖳 *http://www.dh.gov.uk*
BMA: The 'Blue book' and supporting documents *http://www.bma.org.uk*

---

* Improving Patient Questionnaire (IPQ) (charge payable)—🖳 *http://latis.ex.ac.uk/cfep/ipq.htm* or General Practice Assessment Questionnaire (GPAQ)—🖳 *http://www.gpaq.info*

The Personal Medical Services (PMS) contract

Piloting of a new Personal Medical Services (PMS) contract began in April 1998. It was a voluntary option for GPs and other NHS staff to enter locally negotiated contracts as an alternative to the national General Medical Services (GMS) contract. Originally, the key aims of PMS were to:
- Provide greater freedom to address the primary care needs of patients;
- Enable flexible and innovative ways of working, encouraging greater skill mix and a team-based approach to managing patient care;
- Address recruitment problems by providing a GP salaried option and supporting an enhanced role for nurses within general practice;
- Tackle issues of under-resourcing by attracting GPs and nurses to previously under-doctored areas

The GMS contract (🕮 p.34) is a nationally agreed, locally managed contract. The PMS contract is a locally agreed, locally managed contract. It alters the way the primary care providers, not individual doctors, are paid. As decision making is closer to the patient, theoretically PMS contracts can meet local needs better and are freer to innovate to solve problems.

Current situation: >40% of GPs in England now work under PMS contracts. Even though the GMS contract has recently undergone radical reform, the option to become or remain a PMS practice will remain as an alternative contracting arrangement. PMS is no longer a pilot scheme.

Benefits of PMS: External evaluation of the PMS pilots demonstrated the new arrangements provided greater opportunities for reforming the delivery of primary care.

Elements of the PMS contract: PMS contracts do not necessarily contain all the elements of the GMS contract and may contain others in addition. Practices do not claim for each individual service but are paid to provide a package of services. How the practice provides those services is up to the practice. Most PMS budgets consist of:
- *Core services:* Usually services patients would expect to receive from any GP (equivalent to GMS contract essential services).
- *Additional services:* Both those usually expected from a GP (e.g. maternity, minor surgery, contraception) and those usually provided by community or secondary care services (e.g. community nursing, community based specialist services such as endoscopy, ultrasound etc.) (PMS Plus). These are roughly equivalent to additional services (🕮 p.34) and enhanced services (🕮 p.35) under the GMS contract.
- *Prescribing budget* (optional).

New benefits brought in with the new GMS contract in April 2004 also
apply to PMS contract holders:
- Ability to opt out of out-of-hours care provision (📖 p.52)
- Increased seniority pay (📖 p.37)
- Improved pension benefits
- Human resources improvements
- Increased investment in information technology (📖 p.76)

The quality framework and the PMS contract: Mechanisms for
quality delivery and the quality framework are broadly comparable for
GMS and PMS practices (📖 p.40). PMS practices can apply for aspiration
payments and achievement payments (📖 p.36) in the same way as GMS
practices. However, in order to reflect the local nature of the contracts,
standards PMS practices are working to do not have to be the same as
those contained in the National Quality Framework. Nevertheless, all
standards must be: rigorous; evidence-based; monitored fairly; assessed
against criteria agreed between PCOs and providers; and paid at appropriate and equitable rates.

Specialist PMS: Medical services provided by PMS practices to meet
the needs of specialist groups. The need for patients to be registered for
all 'core' primary care services with that practice has been removed. This
enables practices to develop innovative bespoke models of service delivery tailored to specific needs of groups poorly served in the established
primary care system. Some examples are:
- Primary care services for vulnerable groups e.g. the homeless; refugees.
- Specialist services normally provided in secondary care sector but
  which could equally well be provided in the community e.g. out-patient
  elderly care; home-based palliative care; dermatology; ultrasound.
- Specific service provision e.g. services for violent patients; OOH care;
  teenage contraceptive services; sexual health clinics.

Practice-based commissioning: Plans have been announced to
introduce a system by which practices can purchase services for their
patients directly from service providers. Participating practices will be
given an 'indicative budget' they can use to improve variety, quality and
convenience of services by providing services otherwise based in a hospital; by commissioning treatments not provided by the PCO from other
trusts or local hospitals; or, by buying in services from the private sector.

Further information
DoH 🖥 http://www.dh.gov.uk

The consultation

Good communication is an essential for all aspects of a GP's work.

Potential barriers to effective communication: Lack of time; language problems; differing gender, age, ethnic; or social background of doctor and patient; 'sensitive' issues to address; 'hidden' or differing agendas; prior difficult meetings; lack of trust between doctor and patient.

The consultation: Cornerstone of general practice. Various models exist (📖 p.46). Focuses on successful information exchange. There is no 'correct' way to perform a consultation. Approach will vary according to situation and participants.

'Patient centredness': The patient's viewpoint is considered and integrated into the diagnosis and decision making process. Seems to improve patient satisfaction and may improve health outcomes. Consists of 6 interactive components[*]:
- Exploring the disease and illness experience
- Understanding the whole person in context
- Finding common ground regarding management
- Incorporating prevention and health promotion
- Enhancing the doctor-patient relationship
- Being realistic

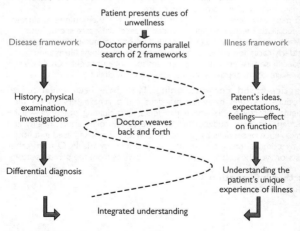

Figure 1.3 The patient centred process*

* Source: Stewart et al. (1995) *Patient-centered medicine: transforming the clinical method.* Sage.

Consultation length: Average consultation length (face to face time) in the UK is 7min (for '10min appointments', face to face time is 8min). Consultation length has ↑ over the last 30y. but is still shorter in the UK (~½ the length) than in Canada or New Zealand. Personality and attitudes influence consultation length—female GPs, older GPs, those with MRCGP, and those with a +ve attitude to mental health problems tend to have longer consultations.

Beneficial effects of longer consultation times:
● ↑ patient and doctor satisfaction;
● improved doctor-patient communication;
● ↑ identification of psychosocial problems and health promotion;
● ↓ reconsultation rates and prescriptions for minor illnesses.

However, as the length of time allocated ↑, the proportion of face to face time ↓.

Consultation rate: Average number of consultations per registered patient per year is 2.5–6.

Factors affecting the consultation rate:
● list size (↑ list size → ↓ rate);
● personal lists (↓ rate);
● new and elderly patients (↑ rate);
● not prescribing for minor ailments (↓ rate);
● social deprivation (↑ rate);
● time of year (↑ in winter);
● ↑ health promotion (↑ rate).

Time keeping: Running late is stressful and frustrating for patients. General practice does not fit conveniently into 10min (or any other size) chunks. Even the best time keepers occasionally run late. Tips:
● *Endeavour to run to time*—start on time; make appointments long enough (e.g. book double appointments for difficult problems, schedule catch up slots in the middle of surgeries, change to longer appointments); break difficult problems or multiple problems up into chunks.
● *If you are running late*—ask reception staff to apologize to patients as they check in and tell them the expected delay.

Consultation models

The consultation process has been extensively studied and many models have been produced—all view it from a slightly different perspective. A brief overview of each is presented here—for more information consult the original texts.

The medical model: Traditional model. History taking → Examination → Investigation → Diagnosis → Treatment → Follow-up. Does not recognize the complexity and diversity of the consultation in general practice.

Balint, 1957: *The Doctor, His Patient and The Illness*—a philosophy rather than a consultation model.
• Psychological problems are often manifested physically.
• Doctors have feelings. Those feelings have a role in the consultation.
• Doctors need to be trained to be more sensitive to what is going on in the patient's mind during a consultation.
Reference: Churchill Livingstone (2000) ISBN: 0443064601

Berne, 1964: *Games People Play*—describes how to recognize behaviours ('games') patients might use and roles patient and doctor might adopt—'Parent, Adult and Child'.
Reference: Penguin Books (2004) ISBN: 0140027688

Becker and Maiman, 1975: Health Belief Model—involves exploration of concerns, beliefs, and expectations of the patient. 5 elements:
• Health motivation
• Perceived vulnerability
• Perceived seriousness
• Perceived costs and benefits of a particular action
• Cues to action—stimuli and triggers for beliefs
Reference: Med Care (1975) **13**:10–24

Heron, 1975: Six Category Intervention Analysis—6 types of intervention a doctor could use with a patient:
1. Prescriptive
2. Informative
3. Confronting
4. Cathartic
5. Catalytic
6. Supportive
Reference: University of Surrey, 1975

Byrne and Long, 1976: *Doctors Talking to Patients*—6 aspects:
1. Doctor establishes a relationship with the patient
2. Doctor attempts to/actually discovers the reason for attendance
3. Doctor conducts verbal ± physical examination
4. Doctor or doctor + patient or the patient consider the condition
5. Doctor (occasionally the patient) detail treatment and investigation
6. Consultation is terminated—usually by the doctor.
Reference: RCGP (1984) ISBN: 0850840929

RCGP, 1976: The consultation can be divided into 'physical, psychological, and social' aspects i.e. in general practice doctors should address emotional, family, social, and environmental factors in addition to the traditional 'organic' medical approach.
Reference: JRCGP (1977) **27**:117

Stott and Davis model, 1979: 'Exceptional potential of the consultation'. 4 tasks:
- Management of presenting problems
- Management of continuing problems
- Modification of help-seeking behaviour
- Opportunistic health promotion
*Reference: JRCGP (1979) **29**:201–5*

Helman's folk model, 1981: Disease vs. illness in general practice
- What has happened?
- Why has it happened?
- Why to me?
- Why now?
- What would happen if nothing where done about it?
- What should I do and who should I consult for further help?
*Reference: JRCGP (1981) **31**:548–52*

Pendleton et al., 1984: *The doctor's tasks:*
- Define the reason for patient's attendance
- Consider other problems (continuing problems and at-risk factors)
- Choose an appropriate action for each problem (involves negotiation between doctor and patient)
- Achieve a shared understanding of the problem (doctor and patient)
- Involve the patient in the management and encourage the patient to accept appropriate responsibility
- Use time and resources appropriately
- Establish and maintain a relationship between doctor and patient
Reference: The New Consultation. Oxford University Press (2003) ISBN: 0192632884

Neighbour, 1987: *The Inner Consultation Checkpoints:*
- Connecting (doctor establishes rapport with the patient)
- Summarizing (doctor clarifies the patient's reason for consulting)
- Handing over (doctor and patient negotiate and agree a management plan)
- Safety netting (doctor and patient plan for the unexpected—managing uncertainty)
- Housekeeping (doctor is aware of his/her own emotions).
Reference: Petroc Press (1999) ISBN: 1900603675

Fraser, 1992: *Areas of competence*
1. Interviewing and history taking
2. Physical examination
3. Diagnosis and problem solving
4. Patient management
5. Relating to patients
6. Anticipatory care
7. Record keeping
Reference: Clinical Method: A general practice approach. Butterworth Heinemann (1999) ISBN: 0750640057

Kurtz and Silverman, 1996: *Calgary—Cambridge Observation Guide.*
5 tasks:
- Initiating the session
- Gathering information
- Building the relationship
- Giving information—explaining and planning
- Closing the session
*Reference: Medical Education (1996) **30**:83–9*

Patient records

General principles

- Be factual, consistent, and accurate. Write records in an indelible fashion as soon as possible after an event/encounter has occurred. Ensure logical sequence; be clear, unambiguous, legible, and concise. Use standard coding techniques if using an electronic record. Wherever possible write notes openly whilst patients/carers are present, in terms they can understand. Date, time, and sign (or otherwise identify yourself) all entries.
- Be relevant and useful:
  - *Information you have on which to base your decisions:* Problems presented to you by the patient; relevant aspects of past and family history; examination findings and test results you already have.
  - *Your impression of the situation:* How you see the problem—may include diagnosis, differential diagnosis, prognosis.
  - *Plan of action:* Negotiated between patient and doctor—may include tests requested, prescriptions given, referrals made.
  - *Information shared and advice given:* Relevant worries or concerns voiced by the patient; information provided to the patient; advice given—especially contingency plans if things don't go to plan; and review/follow-up arrangements.
  - *Include other essential information:* e.g. correspondence to and from other agencies; whether a sickness certificate was issued and, if so, for how long and the reason stated on the certificate; if consent for disclosure of information (📖 p.62) or treatment/examination (📖 p.60) was given.
- Do not include: Abbreviations (especially unconventional ones); jargon; personal views about behaviour or temperament, unless they have bearing on management.

Electronic patient records: 📖 p.76

Confidentiality: 📖 p.62

Amending records: Rectify errors of fact or judgement. Any alterations or additions should be dated, timed, and signed in such a way that the original entry can still be seen. Patients may request correction of information they believe is incorrect—you must record the patient's view. Highlight amendments and reasons for them.

Access to records: Under the Data Protection Act 1998, patients have a right of access to health records which:
- Are about them and from which they can be identified;
- Consist of information relating to their health or condition; and
- Have been made in connection with their care.

⚠ Most doctors' records are included—whenever they were made.

Who can seek access?

- Any competent person may seek access to their own health records including competent children (📖 p.62).
- Any person with parental responsibility may apply for access to records of a child (<18y. or <16y. in Scotland). Where >1 person has parental responsibility, each may apply independently without consent of the other parent.
- Where the patient is incapable of managing his affairs, a person appointed by a court may access records necessary for the appointee to carry out his/her functions.
- A 3rd party authorized by a competent person may seek access to that person's records (but proof of authorization must be provided). If there is doubt, contact the patient to verify consent has been given (📖 p.62).

Access to dead patients' records: 📖 p.62

Requests for access: Nothing prevents doctors from giving patients access to their records on an informal basis provided there is no reason preventing disclosure. Information must *not* be disclosed if it:
- is likely to cause serious physical or mental harm; *or*
- relates to a 3rd party who has not given consent for disclosure (where that 3rd party is not a health professional who has cared for the patient).

If unsure take advice from the BMA or your defence organization.

Formal applications for access must be in writing and accompanied by the appropriate fee. Patients are entitled to a permanent copy of information (e.g. photocopy, print out) which must be accompanied by an explanation of any unintelligible terms. Access must be given within 40d. of receipt of the fee and request. Contact BMA for current fees.

Security of records: Do not leave records (electronic or manual) unattended in easily accessible areas. When not in use, ideally store all files and portable equipment under lock and key. Query the status of strangers. Highlight any concerns to the practice/security manager. Do not reveal how security systems operate.
- *Manual records:* Store files closed and in logical order. Use tracking system to monitor whereabouts of files and return as soon as no longer required.
- *Electronic records:* Do not leave a terminal unattended and logged-in. Do not share log-ins or reveal your password to others. Change passwords regularly and avoid using short or obvious ones. Always clear the screen of a previous patient's information before seeing another. Use a password-protected screensaver to prevent casual viewing of patient information by others.

Further Information

Access to health records by patients. BMA. 🖥 http://www.bma.org.uk
GMC: Guidance on good practice—confidentiality. 🖥 http://www.gmc-uk.org

Telephone consultations, home visits, and referral letters

Telephone consultations

Routine calls: The telephone is a useful way to answer simple queries without wasting valuable surgery time. Most GPs now run telephone clinics where patients are free to ring with their problems, have telephone message books and/or bookable telephone slots in surgery time. Before giving advice, always ensure you have sufficient information upon which to base your judgement. If examination is needed, see the patient.

Emergency calls: Nearly all requests for emergency care are made by telephone. *General rules:*

- *Train surgery staff* to handle distressed callers, recognize serious problems, and act appropriately when such calls are received.
- *Where possible use a single number for patients to access help.* If using an answering machine, ensure the message is easily heard and contains clear instructions. Worried patients find it difficult to cope with complicated telephone referral systems or messages.
- *Take the name and address of the patient.*
- *If a call is from a public telephone box*—take the number.
- *Appear helpful* rather than defensive from the outset. Keep calm and friendly—even in the event of provocation. Worried callers often appear abrupt or demanding.
- *Record* the time of the call, date, patient's name, address and a contact telephone number, brief details of the problem, and action taken (even if calls are being recorded).
- *Collect only information you need to decide whether a visit is necessary.* If a visit is necessary, collect enough information to decide how quickly the patient should be seen and whether extra equipment or help is needed. If a visit is not necessary, decide whether other action would be more appropriate.
- *If giving advice*—make it simple and in language the patient can understand. Repeat to make sure it has been understood. Consider asking the patient/carer to repeat what you've told them. Always tell callers to ring back if symptoms change or they have further worries.
- *If a visit is indicated*—ensure the address is right and ask for directions if you are not sure where to go. Try to give a rough arrival time.
- *In some cases* (e.g. major trauma, large GI bleeds, MI, burns, overdoses) call 999 for an ambulance at once.
- *If a call seems inappropriate*—consider the reason for it (e.g. depression might provoke recurrent calls for minor ailments).

⚠ If in doubt—see the patient

Home visiting: Home visits may be routine checks for housebound patients or emergency visits for patients temporarily unable to get to the surgery. Home visits done in working hours are usually done by practices under their GMS/PMS contract with the local PCO, but in some areas home-visiting services are provided by the PCO and practices are able to 'opt out'.

Safety and security
- In all cases, ensure someone else knows where you are going, when to expect you back, and what to do if you don't return on time.
- If going to a call you are worried about either take someone with you to sit in the car outside or call the police to meet you there before going in.
- If you reach a call and find you are uncomfortable, make sure you can get out.
- Note the layout of the property and make sure you have a clear route to the door.
- Set up your mobile phone to call the police or your base at a single touch of a button.
- Consider carrying an attack alarm.
- If possible, have separate bags for drugs and consultation equipment.
- Leave the drug box locked out of sight in the boot of the car when doing a visit.

Routine visits: Conducted in much the same way as ordinary surgery consultations. Seeing patients in their own environment often gives valuable additional information.

Emergency visits: See emergency calls opposite.
- Try to stick to the problem you've been called about.
- Take a concise history and examine as appropriate.
- Make a decision on management and explain it to the patient and any carers in clear and concise terms they can understand. Repeat advice several times.
- Record history, examination, managements suggested, and advice given in the patient's notes.
- Always invite the patient and carers to ring you again should symptoms change, situation deteriorate, or further worries appear.
- For inappropriate calls, take time to educate the patient and/or carers about self-management and use of emergency GP visiting services.
- Always consider hidden reasons for seemingly unnecessary visits.

Referral letters: Good communication is essential when referring patients to other doctors and agencies. Ensure all referral letters include:
- Address of the referrer (including telephone number if possible)
- Name and address of registered GP, if not the referrer
- Date of referral
- Name, address, and date of birth of the patient (and any other identifiers available e.g. hospital or NHS number)
- Name of the person to whom the patient is being referred (or department if not a named individual)
- Presenting condition—history, examination, investigations already performed with results, treatments already tried with outcomes
- Relevant past medical history and family history
- Current medication and any intolerances/allergies known
- Reason for referral (what you want the recipient of the letter to do) e.g. to repair a hernia, to investigate symptoms, to reassure parents
- Any other relevant information e.g. social circumstances
- Signature (and name in legible format) of referrer

Organization of out-of-hours services

Definition: Out-of-hours (OOH) is defined as 6.30 p.m.–8.00 a.m. on weekdays, the whole weekend, Bank Holidays, and public holidays.

GPs have increasingly moved away from the traditional model of personally providing care 'around the clock'. There are several reasons for this:

- *Changed attitudes of GPs:* GPs find frequent on-call cover too onerous and an unacceptable intrusion into family life.
- *Daytime workload:* the role of the GP has shifted and ever more work comes the GP's way.
- *Number of out-of-hours contacts:* Today, society has a '24-hour' culture. Consequently, the number of GP out-of-hours contacts has risen, as has 'inappropriate' use of A&E services.

Since December 2004, PCOs have taken full responsibility for making sure there is effective OOH provision in the UK.

'Opting out' of OOH: Both PMS and GMS practices can 'opt out' of providing an OOH service. The decision must be made for the whole practice—individual doctors within a practice cannot 'opt out' alone. The cost of opting out for a practice is 7% of the global sum (📖 p.36) (or PMS equivalent).

Provision of services during the OOH period by 'opted out' practices: There is nothing to stop practices that have opted out from offering surgeries or consultations within the time periods specified as OOH. These services can be paid for through the practice global sum (📖 p.36) or, by agreement with the PCO, may be paid for as an enhanced service.

Choice of OOH provider: PCOs can consider a range of alternative OOH care providers, as long as accreditation standards are met. Only where a practice is exceptionally remote will the PCO be able to require a practice to continue providing OOH care. Special arrangements for payment then exist. Several schemes operate side by side:

In-practice rotas: Traditional model of cover. Usually organized in a rota between practice GPs. Largely based on home visiting.

Extended rotas: GPs from a small group of practices on call in rotation.

GP co-operatives: GPs grouped together (often >100 in a co-op) within a district to cover OOH care between themselves. Often, several GPs are on call at any time—1 doing visits; 1 taking calls; 1 seeing patients in a central clinic.

Hospital-based OOH cover: GPs and primary care nurses in A&E departments.

Commercial OOH services: OOH provided by a commercial profit-making organization employing GPs and specialist nurses.

NHS Direct/NHS24: 24h., nurse-led telephone advice service available throughout the UK. It is designed as a first-line service and aims to have links to local primary care and OOH services. There is also an NHS Direct web site and advice booths in public places.

NHS walk-in centres: Walk-in clinics tend to offer nurse consultation and use NHS Direct algorithms. Most are sited in urban areas. They aim to provide easier access to medical care and are increasingly used to cover the OOH period.

Enhanced paramedic services: Providing initial assessment of patients who are not able to get to OOH centres and/or patient transport to OOH centres.

Enhanced community nursing teams: Providing care to patients terminally ill and initial assessment of patients who do not feel able to get to an OOH centre for other reasons.

The future of NHS OOH care: There is a move towards an integrated model of OOH care. One suggestion is that all OOH calls are routed through NHS Direct which will act as a triage system—giving advice or directing callers to the appropriate service (e.g. A&E, ambulance call, GP OOH cover, or routine GP appointment). The use of patient-held 'smart cards' on which each patient's medical record could be stored will allow freer movement of patients between services without the danger of vital information being missed.

Further information

Continuity of care—📖 p.11
DoH: The GMS contract. 🖥 *http://www.dh.gov.uk*
NHS Direct. ☎ 0845 4647. 🖥 *http://www.nhsdirect.nhs.uk* (Separate services for Scotland and Wales can be accessed via this website.)

The doctor's bag

⚠
- The GP's bag must be lockable and not left unattended during home visits.
- Keep the bag away from extremes of temperature.
- If left in the car, keep the bag locked, out of sight—preferably in the boot.

Consider including the following (exact contents will vary according to location and circumstances):

Diagnostic

Stethoscope
Sphygmomanometer
Thermometer
Gloves, jelly, and tissues
Torch
Otoscope
Ophthalmoscope
Tongue depressors
Peak flow meter
Fluorescein sticks
Needles
Syringes
Urine and blood dipsticks
Tourniquet
Sharps box
Patella hammer
Swabs
Specimen containers
Vaginal speculum
Foetal stethoscope/doppler

Administrative

Mobile telephone
Controlled drugs record book
Envelopes
Headed notepaper
Local map
Pathology forms
Prescription pad
List of useful telephone numbers
BNF/Mimms
Obstetric calculator
Peak flow chart/wheel
Continuation cards/adhesive
  strips for notes
Temporary resident records
List of local chemists and OOH
  opening times.

Therapeutic[*]

Injectables

Adrenaline (epinephrine)
Atropine
Amiodarone
Benzylpenicillin injection
Diazepam
Antiemetic e.g.
  prochlorperazine,
  metoclopramide
Antihistamine e.g.
  Chlorphenamine
Hydrocortisone injection
Diuretic e.g. furosemide
Ergometrine
Glucagon ± IV glucose
Opiate analgesic e.g.
  diamorphine, pethidine
Naloxone
Major tranquilliser e.g.
  haloperidol, chlorpromazine
NSAID e.g. diclofenac
Local anaesthetic e.g. lidocaine

Oral drugs

Antacid
Antibiotics (adult tablets
  and paediatric sachets)
Antihistamine
Rehydration tablets/sachets
Aspirin
Paracetamol tablets
Paracetamol suspension
Prednisolone tablets
Diazepam tablets
NSAID e.g. ibuprofen

Other drugs

GTN spray
Bronchodilator for nebuliser
Salbutamol inhaler
Antibiotic eye drops
Glycerol suppositories
Hypostop glucose gel
Rectal diazepam

Other equipment

Airway ± Laerdal mask
Oxygen cylinder and mask with
  reservoir bag
Automated external defibrillator
Nebuliser
Volumatic spacer device
IV cannula
IV giving set and fluids
Antiseptic sachets
Dressing pack
Bandages
Gauze swabs
Adhesive plasters
Scissors
Steristrips
Suturing equipment
Urinary catheter and bag
Thrombolytic therapy (if >½ h.
  from nearest acute hospital and
  have training)

Drugs given from the doctor's bag should be:

In a suitable container *and*
properly labelled with:
• patient's name
• drug name
• drug dosage
• quantity of tablets
• instructions on use
• relevant warnings
• name and address of the
  doctor
• date
• warning 'Keep out of reach of
  children'

⚠ Record origin, batch number and
expiry date of *all* drugs.

⚠ Check drugs 2x/y. to see they
are still in date and usable.

* DTB (2000) **38** (9): 65–8.

The primary healthcare team (PHCT)

The GP does not function alone. Doctors within general practice are an integral part of a team of professionals that care for patients in the community—the primary healthcare team.

Composition of the PHCT: Precise composition depends on overall aims of the team, needs of the practice population, and practice characteristics. Team members include the GPs and:

Practice manager: General manager of the practice, working in liaison with the Partners. Roles include: staff appointments, supervision, training, and dismissals; duty rotas; liaison with outside organizations (e.g. PCO) and other primary healthcare team members (e.g. community nurses and health visitors); maintenance of premises and equipment; and financial planning. Most practice managers have management qualifications.

Practice nurse: Duties can vary but include 'traditional' nursing tasks; health promotion; immunizations; new registration checks; specialist clinics (e.g. asthma, DM, etc.); administration and audit.

Nurse practitioner: Specially trained nurse who takes on clinical responsibility for specific aspects of care she has been trained for (e.g. filtering OOH calls). Seen as a way to alleviate pressure on GPs. Nurse practitioners are at least as effective as GPs in the roles they perform.

District nurse: Qualified nurse who has a community nursing qualification recognized by the Nursing and Midwifery Council. Most work is conducted in patients' homes, particularly in looking after the chronically ill, or those recently discharged from hospital. District nurses are usually employed by local community trusts or PCOs and coordinate their own team of community nurses.

Health visitor: Works with individuals, families, and groups in preventive medicine, health promotion, and education. Health visitors visit all babies after the midwife ceases to attend, carry out developmental assessment checks, and advise on general care and immunization. Some health visitors have a role exclusively for the elderly. Health visitors must be trained nurses and registered as health visitors with the Nursing and Midwifery Council.

Midwife: Important link between hospitals, GPs, and other members of the primary healthcare team in obstetric care. May practice independently when dealing with uncomplicated pregnancies, but are obliged to refer to a doctor in the event of complications. Midwives must be registered with the Nursing and Midwifery Council.

Administrative and clerical staff: Perform all the non-clinical tasks necessary to keep the practice running. Training varies.

Receptionists: Perform an essential role as the interface between the general public and the GPs and nursing staff. Good interpersonal skills are essential. Training varies.

Community pharmacist: Increasing role within practices-managing repeat prescribing, monitoring prescribing practices, and advising on prescribing policy.

Social worker: Helps people live more successfully within the local community by helping them find solutions to their problems. Social workers tend to specialize in either adult or children's services:

- *Adult services:* Roles include working with people with mental health problems or learning difficulties in residential care; working with offenders, by supervising them in the community and supporting them to find work; assisting people with HIV/AIDs; and working with older people at home, helping to sort out problems with their health, housing, or benefits.
- *Children/young people services:* Roles include providing assistance and advice to keep families together; working in children's homes; managing adoption and foster care processes; providing support to younger people leaving care or who are at risk or in trouble with the law; and helping children who have problems at school or are facing difficulties brought on by illness in the family.

Other team members might include dieticians, occupational therapists, physiotherapists, and/or complementary therapists (such as counsellors).

Further information

Association of Medical Secretaries, Practice Administrators and Receptionists (AMSPAR) ☎020 7387 6005 ▣ http://www.amspar.co.uk
Nursing and Midwifery Council (NMC) ☎020 7637 7181 (registrations: ☎020 7333 9333) ▣ http://www.nmc-uk.org
Royal College of Nursing ▣ http://www.rcn.org.uk
Royal College of Midwives ▣ http://www.rcm.org.uk
Community Practitioners' and Health Visitors' Association ▣ http://www.msfcphva.org
British Association of Social Workers ▣ http://www.basw.co.uk

Complaints

Sadly, complaints are a fact of life for most GPs. The most constructive and least stressful approach is to view them as a learning experience and a chance to improve practice risk management strategy. Always contact your local LMC ± defence organization if you are directly implicated in a complaint. Patients who complain generally want:

- Their complaint to be heard and investigated promptly
- Their complaint to be handled efficiently and sympathetically
- To receive a genuine apology if mistakes have occurred
- To be assured that steps will be taken to prevent a recurrence

Time limits for complaints: NHS complaints can only be accepted <1y. after the incident which is the subject of the complaint *or* <1y. after the date at which the complainant became aware of the matter. After that time complaints can only be accepted if there is good reason for delay and it is possible to effectively investigate. A 3y. time limit after the incident (or after the date upon which the claimant became aware that the incident might have caused harm) is placed on civil clinical negligence cases—except for children, who may claim until their 21st birthday.

Conciliation: A way of dealing with complaints that helps to avoid adversarial situations. Either party can ask the local PCO for conciliation, but both parties must agree to it taking place. By bringing the 2 sides together with a neutral conciliator, it aims to:

- explain and clarify matters for both parties
- ensure both parties are really listening to each other
- ensure the process is unthreatening and helpful

Records of complaints: A file on the complaint, including a copy of all correspondence, should be kept separate from clinical records of the patient and, if the patient leaves the practice, should not be sent on with the clinical notes.

Private sector: Most private sector healthcare providers have their own complaints resolution procedures. Patients should contact the organization concerned for details. If dissatisfied when local complaints resolution procedures are exhausted, patients may complain via CHAI (📖 p. 18).

Disciplinary procedures: There is no direct connection between complaints procedures and disciplinary action. If a complaints procedure reveals information indicating the need for disciplinary action, it is the responsibility of the PCO to act or, if there are performance concerns, refer to the NCAA (📖 p.20). If they decide there has been a breach of the terms of service, the PCO can fix a penalty, if appropriate.

Further information

Risk management: 📖 p.73
BMA: 🖳 http://www.bma.org.uk
Medical defence organizations: 📖 p.78

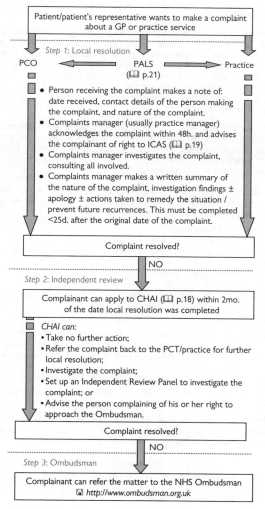

Patient/patient's representative wants to make a complaint about a GP or practice service

Step 1: Local resolution

PCO ◄──── PALS ────► Practice
(📖 p.21)

- Person receiving the complaint makes a note of: date received, contact details of the person making the complaint, and nature of the complaint.
- Complaints manager (usually practice manager) acknowledges the complaint within 48h. and advises the complainant of right to ICAS (📖 p.19)
- Complaints manager investigates the complaint, consulting all involved.
- Complaints manager makes a written summary of the nature of the complaint, investigation findings ± apology ± actions taken to remedy the situation / prevent future recurrences. This must be completed <25d. after the original date of the complaint.

Complaint resolved?

NO

Step 2: Independent review

Complainant can apply to CHAI (📖 p.18) within 2mo. of the date local resolution was completed

CHAI can:
- Take no further action;
- Refer the complaint back to the PCT/practice for further local resolution;
- Investigate the complaint;
- Set up an Independent Review Panel to investigate the complaint; or
- Advise the person complaining of his or her right to approach the Ombudsman.

Complaint resolved?

NO

Step 3: Ombudsman

Complainant can refer the matter to the NHS Ombudsman
🖥 http://www.ombudsman.org.uk

Figure 1.4 The NHS complaints procedure for general practice

Consent

Consent: Implies willingness of a patient to undergo examination, investigation, or treatment (collectively termed 'procedure' on this page). It may be expressed (i.e. specifically says yes or no/signs a consent form) or implied (i.e. complies with the procedure without ever specifically agreeing to it—use with care). For consent to be valid patients:
- Must be competent to make the decision;
- Have received sufficient information to take it;
- Not be acting under duress.

⚠ Under 'common law', touching a patient without valid consent may constitute the civil or criminal offence of battery and if the patient suffers harm as a result of treatment, lack of consent may be a factor in any negligence claim. Never exceed the scope of the authority given by a patient, except in an emergency.

If you are the doctor carrying out a procedure, it is *your responsibility* to discuss it with the patient and seek consent. The task may be delegated but the responsibility *remains yours.*

Information to include
- Reasons why you want to perform the procedure;
- Nature, purpose, and side-effects (common and serious) of proposed procedure;
- Name of the doctor with overall responsibility;
- Whether students or other 'trainees' will be involved;
- Reminder that patients have a right to seek a 2nd opinion and/or can change their minds about a decision at any time.

And for therapeutic procedures/treatments:
- Details of diagnosis and prognosis (if treated and if untreated);
- Management options—including the option not to treat—and for each option an estimation of likely benefits and risks, and probability of success;
- Details of follow-up in order to monitor progress or side-effects.

❶ Document if a patient does not want to be fully informed before consenting.

Written consent: It is good practice to seek written consent if:
- The procedure is complex or involves significant risks ('risk' means any adverse outcome including complications and side-effects);
- The procedure involves general/regional anaesthesia or sedation;
- Providing clinical care is not the primary purpose of the procedure;
- It has consequences for employment, social, or personal life of the patient;
- The procedure is part of a project or programme of approved research.

Establishing capacity to make decisions: No-one may make decisions on behalf of a competent adult. Consult guidance issued by the BMA if you need to assess a patient's capacity to make a decision (e.g. dementia, major psychiatric illness, mental handicap). If in doubt, seek legal advice.

Mentally incapacitated adults: No-one can give or withhold consent to a procedure on behalf of a mentally incapacitated adult[*]. First assess the patient's capacity to make an informed decision about the procedure. If the patient lacks capacity to decide, provided they comply, you may carry out any procedure you judge to be in their best interests, unless it has been refused in a valid and applicable advance directive. If the patient does not comply, you may compulsorily treat only within the safeguards laid down by the Mental Health Act 1983 (📖 p.986).

Advance statements: 📖 p.207

Children (<16y.): A competent child is able to understand the nature, purpose, and possible consequences of a proposed procedure, as well as the consequences of not undergoing that procedure. This is termed 'Gillick competence' after the court case in which the principle was established (Gillick v West Norfolk and Wisbech AHA [1986] FLR 224).

A competent child may consent to treatment . However, if treatment is refused, a parent or court may authorize procedures in the child's best interests[**]. Where a child is not judged competent, *only* a person with parental responsibility may authorize/refuse investigations or treatment. If in doubt, seek legal advice.

Emergencies: When consent cannot be obtained, you may provide medical treatment, provided it is limited to what is immediately necessary to save life or avoid significant deterioration in the patient's health. Respect the terms of any advance statement/living will you are aware of.

Further information

DoH Guidance: 🖥 http://www.dh.gov.uk
BMA: Consent toolkit. Available from 🖥 http://www.bma.org.uk
GMC. Seeking patients' consent: the ethical considerations:
🖥 www.gmc-uk.org/standards/consent.htm
BMA/Law Society. Assessment of mental capacity: guidance for doctors and lawyers.
Available from 🖥 http://www.bma.org.uk.

---

[*] In Scotland, a 'tutor-dative' with appropriate authority may make medical decisions on behalf of a patient.
[**] In Scotland, parents do not have this power to overrule a competent child's decision.

Confidentiality

The Human Rights Act (1998) establishes a right to 'respect for private and family life' and creates a general requirement to protect the privacy of individuals and preserve confidentiality of their health records. Respect for confidentiality is also an essential requirement for the preservation of trust between patient and doctor. Failure to comply with standards can lead to disciplinary proceedings and even restriction/cessation of practice.

Caldicott principles for disclosure of patient information

- *Justify the purpose:* Patients may voluntarily agree to identifiable information about themselves being released to specific individuals for known purposes. Implied consent occurs when a patient is aware their personal information may be shared and of their right to refuse, but makes no objection. Patients must have had a realistic opportunity to refuse. If patients refuse, it should be clearly documented and respected.
- *Don't use patient identifiable information unless it is absolutely necessary:* It is not necessary to seek consent to use anonymous information. If in doubt, seek advice from the BMA or your defence organization. Health information used for $2°$ purposes (e.g. planning, teaching, audit) should, wherever possible, be anonymous
- *Use the minimum necessary patient identifiable information*
- *Access to patient identifiable information should be on a strict 'need to know' basis*
- *Everyone should be aware of their responsibilities*
- *Understand and comply with the law* (see opposite)

Special circumstances

- *Children:* Disclosure can be authorized by a person with parental responsibility. Young people mature enough to understand the implications can make their own decisions and have a right to refuse parental access to their health record.
- *Mentally incapacitated adults:* Capacity must be judged in relation to the decision to be made. People with a mental disability can authorize or prohibit sharing of information if they broadly understand its implications. If a patient lacks the ability to understand, decisions must be based on an evaluation of the person's best interests and reflect the individual's expressed wishes and values. A 3rd party appointed by a court may authorize disclosure.
- *The deceased:* Legislation covering records made since 1st November 1991 permits limited disclosure in order to satisfy a claim arising from death. Where there is *no* claim, there is *no* legal right of access to information.

Breaching confidentiality: Only breach confidentiality in exceptional cases and with appropriate justification. This includes discussing a patient with another health professional not involved currently with that patient's care. Wider disclosure to people loosely associated with care (e.g. support staff in residential care settings) requires patient consent.

Situations where breach of confidentiality may be justified

- *Emergencies:* Where necessary to prevent or lessen a serious and imminent threat to the life or health of the individual concerned or another person (unless previously forbidden by the patient).
- *Statutory requirement:* Ask under which legislation it is sought—check the legislation before disclosing if unsure.
- *The public interest:* What is in the public interest is not defined. The BMA has produced guidance.
- *Public health:* Reporting notifiable diseases (statutory duty—📖 p.481).
- *Required by court or tribunal*
- *Adverse drug reactions:* Routine reporting to the Medicines and Healthcare Products Regulatory Agency (📖 p.128).
- *Complaints:* As part of GMC performance procedures involving doctors.

Legal considerations

- *Human Rights Act:* Compliance with the Data Protection Act and common law of confidentiality should satisfy requirements.
- *Common law of confidentiality:* Built up from case law where practice has been established by individual judgements. The key principle is that information confided should not be used or disclosed further, except as originally understood by the confider, or with their subsequent permission, except in exceptional circumstances (see breach of confidentiality—above).
- *Data Protection Act (1998):* Imposes constraints on processing of personal information. Also requires personal data to be protected against unauthorized/unlawful processing and accidental loss, destruction, or damage. Also applies to personnel records.
- *Administrative law:* The extent the NHS can access confidential information to perform its functions is set down in statutes.
- *Health and Social Care Act (2001):* Allows for certain exceptions to confidentiality laws to be made (e.g. for use in cancer registries).
- *Freedom of information Act (2000):* Applies to all NHS bodies, including GP practices. Practices are required to produce a publication scheme detailing all information routinely published by the practice. In addition, members of the public can make written requests to see any information recorded by the practice in any format. These rights are restricted by certain exemptions (e.g. personal data).

Further information

DoH: Confidentiality guidance. 🖥 *http://www.dh.gov.uk*
BMA: Confidentiality and people under 16. 🖥 *http://www.bma.org.uk*
GMC: Guidance on good practice—confidentiality. 🖥 *http://www.gmc-uk.org*
Data Protection Act: 🖥 *www.informationcommissioner.gov.uk*

Removal from the practice list

Removal of a patient from a practice list can be distressing for both patient and GP. In England and Wales ≈ 53,000 patients/y. are transferred by PCOs at the request of the GP; ≈ 1,000/y. because of an act or threat of violence.

❶ Practice policies for removing patients and dealing with threats/ violence should be stated in practice leaflets.

Situations which justify removal
- **Violence**—Physical violence or verbal abuse towards doctor, practice staff, premises, or other patients. Includes violence or threatening behaviour by other household members not registered with the practice and/or pets (e.g. dogs).
- **Crime and deception**—Deliberate deceit to obtain a service or benefit; obtaining drugs under false pretences for non-medical reasons; use of the doctor to conceal or aid criminal activity; stealing from practice premises.
- **Distance**—New residence outside the designated practice area with failure to register with another GP.

Situations which never justify removal
- **Costly treatment**—GPs can apply for an ↑ in their prescribing budget to allow for this.
- **Particular conditions**—If a particular condition demands costly treat-ment, out of area referrals, or expensive equipment, accommodation can be made at PCO level.
- **Age**—General practice is about looking after patients from cradle to grave. Although patients >75y. do incur higher costs, this is reflected in allocation of funds to the practice.

Situations which do not normally justify removal:
- **Disagreement with the patient's views**—Patients must have freedom to choose whether to accept a GP's advice. The GP can try to influ-ence the view but should not remove a patient if he or she fails to concur.
- **Critical questioning and/or complaints**—Complaints to the practice via normal in-house channels can be constructive and help improve ser-vices and do not usually justify removal of the patient from the practice list. However, personal attacks on a doctor or allegations that are clearly unfounded indicate a serious breakdown in doctor-patient rela-tionship and could justify removal (see opposite).

Patients' rights to change doctor: Patients also have a right to change their doctor. They are not required to give reasons or any period of notice and there is no requirement for the GP to be notified.

Other family members: Removal of other family members should not automatically follow removal of a patient from a practice list unless removal of that patient makes ongoing care of the rest of the household impossible.

Irretrievable breakdown of the doctor-patient relationship
The most contentious reason for removal from a practice list. Causes the most problems. As good doctor-patient relationship is fundamental to successful care, it is in the interest of both patient and GP that the patient moves to another practice list if that relationship breaks down. Difficulty arises when the patient sees matters differently.

- *Inform appropriate members of the practice*—Discuss reasons for breakdown in relationship (e.g. chronic stress, mental illness, cultural differences) and factors that contribute to the situation; consider solutions/alterations in procedures which might help.
- *Inform the patient*—Consider arranging a meeting to discuss matters (can be done through the in-house complaints framework). Explain the nature of the problem and elicit the patient's perspective; be prepared to give ground and compromise.
- *If discussion fails to resolve the problem*—Suggest the patient sees another GP within the practice (though discuss the patient's feelings about the possibility of being treated by the ex-GP in an emergency). Consider giving advice about alternative practices in the area. If the situation continues, then consider removal from the practice list.

Removing patients from the practice list
- *Warn the patient*—A practice can only request removal of a patient from a practice list if, within 12mo. prior to the date of its request to the PCO for removal, it has warned the patient that he/she is at risk of removal and explained the reasons for that. Exceptions to this are violent patients, patients who have moved outside the practice area, and those for whom it would not be safe or be impractical to issue a warning.
- *Inform the PCO* (or Health Board/Central Services Agency) in writing of your decision. Give full patient details. Except in the case of violent patients (see below), removal will not take effect until the 8th day after the request is received by the PCO, unless the patient is accepted by, allocated, or assigned to another GP sooner than this. The patient is always notified by the PCO.
- *Write to the patient* about the decision and reason for removal (take advice from your medical defence organization). Include information on how to register with another practice and reassurance that the patient will not be left without a GP. Take care to ensure reasons given are factual and the tone of the letter is polite and informative.

Immediate removal of any patient who has committed an act of violence: Includes actual or threatened physical violence or verbal abuse leading to fear for a person's safety.

- *Notify the police* (or in Scotland, either the police or the Procurator Fiscal) about the violent behaviour.
- *Notify both the PCO and the patient of the removal in writing*— The PCO has a duty to provide alternative primary medical care services by commissioning specialized directed enhanced services (e.g. GPs with secure facilities for consulting).

Further information
RCGP ⓘ http://www.rcgp.org.uk.
BMA ⓘ http://www.bma.org.uk

Eligibility for free primary medical care for people travelling to and from the UK

Eligibility to receive primary medical care in the UK

- Is determined by whether a person is resident in the UK and not related to nationality or payment of NI/taxes.
- Entitlement to free treatment begins on arrival in the UK—there is *no* qualifying period of residency before free treatment starts.
- Anyone coming to the UK intending to stay for <6mo. does not fulfil these criteria.
- A British resident on extended holiday or a business trip would still count as ordinarily resident.
- Someone who has emigrated, but returns from time to time to take advantage of free NHS care, would not.
- Persons leaving the UK for >3mo. should *not* continue to be registered with a GP. The onus is on the patients to inform the relevant authorities and surrender their medical cards.
- Treat UK nationals resident abroad like any other overseas visitor (unless embassy staff, merchant seamen, or in the armed forces).
- Doctors should *not* provide NHS scripts for conditions that might arise whilst the patient is away e.g. traveller's diarrhoea.
- Prescribing interval for any repeat medication should be related to the next time that medication would normally be reviewed. Generally, this should not be >13wk.
- The prescribing doctor retains medico-legal responsibility for the duration of the prescription.
- If the doctor does decide to prescribe for the patient's stay abroad (e.g. if repeat supplies cannot be obtained at the destination or the drug prescribed has a narrow therapeutic index), it is essential to inform the patient of the need for any regular monitoring, as well as the need to consult a doctor in the event of any unforeseen complications or symptoms.

General rules for treatment of overseas visitors to the UK

- *Emergency or immediately necessary treatment:* Must be offered to overseas visitors free of charge for a period of ≤14d. There is no obligation to provide non-emergency treatment. It is the decision of the GP whether care is deemed necessary. Includes pre-existing conditions that have become worse, oxygen, and renal dialysis.
- *Non-emergency care:* Provide only on a private, paying basis.
- *Forms E111, E112, and E128:* See opposite.
- *Reciprocal healthcare arrangements:* Treat in the same way as nationals from other countries.
- *Refugees* (whether or not awarded leave to stay) are regarded as ordinarily resident.

- *Hospital admission:* A&E services are free, as is compulsory psychiatric treatment and treatment for certain communicable diseases. Testing for the HIV virus and counselling following a test are both free of charge, but any necessary subsequent treatment and medicines may have to be paid for.
- *NHS prescriptions:* Can be issued but quantities supplied should be no more than necessary for immediate purposes. Overseas visitors are charged normal NHS fees.

General rules for British patients traveling abroad: <60 countries worldwide have any sort of healthcare agreements with the UK. When travelling abroad, always have comprehensive medical insurance.

Treatment in the European Economic Area (EEA): Consists of the member states of the European Community plus Iceland, Liechtenstein, and Norway. Free or ↓ cost emergency treatment is available—in most cases on production of a valid Form E111 (see below). Only state-provided emergency treatment is covered. Advise patients to keep a photocopy of the E111 form with the original. Each country has its own rules—details for individual countries are available on the DoH travel advice website. British citizens moving to another EEA country are not entitled to use form E111.

Other reciprocal agreements: The UK has reciprocal agreements with certain countries for the provision of urgently needed medical treatment at ↓ cost or free. Countries and the services available are listed on the DoH travel advice website (🖥 *http://www.dh.gov.uk*). Only urgently needed treatment is provided on the same terms as for residents of that country. Proof of British nationality or UK residence is required.

Forms

E111: Available to any EEA resident and entitles the holder to free emergency medical care in any other EEA country.

E112: Used for referral of a patient from one EEA country to another for specific treatment of a particular condition (e.g. organ transplant, monitoring of an obscure condition).

E128: Applies to 2 groups of EEA nationals only:
- Workers posted temporarily to another member state and members of their families who accompany them.
- Students temporarily in another member state to study and members of their families who accompany them.

❶ Form E128 entitles the holder to free healthcare under the NHS for any condition and is not restricted to emergency or immediately necessary care. Check names, dates of validity, country of validity, and official stamp carefully.

Further information
Health service circular HSC 1999/018 🖥 *http://www.dh.gov.uk*

Practice staff

Practices employ an array of staff. Staff costs are included in the global sum (📖 p.36) paid to a practice.

Recruiting staff
- Review the post—does the post need to be filled or the duties changed?
- Prepare a job description stipulating duties and hours of work.
- Prepare a profile of the person required.
- Decide on a salary range. BMA can give advice.
- Advertise the post.
- Set a closing date for applications.
- Short-list candidates
- Interview—decide who will interview, what points must be covered, and who will ask questions. Ask similar questions to all candidates and score the responses at the time.
- Make a decision on the preferred candidate—if in doubt, defer the appointment or re-interview preferred candidates.
- Confirm the job offer by letter, asking for a formal letter of acceptance in return.
- Plan an induction course for the new employee. A probationary period can be helpful for both employer and employee.
- Produce a contract of employment (see below).

Employment law: Very complex field which changes rapidly. If in doubt, contact your local BMA office for advice. Major points:

Contract of employment: Sample contracts are available from the BMA. All employees must have a written statement of main particulars of employment <2mo. after their start date. Includes: pay, hours, holidays, notice period, disciplinary and grievance procedures.

Pay: Workers must be paid ≥ the national minimum wage for every hour worked. Deductions can only be made if authorized by legislation, contract of employment, or in advance, in writing, by the employee. All employees must receive an itemized pay statement at or before the time they are paid, including all deductions.

Notice: After 1 mo. employment, an employee must give ≥1wk. notice. An employer must give an employee ≥ 1w. notice after 1mo., 2wk. after 2y., 3wk. after 3y., and so on up to 12wk. after ≥12y. unless other notice periods are specified in the contract of employment.

Redundancy pay: After 2y. continuous employment, employers must make 'redundancy payments' related to employee's age, length of continuous service with the employer (up to a maximum of 20y.), and weekly pay.

Pensions: All employees must belong to a pension scheme. The NHS pension scheme is available to practice employees.

Working time: Parents of children <6y. old or disabled children <18y. old may request flexible working patterns and employers have a duty to consider their requests. Working Time Regulations (1998) apply to agency workers and freelancers, as well as employees, and include:

- Average working week ≤48h. (though individuals can opt to work longer)
- 1d. off each week
- A minimum of 4wk. paid annual leave
- In-work rest break if working day ≥6h.
- 11 consecutive hours' rest in any 24-h. period (night workers must work ≤ 8h/d.)

Time off: Employees are entitled to time off for illness; antenatal care; emergencies involving a dependant; certain public duties (e.g. jury service); to look for another job; and approved trade union activities.

Maternity leave: All pregnant employees are entitled to 26wk. ordinary maternity leave, regardless of length of service. Employees with ≥26wk. continuous service by the beginning of the 14th week before the EDD are entitled to 26wk. additional maternity leave (i.e. 1y. in total). Women are entitled to return to their own or an equivalent job after their leave. Similar arrangements exist for adoptive mothers.

Paternity leave: Employees who have worked for their employer for ≥26wk. by the 15th wk. before the baby is due and up to the birth of the child are entitled to 1–2wk. paternity leave, which must be completed within 56d. of the birth.

Parental leave: After 1y. employment, employees are entitled to 13 wk. unpaid parental leave for each child born or adopted up to the child's 5th birthday (or 5y. after adopted). Parents of disabled children can take 18wk. up to the child's 18th birthday.

Health and safety of staff: p.71.

Discrimination: Employers must not either directly or indirectly discriminate against their staff on the basis of race, sex, or disability.

Unfair dismissal: Employees of >1y. standing (or on maternity or adoption leave) are entitled to a written statement of reasons for dismissal. Employers must not dismiss an employee unfairly.

Useful information

Department of Trade and Industry: Individual rights of employees: a guide for employers and employees (PL716 Rev 10). ☐ http://www.dti..gov.uk
Disability Rights Commission ☐ http://www.drc-gb.org/drc
Equal Opportunities Commission ☎ 0161 833 9244 ☐ http://www.eoc.org.uk.
Commission for Racial Equality ☐ http://www.cre.gov.uk

GP premises

GPs can either own or rent the property in which they practice:

- **GPs who own surgeries:** GPs may own surgeries by themselves or in partnership. They receive a payment (known as 'notional rent'), based on the estimated value of the property, for allowing their private buildings to be used for NHS purposes. When a new GP joins a practice as a partner, he or she will be expected to buy into the practice in order to contribute a share of previous investment in the practice premises and equipment.
- **GPs who rent surgeries:** Can claim reimbursement from their PCO/health board for the rent they pay as long as it is 'reasonable' as assessed by the District Valuer.
- **The cost rent scheme:** GPs may build or renovate a property for use as a surgery. The principal is that the Partners raise the finance and the PCO meets interest payments on the loan. Complex area—consult the BMA and PCO for further details.
- **Improvement grants:** Available via PCO in some circumstances.

All new premises/refurbishments must meet national minimum standards.

Disabled access: The Disability Discrimination Act (1995) gives disabled people rights of access to goods, facilities, and services. A disabled person is defined as 'someone who has a physical or mental impairment that has a substantial and long-term adverse effect on his or her ability to carry out normal day-to-day activities'. Since October 1999, practices:

- Have not been able to refuse to take disabled people onto a practice list, or provide a lower standard of service, due to their disability.
- Must consider making reasonable adjustments to the way they deliver their services so that disabled people can use them.

Since October 2004, service providers have also been required to take reasonable steps to tackle physical barriers to the use of services including features of premises, like steps or narrow doorways, that prevent, or make it difficult for, a disabled people to access their services. Exactly what individual practices need to do depends on their individual situation and the needs of their disabled clients.

Building regulations and access for disabled patients: The Building Regulations exist to ensure the health and safety of people in and around all types of buildings. Part M deals with access and facilities for disabled people. Until recently their aim was that all new buildings were accessible to and useable by disabled people. An amended Part M came into force in May 2004 which extended the provisions to alterations on existing buildings and introduced the concept of access and use for all—not simply for those with recognized disabilities.

Health and safety: The basis of British health and safety law is the Health and Safety at Work Act 1974. The Act sets out the general duties employers have towards employees and members of the public, and employees have to themselves and to each other.

Responsibilities of GPs as employers: The Management of Health and Safety at Work Regulations 1992 (the Management Regulations) give clear guidance about employers' duties towards their staff.

1. Employers with ≥5 employees must carry out a risk assessment and record the significant findings. HSE leaflet '5 Steps to Risk Assessment' gives more information;
2. Make arrangements for implementing the health and safety measures identified as necessary by the risk assessment;
3. Appoint competent people (usually the practice manager) to help implement the arrangements;
4. Set up emergency procedures (e.g. fire drills);
5. Provide clear information and training to employees;
6. Work together with other employers sharing the same workplace.

Other important pieces of health and safety legislation

- *Employers' Liability (Compulsory Insurance) Regulations 1969:* require employers to take out insurance against accidents and ill health to their employees and to display the insurance certificate.
- *Health and Safety Information for Employees Regulations 1989:* require employers to display a poster telling employees what they need to know about health and safety.
- *Workplace (Health, Safety, and Welfare) Regulations 1992:* cover a wide range of basic health, safety and welfare issues such as ventilation, heating, lighting, and seating.
- *Reporting of Injuries, Diseases, and Dangerous Occurrences Regulations 1985 (RIDDOR):* require employers to notify certain occupational injuries, diseases and dangerous events.
- *Health and Safety (Display Screen Equipment) Regulations 1992:* set out requirements for work with visual display units (VDUs).
- *Personal Protective Equipment (PPE) Regulations 1992:* require employers to provide appropriate protective clothing and equipment.
- *Provision and Use of Work Equipment Regulations (PUWER) 1992:* require that equipment provided, including machinery, is safe.
- *Manual Handling Operations Regulations 1992:* cover moving of objects by hand or bodily force.
- *Health and Safety (First Aid) Regulations 1981:* cover requirements for first aid.
- *Control of Substances Hazardous to Health Regulations 1994 (COSHH)* requires employers to assess the risks from hazardous substances and take appropriate precautions.
- *Gas Safety (Installation and Use) Regulations 1994:* cover safe installation, maintenance, and use of gas systems and appliances in domestic and commercial premises.

Further information

NHS estates primary care ⊑ *http://www.nhsestates.gov.uk/primary_care*
Health and Safety Executive ☎08701 545500 ⊑ *http://www.hse.gov.uk*

GPs as managers

'If you have time to do something wrong; you have time to do it right'
W. Edwards Deming

GP partners in a practice have dual roles as both clinicians and managers of small businesses. As such, they must cooperate with their partners and practice manager to run the business side of the practice and with primary healthcare team members to cover all aspects of the clinical work.

Definition: Management is the process of designing and maintaining an environment in which individuals, working together, efficiently accomplish selected aims. The manager coordinates individual effort towards the group goal. To do this, he needs technical skill (knowledge specific to the business of the organization); human skill (ability to work with people); conceptual skill (ability to see the 'big picture'); and design skill (ability to solve problems). There are 5 managerial functions:

- *Planning:* Involves selecting missions and objectives and the actions to achieve them—requires decision making.
- *Organizing:* Defining roles—ensuring all tasks necessary to accomplish goals are assigned to those people who can do them best.
- *Staffing:* Ensuring all positions in the organizational structure are filled with people able to fulfil those roles.
- *Leading:* Influencing people so that they will contribute to organization and group goals.
- *Controlling:* Measuring and correcting individual and organizational performance to ensure events conform to plans.

Management and teamwork: Key features which contribute to successful teamwork are:

- *Communication:* Information sharing, feedback, and grievance airing.
- *Clear team rules:* Especially with regard to responsibility and accountability. Make sure these are understood by everyone.
- *Sympathetic leadership:* Any team needs a co-coordinator to direct its efforts. A weak leader may allow the team to drift but an autocratic leader may be too directive and diminish the status of other team members thus ↓ the effectiveness of the team.
- *Clear decision-making process:* Especially if differences of opinion.
- *Pooling:* Knowledge, experience, skills, resources, and responsibility for outcome.
- *Specialization of function:* Team members must understand and respect the role and importance of other team members.
- *Delegation:* Work of the team is split between its members. Each member leaves the others to carry out functions delegated to them.
- *Group support:* Team members share and are committed to a common, agreed purpose or goal which directs their actions.

Practice meetings: Essential to ensure necessary decisions are made; review policies and agree standards of care; review the financial position of the practice; educate and inform practice members; aid communication; and improve morale of practice members.

Risk management: Primary care is about risk and uncertainty, but sometimes we take unnecessary risks and cause ourselves and our patients unnecessary harm. Defence organization records suggest ~½ of all successful negligence claims reflect poor clinical judgement on the doctor's part; the other ½ represent avoidable mishaps which would be susceptible to risk management approaches—often failures in simple administrative systems, communication failures, inadequate records, or lack of training. Risk management is the process of taking steps to minimize risk and keep ourselves and others as safe as possible. All the major defence organizations run risk management programmes for their members. 4 stages:

1. Identify the risk: Through analysis of complaints and comments from GPs, other practice staff, or patients; through significant event audit (📖 p.91); or by using material provided by the defence organizations to identify common pitfalls.
2. Assess frequency and severity of the risk.
3. Take steps to reduce or eliminate the risk.
4. Check the risk has been eliminated.

Categories of risk relevant to general practice
- Clinical care e.g. prescribing errors;
- Non-clinical risks to patient safety e.g. security and fire hazards;
- Risks to the health of the workforce e.g. Hepatitis b;
- Organizational risks e.g. failure to safeguard confidential information and unlicensed use of computer software.

Key safety issues for primary care:
- *Diagnosis*: 28% reported errors.
- *Prescribing*: Prescribing problems occur at a rate of 3–5% of all prescriptions. 9% hospital admissions are due to potentially avoidable problems with prescribed drugs. 4% of drugs are incorrectly dispensed each year.
- *Communication*: Poor communication is a major cause of complaints. 40% of patients have been found to have discrepancies between the drugs prescribed at hospital discharge and those they receive in the community.
- *Organizational change*: In industry, better teamwork, communication, and leadership ↓ adverse incidents.

In each case consider
- *Organizational and management factors:* Financial resources/constraints; practice policies and organization.
- *Work environment factors:* Staffing levels skill mix; work load; equipment.
- *Team factors:* Team structure; communication; supervision.
- *Individual (staff) factors:* Knowledge and skills; competence; physical and mental health.
- *Task factors:* Availability and use of protocols/guidelines; availability and accuracy of test results.
- *Patient factors:* Condition (complexity and seriousness); language and communication; personality and social factors.

Partnership agreements

Partnership disputes are common. A properly drafted partnership agreement may prevent disputes and, if they do occur, may lessen their impact.

Partnership at will: A partnership without an up-to-date written agreement is a 'partnership at will', governed by the 1890 Partnership Act. A 'partnership at will' is a very unstable situation as:
- All partners are deemed to have equal profit shares unless there is clear evidence to the contrary.
- Decisions are made by simple majority.
- Notice may be served by any partner on the others without their prior knowledge or consent.
- Dissolution of the partnership may take immediate effect and no reason need be given to justify it.
- Dissolution may result in the forced sale of all partnership assets (including the surgery premises) and redundancy of all staff.
- There is nothing to prevent any partner, or group of partners, from immediately forming a new practice/partnership to the exclusion of the other partner(s) once the practice is dissolved.

Partnership agreements: Should be drawn up every time a new partner joins a practice. Employed doctors and retainers also require contracts of employment (see below). An agreement checklist is included opposite. Detailed guidance is produced by the BMA and further guidance can be obtained from local BMA offices and LMCs.

Partnership disputes: However good a partnership agreement, disputes still occur. Advice on partnership and employment matters is available from the BMA and LMC and the BMA also provides conciliation services (contact local office). Legal battles are expensive and the BMA will not fund partnership disputes. Try to resolve matters amicably.

Discrimination: It is unlawful for any partnership to discriminate on grounds of sex, marital status, colour, race, nationality (including citizenship), ethnic or national origins when appointing a new partner or in the way they treat an existing partner. The BMA will consider backing GPs to take such matters to industrial tribunals—contact local office. Applications should be made on forms available via local Job centres and must be made within 3mo. of the last act of discrimination.

Contracts of employment for salaried GPs: Model terms and conditions of service for a salaried GP and a model offer letter of employment are available from the BMA or DoH websites. Nationally agreed salary scales apply and are compulsory for GMS but not PMS practices. Responsibilities towards employed GPs—📖 p.68

Partnership agreement checklist

- *Business detail:* Purpose of the business; premises (and basis of occupation). If premises are owned by the partners, state procedure for valuation, payment of the retiring partner, and investment of the incoming partner.
- *Assets:* Specify assets, their ownership, arrangements for valuation, and interest payments. It is illegal to sell goodwill in NHS practices.
- *Income and allowances:* Definition of practice income; allowable expenses.
- *Profit sharing:* Distribution of fees and allowances specified in the SFA and other NHS allowances; distribution of income from non-NHS work.
- *Accounting:* Accounting and banking arrangements; cheque signing; access to accounts and bank statements.
- *Taxation:* Arrangements for paying tax; obligations of each partner.
- *Superannuation*
- *Retirement/suspension/expulsion:* Reasons for suspension or expulsion; process of suspension/expulsion; mechanisms of voluntary leaving/retirement; division of assets in the event of retirement. May include a restrictive covenant preventing the outgoing doctor working in the practice area for a period of time after leaving—seek legal advice.
- *Leave:* Holiday entitlement; basis of deciding who has holiday when; study leave; sabbatical leave; sick leave; maternity, paternity, and adoption leave; compassionate leave.
- *Obligation:* NHS obligations; non-NHS work within the practice; other work outside the practice; educational activities; obligations to each other; hours of work.
- *Decisions and disputes:* Decision-making process; process to manage disputes; process to dissolve partnership. Ensure who pays legal fees for who in the event of a dispute is included.
- *Correct procedure:* Ensure each partner has signed and dated the agreement and that their signature has been witnessed. It is recommended that each partner should take independent legal advice and not rely on the 'practice solicitor' for sole advice.

Further information

DoH ⊠ http://www.dh.gov.uk
BMA ⊠ http://www.bma.org.uk
Disability Discrimination ⊠ http://www.disability.gov.uk and ⊠ http://www.drc-gb.org/drc
Equal Opportunities Commission ☎ 0161 833 9244. ⊠ http://www.eoc.org.uk
Commission for Racial Equality ⊠ http://www.cre.gov.uk

Computers and classification

Under the new GMS contract (📖 p.34), PCOs directly fund 100% of IT costs. Almost all practices now use computers on a daily basis. All specialist GP systems must be approved by the DoH. The software covers all aspects of practice from appointment systems through clinical care to audit and reporting.

Table 1.6 Major software systems currently in use

System	Web address for more information
EMIS	http://www.emis-online.com
GPASS (General Practice Administration System for Scotland)	http://www.gpass.demon.co.uk
Healthy Software	http://www.healthysoft.com
In Practice Systems Ltd. (Vision)	http://www.inps.co.uk
Microtest (Practice Manager)	http://www.microtest.co.uk
Protechnic Exeter (Profiles)	http://www.protechnic.co.uk
Torex Meditel (Ganymede)	http://www.meditel.co.uk
The Phoenix Partnership (TPP, SystemOne)	http://www.thephoenix.co.uk
SEETEC (GP Enterprise)	http://www.seetec.co.uk/gpenterprise
UCL Chime (GP Care)	http://www.chime.ucl.ac.uk

Read codes and SNOMED clinical terms (CT): Read codes are the system used to code general practice in the UK to date. They code history, examination, investigations, diagnosis, interventions, administrative tasks and many other aspects of patient care. Due to incompatibility of different clinical coding systems, a universal coding system, SNOMED CT, has been developed and the aim is to switch over from Read codes to SNOMED CT from 2006. The final version of the Read codes will be issued in January 2006—though they will continue to be used as long as data exists with a Read code in it—but there will be no further changes/updates made after January 2006 and support calls will receive low priority.

Electronic GP records: Since 2000, GPs in England have been able to maintain all records on computer if they gain approval of their PCO—i.e. to be 'paperless'. DoH/BMA good practice guidelines are regularly updated (see opposite).

Information for Health Strategy (1998): Aims to provide:
• A lifelong electronic health record for every person in the country;
• Online 24h. access to records and information about best clinical practice for all NHS clinicians;
• Electronic communication between general practice and hospitals;
• ↑ public access to information and services through online or telephone services;
• New ways of delivering services and care through telemedicine.

NHSnet: Network connecting NHS organizations which is protected from the internet by a firewall. This enables NHS users to access the internet but outside users cannot access NHS web sites (though they can send e-mail to NHS users). By March 2002, all GP practices in the UK had been connected to the NHSnet enabling e-mail, internet access, electronic exchange of information about appointments and test results, shared learning resources, computer-based training packages, discussion forums, and many other benefits. Many practices now receive all lab results electronically, and this is likely to extend to clinic appointment letters in the near future.

NHS Directory: Lists of NHS organizations, departments, and personnel together with biographical details. Will be used to authenticate individuals using the system in order to control access to restricted areas of the NHSnet and ensure confidential data is not transferred into the wrong hands—an essential factor in the development of national electronic records systems for both staff and patients. It will also be used, together with the NHSmail system, to aid communication between NHS staff.

Use of e-mail in the surgery: ~60% of the UK population now has access to e-mail, and its use is increasing rapidly worldwide. National surveys show that patients want to be able to communicate with healthcare professionals by e-mail, but e-mail has been used relatively little to date in healthcare settings due to concerns over quality of content, confidentiality, and liability. Its use is likely to develop further.

PRODIGY: Computer-based decision and learning support tool for GPs, offering a series of recommendations for the treatment of a condition. Used during the consultation, the GP enters a diagnosis, in response to which PRODIGY can suggest management options and provide patient information leaflets. There is also a wealth of clinical background information for use outside the consultation as reference or learning material.

Electronic transmission of prescriptions: Transmission of prescriptions between GPs, community pharmacies, and the Prescription Pricing Authority (PPA). 3 pilot projects ended in 2003. It is expected that a national programme will start once evaluation is complete.

Electronic secondary care appointment booking: Several pilots of electronic appointment booking are underway. Preliminary feedback suggests this is an efficient system which ↑ doctor and patient satisfaction, ↓ waiting times, and ↓ the number of patients who do not arrive at their appointments.

Further information
NHS Information Authority ▣ http://www.nhsia.nhs.uk
DoH: ▣ http://www.dh.gov.uk
- Good practice guidelines for general practice electronic patient records (v.3)
- Information for Health: an information strategy for the modern NHS 1998–2005
- Electronic transmission of prescriptions
Prodigy ▣ http://www.prodigy.nhs.uk
British Computer Society, Primary Healthcare Specialist Group ▣ http://www.bcs.org.uk

Useful websites for GPs

Table 1.7

Website	Description
Organizations	
http://www.nhs.uk	NHS
http://www.dh.gov.uk	Department of Health
http://www.gmc-uk.org	GMC
http://www.bma.org.uk	BMA
http://www.jcptgp.org.uk	JCPTGP
http://www.rcgp.org.uk *http://www.rcplondon.ac.uk* *http://www.rcog.org.uk* *http://www.rcpsych.ac.uk* *http://www.rcn.org.uk*	Royal Colleges
http://www.the-mdu.com *http://www.mps.org.uk* *http://www.mddus.com*	UK Medical Defence Organizations
http://www.bhia.org	British Healthcare Internet Association
Books/journals/evidence-based medicine	
http://www.nelh.nhs.uk	National Electronic Library for Health
http://www.york.ac.uk/inst/crd/ehcb.htm *http://www.york.ac.uk/inst/crd/em.htm*	NHS Centre for Reviews and Dissemination
http://www.sign.ac.uk	Scottish Intercollegiate Guidelines Network
http://www.jr2.ox.ac.uk/bandolier	Bandolier
http://www.npc.co.uk/merec_index.htm	National Prescribing Centre—MeReC Bulletin
http://www.prodigy.nhs.uk	PRODIGY
http://www.bnf.org	BNF
http://www.merck.com/pubs/manual	Merck Manual Textbook of Medicine
http://www.gpnotebook.co.uk	On-line GP encyclopaedia
http://www.bmj.com *http://bmjjournals.com*	BMJ and other BMJ Group journals
http://www.freemedicaljournals.com	Portal to free medical journals on-line
http://www.freebooks4doctors.com	Portal to free medical books on-line

Table 1.7 (cont.)

Website	Description
Other useful medical sites	
http://www1.doctors.net.uk	Doctors net
http://www.medic8.com	Doctors information site
http://www.emedicine.com/	Doctors information site
http://www.adviceguide.org.uk	Citizen's Advice Bureau
http://www.nhsdirect.nhs.uk	NHS Direct
http://www.hon.ch	Index of health information
http://drsdesk.sghms.ac.uk/	Primary care website
http://www.healthcentre.org.uk *http://www.medinfo.co.uk/*	Health information
Useful non-medical sites	
http://www.excite.co.uk/ *http://www.lycos.co.uk* *http://www.google.com*	Search tools
http://www.bt.com *http://www.yell.com*	Telephone directories
http://www.royalmail.com	Post code finder
http://www.inlandrevenue.gov.uk	On-line self-assessment tax form
http://www.rac.co.uk	On-line travel information—roads
http://www.thetrainline.com	Trains—tickets and timetables
http://www.streetmap.co.uk	Maps
http://www.amazon.co.uk	On-line bookshop
http://www.bbc.co.uk	General information; news
http://www.lastminute.com	Travel, gifts, and leisure

Useful books

Wyatt (2001) *Clinical Knowledge and Practice in the Information Age: A Handbook for Health Professionals.* Royal Society of Medicine Press Ltd

Tyrell (2002) Using the Internet in Healthcare. Radicliffe Medical Press

Clinical governance

Clinical governance is a far-reaching quality initiative. It is defined as:
> '*a framework through which NHS organizations are accountable for continuously improving the quality of their services and safeguarding high standards of care by creating an environment in which excellence in clinical care will flourish.*' DoH (1999)

Although the onus is on NHS organizations to make these changes, the legislation makes it clear that all health professionals, guided by their professional bodies, are expected to adhere to the concept.

Essential elements of clinical governance: Figure 1.5

What does clinical governance entail at practice/PCO level?
- Every PCO must appoint a health professional as clinical governance lead.
- PCOs must publish routine reports and an annual progress report on the local implementation of clinical governance.
- Within practices, individual doctors must consider their own professional development and educational needs.
- Regular assessment must be made of performance and development of other health professionals engaged by practices.
- Within practices, there must be continuous review and appraisal of procedures and standards: RAID—Review (gather all stake holders together to look at a particular topic); Agree (strategy to take forward); Intervene (make changes decided upon); Demonstrate (the effect of changes through audit (📖 p.90), patient satisfaction questionnaire, prescribing data, etc.). External peer review should be encouraged.
- Deficiencies in knowledge, skills, or experience must be acted upon through appropriate education and professional development.
- Resources should be provided to help develop clinical governance— time out for audit, PCO meetings, and to address educational needs; funding for courses and educational activities to address deficiencies and enable more effective assessment of standards and performance.

⚠ **Concerns about performance:** In the first instance, any GP with concerns about their own, or a colleague's, performance should discuss the matter confidentially with the Secretary of their LMC, with the clinical governance lead/performance information manager of their PCO, or with the GMC.

Further information
Starey *What is clinical governance*
📖http://www.evidence-based-medicine.co.uk/ebmfiles/WhatisClinGov.pdf
Clinical governance: Quality in the new NHS HSC 1999/065* (16 March 1999)
📖 http://www.dh.gov.uk
Clinical governance support: 📖 http://www.cgsupport.org

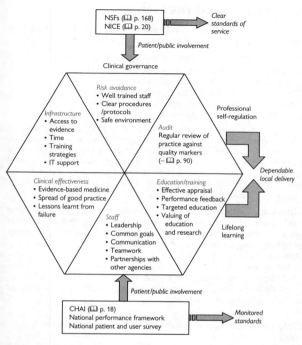

Figure 1.5 Model of clinical governance within the NHS quality improvement framework

Evidence-based medicine

Definition: Conscientious, explicit, and judicious use of current best evidence in making decisions about the care of individual patients.

The 5 steps of evidence-based medicine (EBM) are:

1. Convert clinical information needs into answerable questions
2. Track down the best evidence with which to answer them
3. Critically appraise that evidence for its validity and usefulness
4. Apply the results of this appraisal in clinical practice
5. Evaluate your clinical performance e.g. through audit (📖 p.90)

Practicing EBM involves integrating individual clinical expertise with the best available external clinical evidence from systematic research. The problem for the clinician on the ground is finding and interpreting the appropriate evidence for the clinical situation. If good—quality evidence is out there (and there are many under-researched areas in medicine)—How do you access it? When do you find the time to search for it? How do you assess its quality and relevance?

Critical appraisal: The process of assessing and interpreting evidence by systematically considering its validity, results, and relevance. Essential to avoid misinterpretation and misuse of evidence in practice. In all cases, before integrating evidence into practice consider:

• Are the results of the study valid?
• What are the results?
• Will they help me in caring for my patients?

Critical Appraisal Skills Programme (CASP) appraisal tools are available from 🖥 http://www.phru.nhs.uk/casp

Table 1.8 Classification and grading of evidence—Most → least reliable

Grade	Evidence level	Definition: Evidence obtained from...
A	Ia	Meta-analysis of randomized controlled trials.
	Ib	At least one randomized controlled trial.
B	IIa	At least one well-designed controlled study without randomization e.g. case-controlled study; cohort study.
	IIb	At least one other type of well-designed quasi-experimental study.
	III	Well-designed non-experimental descriptive studies, such as comparative studies, correlation studies, and case studies.
C	IV	Expert committee reports or opinions and/or clinical experience of respected authorities.

Table 1.9 Useful web resources

	Website
General information	
National Electronic Library for Health	www.nelh.nhs.uk (has guidelines index and numerous links to EBM websites)
Bandolier	www.jr2.ox.ac.uk/bandolier
Evidence-based medicine	ebm.bmjjournals.com
ScHARR	www.shef.ac.uk/~scharr/ir/netting/
Guidelines	
NICE	www.nice.nhs.uk
Scottish Intercollegiate Guidelines Network (SIGN)	www.sign.ac.uk
EGuidelines	www.eguidelines.co.uk (registration needed)
Primary Care Clinical Practice Guidelines (US)	www.medicine.ucsf.edu/resources/guidelines
National Guidelines Clearing House (US)	www.guideline.gov
New Zealand Guidelines Group	www.nzgg.org.nz
Systematic reviews	
Cochrane Library	www.nelh.nhs.uk/cochrane
Clinical Evidence (BMJ Publishing)	www.clinicalevidence.com
Health Technology Assessment	www.hta.nhsweb.nhs.uk
Drugs and Therapeutic Bulletin (*Which*)	www.which.net/health/dtb (subscription required)
MeReC Bulletin	www.npc.co.uk/merec_index.htm
NHS Centre for Reviews and Dissemination	www.york.ac.uk/inst/crd
Effective Health Care	www.york.ac.uk/inst/crd/ehcb
Effectiveness Matters	www.york.ac.uk/inst/crd/em.htm
PubMed*	Access via BMJ website (www.bmj.com) or National electronic library for health (www.nelh.nhs.uk)

* When searching, aim to retrieve all the most relevant citations with a minimum of junk.
A useful tip is to use the clinical queries or systematic reviews filter to restrict the amount of information retrieved.

Essential reading

Sackett *et al.* (2005) *Evidence based medicine.* Churchill Livingstone ISBN: 04403074445
Kinloch (1996) *The Pocket guide to critical appraisal.* BMJ Books ISBN: 072791099X
Greenhalgh (2000) *How to read a paper* BMJ Books ISBN: 0727915789

Glossary of terms used in evidence-based medicine

Absolute risk reduction/increase: The absolute arithmetic difference in rates of bad outcomes between experimental and control participants in a trial, calculated as the difference in experimental event rate (EER) and control event rate (CER).

Bias: Systematic disposition of certain trial designs to produce results consistently better or worse than other trial designs. Always consider whether a study is biased before accepting its conclusions. Further information: 🖳 *http://www.jr2.ox.ac.uk/bandolier/Extraforbando/Bias.pdf*

Case-control study: Involves identifying patients who have the outcome of interest (cases) and control patients without the same outcome, and looking back to see if they had the exposure of interest.

Cohort study: Involves identification of two groups (cohorts) of patients—one which received the exposure of interest, and one which did not—and following these cohorts forward for the outcome of interest.

Confidence interval (CI): Quantifies uncertainty in measurement. Usually reported as 95% CI, which is the range of values within which we can be 95% sure that the true value for the whole population lies.

Control event rate (CER): The rate at which events occur in a control group. It may be represented by a percentage (e.g. 10%) or proportion (e.g. 0.1).

Cost-benefit analysis: Assesses whether the cost of an intervention is worth the benefit by measuring both in the same units—usually monetary units. Further information: 🖳 *http://www.jr2.ox.ac.uk/bandolier/painres/download/whatis/Cost-effect.pdf*

Cross-sectional study: Observation of a defined population at a single point in time or time interval.

Experimental event rate (EER): The rate at which events occur in an experimental group. May be expressed as a percentage or proportion (see CER).

False negative/positive: 📖 p.159

Likelihood ratio (LR): Likelihood that a given test result would be expected in a patient with the target disorder compared with the likelihood that the same result would be expected in a patient without the target disorder. Gives an indication of accuracy of a clinical test. The higher the likelihood ratio, the better the test at detecting the disorder.

Meta-analysis: Systematic review that uses quantitative methods to summarize the results. Further information: 🖳 *http://www.jr2.ox.ac.uk/bandolier/painres/download/whatis/Meta-An.pdf*

Number needed to treat (NNT): A measure of the difference between active treatment and control treatment. An NNT of 1 describes a situation where an event occurs in every patient given the active treatment but no patient in the comparison group. There are few circumstances in which a treatment is 100% effective and placebo completely ineffective, so NNTs of 2–3 indicate an effective intervention.

Number needed to harm (NNH): Compares the number having a side-effect in the intervention group against the number having that side-effect in the comparison group. If no-one in the control group and no-one in the comparison group has an unwanted effect, the NNH will be infinity. Therefore, the NNH should be as large as possible.

Odds ratio (OR): Odds of an event are calculated as the number of events divided by the number of non-events. The odds ratio is the ratio of the odds in the experimental group compared to the control group. For epidemiological studies looking for factors causing harm, an odds ratio >1 indicates the factor the experimental group was exposed to caused harm. For experimental studies looking for a decrease in events through treatment, an odds ratio <1 indicates a positive result. Often expressed as a percentage.

Positive predictive value: 📖 p. 159

Relative risk or risk ratio (RR): Ratio of risk in the treated group (EER) to risk in the control group (CER). RR = EER/CER. Is used in randomized trials and cohort studies. If the RR=1 there is no difference between the two groups for that measure.

Relative risk reduction (RRR): Difference between the EER and CER (EER-CER) divided by the CER. Usually expressed as a percentage.

Sensitivity: 📖 p. 159

Specificity: 📖 p. 159

Systematic review: Summary of the medical literature that uses explicit methods to perform a thorough literature search and critical appraisal of individual studies and uses appropriate statistical techniques to combine results of studies of acceptable quality.

Clinical guidelines, protocols, and integrated care pathways

Clinical guidelines: User-friendly statements that bring together the best external evidence and other knowledge necessary for decision making about a specific health problem. Over recent years, there has been a dramatic ↑ in publication of guidelines and protocols. They aim to ↓ harmful or expensive variations in clinical practice, improve healthcare outcomes, and encourage rapid dissemination of useful innovations. Good clinical guidelines have 3 properties:

1. Define practice questions and identify all their decision options and outcomes.
2. Identify, appraise, and summarize best evidence about prevention, diagnosis, prognosis, therapy, harm, and cost-effectiveness.
3. Identify the decision points at which the evidence needs to be integrated with individual clinical experience and clinical circumstances in deciding a course of action.

Advantages and disadvantages of guidelines

Advantages

• Provide guidance for busy clinicians—a consistent basis for decision making
• Practical framework for common problems and chronic disease
• Summarizes the available research evidence
• Can be used as a basis for continuing medical education
• Justification for expenditure—can aid cost-effective use of limited resources
• Facilitate the audit cycle

Disadvantages

• Poor quality guidelines can reinforce poor practice
• Lack of relevance of the guidelines to the clinical setting—much of the 'evidence' used to develop guidelines comes from secondary care and may not reflect the situation in primary care
• Tendency to uniformity—can stifle innovation
• Resistance to change—new methods may not be considered until a new guideline is produced
• Increased risk of litigation
• Cost—they are time consuming to develop and update
• Lack of ownership—guidelines developed by others may not feel relevant
• Difficulties in implementation—guidelines that are not user-friendly and well disseminated will not be used

Before starting to use a guideline: Always ask:

• Is this guideline valid, important, and applicable in your practice?

If the answer is yes, then consider:

• What barriers exist to implementation?
• Can they be overcome?
• Can you enlist collaboration of key colleagues?
• Can you meet the educational and administrative conditions that are likely to determine the success or failure of implementing the strategy?

Protocol: The term reserved for guidelines at the more rigid end of the spectrum. These are very specific guidelines which are expected to be followed in detail, with little scope for variation e.g. resuscitation protocols.

Integrated care pathway (ICP): ICPs amalgamate all the anticipated elements of care and treatment of the multidisciplinary team, for a particular patient group, in order to achieve agreed outcomes. Any deviation from the plan is documented as variance—the analysis of which provides information for the review of current practice. ICPs aim to:
- Facilitate introduction of guidelines and systemic audit into clinical practice
- Improve multidisciplinary communication and care planning
- Reach or exceed existing standards
- ↓ unwanted practice variation
- ↑ clinician—patient communication and patient satisfaction
- Identify research and development questions
- Cross the interface between primary, secondary and social care.

Grading/classification of evidence: 📖 p.82

Further information

National Electronic Library for Health—guidelines database, integrated care pathways database, and useful information on development of guidelines. 🖥 http://www.nelh.nhs.uk
NICE: 🖥 http://www.nice.nhs.uk
Scottish Intercollegiate Guidelines Network: 🖥 http://www.sign.ac.uk
eGuidelines: 🖥 www.eguidelines.co.uk (free registration required)
Primary Care Clinical Practice Guidelines: US Primary Care Guidelines
    🖥 http:// www.medicine.ucsf.edu/resources/guidelines
National Guidelines Clearing House: 🖥 http://www.guideline.gov
New Zealand Guidelines Group: 🖥 http://www.nzgg.org.nz

Outcomes in general practice

Within the NHS there are ↑ demands for accountability and improvements in quality of care. In general practice, the outcome measures used to judge 'quality of care' are a matter of some debate. Possible measures are:

Patient satisfaction: The definition of satisfaction is not uniform. It implies, to a varying degree, meeting both the wants and the needs of the patient. Questionnaires often have low validity and reliability and satisfaction scores are closely related to the psychological health of a patient i.e. someone who is depressed is less likely to be satisfied with services. Nevertheless, satisfaction measures are increasingly being used to judge the effectiveness of the NHS. In the surgery, patient satisfaction audits (e.g. of the appointments system), are a useful way of identifying deficiencies in the system from the user's perspective, which can then be improved. 2 surveys are approved for use in the 'patient experience' domain of the quality standards framework (📖 p.40):

- **Improving Patient Questionnaire (IPQ):** ❶ charge payable.
  💻 http://ex.ac.uk/cfep/ipq.htm
- **General Practice Assessment Questionnaire (GPAQ):**
  💻 http://www.gpaq.info.

Surveys of satisfaction show ~80% of patients are, overall, satisfied with GP care. However, if questioned more specifically about different components of care (e.g. information provided, communication), <½ are completely satisfied.

Patient recall: Many studies suggest that >50% (some estimate up to 90%) of information has been forgotten within a few minutes of leaving the surgery. Characteristics of memorable information:

- The patient perceives it as important;
- The patient understands it (avoid the use of jargon and medical terms, keep language brief and simple, support information with sketches/diagrams ± patient information sheets);
- The information is given early in the consultation;
- The information is given in small chunks (not too much at once).

Patient concordance or compliance: Another measure of the effectiveness of a consultation is the degree to which the patient complies with advice and uses medication supplied as directed. In general practice ~1/3 follow advice closely enough to make it effective; ~1/3 follow some advice but not closely enough to make it effective; ~1/3 follow no advice at all— 📖 p.124.

Prescribing rates: There are wide variations in prescribing rates e.g. variation in the rate of statin prescription cannot be accounted for by population characteristics; prescription rates for antibiotics for minor illness vary widely between GPs. Whether and how these reflect quality of care is controversial.

Referral rates: There are wide variations in referral rates (~3–12/100 consultations) not accounted for by population characteristics. Referral rates are not related to age or GP experience, use of investigations, or postgraduate qualifications. Experience in a specialty ↑ referrals to that speciality implying high referrers are not necessarily inadequate. Attempts have been made to judge appropriateness of referrals but the assessor is often not aware of the full circumstances of the referral e.g. it is appropriate to refer a child for a paediatric opinion purely to allay parental anxiety but the referral might be deemed inappropriate on clinical grounds.

Doctors' ability to detect illness: There are wide variations between GPs in their ability to detect certain illnesses e.g. mental illness. GPs adept at identifying mental health: have empathy, make early eye contact, use directive rather than closed questioning, clarify the complaint at an early stage. Whether this is a marker of quality of care or just the diversity of general practice is debatable.

Performance of procedures: Comparisons of procedure outcome (e.g. inadequate smear rates, diabetic outcome measures, immunization rates) between practices can be a way to identify practices or GPs clearly performing less well than others. The reasons for the discrepancy must then be investigated.

Audit

Audit is defined as 'the systematic critical analysis of quality of health care'. Its purpose is to appraise current practice (*What is happening?*) by measuring it against pre-selected standards (*What should be happening?*), to identify and implement areas for change (*What changes are needed?*), and thus improve performance.

Audit differs from research as research aims to establish what best practice is globally; audit aims to discover how close practice is to best practice on a local level and identify ways of improving care.

Audit is a continual process and an integral part of clinical governance (☐ p.80). All practices in the UK are involved in audit in some way.

Aims of audit
- Improved care of patients
- Enhanced professionalism of staff
- Efficient use of resources
- Aid to continuing education
- Aid to administration
- Accountability to those outside the profession

The audit cycle: The process of identifying areas of care to be audited, implementing any necessary changes, and then periodically reviewing the same issues is known as the audit cycle—see Figure 1.6

Choosing a topic: Any practice matter—clinical or administrative. Make sure the topic is important, manageable, clearly defined, and data is available to assess the criteria chosen. Good starting points are significant events, quality and outcomes framework targets, complaints, NSF or clinical guideline topics, personal observations.

Choosing criteria: Criteria are specific statements of what should be happening. Criteria might be those laid down for quality payments, 'gold standard' care as defined in guidelines, or generated within the practice. Use evidence-based criteria wherever possible. All criteria have to be measurable—ideally with data already collected.

Setting standards: Standards are minimum levels of acceptable performance for a criterion. 100% achievement of standards is unusual, so set realistic standards based on quality framework levels and standards achieved by other practices (e.g. comparative practice data, audits from other practices) or previous audits within the practice.

Observing practice: You can collect information from: computer registers; medical records; questionnaires—patients, staff—or GPs; data collection sheets (e.g. drugs in doctor's bag are all in date).

Comparing results with standards: Consider why standards have not been met—What should be done? Who's going to do it? When? How?

Repeating the audit cycle: to ensure action taken is effective.

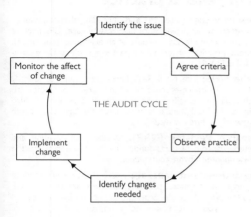

Figure 1.6 The audit cycle.*

Significant event audit: Process in which individual episodes (when there has been a significant occurrence either beneficial or deleterious) are analysed, in a systematic and detailed way, to ascertain what can be learnt about the overall quality of care, and to indicate changes that might lead to future improvements. Significant event audit is a useful learning tool and essential to achieve maximum quality points (📖 p.40). Detailed guidance on the procedure to follow and categories of event suitable to obtain quality points is available from the DoH website (🖥 http://www.dh.gov.uk)

Further information
NICE Best practice in clinical audit. 🖥 http://www.nice.org.uk/pdf/BestPracticeClinicalAudit.pdf
Hardman E., and Joughin C.(1998) FOCUS on Clinical Audit in Child and Adolescent Mental Health Services. Gaskell publications, Chapter 1. 🖥 http://www.rcpsych.ac.uk/publications/gaskell
i-medicine.info: 🖥 http://www.miart.co.uk/i-medicine.info

Research in general practice

Discovery of new knowledge (*research*) and spreading that knowledge (*dissemination*) is essential for provision of high-quality care. GPs may be involved in research at many levels—as part of an academic department, in a research general practice, or just taking part in a project. Drug company research—📖 p.130–1.

Research in the NHS: The NHS R&D Programme aims to identify NHS needs and commission research. Some funds are also available to improve research capacity e.g. fellowships and primary care awards. Also regulates scientific and ethical standards in research through its research governance framework. 🖥 *http://www.dh.gov.uk*

National Research Register (NRR): Database of ongoing and recently completed research projects funded by, or of interest to, the NHS. 🖥 *http://www.update-software.com/national*

University departments of general practice: Every UK medical school has a department of general practice, but there are very few GP academic posts. However, these departments are invaluable sources of advice and support if you contemplate doing any original research of your own.

RCGP: Supports research by giving advice to GPs, providing research training fellowships and research funding through the Scientific Foundation Board, sponsoring 2 research units and 1 research practice, and administering a quality assessment scheme for research practices. 🖥 *http://www.rcgp.org.uk*

Regional research networks: Support GPs wishing to do their own research (or to participate in other people's projects) with courses, newsletters, library facilities, administration, and contact with other like-minded practices. A full list is available from the RCGP.

Ethics: An ethics committee must pass all medical research involving human participants. Permission must be sought from all local ethics committees (LRECs) responsible for the area in which research will take place or, if >4 LRECs, the multi-centre ethics committee (MREC). Information, contacts, and application forms are available from COREC (Central Office for Research Ethics Committees) 🖥 *http://www.corec.org.uk*

Funding: Numerous sources of funding for primary care research are available (including NHS, RCGP, Medical Research Council, and Wellcome Trust) but all are keenly fought for. Take time preparing your protocol. Ask advice. It helps to have an experienced researcher as co-applicant on the application form or as project supervisor. 🖥 *http://www.redinfo.org.uk*

Essential reading

Bowling A. (2002) *Research Methods in Health: Investigating Health and Health Services.* Open University Press

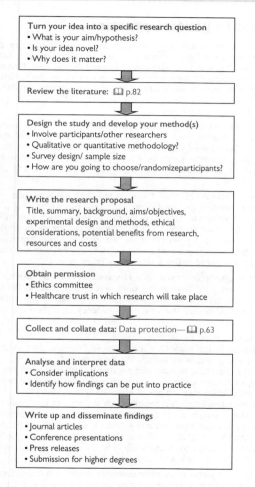

Turn your idea into a specific research question
• What is your aim/hypothesis?
• Is your idea novel?
• Why does it matter?

Review the literature: 📖 p.82

Design the study and develop your method(s)
• Involve participants/other researchers
• Qualitative or quantitative methodology?
• Survey design/ sample size
• How are you going to choose/randomizeparticipants?

Write the research proposal
Title, summary, background, aims/objectives,
experimental design and methods, ethical
considerations, potential benefits from research,
resources and costs

Obtain permission
• Ethics committee
• Healthcare trust in which research will take place

Collect and collate data: Data protection— 📖 p.63

Analyse and interpret data
• Consider implications
• Identify how findings can be put into practice

Write up and disseminate findings
• Journal articles
• Conference presentations
• Press releases
• Submission for higher degrees

Figure 1.7 The research process

Stress in general practice

Increasing stress is a feature of society as a whole. GPs score 2x the national average on stress test scores. Similar figures are seen if anxiety scores are used and 1 in 4 GPs are classed as suffering from depression if depression screening tools are used. Burnout describes the syndrome of emotional exhaustion, depersonalization, low productivity, and feelings of low achievement. A study of British GPs found significant numbers of GPs in all age groups are affected.

Causes of stress in general practice: Insecurity about work (particularly complaints), isolation, poor relationships with other doctors, disillusion with the role of GPs, changing demands, work-home interface, demands of the job—particularly time pressure, problem patients, and emergencies during surgery hours, patients' expectations, and practice administration.

Roots of stress: Many of the main stressors for GPs appear to be created or perpetuated by doctors' own policies: overbooking patients, starting surgeries late, accepting commitments too soon after surgeries are due to finish, making insufficient allowances for extra emergency patients, and allowing inappropriate telephone or other interruptions. Higher than average pressure scores occur in doctors with fast consultation rates compared to those with slower rates.

General characteristics of a stressed person at work Lack of concentration, poor timekeeping, poor productivity, difficulty in comprehending new procedures, lack of cooperation, irritability, aggressiveness, withdrawal behaviour, resentment, ↑ tendency to make mistakes, and resistance to change.

Effects of stress: Poorly documented.
- **Effects on clinical work:** One study showed frustrated doctors are more willing to take undesirable short cuts in treating patients; another, that those doctors with negative feelings of tension, lack of time, and frustration have poor clinical performance (measured by a ↑ prescription rate and lack of explanation to patients).
- **Effects on practice:** Stress has effects on the practice too, resulting in mistakes, arguments, or angry outbursts, poor relationships with patients and staff, increased staff sickness and turnover, and accidents.
- **Effects at home:** Stressed GPs may develop problems in their relationships with their partners and family at home, becoming uncommunicative at home or work, and more withdrawn and isolated.

Experience of stress does not necessarily result in damage. Extent of stress necessary to ↓ performance or satisfaction levels will depend on the doctor's personality, biographical factors, and coping methods, but a concurrent illness or co-existing life event may have additive effects, and can ↑ vulnerability to stress or ↓ ability to cope.

Alcohol: Doctors commonly use alcohol as a coping method for stress. The BMA estimates 7% of doctors are addicted to alcohol and/or other chemical substances, with ½ of those addicted to alcohol alone.

Interventions and solutions:

- *Improve your working conditions:* e.g. longer booking intervals for patient consultations; develop a specialist clinical or academic interest within or outside the practice; learn to decline extra commitments. GPs with high stress levels do not necessarily have low morale but there is a close correlation between levels of job satisfaction and morale—job satisfaction seems to protect against stress.
- *Look at your own behaviour and attitudes:* Stop being a perfectionist; resist the desire to control everything; don't judge your mistakes too harshly.
- *Look after your own health and fitness:* Set aside time for rest and relaxation; make time for regular meals and exercise.
- *Allow time for yourself and your family:* Do not allow work to invade family time. Consider changes in working arrangements to allow more time for leisure and family.
- *Don't be too proud to ask for help:* As well as formal channels for seeking help, there are several informal doctor self-help organizations and counselling services (see below).

Chronic stress: 📖 p.966

Useful contacts

BMA Stress Counseling Service: Service provided by the BMA to members and their families. 24-hour confidential telephone counselling service for all personal, emotional, work or study related problems. ☎0845 9200169.

BMA Doctors Support Line: Callers speak directly to doctors instead of counsellors. Not a 24-hour service. Details of precise hours are on the answerphone message. ☎0870 765 0001.

British Doctors and Dentists Group: Support group of recovering medical and dental drug and alcohol users. Students are also welcomed. Gives confidential help and advice through a local recovering doctor or dentist. National contact (via the Medical Council on Alcohol): ☎0207 487 4445.

National Counselling Service for Sick Doctors: Confidential independent advisory service for sick doctors. 24-hour helpline: ☎0870 241 0535 🖥 http://www.ncssd.org.uk

Sick Doctors Trust: A confidential intervention and advisory service for alcohol and drug ad- dicted doctors, run by doctors, for doctors. 24-hour helpline: ☎0870 444 5163 🖥 http://www.sick-doctors-trust.co.uk

Benefits and aids

⚠ Information in this chapter is up to date at the time of going to press, but issues relating to benefits change rapidly.

Benefits

Millions of pounds of benefits go unclaimed every year. This chapter is a rough guide to the benefits available to enable GPs to point their patients in the right direction. It is not intended as a comprehensive reference.

Table 2.1 Guide to agencies involved in delivering benefits to patients

Agency	Function	Website: http://www. + suffix	Telephone
Department of Work and Pensions (DWP)	Administers all benefits *except:* Tax credits (inland revenue) Statutory sick pay (employer) Housing benefit (local authority) Council tax benefit (local authorities)	dwp.gov.uk	*Benefits enquiry line*—0800 882200 *Help with form completion*—0800 441144 *Information for employers and the self-employed*— 0845 7143143
Jobcentre Plus	Helps people of working age to find work and get any benefits they are entitled to	jobcentreplus. gov.uk	Contact local office (list available on website)
Child Support Agency (CSA)	Administers the Child Support scheme	csa.gov.uk	Enquiry line— 0845 713 31 33
Pension Service	Provides services and support for pensioners and people looking into pensions and retirement	Thepension-service.gov.uk	Contact area office (list available on website)
Inland Revenue	Administers tax credits	inlandrevenue. gov.uk	Tax credit enquiry line—0845 300 3900
Disability and Carers Service	Delivers a range of benefits to disabled people and their carers	disability.gov.uk	Contact local disability benefits office (list available on DWP website)
Appeals Service	Provides an independent tribunal body for hearing appeals	appeals-service. gov.uk	N/A

❶ 0800 numbers are free; 0845 numbers are charged at local rate.

⚠ **Benefit fraud:** Members of the public can telephone the DWP, in confidence, to give information about benefit fraud.
☎ Freefone 0800 85 44 40

Further information for health professionals
Department of Work and Pensions (DWP)
🖳 http://www.dwp.gov.uk

Further information for patients and carers
Government information and services 🖳 http://www.direct.gov.uk
Citizens Advice Bureau 🖳 http://www.adviceguide.org.uk
Age Concern: ☎0800 00 99 66 🖳 http://www.ageconcern.org.uk
Help the Aged: ☎0800 800 65 65 🖳 http://www.helptheaged.org.uk
Counsel and Care ☎0845 300 7585 🖳 www.counselandcare.org.uk

Pensions and bereavement benefits

War pensions: For people injured whilst serving in the armed forces and their dependants (if injury caused or hastened death). Administered by the Veterans Agency, MoD. No time limit for claims.

War disablement pension

- *Basic benefits:* Based on percentage disablement
    - If <20% disabled—lump sum
    - If >20% disabled—weekly sum (pension)
- *Other benefits:* Allowances if severely disabled, e.g.:
    - War Pensioners' Mobility Supplement—for walking difficulty. Holders can apply for the motability scheme and road tax exemption.
    - Constant Attendance Allowance—for high levels of care.

Medical treatment: Some services and appliances may be paid for by the Veterans Agency (includes prescription charges, nursing home fees).

War widows' and widowers' pensions: Payable if spouse's death was as a result of service or, in certain circumstances, if spouse received a war pension prior to death.

Further information

Veterans Agency ☎0800 169 22 77 🖳 http://www.veteransagency.mod.uk

Retirement pension: A state retirement pension is payable to women aged ≥60y. and men aged ≥65y.—even if still working. Claim forms should be received automatically; if not, request one through the local Jobseeker Plus office. Pensions are taxable.

Basic pension: Flat rate amount—different for single people and married couples. If not enough National Insurance (NI) contributions have been paid, amounts may ↓ >80y. higher rate payable which is not dependant on NI contributions.

Increase for dependants: Paid if:
- The claimant's spouse is <60y. and earns under a set amount/does not receive certain other benefits.
- The claimant has children (if claim made before April 2003).

Additional pension: State second pension (replaced SERPS). Based on NI contributions and earnings. Workers can opt out of the additional pension scheme, pay into a private or company scheme instead, and pay lower NI.

Graduated pension: Some people may be entitled to a graduated pension. This is based on earnings between 1961 and 1975.

Extra pension: For a person who defers claiming retirement pension for up to 5y. Extra pension is payable when retirement pension is claimed.

❶ If hospitalized, retirement pension is payable for 1y. at full rate, after which basic pension is ↓ but additional pension stays the same.

Other benefits for pensioners

- *Pension Credit*— 📖 p.102
- *Free colour TV licence:* All pensioners >75y.
- *Winter fuel payment:* Annual payment to all pensioners >60y.
  Freephone advice service ☎0800 22 44 88

Home Responsibilities Protection (HRP): Scheme which protects basic state pension for people who don't work or have low income and are caring for someone. 🖥 *http://www.thepensionservice.gov.uk*

Christmas bonus: One-off payment made a few weeks before Christmas to people receiving a retirement pension or income support.

Bereavement benefits: Payable to men and women whose spouses have died (co-habitation does not count except in Scotland). Bereavement Payment (BPT) is paid where the late spouse has paid enough NI contributions or their death was caused by their employment. Application should be made as soon as possible after death. If the widow/widower remarries or co-habits, benefits are forfeited. Benefits available:

Bereavement payment: Lump sum payable if spouse was not entitled to full basic retirement pension at the time of death.

Widowed parent's allowance: Paid to widows/widowers with children or if pregnant.

Bereavement allowance: Paid for 52wk. from the date of bereavement for spouses >45y. old, not bringing up children, and under retirement age.

Other benefits for widows/widowers

- *Funeral payment*— 📖 p.104.
- *War widows/widowers*—contact Veterans Agency (see opposite).

Cold weather payment: 📖 p.104.

Benefits for people with low income

Table 2.2 Benefits for people with low income

	Eligibility	How to apply	Benefits received
Income Support (IS)	• ≥18y, (16y. in some circumstances) and <60y. • Low income, <£8000 in savings (£16000 if in residential care) and not in receipt of JSA. • <16h. paid work/wk. (and partner <24h./wk.)	Form A1 from local Jobcentre Plus office.	**Money**—depends on circumstances **Other benefits**—housing benefit, community tax benefit, health benefits, and social fund payments. Children <5y. and pregnant women—free milk and vitamins. Children >5y.—free school meals and, in some areas, uniform grants. **Christmas bonus** 🕮 p.101
Job Seekers Allowance (JSA)	• ≥19y. and <60y. (women) or <65y. (men) • Unemployed or working <16h./wk. • Capable of and available for work • Have a Job Seekers agreement that contracts the recipient to actively seek work	Apply by visiting local Job Centre.	**Contributions-based Job Seekers Allowance**—can claim for up to 26wk. Age-dependent fixed weekly payment. **Income-based Job Seekers Allowance**—allowance dependent on circumstances. Entitles claimants to same benefits as income support (see above). **Hardship payments**—available to people disallowed JSA
Pension Credit	**Guarantee credit**— ≥60y. and income below the 'appropriate' amount. Appropriate amount varies according to circumstances. Capital (excluding value of own home) >£6000 is deemed to count as income at the rate of £1/wk./£500 capital. **Savings credit**— ≥65y. and income >savings credit starting point—currently >£82.05/wk. for a single person or >£131.20 if one of a couple. Depends on level of income and circumstances.	Apply on form PC1 ☎0800 991 234	**Money**—depends on circumstances. **Other benefits**—if receiving guarantee credit: automatically eligible for housing benefit, community tax benefit, and social fund payments.

Working Tax Credit (WTC)	• Age ≥16y., working ≥16h./wk., and responsible for a child (<16y. or 16–19y. in full-time education) • Age ≥16y., working ≥16h./wk., and has a disability • Age ≥50y., working ≥16h./wk., and has started work after ≥6mo. of receiving 1 of certain benefits • Age ≥25y. and working ≥30h./wk.	Apply to Inland Revenue: ☎ 0845 300 3900 🖳 http://www.inlandrevenue.gov.uk	**Tax credits**—depends on adding together elements: • Basic element—paid to everyone entitled to WTC • Second adult element • Lone parent element • Working >30h./wk. (can combine both parents hours' if have children) • Disability (if working >16h./wk.) • Severe disability (if working >16h./wk.) • Aged ≥50y. and in receipt of certain benefits before resuming work • Childcare—up to 70% childcare costs
Children's Tax Credit (CTC)	• Age ≥16y. and Responsible for ≥1 child (<16y. or 16–19y. in full-time education) • Family income <£50,000 p.a.	Apply to Inland Revenue: ☎ 0845 300 3900 🖳 http://www.inlandrevenue.gov.uk	**Tax credits:** • Family element—credit for any family eligible—if there is a child <1y. old in the family • Child element—credit for each individual child in the family—if the child is disabled/severely disabled
Health benefits	**Automatic entitlement:** • Age >60y. or <16y. (19y. if in full-time education) • Claiming IS or income-based JSA • Pregnant or within 1y. of childbirth **By application:** • Low income and • Savings <£8000	If automatic exemption, no need to claim. If not, claim using form HC1 available from pharmacies, GP surgeries, and local Jobcentre Plus offices. Pregnancy—🕮 p.112 Free prescriptions—🕮 p.119	**Free:** • Prescriptions • NHS dentistry • NHS eye tests and glasses • NHS wigs and fabric supports • Travel to hospital • Milk and vitamins for pregnant and breast-feeding women, and children <5y.

Table 2.2 (cont.)

	Eligibility	How to apply	Benefits received
Housing Benefit	Low income, living in rented housing. *Exclusions:* Full-time students without dependants, people in residential care or with savings >£16,000.	Via local authority	Pays rent for up to 60wk. Then need to reapply.
Council Tax Benefit and second adult rebate	• **Council tax benefit:** Low income. Exclusions as for housing benefit. • **Second adult rebate:** Payable if someone who lives with you is aged >18y, does not pay rent or council tax, and has low income. • **Council tax reduction:** If single occupier or disabled. • **Disregarded occupants:** Certain people including students, carers, and children, are not counted in calculating the number of people living at a property.	Via local authority	**Council tax benefit:** Pays council tax. **Council tax reductions:** • single occupier—25% discount • all disregarded occupants—50% • disabled—reduction to next lowest council tax band.
The 6 Social Fund payments	• **Crisis loan:** Anyone except students and people in residential care can apply. • **Budgeting loan:** For large purchases. Must receive IS, pension credit, or income-based JSA. • **Funeral payments:** Must receive low income benefit and be responsible for the funeral. • **Cold weather payments:** Average temperature <0°C for ≥7d. Must receive IS, pension credit, or income-based JSA and live with a pensioner, child <5y., or disabled person. • **Maternity grant:** 📖 p.112 • **Community care grant:** 📖 p.106	Cold weather payments should be automatic. All others, claim via local Jobcentre Plus office or 🖥 http://www.dwp.gov.uk	• **Crisis loan:** Up to £1000—interest-free loan repayable when crisis finished, over 78wk. • **Budgeting loan:** As crisis loan. • **Funeral expenses:** Sum towards cost of funeral—usually does not cover full expenses. • **Cold weather payments:** £8.50/wk.

Benefits for disability and illness

Table 2.3 Benefits for disability and illness

	Eligibility	How to apply	Amount
Statutory sick pay	• Employee age ≥16y, and <65y. • Incapable of work due to sickness or disability • Earning ≥ NI lower earnings limit • Unable to work ≥4d. and <28wk. (inc. days when would not normally work) • Those ineligible may be eligible for incapacity benefit or maternity allowance	Notify employer of illness—self-certification first 7d. (SC2 □ p.201); Med 3 after that time (□ p. 201)	£68.20/wk. Some employers have more generous arrangements. Paid through normal pay mechanisms.
Incapacity Benefit	• Not entitled to statutory sick pay (includes self-employed) • Unable to work (Med 3 certification until Personal Capability Assessment is applied when GP may be asked for short factual report or Med 4 □ p.201) • < pensionable age • Sufficient NI contributions (unless aged <20y.)	Form SC1 available from GP surgeries, hospitals, and local social security offices. If employed and unable to claim SSP—apply on form SSP1 supplied by employer.	1–28wk.—£55.90/wk. 29–52wk.—£66.15/wk. >52wk.—£74.15/wk. Plus additions for dependants
Community Care Grant	Receiving Income Support or income-based JSA *and*: • Want to re-establish or help the applicant or a family member stay in the community • Want to ease exceptional pressure on the applicant or a family member • Want to help with certain travel costs	Form SF300 from local social security offices or ⃞ http://www.dwp.gov.uk	Minimum payment £30; no maximum amount.
Disabled Facilities Grant	For work essential to help a disabled person live an independent life. Means tested.	Apply via local housing department.	Any reasonable application for funds is considered.

Disability Living Allowance (DLA)*	• Disability >3mo. and expected to last >6mo. more** • <65y. at time of application **Mobility component:** Help needed to get about outdoors *Higher rate*—unable/virtually unable to walk (age >3y.) *Lower rate* —help to find way in unfamiliar places (age >5y.) **Care Component:** Help needed with personal care • *Lower rate*—attention/supervision needed for a significant proportion of the day or unable to prepare a cooked meal • *Middle rate* —attention/ supervision throughout the day or repeated prolonged attention or watching over at night • *Higher rate* —24-h. attention/supervision day or terminal illness**	☎0800 882 200 (0800 220 674 in Northern Ireland) or Leaflet DS704 available from post offices or Using claim packs available at CAB and social security offices or 🖥 http://www.dwp.gov.uk	**Mobility component:** *Higher rate*—£41.05/wk. *Lower rate*—£15.55/wk. **Care component:** *Higher rate*—£58.80/wk. *Middle rate*—£39.35/wk. *Lower rate*—£15.55/wk.
Attendance Allowance (AA)*	• Disability >3mo. and expected to last >6mo. more** • Aged ≥65y. • Not permanently in hospital or accommodation funded by the local authority • Needs attention/supervision—higher rate if 24h. care required/terminal illness	☎0800 882 200 (0800 220 674 in Northern Ireland) or Leaflet DS704 available from post offices or 🖥 http://www.dwp.gov.uk	*Lower rate*—£39.35 *Higher rate*—£58.80 (for people who need day and night care or are terminally ill)

* No need to receive help to apply. Not means tested.

**Terminal illness (not expected to live >6mo.)—claim under special rules. Claims are processed much faster and the highest care rate is automatically awarded. GP or hospital specialist fills in form DS1500 to provide clinical information to support application (fee can be claimed).

Table 2.3 (cont.)

	Eligibility	How to apply	Amount
Carer's Allowance	• Aged ≥16y, and • Spends ≥35h/wk. caring for a person with a disability who is getting AA or constant attendance allowance or middle or higher rate care component of DLA and • Earning ≤£77.00/wk. after allowable expenses • Not in full-time education	Complete form in leaflet DS700 available from local social security offices or 🖥 http://www.dwp.gov.uk	£43.15/wk. Plus additions for dependants (❶ No new claims for dependent children have been accepted since April 2003)

❶
• People who need someone's help to get out of the house are entitled to free prescriptions—📖 p.119
• Severe Disablement Allowance is still paid to those who applied prior to April 2001

Other useful pages
• Visual impairment/blindness—📖 p.942
• Deafness—📖 p.924
• War pensions—📖 p.100
• Mobility—📖 p.109
• Equipment and adaptations—📖 p.110
• Mothers and children—📖 p.112
• Working Tax Credit—📖 p.103

Mobility for disabled and elderly people

Table 2.4 Mobility for disabled and elderly people   ❶ Local public transport schemes also exist

	Eligibility	How to apply	Benefits received
Blue Badge Scheme	• Age >2y, and ≥1 of the following: • War Pension Mobility Supplement • Higher rate of the mobility component of DLA • Motor vehicle supplied by a government health department • Registered blind • Severe disability in both upper limbs preventing turning of a steering wheel • Permanent and substantial difficulty walking	Apply through local social services department. ❶ In most circumstances the disabled person does not have to be the driver. The badge should not be used if the disabled person is not in the car. 🖳 http://www.dft.gov.uk	Entitles holder to park: • in specified disabled spaces • free of charge or time limit at parking meters or other places where waiting is limited • on single yellow lines for up to 3h. (no time limit in Scotland)
Motability Scheme	• Higher rate mobility component of DLA or • War Pension Mobility Supplement ❶ Driver may be someone else	Contact Motability. Application guide available at 🖳 http://www.motability.co.uk	Registered charity. Mobility payments can be used to lease or hire-purchase a car, powered scooter, or wheelchair. Grants may also be available for advance payments, adaptations, or driving lessons.
Road Tax exemption	• Higher rate mobility component of DLA or • War Pension Mobility Supplement or • Person nominated as someone who regularly drives for a disabled person or • Certain types of powered invalid carriages	Usually received automatically. If not, and claiming DLA, ☎0845 7123456. If claiming War Pension ☎0800 1692277	Exemption from Road Tax.
Seatbelt exemption	Certain medical conditions e.g. colostomy See 🕮 p.202	Medical practitioner must complete exemption certificate	Exemption from wearing seatbelt.

Adaptations and equipment for elderly and disabled people

Table 2.5 Adaptations and equipment for elderly and disabled people ❶ All purchases related to disability are VAT exempt.

	Eligibility	How to apply	Benefits received
Wheelchairs	Anyone requiring a wheelchair(s) for >3mo. Short-term loan of equipment is often available via the Red Cross.	Referral by GP or specialist to wheelchair service centre. Directory service centres available at: 🖳 http://www.wheelchairmanagers.nhs.uk	Provision of suitable wheelchair. Vouchers enable disabled patients to purchase their chairs privately.
Occupational therapy (OT) assessment	All elderly or disabled people	Request needs assessment by occupational therapist via local social services department.	Enables provision of equipment and adaptations necessary to maintain an independent lifestyle.
Disabled Living Centres/ Disability Living Foundation	All elderly or disabled people	49 **Disabled Living Centres** in the UK— list available at 🖳 http://www.dlcc.co.uk **Disabled Living Foundation:** 🖳 http://www.dlf.org.uk.	**Disabled Living Centres**—Look at and try out equipment with OTs on hand to advise **Disabled Living Foundation**—Information on aids and adaptations
Telephone	People who have physical difficulty using the telephone or communication problems	British Telecom produce a booklet 'Communication solutions' obtainable from ☎0800 800150 or 🖳 http://www.bt.com If difficulty using a telephone directory, register to use directory enquiries free ☎0800 587 0195	Gadgets and services that make it easier for disabled or elderly people to use the telephone.
Alarm systems	Any disabled or elderly person who is alone at times, at risk, and mentally capable of using an alarm system	Arrange via local social services or housing department. Alternatively, charities for the elderly have schemes (Help the Aged— seniorlink ☎01255 473 999; Age Concern—Aid-Call ☎0800 772266).	Enables a call for help when the phone cannot be reached.

Benefits for mothers and children

Table 2.6 Benefits for mothers and children

	Eligibility	How to apply	Benefits received
Child Benefit	Anyone responsible for the upbringing of a child aged <16y.	Application form from local social security office or ☐ http://www.dwp.gov.uk	*Oldest child*—£16.50/wk. *Other children*—£11.05/wk.
Statutory Maternity Pay (SMP)*	• Worked for the same employer for 26wk. into the 15th week before the baby is due • Pregnant at (or have had the baby by) the 11th week before the baby is due • Earning ≥ NI lower earnings limit in the relevant period	• Inform employer at least 28d. before starting leave • Mat B1 form—☐ p.201 & p.775	Paid for up to 26wk. (Maternity Pay Period—MPP)—can start any time from 11th week before the baby is due until the week of birth. • 1st 6wk—90% usual average earnings • 6–26wk—90% of usual earnings or £102.80/wk.—whichever is lower.
Maternity Allowance (MA)*	• Employed/self-employed for ≥26w. in the 66w. preceding the baby's due date (test period). • Average weekly earnings of ≥£30/wk. for at least 13w. of the test period • Do not qualify for SMP (e.g. changed jobs, become unemployed, self-employed).	• Apply >26/40 and within 3mo. of date MA due to start. Need: • Form MA1 (available from social security offices, employer, or DWP ☐ http://www.dwp.gov.uk • MATB1; and, if employed • Form SMP1 from employer.	Paid for 26wk. (Maternity Allowance Period—MAP)—can start any time from 11th week before the baby is due until the day after birth. 90% of usual earnings or £102.80/wk.—whichever is lower.

| Sure Start Maternity Grant | • From 11w. before baby is due to <3mo. after birth/adoption
• Claiming IS or income-based JSA; Child Tax Credit at a higher rate than the maximum family element or Working Tax Credit with a disability or severe disability element | Form SF100 from social security offices. | £500 payment |

❶ Free prescriptions/dentistry are available to all children <16y., mothers while pregnant and <1y. after birth, and families with low income—📖 p.119.

* Incapacity benefit and income support may be available for women unable to claim SMP or MA—📖 p.106; Statutory paternity pay is paid if gross weekly earnings are ≥ £79/wk. for 1–2 consecutive weeks at £102.80/wk. or 90% of average weekly earnings if less.

Occupational illness and criminal injury

Occupational illness: If a patient develops an occupational disease, a doctor is obliged to notify their employer in writing with the patient's consent. The doctor does not need to make a judgment about whether the disease is, in that particular case, caused by the occupation.

Employers must then inform the Reporting of Injuries, Diseases and Dangerous Occurrences Regulations (RIDDOR) incident contact centre (☎0845 300 99 23 🖥 http://www.riddor.gov.uk). Self-employed patients must contact RIDDOR themselves.

Patients who do not give consent for the doctor to notify his/her employer may allow the doctor to inform the employer's occupational health department or RIDDOR directly instead.

Notifiable industrial diseases ❶ This is not a complete list

- Poisoning by industrial agents e.g. lead, arsenic, mercury
- Repetitive strain injury
- Vibration white finger
- Bursitis e.g. housemaid's knee
- Occupational asthma
- Folliculitis and acne (associated with work with tar, pitch, or oils)
- Occupational infection e.g. hepatitis B in healthcare workers, anthrax in farmers
- Chrome ulceration
- Irritant dermatitis e.g. hairdressers' dermatitis
- Tenosynovitis e.g. as a result of repeated movements of the hand/wrist.
- Pneumoconiosis
- Extrinsic allergic alveolitis
- Occupational deafness
- Occupational cancers e.g. nasopharyngeal cancer in woodworkers; bladder cancer in plastic workers; cancers as a result of ionizing radiation; mesothelioma due to asbestos exposure

---

Industrial injury: Injured employees should always report details of the accident to their employer and record them in the accident book as soon as possible—however trivial the injury. Employers must inform RIDDOR of:

- dangerous incidents—even if no-one was hurt
- incidents where death or serious injury occurs
- incidents resulting in injury requiring >3d. absence from work
- incidents involving gas

Industrial injuries disablement benefit: Available to employed earners for injuries resulting from accidents or certain (prescribed) illness arising as a result of employment, even if the employee was either part or wholly to blame. 'Industrial' covers virtually all forms of work. For accidents, claims can be made at any time after the event but benefit is paid only if there are still effects of the injury after the 91st day.

Prescribed industrial disease: Disease for which benefit is paid if the applicant worked in a job for which that disease is 'prescribed' and it is likely the employment caused the disease. Claims may be made at any time with the exceptions of occupational deafness (claim <5y. after leaving employment) and occupational asthma (claim <10y. after leaving employment). The list of prescribed diseases is similar to but *not* the same as the list of notifiable diseases.

Benefits that may be payable

Disablement benefit: If the person was a paid employee at the time of the accident or when s/he contracted the disease; *and* disability is assessed at ≥14% (exceptions: occupational deafness >20%; dust-related lung disease—no level). If a patient claims benefit for >1 industrial accident or disease, assessments may be added together and benefit awarded on the total.

Reduced earnings allowance: Accident occurred/disease contracted prior to 1st October 1990; disablement assessment of ≥1%; *and*
- unable to work; *or*
- unable to work at normal job; *or*
- working less hours at normal job.

Retirement allowance: Reduced earnings allowance becomes retirement allowance at age 60y. (woman) or 65y. (man). It is paid at 25% the rate of reduced earnings allowance when a claimant stopped work.

Constant attendance allowance: For people so disabled they need constant care and attention and who are getting disablement benefit for disability assessed at 100%. 4 rates of benefit.

Exceptionally severe disablement allowance: For people who get constant attendance allowance at high rate and where need for attendance is likely to be permanent.

❶ People who suffer from industrial diseases or have suffered disability as a result of an industrial accident are also eligible to apply for benefits available for any disabled individuals—📖 p.106–10.

Making claims: Through local Jobcentre Plus or social security office. A full list of prescribed industrial diseases is also available from these places. Some claims can be made on-line: 🖥 http://www.jobcentreplus.gov.uk

Criminal injuries: Compensation may be available for victims of violent crimes—even if the attacker is not identified. Compensation is paid for the injury, loss of earnings, and expenses. Contact Criminal Injuries Compensation Authority 🖥 http://www.cica.gov.uk

Useful contacts

RIDDOR: Incident Contact Centre ☎0845 300 99 23 🖥 http://www.riddor.gov.uk
Health and Safety Executive: ☎0870 1545500 🖥 http://www.hse.gov.uk
Jobcentre Plus 🖥 http://www.jobcentreplus.gov.uk
Trade Unions

Prescribing

Further information

British National Formulary (BNF) 🖥 *http://www.bnf.org*

NHS prescriptions (1)

> *'A doctor is a man who writes prescriptions till the patient either dies or is cured by nature'*
> John Taylor (1694–1761)

At any one time, 70% of the UK population is taking medicines. ¾ of people >75y. are taking prescribed medicines and 36% of older people take ≥4 different medications on a regular basis. 1.7 million prescriptions are dispensed daily within the NHS to prevent illness, cure existing illness, and give symptomatic relief, costing >£6 billion/y. (>10% NHS costs).

Prescribing forms a major part of any GP's workload. Bad prescribing wastes resources, deprives patients of the chance to benefit, and may cause illness. Medicines should be prescribed only when necessary and, in all cases, benefits of prescribing should be weighed against risks.

Prescription pre-payment certificate (PPC): If not entitled to free prescriptions but needing a lot of medication (>5 prescriptions/4mo. or >14/y.) it is cheaper for a patient to purchase a 'pre-payment certificate'. There are 4 ways to purchase a PPC:

• Internet 🖳 http://www.ppa.org.uk
• Telephone ☎0845 850 00 30
• Post—form FP95 available from doctors' surgeries and pharmacists or 🖳 http://www.dh.gov.uk. Send completed form to PPC Issue Office, PO Box 854, Newcastle-upon-Tyne NE99 2DE
• From a pharmacy registered to sell PPCs. List available at 🖳 http://www.ppa.org.uk

Refunds: Send PPC and letter explaining the reason for refund to PPC Issue Office (address above). Full refund may be claimed if <1mo. after purchase the holder becomes entitled to free prescriptions or dies. Partial refund may be claimed if the holder dies >1mo. after issue or if the holder becomes entitled to free prescriptions 1–4mo. after issue.

Reclaiming money spent whilst awaiting exemption certificate or PPC: Ask for official receipt at pharmacy when drug is paid for (FP57 England/EC 57 Scotland). Claim money back within 3mo.

Drugs cheaper OTC: The Consumer's Association publishes a list of drugs with recommended retail price < the prescription charge and circulates it periodically with *Drugs and Therapeutics Bulletin*. Copies can be obtained from: Dept. DTB, Consumer's Association, Castlemead, Gascoyne Way, Hertford, SG14 1LH.

❶ Prescriptions currently cost less in Wales, and the aim of the Welsh Assembly is to abolish prescription charges completely by 2007.

Table 3.1 Free prescription entitlement

Free prescription entitlement	Action needed
• Prescription for contraception • >60y, or <16y, or 16–18y, of age in full-time education • Patient or family receiving IS or income-based JSA	Tick box on reverse of prescription form
Pregnant women and women who have had a baby <12mo. ago (MatEx)	Fill in form FW8 as soon as pregnancy confirmed—exemption certificate lasts 1y, from EDD. If form not completed until after baby is born exemption certificate lasts 12mo. after date of birth. Includes dentists' charges.
Certain conditions (MedEx): • DM (unless diet controlled only) • Myxoedema/requirement for thyroxine or hypoparathyroidism • Epilepsy requiring continuous anticonvulsants • Permanent fistula (e.g. colostomy) needing stoma dressing/appliance • Hypoadrenalism (inc. Addison's disease) needing replacement therapy • Hypopituitarism including diabetes insipidus • Myasthenia gravis • Unable to go out without the help of another person due to a continuing physical disability	Fill in form FP92A (available from doctors' surgeries). Requires a doctor's signature to confirm condition when applying for exemption. Certificate lasts 5y, or until 60th birthday if sooner.
War pensioners—prescriptions related to pensionable condition only	Apply through Veterans' Agency ☎0800 169 22 77
Low income and <£8000 savings (higher if in residential care or aged ≥60y,), or pending application for any benefit listed above	Students are eligible. Includes opticians' and dentists' charges. Apply through NHS low income scheme (LIS) on form HC1 ☎0845 850 1166 or 🖳http://www.ppa.org.uk/ppa/HC1_form_intro.htm

❶ Leaflet HC11 (Help with Health Costs) is available from Post Offices, some pharmacies, GP surgeries, or Department of Health, PO Box 777, London SE1 6 X H.

NHS prescriptions (2)

⚠ Legal responsibility for prescribing lies with the person who signs the prescription form

British National Formulary (BNF): contains a list of all drugs which a registered medical practitioner can prescribe on NHS prescription. Does not include homeopathic drugs which can be prescribed on NHS prescription or aids and appliances. Dentists and nurses have their own limited formulary. ▣ http://www.bnf.org

Claiming for items dispensed by a non-dispensing GP: All GPs may claim payment for dispensing certain items which are supplied and personally administered by the GP or practice staff on their behalf. Claims are made on form FP10 (GP10) to the PPA and must state the name of the patient, item dispensed, and manufacturer of the item. Claimable items are:

- Vaccines
- Anaesthetics
- Injections
- Sutures
- Skin closing strips
- IUCDs
- Contraceptive caps/diaphragms
- Diagnostic reagents
- Pessaries which are appliances (e.g. ring pessary)

❶ Different arrangements apply for high-volume vaccines e.g. influenza

Prescription writing: NHS prescriptions are written on form FP10 (GP10 in Scotland). They should be legible and in indelible ink. They are valid for 13wk. from the date written on them. Include:
- Patient details—full name, address, and age/date of birth if <12y.
- Date
- Full name of drug (not abbreviated) with quantity to be supplied and dose interval (avoid the use of decimal points e.g. quantities <1g, write in mg). If you want a description of the drug included on the label, write it on the prescription.
- Deletion of any unused space (e.g. by striking through)
- Signature of the prescriber in ink
- Name and address of the prescriber

❶ Special rules apply for controlled drugs—▢ p.132

Computer issued prescriptions (form FP10(C)): Should contain the same information as their hand-written equivalents. They must still be signed in ink by the responsible GP. Prescriptions for controlled drugs (with the exception of phenobarbitone) must not be printed from computer—blank forms may be printed, but details apart from the name and address of the GP and their health authority and prescribing number must be handwritten. Prescriptions for phenobarbitone can be computer generated but the date must be handwritten.

Guidelines are available from the Joint Computing Group of the GPC and RCGP (summary is available in the BNF ▣ http://www.bnf.org)

Non-NHS prescriptions: The same rules apply to the writing of private prescriptions as NHS prescriptions but private prescriptions should not be written on FP10 forms (normally headed note paper is used). There are no restrictions upon which drugs can be prescribed.

Nurse prescribers: (*BNF*—Appendix NPF). List of preparations approved by the Secretary of State which may be prescribed on form FP10P (form HS21(N) in Northern Ireland, form GP10(N) in Scotland, forms FP10(CN) and FP10(PN) in Wales) by nurses for NHS patients. Nurses who have undergone additional training can prescribe from the nurse prescribers' extended formulary list.

Dentists: (*BNF*—Appendix DPF). Can prescribe medication for dental conditions to their NHS patients on form FP10 (D) (GP14 in Scotland).

Emergency supply of medicines by pharmacists: In emergency situations, pharmacists can dispense prescription only medicines (POM). In general, ≤5d. supply can be dispensed.

Patient information: Since 1994, all newly licensed/relicensed medicines dispensed in an original pack must be accompanied by a patient information leaflet (PiL). Despite the fact most drugs are now supplied with PiLs, doctors should make patients aware of 'substantial or special risks when offering treatment'. How much information to give is unclear. Information regarded as important by patients is: name of the drug; what to do if a dose is missed; purpose of treatment; precautions (e.g. effect on driving); when and how to take the medicine; problems with alcohol and other drugs; unwanted effects and what to do about them.

Security of prescriptions: Prescription theft and fraud is common and wastes valuable NHS resources. *Basic precautions:*
- *Prescriptions*—should not be left unattended at reception desks; should not be left in a car where they might be visible; and, when not in use, should be kept in a locked drawer, both at the surgery and at home.
- *Writing prescriptions*—draw a diagonal line over the blank part of the form under the prescription; write the quantity in words and figures for drugs prone to abuse (even if not controlled drugs); make alterations clear and unambiguous and add your initials against any altered items.

If prescription fraud is suspected ☎08702 400 100

Further information

Counter Fraud and Security Management Service (CFSMS) ⌨ *http://www.cfsms.nhs.uk*

Cost-effective prescribing

Generic prescribing: Use of generic names when prescribing is one of the simplest ways to ↓ cost of drugs to the NHS, but only 63% drugs prescribed by GPs in the UK are prescribed generically.

Every marketed drug has a chemical name, generic name, and a proprietary or brand name. For as long as the drug's patent is valid, the company that developed the drug will derive income from prescriptions, whatever the name on the prescription. Once the patent has expired, competitors can manufacture the drug and market it under its generic or an alternative brand name. If the drug is prescribed generically, the pharmacist decides which brand to supply and market forces drive price ↓.

Advantages of generic prescribing: Cost ↓, professional convenience (there are often several brand names for one drug—using generic names, everyone knows they are talking about the same thing), ↓ inconvenience to the patient (pharmacists do not stock each brand of a given drug and, if prescribed by brand name, may have to order a supply; usually generic preparations of all commonly used drugs are available).

Reasons not to prescribe generically

- *Drugs with a low therapeutic index:* e.g. lithium, carbamazepine, phenytoin, ciclosporin—dosage is carefully titrated against plasma concentration or response. Small differences in plasma concentrations can be clinically significant.
- *Modified release formulations:* e.g. diltiazem, nifedipine, amino phylline, or theophylline products. Composition and pharmokinetic properties are very difficult to standardize.
- *Formulations containing ≥2 drugs:* Some do have generic names (e.g. co-amilofruse 5/40, co-proxamol); others do not. Don't make up a generic name if there isn't one.

Evidence-based prescribing: Decisions on what to prescribe and when, were, in the past, largely based on guess work or faith. With the advent of information from randomized controlled trials and their evaluation using systematic reviews and other techniques, such decisions can now be based (at least in part) on scientific evidence. Failure to do this may cause patients to suffer unnecessary side-effects of ineffective drugs, deprive patients of the chance to benefit from effective treatments, and waste valuable resources. *Sources of information:* 📖 p.82–3.

NICE: 📖 p.20

Rationing: 📖 p.11

Practice formularies: An agreed practice formulary is an effective way to limit prescribing and costs of prescribing. Compiling a formulary from scratch is a daunting prospect but there are many formularies available, which can then be modified according to evidence that emerges and review within a practice (contact PCO prescribing lead). When compiling or reviewing a formulary consider: evidence of efficacy; safety; cost effectiveness; local policy.

Prescription Pricing Authority (PPA): Special health authority with 4 functions:
1. To scrutinize pricing and payment to contractors for dispensing of NHS prescriptions
2. Prevention of prescribing and dispensing fraud in the NHS
3. Provision of prescribing and dispensing information to the NHS (excluding hospital dispensing)
4. Management of the NHS low income scheme.

PACT data: Since 1988, the PPA has provided GPs in England and Wales with regular information on their prescribing habits and costs through *Prescribing analysis and cost* (PACT). 2 levels of information:
- *Standard report:* Sent to each GP with a prescribing number on a quarterly basis. Outer pages—practice or GP level details of cost and number of prescriptions for that quarter; top 20 drugs which drive the GP's prescribing costs; top 40 BNF sections; and average cost/prescription. Centre pages—information on a topical aspect of prescribing and related practice-specific feedback.
- *Prescribing catalogue:* Issued only at the request of the prescriber. Full inventory of prescriptions during the period specified (1–24mo.).

It can be used to improve prescribing habits, ↓ prescribing costs, and to produce formularies and prescribing policies.

A similar scheme operates in Scotland (Scottish Prescribing Analysis—SPA).

Further information
UK Medicines information: 🖳 *http://www.ukmi.nhs.uk*
Electronic medicines compendium: 🖳 *http://www.medicines.org.uk*
Prescription Pricing Authority: 🖳 *http://www.ppa.org.uk*

Medicines management and concordance

Medicines management: Defined as 'facilitating the maximum bene-fit and minimum risk for medicines for individual patients'. Encompasses the way medicines are selected, procured, delivered, prescribed, administered, and reviewed to optimize use. *Components are:*
- Optimizing a medication regime (right drug at right time);
- Facilitating adherence to medication, including beliefs and fears as well as physical problems;
- Organizing supply and administration support, such as repeat dispensing systems;
- Providing monitoring and feedback systems.

Concordance: Is a process of prescribing and medicine taking based on partnership. Patient concordance (or rather lack of it) is a major challenge in general practice. For drugs to be optimally effective they should be taken as directed by the prescriber. Concordance sufficient to attain therapeutic objectives occurs about ½ the time—1:6 patients take medication exactly as directed; 1:3 take medication as directed 80–90% of the time; 1:3 take medication 40-80% of the time; the remaining 16–17% take medication as directed <40% of the time. 20% prescriptions are never 'cashed'.

'White-coat concordance': Phenomenon in which 90% of patients take regular medication as directed for a period before a check up—may mask effects of non-concordance.

Consequences of non-concordance: Failure to attain therapeutic targets e.g. failure to take antihypertensive medication ↓ reduction of stroke by 30–50%; wastage of precious resources (~£230 million worth of medicines are returned to pharmacies each year for disposal—the true quantity wasted is many times that).

Causes of non-concordance
- *Patient beliefs*: Strongest predictor of compliance—how natural a medicine is seen to be, the dangers of addiction and dependence, the belief that constant use may lead to ↓ efficacy have all been shown to influence compliance.
- *Lifestyle choices*
  - Unpleasant side-effects (especially if not pre-warned)
  - Inconvenience (e.g. multiple daily dosage regimes—though little difference between od and bd dosage)
  - No perceived benefit
- *Information:* Instructions not understood or poor understanding of the condition/treatment.
- *Practical:* Forgetfulness; inability to open containers.
- *Professional*
  - Doctor-patient relationship (link between patient satisfaction with consultation and subsequent concordance).
  - Inappropriate prescribing; mistakes in administration/dispensing.

Improving concordance: ~70% patients want to be more involved in decisions about treatment. Doctors underestimate the degree to which they instruct and overestimate the degree to which they consult and elicit their patients' views. The doctor's task is, by negotiation, to help patients choose the best way to manage their problem. Patients are more likely to be motivated to take medicines as prescribed when they:
- Understand and accept the diagnosis
- Agree with the treatment proposed
- Have had their concerns about the medicines specifically and seriously addressed.

Ways to improve concordance

- Use simple language and avoid medical terms.
- Discuss reasons for treatment and consequences of not treating the condition ensuring information is tailored, clear, accurate, accessible, and sufficiently detailed.
- Seek the patient's views on their condition.
- Agree course of action before prescribing.
- Explain what the drug is, its function, and (if known and not too complex) its mechanism of action.
- Keep the drug regime as simple as possible—od or bd dosing preferable, especially long-term.
- Seek the patients views on how they will manage the regime within their daily schedule and try to tie in with daily routine (e.g. take one in the morning when you get up).
- Discuss possible side-effects (especially common or unpleasant side-effects).
- Give clear verbal instructions and reinforce with written instructions if complex regime, elderly, or understanding of patient is in doubt.
- Deal with any questions the patient has.
- Repeat information yourself and also ask patients to repeat information back to you to reinforce.
- If necessary, arrange review within short time of starting medicine to discuss progress or queries, or arrange follow-up by another member of the primary healthcare team (e.g. asthma nurse to check inhaler technique 2–3wk. after starting inhaler).
- Address further patient questions and practical difficulties at follow-up.
- Monitor repeat prescriptions.

Further information

Medicines Partnership: from compliance to concordance. ⊡ *http://www.concordance.org*
Managing Medicines: ⊡ *http://www.managingmedicines.com*

Repeat prescribing

80% of NHS prescriptions are for repeat medication. Good practice is essential to ensure wastage (>10% of total prescribing costs) is kept to a minimum. *Essential elements are:*

- *Written explanation*—repeat prescribing process for patients and carers
- *Practice personnel with dedicated responsibility*—ensure patient recall and regular medication review
- *Agreed practice policies*—for repeat prescriptions e.g. duration of supply; procedure if someone 'runs out' but isn't authorized to have more
- *Authorization check*—each time a prescription is signed
- *Compliance check*—for under or over-use (prescription frequency)
- *Equivalence check*—all regular prescriptions are for the same duration of treatment so that prescription requests can be synchronized
- *Regular housekeeping*—keep records of medication up to date (including dosage instructions); particular care after hospital discharge when medication could have been substantially changed
- *Training of practice staff*

Review process: Invite patient ± carer. *Areas to cover:*
- *Explain* what you want to do in the review and the reasons for it
- *Compile* a list of all medicines being taken/used including: prescribed medication; OTC drugs; herbal/homeopathic medicines; illicit drugs; and medicines borrowed from others, and *compare* the list of drugs generated with the prescription record
- *Concordance*—find out whether and how medication is taken
- *Explore* understanding of purpose of medication and consequences of not taking it, and how much, how often, when
- *Discuss* misconceptions/queries
- *Ask* about side-effects
- *Review relevant monitoring tests* e.g. TFTs; INR; HbA$_{1c}$
- *Review practical aspects*—problems ordering/receiving repeat prescriptions; using medicines e.g. problems opening containers; with formulations e.g. difficulty swallowing tablets; reading labels—can request large print; remembering to take medication—consider reminder chart, Dossett box, altering times of doses to fit in better with daily schedule
- *Check* necessity and appropriateness of all prescriptions (see Figure 3.1)

Further information

Cantrill *et al.* (1998) Quality in Health Care; **7**: 130–5.
DOH: Medicines and older people. 🖳 http://www.dh.gov.uk
UK medicines information: 🖳 http://www.ukmi.nhs.uk
Electronic medicines compendium: 🖳 http://www.medicines.org.uk

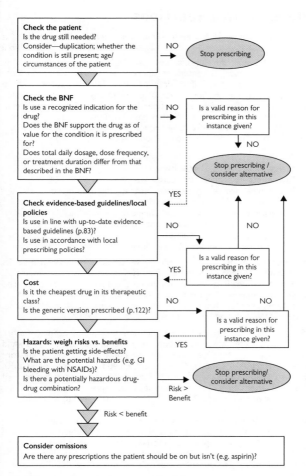

Check the patient
Is the drug still needed?
Consider—duplication; whether the condition is still present; age/circumstances of the patient

NO → Stop prescribing

Check the BNF
Is use a recognized indication for the drug?
Does the BNF support the drug as of value for the condition it is prescribed for?
Does total daily dosage, dose frequency, or treatment duration differ from that described in the BNF?

NO → Is a valid reason for prescribing in this instance given?

↓ NO

Stop prescribing / consider alternative

YES

Check evidence-based guidelines/local policies
Is use in line with up-to-date evidence-based guidelines (p.83)?
Is use in accordance with local prescribing policies?

NO → Is a valid reason for prescribing in this instance given?

NO

YES

Cost
Is it the cheapest drug in its therapeutic class?
Is the generic version prescribed (p.122)?

NO → Is a valid reason for prescribing in this instance given?

NO

YES

Hazards: weigh risks vs. benefits
Is the patient getting side-effects?
What are the potential hazards (e.g. GI bleeding with NSAIDs)?
Is there a potentially hazardous drug-drug combination?

Risk > Benefit → Stop prescribing/consider alternative

Risk < benefit

Consider omissions
Are there any prescriptions the patient should be on but isn't (e.g. aspirin)?

Figure 3.1 Deciding whether a prescribed drug is appropriate

Adverse drug reactions

'I don't want two diseases—one nature-made and one doctor-made'
Napolean Bonaparte, St. Helena, 1820

In 5–17% hospital admissions, an adverse drug reaction is implicated. Any drug may produce unwanted or unexpected effects. Common side-effects are listed in the BNF or drug data sheet but any patient can have an allergic reaction or idiosyncratic response to any drug. The possibility of rare (<1:5000) or delayed reactions means that safety of new medicines cannot be established until they have been used for some time in a large population. A 24h. freefone service is available for information and advice about suspected adverse reactions (☎0800 731 6789).

Classification:
- *Allergy*—anaphylaxis, allergic rash
- *Toxic effect*—e.g. ataxia with carbamazepine if dose too high
- *Predictable*—well recognized side-effect e.g. dry mouth with amitriptyline, GI bleeding with aspirin
- *Idiosyncratic*—unpredictable and unique to the individual
  - *Type A:* common and relates to the pharmacology of the drug e.g. constipation with opiates
  - *Type B:* rare, unpredictable, and often serious

Defective medicines: A medicine which does not conform to its specification is deemed defective. Report suspected defective medicine, with as much detail as possible on product and nature of defect to: The Defective Medicines Report Centre, Medicines and Healthcare Products Regulatory Agency, Room 1801, Market Towers, 1 Nine Elms Lane, London SW8 5NQ ☎020 7273 0574 or 020 7210 3000.

Suspected adverse reactions: To any therapeutic agent (whether OTC, herbal/alternative medication, or prescribed by a doctor) should be reported to the Medicines and Healthcare Products Regulatory Agency (MHRA—formerly MCA—CSM Freepost, London SW8 5BR). Forms ('Yellow cards') are available from that address or in the back of the BNF. Alternatively, report online at 🖳 *http://www.mca.gov.uk*
- *For new drugs* (marked ▼ in BNF): Doctors are asked to report all reactions whether or not causality is clear.
- *For established drugs:* Doctors are asked to report all reactions in children; all serious suspected reactions, even if the effect is well documented (e.g. anaphylaxis, blood disorders, renal or liver impairment, drug interactions) *but not* well-known; relatively minor side-effects (e.g. constipation with opioids, insomnia with SSRIs).

Prevention of adverse reactions
- Never use a drug unless there is a good indication.
- Ask the patient if they have had reactions previously to a drug, before prescribing.
- Ask about other drugs the patient is taking (including self-medication). Consider interactions.
- Consider the effects of age and hepatic or renal impairment.
- Prescribe as few drugs as possible (the more drugs, the more likelihood of interactions).
- Give clear instructions about how to take the drug.
- Wherever possible, use a drug you are familiar with. If using a new drug, be alert to side-effects.
- Warn the patients about potentially serious side-effects (e.g. risk GI ulceration with NSAIDs).

Consumer Protection Act (1987): If a patient is damaged by a defective product, liability falls on the producer (unless outside the EC, when it falls to the importer). If the importer cannot be identified, liability falls on the supplier. This is important for GPs. Those who dispense are at greatest risk, but all GPs occasionally supply drugs in an emergency or for procedures within the surgery (vaccinations, minor surgery, contraception). Always record manufacturer, batch number, and expiry date when using such drugs and keep records of storage of drugs and maintenance of equipment.

Poisoning: 📖 p.1078

Poisons information

UK National Poisons Information Service ☎0870 600 6266
TOXBASE poisons database 🖥 *http://www.spib.axl.co.uk*

Licensing

In the UK, the Medicines Act (1968) makes it essential for anyone who manufactures or markets a drug for which therapeutic claims are made, to hold a licence. The Licensing Authority, working through the Medicines and Healthcare Products Regulatory Agency (MHRA), can grant both manufacturer's licence and marketing authorization (which allows a company to market and supply a product for specified indications). Although doctors usually prescribe according to the licensed indications, they are not obliged to.

Prescribing outside licence: There may be occasions when a doctor feels it is necessary to prescribe outside a drug's licence:
- *Generic formulations* for which indications are not described. The prescriber has to assume the indications are the same as for branded formulations.
- *Use of well-established drugs for proven but not licensed indications* e.g. amitriptyline for neuropathic pain.
- *Use of drugs for conditions where there are no other treatments* (even if the evidence of their effectiveness is not well proven). This often occurs in secondary care when new treatments become accepted. GPs may become involved if a patient is discharged to the community and the GP is asked to continue prescribing. ❶ The person signing the prescription is legally responsible.
- *Use of drugs not covered by their licensed indications.* Frequently occurs in paediatrics.

⚠ Before prescribing any medication (whether within or outside the licence), weigh risks against benefits. The more dangerous the medicine, and the flimsier the evidence-base for treatment, the more difficult it is to justify the decision to prescribe.

When prescribing licensed drugs for unlicensed indications inform patients and carers of what you are doing and why. Explain that the patient information leaflet (PiL) will not have information about the use of the drug in these circumstances. Record in the patient's notes your reasons for prescribing outside the licensed indications for the drug.

Clinical trials: Drug discovery and development is a protracted process (>10y.) costing huge sums of money (≈£100 million). Clinical testing is conventionally divided into 5 stages:
- *Phase I trials:* clinical pharmacology in normal volunteers.
- *Phase II trials:* preliminary small-scale studies.
- *Phase III trials:* large-scale trials (several thousand patients often). Once complete, application is made for a licence to sell the drug.
- *Phase IV trials:* post-marketing surveillance—large-scale follow-up of patients using the drug to establish evidence of long-term efficacy and safety.
- *Phase V trials:* further trials to compare efficacy and safety with other marketed compounds and explore new indications.

GPs are unlikely to be involved before phase III. Taking part in trials can benefit both patients and practice, but consider proposals carefully before embarking on a project (see below).

Research in general practice: 📖 p.92

Questions to ask before agreeing to take part in a clinical trial

- Are the aims and objectives of the study defined?
- What is the design?
- Which drug is to be tested?
- What are the end-points?
- Are the criteria for identifying patients clear and explicit?
- Are the numbers to be recruited specified and feasible?
- Are the observations to be made clearly and vigorously defined?
- Are the arrangements for providing information to patients and for obtaining informed consent satisfactory?
- Has ethical approval of the study been obtained?
- Are the financial arrangements clearly set out (minimum— reimbursement of patients' expenses and practice expenses)?
- Has adequate provision been made for compensation in the event of injury to patients in the course of the study?

Controlled drugs (CDs)

Prescriptions ordering CDs in schedules 2 or 3 must be hand written (with the exceptions of temazepam capsules and phenobarbitone—for which date must be handwritten) and signed and dated by the prescriber. *Prescriptions must state:*

- Name and address of the patient
- Form and strength of the preparation
- Total quantity of the preparation or number of dose units in words and figures
- Dose the patient should take

For example: Morphine sulphate 10mg (ten milligram) tablets, one to be taken twice daily. Please supply 60 (sixty) tablets, total 600 (six hundred) milligrams.

A prescription may request the drug to be dispensed in instalments, when the amount in each instalment and interval between instalments should be stated.

Prescriber's responsibilities

- To avoid creating dependence by unnecessarily introducing CDs to patients.
- Careful monitoring to ensure the patient does not gradually ↑ the dose of drug to a point where dependence becomes more likely.
- To avoid being an unwitting source of supply for addicts. If you suspect an addict is going round surgeries with intent to obtain supplies, contact your PCO so that they can issue a warning to other practices.

Notification of drug misusers: Doctors are expected to report, on a standard form, cases of drug misuse to their regional or national drug misuse database or centre. All types of problem drug misuse should be reported. Databases cannot be used as a check on multiple prescribing as data are anonymized.

Table 3.2 Regional and national drug misuse databases/centres

Region	Area code telephone number (fax)
South East (West) and Eastern	01865 226734 (226652)
Thames and South East (East)	020 7594 0811 (7594 0866)
Merseyside and Cheshire	0151 231 4319 (231 4320)
North Western	0161 772 3782 (772 3445)
Northern and Yorkshire	0113 295 1337 (295 1310)
South West	0117 918 6880 (918 6883)
Trent	0116 225 6360 (225 6370)
West Midlands	0121 580 4331 (525 7980)
Scotland	0131 551 8715 (551 1392)
Wales	029 2082 6260 (2082 5473)
Northern Ireland	028 9052 2421 or 9052 0532

Misuse of Drugs Act (1971): Controls manufacture, supply, and possession of CDs. Penalties for offences are graded according to perceived harmfulness of the drug into 3 classes:
- *Class A:* e.g. cocaine, diamorphine (heroin), methadone, LSD, ecstasy
- *Class B:* e.g. oral amphetamines, barbiturates
- *Class C:* e.g. most benzodiazepines, androgenic and anabolic steroids, cannabis (recent downgrading)

Misuse of Drugs Regulations (1985): Defines persons authorized to supply and possess CDs while carrying out their professions and describes the way in which this is to be done. 5 schedules of drug:
- *Schedule 1:* Drugs not used for medicinal purposes e.g. LSD. Possession and supply prohibited except with special licence.
- *Schedule 2:* Drugs subject to full CD controls (written dispensing record, kept in locked container, CD prescription regulations) e.g. diamorphine, cocaine, pethidine.
- *Schedule 3:* Partial CD controls (as schedule 2 but no need to keep register—some drugs subject to safe custody regulations) e.g. barbiturates, temazepam, meprobamate, buprenorphine.
- *Schedules 4 and 5:* Most benzodiazepines, anabolic and androgenic steroids, HCG, growth hormone, codeine. Controlled drug prescription requirements do not apply, nor do safe custody requirements.

❶ For patients or doctors travelling abroad with schedule 2 or 3 drugs, an export licence may be required. Further details can be obtained from the Home Office (☎020 7273 3806). Patient applications must be accompanied by a doctor's letter giving details of: patient's name and current address; quantities of drugs to be carried; strength and form of drugs; dates of travel. For clearance to import the drug into the country of destination, it is advisable to contact the Embassy or High Commission of that country prior to departure.

Prescribing for addicts: Only practitioners who hold a special licence from the Home Office may prescribe diamorphine, diconal (dipipanone), or cocaine for the treatment of drug addiction (though any doctor can prescribe these drugs for addicts if they need them for relief of pain). Management of drug addiction—📖 p.240.

Prescribing for special groups (1)

Palliative care: 📖 p.999–1014
Children

⚠ Keep all medicines out of the reach of children (and preferably in a locked cupboard).

- Children differ from adults in their response to drugs. Consult BNF or Paediatric Vade Mecum before prescribing unfamiliar drugs. Always check dose carefully. Many drugs are not licensed for use with children.
- Paediatric suspensions often contain sugar. For long-term use or children having frequent prescriptions consider sugar-free versions.
- Do not advise adding medicines to infant feeding bottles—they may interact with milk and dose will be ↓ if not all the contents are drunk.
- Information on drugs used to treat rare paediatric conditions: Alder Hey Children's Hospital (☎0151 252 5381) or Great Ormond Street Hospital (☎020 7405 9200).
- Report *all* adverse reactions on Yellow Cards—📖 p.128

The elderly: Use of medicines ↑ as people get older. Medicine-related problems are assessed as part of the joint social and healthcare assessment procedure, prompting specialist assessment if problems are identified. Prescribing for the elderly is a priority area highlighted in the NSF for older people (📖 p.992). It sets targets that all people ≥75y. should have their medication reviewed annually, with those taking ≥4 medicines having a 6mo. review. By 2004, all PCOs should also have schemes in place to ensure older people get more help from pharmacists in using their medicines. Problems commonly encountered:

- *Polypharmacy:* Elderly people often have multiple problems—it is easy to keep adding drugs for each new problem leading to confusion, poor compliance, and multiple interactions and side-effects. Review repeat medication regularly and stop ineffective or redundant drugs (📖 p.127). Before prescribing a new drug, consider whether it is necessary and, if so, whether the drug regime can be simplified.
- *Specific medicines:* Need close monitoring e.g. warfarin, NSAIDs, diuretics, digoxin, hypnotics, psychotropics.
- *Form of the medicine:* Swallowing tablets can be difficult for elderly people. Consider using liquid preparations or, if no suitable preparation is available and the drug is in tablet form, crushing it with a spoonful of semi-solid ice cream.
- *Confusion post-discharge:* Up to ½ all patients are inadvertently prescribed the wrong medication after hospital discharge.
- *Drug hoarding/self-medication:* Especially if there have been recent changes in medication, it is common for elderly people to have a back stock of drugs and to continue taking their old drugs alongside new ones. Many elderly people also self-medicate extensively with OTC preparations. If necessary, do a home visit to sort out the drugs.

- **↑ susceptibility to side-effects:** Common. Sometimes due to impaired renal function (always assume any elderly person has moderate impairment if renal function is not known). Elderly people also tend to be hypersensitive to effects of CNS drugs e.g. benzodiazepines—use with care.
- **Social and personal factors:** Low level of home support; physical factors e.g. poor vision, poor hearing, or poor manual dexterity; and mental state e.g. confusion/disorientation, depression—can all affect the ability of an older person to take medication.

Guidelines for prescribing for the elderly

- **Limit the range of drugs you use:** Prescribe from a limited array of drugs that you know well.
- **Repeats and disposal:** Tell patients how to get more tablets and what to do with any left over if a drug is stopped. Monitor the frequency of repeat prescriptions. Review repeat prescriptions regularly (📖 p. 126).
- **↓ the dose:** Start with 50% of the adult dose. Avoid drugs likely to cause problems (e.g. long-acting antidiabetic agents such as glibenclamide).
- **Review regularly:** Consider whether each drug could be stopped or the regime simplified. Consider lowering dosage of drugs if renal function is deteriorating. Involve carers if appropriate.
- **Simplify regimes:** Use od or bd regimes wherever possible.
- **Explain clearly:** Put precise instructions on the drug bottle; when prescribing give written instructions about how the drug should be taken. Ensure explanations are given to carers as well as patients, where appropriate.
- **Consider method of administration:** Bottles with child-proof tops are often impossible for arthritic hands to open. Suggest the patient asks the chemist for a standard screw cap. Drug administration boxes in which the correct tablets are stored in slots marked with the day and time of administration can be helpful. They are available from pharmacists and can be filled by the patient, a carer, friend, or relative. Medication reminder charts can also be helpful.

Further information

Zermansky et al. (2001) BMJ **323**: 1340–4

DOH: Pharmacy in the future: Implementing the NHS Plan—a programme for pharmacy in the National Health Service. 🖥 http://www.dh.gov.uk

DOH: Medicines and older people. 🖥 http://www.dh.gov.uk

UK medicines information: 🖥 http://www.ukmi.nhs.uk/

Electronic medicines compendium: 🖥 http://www.medicines.org.uk

Prescribing for special groups (2)

Borderline substances: *BNF* Appendix 7

For certain conditions, foods and toilet products can be regarded as drugs and prescribed under the NHS (e.g. gluten-free foods for coeliac disease, nutritional supplements for disease-related malnutrition). The Advisory Committee on Borderline Substances advises on which products are available for certain specified conditions. Products should not be prescribed for any other condition. Use form FP10 (GP10 in Scotland) and endorse with the letters ACBS.

Pregnancy: Drugs taken by the mother can harm the foetus at any stage in pregnancy. *Mechanisms:*
- *1st trimester:* Teratogenesis causing congenital malformations. Greatest risk—wk. 3–12.
- *2nd and 3rd trimesters:* Toxic effects; effects on growth/development.
- *Around labour:* May affect labour or have adverse effects on the newborn baby.

Only prescribe if essential, especially in the 1st trimester. Stick to tried and tested drugs when possible (see *BNF* Appendix 4 for list of drugs with known affects); use smallest effective-dose; avoid new drugs.

Further information
BNF Appendix 4; National Teratology Information Service ☎0191 232 1525.

Breast-feeding: Drugs taken by a breast-feeding mother can affect the child by inhibiting lactation or entering the milk and causing toxicity to the infant. Therapeutic doses in the mother can cause toxicity in the infant if the drug is concentrated in milk (e.g. iodides). Avoid prescribing wherever possible. Stick to tried and tested drugs (see *BNF* Appendix 5).

Renal impairment: Renal function ↓ with age but may not be reflected by raised creatinine due to ↓ muscle mass. Always assume mild–moderate renal failure if prescribing for the elderly. Renal impairment can change the effects of drugs by:
- *Inability to excrete drug:* May cause toxicity. Dose reduction or increase in interval between doses may be necessary.
- *Increased sensitivity to drugs:* (even if elimination is unimpaired).
- *Poor tolerance of side-effects:* Nephrotoxic drugs may have more serious side-effects.
- *Lack of effectiveness:* When renal function is reduced.

❶ In general practice, serum creatinine is a rough guide to renal function:
- Mild renal impairment—creatinine 150–300µmol/l
- Moderate renal impairment—creatinine 300–700µmol/l
- Severe renal impairment—creatinine >700µmol/l

Further information
BNF Appendix 3; patients on dialysis—consult local renal unit.

Hepatic impairment: Problems don't tend to arise until late stages of liver failure when there is jaundice, ascites, or evidence of encephalopathy. Problems are due to:

- **Impaired drug metabolism:** Many drugs are metabolized by the liver. In severe liver failure, dose may need to be ↓ +/− dosage interval ↑. A few drugs are excreted in the bile unchanged and may accumulate in patients with obstructive jaundice (e.g. rifampicin, fusidic acid).
- **Hypoproteinaemia:** Liver failure is invariably associated with low plasma protein. This affects binding of drugs. Highly protein-bound drugs (e.g. phenytoin, prednisolone) can become toxic in normal dosage.
- **Hepatotoxicity:** Liver toxicity will have increased effect if hepatic reserve is already reduced.
- **Clotting:** Blood clotting factors are made in the liver. In liver disease, effects of oral anticoagulants are increased.
- **Encephalopathy:** Drugs that depress cerebral function (e.g benzodiazepines, opiates) can precipitate encephalopathy due to severe liver failure.
- **Fluid retention:** Drugs causing fluid retention (e.g. NSAIDs) make oedema and ascites worse.

Further information
BNF Appendix 2 (list of drugs to be avoided/used with caution).

Driving whilst taking drugs: 📖 p.202 or
🖥 *http:// www.dvla.gov.uk/at_a_glance/content.htm*

Further information
UK medicines information 🖥 *http://www.ukmi.nhs.uk*
Electronic medicines compendium 🖥 *http://www.medicines.org.uk*

Drugs and sport

Most sport regulating bodies have strict codes regarding drug use by participating sportsmen. Although broadly similar, regulations may differ in detail.

Prohibited classes of drugs
- *Stimulants*—e.g. amphetamine, caffeine (above 12mcg/ml), ephedrine, certain β_2 agonists.
- *Narcotics*—e.g. diamorphine, pethidine, methadone.
- *Anabolic agents*—e.g. nandrolone, DHEA, testosterone.
- *Diuretics*—e.g. frusemide, bendrofluazide.
- *Peptide and glycoprotein hormones and analogues*—e.g. growth hormone, erythropoietin.

Classes of drugs subjected to restrictions
- *Alcohol and marijuana*—restricted in certain sports.
- *Local anaesthetics*—local or intra-articular injection only (provide written notification of administration for relevant medical authority).
- *Corticosteroids*—topical, inhaled, or local/intra-articular injection only (provide written notification of administration for relevant medical authority).
- *β-blockers*—restricted in certain sports.

Anabolic steroid misuse: Significant problem in the UK (5% in gyms and fitness clubs). Drugs are often used in complicated regimes at high doses to ↑ lean muscle mass and ↓ body fat. *Side-effects include:* ↑ cholesterol, ↑ BP, gynaecomastia, ↑ LFTs, testicular atrophy, baldness, acne, and mood changes. Other drugs may be taken in conjunction with anabolic steroids to ↓ these side-effects.

⚠ Doctors who prescribe or collude in the provision of drugs or treatment with the intention of improperly enhancing an individual's performance in sport risk losing their GMC registration. This does not preclude the provision of any care or treatment where the doctor's intention is to protect or improve the patient's health.

Further information
UK Sport Produces a card giving more detailed information. Available from UK Sport, 40, Bernard Street, London WCA 1ST ☎020 7211 5100 ▣ *http://www.uksport.gov.uk* (information resources). Status of a particular medicine may be checked on the Drug Information Line ☎0800 528 0004 or ▣ *http://www.uksport.gov.uk/did*

Table 3.3 Treatment of common conditions for sportsmen

	Allowed	Banned
Asthma	Sodium cromoglycate, theophylline. Inhaled salbutamol, terbutaline, salmeterol, beclomethasone, or fluticasone. Provide written notification of administration for relevant medical authority.	Products containing sympathomimetics e.g. ephedrine, isoprenaline, fenoterol, rimiterol, orciprenaline.
Cold/cough	All antibiotics, steam and menthol inhalations, permitted antihistamines, terfenadine, astemizole, pholcodine, guaiphenasin, dextromethorphan, paracetamol.	Products containing sympathomimetics e.g. ephedrine, pseudoephedrine, phenylpropanolamine.
Diarrhoea	Diphenoxylate, loperamide, products containing electrolytes (e.g. Dioralyte).	Products containing opioids e.g. morphine.
Hayfever	Antihistamines, nasal sprays containing a corticosteroid or xylometazoline, eye-drops containing sodium cromoglycate.	Products containing ephedrine or pseudoephedrine.
Pain	Codeine, paracetamol, all NSAIDs, dextropropoxyphene.	Products containing opioids, caffeine.
Vomiting	Domperidone, metoclopramide, prochlorperazine, cinnarizine.	

Complementary medicine

Complementary medicine

In the UK ~90% of the population have tried complementary or alternative medicine (CAM) at some time. But, although CAM undoubtedly helps many individuals, its use remains controversial.

Reasons for caution

- *Lack of evidence of effectiveness:* There are many anecdotal reports and small-scale observational studies of the positive effects of complementary therapies but large-scale, high-quality studies tend to be –ve.
- *Lack of regulation of practitioners:* Anyone can call themselves a therapist and practice. It is always important to find a reputable practitioner with accredited training who is a member of a recognized professional body It is also important to ensure any practitioner used carries professional indemnity insurance.
- *Lack of regulation of products:* Most complementary 'medicines' are sold as foods rather than medicines and do not hold a product licence. No licensing authority has assessed efficacy, safety, or quality and interactions with conventional medicines are unknown. Complementary medicines can, and do, cause adverse effects—just because they are natural does not mean they are safe.

Legal position of GPs

Practising complementary medicine: Conventionally trained doctors can administer any unconventional medical treatments they choose. The 'Bolam test' applies—in other words, if a doctor has undergone additional training in a complementary discipline and practises in a way that is reasonable and would be considered acceptable by a number of other medically qualified complementary practitioners, his or her actions are defensible.

Referring to complementary medicine practitioners

- *Delegation to non-medically qualified practitioner:* Ask yourself:
  - *Is my decision to delegate to this complementary therapy appropriate?* Evidence-based decisions are most persuasive; commonly accepted but unproven indications are also acceptable.
  - *Have I taken reasonable steps to ensure that the practitioner is qualified and insured?* Usually sufficient to ensure s/he is a member of the main professional regulatory body responsible for that discipline. Main bodies require members to be fully indemnified.
  - *Has my medical follow-up been adequate?* Continue following-up chronic conditions as usual. Don't issue repeat prescriptions without having sufficient information to ensure safe prescribing.
- *Referral to medically qualified practitioner/state registered osteopath or chiropractor:* Same legal situation as when referring to another conventional healthcare practitioner for any other service. As long as the decision to make the referral is appropriate (see above), all further responsibility is taken over by the practitioner providing the specialist service.

Further information

Bandolier 🖳 *http://www.jr2.ox.ac.uk/bandolier/booth/booths/altmed.html*

Acupuncture

Acupuncture means 'piercing with a sharp instrument'. Needles are used to alleviate symptoms or cure disease. Mechanism of action remains unclear. Broadly, 2 forms exist—traditional/Chinese and modern/Western. There is no 'right way' to practice as there is no scientific data comparing the two.

Traditional acupuncture: Based on Chinese medicine where health is a balance between 'ying' and 'yang', illness is imbalance, and treatment aims to restore balance. Needles are inserted into channels representing 12 organs recognized in Chinese medicine to stimulate or sedate the flow of chi, an energy force flowing in these channels (meridiens) and sustaining life in parallel to blood. In most cases, a number of needles are inserted and left for up to 20min.

Modern acupuncture: Uses modern anatomy and physiology and ignores the rules of traditional Chinese medicine. Traditional acupuncture points are still used for some illnesses but often the acupuncturist makes use of trigger points—areas, usually in muscle, which hurt when pressed and may cause pain to radiate to other places. Needling the trigger point relieves pain.

Use and evidence: Acupuncture has been used to treat all conditions but is commonly used in Europe and the USA to treat musculoskeletal problems and chronic disease. Although Table 4.1 reports the overall outcome of systematic reviews and good quality randomized controlled trials for various applications of acupuncture, it should be used with caution as there are very few large, good-quality trials in existence and almost all are –ve.

Table 4.1 Evidence for common uses of acupuncture

Largely +ve	Inconclusive	Largely –ve
Back pain[S]	Chronic pain[S]	Cocaine addiction[R]
Idiopathic headache[C]	Neck pain[S]	Smoking cessation[C]
Post-operative nausea and vomiting (adults)[S]	Fibromyalgia[S*]	Stroke[S]
	Osteoarthritis[S]	Carpal tunnel syndrome[C]
	Rheumatoid arthritis[C]	Hot flushes[S]
	Tennis elbow[C]	Tinnitus[S]
	TMJ dysfunction[S]	
	Weight reduction[S]	
	Asthma[C]	
	Labour pain[C]	

* Some evidence acupuncture causes exacerbation of symptoms for some patients.

Contraindications: Unwilling or frightened patient, pregnancy (especially 1st trimester, as anecdotal evidence suggests ↑ risk of miscarriage), bleeding disorders and anticoagulant use (relative contraindication), skin infections or diseased skin, disorders of the immune system, valvular heart disease (only if indwelling needles are used).

Side effects: Rare (1:1000 treatments)
- Infection (ONLY go to practitioners using disposable needles)
- Bruising/haemorrhage
- Anatomical damage (pneumothorax most common)
- Needle fracture or needles left in situ
- Fainting
- Sweating
- Convulsions
- Miscarriage (anecdotal)

Variants of acupuncture

Auriculotherapy: Microsystem of acupuncture based on a 'homunculus' or map of the body on the ear. Stimulation of points on the ear representing an area in pain produces analgesia. Best known for treatment of addiction, especially smoking. No good-quality evidence of effectiveness. Often practised using semi-permanent needles in an attempt to prolong its effects at the risk of infection at the needle site. Should not be used for patients with artificial heart valves, valvular heart disease, or immune deficiency.

Transcutaneous electrical nerve stimulation (TENS): Electrodes are placed on the skin over the painful area or at other locations e.g. over cutaneous nerves, trigger points, acupuncture sites. The TENS unit passes electrical current through the electrodes. The patient can control strength of current and pulse interval. Widely used by midwives, physiotherapists, and in hospitals. No good evidence of effectiveness.

Reflexology: A representation of the body is found on the foot. Diagnosis is through palpation of the sole of the foot for tender points. These correspond to the area of the body where there is pain. Treatment consists of massaging these points or applying acupressure to relieve symptoms. No good-quality evidence of effectiveness but unlikely to do any harm.

Professional organizations

British Medical Acupuncture Society ☎01925 730727; *Fax:* 01925 730492
   ▣ *http://www.medical-acupuncture.co.uk*
British Acupuncture Council ☎020 8735 0400 ▣ *http://www.acupuncture.org.uk*
Acupuncture Association of Chartered Physiotherapists ☎01747 861151 *Fax:* 01747 861717
   ▣ *http://www.aacp.uk.com*
Association of Reflexologists ☎0870 5673320 ▣ *http://www.aor.org.uk*

Further reading

Effective health care (2001) Acupuncture **7**(2) ▣ *http://www.york.ac.uk/inst/crd/ehcb.htm*

Homeopathy

From the Greek meaning 'treatment by similars'

Theory of homeopathy: Homeopathy works on the principle that like cures like. The majority of homeopathic remedies are derived from plants, although chemical and animal sources are also used. A remedy is chosen that mimics the symptoms displayed by the patient e.g. homeopathic ipecacuanha is used to treat nausea and vomiting. Most remedies are serially diluted in steps of 1:10 (decimal x) or 1:100 (centesimal c).

⚠ Some lay practitioners believe conventional drugs ↓ efficacy of homeopathy. It is important that users of homeopathic drugs do not stop taking conventional medicines unless advised to by the doctor who prescribed them.

Use: Often used to treat symptoms of acute self-limiting illness. Also used widely for chronic conditions e.g. eczema, stress, depression and chronic fatigue. Homoeopathic treatment is slow. The 'rule of 12' states 1mo. of treatment is required for each year the patient has the problem.

Availability of drugs: Manufacture of homeopathic medicine is controlled by the Medicines Act (1968). Homeopathic drugs can be purchased OTC at pharmacies and health food shops or prescribed on NHS prescription.

⚠ Legal responsibility for prescribing lies with the person who signs the prescription form.

Side effects/contraindications: Homeopathic remedies of sufficient dilution (>30x or 12c) and obtained from a reputable manufacturer are unlikely to cause adverse effects or interact with conventional medicines. Homeopathy also appears to be safe in women who are pregnant/ breastfeeding, but should not be used to treat serious conditions for which there is a proven conventional therapy.

Evidence: With higher dilutions (>12c), a theoretical problem arises as the solution may not contain any molecules of the mother substance. Nevertheless, homeopaths claim more dilute solutions are *more* effective. Meta-analysis[1] published in 1997 pooled all studies comparing homeopathy against placebo and concluded that, overall, homeopathy works. However, there is insufficient information about use of homeopathy in most clinical situations to decide when, and if, homeopathy is a credible adjunct or alternative to conventional treatment.

1 Linde et al. (1997) *Lancet* **350**: 834–43.

Table 4.2 Evidence for common uses of homeopathy

Largely +ve	Inconclusive	Largely −ve
Post-operative ileus[S]	Atopic eczema[S]	Bruising[S]
Dandruff and seborhhoeic dermatitis[R]	Chronic asthma[C]	Osteoarthritis[S]
	Ocular symptoms of hayfever[r,S]	Rheumatoid arthritis[S]
	Influenza[C]	Headache[S]
	Dementia[S]	Delayed-onset muscle soreness[S]
	Pre-menstrual syndrome[R]	
	Low back pain[R]	Migraine prophylaxis[S]
	Otitis media[R]	
	Acute sinusitis[R]	
	Labour pain[C]	

Professional organizations

British Homoeopathic Association ☎0870 444 3950 *Fax:* 0870 444 3960
🖳 *http://www.trusthomeopathy.org*
Society of Homeopaths ☎01604 621400 *Fax:* 01604 622622 🖳 *http://www.homeopathy-soh.org*

Herbal medicine

Use of plants or plant parts for medicinal purposes. Conventional medicine uses many drugs derived from herbal substances e.g. digoxin, aspirin, and morphine. Herbal medicine uses plant extracts, not isolated constituents. Herbalists believe different compounds contained in a herbal preparation act synergistically.

Availability of herbal medicine: Widely available in the UK. Most products are unlicensed and sold as foods. *Problems:*
- Quality assurance
- Accidental contamination
- Botanical quality
- Unknown optimum dose/dosage range
- Lack of data on drug interactions

⚠ Report all adverse herbal medicine reactions and drug interactions using the yellow card scheme (p.128). Keep a sample of the implicated herbal medicine.

Uses and evidence: Used for a wide range of conditions, often with little evidence of efficacy. See Table 4.3.

Aromatherapy: Use of aromatic plant oils (usually by inhalation or application to the skin) for benefit. No good evidence of effectiveness. Oils used are extremely concentrated. *Uses:*
- Lavender oil
- Tea tree oil
- Geranium oil
- Eucalyptus oil
- Thyme oil
- Rosemary oil
- Peppermint oil
- Valerian oil
- Burns, blisters, insomnia
- Headlice, athlete's foot, wound infection
- Calming, antidepressant
- Clear blocked noses (Vicks Vaporub®)
- Antiseptic—used for colds and flu
- Antiseptic and soothing—good for sinus infections
- Headache, indigestion
- Anxiety and insomnia

Cautions, side-effects, and contraindications: Volatile oils are readily absorbed through mucus membranes and may be as potent as any drug. Sold as unlicensed products—quality, safety, interactions, and efficacy have not been assessed. Can be poisonous if ingested.

Professional organizations
British Herbal Medical Association: ☎01202 433691
Fax: 01202 417079 🖳 *http://www.ex.ac.uk/phytonet/bhma.html*
National Institute of Medical Herbalists: ☎01392 426022 *Fax:* 01392 498963
🖳 *http://www.nimh.org.uk*
International Federation of Professional Aromatherapists: ☎01455 637987
🖳 *http://www.ifparoma.org*
Aromatherapy Organizations Council: ☎0870 7743477 🖳 *http://www.aocuk.net*

Table 4.3 Herbal products with evidence of efficacy

Herb	Side-effects	Evidence
Saw palmetto	Dizziness and mild GI effects. Rare: pruritus, headache, ↑ BP.	BPH. Improvement in symptoms when used for >1–2mo. Side-effects <finasteride[C].
Echinacea	Nausea, dizziness, SOB, dermatitis, pruritus, and hepatotoxicity. Rare: allergy ⚠ Advise patients NOT to take for >8wk. as can cause immune suppression	Prevention and treatment of common cold— majority of studies +ve[C]. Theoretically, may ↓ effects of immuno-suppressants and be harmful in autoimmune disease and HIV.
St. John's Wort	Dry mouth, GI symptoms, fatigue, headache, dizziness, skin rash, and ↑ sensitivity to sunlight. Drug interactions: ↓ effect of anti-convulsants, warfarin, ciclosporin, digoxin, theophylline, and COC pill. Serotonergic effects (sweating, shivering, muscle contractions) with triptans and antidepressants. ⚠ DO NOT use concurrently with prescription antidepressants.	Depression—effective treatment[S]. Discontinue 2wk. prior to surgery as theoretical risk of interaction with anaesthetic agents.
Gingko biloba	Spontaneous bleeding. Drug interactions: ↑ effect of warfarin and antiplatelet agents.	Effective for improving cerebral blood flow[S] and intermittent claudication[S]. May help tinnitus[S].
Feverfew	May cause breakthrough menstrual bleeding. Caution with anticoagulants.	Migraine prophylaxis— probably effective[C].
Chinese herbal medicine	Serious blood dyscrasias and hepatotoxicity have been reported.	Effective for childhood eczema[S] and irritable bowel syndrome[R].

Other products for which there is evidence of effectiveness

- Aloe vera (psoriasis[S] and genital herpes[S])
- Oil of evening primrose (rheumatoid arthritis[C])
- Kava (anxiety[S])
- Valerian (insomnia[S])
- Peppermint oil (irritable bowel syndrome[S])
- Horse chestnut seed extract (chronic venous insufficiency[C])
- Yohimbine (erectile dysfunction[S])

Further information

Herbmeda 🖥 http://www.herbmed.org

Dietary manipulation and supplementation

'Let your food be your medicine'
Hippocrates (460–377 BC)

Healing foods: Branch of herbal medicine. Common examples for which there is some evidence of effectiveness include:
- *Chondroitin:* ↓ pain and symptoms of OA[S].
- *Cranberry juice:* Trial evidence for effect in prevention or treatment of UTI[R] not supported by Cochrane review[C].
- *Fish oil:* Cardioprotective effects[R]; ↓ pain and symptoms of RA[S].
- *Garlic:* ↓ cholesterol[S]; antithrombotic/fibrinolytic effects[S]. May have a role in cancer prevention.
- *Ginger:* ↓ nausea in a variety of situations[S].
- *Honey:* Wound dressing—improves healing[S].
- *Soya:* ↓ menopausal symptoms[S].
- *Yoghurt:* No evidence for treatment of vaginal infection or prevention of recurrence[S]. Mixed evidence[R] and no systematic reviews for treating diarrhoea with yoghurt.
- *Xylitol:* Some evidence in vitro and animal studies that ↓ bacterial infection. Currently under investigation for effects in minor illness e.g. sore throat.

Nutritional medicine: Involves prescribing vitamins, minerals, amino acids, and essential fatty acids. Prescription is based on investigations into the individual's nutritional state by history taking, nutritional diaries, and analysis of samples of blood, sweat, and hair. Evidence of effectiveness:
- *Calcium supplements ± vitamin D:* ↓ incidence of osteoporosis and osteoporotic fracture[CS]. Calcium may ↓ BP[S].
- *Folate supplements:* Taken preconceptually ↓ incidence of neural tube defect[R].
- *Glucosamine:* ↓ pain and symptoms of OA[C]. ⚠ Some products are derived from marine sources—patients allergic to shellfish should ensure product is synthetically manufactured.
- *Selenium:* Suggestion of protective effect against gastro-oesophageal cancer. No good-quality evidence and recent epidemiological data suggest supplements may be harmful.
- *Vitamin A:* Cancer prevention[S]. ⚠ Patients should NOT take supplements in pregnancy.
- *Vitamin B$_6$:* May be effective for premenstrual syndrome[S] but excessive ingestion (>2000mg/d.) causes peripheral neuropathy. Possible effect on autism[S].
- *Vitamin B$_{12}$:* No evidence of beneficial effect on cognition[C].
- *Vitamin C:* ↓ duration of symptoms of common cold if used in high doses[C]. May ↓ BP[S].
- *Vitamin E:* May have a role in prevention of cardiovascular disease[S]. Unclear whether helpful for dementia[C] and intermittent claudication[C].
- *Zinc:* Inconclusive evidence shortens duration of common cold[C].

Probiotics: Probiotics are orally administered microbial cell preparations or components of microbial cells that may have a beneficial effect on the health and well-being of the host. There is some evidence of efficacy in treating a variety of medical problems including infectious diarrhoea[C], other gastrointestinal conditions (including inflammatory bowel disease and irritable bowel syndrome), and atopy[S]. There is increasing interest in the use of probiotics in mainstream medicine and the evidence base for or against the use of these preparations is likely to increase over the next few years.

Environmental medicine: Based on the premise that individuals develop adverse responses to environmental substances, most commonly foods, which manifest as disease. Adverse reactions are termed 'allergies' or intolerance. This is a different use of the term allergy than that used in conventional medicine. In environmental medicine it means a reaction with insidious onset that is not predictable and does not trigger the immune pathways responsible for allergy.

Investigations involve diagnostic use of elimination diets or substance avoidance; challenge testing by exposure to the substance, and the coca pulse test (speeding or slowing of the pulse by >10bpm after exposure).

❶ Allergy testing machines based on electrical skin resistance are in common use, though they produce inconsistent results and there is no evidence they are predictive of intolerance.

Food intolerances are generally multiple with 1 or 2 'major' foods and several more 'minor' foods responsible for triggering effects. Common examples are: caffeine, milk, gluten, citrus fruit. Beware that patients on multiple exclusion diets do not become malnourished. There is very little evidence of effect—Cochrane review of use for recurrent childhood abdominal pain and systematic review of use for childhood eczema were both inconclusive.

Professional organizations
British Herbal Medical Association: ☎01202 433691 🖳 http://www.ex.ac.uk/phytonet/bhma.html
Society for Environmental Therapy (SET): ☎01473 723552

Physical therapies

Osteopathy and chiropractic: Physical treatments aimed at restoring alignment of the joints and improving functioning of the body. In the UK, both are distinguished from other complementary therapies by being under statutory regulation. All osteopaths and chiropractors have to undergo training lasting 4–5y.. After that time, they are registered with their governing body which enforces a code of standards and discipline. They must have professional indemnity insurance.

Osteopathy: From Greek meaning 'bone disease'. Operates on the theory that if structure is improved, improvement in function follows.

Chiropractic: Diagnosis, treatment, and management of conditions due to mechanical dysfunction of the joints and their effects on the nervous system. Chiropractors aim to restore normal alignment of joints.

McTimoney chiropractic: Branch of chiropractic that uses slightly different, gentler techniques than conventional chiropractic treatment.

Method: Osteopaths and chiropractors use standard orthopaedic techniques and may perform investigations including X-rays. They like to work closely alongside conventional physicians, referring back to them any problems they detect outside their field of expertise. Treatment is usually physical, using massage and joint manipulation. Both treat the whole patient, giving advice on posture, lifestyle, and prevention of musculoskeletal and other problems.

Evidence: Some good evidence of effectiveness especially for back pain[R].

Massage: If we hurt ourselves, we rub it better. There are many different variants of massage, but the most common seen in the UK are 'Swedish massage' and 'Shiatsu' (or Japanese massage). Shiatsu uses a variant of acupressure (allied to acupuncture but using pressure on key points rather than needles) to enhance its effect.

Evidence: ↑ mobility[R], ↑ blood flow[R], ↑ expiratory volume[R], ↓ musculoskeletal and phantom limb pain[R], ↓ lymphoedema[R]. No convincing systematic review evidence of effect.

Yoga: Ancient art involving a sequence of physical stretches involving the whole body over a session. It is done slowly and in silence. Whilst performing the moves, participants breath slowly and deeply, fixing their minds on the activity they are doing. Yoga should be taught by an experienced instructor.

Evidence: ↓ seizure frequency for epileptics[C].

Tai chi chuan: Variously translated as 'supreme boxing' and the 'root of all motion'. It is considered a martial art but is not combative. It is based on fluidity and circular movements.

Evidence: ↓ falls and fear of falls in the elderly[R].

Physiotherapy: Physiotherapy is a healthcare profession concerned with maximizing potential, enhancing bodily function, and preventing future problems. It uses mainly physical approaches to achieve this including:

- Manipulation
- Exercise
- Posture
- Massage
- Relaxation
- Ultrasound

Often physiotherapists also use other complementary therapies during the course of their work e.g. acupuncture, aromatherapy, TENS.

Physiotherapists work in many health settings and are widely used and appreciated by patients in the community for conditions ranging from stress incontinence, and chest disease to musculoskeletal problems. They are an integrated part of the healthcare team and work closely with other members of the team.

Evidence: There is an extensive evidence base for the effectiveness of physiotherapy in a wide variety of conditions.

Pilates: Method of exercise involving physical movement designed to stretch, strengthen, and balance the body, together with focused breathing patterns.

Evidence: No specific evidence, though probably has the same benefits as general exercise—📖 p.232.

Professional organizations

General Osteopathic Council ☎020 7357 6655 🖳 http://www.osteopathy.org.uk
British Chiropractic Association ☎0118 950 5950 🖳 http://www.chiropractic-uk.co.uk
The Shiatsu Society ☎0845 130 4560 🖳 http://www.shiatsu.org
The British Wheel of Yoga ☎01529 306 851 🖳 http://www.bwy.org.uk
Tai Chi Union ☎0141 810 3482 🖳 http://www.taichiunion.com
Chartered Society of Physiotherapy ☎020 7306 6666 🖳 http://www.csp.org.uk
UK Pilates Foundation ☎07071 781 859 🖳 http://www.pilatesfoundation.com
Pilates Institute ☎020 7253 3177 🖳 http://www.pilates-institute.com

Other complementary therapies

Alexander Technique: Practical method for improving the way we 'use' ourselves in the activities of everyday life. No evidence of effectiveness but unlikely to be harmful.

Art therapy: Use of art as a therapeutic activity. Review of role in treatment of schizophrenia inconclusive[C].

Autogenic training: A kind of relaxation technique which involves passive concentration and psychophysiological stimuli. There are 6 standard exercises to aid relaxation, ↑ warmth in the abdominal region, and cool the cranial region. The technique takes ~ 8wk. to learn effectively and sessions 3x/d. are encouraged. It is used for a variety of conditions, including the treatment of hypertension. No evidence of effectiveness.

Ayurveda: Practised primarily in the Indian subcontinent for 5000y. Ayurveda includes diet and herbal remedies and emphasizes the use of body, mind, and spirit in disease prevention and treatment. No good evidence of effectiveness.

Cognitive behaviour therapy: 📖 p.958

Counselling: 📖 p.958

Faith healing: Healing is an ancient art, practised by most civilizations, and given much prominence by the ancient Greeks. During the healing process, the healer transmits an 'energy' which produces a harmonizing and healing effect. This energy is transmitted in different ways according to the type of healer consulted. No good-quality evidence of effect, though one study did show prayer ↓ mortality in a cardiac unit[R].

Hypnotherapy: Hypnosis can be defined as a state of heightened suggestibility or altered state of consciousness where the subject feels very relaxed. In medical hypnotherapy, the patient is not controlled or manipulated and can normally remember what has taken place after the session has ended. Hypnotherapy consists of training the patient to relax very deeply—often with a focus, a scene, smell, touch sensation, or colour to aid this process. *Evidence:* No evidence of effectiveness for smoking cessation[C] or weight loss[C]. May be helpful for pain relief in labour[C] and to ↓ symptoms of IBS[S].

Meditation: The instructor gives each individual a phrase or word—the *mantra*—which must not be divulged. The process involves siting quietly with eyes closed repeating the mantra for 20min. at a time 1 or 2x/d. The mantra focuses the mind on a single idea. If distractions occur, they are observed and put out of mind. No good evidence of effectiveness.

Reiki: Japanese word representing universal life energy. Reiki is based on the belief that when spiritual energy is channelled through a Reiki practitioner, the patient' spirit is healed, which in turn heals the physical body. No evidence of effectiveness.

Relaxation: Can either be done with a therapist or alone. A number of good relaxation tapes exist. It must be done in a quiet environment.
- The patient starts in a comfortable position.
- S/he is asked to close his/her eyes and then focus on each part of the body in turn, from toes upwards, for a period of about 10sec. at each location.
- Often the patient is asked to feel the part of the body being focused on becoming heavy.
- After this has been done, the patient is asked to visualize an idyllic scene—to breath the smells, hear the sounds, and feel the textures.
- An image can be provided such as a perfect evening on a warm, deserted beach.

Relaxation training is widely used throughout medicine. No convincing evidence of effect but unlikely to be harmful.

Professional organizations

Society of Teachers of the Alexander Technique ☎020 7284 3338 ▣ http://www.stat.org.uk
British Autogenic Society ☎020 7383 5108 ▣ http://www.autogenic-therapy.org.uk
National Federation of Spiritual Healers ☎0845 1232777 ▣ http://www.nfsh.org.uk
The Hypnotherapy Association ☎01257 262124 ▣ http://www.thehypnotherapyassociation.co.uk
UK Reiki Federation ☎01264 773774 ▣ http://www.reikifed.co.uk

Prevention

❶ All patients aged 16–75y. are entitled to request a routine health check if they haven't been seen, for health reasons, in the practice in the past 3y.
❶ All patients aged >75y. are entitled to a routine health check if they haven't been seen, for health reasons, in the practice in the past year.

Prevention and screening

In all disease, the goal is prevention.

Definitions

- *Primary prevention:* Prevention of disease occurrence.
- *Secondary prevention:* Controlling disease in early form (e.g. carcinoma in situ).
- *Tertiary prevention:* Prevention of complications once the disease is present (e.g. DM).

Barriers to prevention

- *Patient:* Blinkering ('It'll never happen to me'); rebellion ('I know it's bad—but it's cool'); poor motivation (path of least resistance).
- *Doctor:* Time; money—health promotion takes time and personnel; motivation—health promotion is repetitive and boring.
- *Society:* Pressure from big business (e.g. cigarette advertising and Formula 1); other priorities; ethics (e.g. public uproar at threats not to offer cardiac surgery to smokers).

Screening: The idea of screening is attractive—the ability to diagnose and treat a potentially serious condition at an early stage when it is still treatable. An ideal screening test should pick up all those who have the disease (have high sensitivity) and must exclude those who do not (high specificity). It must detect *only* those who have a disease (high positive predictive value—Table 5.1) and should exclude *only* those who do not have the disease (high negative predictive value).

The Wilson–Jungner criteria*: All screening tests should meet the following criteria before they are introduced to the target population:
- The condition being screened for is an important health problem
- Natural history of the condition is well understood
- There is a detectable early stage
- Treatment at early stage is of more benefit than at late stage
- There is a suitable test to detect early stage disease
- The test is acceptable to the target population
- Intervals for repeating the test have been determined
- Adequate health service provision has been made for the extra clinical workload resulting from screening
- Risks, both physical and psychological, are < benefits
- Costs are worthwhile in relation to benefits gained

UK screening programmes

- Cervical cancer 🕮 p.716
- Diabetic retinopathy 🕮 p.415
- Breast cancer 🕮 p.516
- Genetic 🕮 p.770
- Antenatal 🕮 p.770–3
- Neonatal hearing 🕮 p.827
- Haemoglobinopathy 🕮 p.773
- Child health surveillance 🕮 p.814

* Wilson and Jungner (1968) *Principles and practice of screening for disease* (Public Health Paper Number 34). Geneva: World Health Organization.

Table 5.1 Performance of screening tests

		Disease	
		Present	**Absent**
Test	**Positive**	True positive (a)	False positive (b)
	Negative	False negative (c)	True negative (d)

Sensitivity $= \dfrac{a}{(a+c)}$ Negative predictive value $= \dfrac{D}{(c+d)}$

Specificity $= \dfrac{d}{(b+d)}$ Positive predictive value $= \dfrac{a}{(a+b)}$

Screening in the future: 📖 p.160

Performance of screening tests: For a screening programme to be effective and ↓ morbidity and mortality, there must be:
- Adequate participation of the target population.
- Few false negative or false positive results (Table 5.1).
- Screening intervals shorter than the time taken for the disease to develop to an untreatable stage.
- Adequate follow-up of all abnormal results.
- Effective treatment at the stage detected by screening.

⚠ There is no ideal screening test. Always explain:
- Purpose of screening
- Likelihood of positive/negative findings and possibility of false positive/negative results
- Uncertainties and risks attached to the screening process
- Significant medical, social, or financial implications of screening for the particular condition or predisposition
- Follow-up plans, including availability of counselling and support services.

Table 5.2 Benefits and disadvantages of screening

Benefits	Disadvantages
• Improved prognosis for some cases detected by screening.	• Longer morbidity in cases where prognosis is unaltered.
• Less radical treatment for some early cases.	• Overtreatment of questionable abnormalities.
• Reassurance for those with negative test results.	• False reassurance for those with false negative results.
• Increased information on natural history of disease and benefits of treatment at early stage.	• Anxiety and sometimes morbidity for those with false positive results.
	• Unnecessary intervention for those with false positive results.
	• Hazard of screening test.
	• Diversion of resources to the screening programme.

Screening in the future

Prostate cancer: 2nd most common cause of death from cancer in UK men. Prevalence is rising. *Problems with screening:*

- Incidental post-mortem evidence of prostate cancer is high (≈75% men >75y.), very few become clinically evident → many more men would be found by screening with prostate cancer than would die or have symptoms from it;
- Natural history of prostate cancer is not understood—there is no means to detect which 'early' cancers become more widespread;
- Inadequate screening tests (see below);
- It is not clear if early treatment enhances life expectancy;
- Peak incidence of morbidity and mortality is in old age (75–79y.), so potential years of life saved by screening are small.

Screening tests

- **Prostate specific antigen (PSA):** Routinely measured in men with urological symptoms. Abnormal PSA is a common reason for referral to a urologist. Its sensitivity and specificity are poor. Other reasons for ↑ PSA:
  - Acute and chronic prostatitis
  - BPH
  - Physical exercise
  - Instrumentation
  - Ductal obstruction

❶ PSA may be *normal* when early prostate cancer is present.

There is considerable demand for PSA testing amongst men worried about the disease. The Government has introduced a PSA Informed Choice Programme. A key element is information provision for men requesting the test to enable them to decide whether or not to take it.

- **Digital rectal examination (DRE):** Operator-dependant; fails to detect early prostate cancers; and lacks specificity. Annual screening in the USA and Germany has not ↓ mortality.
- **Transrectal ultrasound (TRUS):** Too expensive for widespread use.

The most effective screening regime involves DRE and PSA testing followed by TRUS for suspicious lesions[s]. Optimal screening interval is unknown but serial screening ↑ detection.

Ovarian cancer: 4th most common cause of cancer death in women. Confined to 1 ovary ≈90% 5y. survival but 80% are picked up at later stages when 5y. survival is ≈10%. No reliable screening test. Options are USS, measurement of CA125, and genetic screening. USS and CA125 have low sensitivity/specificity. Genetic screening can only detect a few familial cases. If an abnormality is found on screening, laparotomy is required to exclude cancer, and there is a lack of evidence that treatment at an early stage ↓ mortality. Further information is expected when a large trial of screening for ovarian cancer reports in 2010.

Colorectal cancer: Common cause of death with well-defined premalignant phase (adenomatous polyp). Prognosis depends on stage at diagnosis. Patients with strong FH of large bowel cancer, or ulcerative colitis are screened already with colonoscopy with proven benefit, but colonoscopy is too expensive for use in a universal screening programme. Possible alternatives:

- **Faecal occult bloods (FOBs):** +ve in 56–78% patients with asymptomatic colorectal cancer. Malignancies detected are less advanced. *Problems:* 40% cancers are missed and high false +ves—but does ↓ mortality. Very short lead time, so frequent screening is needed. Completed pilot study recommended introduction of a national screening programme[1].
- **DRE:** <40% within reach.
- **Sigmoidoscopy:** Could detect 60% cancers. May be protective for up to 10y. *Problems:* overtreatment (some polyps may never become malignant), acceptability of test, cannot detect proximal tumours.

Table 5.3 Screening programmes currently under evaluation in the UK

Screening under evaluation	Page	Notes
Abdominal aortic aneurysm	p.358	Initial pilot +ve; larger pilot underway
Ovarian cancer	p.160	Pilot will report in 2010
Lung cancer	p.388	US pilot results awaited
Bladder cancer	p.700	For high-risk groups only
Genital chlamydia	p.743	National programme planned
Glaucoma	p.948	
Oral cancer	p.910	
HPV infection	p.744	Pilot findings awaited
Cystic fibrosis (neonatal)	p.394	New programme agreed
Cystic fibrosis (antenatal)	p.394	HTA report recommended screening[2]
Colorectal cancer	p.161	+ve findings from large-scale pilot
Type 2 diabetes	p.405	
Thyroid disease	p.422	Pilot project underway
Prostate cancer	p.160	Prostate cancer risk management programme started

Further information
National Electronic Library for Screening ⬚ http://www.nelh.nhs.uk/screening
NHS Cancer Screening Programmes ⬚ http://www.cancerscreening.nhs.uk
DoH ⬚ http://www.dh.gov.uk
UK Newborn Screening Programme Centre ⬚ http://www.newbornscreening-bloodspot.org.uk

1 Available on ⬚: http://www.cancerscreening.nhs.uk/colorectal/finalreport.pdf
2 HTA (1999), vol. 3, no. 8

Accident prevention

'A safe, secure and sustainable environment is a prerequisite for a healthy nation'

Department of Health, 'Our Healthier Nation', 1998

Accidents are the most common cause of death in children >1y. They also cause death and permanent disability for thousands of adults and elderly people every year. High-risk groups are children ≤4y.; elderly people; alcoholics; and teenage males.

Drowning: 3rd most common cause of accidental death among the under 16s. > ½ those who drown can swim. 44% of drownings occur in rivers or streams; 3% in garden ponds; 2% in swimming pools; and 5% in home baths. Alcohol is a contributory factor in 14% cases. The best way to ↓ drowning is prevention—spot the dangers; take safety advice; don't go near water alone; learn how to help others.

Road safety: Responsible for 30–40% of all fatal accidents. *Prevention:*
- Avoid alcohol or any other drugs that hamper driving performance when driving
- Keep speed down
- Do not drive if tired or ill
- Wear seatbelts and appropriate protective clothing (e.g. helmet if riding a pedal or motor cycle)
- Ensure children are properly strapped in
- Keep vehicles well maintained
- When cycling, use cycle tracks if available
- Supervise children close to roads; teach them the Green Cross code

Home safety: Every year >4000 people die due to accidents in the home and nearly 3 million seek treatment in A&E departments. Inside the home, most accidents occur in the living/dining room, followed by the kitchen. Accidents inside the home include fires, choking/suffocation, drowning, falls, poisoning, injury by hot substances, and electrical injuries. *Prevention:* Spot the dangers; take safety advice (e.g. from HV if young children in the house); fit smoke alarms and safety devices (e.g. stair gates for toddlers); ensure adequate supervision of children or elderly confused people; maintain equipment correctly.

Prevention of falls: Falls are one of the biggest risk factors for fracture. Tendency to fall ↑ with age. All elderly people should have their risk of falls assessed regularly—whether or not they have osteoporosis.

Is a falls assessment needed? Ask if patients fall—they may not volunteer the information spontaneously.
- The 'Get up and go' test—people who can get up from a chair without using their arms, walk several paces, and return with no difficulty or unsteadiness are at low risk of falling.
- People who have difficulty with the 'Get up and go' test, have to stop walking while talking, present following a fall, or who have recurrent falls, need a falls assessment.

Falls assessment: If available, refer to a specialist falls service. Record:
- Frequency and history of circumstances around any previous falls
- Drug therapy: polypharmacy, hypnotics, sedatives, diuretics, antihypertensives may all cause falls
- Assessment of vision
- Examination of gait and balance, including abnormalities due to foot problems or arthritis, and motor disorders e.g. stroke, PD
- Examination of basic neurological function, including mental status (impaired cognition and depression), muscle strength, lower extremity peripheral nerves, proprioception, and reflexes
- Assessment of basic cardiovascular status including BP (exclude postural hypotension), heart rate, and rhythm
- Assessment of environmental risk factors e.g. poor lighting (particularly on the stairs), loose carpets or rugs, badly fitting footwear or clothing, lack of safety equipment such as grab rails, steep stairs, slippery floors, or inaccessible lights or windows

Measures to ↓ risk of falls and damage from falling
- Modify identified hazards or risk factors
- Assess and correct vision, if possible
- Correct postural hypotension—alter medication; consider compression stockings (but many elderly people cannot themselves apply stockings tight enough to be of any use)
- Treat other medical conditions e.g. refer to cardiology if arrythmia
- Review medication and discontinue/alter inappropriate medication
- Remove environmental hazards—arrange bath at a day centre, refer to OT to identify and correct hazards in the home e.g. remove loose carpets, wheeled trolley for use indoors, commode or urine bottle for night time use, moving the bed downstairs
- Refer to OT to identify and correct hazards in the home
- Liaise with other members of the primary healthcare team and social services to provide additional support if needed; refer to local council for 'carephone' or alarm system to call for help if any further falls
- Refer to rehabilitation/physiotherapy to improve confidence after falls and for weight-bearing exercise (focusing on strength and flexibility) and balance training (↓ risk of falls)
- Use of hip protectors ↓ fracture risk in patients at high risk, but compliance is a problem[c]

Falls amongst the elderly: 📖 p.996

Osteoporosis and prevention of fracture: 📖 p.568

Medicines: Warn patients to keep all medicines out of the reach of children. Advise patients to dispose of unwanted medicines by returning them to a supplier/GP surgery for destruction.

Further information
The Royal Society for the Prevention of Accidents *Email:* help@rospa.co.uk
🖥 *http://www.rospa.com*
SIGN (2002) Prevention and management of hip fracture in older people 🖥 *http://www.sign.ac.uk*

Chronic disease management

Chronic disease

The predominant disease pattern in the developed world is one of chronic or long-term illness. In the UK, 17.5 million adults are currently living with a chronic disease.

Long-term conditions frequently seen and managed in general practice are: DM, arthritis (of all types), cancer, back pain, asthma and other chronic lung disease, irritable bowel syndrome, chronic inflammatory bowel disease, stroke, Parkinson's disease, multiple sclerosis and other neurological conditions, hypertension, heart disease, hypercholesterol-aemia, dementia, depression, renal and liver failure.

Although details of chronic illness management depend on the illness, people with chronic diseases of all types have much in common with each other. They all:
- Have similar concerns and problems (📖 p.170)
- Must deal not only with their disease(s) but also the impact it has on their lives and emotions

Common elements of effective chronic illness management

- **Involvement of the whole family:** Chronic diseases do not only affect the patient but everyone in a family.
- **Collaboration between service providers and patients/carers:**
  - Negotiate and agree a definition of the problem
  - Agree targets and goals for management
  - Develop an individualized self-management plan
- **Personalized written care plan:** Take into account patient/carers' views and experience and the current evidence base.
- **Tailored education in self-management:** A diabetic spends ~3h./y. with a health professional—during the other 8757h. he manages his own condition. Helping patients with chronic disease to understand and take responsibility for their condition is imperative. User-led (i.e. led by someone who suffers from the condition) self-management education programmes are most effective.
- **Planned follow-up:** Pro-active follow-up according to the care plan—use of disease registers and call-recall systems is important.
- **Monitoring of outcome and adherence to treatment:**
  - Use of disease and treatment markers
  - Monitoring of compliance e.g. checking prescription frequency (📖 p.124)
  - Medicine management programmes (📖 p.124)
- **Tools and protocols for stepped care:**
  - Provide a framework for using limited resources to greatest effect
  - Step professional care in intensity
  - Start with limited professional input and systematic monitoring
  - Augment care for patients who do not achieve an acceptable outcome
  - Initial and subsequent treatments are selected according to evidence-based guidelines in light of a patient's progress (📖 p.86)

- *Targeted use of specialist services:* For those patients who cannot be managed in primary care alone.
- *Monitoring of process:* Continually monitor management of patients with chronic disease through clinical governance mechanisms (📖 p.80). Ensure changes are made promptly to optimize care.

Essential reading

Von Korff *et al.* (2002) Organising care for chronic illness. *BMJ* **325**: 92–4

National Service Frameworks

National Service Frameworks (NSFs) are models of how services should be provided. They were developed to improve patient care and address variations in service provision across the country and are a key part of NHS quality initiatives. They cover all areas of service delivery—not just clinical practice. There will usually be one new framework each year.

Table 6.1 NSFs in existence/preparation

Topic	Date of publication
Mental Health	September 1999
Coronary Heart Disease	March 2000
Older People	March 2001
Diabetes	December 2001/January 2003
National Cancer Plan	September 2000
Renal Services	January 2004/February 2005
Children's Services	September 2004
Long-term conditions (focusing on neurological conditions)	March 2005

❶ Full text of all published NSFs is available on the DoH website 🖳 http://www.dh.gov.uk

Aims

- To set national standards
- To define service models and identify key interventions for specific service or care groups
- To put in place programmes to support implementation
- To establish performance measures against which progress within an agreed timescale will be measured

What can the PCO do?

- Consider employing a nurse with specialist skills to work across the PCO (e.g. cardiology nurse) and explore ways of supporting GPs to develop 'special interests' in an NSF-related disease area (📖 p.32)
- Work with voluntary agencies and others to commission user-led self-management programmes
- Support practices with installation of disease management templates
- Set clear standards/guidelines for repeat prescribing
- Work with local secondary care trusts on prescribing issues
- Explore different ways of providing services to help practices cope with rising demand (e.g. phlebotomy support)
- Ensure effective leadership in major disease areas/clinical governance
- Encourage sharing of approaches and good practice across the PCO

What can the practice do?
- Set up chronic disease management clinics for conditions/patient groups covered by the NSFs
- Develop nursing skills within the practice to improve patient education and self-management, and allow nurse prescribing
- Provide information about/access to self-management programmes and information and advice on self-monitoring for patients with chronic diseases
- Make effective use of computer-based disease management templates
- Implement NICE guidelines on drugs and review prescribing practice to ensure it reflects NSF objectives
- Ensure there is a suitable forum for learning from others' experiences across the practice e.g. how a difficult or unusual case/presentation was handled

Monitoring NSF standards: The Healthcare Commission (or CHAI—☐ p.18) is the main organization responsible for monitoring NSF standards. Other organizations are: National Performance Framework and National Patient and User Survey.

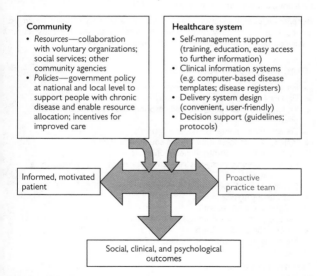

Community
- *Resources*—collaboration with voluntary organizations; social services; other community agencies
- *Policies*—government policy at national and local level to support people with chronic disease and enable resource allocation; incentives for improved care

Healthcare system
- Self-management support (training, education, easy access to further information)
- Clinical information systems (e.g. computer-based disease templates; disease registers)
- Delivery system design (convenient, user-friendly)
- Decision support (guidelines; protocols)

Informed, motivated patient

Proactive practice team

Social, clinical, and psychological outcomes

Figure 6.1 Model for chronic disease care

The expert patient

Most doctors acknowledge that many of their patients with chronic conditions know their own condition best. Expert patient programmes (or patient self-management programmes) utilize this fact to improve patient care. The aim is to promote effective partnerships in management of chronic disease by combining the expertise of patient and doctor (see Fig. 6.2).

Chronic disease self-management programmes: developed over the last 20y. These are a system of patient education and empowerment. As well as using health professionals, they use trained lay people with chronic illness as tutors. The 5 core self-management skills are:
- Problem solving
- Decision making
- Resource utilization
- Formation of a patient-professional partnership
- Taking action

But none of these is in itself the key to effective self-management. The key is the change in the individual's confidence and belief that they can take control over their disease and their life.

Benefits include: ↓ severity of all symptoms; ↓ severity of pain; improved life control and activity; improved resourcefulness and life satisfaction; enhanced doctor-patient relationship; ↓ use of health services.

Common patient concerns

- Finding and using health services
- Finding and using other community resources
- Knowing how to recognize and respond to changes in a chronic disease
- Dealing with problems and emergencies
- Making decisions about when to seek medical help
- Using medicines and treatments effectively
- Knowing how to manage stress and depression that accompany a chronic illness
- Coping with fatigue, pain, and sleep problems
- Getting enough exercise
- Maintaining good nutrition
- Working with your doctor(s) and other care providers
- Talking about your illness with family and friends
- Managing work, family, and social activities

Essential reading

DOH (2001) The expert patient: a new approach to chronic disease management for the 21st century. ▨ *http://www.dh.gov.uk*

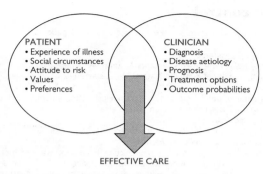

EFFECTIVE CARE

Figure 6.2 The patient–professional partnership

Pain control

Pain is always subjective, so take it at face value in *all* patients.

History: Consider:
- *Site of pain:* Where? Any radiation? Numbness where pain felt?
- *Onset:* How long? How did it start? What started it? Change over time?
- *Character of pain:* Type of pain—burning, shooting, stabbing, dull, etc.
- *Radiation:* Does the pain go anywhere else?
- *Associated features*
- *Timing/pattern:* Is it worse at any time of day? Is it cyclical?
- *Exacerbating and relieving factors*
- *Severity:* Record, especially if pain is chronic and you want to measure change over time. Consider patient diary. Ask about:
  - Pain intensity e.g. none–mild–moderate–severe; rank on 1–10 scale
  - Record interference with sleep or usual activities
  - Pain relief e.g. none–slight–moderate–good–complete
- *Previous treatments tried and result*

Acute pain: Cause is usually obvious—amount of pain is not related to severity of cause. Remember, fear makes pain worse.

Chronic pain: >3–6mo.—7% adults in UK. Usually multifactorial. Be aware of 2° gain from pain if symptoms seem out of proportion (outstanding compensation claims are a significant factor in success of pain management). Set realistic targets—abolition of pain may be impossible (70% have pain despite analgesia). If analgesia is not helping, stop it. The aim is often rehabilitation with ↓ in distress/disability. A multidisciplinary approach is essential.

Strategies for pain management
- *Prevention:* e.g. wrist splints for carpal tunnel syndrome; analgesia prior to minor surgery.
- *Removal of cause:* Treat medical causes of pain e.g. infection, ↓ blood sugar (diabetic neuropathy). Refer surgical causes for surgery if surgery is appropriate e.g. OA—joint replacement.
- *Pain-relieving drugs:* Start with a single drug at low dose and step up dose or add another drug as needed—see Fig. 6.3. Especially in situations of acute pain, step down if pain diminishes (📖 p. 174–5).
- *Physical therapies:* Acupuncture (📖 p.144), physiotherapy (📖 p.153), or TENS (📖 p.145).
- *Nerve blocks:* Consider referral for epidural (low back pain), local nerve block, or sympathectomy (e.g. vascular rest pain).
- *Modification of emotional response:* Psychotropic drugs e.g. anxiolytics, antidepressants.
- *Modification of behavioural response:* e.g. back pain—consider referral.

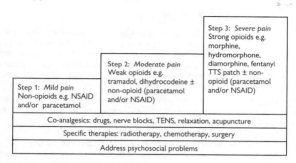

Figure 6.3 WHO analgesics ladder

Neuropathic pain: Sharp or burning pain. Typically does not respond well to ordinary analgesia. Tends to be associated with numbness around the area of pain and may be less troublesome when the patient is distracted.

• Try antidepressants (e.g. amitriptyline, 10–25mg nocte increasing as needed every 2wk. to 75–150mg)—treatment should start to have an effect within 2wk.
• If unsuccessful, consider anticonvulsants (e.g. gabapentin, carbamazepine, phenytoin, sodium valproate, or clonazepam) at standard anticonvulsant dosages.
• Local treatments are sometimes helpful e.g. capsaicin cream.

Trigeminal neuralgia—p.599

Referral: If unable to remove cause and unable to achieve adequate pain relief, consider referral to a specialist pain control clinic (or palliative care team if more appropriate).

Essential reading
Moore *et al.* (2003) *Bandolier's Little Book of Pain.* OUP. ISBN: 0192632477

Further information
The Oxford Pain Internet Site 🖳 *http://www.jr2.ox.ac.uk/bandolier/booth/painpag*

Pain-relieving drugs

Paracetamol: As effective a painkiller as ibuprofen. No anti-inflammatory effect but potent antipyretic. Drug of choice in OA where inflammation is absent. Side-effects are rare. Dose 1g qds. Overdose (>4g/24h.) can be fatal causing hepatic damage sometimes not apparent for 4–6d. Inadvertent overdosage is easy due to presence of paracetamol in most OTC cold preparations—refer to A&E.

NSAIDs: Anti-inflammatory, analgesic, antipyretic. Start at lowest recommended dose and don't use >1 NSAID concurrently. 60% respond to any NSAID—for those who don't, another may work. *Side-effects:*
- *GI side-effects:* Common (50%) including GI bleeds (¼ GI bleeds in UK). ↑ with age. Risks are dose-related and vary between drugs.
  - For the elderly, those on steroids, or with past history of GI ulceration or indigestion, protect the stomach with misoprostol or PPI.
  - Selective inhibitors of cyclo-oxygenase-2 (COX2) are equally effective and safer. Consider in high-risk patients[N] at low risk of cardiovascular disease. ❶ COX2 inhibitors have NO effect on platelet aggregation; they have no benefit if used in patients on continuous low-dose aspirin; and there is no evidence combining a COX2 inhibitor with PPI/misoprostol gives extra stomach protection. Do not use for patients with a past history of cerebrovascular or ischaemic heart disease.
- *Other side-effects:* Hypersensitivity reactions (5–10% asthmatics develop bronchospasm); fluid retention (relative contraindication in patients with ↑BP/cardiac failure); renal failure (rare—more common in patients with pre-existing renal disease); hepatic impairment (particularly diclofenac).

Topical NSAIDs: Of proven benefit for acute and chronic conditions and can be as effective as oral preparations. They have lower incidence of GI and other side-effects, though these still occur.

Table 6.2 Commonly used NSAIDs

Drug	Dosage	Features
Ibuprofen	1.2–1.8g/d. in 3–4 divided doses	Fewer side-effects than other NSAIDs. Anti-inflammatory properties are weaker. Don't use if inflammation is prominent e.g. gout.
Naproxen	0.5–1g/d. in 1–2 divided doses	Good efficacy with a low incidence of side-effects.
Diclofenac	75–150mg/d. in 1–2 divided doses	
Mefenamic acid	500mg tds	Minor anti-inflammatory properties. Tends to be used for dysmenorrhoea (📖 p.726). Occasionally associated with diarrhoea and haemolytic anaemia—discontinue.
Meloxicam	7.5–15mg od	Selective COX2 inhibitors. As effective as non-selective NSAIDs and share side-effects but risk of serious upper GI events is lower. Only use if high risk of GI side effects[N] and low cardiovascular risk.
Celecoxib	200mg od or bd	

Combination analgesics

- Combining 2 analgesics with different mechanisms of action enables better pain control than using either drug alone at that dose.
- Combinations have ↓ dose-related side-effects but the range of side-effects is ↑ (additive effects of 2 drugs).
- In general practice, the most common combinations are aspirin or paracetamol with a mild opiate (e.g. co-codamol, co-dydramol). These combinations are no more effective than paracetamol alone but have more side-effects and are more dangerous in overdose.
- Combinations using full-dose opiate (e.g. solpadol) are more effective than paracetamol alone but it is cheaper and more flexible if constituents are prescribed separately.

Opioids: Chronic pain may not respond to an opiate. Give for a 2wk. trial and only continue if of proven benefit. Worries of tolerance/addiction are unfounded for patients with true opioid-sensitive pain.

Use of morphine

- *Starting:* Give clear instructions—starting dose 2.5mg or 5mg 4 hrly; ↓ starting dose if renal/hepatic failure. Regular administration and breakthrough top-ups as required. Start with short-acting morphine 4 hrly and slowly titrate up dose. Warn about side-effects. *Driving*—advise that when on regular stable dose, can drive.
- *Prevention of side-effects:* Provide prophylactic laxatives to prevent constipation. Nausea (40%)—use antiemetic e.g. haloperidol 1.5–3mg nocte; usually resolves in <2wk. Subacute overdosage (slowly progressive somnolence and respiratory depression—common in patients with renal failure)—withhold drug for 1–2 doses, then reintroduce at 25% lower dose.
- *Titration:* ↑ by 30–50% daily until pain is controlled/side-effects prevent further ↑. Give the same dose as is being used 4 hrly as prn dose for breakthrough pain. (If using slow-release preparation, calculate equivalent short-acting 4 hrly dose.)
- *Maintenance:* Once pain is controlled, consider long-acting preparation of equivalent dosage (e.g MST bd or MXL od). If dose ↑ is then necessary, use $1/3$–$1/2$ dose increments. ↑ dose rather than frequency, as tablets are designed for od or bd dosing.
- *Other routes of administration:* If po administration is impossible consider diamorphine syringe driver ($1/3$–$1/2$ dose oral morphine/24h.), rectal morphine, or a fentanyl patch:
  - Morphine salt 90mg/d. ≡ fentanyl '25' patch
  - Morphine salt 180mg/d. ≡ fentanyl '50' patch
  - Morphine salt 270mg/d. ≡ fentanyl '75' patch
  - Morphine salt 360mg/d. ≡ fentanyl '100' patch
- *Trouble shooting*
  - *Continuing pain and frequent prn doses*—↑ regular dose.
  - *Persisting side-effects* (drowsiness, jerking, vomiting, confusion)—↓ dose.
  - Considerable pain despite marked side-effects—use alternative.

Rehabilitation

'Use strengthens, disuse debilitates'
Hippocrates (460–357 BC)

13–14% of the population have some disability. This is increasing as populations age and people survive longer with disability. Most patients are best managed by a multidisciplinary team in their home environment (if practicable) with a problem-oriented approach. Good interdisciplinary communication and coordination is essential and many patients benefit from specialist rehabilitation services. Psychological and socio-cultural aspects are as important as medical aspects.

Principles of rehabilitation:

- *Use of assessments/measures:* Central to management of any disability. Use validated measures accepted by all team members (e.g. Barthel index—📖 p.628). Reassess regularly.
- *Teamwork:* Good outcomes are associated with clinicians working as a team towards a common goal with patients and their families (or carers) included as team members.
- *Goal-setting:* Goals must be meaningful, challenging, but achievable. Use short- and long-term goals. Involve the patient ± carer(s). Regularly renew, review, and adapt.
- *Underlying approach to therapy:* All approaches focus on modification of impairment and improvement in function within everyday activities. Patients derive benefit from therapy focused on the management of disability.
- *Intensity/duration of therapy:* How much therapy is needed? Is there a minimum threshold below which there is no benefit at all? Studies on well organized services show it is rare for patients to receive >2h. therapy/d. No-one knows what is ideal.

Role of the GP:
Maintain an open door policy and encourage patients and carers to seek help for problems early. Try to become familiar with a patient's disease, even if it is rare. It is impossible to plan care without knowledge of course and prognosis and an easy way to lose a patient's confidence is if you appear ignorant of their condition.

The GP of any patient receiving rehabilitation in the community is a team member and may be the key worker who coordinates care. Information alone can improve outcome. Consider:
- Can physical symptoms be improved?
- Can the psychological symptoms be improved (including self-esteem)?
- Can functioning within the home be improved? (aids and adaptations within the home, extra help)?
- Can functioning in the community be improved (mobility outside the home, work, social activities)?
- Can the patient's or carer's financial state be improved?
- Does the carer need more support?

If progress is slower than expected, or stalls, consider other medical problems (e.g. anaemia, hypothyroidism, dementia), a neurological event, depression, and communication problems (e.g. poor vision/hearing).

Multidisciplinary working: A multidisciplinary approach is ideal e.g.
- *DNs* provide nursing care and equipment, advice on all aspects of nursing care, and teach carers how to do everyday tasks (e.g. emptying catheter bags, lifting). They are sources of information on local services and provide support for carers of patients on their caseload.
- *Health visitors for the elderly* (where available) provide general support for patients/carers and have good local knowledge.
- *Community physiotherapists* are invaluable sources of help, advice, and equipment for practical problems relating to mobility.
- *OTs* can help patients and carers cope with difficulties in everyday living caused by disability by providing aids and appliances and arranging alterations; font of knowledge on ways to help with every day activities of living.
- *Speech therapists* can help with communication problems.

Referral
- *Medical opinion:* for clarification of diagnosis (e.g. if diagnosis is in doubt or patient has symptoms/signs incongruous with diagnosis).
- *Specialist rehabilitation services:* new or deterioration in existing impairment, disability, or handicap or advances in management that warrant re-referral for specialist care.
- *Social services:* for assessment of the home for modification, assessment to allow application for mobility aids or services to help the disabled person and/or carer to cope.
- *Voluntary organizations and self-help groups:* useful sources of support for patients and carers.
- *Citizen's Advice Bureau:* for independent advice on benefits and services.
- *Disabled Living Foundation:* for independent advice on equipment and appliances—see below

Common neurological rehabilitation problems: p.626

Equipment and adaptations: p.110

Driving: p.202   **Benefits:** p.98–115

Employment: p.201   **Carers:** p.178

Patient information and support
Disabled Living Foundation: Advice about equipment and appliances ☎0845 130 9177 📖 http://www.dlf.org.uk
Age Concern: Wide range of information and factsheets ☎information line 0800 00 99 66 📖 http://www.ageconcern.org.uk
Royal Association for Disability and Rehabilitation (RADAR) ☎020 7250 3222 📖 http://www.radar.org.uk
Disablement Information and Advice Line (DIAL) ☎01302 310123 📖 http://www.dialuk.info

Care of informal carers

In the UK there are 6 million informal carers who are vitally important to the well-being of disabled people in the community. Most are relatives or friends of the person being cared for. Many are elderly with health problems themselves. There is good evidence their health suffers as a result of caring—52% report treatment for a stress-related illness since becoming a carer and 51% report being physically injured as a result of caring. GPs and their primary care teams are often the 1st point of access for any help needed and 88% carers have seen their GP in the past 12mo. Carers see the GP as the professional most able to improve their lives, but few GPs have had any training about their problems and 71% carers believe their GPs are unaware of their needs.

Physical help: Record whether a patient is a carer in their notes.
- *Practical advice on nursing skills*—ask DNs to review problems.
- *Advice on management*—specialist nurses (Macmillan nurses, diabetic liaison nurses, etc.) provide special expertise.
- *Additional help*—social services can provide home care. Voluntary organizations provide sitting services e.g. Marie Curie nurses, Crossroads schemes. Every carer has a right to ask for a full assessment of their needs by the social services.
- *Home modification*—local authorities can arrange modifications. DNs have access to equipment needed for nursing. The Red Cross loans commodes, wheelchairs, etc.
- *Respite*—hospitals, hospices, and local authorities provide day care (to give regular breaks each week) and respite care (for a week or more at a time).

Emotional support
- *Self-help carers groups*—opportunity to share experiences with people in similar situations.
- *Always ask the carer how they are when visiting*—even if they themselves are not your patient.
- *If the patient and/or carer have a religion, the clergy will often provide ongoing support.*
- *Maintain good lines of communication*—treat the carer as a team member. Make sure you inform both carer and patient fully. Make appointments for review. Don't be short with a carer, patronizing, or impossible to contact.

Financial support: Many patients who have carers are entitled to Attendance Allowance or Disability Living Allowance (🕮 p.107). If the patient is not expected to live >6mo. they are entitled to claim under Special Rules. This benefit is *not* means tested. Other benefits:
- *Low income*—🕮 p.102–4.
- *Given up work to look after the patient*—may be eligible for Carer's Allowance—🕮 p.108.
- *Substantial modification to home*—Council Tax may be payable at lower rate (consult local council).

Support organizations

Carers UK 🖳 http://www.carersonline.org.uk ☎020 7490 8818

Princess Royal Trust for Carers 🖳 http://www.carers.org ☎020 7480 7788

Support organizations for the patient's condition (e.g. Stroke Association—📖 p.607)

Department of Work and Pensions 🖳 http://www.dwp.gov.uk
  ☎*Benefits Enquiry Line*—0800 882200; 0800 243355 (minicom facility); 0800 441144 (for help with form completion)

Citizen's Advice Bureau 🖳 http://www.adviceguide.org.uk

Age Concern ☎0800 00 99 66 🖳 http://www.ageconcern.org.uk

Help the Aged ☎0800 800 65 65 🖳 http://www.helptheaged.org.uk

Counsel and Care ☎0845 300 7585 🖳 http://www.counselandcare.org.uk

Minor surgery

'*A minor operation: one performed on someone else*'
Unaccredited
Penguin Dictionary of Humerous Quotations (2001)

Providing minor surgery

Under the new GMS contract, minor surgery can be provided as an additional service or directed enhanced service (📖 p.35).

Minor surgery as an additional service: Includes curettage and cautery and—in relation to warts, verrucae, and other skin lesions—cryocautery. In all cases, a record of consent of the patient to treatment and a record of the procedure itself should be kept. Payment is included within the global sum payment. If a practice does not want to provide this service it must 'opt out' and global sum payment is ↓ by 0.6%.

Minor surgery as a directed enhanced service: Extends the range of procedures beyond those practices are expected to do as an additional service. For the purpose of payment, procedures have been divided into 3 groups:
- Injections—muscles, tendons, and joints
- Invasive procedures—including incisions and excisions
- Injections of varicose veins and piles

Payment: Treatments are priced according to the complexity of the procedure, involvement of other staff, and use of specialized equipment. Terms for this must be negotiated locally. Typical figures in 2004/5 are £40 for a joint injection or £80 for a simple excision.

Qualification to provide the service: Practices can provide this service if they can demonstrate they have the necessary facilities and personnel (partner, employee, or sub-contractor) with the necessary skills. This includes:
- Adequate equipment
- Premises compliant with national guidelines as contained in Health Building Note 46: General Medical Practice Premises (DoH)
- Nursing support
- Compliance with national infection control policies—sterile packs from the local CSSD, disposable sterile instruments, using approved sterilization procedures, etc.
- Ongoing training in minor surgery, related skills, and resuscitation techniques
- Regular audit and peer review to monitor clinical outcomes, rates of infection, and procedure.

Minor surgery in PMS practices: PMS contracts are negotiated on an individual basis with the local primary care organization. In most cases however, the contract provides for similar arrangements and payments to those in place for GMS practices.

⚠ Never attempt a procedure if you are unsure about it—know the boundaries of your experience and abilities.

Location and equipment: A suitable room, adequate lighting, the appropriate equipment, and sufficient uninterrupted time is needed for successful minor surgery. An experienced assistant is also a great help. Sterile instruments and gloves and aseptic technique are essential.

- *Basic minor surgery sets:* Scalpel; several sizes of blade (e.g. size 11 and 15); toothed forceps; needle holder; fine scissors; artery forceps; skin hook; curette.
- *Additional equipment required:* Skin preparation liquid (e.g. chlorhexadine); local anaesthetic (e.g. lignocaine 1%); suitable sized needles and syringes; sterile towels; swabs; sterile specimen pots; suture materials and dressings for the wound. For joint injection, ensure you have steroid and local anaesthetic drawn up and suitable sized needles available before starting.

⚠ Always make sure you know how many blades, sutures, needles, and swabs you have and ensure that you have accounted for and safely disposed of them at the end of the procedure.

Consent: Patient consent for the procedure must be sought and recorded in the notes. This involves giving enough information about the procedure and other possible treatment options to allow the patient to make an informed decision about whether to proceed; the patient and consenting doctor should then both sign the consent form and the form should be filed in the patient's medical records (📖 p.60)

Histological examination: All tissue removed by minor surgery should be sent for histological examination unless there are exceptional or acceptable reasons for not doing so.

Documentation: Maintain full, legible, accurate records. Include:
- History of the complaint
- Examination findings
- Diagnosis
- Full details of the procedure undertaken—include dose, batch number, expiry date, and quantities of drugs; size and number of sutures
- Follow-up arrangements.

If the patient is not registered with the practice undertaking the minor surgery, then a complete record of the procedure must be sent to the patient's registered practice for inclusion in the GP notes.

Follow-up and outcome: Should be recorded in the patient's notes. Advise the patient as to what to expect after the procedure, precautions to take, when to return for suture removal, signs that would indicate the need for reconsultation, and the expected recovery/healing time. Arrange a follow-up appointment for all but the most straightforward procedures.

Basic techniques

Local anaesthesia: 0.5–2% lidocaine, xylocaine, and procaine are the most commonly used preparations. Epinephrine (1:200,000) added to local anaesthetic ↓ bleeding and prolongs anaesthesia, but do not use epinephrine in areas supplied by end arteries (i.e. fingers, toes, penis, ear, nose). The safe maximum dose of local anaesthetic in adults is 20ml of 1% solution (less in elderly and children)—overdose causes fits or cardiac arrhythmias.

Administering local anaesthetic

- Pre-warn patients that local anaesthetic stings before numbing and that they will still be able to feel pressure—but not pain. If pain is felt, more anaesthetic is needed.
- Clean the skin, insert a small needle intradermally, and raise a small bleb before infusing more deeply.
- Always pull back on the syringe plunger before injecting to check that you are not in a blood vessel.
- Anaesthetic must be infused all around the excision site. This may require several needle insertions—try to do this through an already numb area to ↓ discomfort for the patient.
- Allow time for the anaesthetic to take effect (2–5min) before proceeding.

Suturing: Various techniques for suturing and knot tying can be used (e.g. interrupted, continuous, subcuticular). Always make a careful record of the number of stitches and when they should be removed. Usually stitches need removal after 3–5d., on the face, 7–14d. on the back and legs, and 5–7d. elsewhere. Steristrips can be used instead of or in addition to stitches in some circumstances.

Cautery: Chemical (silver nitrate) or electrocautery are used alone, or in combination with other methods (e.g. curettage), to secure haemostasis or destroy tissue. *Suitable conditions:* nose bleeds (📖 p.1042), spider naevi, telangiectasia.

⚠ *Do not* use electrical cautery for patients with a cardiac pacemaker.

Implants: Subcutaneous implants are prescribed for several conditions (e.g. prostate cancer). Most implants come pre-packaged with an insertion cannula and information leaflet—always read and follow the instructions if administering a new product and ensure position of implant and timing of administration is correct.

Suture types

- *Absorbable* e.g. catgut, dexon, vicryl—used to stitch deep layers to help ↓ tension.
- *Non-absorbable* e.g. silk, prolene, nylon—used for closure of skin wounds after minor surgery.

Needle types: straight, curved, cutting, or round bodied. Surgical site and personal preference dictate which to use—a cutting needle is usually used for skin.

Suture thickness (gauge): indicated by a number (10/0 is fine and 2/0 thick). For skin closure: 6/0 or 5/0 is usually used for the face, 3/0 on legs and back, and 4/0 elsewhere.

Removal of skin lesions

Ensure that you have had training in the techniques—learning by experience is much better than from a book. There are many courses available.

- **Only** remove benign lesions—refer suspicious lesions to a specialist for expert management.
- **Only** remove lesions that you are confident that you can cope with (take special care with lesions on the face or lip margin—the scar may be very noticeable).
- **Send all** excised lesions for histology—place in formalin and carefully label with the site and side.

Excision of skin lesions

- Gain written consent—ensure you have warned the patient about the likely size of the scar and the possibility of keloid (especially if the lesion is on a risk area e.g. upper back and chest).
- Work out the direction of the skin contour lines, clean and anaesthetize the area (📖 p.184).
- An elliptical incision—≈3x as long as it is wide—is suitable for most lesions. Place the incision in the skin contour lines if possible (marking the incision line can be helpful).
- Cut through the skin at right angles to the surface with a smooth sweep of the blade.
- Use a skin hook to lift the skin from one end of the ellipse.
- Use the scalpel blade to remove the skin from the subcutaneous fat.
- Save the excised specimen for histology.
- Close the wound by carefully apposing the edges (slightly everted) using interrupted non-absorbable sutures. Avoid tension in the sutures and knot securely. Large wounds may benefit from the use of deep absorbable sutures to reduce skin tension.

Curettage: Useful for seborrhoeic warts, pyogenic granuloma, keratoacanthoma, or single viral warts. Not suitable for naevi. Use only if the diagnosis is certain—scrapings can be sent for histology but the architecture of the lesion is lost. Numb the area with local anaesthetic and remove the lesion with gentle scooping movements using a curette spoon. Finally, cauterize the base of the lesion.

Cryotherapy: Liquid nitrogen can be used to treat viral and seborrhoeic warts and solar keratoses. Local arrangements for delivery of liquid nitrogen differ—often a clinic session to treat all suitable lesions at the same time is helpful. If diagnosis is uncertain, excise the lesion or take a biopsy prior to freezing. A cotton wool bud or nitrogen spray gun can be used to apply liquid nitrogen for ~10s. until a thin frozen halo appears at the base of the lesion. A blister forms <24h. after treatment; the lesion then falls off with the blister. Repeat treatment may be needed after 4wk.

Side-effects: Pain, failure to remove the lesion, skin hypo-pigmentation, ulceration of lower leg lesions (especially in elderly patients).

Joint and soft tissue injections

Steroids can have a potent local anti-inflammatory effect and dramatically improve certain musculoskeletal problems. Most joint injections are straightforward and can be undertaken within a general practice setting.

General rules

- Always use aseptic technique.
- Do not inject if there is local sepsis (e.g. cellulitis) or any possibility of joint infection.
- Never inject into the substance of a tendon—this may cause rupture (in tenosynovitis, steroid is injected into the tendon sheath).
- Injections should not require pressure on the syringe plunger—if so, the needle is probably not correctly located (tennis elbow is an exception).
- Undertake as few injections as possible to settle the problem—often 1 is sufficient. If no improvement after 2 or 3, then reconsider the diagnosis.
- Do no more than 3 or 4 injections/patient/appointment and no more than 3 or 4 in any single joint/y.—more than this ↑ risk of systemic absorption and joint damage.

Preparation for the procedure

- Take a history, make a careful examination, and have a clear diagnosis before considering injecting steroids.
- Gather the needles, syringes, a sterile container (for sending aspirated fluid), steroid, local anaesthetic, skin preparation fluid (e.g. chlorhexidine), cotton wool, and elastoplast beforehand.
- The injected joint should be rested for 2–3d. afterwards if possible—certainly avoid heavy activity. Make sure the patient is comfortable, has given informed consent, and knows what to expect.

Steroid preparations: (↑ order of potency)—hydrocortisone acetate, methylprednisolone acetate, triamcinolone hexacetonide.

Local anaesthetic (LA): e.g. lidocaine 1% can be mixed with the steroid for some injections—LA effect occurs immediately and lasts 2–4h.. The patient may then experience some return of symptoms (pain) before the steroid takes effect—warn the patient.

Follow-up

- Some injections are painful at administration—this is normal for tennis elbow and plantar faciitis.
- Severe or increasing pain ~48h. after injection may indicate sepsis—advise the patient to return urgently if this occurs.
- If steroid is injected close to the skin surface (as in tennis elbow), skin dimpling and pigment loss can occur—warn the patient.

Further information

Silver T. *Joint and soft tissue injection: injecting with confidence.* Radcliffe Medical Press

❶ Most hospital Rheumatology Departments have a joint injection clinic and are happy to allow GPs to watch to gain experience

Patient information

Arthritis Research Campaign (ARC) Patient information leaflet: 'Local steroid injections'
☎0870 850 5000 🖳 http://www.arc.org.uk

Lower limb injections

The knee: Joint effusions are common (e.g. trauma, ligament strains, OA, RA, gout). Aspiration of fluid can:
- help make a diagnosis e.g. gout
- be a therapeutic procedure—draining a tense effusion can relieve pain
- precede administration of steroids e.g. RA flare

Aspirated fluid should be clear or slightly yellow and not purulent. If aspirating an effusion, send the fluid for analysis. Any sign of infection within the joint prohibits steroid use.

Technique for aspiration and joint injection
- Lie the patient on couch with knee slightly bent (place a pillow under the knee as this relaxes the muscles).
- Palpate the joint space under the lateral or medial edge of the patella and inject/aspirate just below the superior border of the patella with the needle horizontal—Figure 7.1.
- Use a green (21 gauge) needle.
- If aspirating and then injecting steroids, maintain the needle in position and swap the syringe.
- Normal doses of steroid are triamcinolone 20mg or methylprednisolone 40mg.
- In prepatella bursitis, aspiration and injection of hydrocortisone 25mg into the bursa can help settle inflammation.

Plantar faciitis: Painful area in the middle of the heel pad can be helped by steroid injection into the most tender spot—it hurts, so advise analgesia. Mixing lidocaine 1% with the steroid (e.g. triamcinolone 10–20mg) can help. Two methods are commonly used: injection through the tough skin of the sole of the foot (more accurate) or a lateral approach (less painful)—Figure 7.2. Rest the foot for several days and use an in-shoe heel pad. Rupture of the plantar fascia is a rare complication.

Tenosynovitis: Causes pain and stiffness in the line of the tendon and crepitus over the affected tendon. The most common site is the base of the thumb (DeQuervain's tenosynovitis). Injecting steroid and local anaesthetic (e.g. hydrocortisone 25mg and 1ml 1% lignocaine) into the space between the tendon and the sheath can help.
- Insert the needle along the line of the tendon just distal to the point of maximum tenderness.
- Advance the needle proximally into the tendon (felt as a resistance) and then slowly withdraw until the resistance disappears. The tip of the needle is now in the tendon sheath.
- It is now safe to inject—the tendon sheath may swell.   •
- Advise the patient to rest the affected area for several days and avoid the precipitating activity.

(a) (b)

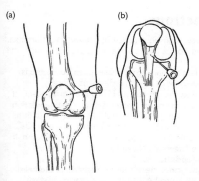

Figure 7.1 Knee joint injection. (Reproduced with permission from *Oxford Handbook of Clinical Specialties* (2003), Oxford University Press, Oxford.)

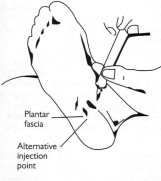

Plantar fascia

Alternative injection point

Figure 7.2 Injection of plantar fasciitis

Upper limb injections

Carpal tunnel syndrome: Can be relieved by steroid injection. Pain may worsen after injection for ≤48h. before it improves—warn the patient. *Technique:*

- Sit the patient with hand resting on a firm surface, palm up. Palmaris longus tendon can be seen by wrist flexion against resistance.
- Insert the needle at the distal skin crease, at 45° to the horizontal, pointing towards the fingers, just radial (thumb-side) to the palmaris tendon. Palmaris longus is absent in 10%—inject between the tendons of flexor digitorum superficialis and flexor carpi radialis—Figure 7.3.
- Use a green (21 gauge) needle and advance it to about ½ its length. If there is sudden pain in the fingers you have hit the median nerve—withdraw the needle and reposition it.
- Inject steroid e.g. 10mg triamcinolone. If there is resistance, the needle is not in the right place. Don't use LA as it causes finger numbness.
- Rest the hand for several days afterwards.

Shoulder: Injection can help rotator cuff problems, frozen shoulder, subacromial bursitis and rheumatoid arthritis. There are several approaches (anterior, posterior, subacromial, or lateral)—the joint space communicates in most cases, so steroid will reach the whole joint whichever approach is used. *Anterior approach:*

- Sit patient with the arm relaxed at the side and slightly externally rotated. Palpate the space between the head of humerus and the coracoid process.
- Insert the needle (green, 21 gauge) horizontally into that gap ensuring the needle is lateral to the coracoid process—Figure 7.4. The needle will need to be inserted for most of its length to reach the joint space.
- Typical dose is 1ml steroid e.g. triamcinolone 20mg + 1ml 1% lidocaine.
- There should be no/little resistance to injecting the fluid. If there is, the needle is wrongly positioned.

AC joint injection: Can help the pain of OA. Palpate the joint space—the needle can be inserted anteriorly or superiorly. If you push the needle too far you may enter the shoulder joint. Small joint space means only 0.2–0.5ml can be injected, Use a blue (23 gauge) needle and don't add LA.

Elbow: Tennis or golfer's elbow respond well to steroid injection. Steroid is infiltrated into the tender spots at the tendon insertion, rather than into a joint space. Thus, there is resistance on injection and it can be quite painful, warn the patient. The steroid is injected relatively superficially—so warn the patient about the possibility of skin dimpling or pigment loss.

- Sit the patient with the elbow flexed to 90° and palpate the most tender spot.
- Insert the needle into that spot and inject 0.1–0.2ml of steroid (e.g. hydrocortisone 25mg/1ml). Then, without making a new skin puncture, move the needle in a fan shape around the area injecting small amounts of steroid. Try to inject all the tender area—Figure 7.4.
- Pain of injection may last 48h.—advise resting the arm and analgesia.

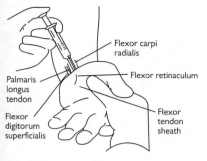

Figure 7.3 Injection of the carpal tunnel

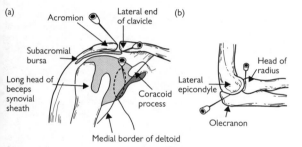

Figure 7.4 Injection of shoulder joint and elbow joint. (Reproduced with permission from *Oxford Handbook of Clinical Specialties* (2003), Oxford University Press, Oxford.)

Miscellaneous topics

Complications of surgery and injury that might be seen in general practice

Wound infection

Risk factors
- Malnutrition
- DM
- Carcinomatosis
- Steroid therapy
- Infection near the site of incision
- Contamination of the wound

Presentation: Suspect if a wound becomes painful. Look for swelling, erythema, wound tenderness, ± pus.

Management: If pus is present, send a swab for M,C&S:
- If the wound is indurated and infection localized to the wound, suspect Staphylococcus infection. Treat with flucloxacillin 250–500mg qds (or erythromycin 250–500mg qds if penicillin allergy).
- If there is cellulitis around the wound, suspect Streptococcus. Treat with penicillin V 250–500mg qds or erythromycin 250–500mg qds.
- If foul smelling, suspect anaerobes. Treat with metronidazole 400mg tds.

Give adequate analgesia; dress the wound frequently; review regularly; allow pus to drain. Refer back to the operating surgeon if simple measures are ineffective.

Wound dehiscence: Breakdown of a surgical wound—usually abdominal. May be partial or complete.
- *Partial breakdown*—skin remains intact but muscle layers break down → incisional hernia. Typically, the patient feels something 'give' ± sudden ↑ in pain and pink fluid discharge. Refer for urgent reassessment by the operating surgeon.
- *Complete dehiscence*—wound breaks down entirely. The patient becomes shocked and distressed. Lie flat; give strong opiate analgesia; cover the wound with a sterile pack soaked in saline; admit as a '999' emergency.

Risk factors
- Malnutrition
- Obesity
- ↑ intra-abdominal pressure e.g. from coughing
- Wound infection
- Haematoma formation
- Ascites draining through a wound

Fistula formation: Abnormal communication forms between one organ and another—see Table 8.1. Refer any suspected case urgently back to the operating surgeon.

Risk factors
- Malnutrition
- Carcinomatosis
- Wound infection
- Distal obstruction

DVT: 📖 p.364

Pulmonary embolus: 📖 p.1054

Table 8.1 Presentation of fistula

Connection	Presentation
Bowel → skin	Faecal discharge through wound
Bladder/ureters → skin	Clear, watery discharge which smells of urine
Bowel → vagina	Faeculent material in vagina
Bladder → vagina	Leakage of urine per vaginum
Bowel → bladder	Air or faeculent material in urine; recurrent UTI

UTI: Common after any procedure in which the bladder has been instrumented. Send an MSU if suspected. If symptoms are unpleasant, treat with trimethoprim 200mg bd for 7d. without waiting for the result. Dysuria and ↑ frequency are common for 2–3wk. after TURP. Suspect UTI if symptoms worsen >1wk. post-op.

Acute retention of urine: 📖 p.690.

Subphrenic abscess: Rarely follows 7–21d. after generalized peritonitis—particularly after acute appendicitis.

Presentation: General malaise, swinging fever, nausea, and loss of weight ± pain upper abdomen which radiates to the shoulder tip. Breathlessness can be associated due to reactive pleural effusion or lower lobe collapse. Examination may reveal subcostal tenderness ± liver enlargement.

Investigations: FBC (leucocytosis); CXR; USS.

Management: If suspected, admit acutely for surgical assessment.

Compartment syndrome: Crush injury, fracture, prolonged immobility or tight splints, dressings or casts can result in ↑ pressure within muscle compartments → vascular occlusion, hypoxia, necrosis and further ↑ pressure. *Signs:* swelling, severe pain, distal numbness, redness, mottling, blisters. Refer as an emergency for orthopaedic assessment—a fasciotomy may be needed to relieve the pressure.

Reflex sympathetic dystrophy (algodystrophy, complex regional pain disorder): Pain ± vasomotor changes in a limb → loss of function. Most common in the hand and wrist. Usually follows trauma (but the trauma may be trivial and signs may appear weeks or months later). *Signs:* Pain at rest exacerbated by movement and light touch, swelling, discoloration, temperature changes, abnormal sensitivity, sweating, and loss of function. X-ray may show osteopoenia.

Management: Physiotherapy (improves prognosis if started early); analgesia (NSAIDs). Refer to pain clinic and/or rheumatology for IV bisphosphonates (responds well if treated early) and 'mirror' therapy.

Time off work

The longer a patient is off work, the lower the chances of returning—
<50% of people who have been absent for >6mo. ever return to work.
- Wherever possible, suggest work adjustments rather than signing
  the patient off work. Can be done through the 'remarks' section of the
  Med3 form (📖 p.201)
- Suggest work adjustments if the patient is off sick to enable early
  return to work (can be done in the remarks section of the Med3 form)
- Suggest graduated work/transitional arrangements to ease the patient
  back into work.
- Involve occupational health professionals

Post-operative time off work: See Table 8.2

❶These are not hard and fast rules—alter them to fit individual circumstances (e.g. laparoscopic procedures often entail less time off than open
procedures; patients performing hard manual jobs may require more
time off work)

Time off work for emergencies: In many cases, patients have the
right to take time off work to deal with an emergency involving someone
who depends on them, but they may only be absent for as long as it
takes to deal with the immediate emergency.

Dependants include spouse or partner, children, parents, or anyone living
with the patient as part of their family. Others who rely wholly on the
patient for help in an emergency may also qualify.

Emergencies include situations in which a dependant:
- is ill and needs help
- is involved in an accident or assaulted
- needs the patient to arrange their longer-term care
- needs the patient to deal with an unexpected disruption or breakdown
  in care, such as a childminder or nurse failing to turn up
- goes into labour
- dies and the patient needs to make funeral arrangements or to attend
  the funeral.

The legal right only covers emergencies and employers do not have to
pay for time taken off.

Certification of time off work: 📖 p.200

Table 8.2 List of expected time off work for uncomplicated procedures

Operation	Minimum expected (wk.)	Maximum expected if no complications (wk.)
Angiography/angioplasty	<1	4
Appendectomy	1	3
Arthroscopy	<1	<1
Cataract surgery	2	4
Cholecystectomy	2	5
Colposcopy ± cautery	<1	<1
CABG or valve surgery	4	8
Cystoscopy	<1	<1
D&C, ERPC, or TOP	<1	<1
Femoro-popliteal grafts	4	12
Haemorrhoid banding	<1	<1
Haemorrhoidectomy	3	6
Hysterectomy	3	7
Inguinal or femoral hernia	1	3
Laparoscopy ± sterilization	<1	<1
Laparotomy	6	12
Mastectomy	2	6
Pacemaker insertion*	<1	<1
Pilonidal sinus**	<1	<1
Retinal detachment	<1	Avoid heavy work, lifelong
Total hip or knee replacement	12	26
TURP	3	6
Vasectomy	<1	<1

* Driving—see 📖 p.203.
** If time off for dressings is allowed.

Certifying fitness to work

Own occupation test: Applies to those claiming for the first 28wk. of their illness:
- statutory sick pay from their employer
- incapacity benefit if the patient has done a substantial amount of work in the 21wk. prior to the illness

The doctor assesses whether the patient is fit to do their *own* job.

Personal capability assessment (formerly the 'All work test'): Assesses a patient on a variety of different mental and physical health dimensions for ability to work. Not diagnosis dependant. Applies to:
- everyone after 28wk. incapacity
- those who do not qualify for the own occupation test from the start of their incapacity

Claimants are sent form IB50 to complete themselves and are asked to obtain form Med4 from their GP. If the Department of Work and Pensions (DWP) is not happy to continue paying their benefit on the basis of these reports, the applicant is called for a medical examination. Conditions which exempt patients from further examination are:
- Receipt of highest rate care component of Disability Living Allowance (DLA), Constant Attendance Allowance, or >80% disabled for other benefit purposes
- Terminal illness
- Tetraplegia or paraplegia, hemiplegia, progressive neurological or muscle wasting disease
- Registered blindness
- Persistent vegetative state
- Severe mental illness or dementia
- Progressive immune deficiency (including AIDS)
- Severe learning disabilities
- Active and progressive polyarthropathy
- Severe progressive cardio-respiratory disease which persistently limits exercise tolerance.

Private certificates: Some employers request private certificates in the 1st week of sickness absence. They should request them in writing. If the GP chooses to provide the service, (s)he may charge both for a private consultation and the provision of a private certificate. The company should accept full responsibility for all fees incurred by the patient.

Permitted work: Incapacity benefits do allow very limited work—therapeutic work (must be done as part of a treatment programme and in an institution which provides sheltered work for people with disabilities); voluntary work; local authority councillor; disability expert on an appeal tribunal or member of the Disability Living Allowance advisory board (not >1d./wk.).

Disability Discrimination Act 1995: Some circumstances require employers to make reasonable adjustments for an employee with a long-term disability. Advise patients to seek specialist advice.

Disability employment advisors: Provided by the Employment Service to assist disabled patients to get back to work. Contacted by:
• writing a comment to the effect that intervention would be helpful in the comments box on form Med3 *or*
• writing to the local Jobcentre (with the patients' permission)

Useful information

Department of Work and Pensions. Medical evidence for statutory sick pay, statutory maternity pay, and social security incapacity benefit purposes: A guide for registered medical practitioners. IB204. June 2004. ▣ *http://www.dwp.gov.uk*
Disability Discrimination Act. ▣ *http://www.disability.gov.uk*

Forms for certifying incapacity to work

SC1—self-certification form for people not eligible to claim statutory sick pay who wish to claim incapacity benefit. Certify first 7d. of illness. Available from local Jobcentre Plus offices and GP surgery.

SC2—as SC1 but for people who can claim statutory sick pay. Available from employer, local Jobcentre Plus offices, and GP surgery.

Med 3—filled in by GP or hospital doctor who knows the patient. For periods of incapacity to work likely to be >7d. If return within 14d. is forecast, give fixed date of return ('closed certificate'). If longer, specify a period of time (e.g. 2mo.) ('open certificate'). Before the patient returns to work, reassess and give further certificate with fixed date of return. Only one Med3 can be issued per patient per period of sickness. If mislaid, reissue and mark 'duplicate'.

Med 4—see personal capability assessment (opposite). Only completed once for any period of incapacity from work.

Med 5—can be used if:
• a doctor has not seen the patient but on the basis of a recent (<1mo.) written report from another doctor is satisfied that the patient should not work—the certificate should not cover a forward period of >1mo.;
• the patient returned to work without receiving a closed certificate (see Med3 above);
• >1d. since the patient was seen (so Med3 or Med4 cannot be issued) but it is clear the disability is ongoing.

Med 6—when it is felt that putting a diagnosis on a Med3/Med4 would be harmful either directly to a patient or through their employer knowing their diagnosis. A vague diagnosis is put on the form and a Med6 completed which requests the Department of Works and Pensions (DWP) to send a form to obtain more precise details.

RM 7—form sent to DWP which requests review of the patient by them sooner than would usually be undertaken.

Mat B1—signed by doctor or midwife. Provided to pregnant women once within 20wk. of EDD. Enables her to claim statutory maternity pay and other benefits (▭ p.112).

Fitness to drive

⚠ Driving licence holders (or applicants) have a legal duty to inform the DVLA of any disability likely to cause danger to the public if they were to drive.

Driving licence types

- **Group 1**—ordinary licence for driving a car/motorcycle. Old licences expire at 70th birthday and then must be renewed 3yrly. Applicants are asked to confirm they have no medical disability. If so, no medical examination is necessary. New photocard licences are automatically renewed 10yrly until age 70y. Minimum age 17y. (16y. if disabled).
- **Group 2**—enables holders to drive lorries and buses. Min. age 21y. Initially valid until 45th birthday, then renewable every 5y. until 65th birthday. >65y., renewable annually. Medical examination is needed to renew Group 2 licences. Applicants must bring form D4 (available from post offices) with them. Examinations take ~½ h. A fee may be charged by the GP.

Determining fitness to drive: Patients with any disorder which may cause danger to others if they drove, should be advised not to drive and contact the DVLA. The DVLA gives advice on when they can restart.

Driving after surgery: Drivers do not need to notify the DVLA unless a condition likely to affect safe driving persists >3mo. (certain exceptions apply for neurological and cardiovascular disorders). It is the responsibility of the driver to ensure that he/she is in control of the vehicle at all times. It might also be advisable for the driver to check with his/her insurer before returning to drive after surgery. *Consider:*
- Recovery from the surgical procedure
- Recovery from anaesthesia (sedation and cognitive impairment)
- Distracting effect of pain
- Impairment due to analgesia (sedation and cognitive impairment)
- Physical restrictions due to the surgery or the underlying condition

Disabled drivers who want to learn to drive or return to driving following onset of their disability should have an assessment of their driving ability and/or advice on controls and adaptations needed. Licences may be limited to adapted vehicles. A list of driving assessment centres can be obtained from the DVLA website. Information sheets are available from: MAVIS ☎01344 661 000 🖳 *www.dft.gov.uk/access/mavis*

Seatbelt exemption: GPs can sign a form to exempt patients (e.g. those with colostomies) from having to wear a seatbelt. Consider very carefully the reasons for exemption in view of the weight of evidence in favour of seatbelts. A fee can be charged for this service.

❶ Patients on low income can apply for a free medical examination on a form available from: Department for Transport, Road Safety Division 1, Zone 2/11, Great Minster House, 76 Marsham Street, London SW1P 4DR ☎020 7944 2046.

Breaking confidentiality: When a patient continues to drive despite advice by a doctor to stop, a doctor has an *obligation* to breach confidentiality and inform the DVLA.

- If the patient does not understand the advice to stop driving, inform the DVLA.
- If the patient does understand, explain your legal duty to inform the DVLA if they do not stop driving. If they still refuse, offer a second medical opinion (on the understanding they stop driving in the interim).
- If the patient still continues driving, consider action such as recruiting next-of-kin to the cause (but beware of breach of confidentiality).
- If all else fails, inform the DVLA in confidence. Before doing this, write to the patient to inform him/her of your intended actions. Once the DVLA has been informed, you should also write to the patient, to confirm that a disclosure has been made. Consider contacting your medical defence organization for advice.

Further information

DVLA *At a glance guide to the current medical standards of fitness to drive for medical practitioners,* Available from ⌨ www.dvla.gov.uk

Medical advisers from the DVLA can advise on difficult issues. Contact: Drivers Medical Unit, DVLA, Swansea SA99 1TU or ☎01792 761119

Mobility Advice and Vehicle Information Service (MAVIS) ⌨ www.dft.gov.uk/access/mavis

Certificates of exemption from compulsory seatbelt wearing can be obtained from: Department of Health, PO Box 777, London SE1 6XH; ☎08701 555455 (NHS Responseline); *Email:* doh@prologistics.co.uk

Brief guide to DVLA fitness to drive criteria

⚠ Any person driving (or attempting to drive) on the public highway or other public place whilst unfit due to any drug, whether prescribed or illicit, is liable to prosecution.

Neurology

- *Single seizure/fit/epilepsy/undiagnosed loss of consciousness:* Licence revoked. Specified seizures with identifiable non-recurring, proking cause (e.g. at the time of stroke or intracranial surgery) may be dealt with on a case-by-case basis by the DVLA.
  - *Group 1*—seizure free for 1y. to regain licence.
  - *Group 2*—seizure free without medication for 10y. to regain licence (or 5y. if cause of collapse unknown).
- *Withdrawal of antiepileptic medication:* Licence not revoked but no driving during period of withdrawal and for 6mo. without medication.
- *Single CVA/TIA/episode amaurosis fugax:*
  - *Group 1*—1mo. off driving. Restart when clinically fit thereafter.
  - *Group 2*—licence revoked. Review after 5y.
- *Recurrent CVA/TIA/amaurosis fugax:*
  - *Group 1*—stop driving until attacks controlled for 3mo.
  - *Group 2*—licence revoked.

Cardiovascular disease

- *Hypertension:* If asymptomatic, continue driving.
  - *Group 2*—stop driving if systolic >180 or diastolic >100mmHg until BP controlled.
- *Arrythmia:* Stop driving.
  - *Group 1*—until attacks controlled.
  - *Group 2*—licence revoked until arrythmia controlled >3mo. and renewed only if the left ventricular ejection fraction is >0.4.
- *Pacemaker insertion*—(includes box change):
  - *Group 1*—stop driving for 1wk.
  - *Group 2*—stop driving for 6wk.
  Other implantable defibrillator devices—see DVLA guidance.
- *Stable angina:*
  - *Group 1*—stop driving if attack whilst at the wheel until symptoms controlled.
  - *Group 2*—licence revoked until symptom free >6wk. Renewal requires medical examination and exercise ECG.
- *Unstable angina/MI/CABG:*
  - *Group 1*—stop driving for 1mo. Restart when clinically fit thereafter.
  - *Group 2*—licence revoked. Reviewed after 6wk. with medical examination and exercise ECG.
- *Coronary angioplasty:*
  - *Group 1*—stop driving for 1wk. Restart when clinically fit thereafter.
  - *Group 2*—licence revoked. Reviewed after 6wk. with medical examination and exercise ECG.
- *Postural hypotension/syncope:* If cause is clear and not sudden or disabling, continue driving.

Diabetes mellitus

- **Controlled by diet/oral hypoglycaemics:** Continue driving if adequate control, unless related problems (e.g. loss of visual acuity, CHD, CVA).
- **Controlled with insulin:** Stop driving if poor control, related problems that prevent driving, frequent hypoglycaemic episodes, or inability to recognize hypoglycaemia.
  - Group 2—if issued after 1.4.1991, licence revoked. If issued before then, DVLA considers each case individually.

Psychiatric conditions

- **Dementia:**
  - Group 1—stop if pose danger to public. Annual review.
  - Group 2—licence revoked.
- **Anxiety, depression, other neuroses:**
  - Group 1—unless severe, continue driving. Stop if severe (especially if suicide at the wheel might be a possibility) or if medication inhibits ability to drive.
  - Group 2—licence revoked if serious acute mental illness. Restored if symptom free and stable for ≥6mo.
- **Psychosis:**
  - Group 1—licence revoked. Restored if well and stable for ≥3mo., compliant with treatment, free from adverse drug effects which would impair driving. Specialist report required.
  - Group 2—licence revoked for 3y. Restored if stable and off antipsychotic medication which might affect ability to drive. Specialist report required.
- **Drug or alcohol misuse or dependency:** DVLA arranges assessment prior to licence restoration.
  - Group 1—6mo. off driving (1y. after alcohol or drug-related seizure or detoxification for alcohol, opiate, cocaine, or benzodiazepine dependence).
  - Group 2—licence revoked for 1y. (3y. if alcohol dependence or misuse of opiates, cocaine, or benzodiazepines; 5y. if alcohol- or drug-related seizure).

Conditions affecting vision

- **Visual acuity:**
  - Group 1—able to read in good light (with glasses or contact lenses) a number plate containing figures 79mm high and 57mm wide at a distance of 20.5m (20m where the characters are 50mm wide).
  - Group 2—corrected vision of 6/9 (best eye) and 6/12 (other eye). Stop driving if uncorrected acuity in either eye <3/60.
- **Night blindness:** Stop driving.
- **Colour blindness:** No restrictions.
- **Visual field defects:** Stop driving.
  - Group 1—restore if able to meet DVLA criteria.
- **Diplopia:** stop driving.
  - Group 1—can resume if controlled (e.g. by wearing patch).

Miscellaneous

- **Sleep apnoea:** Stop driving. Restart when symptoms adequately controlled.

Fitness to make decisions

A GP asked to give an opinion on a patient's mental capacity, should:
- Have access to the patient's records and ideally know the patient
- Seek information from friends, relatives, and carers
- Examine the patient, assess type and degree of deficit and ability to comply with the specific requirements listed for each situation
- Decide if assessment should be postponed while measures are taken to improve capacity
- Record all the above information

Even if a doctor thinks a proposed action is in the patient's best interests, he/she must not judge the patient capable if that is not clearly the case. If in doubt, seek a second opinion.

Power of attorney: Covers financial matters only.
- **Ordinary power of attorney:** Ceases to have effect if the patient (donor) becomes mentally incapable; the donor must understand the nature and effect of what he or she is doing.
- **Enduring power of attorney (EPA):** Continues if the donor is mentally incapable, provided it is registered with the Court of Protection. The donor must understand that the:
  - Attorney will be able to assume complete authority over the person's affairs and do anything with the donor's property that the donor could have done;
  - Authority will continue if the donor becomes mentally incapable and is irrevocable while the donor remains incapable.

❶ In Scotland, an ordinary power of attorney signed after January 1991 remains valid even if the donor becomes mentally incapable.

Court of Protection: If a person, by reason of mental disorder, becomes incapable of managing his or her affairs but has not previously signed an EPA, it may be necessary for someone, usually the nearest relative, to apply to the Court of Protection for the appointment of a 'receiver' to do so. The medical practitioner will be asked to complete form CP3. Alternatively, if the patient's affairs are simple (e.g. state pension), direct arrangements can be made with relevant authorities.

Testamentary capacity: The capacity to make a will. Anyone can make a will provided:
- They understand the nature and effect of making a will, extent of property being disposed of, and claims others may have on that property;
- The decision is not the result of their condition (e.g. due to a delusion).

❶ Decisions don't have to seem rational to others, especially if consistent with premorbid personality.

Capacity to consent to medical treatment: 📖 p.60

Advance directives: Statements in which a person makes a decision about medical treatment in case he or she becomes incapable of making that decision later.

- Respect any refusal of treatment given when the patient was competent, provided the decision is clearly applicable to present circumstances, and there is no reason to believe that the patient has altered that decision.
- It is legally binding if it is clearly established, applicable to the current situation, and was made without undue pressure from others.
- The BMA recommends doctors should *not* withhold 'basic care' (e.g. symptom control) even in the face of a directive which specifies that the patient should receive no treatment.
- Where an advance statement is not available, take patients' known wishes into consideration.

Further information

The Law Society and the BMA (1995) *Assessment of mental capacity; guidance for doctors and lawyers.* BMA.
BMA local offices.
Medical defence organizations: 📖 p.79

Fitness for other activities

Fitness to fly: Passengers are required to tell the airline at the time of booking about any conditions that might compromise their fitness to fly. The airline's medical officer must then decide whether to carry them or not.

Hazards of flying
- Cabin pressure—oxygen levels are lower than at ground level and gas in body cavities expands 30% in flight
- Inactivity and dehydration
- Disruption of routine
- Alcohol consumption
- Stress and excitement

Contraindications to flying
- *Respiratory disease*—
  - Suspected pneumothorax/pneumomediastinum—patients should not fly for 14d. after complete resolution of pneumothorax.
  - Chronic lung disease—if a patient can walk >50m. without getting breathless, s/he should be fit to fly. Supplementary oxygen can be provided in flight for patients unable to walk this far but the patient must pre-book this with the airline and there is usually a charge.
- *Heart disease*—Patients should not travel if they have unstable angina, poorly controlled heart failure, or an uncontrolled arrythmia, Patients should also refrain from travelling <10d. post uncomplicated MI (3–4wk. if complicated recovery) and for 3–5d. post angioplasty.
- *Thrombo-embolic disease*—Patients should not travel with a DVT before established on anticoagulants.
- *Neurological disease*—Patients should not travel for 3d. post stroke or, if epileptic, within 24h. of a grand mal fit.
- *Infectious disease*—Patients must not travel with untreated infectious disease.
- *Psychiatric illness*—Patients should not travel if they have disturbed or unpredictable behaviour that could disrupt the flight.
- *Fractures*—Flying restricted for 24–48h. (depending on the length of the flight) after the plaster cast has been fitted.
- *Haematological disease*—Anaemia (<7.5g/dl) and recent sickling crisis may restrict flying.
- *Pregnancy*—Most airlines will not carry women >36wk. pregnant (3rd trimester if multiple pregnancy), or with history of premature delivery, cervical incompetence, bleeding, or ↑ uterine activity.
- *Ear problems*—Flying with otitis media or sinusitis can result in pain ± perforation of the ear drum. Patients are advised not to fly until symptoms resolve.
- *Babies* <2d. old should not fly (preferably <7d. old).
- *Surgery*—Patients should not travel <10d. post surgery to the chest, abdomen, or middle ear. Any other procedure where gas is introduced into the body also needs careful consideration.

Precautions

- Carry all regular medication, especially relief medications (e.g. salbutamol, GTN spray) in the cabin;
- For people who have to time their medication carefully, keep to times medication was taken at home for duration of flight (e.g. diabetics—take snacks to eat and take insulin at normal times);
- Drink plenty of liquid (non-alcoholic) to prevent dehydration;
- Do calf exercises/get up and walk and down at intervals to prevent venous stasis in legs (for those at risk of venous thromboembolism, worth using prophylactic aspirin 75mg od and compression stockings for flight);
- Pre-warn airlines of special needs so that they can accommodate them (e.g. extra leg room, special diet, oxygen in-flight, transport to and from plane).

Fitness to perform sporting activities: GPs are commonly asked to certify fitness to perform sports. Normally, the patient will come with a medical form. If there is a form, request to see it before the medical. If there is no form and you are unsure what to check, telephone the sport's governing body or the event organizer. A fee is payable by the patient.

Many gyms and sports clubs also ask older patients and patients with pre-existing conditions or disabilities to check with their GP before they will sign them on. Assuming that a suitable regime is undertaken, most people can participate in some form of sporting activity. Consider the patient's baseline fitness, check BP and medications, and recommend a gradual introduction to any new forms of exercise. HOCM (📖 p.352) can cause sudden death during sport. It is difficult to exclude on clinical examination—if there is a FH or systolic murmur refer to cardiology before recommending new intense activity.

Pre-employment certification: It is becoming increasingly common for GPs to be asked about the 'medical' suitability of candidates to perform a job. This is not part of the GP's terms of service and, therefore, a GP can refuse to give an opinion. In all cases where an opinion is given, a fee can be claimed. Common examples are:

- Ofsted forms for childminders
- Care home staff—proof of 'physical and mental fitness'
- Food handlers—certificates of fitness

⚠ Remember—signing a form may result in legal action against you should the patient NOT be fit to undertake an activity.

Where possible include a caveat e.g. 'based on information available in the medical notes, the patient appears to be fit to ... although it is impossible to guarantee this.'

If unsure, consult your local LMC or medical defence organization for advice.

Confirmation and certification of death

⚠ The death certification process in England and Wales is currently under review and likely to change in the near future.

English law *does not* require a doctor:
- To confirm death has occurred or that 'life is extinct'. A doctor is only required to certify what, in their opinion, was the cause.
- To view the body of a deceased person. There is no obligation to see/examine a body before issuing a death certificate.
- To report the fact that death has occurred.

English law *does* require the doctor who attended the deceased during the last illness to issue a certificate detailing the cause of death. Certificates are provided by the local registrar of births, marriages, and deaths. A special certificate is needed for infants of <28d. old.

Death in the community: ¼ occur at home.

Expected deaths: In all cases, advise to contact the undertakers and ensure the patient's own GP is notified.
- *Patient's home:* Visit as soon as practicable.
- *Residential/nursing home:* If possible, the GP who attended during the patient's last illness should visit and issue a death certificate.
The 'on-call' GP is often requested to visit. There is no statutory duty to do this, but it is reassuring for the staff at the home and often necessary before staff are allowed to ask for the body to be removed.

Unexpected and/or 'sudden' death: If called, advise the attendant to call 999. Visit and take a rapid history from any attendants. Then:
- *Resuscitate if appropriate:* Drowning and hypothermia can protect against hypoxic neurological damage; brains of children <5y. old are more resistant to damage.
- *Report the death to the coroner:* If any suspicious circumstances or circumstances of death are unknown/unclear, call the police.

Alternatively, if police or ambulance service is already in attendance and death has been confirmed, suggest the police surgeon is contacted.

Cremation: The Cremation Acts of 1902 and 1952 require 2 doctors to complete a certificate to establish identity and that the cause of death is not suspicious before a person can be cremated. A fee is payable to each doctor by the person arranging the funeral. It has 2 parts:
- *Part B:* Completed by the patient's usual medical attendant—usually his/her GP.
- *Part C:* Completed by another doctor who must have held full GMC registration (or equivalent) for ≥5y. and is not connected with the patient in any way, nor directly connected with the doctor who issued part B—usually a GP from another practice.

⚠ Pacemakers and radioactive implants must be removed from the deceased before cremation can take place.

Further information on completing cremation forms
Home Office ⧉ *http://www.homeoffice.gov.uk/docs2/compcrembc.html*

Deaths which must be reported to the coroner
- Sudden or unexpected deaths
- Accidents and injuries
- Industrial diseases e.g. mesothelioma
- Service disability pensioners
- Deaths where the doctor has not attended within the past 14d.
- Deaths arising from ill treatment e.g. abuse, neglect, starvation, hypothermia
- Cause of death unknown
- Deaths <24h. after hospital admission
- Poisoning (chronic alcoholism and its sequelae are no longer notifiable per se)
- Medical mishaps (including anaesthetic complications, short- or long-term complications of operations, drugs—whether therapeutic or addictive)
- Abortions
- Prisoners
- Stillbirths (when there is doubt about whether the baby was born alive)

Notification of death to the coroner: The coroner can be contacted via the local police. Reporting to the coroner does not automatically entail a post-mortem. The coroner, once circumstances of death are clear, may advise the GP to tick and initial box A on the back of the certificate, which advises the Registrar that no inquest is necessary. Deaths which *MUST* be reported to the coroner are listed in the box above.

❶ In Scotland, deaths are reported to a procurator fiscal. The list of reportable deaths is the same, with the addition of deaths of foster children and the newborn.

Recording deaths at the practice: Death registers are useful. Routine communication of deaths to all members of the primary health-care team and other agencies involved with the care of that patient (e.g. hospital consultants, social services) avoids the embarrassing and distressing situation of ongoing appointments and contacts being made for that patient. Record the death in the notes of any relatives/partner registered with the practice.

Benefits available after a death
- For widows/widowers: 📖 p.101
- Funeral payment: 📖 p.104

Patient advice and support
Department of Work and Pensions (DWP)
- Leaflet D49: 'What to do after a death in England and Wales'. Available from 🖳 http://www.dwp.gov.uk/publications/dwp/2003/d49_oct.pdf
- Funeral payment: information and on-line application form 🖳 http://www.jobcentreplus.gov.uk
Scottish Executive 'What to do after a death in Scotland'. Available from 🖳 http://www.scotland.gov.uk/library5/social/waad-00.asp
Office of Fair Trading. 'Arranging funerals'. 🖳 http://www.oft.gov.uk

Organ donation

>5500 people in the UK are waiting for an organ transplant that could save or dramatically improve their life, but <3000 transplants are carried out each year. There is a desperate need for more donors. In 2003, ~400 people died while waiting for a transplant.

Absolute contraindications to any organ donation

- Untreated systemic infection
- HIV
- Hepatitis B or C
- Alzheimer's disease and other diseases of unknown aetiology (e.g. MS, motor neurone disease)
- Creutzfeld–Jacob disease
- Any high-risk factor for HIV (defined by DoH as: homosexual men, prostitutes, history of IV drug abuse, haemophiliacs, people who have had sexual relations with local people from Africa south of the Sahara since 1977, sexual partners of people in these groups)

Donor cards and the NHS Organ Donor Register: Potential donors should always discuss their wishes with their relatives. They can register their desire to donate their organs after death by adding their names to the NHS Organ Donor Register and/or obtaining an organ donor card. Contact the NHS Organ Donor Line ☎0845 60 60 400 or sign up on-line at 🖳 www.uktransplant.org.uk

Live donation: Certain tissues can be donated whilst a donor is alive:
- **Blood:** Contact the Blood Transfusion Service ☎0845 7 711 711 🖳 http://www.blood.co.uk (in South, Mid, East, and West Wales ☎0800 25 22 66 🖳 http://www.welshblood.org.uk). New donors age 17–59y. are accepted and donors can continue giving blood until age 70.
- **Bone marrow:** Contact the British Bone Marrow Registry ☎0845 7 711 711 🖳 http://www.blood.co.uk (in South, Mid, East, and West Wales contact the Welsh Bone Marrow Registry ☎0800 371 502 🖳 http://www.welshblood.org.uk). A blood sample is taken on registration to allow tissue matching. Donation involves a small operation in which bone marrow is harvested—usually from iliac crests.
- **1 kidney, part of lung, liver, or SI:** Usually close relatives. Removal of the organ/part-organ involves a major operation for the donor. Risks to donor must be weighed vs. benefits to recipient.

Donation after death: Table 8.3
- **Heart-beating donation:** Donors must be maintained on a life-support machine at the time of death and until the organs are removed. The role of the GP in these situations is pre-emptive (information about organ donor register/donor cards) and to support families in making the decision whether to donate. Organs that can be donated are: kidneys, hearts, livers, lungs, pancreases, corneas, heart valves, bone, and skin.

- ***Non-heart beating donation:*** The most important group for GPs, as donation can occur even if the patient dies in the community. The GP must initiate removal of tissues by contacting the local organ transplant coordinator or the national blood services tissue division ☎07693 086823.
- ***Donation of whole body for medical education:*** Contact HM Inspector of Anatomy (☎020 7972 4342/4551). Relatives should contact the medical school with which the donor has made arrangements after their death. Medical schools arrange collection of the body and a simple funeral. Not all bodies are accepted. The donor *must* give authorization for donation prior to death.
- ***Tissue donation after death for research purposes:*** Can be done in addition to donation for transplantation—organs for transplant are taken first. 🖳 *http://www.bodydonation.org.uk*

Approach to relatives: Many families find the act of donation a source of comfort. Even with a signed donor card, the relatives of the patient must give their consent to organ donation post-mortem.

The Coroner: For any patient normally referred to the Coroner, Coroner's permission must be gained before tissues are removed.

Further information

United Kingdom Transplant 🖳 *http://www.uktransplant.org.uk*

Table 8.3 Organs suitable for non-heart beating donation

Organ	Criteria for donation	Specific contraindications
Corneas	>1y. old; no upper age limit	Scarring/ulceration of cornea
	May be retrieved up to 24h. after death	Leukaemia/certain lymphomas
		Malignancy otherwise is *not* a contraindication, neither is poor eye sight
Heart valves	3mo.–60y.	Congenital valve defect
	May be retrieved up to 48h. after death	Rheumatic heart disease
		Cardiac arrest/MI and malignancy are *not* contraindications
Skin	16–85y.	Prolonged steroid therapy
	>1.7m tall and >70kg weight	Chronic skin disease e.g. psoriasis
	May be retrieved up to 48h. after death	Malignancy
Bone	≥16y.; no upper age limit	Any history of malignancy
	May be retrieved up to 24h. after death	Osteomyelitis
		Rheumatoid arthritis
		Traumatic bone fractures

Bereavement, grief, and coping with loss

Models of grief

Traditional model: The bereaved person moves through phases until 'recovery':

- *Initial shock:* Sense of unreality, detachment, disbelief, or 'numbness'. Lasts from hours to days.
- *Yearning:* Pangs of grief, episodes of intense pining, and a desire to search interspersed with anxiety, guilt, and self-reproach.
- *Despair:* The permanence of the loss is realized. Despair and apathy, social withdrawal, poor concentration, pessimism about the future.
- *Recovery:* Rebuilding of an identity and purpose in life.

Recent models: Grief represents an oscillation between loss and restoration—focused behaviour, demonstrated by swings in mood, thoughts, and behaviour between memories of the dead person and 'getting on with life'. Avoidance or denial of the loss is common and a part of the process.

Health consequences of bereavement

- ↑ *mortality* (↑ deaths from CHD, cirrhosis, suicide, accidents)— particularly in first 6mo. *Risk factors:* ♂>♀, age <65y., lower social class.
- *Mental health problems:* Depression, anxiety, ↑ risk of suicide, substance abuse, identification reaction (hyperchondriacal disorder— symptoms mimic those of deceased e.g. chest pain if died from MI), insomnia, self-neglect.
- *Physical problems:* Fatigue, aches and pains (e.g headaches, musculo-skeletal pain), appetite change, GI symptoms, ↓ immune response (↑ minor infection).
- *Others:* Interference with family life, education, and employment, social isolation/loneliness, ↓ income.

Role of the primary care team: Develop a practice policy for dealing with bereaved patients. Flag notes. Consider staff training and active follow-up of bereaved patients. If the person who has died is registered with the practice, ensure all medical referrals/appointments are cancelled.

Bereaved children: Children understand what death is by 8y. and even children of 2–3y. have some understanding of death. Exclusion makes children isolated and often makes the death of someone they have known more, not less, painful. Prepare children for a death, if possible, and give them a chance to have their questions answered. If a child has problems, seek specialist help.

Benefits for widows/widowers: p.101

Abnormal grief reactions: Whether a grief reaction is normal or abnormal depends on individual circumstances—personality, situation surrounding death, and cultural expectations. Recognized patterns of abnormal grief are:

• Inhibited grief—grief is absent or minimal
• Delayed grief—late onset *and*
• Prolonged or chronic grief—inability to rebuild life in any way

If abnormal grief is suspected:

• Monitor carefully
• Consider referral for bereavement counseling e.g. to CRUSE
• Consider clinical depression (📖 p.968) or post-traumatic stress disorder (📖 p.963)
• If symptoms are persistent or worsening despite treatment, or if there is suicidal risk, refer to psychiatry for specialist advice

---

Risk factors for poor outcome after bereavement

Predisposing factors
• Multiple prior bereavements
• History of mental illness (e.g. depression, anxiety, suicidal attempts or threats)
• Ambivalent or dependent relationship with the deceased
• Low self-esteem
• Being male
• Poor social or family support

Situations where the circumstances of death may cause particular problems for the bereaved
• Sudden or unexpected death
• Death of parent when child or adolescent
• Multiple deaths (e.g. disasters)
• Miscarriage, death of baby, child, or sibling
• Cohabiting partners, same sex partners, extra-marital relationship
• Death due to aids, suicide
• Deaths where those bereaved may be responsible
• Deaths from murder, high media profile, or involving legal proceedings
• Where a post-mortem and/or inquest is required

Useful contacts

CRUSE ☎0870 167 1677 🖥 http://www.crusebereavementcare.org.uk
Royal College of Psychiatrists information leaflet. Available at 🖥 http://www.rcpsych.ac.uk
National Association of Widows ☎024 7663 4848 🖥 http://www.widows.uk.net

Breaking bad news

It is never easy to break bad news. GPs do it frequently.

Why is breaking bad news hard?

- *Admission of failure:* When we tell patients bad news, it is often an admission that we have failed. When we fail, we naturally question what we have done and, when looking at our practice in retrospect, it is easy to find fault. Feelings of guilt are common.
- *Fear of the reaction of the patient:* We all have a desire to avoid unpleasantness but sharing information with patients may be a positive way forwards. Even if news is bad, it gives the patient control of the situation.

Guidelines for sharing bad news with a patient

DO

- Plan the consultation as far as possible. Check the facts first and ensure you have all the information. Ensure privacy and freedom from interruption.
- Set aside enough time.
- Ask if the patient would like a relative or friend with them. Make sure you introduce yourself and find out their name and relationship to the patient.
- Make eye contact—watch for non-verbal messages. Sit at the same level as the patient.
- Use simple and straightforward language.
- Allow silence, tears, or anger.
- Be prepared to go over facts again.
- Answer questions.
- Reflect on what the patient or relative have said to allow you to modify your understanding of their feelings.
- Take into account the patient's current health e.g. if in pain, then sort out the pain and schedule a further discussion when the patient is more comfortable.
- Offer ongoing support

DON'T

- Lie or fudge the issue.
- Get your facts wrong.
- Break bad news in public.
- Give the impression of being rushed or distant.
- Give too much information. It is better to be concise—the finer points can be filled in later.
- Interrupt or argue.
- Say that 'nothing can be done'—there is always something that can be done.
- Meet anger with anger.
- Say, you 'know how they feel'—you don't.
- Be frightened to admit you don't know something.
- Use medical jargon
- Leave the patient with no follow-on contact.
- Agree to withhold information from the patient.

Common problems

- *What if the relatives don't want you to tell the patient?* With adults of sound mind, information is confidential to the patient and can only be released, even to close relatives, with the patient's permission. Relatives who say they don't want the patient to know often do so to protect their relative. It is important to recognize that they know your patient best. First, explore their worries and point out the difficulties of the patient not knowing. Often, once a relative realizes that the patient knows things are not right and needs help and support to face the situation, they come round to the patient being told. Stress that you will not lie to a patient if asked a direct question.

- *How do you know if the patient wants to know?* Most people (80–90%) *do* want to know. Assume this is the case and then feel your way carefully. Give the patient ample opportunity to say they don't want to know.

- *How do you respond to questions you cannot answer?* The best way to deal with this is to say you don't have all the answers but will answer when you can, find out what you can, and say when you don't know.

Assault and accidents

Domestic violence: 📖 p.220

Victims of crime or accidents: Victims need treatment of injuries and emotional support. Record information carefully, as it may be needed for legal cases. Note the date, time, and place of the event. Record injuries in detail (physical and psychological)—including measuring the size of lacerations and bruises. Arrange for photos to be taken (police may arrange this). Encourage reporting of the incident to the police (the patient will not be eligible for criminal injury compensation if it is not reported). Give patient details of local victim support groups. If the patient's safety is an issue, contact the duty social worker for a place of safety.

Rape and indecent assault: If a patient reports rape or indecent assault and is willing to report the matter to the police, do not examine her/him. The case against the assailant could be won or lost on the basis of evidence gained by examination of an alleged victim, so it is best done by a doctor trained and experienced in such work.

If the patient will not report the matter to the police, take a full history and note LMP, contraception, sexual history. Make a note of any injuries and take photographs, if possible and appropriate. Do not insist on examination if the patient is unwilling. Ensure a chaperone is present if any examination is attempted. Discuss the need for emergency contraception, prophylactic antibiotics (e.g. ciprofloxacin 250mg po stat), blood tests at 3mo. to exclude transmission of syphilis and 3–6mo. for exclusion of seroconversion for HIV.

If at high risk for HIV transmission, refer to A&E for consideration of prophylaxis (📖 p.499). Discuss the need for counselling and inform the patient about the victim support scheme and rape crisis centres. Arrange follow-up in 2–3wk.

Criminal injuries compensation: For victims of violent crimes—even if the attacker is not identified. Compensation is paid for the injury, loss of earnings, and expenses. Claim by contacting the Criminal Injuries Compensation Authority, Tay House, 300, Bath Street, Glasgow G2 4LN ☎0800 358 3601 🖥 *http://www.cica.gov.uk*

Post-traumatic stress disorder (PTSD): 23% assault victims and 80% rape victims develop PTSD. ♀:♂ ≈ 2:1. Defined as significant symptoms 1mo. after the event i.e. flashbacks, nightmares, survivor guilt, mood changes, detachment, poor concentration, insomnia, anxiety, and depression. Alcohol abuse and work and relationship problems are common. Symptoms may last years. See 📖 p.963.

Accident prevention: 📖 p.162

Child abuse: 📖 p.886

Elder abuse: 📖 p.221

Further information

Victim Support Treating victims of crime: *Guidelines for health professionals.* (National office: Cranmer House, 39 Brixton road, London SW9 6DZ. ☎020 7735 9166 🖳 http://www.victimsupport.org)

Patient information and support

Victim support: ☎0845 3030 900; 🖳 http://www.victimsupport.org
Rape Crisis UK and Ireland: 🖳 http://www.rapecrisis.org.uk
Survivors UK: Provides resources for men who have experienced any form of sexual violence ☎0845 122 1201 🖳 http://www.survivorsuk.org.uk

Domestic violence

Used to describe physical, emotional, and mental abuse of women by male partners. Affects ~1:4 women—the most common form of interpersonal crime. 60%—current partner; 21%—former partners. ½ suffer >1 attack; $\frac{1}{3}$ have been attacked repeatedly.

General practice is often the first place in which women seek formal help but only ¼ actually reveal they have been beaten. Without appropriate intervention, violence continues and often ↑ in frequency and severity. By the time the woman's injuries are visible, violence may be a long-established pattern. On average, a woman will be assaulted 35 times before reporting it to police.

Effects: High incidence of psychiatric disorders, particularly depression, and self-damaging behaviours including drug and alcohol abuse, suicide, and parasuicide.

Factors preventing the woman leaving the abusive situation: Loss of self-esteem makes women think they are to blame; fear of partner; disruption of the family and her children's relationship with their father; loss of intimate relationship with partner; fall in income; risk of homelessness; fear of the unknown.

Guidelines for care

- Consider the possibility of domestic violence—ask directly.
- Emphasize confidentiality.
- Document—accurate, clear documentation, over time at successive consultations, may provide cumulative evidence of abuse and is essential for use as evidence in court, should the need arise.
- Assess the present situation—gather as much information as possible.
- Provide information and offer help in making contact with other agencies.
- Devise a safety plan—give the phone number of local women's refuge; advise to keep some money and important financial and legal documents hidden in a safe place in case of emergency; help plan an escape route in case of emergency.

Do not pressurize women into any course of action. If the patient decides to return to the violent situation, she will not forget the information and support given. In time, this might give her the confidence and back up she needs to break out of her situation.

⚠ If children are likely to be at risk you have a duty to inform social services or police, preferably with the patient's consent (📖 p.885).

Assaults and accidents: 📖 p.218
Child abuse: 📖 p.886

Elder abuse: Defined as: 'A single or repeated act or lack of appropriate action, occurring within any relationship where there is an expectation of trust, which causes harm or distress to an older person'.

Older people may report the abuse, but often do not. May take several forms which may co-exist:

- *Physical* e.g. cuts, bruises, unexplained fractures, dehydration/malnourishment with no medical explanation, burns
- *Psychological* e.g. unusual behaviour, unexplained fear, appears helpless or withdrawn
- *Financial* e.g. removal of funds by carers, new will in favour of carer
- *Sexual* e.g. unexplained bruising, vaginal or anal bleeding, genital infections
- *Neglect* e.g. malnourished, dehydrated, poor personal hygiene, late requests for medical attention

Prevalence (in own home): physical abuse—2%; verbal abuse—5%; financial abuse—2%.

Signs: Inconsistent story from patient and carer, inconsistencies on examination; fear in presence of carer; frequent attendance at A&E; frequent requests for GP visits; carer avoiding GP.

Management: Talk through the situation with the patient, carer, and other services involved in care. Assess the level of risk. Consider admission to a place of safety—contact social services and/or police as necessary; seek advice from Action on Elder Abuse.

Further information

Department of Health. *Domestic violence: a resource manual for health care professionals.* Available from ▣ http://www.dh.gov.uk
Home Office: ▣ http://www.homeoffice.gov.uk/crime/domesticviolence
RCGP. *Domestic violence.* ▣ http://www.rcgp.org.uk
Ramsay J. et al. (2000) *Should health professionals screen women for domestic violence? Systematic review.* BMJ 325; 314

Useful contacts

Womens' Aid: ☎0808 2000 247 ▣ http://www.womensaid.org.uk
Action on Elder Abuse ☎0808 808 8141 ▣ http://www.elderabuse.org.uk
Police domestic violence units ☎0845 045 45 45
Local authority social services departments
Local authority housing departments

Social factors in general practice

'The task of medicine is to promote health, to prevent disease and to treat the sick … These are highly social functions'
H.E. Sigrist, *Civilization and Disease*, 1943

Deprivation: Social deprivation is linearly associated with death from all causes, with no threshold and no upper limit. The most pronounced effect is with circulatory and other smoking-related disease. A similar trend is seen with infant mortality, morbidity from chronic illness (particularly musculoskeletal, cardio-vascular, and respiratory conditions) and teenage pregnancy.

This is not a new problem, nor one unique to the UK. Suggestions it is due to smoking and eating habits may be partly correct, but this disparity was in evidence 80y. ago when those of social classes I and II were more likely to smoke, eat foods high in saturated fats, and take less exercise. Disparity in health is closely related to income. In the UK an ↑ proportion of the population is now living on <50% of average income than 20y. ago—the mortality gap has grown proportionately.

Impact on general practice: Higher incidence of illness → ↑ requirement for primary care team services and ↑ use of out-of-hours and A&E services amongst deprived communities. This is recognized in the UK in the Carr–Hill Index which allocates funds to practices (📖 p.38).

Homelessness

Bed and breakfast accommodation: Adverse effects of living in temporary bed and breakfast accommodation are well documented:
- Adults have an ↑ incidence of depression than people of similar social standing in their own homes;
- Homeless women are 2× as likely to have problems in pregnancy and 3× as likely to require admission in pregnancy;
- ¼ of babies born to women living in bed and breakfast accommodation are of low birth weight (national average <1:10);
- Children from these families are less likely to receive their immunizations, more likely to have childhood accidents, and have higher incidence of minor and diarrhoeal diseases.

Sleeping rough: Poor diet, poor accommodation, and lack of access to medical services are universal problems in this group. A study done in 1986 in London found ⅓ are psychotic; ¼ have severe physical problems; ⅔ have no contact whatsoever with medical services. Evidence shows that if services are provided, homeless people will use them.

Divorce: Divorcees of all ages are at greater risk of premature death (2× ↑ for men aged 35–42y.) than married people—mainly from cardio- and cerebrovascular disease, cancer, suicide, and accidental death. There is also a similar ↑ in morbidity. Children of divorced parents have ↑ risk of ill health from the time of separation until adult life, with children <5y. old when their parents separate being particularly vulnerable. They are also more prone to psychiatric illness later in life and are more likely to become divorced themselves.

Employment and unemployment: Effects of work have been compared to effects of vitamins—we need a certain amount to be healthy; then there is a plateau, where extra doesn't help, and too much is harmful. There is good evidence that unemployment causes both ↑ mortality (from coronary vascular disease, cancers, suicide, violence, and accidents) and ↑ morbidity (depression, IHD). Threat of unemployment alone can cause morbidity—in 1 study GP consultation rates rose by 20% and referral rates by 60% after it was announced a factory would close. Increases were found in other family members too.

Refugees and asylum seekers: The Geneva Convention defines a refugee as any person who 'owing to well-founded fear of being persecuted for reasons of race, religion, nationality, membership of a particular social group or political opinion, is outside the country of his nationality and is unable or, owing to such fear, is unwilling to return it.' Refugees are entitled to free healthcare in the UK. Consider:

- *Cultural and religious issues*—📖 p.225.
- *Physical needs*—Health needs are diverse, depending on country of origin and previous level of healthcare. Always consider infectious diseases e.g. hepatitis B, HIV, TB, and malaria. Ensure refugees claim all health-related benefits available to them e.g. free prescriptions.
- *Psychological needs*—Depression, anxiety, panic attacks, agoraphobia, and poor sleep are common. Symptoms are often reactions to past experiences and current situation. Social isolation, hostility, and racism compound them. Use medication, if appropriate, but also address other issues.

⚠ Although telling their story is helpful for some refugees—'active forgetting' is the way people cope with their difficulties in some cultures.

- *Victims of torture*—May present with many non-specific health problems. Some are the result of physical trauma; most are of mixed physical and psychological origin. Considerable time and patience is needed to manage them, but it is worth it. Advice and support is available from the Medical Foundation for the Care of Victims of Torture (🖥 www.torturecare.org.uk).
- *Family*—Many will have left other family members behind. They may not know their whereabouts, or even if they are alive or dead. The Red Cross or Red Crescent can help with tracing (🖥 www.redcross.org.uk).

Useful contacts

Shelter advice for homeless people ☎0808 800 4444 🖥 http://www.shelter.org.uk
RELATE relationship counselling ☎0845 1 30 40 16 (cost of telephone counselling—£45/h. in Summer 2004) 🖥 http://www.relate.org.uk
Couple Counselling Scotland ☎01382 640340 (Thursday 2–4 p.m.) 🖥 http://www.couplecounselling.org
The Refugee Council 🖥 http://www.refugeecouncil.org.uk
Asylum Aid ☎0207 247 8741 🖥 http://www.asylumaid.org.uk

Multicultural medicine

Britain is a multicultural and multifaith society. It is important that providers of care take into account cultural and spiritual needs.

⚠ Table 8.4 is a rough guide to religious differences which affect health care. It is forcibly brief and cannot address all the many variations. Everyone is an individual, and there is a real danger of 'pigeon-holing' patients by religion or ethnic background and making incorrect assumptions as a result. Always ask patients/family about their own preferences.

Communication: Effective communication is essential.

Do not assume English proficiency: It is important to ascertain that you understand the patient and that the patient understands you.
- Ask the patient to let you know if s/he doesn't understand. Consider using an interpreter (see below).
- Speak clearly and slowly and repeat important information. Avoid jargon, confusing phrases, double negatives, and rhetorical questions.
- Ask patients to tell you what you have said, to check comprehension.
- Be wary of sounding condescending—English skills are not a reflection of a hearing disorder or level of intelligence.

Respect beliefs and attitudes: People have different reactions towards illness, life, and death. Ask patients to provide you with information about their own ideas e.g for newly arrived immigrants, ask: 'Could you tell me what would happen to you if you were in your country?'

Using interpreters: Interpreters are an important resource in providing a voice for patients whose proficiency in English is poor or insufficient for the situation. In general, anyone who has been in an English-speaking country for <2y. will need an interpreter. Sometimes a friend or another family member can be used, but if sensitive issues have to be discussed or it is essential that the information is translated accurately, use a professional. *General tips:*
- Anticipate an interpreter will be needed where possible and pre-book someone of the same gender who speaks the same language/dialect and will be ethnically acceptable to the patient.
- Explain that the interpreter is bound to maintain confidentiality.
- Face and speak in the first person directly to the patient, not the interpreter. Interpreters are solely there to convey information in a language both patient and doctor can understand—not to analyse information, or decide what should or should not be conveyed.

Useful contacts

Ethnologue language guide 🖳 *http://www.ethnologue.com/country_index.asp*
Interpreter services (fees payable): Language line ☎0800 169 2879;
National Interpreting Service ☎0800 169 5996
Babel Tree Project—Health information in 123 languages 🖳 *http://www.adec.org.au/babeltree*
NHS—Direct multilingual health information and advice ☎0845 4647 🖳 *www.nhsdirect.nhs.uk*

Table 8.4 Religious differences important in healthcare

Religion	Dietary restrictions	Fasting	Transfusion/transplant	Family planning	Death
Buddhist	Mainly vegetarian	N/A	No objections	No objections; abortion not allowed	Cremation preferred; no objections to PM
Christian	None	N/A	No objections	Some approve of natural methods only	Burial or cremation; no objections to PM
Hindu	Most do not eat beef; Some are strict vegetarians.	Fasting involves limiting type of foods	No objections	No objections	Strong preference to die at home. The body should not be touched by non-Hindus. All adults are cremated. No PMs unless legally required.
Muslim	No pork. Other meat must have been killed in a special manner (Halal). Alcohol is prohibited.	Fasting sunrise → sunset during Ramadan	Strict Muslims may not consent to transplant	Variable—strict Muslims do not approve	The body should not be touched by non-Muslims. All Muslims are buried. No PMs unless legally required.
Jehovah's witness	No foods containing blood or blood products. No alcohol	N/A	No blood transfusion or organ transplant. Dialysis is usually permitted	No objections	Burial or cremation. No objections to PM
Jewish	No pork, rabbit or shellfish. Meat prepared in Kosher fashion. Liberal Jews may not adhere to dietary restrictions.	Orthodox Jews may fast for Yom Kippur	No objections	Some Orthodox Jews prohibit contraception. Most Jewish boys are circumcised 8d. after birth	Burial is preferred. No PMs unless legally required.
Sikh	No beef. Most are vegetarian. Alcohol is forbidden.	N/A	No objections	Allowed but not openly discussed	Children and adults are cremated.

Diet

The role of the GP and primary care team
- *Screening*—identification of obese patients and patients in need of dietary advice for other reasons.
- *Assessment*—motivation to change and barriers to change.
- *Discussion and negotiation*—exploration of knowledge about diet; negotiation of goals.
- *Goal setting*—2–3 food-specific goals on each occasion. Set a series of mini targets which make them appear more realistic and achievable.
- *Monitoring progress.*

General foods to avoid or decrease
- Fatty meat products (sausages, salami, meat pies)
- ≥140grams/d. (~12–14 portions/wk.) of processed and red meat (beef, lamb, pork)
- High-fat dairy products—full-cream milk, butter, full-fat cheese
- Full-fat spreads
- Crisps
- Cakes and biscuits
- Salted peanuts
- Canned and other pre-prepared food high in salt and sugar

The ideal diet: See Figure 8.1, 📖 p.228
- *Eat a variety of foods* and the right amount to maintain a healthy weight (Figure 8.2, 📖 p.229).
- *Use starchy foods* (e.g. bread, rice, pasta, potatoes) as the main energy source and plenty of fruit and vegetables (>5 pieces of fruit/portions of vegetables/d.). Don't overcook vegetables (steaming is preferable to boiling) and keep the delay between cutting fruit and vegetables to eating them to a minimum.
- *Eat plenty of fibre*—good sources are: high-fibre breakfast cereals, pulses, beans, wholemeal bread, potatoes (with skins), pasta, rice, oats.
- *Eat oily fish* (e.g. mackerel, herring, pilchards, salmon) at least 1–2x/wk. and cut down on cooked red or processed meat; consider substituting meat with vegetable protein (e.g. pulses, soya).
- *Choose lean meat*—remove excess fat/poultry skin and pour off fat after cooking; boil, steam, or bake foods in preference to frying; when cooking with fat, use unsaturated oil (e.g. olive, sunflower), and use cornflour rather than butter and flour to make sauces.
- *Use skimmed milks*—low-fat yoghurts/spreads/cheese (e.g. Edam or cottage cheese).
- *Avoid adding salt or sugar* to foods and cut down on sweets, biscuits, and sticky deserts.
- *Drink at least 4–6 pints (2–3l) of fluid* (preferably not tea, coffee, or alcohol) each day and avoid excessive alcohol intake (<21u/wk. for men and <14u/wk. for women—📖 p.236).

Malnutrition: 50% of women and 25% of men aged >85y. are unable to cook a meal alone. Malnutrition is not only a disease of the 3rd world, it is common amongst the elderly in the UK.

Poor nutritional status: Slows rate of wound healing, ↑ risk of infection, ↓ muscle strength, is detrimental to mental well-being, and ↓ the ability of elderly people to remain independent.

Risk factors
- Low income
- Living alone
- Mental health problems (e.g. depression)
- Dementia
- Recent bereavement
- Gastric surgery
- Malabsorption
- ↑ metabolism
- Difficulty eating and/or swallowing (stroke, neurological disorder, MND)
- Presence of chronic disease (e.g. Crohn's disease, UC, IBS, cancer, COPD, CCF)

Management
- *General nutritional advice:* Encourage to eat more and ↑ consumption of fruit and vegetables; consider using nutritional, vitamin and mineral supplements (e.g. vitamin D supplements for the housebound and institutionalized);
- *Inability to prepare meals/shop:* Consider referral to social services; Meals on Wheels; community dietician; community day centre; local voluntary support organization.
- *Difficulty with utensils:* Consider aids/equipment (cutlery, non-slip mats).
- *Nausea:* Consider antiemetics.
- *Difficulty with swallowing:* Investigate the cause. If none found or unable to resolve the problem, consider pureed food and/or thickened fluids.

Useful information
The Scientific Advisory Committee on Nutrition (SACN): 🖳 *http://www.sacn.gov.uk*
The British Nutrition Foundation: 🖳 *http://www.nutrition.org.uk*

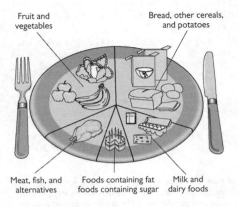

Fruit and vegetables

Bread, other cereals, and potatoes

Meat, fish, and alternatives

Foods containing fat foods containing sugar

Milk and dairy foods

Figure 8.1 The plate model. Developed nationally to communicate current recommendations for healthy eating. It shows rough proportions of the various food groups that should make up each meal

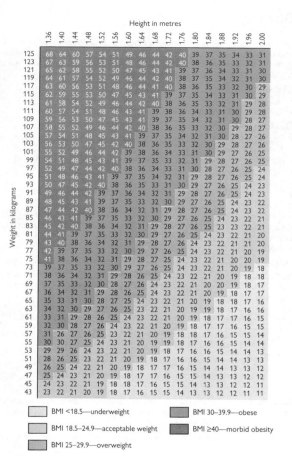

Figure 8.2 BMI ready reckoner

Obesity

Obesity is one of the most important preventable diseases in the UK. The best measure of obesity is body mass index (BMI). Recent evidence shows it is increasing and is set to take over from smoking as the number one preventable cause of disease in the UK.

Classification: BMI (weight in kg ÷ (height in m)^2):
- 18.5–24.9 = normal
- 25–29.9 = overweight
- 30–39.9 = obese
- >40 = morbid obesity

Health risks of obesity
- Death (BMI >30 carries 3x ↑ risk of mortality)
- IHD
- Hypercholesterolaemia
- ↑ BP
- Cerebrovascular disease
- Type 2 DM
- Gallbladder disease
- Complications after surgery
- Sleep apnoea
- Psychological problems
- Cancer of cervix, uterus, ovary, and breast
- Musculoskeletal problems and arthritis
- Ovulatory failure
- Menstrual irregularities
- PCOS
- Complications in pregnancy (gestational DM, ↑ BP, pre-eclampsia), labour, and delivery
- Stress incontinence

Waist circumference: An alternative indirect measurement of body fat that reflects the intra-abdominal fat mass. Strongly correlated with CHD risk, DM, hyperlipidaemia, and ↑ BP. Measured halfway between the superior iliac crest and the rib cage in the mid-axillary line.

Table 8.5 Association of waist circumference with risk of CHD and DM

	Waist circumference ↑ risk of CHD, DM	Substantial risk of CHD, DM
♂	≥94cm (37inches)	≥102cm (40inches)
♀	≥80cm (32inches)	≥88cm (35inches)

Risk factors: Genetic predisposition (accounts for about $\frac{1}{3}$ obesity); previous obesity and successful dieting; physical inactivity; low education; smoking cessation; female gender.

Prevention: Begins in childhood by instilling healthy patterns of exercise and diet.

❶ There is little evidence to show that dietary advice by GPs or practice nurses is heeded. Most influence on diet comes from national food policy, price of food, advertising, general education, and culture.

Treatment: When the body's intake > output over a period of time, obesity results. Management of obesity aims to reverse this trend on a long-term basis:
- ↓ *calorie diets:* All obese people lose weight on a low-energy intake. A realistic goal is weight loss of 1–2lbs (0.5–1kg)/wk. and is achievable

using diets of 1000–1500kcal/d. intake. Rates of weight loss >1kg/wk. involve loss of lean tissue rather than fat. Aim for BMI of 25. There is no health benefit of weight ↓ below this. Weight loss in the first few weeks may be higher due to water and glycogen depletion. If simple diet sheets are not effective, refer to a dietician.

- **Very low-calorie diets** (<800kcal/day): Only limited place in management as this pattern of eating cannot be maintained and rebound weight gain is seen on stopping. Only use to treat morbid obesity under strict supervision.
- **Healthy diet:** ↓ fat intake; ↑ proportion of unrefined carbohydrate; eat 5 portions of fruit and vegetables/d.; ↓ hidden sugars (alcohol, prepared foods); ↑ fibre—📖 p.226 and 228.
- **Exercise:** Regular aerobic exercise helps ↓ weight and improve health. Tailor advice to the individual and local facilities—📖 p.232.
- **Drug therapy** (BNF 4.5): Drugs specifically licensed for the treatment of obesity are orlistat (120mg tds with food) and sibutramine (10–15mg od—monitor BP and pulse rate closely). Consider if BMI >30kg/m^2 or >27kg/m^2 in the presence of co-morbidity e.g. DM. There is little evidence to guide selection but it is logical to choose orlistat for those who have a high intake of fats and sibutramine for those who cannot control their eating. Combination therapy involving >1 anti-obesity drug is contraindicated. NICE has published guidelines on administration—summarized in the BNF.
- **Group therapy:** Group activities e.g. Weight Watchers, seem to have a higher success rate in producing and maintaining weight loss.
- **Behavioural therapy:** Shown to be effective individually and in groups when combined with low-calorie diets. In simplest form, involves advice to avoid situations that tempt overeating.
- **Surgery:** Only consider referral as a last resort if behavioural and dietary modification have failed and BMI >40. Gastroplasty is the most common procedure. Mortality is high.
- **Follow-up** on a regular basis is essential to maintain motivation.

Maintenance of weight loss: Once a patient has lost weight, diet still needs to be monitored. On-going follow-up has been shown to help sustain weight loss. Weight fluctuation (yo-yo dieting) may be harmful.

Essential reading

National Audit Office *Tackling obesity in England* (2001) 🖥 http://www.nao.org.uk

NICE 🖥 http://www.nice.org.uk
- Guidance on the use of sibutramine for the treatment of obesity in adults (2001)
- Orlistat for treatment of obesity in adults (2001)

National Obesity Forum 🖥 http://www.nationalobesityforum.org.uk
- Guidelines on the management of adult obesity and overweight in primary care (2002)
- An approach to weight management in children and adolescents (2–18years) in primary care (2003)

SIGN *Management of obesity in children and young people* (2003) 🖥 http://www.sign.ac.uk

Exercise

'Lack of physical activity is a major underlying cause of death, disease and disability. Preliminary data from a WHO study on risk factors suggest that a sedentary lifestyle is one of the 10 leading global causes of death and disability. More than 2 million deaths each year are attributable to physical inactivity.'

WHO, *Move for Health*, 2002

In the UK, 60% of men and 70% of women are not active enough to benefit their health.

Recommended amounts of activity (DoH)
- *Adults:* ≥30mins. moderate intensity exercise across the day on ≥5d./wk.
- *Children:* ≥1h. moderate intensity exercise across the day every day.

Dimensions of exercise
- **Volume or quantity**—quantity of activity usually expressed as kcal per day or week. Can also be expressed as MET hours per day or week, where 1 MET = resting metabolic rate.
- **Frequency**—number of sessions per day or week.
- **Intensity**—light, moderate, or vigorous. Light intensity = <4 METS (e.g. strolling); moderate = 4–6 METS (e.g. brisk walking); vigorous = 7+ METS (e.g. running).
- **Duration**—time spent on a single bout of activity.
- **Type or mode** e.g. brisk walking, dancing, or weight training.

Exercise is beneficial: Regular physical activity—
- ↓ **risk of:**
  - CHD—physically inactive people have ~2x ↑ risk of CHD and ~3x ↑ risk of stroke[S].
  - DM—through ↑ insulin sensitivity[S].
  - Obesity[S]—📖 p.230.
  - Osteoporosis—↓ risk of hip fractures by ½ [S].
  - Cancer—↓ risk of colon cancer ~ 40%. There is also evidence of a link between exercise and ↓ risk of breast and prostate cancers[S].
- **Is a useful treatment for:**
  - ↑ BP—can result in 10mmHg drop of systolic and diastolic BP; can also delay onset of hypertension[S].
  - Hypercholesterolaemia—↑ HDL, ↓ LDL[C].
  - Post-MI[C]—📖 p.332
  - DM—improves insulin sensitivity and favourably affects other risk factors for DM including obesity, HDL/LDL ratio, and ↑BP.
  - HIV—↑ cardiopulmonary fitness and psychological well-being[C].
  - Arthritis and back pain—maintains function[C].
  - ↓ intensity of depression; ↓ anxiety[S].
- **Benefits the elderly:**
  - Maintains functional capacity.
  - ↓ levels of disability.
  - ↓ risk of falls and hip fracture.
  - Improves quality of sleep[C].

Effective interventions

- *Healthcare*—↑ physical activity for 1° and 2° prevention is effective in the short term; no evidence effects are maintained long-term. Counselling for physical activity is as effective as more structured exercise sessions.
- *Workplace*—interventions to ↑ rates of walking to work are effective.
- *Schools*—appropriately designed and delivered PE curricula can enhance physical activity levels. A whole school approach to physical activity promotion is effective.
- *Transport*—well-designed interventions ↑ walking and cycling to work.
- *Communities*—community-wide approaches to physical activity promotion → ↑ activity.

Negotiating change: It is possible to encourage people to ↑ activity levels. As with all lifestyle interventions, the patient must want to change.
- If exercise levels are satisfactory, congratulate and inform about the benefits of exercise.
- If levels are unsatisfactory, explain the benefits of a higher level of physical activity and support with health education leaflets.
- Once the patient has agreed, advise and agree ways to do that.

You are more likely to be successful if:
- Exercise recommended is moderate, does not require attendance at a special facility, and can be incorporated into daily life routines e.g. walking/cycling to work.
- You suggest a graduated programme of exercise for sedentary patients (there is an ↑ risk of sudden cardiac death associated with sudden vigorous exercise).

Exercise schemes

- *Specialist rehabilitation schemes* (e.g. cardiac, respiratory) are in operation in many areas. They are usually operated in association with specialist services and incorporate exercise and education for patients with specific conditions e.g. post-MI (📖 p.332).
- *Exercise prescription schemes*—collaboration between community medical services and local sports facilities. They offer low-cost, supervised exercise for patients who might otherwise find it unacceptable to visit a gym, and are accessed by GP 'prescription'.
- *Local sports centres*—many sports facilities also offer special sessions both on dry land and in the swimming pool for pregnant women, the over 50s, and people with disability.

Essential reading

DoH: *National Quality Assurance Framework on Exercise Referral Systems* (2001)
🖳 http://www.dh.gov.uk
NICE: 🖳 http://www.publichealth.nice.org.uk
- Improving physical activity
- Guidance on the preventive aspects of the CHD NSF
- Cancer prevention: a resource to support local action in delivering the Cancer Plan
US Surgeon General *Report on Physical Activity and Health*
🖳 http://www.cdc.gov/nccdphp/sgr/sgr.htm

Smoking

Facts and figures: In the UK, 12 million adults (28% ♂; 26% ♀) smoke cigarettes and a further 3 million smoke pipes or cigars. *Prevalence:* highest aged 20–24y. Government targets aim to ↓ smoking to 26% by 2005 and to ≤24% by 2010; surveys of smokers show 70% want to stop and 30% intend to give up in <1y.—but only ~2%/y. successfully give up permanently.

1% school children are smokers when they enter secondary school; by 15y., 22% are smoking. 82% of smokers start as teenagers. Government targets aim to ↓ smoking amongst children to ≤9% by 2010.

Risks of smoking: Greatest single cause of illness and premature death in the UK. ½ all regular smokers will eventually die as a result of smoking—120,000/y. Tobacco smoking is associated with ↑ risk of:
- Cancers: lung (>90% are smokers), lip, mouth, stomach, colon, bladder (~30% ALL cancer deaths)
- Cardiovascular disease: arteriosclerosis, coronary heart disease, stroke, peripheral vascular disease
- DM
- Chronic lung disease: COPD, recurrent chest infection, exacerbation of asthma
- Dyspepsia and/or gastric ulcers
- Thrombosis (especially if also on the COC pill)
- Osteoporosis
- Problems in pregnancy: PET, IUGR, pre-term delivery, neonatal and late foetal death.

Passive smoking is associated with:
- ↑ risk CHD and lung cancer (↑ by 25%)
- ↑ risk of cot death, bronchitis, and otitis media in children.

Nicotine withdrawal symptoms
- Urges to smoke (70%)
- ↑ appetite (70%—average 3–4kg weight gain)
- Depression (60%)
- Restlessness (60%)
- Poor concentration (60%)
- Irritability/aggression (50%)
- Night-time awakenings (25%)
- Light headedness (usually 1st few days after quitting—10%)

Helping people to stop smoking: Advice from a GP about smoking cessation results in 2% of smokers stopping; 5% if advice is repeated[CE].

Aids to smoking cessation: BNF 4.10

⚠ Prescribe *only* for smokers who commit to target stop date. Initially, prescribe only enough to last 2wk. after the target stop date i.e. 2wk. nicotine replacement therapy or 3–4wk. bupropion. Only offer a 2nd prescription if the smoker demonstrates continuing commitment to stop smoking.
❶ If unsuccessful, the NHS will not fund another attempt for ≥6mo.

Nicotine replacement therapy (NRT): ↑ the chance of stopping ~1½ x[N]. All preparations are equally effective[C] and available on NHS prescription. Start with higher doses for patients highly dependent. Continue treatment for 3mo., tailing off dose gradually over 2wk. before stopping (except gum which can be stopped abruptly). Several preparations are now licensed for use in pregnancy if unable to stop without NRT. Contraindicated immediately post MI, stroke, or TIA, and for patients with arrythmia.

Bupropion (Zyban™): Smokers (>18y.) start taking the tablets 1–2wk. before their intended quit day (150mg od for 3d. then 150mg bd for 7–9wk.). ↑ cessation rate >2x.[N] *Contraindications:* epilepsy or ↑ risk of seizures, eating disorder, bipolar disorder, pregnancy/breast-feeding.

Alternative therapies: Some evidence hypnotherapy (📖 p.154) is helpful in some cases[S].

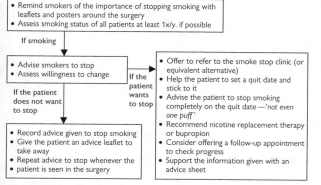

- Remind smokers of the importance of stopping smoking with leaflets and posters around the surgery
- Assess smoking status of all patients at least 1x/y. if possible

If smoking

- Advise smokers to stop
- Assess willingness to change

If the patient does not want to stop

If the patient wants to stop

- Offer to refer to the smoke stop clinic (or equivalent alternative)
- Help the patient to set a quit date and stick to it
- Advise the patient to stop smoking completely on the quit date—'not even one puff'
- Recommend nicotine replacement therapy or bupropion
- Consider offering a follow-up appointment to check progress
- Support the information given with an advice sheet

- Record advice given to stop smoking
- Give the patient an advice leaflet to take away
- Repeat advice to stop whenever the patient is seen in the surgery

Figure 8.3 Management plan for smokers attending the surgery

Essential information

Clinical evidence: Cardiovascular disorders: changing behaviour; smoking cessation
🖳 http://www.nelh.nhs.uk
NICE: (2002) *Nicotine replacement therapy and bupropion for smoking cessation*
🖳 http://www.nice.org.uk
Cochrane: Silagy C. et al. (2004) *Nicotine replacement for smoking cessation*
🖳 http://www.nelh.nhs.uk

Useful contacts

Action on Smoking and Health (ASH) ☎020 7739 5902 🖳 http://www.ash.org.uk
NHS: Smoking helpline ☎0800 169 0 169; pregnancy smoking helpline: ☎0800 169 9 169
🖳 http://www.givingupsmoking.co.uk
Quit: Helpline ☎0800 00 22 00 🖳 http://www.quit.org.uk

Alcohol

Assessing drinking
Suspicious signs/symptoms: ↑ and uncontrolled BP; excess weight; recurrent injuries/accidents; non-specific GI complaints; back pain; poor sleep; tired all the time.

Ask: Assess amount, time of day, socially or alone, daily or in binges, blackouts, situations associated with heavy drinking. Consider using the CAGE questionnaire to assess dependence:
- Have you ever felt you should **C**ut down on your drinking?
- Have people **A**nnoyed you by criticizing your drinking?
- Have you ever felt bad or **G**uilty about your drinking?
- Have you ever had a drink first thing in the morning to steady your nerves or to get rid of a hang over (**E**ye opener)?

Risk factors
- Previous history
- Family history
- Poor social support
- Work absenteeism
- Emotional and/or family problems
- Financial and legal problems
- Drug problems
- Alcohol associated with work e.g. publican

Examination: Smell of alcohol, tremor, sweating, slurring of speech, BP (↑ BP), signs of liver damage.

Investigations: FBC (↑ MCV); LFTs (↑ GGT identifies ~25% of heavy drinkers in general practice; ↑ AST; ↑ bilirubin). Often incidental findings.

Health risk: Continuum—individual risk depends on other factors too (e.g. smoking, heart disease, pregnancy). Recommended safe levels of alcohol consumption are <21u/wk. for men and <14u./wk. for women.

Table 8.6 Health risks associated with levels of alcohol consumption

Health risk	Men (units/wk.)	Women (units/wk.)	
Low	<21	<14	1 unit = 8g alcohol = 1/2 pint of beer (if strong beer, can be as much as 1.75 units), small glass of wine/sherry, 1 measure of spirits (spirit measure in Scotland is 1.2 units).
Intermediate	21–50	15–35	
High	>50	>35	1 bottle of 12% wine = 9 units.

Alcohol-associated problems
Death: ~40,000 deaths/y. in the UK are directly caused by alcohol.

Social
- Marriage breakdown
- Absence from work
- Loss of work
- Social isolation
- Poverty
- Loss of shelter/home

Mental health: Anxiety, depression and/or suicidal ideas; dementia and/or Korsakoffs ± Wernicke's encephalopathy (📖 p.625).

Physical

- ↑ BP
- CVA
- Sexual dysfunction
- Brain damage
- Neuropathy
- Myopathy
- Cardiomyopathy
- Infertility
- Gastritis
- Pancreatitis
- DM
- Obesity

- Foetal damage
- Haemopoietic toxicity
- Interactions with other drugs
- Fatty liver
- Hepatitis
- Cirrhosis
- Oesophageal varices ± haemorrhage
- Liver cancer

- Cancer of the mouth, larynx and oesophagus
- Breast cancer
- Nutritional deficiencies
- Back pain
- Poor sleep
- Tiredness
- Injuries due to alcohol-related activity (e.g. fights)

Beneficial effects of alcohol: Moderate consumption (1–3u./d.) ↓ risk of non-haemorrhagic stroke, angina pectoris, and MI.

Management of alcohol abuse: 📖 p.238

Patient advice and support

Drinkline (government-sponsored helpline) ☎0800 917 8282
Alcohol Concern 🖳 http://www.alcoholconcern.org.uk
Alcoholics Anonymous ☎0845 7697555 🖳 http://www.alcoholics-anonymous.org.uk

Management of alcohol abuse

'An alcoholic is someone you don't like who drinks as much as you do'

Dylan Thomas (1914–1953)

Management strategies: Figure 8.4

Patients drinking within acceptable limits: Reaffirm limits.

Non-dependent drinkers: Brief GP intervention results in ~24% reducing their drinking. Provide information about safe amounts of alcohol and harmful effects of exceeding these. If receptive to change, confirm weekly consumption using a drink diary, agree targets to ↓ consumption, and negotiate follow-up.

Alcohol-dependent drinkers: Suffer withdrawal symptoms if they ↓ alcohol consumption (e.g. anxiety, fits, delirium tremens—📖 p.1068).

- If wanting to stop drinking—refer to the community alcohol team; suggest self-help organizations e.g. AA; involve family and friends in support.
- Detoxification in the community usually uses a reducing regimen of chlordiazepoxide over a 1wk. period (20–30mg qds on days 1 and 2; 15mg qds on days 3 and 4; 10mg qds on day 5; 10mg bd on day 6; 10mg od on day 7; then stop).
- Community detoxification is contraindicated for patients with:
  - Confusion or hallucinations
  - History of previously complicated withdrawal e.g. withdrawal seizures or delirium tremens
  - Epilepsy or fits
  - Malnourishment
  - Severe vomiting or diarrhoea
  - ↑ risk of suicide
  - Poor co-operation
  - Failed detoxification at home
  - Uncontrollable withdrawal symptoms
  - Acute physical or psychiatric illness
  - Multiple substance misuse
  - Poor home environment

If ambivalent/unwilling to change: Provide information; reassess and re-inform on each subsequent meeting; support the family.

Delerium tremens: 📖 p.1068

Vitamin B supplements: People with chronic alcohol dependence are frequently deficient in vitamins, especially thiamine—give oral thiamine indefinitely (if severe, 200–300mg/d.; if mild, 10–25mg/d.)[G]. During detoxification in the community, give thiamine 200mg od for 5–7d.

Relapse: Common. Warn patients and encourage them to re-attend. Be supportive and maintain contact (↓ frequency and severity of relapses[G]). Consider drugs to prevent relapse e.g. acamprosate, disulfiram (specialist initiation only).

Alcohol and driving: 📖 p.205

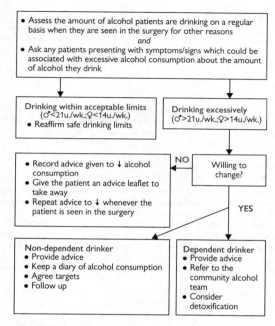

Figure 8.4 Management strategy

Essential reading

(1997) *Addiction and dependence—II: alcohol. BMJ* 315, 358–60
(2000) *Managing the heavy drinker in primary care. DTB* 38(8), 60–64
SIGN (2003) *The management of harmful drinking and alcohol dependence in primary care*
    🖳 *http://www.sign.ac.uk*

Patient advice and support

Drinkline (government-sponsored helpline) ☎0800 917 8282
Alcohol Concern 🖳 *http://www.alcoholconcern.org.uk*
Alcoholics Anonymous ☎0845 7697555 🖳 *http://www.alcoholics-anonymous.org.uk*

Drugs misuse

1:10 adults report using illicit drugs in the last year. Of those presenting for treatment, opioids are the main drugs of abuse (heroin—54%; methadone—13%), but the most frequently abused drugs are cannabis, amphetamine, ecstasy, and cocaine. 3 factors appear important:
• availability of drugs
• vulnerable personality
• social pressures, particularly from peers

Detection: Warning signs suggesting drug misuse:
• *Use of services:* Suspicious requests for drugs of abuse (e.g. no clear medical indication, prescription requests are too frequent).
• *Signs and symptoms:* Inappropriate behaviour; lack of self-care; unexplained nasal discharge; unusually constricted or dilated pupils; evidence of injecting (e.g. marked veins); hepatitis or HIV infection.
• *Social factors:* Family disruption; criminal history.

Assessment: Assess on >1 occasion before deciding how to proceed. Exceptions are severe withdrawal symptoms and/or evidence of an established regime requiring continuation. Points to cover:
• *General information:* Check identification (ask to see an official document); contact with other agencies (including last GP)—check accuracy of report; current residence; family (partner, children); employment; finances; current legal problems; criminal behaviour (past and present).
• *History of drug use:* Current and past usage; knowledge of risks; unsafe sexual practices.
• *Medical and psychiatric history:* Complications of drug abuse (e.g. HIV, hepatitis, accidents); general medical and psychiatric history; overdoses (accidental or deliberate); alcohol abuse.
• *Investigations:* Consider urine toxicology to confirm drug misuse; blood for FBC, LFTs, Hep B, C, and HIV serology (with consent and counselling).

Management: Aims to ↓ risk of infectious diseases; ↓ drug-related deaths, and ↓ criminal activity used to finance drug habits. The GP and PHCT have a vital role—identifying drug misusers; assessing their health and willingness to modify drug abusing behaviour; and routine screening and prevention (e.g. cervical screening, contraception).

General measures: On each meeting consider:
• *Education:* Safer routes of drug administration; risks of overdose; condom use; driving and drug misuse (📖 p.205).
• *Hepatitis B immunization:* For injecting drug misusers not already infected/immune and close contacts of those already infected.
• *Treatment of dependence:* Set realistic goals. Responsibility contracts signed by GP, patient ± community pharmacist can be helpful. Review regularly. Give contact numbers for community support organizations. Seek advice and/or refer to a community substance misuse team as needed.

Specific drugs

- *Opiates:* Refer to substance abuse team. Untreated heroin withdrawal reaches a peak 36–72h. after the last dose (methadone—4–6d.). *Symptoms:* sweating, running eyes/nose, hot and cold turns ± gooseflesh, GI problems (anorexia, nausea, vomiting, diarrhoea, abdominal pain), restlessness and tremor, insomnia, aches and pains, tachycardia ± hypertension. Subside by 5d. (methadone—10–12d.).
- *Benzodiazepines:* Taper dosage over weeks. Seek specialist advice if the patient has any chronic debilitating condition or heart disease. Withdrawal symptoms include rebound anxiety, tremor, tachycardia, tachypnoea, nausea, abdominal and muscular cramps, diarrhoea. Rarely, perceptual disturbances and seizures.
- *Stimulants* (e.g. amphetamines, cocaine, ecstasy): Can be stopped abruptly. Some patients experience insomnia and depression. May require antidepressant drugs after withdrawal.
- *Hallucinogenic drugs* (e.g. LSD): Can be stopped abruptly.
- *Barbiturates:* Admit to hospital for supervised withdrawal. Sudden cessation may cause fits ± death.

Solvent abuse: Common amongst teenagers as solvents are easily obtained and cheap. Initial effects of inhalation are euphoria, incoordination, blurred vision, and slurring of speech. Rarely, the solvent may cause bronchoconstriction or arrhythmia and deaths, when they occur, are usually due to hypoxia, VF, or accidents whilst intoxicated. Symptoms to look for in the surgery are changes in behaviour (e.g. drop in school performance or attendance, irritability, mood swings) and local changes due to inhalation (e.g. cough, headaches, conjunctivitis). If detected, refer to the youth support agencies.

Essential reading

DoH (1999) *Drug misuse and dependence—guidelines on clinical management*
🖳 http://www.dh.gov.uk

Patient advice and support

'Talk to FRANK' (England and Wales): Government-run information, advice, and referral service. ☎(24 hour) 0800 77 66 00 🖳 http://www.talktofrank.com
'Know the Score' (Scotland): ☎0800 587 5879 🖳 www.knowthescore.info
Drugscope: Information about drug abuse and how to get treatment
🖳 http://www.drugscope.org.uk
Drugs-info: Information about substance abuse for families of addicts
🖳 http://www.drugs-info.co.uk
ADFAM: Support for families of addicts ☎020 7928 8898 🖳 http://www.adfam.org.uk
Ecstasy 🖳 http://www.ecstasy.org
Benzodiazepines 🖳 http://www.benzo.org.uk
Solvent abuse ☎0808 800 2345 🖳 http://www.re-solv.org
National Treatment Agency for Substance Abuse 🖳 http://www.nhs.uk
Substance Misuse Management in General Practice (SMMGP)
🖳 http://www.smmgp.demon.co.uk

Insomnia

From the Latin meaning 'no sleep'. Describes a perception of disturbed or inadequate sleep. ~1:4 of the UK population (♀>♂) are thought to suffer in varying degrees. Prevalence ↑ with age, rising to 1:2 amongst the over 65s. Causes are numerous. Common examples include:

- *Minor, self-limiting:* Travel, stress, shift work, small children, arousal.
- *Psychological:* ~½ have mental health problems—depression, anxiety, mania, grief, alcoholism.
- *Physical:* drugs (e.g. steroids), pain, pruritus, tinnitus, sweats (e.g. menopause), nocturia, asthma, obstructive sleep apnoea.

Definition of 'a good's night sleep'

- <30min. to fall asleep
- Maintenance of sleep for 6–8h.
- <3 brief awakenings/night
- Feels well rested and refreshed on awakening

Management: Careful evaluation. Many do not have a sleep problem themselves, but a relative feels there is a problem (e.g. the retired milkman continuing to wake at 4 a.m.). Others have unrealistic expectations (e.g. they need 12h. sleep/d.) Reassurance alone may be all that is required.

For genuine problems

- *Eliminate as far as possible any physical problems preventing sleep* e.g. treat asthma or eczema; give long-acting pain killers to last the whole night; consider HRT for sweats, refer if obstructive sleep apnoea is suspected (📖 p.400)
- *Treat psychiatric problems* e.g. depression, anxiety.
- *Sleep hygiene*—see box.
- *Relaxation techniques:* Audiotapes (borrow from libraries or buy from pharmacies); relaxation classes (often offered by local recreation centres/adult education centres); many physiotherapists can teach relaxation techniques.
- *Consider drug treatment:* Last resort. Benzodiazepines may be prescribed for insomnia 'only when it is severe, disabling, or subjecting the individual to extreme distress.'

Drug treatment: Benzodiazepines (e.g. temazepam), zolpidem, zopiclone, and low-dose TCA (e.g. amitriptyline 25–50mg) nocte are all commonly prescribed for patients with insomnia.

- *Side-effects:* Amnesia and daytime somnolence. Most hypnotics do affect daytime performance and may cause falls in the elderly. Warn patients about their affect on driving and operating machinery.
- Only prescribe a few weeks' supply at a time due to potential for dependence and abuse.

⚠ Beware the temporary resident who has 'forgotten' his/her night sedation.

Complications of insomnia: ↓ quality of life; ↓ concentration and memory affecting performance of daytime tasks; relationship problems; risk of accidents. 10% motor accidents are related to tiredness.

Principles of 'sleep hygiene'

- Don't go to bed until you feel sleepy
- Don't stay in bed if you're not asleep
- Avoid daytime naps
- Establish a regular bedtime routine
- Reserve a room for sleep only (if possible)—do not eat, read, work, or watch TV in it
- Make sure the bedroom and bed are comfortable, and avoid extremes of noise and temperature
- Avoid caffeine, alcohol, and nicotine
- Have a warm bath and warm milky drink at bedtime
- Take regular exercise but avoid late night hard exercise (sex is OK)
- Monitor your sleep with a sleep diary (record both the times you sleep and its quality)
- Rise at the same time every morning regardless of how long you've slept

Patient information and support

Royal College of Psychiatrists: Patient information sheets ⌨ http://www.rcpsych.ac.uk

Symptoms, signs, and laboratory results

In general practice, patients do not come neatly packaged with a diagnosis. Moreover, they do not know what characteristics they must show to be a typical patient with a particular condition—and frequently present atypically.

When confronted with a symptom, sign, or abnormal laboratory result, we need to know what the possible diagnoses are and then, placing that knowledge in clinical context, decide what the best course of action is.

This section is an A–Z catalogue of symptoms and signs seen in general practice and suggestions about their likely causes, it is followed by a catalogue of commonly requested laboratory tests and the likely meaning of abnormal results.

A–Z of symptoms and signs

Laboratory results

A

Abdominal masses: Abdominal masses are distinguished from pelvic masses by the ability to get beneath them.

Causes of solid abdominal mass
- Stool
- Malignancy (any intra-abdominal organ or kidney)
- AAA
- Crohn's mass
- TB mass
- Appendix mass or abscess
- LNs
- Splenomegaly
- Hepatomegaly

Pelvic mass: 📖 p.278

Abdominal distention: Consider the 6F's—
- Fluid—ascites or full bladder
- Fat
- Faeces
- Flatus—intestinal obstruction; air swallowing
- Foetus
- Food (e.g. in malabsorption)

Abdominal pain

Acute abdomen: 📖 p.1066

Acute abdominal pain in pregnancy: 📖 p.796

Colic: 📖 p.253

Table 9.1 Differential diagnosis of abdominal pain

Renal and gynaecological causes	GI causes	Other causes
Renal colic	IBS	Post-herpetic neuralgia
UTI	Constipation	Spinal arthritis
Pyelonephritis	Diverticular disease	Muscular pain
Hydronephrosis	Gallbladder disease	AAA
Ectopic pregnancy	Liver disease	Mesenteric artery ischaemia
Pelvic inflammatory disease	Crohn's	Mesenteric adenitis
Ovarian cyst	UC	MI
Gynaecological malignancy	Gastritis	Pneumonia
	Peptic ulcer	Subphrenic abscess
	Appendicitis	DM
	Meckel's diverticulum	Porphyria
	Pancreatitis	Addison's
	Bowel obstruction	Lead poisoning
	GI malignancy	

History: Consider:
- Site of pain—see Figure 9.1
- Onset: How long? How did it start? What started it? Change over time?
- Character of pain: Type of pain—burning, shooting, stabbing, dull, etc.
- Radiation
- Associated symptoms e.g. nausea, vomiting, diarrhoea
- Timing/pattern e.g. constant, colicky, relationship to food
- Exacerbating and relieving factors
- Severity
- Previous treatments tried and result

Examination: Temperature, pulse, BP, jaundice, anaemia, site of pain (Figure 9.1), guarding/rebound tenderness, rectal/vaginal examination as necessary.

Management: Try to ascertain cause from history and examination (Table 9.1) and treat accordingly.

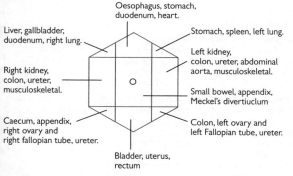

Oesophagus, stomach, duodenum, heart.

Stomach, spleen, left lung.

Liver, gallbladder, duodenum, right lung.

Left kidney, colon, ureter, abdominal aorta, musculoskeletal.

Right kidney, colon, ureter, musculoskeletal.

Small bowel, appendix, Meckel's divertiuclum

Caecum, appendix, right ovary and right fallopian tube, ureter.

Colon, left ovary and left Fallopian tube, ureter.

Bladder, uterus, rectum

Figure 9.1 Site of abdominal pain gives important clues about the organ involved

Absent periods: Amenorrhoea/absent periods—📖 p.728

Absent testis: May be absent because it is undescended, retractile, or has been removed.

Retractile testis: Usually young boys with active cremasteric reflex. No treatment needed. *Examination:* scrotum is usually well developed. Try to find the testis and milk it down into scrotum. May be found anywhere from the scrotum to the internal inguinal ring. If not found or unable to bring down into scrotum, assume undescended.

Undescended testis: 📖 p.840

Acanthosis nigricans: 📖 p.633

Acute abdomen: 📖 p.1066

Acute confusion: 📖 p.976

Acute retention of urine: 📖 p.690

Alopecia: Hair loss or alopecia—📖 p.658

Altered colour or smell of menstrual blood: No known associations.

Anaemia: 📖 p.522

Anal pain: Treat the cause. *Consider:*
- Anal fissure
- Haemorrhoids
- Perianal abscess
- Anal fistula
- Skin infection (e.g. hidradenitis suppurativa)
- Perianal heamatoma (thrombosed pile)
- Pilonidal sinus
- Functional pain (proctalgia fugax)
- Anal carcinoma

Anorexia: Absence of appetite. Non-specific symptom. *Possible causes:*
- Malignancy—GI tract e.g. stomach, colon, or disseminated malignancy from any cause
- Infection e.g. appendicitis, pneumonia
- Inflammatory diseases e.g. Crohn's disease
- Right ventricular failure
- Metabolic disease e.g. uraemia, hypercalcaemia
- Drugs e.g. cytotoxics
- Psychiatric conditions e.g. anorexia nervosa, depression, anxiety

Anosmia

Bilateral anosmia: More common than unilateral.
- *Local causes:* URTI, rhinitis, enlarged turbinates, nasal polyps.
- *Central causes:* CNS tumours (meningioma of the olfactory groove, ethmoid tumours, frontal lobe tumours), after head injury, meningitis, hydrocephalus, Kallman's syndrome.

Unilateral anosmia: One-sided loss of the sense of smell. *Causes:* head injury, frontal lobe lesion (e.g. meningioma of the olfactory groove, frontal lobe tumour).

Anuria: Failure of the kidneys to excrete urine. Classified as:
- *Obstructive:* Urinary tract obstruction—📖 p.690
- *Non-obstructive:* Renal failure—📖 p.680

Anxiety: 📖 p.960–4

Apex beat
- The normal position of the apex beat of the heart is the 5th intercostal space, in (or just medial to) the midclavicular line.
- Infants and children have apex beats which are superior and more lateral to those of adults.
- Apex beat may not be palpable if the patient is obese, has hyperexpanded lungs (e.g. COPD), or a pericardial effusion.
- The apex beat is moved sideways or inferiorly if the heart is enlarged (e.g. CCF) or displaced (e.g. pneumothorax).

Aphasia: Dysphasia—📖 p.257

Arthralgia: Joint pain—📖 p.271

Ascites: Free fluid in the peritoneal cavity. *Signs:* abdominal distention, shifting dullness to percussion, fluid thrill. *Causes:*
- Malignancy—any intra-abdominal organ, ovary, or kidney
- Hypoproteinaemia e.g. nephrotic syndrome
- Right heart failure
- Portal hypertension

Asterixis: Movement patterns (abnormal)—📖 p.275

Athetosis: Movement patterns (abnormal)—📖 p.275

B

Back pain: 📖 p.550

Beliefs (abnormal): Decide whether a belief is normal in the context of the patient. If not, decide if the belief is a:
- **Delusion** i.e. a belief that does not seem to have a rational basis and which is not amenable to argument (📖 p.255) *or*
- **Overvalued idea** i.e. belief that is odd but understandable given the patient's background

Blackouts: Establish what the patient means by blackout:
- **Fall:** 📖 p.996
- **Loss of consciousness:** 📖 p.274
- **Dizziness or vertigo:** 📖 p.256
- **Visual loss:** 📖 p.942

Blistering of the skin: 📖 p.652

Bone pain: *Consider:*
- *Fracture*—due to injury, stress fracture, or pathological fracture
- *Arthritis*—referred pain from affected joints
- *Malignancy*—primary bone malignancy, haematological malignancy e.g. multiple myeloma, or secondaries (usually from breast, prostate, lung, thyroid, kidney—more rarely, bowel melanoma)
- *Benign bone tumour*
- *Osteomyelitis*
- *Metabolic causes*—e.g. hypercalcaemia

Bowel motions (abnormal)

Bloody stool: Find out what the patient means:
- *Is the blood changed or unchanged?* The further proximal the bleed, the more likely the blood will be changed (though a brisk gastric or duodenal bleed can result in red rectal bleeding).
- *Is the bleeding related to passage of stool?* Blood on the toilet paper or in the pan not mixed with stool is often from anal bleeding due to haemorrhoids or an anal fissure.
- *Is blood mixed with stool?* Mixed blood + stool implies bleeding proximal to the sigmoid colon; blood around the stool implies a distal bleed.

Change in bowel habit: 📖 p.251

Constipation: 📖 p.472

Diarrhoea: 📖 p.255

Fresh rectal bleeding: Lower GI bleed—📖 p.1040

Melaena: Upper GI bleed—📖 p.1040

Slimy stool: Caused by overproduction of mucus in the large bowel. Almost always associated with colonic disease or irritable bowel syndrome. Investigate further.

Steatorrhoea: 📖 p.291

Aluminium paint stools: China clay stools—pale cream coloured stools usually caused by pancreatic cancer.

Bradycardia: Heart rate <60bpm—📖 p.312 and 346

Breast
- **Enlargement—men:** Gynaecomastia—📖 p.515
- **Lump:** 📖 p.512
- **Pain:** 📖 p.513

Breathlessness: Dyspnoea—📖 p.258

Breath sounds: Assess character of breath sounds and added sounds:
- *Bronchial breathing:* Breath sounds are harsher than normal—often caused by lung consolidation e.g. due to pneumonia
- ↓ *breath sounds:* Consider: pleural effusion, pneumothorax, emphysema, lung collapse
- *Added sounds:* Pleural rub (📖 p.279); wheeze (📖 p.298); crepitations/crackles (📖 p.254)

C

Cachexia: Severe generalized muscle wasting. *Causes:* Neoplasia, malnutrition, chronic infection (e.g. TB); prolonged inactivity; dementia.

Carotid bruits: May signify stenosis (>30%), often near the origin of internal carotid. Heard best behind the angle of the jaw. *Usual cause:* atheroma.

Carotid artery stenosis: 📖 p.609

Carotid pulse: Pulses—📖 p.283

Change in bowel habit: Once obvious causes (e.g. gastroenteritis, constipation due to opiates) have been excluded, investigate persistent diarrhoea or constipation in all patients, especially those >45y. *Common causes:*

- Carcinoma of the colon
- UC
- Crohn's disease
- Diverticular disease
- Pancreatic disease
- Bowel obstruction

Chest deformity

Barrel chest: AP diameter ↑, expansion ↓. Seen with chronic hyperinflation (e.g. asthma/COPD).

Pigeon chest (pectus carinatum): Prominent sternum with a flat chest. Seen in patients with chronic childhood asthma or rickets.

Funnel chest (pectus excavatum): The lower end of sternum is depressed.

Kyphosis: ↑ forward spinal convexity. Usually affects the thoracic spine.
- *Postural kyphosis* ('drooping shoulders' or 'roundback') is common and voluntarily correctable.
- *Structural kyphosis* cannot be corrected voluntarily. *Common causes:* osteoporosis, Paget's disease, ankylosing spondylitis, and adolescent kyphosis (Scheuermann's disease). May cause a restrictive ventilatory defect.

Scoliosis: ↑ lateral curvature of the spine. Above and below the scoliosis, secondary curves develop to maintain normal position of head and pelvis. In all cases, refer to orthopaedics for assessment.
- *Non-structural scoliosis* ('mobile scoliosis') is usually secondary to an abnormality outside the spine e.g. unequal leg length. It disappears when that is corrected.
- *Structural scoliosis* ('true scoliosis') is non-correctible. *Causes:* Idiopathic, neuromuscular (e.g. cerebral palsy, muscular dystrophy, neurofibromatosis), trauma, osteoporosis, TB of the spine (rare), spinal tumours (rare), congenital abnormalities of the spine (rare).

Harrison's sulcus: Groove deformity of the lower ribs at the diaphragm attachment site. Suggests chronic childhood asthma or rickets. (*E. Harrison(1766–1838)—British physician*)

Chest pain: Common symptom.

⚠ Always think—could this be an MI, PE, dissecting aneurysm, or pericarditis?

If a patient is acutely unwell with chest pain and the cause is not clear, err on the side of caution and admit for further assessment. See 'Acute chest pain'—📖 p.1046

History: Ask about site and nature of pain, duration, associated symptoms (e.g. breathlessness, nausea), provoking and relieving factors, PMH, drug history, smoking history, FH (e.g. heart disease).

Table 9.2 Causes of chest pain

Potentially fatal	Poorly localized	Well localized
MI	Angina	Fractured rib
Aortic dissection	MI	Muscle sprain
PE	Myocarditis	Tietze's syndrome
Oesophageal rupture	Mitral valve prolapse	Pericarditis
	HOCM	Pleurisy
	Pneumonia	PE
	Tracheitis	Shingles
	Reflux oesophagitis	Mastitis
	Oesophageal spasm	Biliary colic
	Peptic ulcer	Da Costa's syndrome
	Cervical spondylosis	Bornholm disease

Examination: Check BP in both arms, general appearance (distress, sweating, pallor), JVP, apex beat, heart sounds, lung fields, local tenderness, pain on movement of chest, skin rashes, swelling or tenderness of legs (?DVT).

Investigations: ECG and CXR may be helpful.

Central chest pain

- *Angina:* Constricting pain. May radiate to one/both arms, neck, or jaw. Can be provoked by exercise (relieved by stopping), cold, or ingestion of food. Often associated with breathlessness and/or palpitations. Rapidly relieved by GTN spray—📖 p.328.
- *MI:* Constricting or crushing pain or intense dull ache lasting >½ h. despite GTN spray. Radiates to either or both shoulders/arms and/or neck/jaw. Associated with dyspnoea, sweating, palpitations, nausea ± vomiting, and often a sense of doom. Admit.
- *Dissecting thoracic aneurysm:* May present with sudden tearing interscapular back pain or pain similar to MI ± radiation through to the back. Often the patient is very unwell and shocked (though not always)—BP is different in the 2 arms. Admit.
- *Pericarditis and pleurisy:* Sharp pain, worse on inspiration ± fever, breathlessness. Treat the cause.
- *Oesophageal pain:* May be very similar to cardiac pain. Suspect if related to food or alcohol ingestion or occurs in bed on lying flat. Relieved by antacids e.g. Gaviscon. Relieved by GTN spray, but less rapidly than angina.

Non-central chest pain: Remember—may still be cardiac.
- *Pleuritic pain/pleurisy:* Sharp pain, usually well localized, prevents deep inspiration ('catches as I breath'). Implies inflammation of the pleura. Treat the cause. *Causes:* chest infection, PE, malignancy e.g. mesothelioma.
- *Fractured rib:* Usually history of injury (though may not be—especially if pathological fracture). Pain well localized and point tenderness over

rib. Pain made worse by light pressure over sternum. Treat with simple analgesia. Heels spontaneously. No need for X-ray except if diagnosis is unsure or unless other pathology is suspected.

- *Musculoskeletal pain:* Common. Sharp or dull pain. Due to radiation of pain from thoracic spine or local muscular injury. Usually made worse by movement and relieved by rest and NSAIDs.
- *Shingles:* Pain (often burning in nature)in a dermatomal distribution. Vesicles appear days later. Treatment—📖 p.494.
- *Gallbladder and pancreatic disease:* May mimic cardiac pain or be felt as atypical chest pain. Management—📖 p.446 and 448 respectively.
- *Functional:* Continuously varying locations, brief stabbing pains (<30sec.). Beware of addicts feigning chest pain to receive opiate analgesia.

Cheyne–Stokes respiration: Breathing becomes progressively deeper and then shallower (± episodic apnoea) in cycles. *Causes:* brainstem lesions/compression (stroke, ↑ ICP); chronic pulmonary oedema; poor cardiac output. It is enhanced by narcotics.

Chorea: Movement patterns (abnormal)—📖 p.275

Chronic retention of urine: 📖 p.691

Clubbing of nails: 📖 p.661

Claudication: 📖 p.360

Clonus: Reflexes—📖 p.285

Coffee grounds vomit: 📖 p.1041

Colic
- **Infantile:** 📖 p.831
- **Colicky abdominal pain:** Pain which comes and goes. Can be the result of obstruction in a viscus (e.g. GI obstruction, renal colic, biliary colic) or IBS.

Compulsion: Forced behaviour repeated in spite of inappropriateness, or unreasonableness and associated discomfort in response to an obsession. Can be disabling e.g. repeated handwashing hundreds of times a day. Obsessive-compulsive disorder—📖 p.965.

Confusion
- **Acute:** 📖 p.976
- **Longstanding:** 📖 p.978

Constipation
- **Adults:** 📖 p.472
- **Children:** 📖 p.856

Coryza: Discharge from the mucous membrane of the nose. Usually due to acute viral URTI. *Other causes:* rhinitis (allergic or vasomotor), prodrome to measles or pertussis.

Cough: Reaction to irritation anywhere from pharynx to lungs.

Acute cough (<3wk.): *Causes:*
- URTI
- Croup
- Tracheitis
- LRTI
- Pneumonia—productive, loose cough
- Acute exacerbation of asthma normally well controlled
- Inhaled foreign body—especially in well children

Reserve CXR for patients with marked focal chest signs or where inhalation of foreign body is suspected.

Management: Treat the cause where possible; advise OTC cough mixture as needed e.g. simple linctus; steam inhalation often eases symptoms temporarily; review if not clearing.

Chronic cough (>2wk.): *Causes:*
- Postnasal drip
- Postviral
- Pertussis
- TB
- Bronchiectasis
- Pulmonary oedema
- Lung cancer
- COPD
- Asthma
- Foreign body
- Vocal cord palsy
- GORD
- LVF
- Drug-induced (e.g. ACE inhibitors)
- Smoker's cough
- Psychogenic

⚠ **Red flags:** Weight ↓, night sweats.

Management: Treat the cause. If no cause is found, refer for medical opinion.

Crackles in the chest: Produced by air flow moving secretions from airways or lung tissue.
- **Fine crackles:** Consider pulmonary oedema (early inspiratory); early pneumonia; fibrosing alveolitis (late inspiratory).
- **Coarse crackles:** Consider TB; resolving pneumonia; bronchiectasis; lung abscess.

Cramp: Painful muscle spasm. Common—especially at night and after exercise. Rarely associated with disease—salt depletion, muscle ischaemia, myopathy. Forearm cramps suggest motor neurone disease. Night cramps in the elderly may respond to quinine bisulfate 300mg nocte twice weekly.

Writer's cramp: 📖 p.259

Crying babies: 📖 p.890

Cyanosis: Dusky blue skin.

Central cyanosis: Cyanosis of mucus membranes e.g. mouth. *Causes:* lung disease resulting in inadequate oxygen transfer (e.g. COPD, PE, pleural effusion, severe chest infection); shunting from pulmonary to systemic circulation (e.g. Fallot's tetralogy, PDA, transposition of the great arteries); inadequate oxygen uptake (e.g. met- or sulf-haemoglobinaemia).

Peripheral cyanosis: e.g. cyanosis of fingers. *Causes:* as for central cyanosis plus: physiological (cold, hypovolaemia); local arterial disease. Feet can be a dusky blue colour due to venous disease too. When occurs without central cyanosis, does not imply abnormal oxygen saturation.

D

Deafness: 📖 p.924

Delayed puberty: 📖 p.282

Delirium
- **Acute confusion**—📖 p.976
- **Delirium tremens**—📖 p.1068

Delusions: Beliefs held unshakably, despite available counter-evidence, and which are unexpected in view of circumstances and background. The belief is usually (but not always) false.
- **Primary delusions:** Belief arrives in the head fully formed. e.g. thought insertion; strongly suggestive of schizophrenia.
- **Secondary delusions:** Belief arises on the basis of experience e.g. someone who has lost their job several times through no fault of their own may believe they are unemployable.

Paranoid delusions: Delusions which concern the relationship between the patient and other people. Associated with schizophrenia, depressive states, and acute and chronic cognitive impairment. Can be:
- Delusions of reference: Ideas of reference—📖 p.292
- Delusions of persecution: 📖 p.293
- Delusions of grandeur: 📖 p.293

Depersonalization: Perceptions (abnormal)—📖 p.278

Derealization: Perceptions (abnormal)—📖 p.278

Diarrhoea
Acute diarrhoea: Usually self-limiting, lasting 2–5d. *Causes:*

- Dietary indiscretion
- Infection e.g. food poisoning, traveller's diarrhoea
- Constipation with overflow
- Pseudomembranous colitis—recent history of oral antibiotics
- Onset of inflammatory bowel disease or other chronic diarrhoea

Management
- **Send a stool sample** for M,C&S if fever, bloody diarrhoea, food worker, recent return from tropical climate, immunocompromised patient, or lasts >7d.
- **Treat with rehydration:** Encourage clear fluid intake ± rehydration salts. Reserve antidiarrhoeals (e.g. loperamide) for patients in whom diarrhoea would be difficult (e.g. immobility, travel, work). Never give children antidiarrhoeal agents.
- **Food:** Stick to a bland diet, avoiding dairy products, until diarrhoea has settled. Babies who are breast fed or have not been weaned should continue their normal milk. Some advocate using half-strength milk for non-breast fed babies, though the benefits of this have not been demonstrated.
- **If dehydrated and unable to replace fluids** e.g. concomitant vomiting, child refusing to drink: Admit.
- **If no cause found and lasts >3wk. or any atypical features:** Refer for urgent investigation or admit.

Chronic diarrhoea: 📖 p.450

Difficulty walking
- Walking difficulty: 📖 p.297
- Gait (abnormal): 📖 p.263

Disturbed behaviour

Acute management: 📖 p.1082

Causes
- *Physical illness:* Infection (e.g. UTI, chest infection); hypoglycaemia; hypoxia; head injury; epilepsy.
- *Drugs:* Alcohol (or alcohol withdrawal); prescribed drugs (e.g. steroid psychosis); illicit drugs (e.g. amphetamines).
- *Psychiatric illness:* Schizophrenia; mania; anxiety/depression; dementia.
- *Personality disorder:* e.g. attention-seeking.

Dizziness and giddiness: Distinguish between true vertigo (the illusion of rotatory movement—the room spinning) and a feeling of unsteadiness or lightheadedness:
- *Vertigo:* 📖 p.928.
- *Imbalance:* Implies difficulty in walking straight (e.g. from disease of peripheral nerves, posterior columns, or cerebellum).
- *Faintness:* The feeling of being about to pass out. Some seizure disorders and a variety of non-neurological conditions (e.g. postural hypotension; vasovagal fainting; hyperventilation; hypoglycaemia; arrythmias; cough syncope). Sometimes 2 or 3 elements co-exist.

Dry eyes: 📖 p.938

Dry mouth: *Causes:* anxiety, drugs, or Sjögrens syndrome. Look for cause and rectify if possible. Prescribe artificial saliva e.g. glandosane.

Dysarthria: Difficulty with articulation due to incoordination or weakness of the musculature of speech. Language is normal. Ask to repeat 'baby hippopotamus' or 'British constitution'. Treat the cause if possible; otherwise support with speech therapy and aids to communication. *Causes:*
- *Cerebellar disease:* Slurring as if drunk. Speech is irregular in volume and scanning in quality.
- *Extrapyramidal disease:* e.g. PD—soft, indistinct, and monotonous.
- *Pseudo-bulbar palsy:* Patients may present with alteration of speech (typically nasal speech sounding like Donald Duck), difficulty swallowing or chewing. The tongue is spastic and jaw jerk ↑. *Causes:* stroke (bilateral); MS; MND.
- *Bulbar palsy:* Loss of function of the tongue, muscles of chewing/swallowing ± facial muscles. *Examination:* flaccid, fasciculating tongue, jaw jerk normal or absent, speech—quiet, hoarse, or nasal. *Causes:* MND, Guillain Barré syndrome, alcoholic brainstem myelinolysis (central pontine myelinolysis), brainstem tumours (1° or 2°), syringobulbia, polio, hyponatraemia.
- *Other lesions:* Neuromuscular junction—myaesthenia gravis; palate paralysis (nasal speech).

Dyslexia: 📖 p.898

Dyspareunia
• **Female:** 📖 p.726.
• **Male:** Usually associated with infection e.g. urethritis, prostatitis.

Dyspepsia or indigestion: 📖 p.432

Dysphagia: Difficulty swallowing food or liquids.

⚠ Refer all patients with dysphagia for urgent endoscopy or to a rapid-access dysphagia clinic if available.

Causes
• *Acute*
  • Sore throat   • Quinsy   • Foreign body in throat
  • Epiglottitis   • Glandular fever   • Acute caustic stricture
• *Progressive*
  • **Within the oesophagus:** 📖 p.434 and 440. Carcinoma of the oesophagus, foreign body, chronic benign stricture, achalasia, pharyngeal pouch, Plummer-Vinson syndrome, oesophageal perforation.
  • **Compression from outside:** Enlarged mediastinal LNs, lung cancer, enlarged left atrium, large retrosternal goitre, thoracic aneurysm.
  • **Other:** Bulbar palsy, myaesthenia gravis, hysteria, anxiety state.

Dysphasia: Impairment of language due to brain damage to the dominant hemisphere. The left hemisphere is dominant for 99% of R-handed people and 60% L-handers. In most cases, due to stroke or brain tumour. Rarely due to head injury or dementia. *Assessment:*
• Is speech fluent, grammatical, meaningful, and apt? If yes, dysphasia unlikely.
• Comprehension—can the patient follow 1, 2, or multiple step commands?
• Repetition—can the patient repeat a phrase after you?
• Naming—can the patient name common and uncommon items?
• Reading and writing? Usually affected too. If not, question the diagnosis of dysphasia.

Classification: Table 9.3. Mixed pictures are common.

Treatment: Speech therapy (may or may not be helpful), support (e.g. dysphasia groups: contact via Stroke Association—📖 p.607), aids to communication (e.g. computers, picture boards).

Table 9.3 Classification of dysphasia

Characteristics of dysphasia	Broca's (expressive)	Wernicke's (receptive)	Conduction	Transcortical
Fluent?	✗	✓	✓	✓ or ✗
Repetition normal?	✗	✗	✗	✓
Understanding impaired?	✗	✓	✗	✓ or ✗

Table 9.4 Causes of dyspnoea

	Acute	Subacute	Chronic
Cardiac disease	Acute LVF Arrythmia Shock	Arrythmia	CCF Mitral stenosis Aortic stenosis
Lung disease	Pneumothorax Acute asthma attack PE Acute pneumonitis e.g. due to inhaling toxic gas	Asthma Infective Exacerbation of COPD Pleural effusion Pneumonia	COPD Fibrosing alveolitis Occupational lung diseases Mesothelioma Lung cancer
Other	Hyperventilation Foreign body inhalation Guillain-Barré syndrome Altitude sickness Ketoacidosis Polio	Aspirin poisoning Myaesthenia gravis Thyrotoxicosis	Kyphoscoliosis Anaemia MND MS

Dyspnoea: Sensation of shortness of breath. Try to quantify exercise tolerance (e.g. dressing, distance walked, climbing stairs).

Speed of onset helps diagnosis: Table 9.4

Combined chest pain and dyspnoea: *Consider:*
- MI
- Pericarditis
- Dissecting aneurysm
- PE
- Oesophageal pain
- Musculoskeletal pain
- Chest infection
- Pulmonary malignancy e.g. mesothelioma, Ca lung

Orthopnoea: 📖 p.277

Paroxysmal nocturnal dyspnoea: 📖 p.278

Exertional dyspnoea: Breathlessness with exercise. Generally, causes are the same as dyspnoea. The New York Heart Association classifies 4 grades of severity:
- *Normal*
- *Moderate:* Walking on the level causes breathlessness.
- *Severe:* Has to stop due to breathlessness when walking on the flat. All but the lightest housework is impossible.
- *Gross:* Slightest effort → severe breathlessness. The patient is almost bed/chair bound.

Dyspraxia: Impairment of performance of complex movements despite preservation of ability to perform their individual components. Test by asking the patient to perform everyday tasks (e.g. dress/undress), copy complex hand movements, and do familiar sequences of movements (e.g. 'head, shoulders, knees, and toes').

Childhood: 📖 p.898

Adults: Most common causes are stroke or SOL. Involve rehabilitation services and OT.
- *Dressing dyspraxia:* Patient is unsure of the orientation of clothes on his/her body.
- *Constructional dyspraxia:* Difficulty in assembling objects or drawing (ask to draw 5-pointed star).
- *Gait dyspraxia:* Gait disorder, although the lower limbs function normally—more common amongst the elderly.

Dystonia: Prolonged muscle contraction producing abnormal postures or repetitive movements.
- *Spasmodic torticollis:* Head is pulled to one side and held there by a contracting sternomastoid muscle. Treat with physiotherapy.
- *Blepharospasm:* Involuntary contraction of the orbicularis oculi.
- *Writer's cramp:* Spasm of the hand and forearm muscles on writing.

Dysuria and urgency: Painful micturition due to urethral or bladder inflammation. *Causes:* UTI, urethral syndrome, inflammation (e.g. interstitial cystitis, radiation induced cystitis), intravesical lesion (tumour, stone), atrophy (menopause).

E

Ear
- **Discharge:** 📖 p.922
- **Pain:** 📖 p.922

Eccymosis: Purpura—📖 p.284

Encoparesis: 📖 p.895

Enuresis: 📖 p.894

Epigastric pain: Treat the cause.

Acute causes
- Peptic ulcer/gastritis
- Gallbladder disease
- Irritable bowel syndrome
- Peritonitis
- Pancreatitis
- GI obstruction
- Ruptured aortic aneurysm
- MI
- Pneumonia or other disease affecting the pleura
- Spinal disease e.g. spondylosis

Chronic causes: Peptic ulcer; gastric cancer; chronic pancreatitis; aortic aneurysm; root pain referred from the spine.

Epistaxis: 📖 p.1042

Erectile dysfunction: 📖 p.702

Erythema: Redness of the skin—usually due to vasodilation. It may be localized (e.g. pregnancy—on the palms) or generalized (e.g. drug eruption, viral exanthem).

Excess hair: Hairiness—📖 p.658

Excess sweating: Hyperhydrosis—📖 p.659

Exertional dyspnoea: 📖 p.258

Exophthalmos: The eyes protrude from the orbit and thus have a staring appearance. Stand at the same level as the patient and look at the patient's eyes. There should be no white of the sclera visible below the iris. If the eye is pushed forward, as in exophthalmos, white sclera is seen below the iris and the patient can look upwards without moving his/her eyebrows (distinguishes from lid retraction).

Bilateral: Caused by Grave's disease.

Unilateral: Caused by Grave's disease, orbital disease (e.g. tumours, cellulitis); vascular disease (e.g. cavernous sinus thrombosis, carotid-cavernous fistula); sinus disease (e.g. tumour).

Eyelid problems: 📖 p.936 and 938

Eye pain: Consider:
- *Painful conditions:* Corneal abrasion, foreign body, keratitis, iritis, scleritis, acute glaucoma, ophthalmic shingles, arc eye.
- *Eye discomfort:* Conjunctivitis, entropion, trichasis, dry eye, episcleritis, optic neuritis.
- *Referred pain:* Tension type headache, migraine, refractive error, trigeminal neuralgia, ophthalmic shingles, giant cell arteritis, ocular muscle imbalance, ↑ ICP.

Eye (red): 📖 p.936

F

Facial flushing: Flushing—📖 p.261

Facial pain: Treat the cause. Common causes:
- Trigeminal neuralgia
- TMJ disorders
- Dental disorders
- Sinusitis
- Migrainous neuralgia
- Shingles and post-herpetic neuralgia

No cause is found in many patients—it is then termed *atypical facial pain*. Atypical facial pain may respond to simple analgesia with paracetamol or a NSAID. If this fails, try nerve painkillers e.g. amitriptyline nocte. Refer those with troublesome symptoms to ENT, maxillofacial surgery, or neurology.

Facial palsy: Paralysis of the facial nerve → facial weakness ± loss of taste in the anterior 2/3 of the tongue. *Assessment:* Check facial movements e.g. ask the patient to screw up his eyes, smile, and blow out his cheeks. Always ask the patient to raise his eyebrows—the brow is spared if unilateral upper motor neurone lesion (e.g. CVA). *Causes:*
- *Unilateral upper motor neurone lesion:* Tumour, CVA.
- *Unilateral lower motor neurone lesion:* Tumour (e.g. acoustic neuroma), CVA, MS, Bells palsy, Ramsay–Hunt syndrome, otitis media, fracture in the temporal bone, parotid tumour, facial laceration (including post-op), sarcoid, HIV.

- *Bilateral:* Rare. Consider Bells palsy, sarcoid, Guillain-Barré syndrome, polio, and other causes of facial weakness e.g. myasthenia gravis, myopathies.

Fainting: Vasovagal attack/simple faint. Common. Peripheral vasodilation, bradycardia, and venous pooling → postural hypotension. Often cause is unclear though ♀>♂. *Known precipitants:* fright (e.g. during venesection) or emotion. *Features:*

- *Prodrome:* Dizziness, visual disturbance, nausea, sweating, ringing in the ears, a sinking feeling, and yawning;
- *Faint:* Extreme pallor, momentary unconsciousness (with fall to the floor if standing ± tonic-clonic jerks if held upright);
- *Rapid recovery.*

Management: Exclude other reasons for loss of consciousness (📖 p.274). No treatment needed—reassure.

Falls: 📖 p.996

Fatigue: 📖 p.582 and p.626

Fever: Pyrexia—📖 p.284.

Flatulence: 400–1300mL of gas are expelled per rectum daily. If this seems excessive to the patient, he may complain of flatulence. Most patients complaining of flatulence have no GI disease. The most likely cause is air-swallowing (aerophagy). Reassure.

Flight of ideas: Thought disorders—📖 p.292

Flushing: Erythema due to vasodilation. Common and usually benign. Tends to affect face, neck, and upper trunk. *Causes:*

- *Physiological:* exertion, heat
- *Emotion* e.g. anger, anxiety, embarrassment
- *Foods* e.g. spices, chillies, alcohol
- *Endocrine* e.g. menopause, Cushing's
- *Drugs* e.g. morphine, tamoxifen, danazol, GnRH analogues, clomifene, nitrates, calcium channel blockers
- *Dermatological:* rosacea (unknown mechanism); contact dermatitis
- *Inflammatory:* SLE, dermatomyositis
- *Infection* e.g. slapped cheek syndrome (5th disease), celluliltis, or erysipelas
- *Tumour:* pancreatic tumours, medullary thyroid cancer, carcinoid, phaeochromocytoma.

Management: Treat cause if possible (e.g. avoid alcohol; HRT). Embarrassing flushing may be helped with a small dose of propranolol (e.g. 40mg od/bd) or clonidine (e.g. 50 mcgm bd).

Foot drop: The patient trips frequently or walks with a high stepping gait. On examination, the patient is unable to walk on his heels and cannot dorsiflex his foot. Check ankle jerk. *Causes:*

- *Common peroneal palsy:* e.g. due to trauma—normal ankle jerk
- *Sciatica:* ankle jerk absent
- *L4, L5 root lesion:* ankle jerk may be absent
- *Peripheral motor neuropathy:* e.g. alcoholic—ankle jerk weak or absent

- *Distal myopathy:* ankle jerk weak or absent
- *Motor neurone disease:* ↑ ankle jerk

Foot pain

Forefoot pain: *Causes:* forefoot pathology (e.g. pes cavus, pes planus), stress fractures, RA, DM, gout, OA, paralytic deformity, post-traumatic syndromes, nerve root pathology, tarsal nerve compression.

Heel pain: *Causes:*
- *Within the heel:* osteomyelitis, tumours, Paget's disease, arthritis of the subtalar joint
- *Behind the heel:* ruptured Achilles tendon, Achilles tendinitis
- *Under the heel:* tender heel pad, plantar faciitis, plantar calcaneal bursitis

Foot pulses: 📖 p.283 and p.361

Frequency: Passage of urine more often than usual. *Causes:*
- UTI
- Urethral syndrome
- Detrusor instability
- Inflammation (e.g. interstitial cystitis)
- Fibrosis (e.g. post-radiotherapy)
- Atrophy (menopause)
- Neurogenic bladder (e.g. MS)
- External pressure (e.g. pregnancy, fibroids)
- Bladder tumour or stone
- Enlarged prostate
- Drugs (e.g. diuretics)
- DM
- Excessive fluid intake
- Habit

Funny turns in small children: *Consider:*

Epilepsy: 📖 p.866

Non-epileptic attacks: Usually self-limiting and harmless but can be very frightening for parents/carers. Parental education about the likely duration and cause of attacks and reassurance that the child will come to no harm are important.
- *Simple blue breath-holding attacks:* Onset usually >6mo. of age. Common. Provoked by frustration or upset. *Signs:* +ve valsalva manoeuvre, cynanosis, stiffening, and coma. No treatment needed—spontaneous recovery. Most children 'grow out' of the attacks by 3y.
- *White reflex asystolic (anoxic) attacks:* May start before 6mo. but most common from 6mo.–2y. Usually triggered by minor injury or anxiety. *Signs:* vagal asystole, pallor, rapid coma, stiffening, upward eye movement ± urinary incontinence. No treatment needed—spontaneous recovery.
- *Reflex syncope:* 'Faints'. Common—📖 p.261
- *Others causes are rare but include:*
  - Benign paroxysmal vertigo
  - Benign myoclonus of infancy
  - Cardiac arrhythmias
  - Sleep phenomena
  - Pseudoseizures
  - Munchhausen syndrome by proxy
  - Hypoglycaemia
  - Hyperventilation

G

Gait (abnormal): Gait means manner of walking.

Abnormal movements: Normal gait is interrupted by abnormal movements e.g. choreiform movements, athetoid movements, or hemi-ballismus (□ p.275).

Antalgic gait: Gait adjusts to try to minimize pain in a joint—usually OA hip. The patient leans towards the affected side and takes a rapid step on that side followed by a slower step on the contralateral side.

Drunken gait: As its name suggests, a drunken gait is the type of gait adopted by someone who is drunk. The other major cause is a cerebellar lesion. *Features:*
- Wide-based gait or reeling gait on a narrow base
- Feet are often raised too high and placed over carefully with the patient looking ahead
- If a cerebellar lesion, the patient falls to the side of the lesion

Foot drop: Patients have a high-stepping gait to prevent scraping the toe on the ground.

Frontal lesions: Marked unsteadiness—the feet appear stuck to the floor causing a wide-based, shuffling gait.

Hemiplegic gait: Style of walking seen in patients with UMN lesions. *Features:*
- Arm adducted and internally rotated, elbow flexed and pronated ± finger flexion
- Foot is plantar flexed and the leg swings in a lateral arc

Parkinsonian gait: Seen in patients with PD and other causes of Parkinsonism. *Features:*
- *Akinesia:* Hesitation in starting walking (may be relieved by placing a line on the floor for the patient to step over).
- *Marche au petit pas:* Small, shuffling steps.
- *Festinant gait:* Flexed posture as if hurrying to keep up with feet.
- *Lack of normal arm swing*
- *Kinesia paradoxica:* Patients can perform fast or energetic movements more easily than slow ones e.g. running may be easier than walking.

Scissor gait: As the name implies, the patient walks as if his legs were like a pair of scissors. Associated with spastic paraplegia:
- Both legs are held rigid with plantar flexion of the ankle, extension of the knee, and adduction/internal rotation of the hips.
- The patient walks on tiptoe and the knees rub together/cross during the walking cycle.
- Often accompanied by complex movements of the upper limbs to assist the walking movements.

Sensory ataxic gait: Loss of proprioception due to peripheral neuropathy or spinal cord disease (e.g. cervical spondylosis, MS, syphilis, combined degeneration of the cord) results in an ataxic gait similar to that seen with cerebellar disease. *Features:*
• Broad-based gait with a tendency to stamp feet down clumsily
• Patient tends to look at feet throughout the walking cycle
• Romberg's sign +ve

Waddling gait: Typically seen in patients with proximal myopathy e.g. due to muscular dystrophy. *Other causes:* pregnancy, CDH. *Features:*
• Broad-based gait in which the pelvis drops to the side of the leg being raised
• The patient moves his body and hips to accommodate this, resulting in a duck-like waddle in the swing phase
• Commonly accompanied by ↑ forward curvature of the lower spine

Galactorrhoea: Hyperprolactinaemia—📖 p.428

Genital ulcers: *Causes:*
• Genital herpes
• Primary syphilis
• Behçet's syndrome.

If history of foreign travel, partner from abroad, or doubt about diagnosis, refer to GUM clinic.

Gingivitis: 📖 p.910

Globus pharyngis (or hystericus): A sensation of a lump/discomfort in the throat. Discomfort is often relieved by eating and there is no obstruction to swallowing of fluids or solids. Probably due to cricopharyngeal spasm. Associated with reflux oesophagitis/peptic ulcer in some patients. Investigate to exclude other pathology e.g. with barium swallow/upper GI endoscopy.

Table 9.5 Differential diagnosis of groin lumps

Position relative to the skin	Groin lump	Position relative to the inguinal ligament	
		Above	Below
In the skin	Lipoma, fibroma, haemangioma, and other skin lumps	✓	✓
Deep to the skin	Femoral or inguinal lymph nodes	✓	✓
	Saphena varix of the femoral vein	×	✓
	Femoral artery aneurysm	×	✓
	Femoral hernia	×	✓
	Inguinal hernia	✓	×

Groin lumps: The inguinal ligament runs from the pubic tubercle medially to the anterior superior iliac spine laterally. Differential diagnosis of groin lumps—Table 9.5.

Guarding: Reflex contraction of abdominal muscles signifying local or general peritoneal inflammation.

Gums

- **Bleeding gums:** Consider periodontal disease (by far the most common cause); pregnancy; leukaemia, bleeding disorders; scurvy.
- **Hypertrophied gums:** Associated with phenytoin use.
- **Blue line:** Along the margin of the teeth—suggests lead poisoning.
- **Gum inflammation:** Gingivitis—🕮 p.910

Gynaecomastia: 🕮 p.515

Table 9.6 Causes of haematuria

Gynaecological	• Menstruation	• Cervical bleeding
	• PMB	• Atrophic vaginitis
	• Bleeding in pregnancy	
Kidney	• Stones	• Infection
	• Tumour	• Glomerulonephritis
Ureter	• Stones	• Tumour (rare)
Bladder	• UTI	• Tumour
	• Stones	• Chronic inflammation
Prostate	• Prostatitis	• Tumour
Urethral inflammation		

H

Haematuria: *Causes*—Table 9.6
- May be frank (visible) or microscopic (up to 20% population).
- Investigate *all* cases of haematuria further.
- Check MSU for M,C&S, check blood for U&E, creatinine. Free Hb and myoglobin make urine test sticks +ve in absence of red cells.
- Urine discolouration can result from beetroot ingestion, porphyria, or rifampicin.
- If cause is identified (e.g. sample taken when menstruating, UTI)— repeat the check for blood in urine once treated/resolved.
- Refer if no cause is found. Rapid access one-stop clinics now operate in most areas.

Haematospermia: Blood in semen. In most cases benign and self-limiting. Persistent symptoms are more likely to be pathological. In ♂<40y. examine testes and epididymes and check MSU to exclude UTI. In ♂>40y. examine testes, epididymes and prostate, check MSU and PSA. May be associated with prostatitis, UTI, minor trauma or rarely prostate cancer. If no cause found and continues, refer to urology.

Haemoptysis: Expectoration of blood or blood-stained sputum. Melaena occurs if enough blood is swallowed. Haemoptysis rarely needs treating in its own right but *always* requires investigation to find the cause. If massive, admit as an acute emergency. If terminal event (e.g. inoperable lung cancer), consider prompt IV morphine ± sedative. *Causes:*

- *Respiratory:* Lung cancer; TB; bronchitis; bronchiectasis; lung abscess; pneumonia; violent coughing; inhaled foreign body; aspergilloma; trauma.
- *Cardiovascular:* PE (blood is not mixed with sputum); mitral stenosis; acute LVF.
- *Other:* Collagen vascular disease (e.g. polyarteritis nodosa); bleeding diathesis; mycoses (e.g. aspergilloma); foreign body.

Hairiness: 📖 p.658 and p.659

Hair loss or alopecia: 📖 p.658

Halitosis: Common after sleep.

Short-term halitosis is associated with acute illness e.g. tonsillitis, appendicitis (foetor oris), gastroenteritis, diabetic ketoacidosis.

Chronic halitosis is usually caused by bacterial putrefaction of food debris and dental plaque and is related to poor oral hygiene. Associated with gingivitis ± peridontitis. Smoking, alcohol, isosorbide dinitrate, and disulfiram exacerbate the problem.

Management
- Examine the mouth and recommend a dental check
- Advise on oral hygiene e.g. regular brushing of teeth and tongue, dental flossing
- Give advice on smoking cessation
- Dietary advice—avoid garlic, onions, curries
- Treat any local infection e.g. gingivitis
- Mouthwashes e.g. 0.2% aqueous chlorhexidine gluconate help ↓ dental plaque

Hallucinations: Sensory experiences in the absence of stimuli. May be visual, auditory, gustatory, olfactory, or tactile.
- *Visual, tactile, and auditory hallucinations* suggest mental illness:
  - Visual and tactile hallucinations suggest organic disorder e.g. dementia, acute confusional state, metabolic encephalopathy, drug abuse.
  - Auditory hallucinations suggest psychosis.
- *Hallucinations experienced when the patient is falling asleep* (hypnagogic hallucination) or waking up (hypnapompic hallucination) are features of narcolepsy.
- *Olfactory and gustatory hallucinations* often occur together. May be suggestive of psychosis but also occur with temporal lobe epilepsy and olfactory bulb tumours

Headache: 📖 p.596

Hearing loss: 📖 p.924

Heartburn: Retrosternal gripping or burning pain occurring in waves and rising towards the neck. Sometimes radiates → back and may be accompanied by reflux of acid into the mouth. Worsened by stooping, lying down, large and/or fatty meals, alcohol, smoking, and/or pregnancy. Generally, heartburn is the result of gastric acid reflux onto the oeso-phageal mucosa. It may be a feature of dyspepsia, but dyspepsia can occur without heartburn. *Causes:*

- No cause found (30%)
- Oesophagitis (24%)
- DU (17%)
- Hiatus hernia (15%)
- Gastritis (9%)
- Duodenitis (6%)
- Gastric ulcer (5%)
- Reflux of bile (0.7%)
- Gastric cancer (0.2%)

❶ 23% patients have ≥2 identifiable causes of heartburn

Management: See dyspepsia 📖 p.432

Table 9.7 Differential diagnosis of heart murmurs

Type of murmur	Description	Causes
Ejection systolic murmur	↑ to reach a peak midway between the heart sounds.	• Flow murmurs e.g. children, pregnancy, with fever, during/after exercise • Aortic stenosis or sclerosis (📖 p.354) • Pulmonary stenosis (📖 p.355) • HOCM (📖 p.352)
Pan-systolic murmur	Uniform intensity between the 2 heart sounds. Merges with 2nd heart sound.	• Mitral valve regurgitation or prolapse (📖 p.354) • Tricuspid regurgitation (📖 p.355) • VSD (📖 p.356) • ASD (📖 p.356)
Early diastolic murmur	Occurs just after the 2nd heart sound. High pitched and easily missed.	• Aortic regurgitation (📖 p.355) • Pulmonary regurgitation (📖 p.355) • Tricuspid stenosis (mitral stenosis co-exists)
Mid-diastolic murmur	Midway between 2nd heart sound of 1 beat and 1st of the next. Rumbling and low pitched.	• Mitral stenosis (📖 p.354) • Aortic regurgitation. (Austin–Flint murmur—📖 p.355).

Heart murmurs

⚠ Red flag symptoms

- Cyanosis
- Breathlessness
- Lethargy and tiredness
- Collapse
- Weight loss (or failure to thrive in children)

Due to abnormalities of flow within the heart and great vessels. Very common. Often incidental findings. Described by:

- Location—where heard loudest
- Intensity—graded out of 6, 1 being virtually undetectable and 6 being heard by an observer without a stethoscope

- Timing—systolic or diastolic, *and*
- Radiation—does the murmur spread elsewhere e.g. to the axilla (mitral regurgitation murmur)?

Always refer for echocardiographic confirmation. Differential diagnosis—Table 9.7 (📖 p.267).

Heart sounds: Low- and medium-frequency sounds (e.g. 3rd and 4th heart sounds) are more easily heard with the bell applied lightly to the skin. High-frequency sounds (e.g. 1st and 2nd heart sounds and opening snaps) are more easily heard with a diaphragm. Interpretation of heart sounds—Table 9.8.

Heat rash: Fine, red, maculopapular rash, most common in small children. Usually on trunk/neck and self-limiting.

Heavy periods: Menorrhagia/heavy periods—📖 p.724

Heel pain: 📖 p.262

Hemiballismus: Movement patterns (abnormal)—📖 p.275

Hepatomegaly: *Causes:*
- *Apparent:* Reidel's lobe, low-lying diaphragm
- *Tumours:* Secondary (most common), primary
- *Venous congestion:* Heart failure, hepatic vein occlusion
- *Haematological:* Leukaemia, lymphoma, myeloproliferative disorders, sickle cell disease
- *Biliary obstruction:* Particularly extrahepatic
- *Inflammation:* Hepatitis, abscess, schistosomiasis
- *Metabolic:* Fatty liver, early cirrhosis, amyloid, glycogen storage disease
- *Cysts:* Polycystic liver, hydatid

Hirsutism: 📖 p.658

Hoarseness: 📖 p.916

Hyperhidrosis: 📖 p.659

Hyperpigmentation: Normally due to hypermelanosis—occasionally, other pigments e.g. iron, carotene. *Causes:*
- *Genetic:* Racial; freckles/lentigo; neurofibromatosis; Peutz-Jeghers syndrome.
- *Drugs:*
  - Amiodarone—blue-grey pigmentation of sun-exposed areas
  - Minocycline—blue-black pigmentation in scars and buccal mucosa
  - Chloroquine—blue-grey pigmentation of face and arms
  - Chlorpromazine—grey pigment in sun-exposed sites
  - Cytotoxics
- *Endocrine:* Addison's disease; chloasma; Cushing's syndrome.
- *Nutritional:* Excess ingestion of carrots (carotinaemia); malabsorption; malnutrition; pellagra.
- *Post-inflammatory:* Eczema; lichen planus; systemic sclerosis.
- *Other:* Benign naevi; malignant melanoma; chronic renal failure; acanthosis nigricans.

Hypertrichosis: 📖 p.659

Table 9.8 Heart sounds, abnormalities, and their causes

Heart sound		Causes
1st heart sound Heard loudest at the apex Caused by closing of the mitral and tricuspid valves	Soft	Mitral regurgitation, low BP, rheumatic carditis, severe heart failure, LBBB
	Loud	AF, tachycardia, atrial premature beat, mitral stenosis
	Variable intensity	Varying duration of diastole, complete AV block
	Split	RBBB, paced beat from the left ventricle, left ventricular ectopics, ASD, Ebstein's anomaly, tricuspid stenosis
2nd heart sound Caused by closure of the aortic (A2) and pulmonary (P2) valves A2 and P2 split on inspiration so that P2 is heard after A2	Soft	A2—calcification of the aortic valve, dilatation of the aortic root P2—pulmonary stenosis
	Loud	A2—↑BP, thin patients P2—pulmonary hypertension, ASD
	Wide splitting	May be the result of early A2 or delayed P2 *Early A2*—mitral regurgitation, VSD *Delayed P2*—RBBB, pulmonary stenosis, ASD, right ventricular failure
	Reversed splitting	A2 is delayed. P2 occurs before A2 so the split between the sounds ↓ on inspiration *Delayed A2*—LBBB, systolic hypertension, HOCM, severe aortic stenosis, PDA, left heart failure
	Single	Calcification of the aortic valve, pulmonary stenosis, Fallot's tetralogy, Ebstein's anomaly, pericardial effusion, large VSD, obesity, emphysema
Clicks and snaps	Early systolic	Caused by opening of the aortic or pulmonary valves *Aortic*—aortic stenosis, bicuspid valve *Pulmonary*—pulmonary stenosis, pulmonary hypertension
	Mid/late systolic	Mitral valve prolapse
	Diastolic	Caused by opening of the mitral or tricuspid valves. Silent in the healthy heart *Mitral*—mitral stenosis, rapid mitral flow e.g. PDA, VSD, severe mitral regurgitation *Tricuspid* (rare)—rheumatic stenosis, ASD
3rd heart sound Heard in diastole after the 2nd heart sound	Right ventricle	Loudest at lower left sternal edge. Never normal. *Causes*—right heart failure, tricuspid regurgitation, ASD, constrictive pericarditis
	Left ventricle	Loudest at the apex when inclined to the left. Can be normal in children and pregnancy. *Other causes:* LVF, mitral regurgitation, anterior MI
4th heart sound Heard in late diastole		Maximal at the apex or lower left sternal edge. Never normal. *Causes*—ventricular hypertrophy or fibrosis and HOCM

Hyperventilation: May be fast (>20 breaths/min) or deep (tidal volume ↑). If inappropriate, results in palpitations, dizziness, faintness, tinnitus, chest pains, perioral and peripheral tingling (due to plasma Ca^{2+} ↓)—most common cause is anxiety; others include PE, early pulmonary oedema, hyperthyroidism, fever, lymphangitis, and weakness of respiratory muscles.

Kussmaul respiration: Deep, sighing breathing that is principally seen in metabolic acidosis e.g. diabetic ketoacidosis and uraemia.

Neurogenic hyperventilation: Hyperventilation produced by stroke, tumour, or CNS infection.

Hypoventilation: Abnormally decreased pulmonary ventilation. Respiration may be too slow or tidal volume ↓. *Causes include:*
- *Respiratory depression* e.g. opiate analgesia, anoxia, trauma
- *Neurological disease* e.g. Guillain-Barré disease, polio, motor neurone disease, syringobulbia
- *Lung disease* e.g. pneumonia, collapse, pneumothorax, pleural effusion
- *Respiratory muscle disease* e.g. myasthenia gravis, dermatomyositis
- *Limited chest movement* e.g. kyphoscoliosis

I

Ideas of reference: Thought disorders—📖 p.292

Illusions: Perceptions (abnormal)—📖 p.278

Impotence: Erectile dysfunction—📖 p.702

Incontinence
- **Faeces:** 📖 p.451
- **Urine:** 📖 p.694

Insomnia: 📖 p.242

Itch: Pruritus—📖 p.281

J

Jaundice: Yellow pigmentation due to excessive bile pigment. Clinical jaundice appears when serum bilirubin >35µmol/l. Always refer for further investigation (pre-hepatic and hepatic jaundice → physician; post-hepatic jaundice → surgeon)—Table 9.9. *Causes:*
- ↑ *production (pre-hepatic jaundice):* Haemolytic anaemia, drug-induced haemolysis, malaria, Gilbert's and Crigler-Najjar syndrome
- *Defective processing (hepatic jaundice):* Hepatitis, cirrhosis
- *Blocked excretion (obstructive jaundice):* Gallstones, carcinoma of the pancreas, primary biliary cirrhosis, primary sclerosing cholangitis, cholangiocarcinoma, sepsis, enlarged porta hepatis (e.g. due to lymphoma)

Table 9.9 Distinguishing different types of jaundice

	Type of jaundice		
	Pre-hepatic	**Hepatic**	**Obstructive**
Tests			
Bilirubin	↑↑	↑↑	↑↑
ALT	Normal	↑↑	↑
Alkaline phosphatase	Normal	↑	↑↑↑
Hb	↓	Normal	Normal
Jaundice	Mild, lemon yellow	Marked jaundice	Deep jaundice
Other symptoms		Tender, enlarged liver. Stools normal colour.	Itching skin, pale stools.

❶ A mixed picture is common and can be confusing.

Joint pain

Pain in 1 joint: Common. Ask:
- **Is the problem articular or periarticular?**
  - Articular disease (e.g. osteoarthritis)—joint line tenderness and pain at the end of the range of movement in any direction.
  - Periarticular problems (e.g. ligamentous injury)—point tenderness over the involved structure, and pain exacerbated by movements.
- **If periarticular**, which structure is causing pain? *Options:* Bursa; tendon; tendon sheath; ligament; soft tissue.
- **If articular**, is the problem inflammatory or mechanical? Look for:
  - Signs of inflammation—warmth, redness, effusions. May indicate joint infection or inflammatory arthritis.
  - Features of a mechanical problem—locking or catching e.g. cartilage tear.

⚠ **Red flags:** Features which should prompt early/urgent referral—
- Inflamed joint with associated fever or constitutional disturbance—beware of infection.
- Any joint which is 'locked' or so painful that movement is impossible.
- Severe pain at rest or at night.
- Pain that gets relentlessly worse over a period of days or weeks.

Pain in multiple joints
- Differentiate between articular or periarticular disease and whether the condition is inflammatory or not, as for pain in 1 joint (above). Screening with blood tests (ESR or CRP, FBC ± autoimmune profile) may help.
- Look for the pattern of disease—joint sites involved and other symptoms/signs.

Common arthropathies:
- Osteoarthritis
- Rheumatoid arthritis
- Ankylosing spondylitis
- SLE
- Reactive arthritis

- Psoriatic arthritis
- Enteropathic arthropathy
- Gout or pseudogout
- Sicca syndrome
- Malignancy

⚠ **Red flags:** Features which should prompt early/urgent referral—
- Severe systemic symptoms—high fevers, significant weight loss, or a very ill patient (suggests rheumatoid arthritis, sepsis, or malignancy).
- Focal systemic signs e.g. rashes, nodules, or GI disturbances.
- Severe pain and/or inability to function.

Jugular venous pressure: Observe internal jugular vein at 45° with head turned slightly to the left. Vertical height is measured in relation to the sternal angle. Raised if >4cm.

Causes of ↑ JVP
- Fluid overload
- Right heart failure and CCF
- SVC obstruction (non-pulsatile)
- Tricuspid or pulmonary valve disease

- Pulmonary hypertension
- Arrythmia—AF or atrial flutter, complete heart block
- ↑ intrathoracic pressure e.g. pneumothorax, PE, emphysema

Kussmaul's sign: The JVP usually drops on inspiration, along with intrathoracic pressure. The reverse pattern is called Kussmaul's sign. Caused by ↑ intrathoracic pressure or constrictive pericarditis. (*A. Kussmaul (1822–1902)—German physician*)

Wave patterns
- *A wave:* Due to right atrial systole; coincides with the 1st heart sound; precedes the carotid pulse.
- *C wave:* Due to transmission of right ventricular pressure before the tricuspid valve closes. Rarely visible.
- *X descent:* Due to relaxation of the right atrium.
- *V wave:* Due to venous blood filling the right atrium whilst the tricuspid valve is closed as the ventricles contract. Occurs at the same time as the carotid pulse.
- *Y descent:* Due to opening of the tricuspid valve when the ventricles relax.

Abnormal wave patterns: Table 9.10

K

Koilonychia: 📖 p.661

Table 9.10 Abnormal JVP wave patterns and their causes

Condition	Abnormal wave pattern
Tricuspid regurgitation	Large systolic wave which replaces the C and V wave with steep Y descent
Tricuspid stenosis	Large A wave, small V wave, slow Y descent
Complete heart block, VT, or other causes of atrio-ventricular dissociation	Cannon waves: very large A waves which occur when the right atrium contracts against a closed tricuspid valve
AF	Absent A wave, C wave normal
Constrictive pericarditis	Kussmaul's sign, steep Y descent

L

Left iliac fossa pain: Treat the cause. *Common causes:*
Acute
- Gastroenteritis
- Ureteric colic
- UTI
- Diverticulitis
- Torted ovarian cyst
- Salpingitis
- Ectopic
- Volvulus
- Pelvic abscess

Chronic/subacute
- Constipation
- Irritable bowel syndrome
- Colon cancer
- Inflammatory bowel disease
- Hip pathology

Left upper quadrant pain: Treat the cause. *Causes:*
- Large kidney or spleen
- Gastric or colonic cancer
- Pneumonia
- Subphrenic or perinephric abscess
- Renal colic
- Pyelonephritis

Leg ulceration: 📖 p.640

Lethargy: Tired all the time—📖 p.582

Leoconychia: 📖 p.660

Lid lag: Lagging behind of the lid as the eye looks down.
- *Lid retraction:* Static state of the upper eyelid traversing the eye above the iris, rather than transecting it.
- *Causes of lid lag and lid retraction:* Thyrotoxicosis and anxiety.

Limping child: 📖 p.872

Loin pain: Pain in the side at the back below the ribs. *Causes:*
- Pyelonephritis
- Pain referred from the back
- Hydronephrosis
- Renal stone
- Renal tumour
- Perinephric abscess

Loss of consciousness (history of): Check the patient lost consciousness, not felt faint or dizzy. *Causes:*

- Vasovagal—fainting 📖 p.261
- Micturition or cough syncope—📖 p.292
- Effort syncope—loss of consciousness on exercise, usually of cardiac origin
- Carotid sinus syncope—loss of consciousness on turning head too far
- Epilepsy—📖 p.618
- Stokes-Adams attacks—📖 p.346
- TIA—📖 p.606
- Hypoglycaemia—📖 p.413 and 1070
- Postural/orthostatic hypotension—📖 p.280

Lumps in the neck: Most neck lumps are reactive LNs—suggested by a short history, soft tender mobile lump, and concurrent infection. Give these a few weeks to settle. If not settling, check FBC and ESR and refer for further investigation. Other lumps—consider history and site.

If superficial to the underlying muscle and fascia: *Consider:*
- Sebaceous cyst
- Lipoma
- Lymphoma
- TB
- Neurofibroma

Midline swelling: *Consider:*
- Dermoid cyst
- Thyroglossal cyst (moves on sticking out tongue)
- Pharyngeal pouch
- Laryngocoele
- Subhyoid bursa
- Plunging ranula
- Carcinoma of the larynx, trachea, or oesophagus

Lateral structures: Reactive LNs are most common. *Other causes:*
- Thyroid swelling
- Branchial cyst
- Cystic hygroma
- Carotid artery aneurysm
- A-V fistula
- Spinal abscess
- Cervical rib
- Carotid body, sternomastoid, or salivary gland tumour

Lymphadenopathy: Palpable enlargement of the LNs
Benign causes
- *Infective*
  - Bacterial—pyogenic, TB, brucella
  - Fungal
  - Viral—EBV, CMV, HIV
  - Toxoplasmosis
  - Syphilis
- *Non-infective:* Sarcoid, connective tissue disease (rheumatoid); skin disease (eczema, psoriasis); drugs (phenytoin); berylliosis.

Malignant: Lymphoma, CLL, ALL, metastases.

Management
- *Adults:* If LNs persist >2wk. check FBC, ESR ± EBV screen. Refer lymphadenopathy >1cm diameter persisting for >6wk. for urgent further investigation.
- *Children:* Refer to paediatrics urgently if:
  - Non-tender, firm/hard LN >3cm diameter
  - Progressively enlarging LNs

- LNs associated with other signs of ill-health (e.g. fever, weight loss)
- Enlarged axillary nodes or supraclavicular nodes in the absence of local infection

Lymphoedema: 📖 p.1013

M

Meningism: Headache, stiff neck, and photophobia. Associated with meningitis. May also be seen with encephalitis and SAH.

Menstrual problems: Period problems—📖 p.279

Mouth ulcers: Treat the cause. *Consider:*
- Apthous ulcers
- Trauma e.g. sharp tooth, false teeth
- Crohn's
- UC
- Coeliac
- Drugs e.g. steroids, gold
- Reiter's disease
- Bechet's disease
- Herpes simplex
- Herpes zoster
- Vincent's angina
- Erythema multiforme
- Self-inflicted e.g. burns

⚠ If a mouth ulcer remains for >3wk, refer to oral surgeons for biopsy.

Sore mouth: 📖 p.290

Movement patterns (abnormal)

Asterixis: Intermittent lapses of an assumed posture. May involve arms, neck, tongue, jaw, and eyelids. Usually bilateral, absent at rest, and asynchronous on each side. *Causes:* Liver failure (flapping tremor), heart failure, respiratory failure, renal failure, hypoglycaemia, barbiturate intoxication.

Athetosis: Slow, confluent, often rhythmic, purposeless movements of hands, tongue, fingers, or face. *Causes:* Cerebral palsy, kernicterus.

Chorea: Non-rhythmic, jerky, purposeless movements (especially hands) with voluntary movements possible in between. *Most common causes:* Cerebral palsy, Huntington's chorea, Sydenham's chorea.

Gait (abnormal): 📖 p.263

Hemiballismus: Large-amplitude, involuntary flinging movements of limbs. May occur after stroke, in Huntington's disease, or with high doses of L-dopa for PD.

Myoclonus: Sudden involuntary focal or general jerks. May be normal, especially if occurs when falling asleep. *Other causes:*
- Neurodegenerative disease (e.g. CJD)
- Myoclonic epilepsy
- Benign essential myoclonus (generalized myoclonus beginning in childhood as muscle twitches; may be inherited as autosomal dominant)
- Asterixis (metabolic flap e.g. liver failure, uraemia)

Treatment: If needed, treat with sodium valproate or clonazepam.

Tardive dyskinesia: Involuntary chewing and grimacing movements due to long-term neuroleptics (metoclopramide and prochlorperazine are also possible causes). Withdraw neuroleptic—if no improvement after 3–6mo. consider tetrabenazine 25–50mg tds po.

Tics: Brief, repeated, and stereotyped movements which are able to be suppressed voluntarily for a while. Common in children and usually resolve spontaneously. Consider clonazepam or clonidine if tics are severe.

Gilles de la Tourette syndrome: 📖 p.891

Myalgia: Isolated myalgia can be a result of overuse or soft tissue injury. Generalized myalgia is associated with many diseases including:
- Infection
- Fibromyalgia
- PAN
- Wegener's granulomatosis

Myoclonus: Movement patterns (abnormal)—📖 p.275

N

Nail changes: 📖 p.660

Nasal obstruction: 📖 p.918. Common symptom experienced by most people from time to time. *Causes:*
- *Mucosal swelling:* Coryza, allergic, or vasomotor rhinitis, iatrogenic, polyps
- *Septal deviation:* Trauma, congenital e.g. 2° to cleft lip
- *Other:* Tumour, enlarged adenoids (associated with glue ear and deafness), foreign body

⚠ **Red flag:** Assume consistent unilateral blockage is neoplastic until proved otherwise. Refer urgently to ENT.

Neck
- Pain: 📖 p.548
- Lumps: 📖 p.274
- Stiffness: Exclude life-threatening causes e.g. meningitis, SAH. Other causes are neck arthritis, painful cervical lymphaedenopathy, upper lobe pneumonia.

Night sweats: *Consider:* TB; lymphoma; leukaemia; solid tumour (e.g. renal carcinoma); menopause; anxiety states.

Nipple discharge: 📖 p.513

Nipple eczema: 📖 p.513

Nodules: Skin lesions—📖 p.289

Nose bleeds: 📖 p.1042

Nystagmus: Involuntary, oscillatory eye movements. Can be congenital or due to labyrinthine or visual system problems. Refer all cases, unless associated with self-limiting labyrinthitis, for assessment.

O

Obesity: 📖 p.230

Obsessions: Thought disorders—📖 p.293

Odd ideas
- **Acute confusion:** 📖 p.976
- **Compulsions:** 📖 p.253
- **Delusions:** 📖 p.255
- **Dementia:** 📖 p.978
- **Flight of ideas:** Thought disorders—📖 p.293
- **Hallucinations:** 📖 p.266
- **Ideas of reference:** Thought disorders—📖 p.292
- **Obsessions:** Thought disorders—📖 p.293
- **Overvalued ideas:** Beliefs (abnormal)—📖 p.249
- **Perceptions (abnormal):** 📖 p.278
- **Thought disorders:** 📖 p.292

Oedema: Abnormal accumulation of fluid in the intercellular spaces. Results from:
- ↓ drainage of the intercellular fluid by the lymphatics e.g. lympho-edema (📖 p.1013)
- ↑ capillary permeability → ↑ intercellular fluid e.g. infection, inflammation
- ↓ capillary hydrostatic pressure due to:
  - ↑ pressure at the arterial end of the capillary
  - ↑ venous back-pressure e.g. DVT, paralysis of a limb, right heart failure
  - ↓ intracapillary protein e.g. hypoalbuminaemia due to cirrhosis, nephritic syndrome, or malignancy

Swelling of the ankles/legs: 📖 p.291

Off legs: Walking difficulty—📖 p.297

Oliguria: Urine output <400ml/24h. *Causes:* dehydration, cardiac failure, ureteric obstruction, acute or chronic renal failure.

Orthopnoea: Dyspnoea on lying flat and relieved by sitting up. Associated with left heart dysfunction e.g. LVF.

P

Painful periods: Dysmennorhoea/painful periods—📖 p.726

Pallor: Non-specific sign which may be racial, familial, or cosmetic. Pathology suggested includes anaemia, shock, Stokes-Adams attack, vasovagal faint, myxoedema, hypopituitarism, and albinism.

Palmar erythema: Associated with pregnancy, liver disease, and polycythaemia.

Palpitations: The uncomfortable awareness of heart beat. Can be physiological (e.g. after exercise, at times of stress) or signify arrhythmia. Ask the patient to tap out the rhythm.
- **Bradycardia:** 📖 p.346
- **Occasional missed beat:** suggests ventricular ectopics—📖 p.342
- **Tachycardia:** 📖 p.342

Papilloedema: *Causes:*
- Intracranial SOL
- Encephalitis
- SAH
- Benign intracranial hypertension
- Malignant hypertension

- Optic neurtitis
- Disc infiltration e.g. leukaemia
- Ischaemic optic neuropathy
- Retinal venous obstruction
- Metabolic causes
  e.g. hypoclacaemia

⚠ Always refer any patient with papilloedema for immediate specialist medical opinion.

Parasternal heave: Detect by placing the heel of the hand over the left parasternal region. When a heave is present, the heel of the hand is lifted off the chest wall with each heart beat. *Causes:* Usually due to right ventricular enlargement; rarely due to left atrial enlargement.

Parkinsonism: 📖 p.610

Paroxysmal nocturnal dyspnoea: Acute form of dyspnoea that causes the patient to awake from sleep. The patient is forced to sit upright or stand out of bed for relief. Associated with pulmonary oedema.

Pelvic mass: Characterized by not being able to get beneath it.

Causes of pelvic mass
- Foetus
- Full bladder
- Fibroids

- Gynaecological malignancy
- Bladder cancer

Pelvic pain: 📖 p.720

Penile discharge: Associated with urethritis e.g. due to Chlamydia or gonorrhoea. Refer to GUM clinic.

Perceptions (abnormal): *Consider:*
- **Illusion:** Misinterpretation of visual or other information e.g. a person seeing a shadow of a tree moving in the breeze might interpret it as a person moving. Can happen if ↓ level of consciousness or occasionally if visual impairment.
- **Hallucination:** False perception i.e. without an external stimulus— 📖 p.266.
- **Pseudohallucination:** Vivid perception which is recognized as not being real e.g. delirium tremens.
- **Depersonalization:** Feeling of being unreal—like an actor playing yourself. Associated with a wide range of mental illness e.g. depression, schizophrenia.
- **Derealization:** Feeling of everything around you being unreal—like in a dream. Often linked to depersonalization.

Perianal pain: Treat the cause. *Consider:*
- Haemorrhoids
- Anal fissure
- Perianal haematoma
- Perianal abscess
- Rectal/anal tumour
- Perianal fistula
- Proctalgia fugax—intense stabbing pain for no apparent cause; aetiology unknown

Period problems
- **Absent/infrequent periods:** 📖 p.728
- **Menorrhagia/heavy periods:** 📖 p.724
- **Dysmenorrhoea/painful periods:** 📖 p.726
- **Infrequent periods:** 📖 p.728
- **Intermenstrual bleeding:** 📖 p.714
- **Postcoital bleeding:** 📖 p.714
- **Postmenopausal bleeding:** 📖 p.713
- **Prolonged menstruation:** 📖 p.280
- **Wish to postpone a period:** 📖 p.748

Perseveration: Thought disorders—📖 p.293

Petechiae: Purpura—📖 p.284

Photophobia: Painful vision in normal light. One of the 3 principle features of meningism. Associated with meningitis. Discomfort in the light can also be a feature of eye disease e.g. conjunctivitis and migraine.

Photosensitivity: 📖 p.662

Pigmentation of skin
- **Hypopigmentation**—📖 p.656
- **Hyperpigmentation**—📖 p.656

Pleuritic chest pain/pleurisy: Chest pain—📖 p.251

Pleural effusion: 📖 p.392

Pleural rub: Creaking sound produced by movement of visceral over parietal pleura when both are inflamed (e.g. pneumonia, infarction).

Polydipsia: Over-frequent drinking of fluid; often associated, for logical reasons, with polyuria. Ask if it is associated with thirst. Take a history of fluid intake. If no history of excess fluid intake and BM/fasting blood glucose is normal, investigate further with U&E, Cr, and Ca^{2+}.

Common causes
- *Change in lifestyle*—may be associated with polyuria but no other symptoms. No history of thirst.
- *DM*—usually accompanied by a history of thirst.

Other causes: Diabetes insipidus, hypercalcaemia, compulsive water drinking (may be a feature of psychotic illness), and phosphorus poisoning.

Polyuria: Passage of excessive urine. Check the patient does not mean frequency of urination. It can be difficult to distinguish the two. Causes are similar to those of polydipsia and the 2 symptoms are related. Take a history of fluid intake. If no history of excess fluid intake and BM/fasting blood glucose is normal, investigate further with MSU (for M, C & S), U&E, Cr, and Ca^{2+}.

Consider
- *DM*—always check a BM and/or fasting blood glucose if a patient complains of polyuria
- *Diabetes insipidus*
- *Hypercalcaemia*
- *Excessive intake*—due to change in lifestyle or psychiatric conditions e.g. schizophrenia
- *Chronic renal failure*
- *Drugs*—diuretics, caffeine, alcohol

Postcoital bleeding: 📖 p.714

Postural hypotension: *At-risk groups:*
- Young women, particularly if pregnant
- The elderly
- Patients taking medication with hypotensive side-effects e.g. β-blockers
- Patients with autonomic neuropathy e.g. 2° to PD or DM

Presentation: Patients complain of falls, faints, or feeling light-headed when they stand up, particularly when getting out of bed or a hot bath.

Examination: Confirm diagnosis by checking BP—lying and then standing. Standing usually causes a slight ↓ in the systolic BP (<20mmHg) and a slight ↑ in the diastolic BP (<10mmHg). In postural hypotension, there is usually a marked ↓ in both systolic and diastolic BP.

Management
- *Review medication*—Stop any non-essential medication contributing to symptoms e.g. night sedation, unnecessary diuretics
- *Optimize treatment* of intercurrent heart disease, PD, or DM
- *Advice*—advise patients to take care when standing, especially when getting up from their beds, on getting out of a hot bath or shower, and after meals

Precocious puberty: 📖 p.282

Priapism: Persistent painful erection not related to sexual desire.
Cause: Intracavernosal injection for impotence, idiopathic, leukaemia, sickle cell disease, or pelvic tumour.

Treatment: Ask the patient to climb stairs (arterial 'steal' phenomenon), apply ice packs. If unsuccessful, refer to A&E for aspiration of corpora. Rarely, surgery is needed.

Prolonged menstruation: Bleeding for >5–6d./cycle. Most loss occurs in the first 3d. . Long periods do not equate to ↑ menstrual loss, so prolonged menstruation *per se* does not need investigation. Frequently goes with menorrhagia—📖 p.724.

Prostatism: Symptoms of prostate enlargement. In all cases consider alternative causes of symptoms. 2 elements:

Irritative symptoms: Urgency, dysuria, frequency, nocturia. *Differential diagnosis:* Enlarged prostate, UTI, polydipsia, detrusor instability, hypercalcaemia, uraemia.

Obstructive symptoms: ↓ size and force of urinary stream, hesitancy and interruption of stream whilst voiding. *Differential diagnosis:* Prostatic enlargement, strictures, tumours, urethral valves, bladder neck contracture.

International prostate symptom score: 📖 p.704

Management of BPH and prostate cancer: 📖 p.686–9

Pruritus: Itch. *Are there skin lesions present?*

Skin lesions present
- *Examine the skin lesion:* Search for unexcoriated lesions.
- *Investigation:* Normally not warranted. Exceptions are patch testing for contact dermatitis and skin biopsy for dermatitis herpetiformis.

Causes

- Urticaria
- Contact dermatitis and allergies to food and drugs
- Prickly heat
- Skin infestations e.g. scabies, pediculosis, insect bites
- Infections—viral e.g. chickenpox; fungal
- Dermatitis herpetiformis
- Lichen planus
- Senile atrophy

❶ Don't forget psychological causes in which excessive excoriation causes lichenification of the skin.

Skin lesions absent: Large differential diagnosis:
- *Examination:* Look for pallor, jaundice, weight ↓, LN enlargement, and abdominal organomegaly.
- *Investigation:* As necessary—consider urinalysis (dipstick and MSU), FBC, ESR, Serum ferritin, LFTs (including alkaline phosphatase), U&E, glucose, serum Ca^{2+} (correct for low albumin), TFTs, and CXR.
- If still undiagnosed, refer.

Causes
- Hepatic—obstructive jaundice, pregnancy
- Endocrine—DM, thyrotoxicosis, hypothyroidism, hyperparathyroidism
- Renal—chronic renal failure
- Haematological—polycythaemia rubra vera, iron deficiency, leukaemia, Hodgkin's disease
- Malignancy—any carcinoma
- Drug allergies
- Psychological—obsessive states, schizophrenia
- Rare causes—diabetes insipidus, roundworm infection

Pruritus ani
- Itch occurs if the anus is moist or soiled e.g. poor personal hygiene; anal leakage or faecal incontinence; fissures; nylon/tight underwear.
- *Other causes:* Dermatological conditions (e.g. contact dermatitis, lichen sclerosus); threadworm infection; anxiety; other causes of generalized pruritus (above).

Management: Treat cause if possible; avoid spicy food; moist wipe post-defaecation.

Pseudohallucination: 📖 p.278

Ptosis: Drooping of the upper eyelid. *Causes:*
- *3rd nerve lesion:* Usually causes unilateral complete ptosis. Look for other evidence of 3rd nerve lesion (opthalmoplegia with outward deviation of the eye, pupil dilated and unreactive to light, and accommodation).
- *Sympathetic paralysis:* Usually causes unilateral partial ptosis. Look for other evidence of sympathetic lesion (constricted pupil, lack of sweating on same side of face—*Horner's syndrome*).
- *Myopathy (dystrophia myotonica, myasthenia gravis):* Usually causes bilateral partial ptosis.
- *Congenital (present since birth):* May be unilateral or bilateral; is usually partial; and is not associated with other neurological signs.
- *Syphilis*

Puberty:
Delayed puberty: No pubertal changes in a girl aged 13y. or boy aged 13½ y. or failure of progression of puberty over 2y. Affects ~2% population. In all cases refer to paediatrics for further investigation. Constitutional delay accounts for 90%. *Other causes:* Chromosomal abnormalities (e.g. Turner's or Klinefelter's syndromes); GnRH deficiency (e.g. pituitary lesions, gonadal failure, hypothyroidism); hypothalamic suppression (e.g. anorexia nervosa, sportsmen, systemic illness).

Precocious puberty: Puberty before the normal age for the population. In the UK this is <8y. for girls and <9y. for boys. In all cases, refer for specialist investigation and advice on management. Precocious puberty may be:
- *True:* Course and pattern are normal, but early. *Causes:* Idiopathic (90% ♀; 50–60% ♂), hypothalamic tumour, other CNS pathology.
- *Pseudo:* Pattern is abnormal e.g. 1 element of puberty occurs (e.g. breast development), but other elements do not. *Causes:* Idiopathic, testicular or ovarian tumour, congenital adrenal hyperplasia, hepatoblastoma, adrenal virilizing tumours, Cushing's syndrome.

Pulmonary oedema: Accumulation of fluid in the pulmonary tissues and air spaces. *Causes include:*

Cardiac/vascular
- Left heart failure
- Mitral stenosis
- MI
- Hypertension

Other
- High altitude
- Kidney failure
- Nephrotic syndrome
- Cirrhosis

- Pulmonary venous obstruction
- IV fluid overload

Lung
- Pneumonia
- Pneumonitis due to inhalation of toxic substances e.g. gases or radiation

- Lymphatic obstruction e.g. due to tumour

- PE

Pulses: When assessing the pulse, consider:

Rate
- *Tachycardia*: >100bpm—📖 p.342
- *Bradycardia*: <60bpm—📖 p.346

Rhythm
- *Irregularly irregular*: AF, multiple ectopics
- *Regularly irregular*: 2nd degree heart block

Character and volume: Assess with a central pulse e.g. carotid or femoral.
- *Small volume:* Shock, pericardial tamponade, aortic stenosis (slow-rising).
- *Large volume:* Hyperdynamic circulation (e.g. pregnancy), aortic incompetence (water-hammer, collapsing pulse), PDA.
- *Pulsus paradoxus:* Pulse weakens in inspiration by >10mmHg—asthma, cardiac tamponade, pericarditis.

Foot pulses: 📖 p.361.

Pupil abnormalities: Pupils are normally central, of equal size, and react equally to light and accommodation. *Pupil abnormalities:*

Fixed dilated pupil: *Causes:* trauma (e.g. blow to the iris), mydriatics, acute glaucoma, 3rd nerve palsy, coning.

Afferent pupillary defect: Pupils are the same size but there is an absent constriction response to light in the affected eye. Constriction does occur if light is shone into the other eye (consensual response). *Causes:* optic neuritis, retinal disease.

Argyll–Robertson pupil: Occurs in patients with DM and neurosyphilis. Bilateral small irregular pupils with no light response. (*D. Argyll Robertson (1837–1909)—Scottish ophthalmologist*)

Holmes–Adie pupil: Accommodation is partially paralysed causing blurring of near vision, slight pupil dilation, and a very slow pupil response to light and accommodation (minutes). Occurs unilaterally in young adults. It is not associated with serious neurological disease. (*G.M. Holmes (1876–1965)—Irish neurologist; W.J. Adie (1886–1935)—British neurologist*)

Horner's syndrome: Sympathetic nerve disruption to the iris causes a small (miotic) pupil, partial lid ptosis, and lack of pupil dilation in the dark. *Causes:* Pancoast tumour, aortic aneurysm, MS, posterior inferior artery or basilar artery occlusion, cervical cord or mediastinal tumour, hypothalamic lesions, syringomyelia. (*J. F. Horner (1831–1886)—Swiss ophthalmologist*)

Purpura: Blue-brown discolouration of the skin due to bleeding within it. Petechiae are small dot-like purpura, whilst ecchymoses are more extensive. Treat the cause. *Causes:*
- **Idiopathic:** e.g. idiopathic pigmented purpura (brownish punctate lesions on the legs).
- **Vessel wall defects:** Vasculitis; paraproteinaemia; infection (e.g. meningococcal meningitis, septicaemia, EBV); ↑ intravascular pressure (e.g. venous disease).
- **Clotting defects:** Abnormal platelet function; thrombocytopoenia; anticoagulant therapy; coagulation factor deficiency.
- **Defective dermal support:** Dermal atrophy (e.g. ageing, steroids, disease); scurvy (vitamin C deficiency).

⚠ Admit any patient with new purpura who is unwell as a 999 emergency.

Henoch–Schönlein purpura (HSP): Presents with a purpuric rash over buttocks and extensor surfaces. Often follows a respiratory infection. Commoner in children than adults; ♂ > ♀. *Other features:*
- Urticaria
- Abdominal pain (± intussusception)—may mimic an acute abdomen
- Nephritis
- Platelet count is normal
- Joint pains

Prognosis: Most recover fully over a few months.
(E. Henoch (1820–1910) and J. Schönlein (1793–1864)—German physicians)

Pyrexia: Oral temperature raised above 37.5°C. Normal range varies according to where the temperature is measured—Table 9.11. *Common causes:*

Infection: By far the most common cause in general practice.
- Viral infection (e.g. EBV, URTI, influenza)
- UTI
- Chest infection
- Tonsillitis
- OM
- Sinusitis
- Cholecystitis
- Cellulitis

❶ Don't forget tropical diseases e.g. malaria in patients returning from abroad. Think of TB and SBE—especially in high-risk patients.

Cancer: Lymphoma; leukaemia; solid tumours (e.g. hypernephroma).
Immunogenic causes: Connective tissue disease and autoimmune disease (e.g. RA, SLE, PAN, polymyalgia rheumatica); sarcoidosis.
Thrombosis: DVT; PE   **Drugs:** e.g. antibiotics

Table 9.11 Normal temperature as measured in different locations

Place of measurement	Normal range
Oral	35.5–37.5°C (95.9–99.5°F)
Rectal	36.6–38.0°C (97.9–100.4°F)
Axillary	34.7–37.3°C (94.5–99.1°F)
Ear	35.8–38.0°C (96.4–100.4°F)

Pyrexia of unknown origin: Defined as a fever (either intermittent or continuous) which has lasted for >3wk. and for which no cause has been found. Re-check history. Re-examine carefully. Check FBC; monospot (depending on age of the patient); ESR; LFTs; urine (M,C&S); viral titres and blood cultures; and CXR. If cause does not become obvious, refer urgently for further investigation.

R

Rash: Skin eruption—📖 p.288

Rebound abdominal pain: Present if, on the sudden removal of pressure from the examiner's hand, the patient feels a momentary increase in pain. It signifies local peritoneal inflammation.

Rectal bleeding in adults: 📖 p.1040

Rectal bleeding in children: 📖 p.856

Red eye: 📖 p.936

Reflexes: A reflex is an automatic response to a stimulus. The pathway a reflex follows (reflex arc) goes from the stimulus, via a sensory nerve, to the spinal cord, and then back along a motor nerve to cause muscle contraction, without involvement of the brain.

Absent or ↓ reflex: Implies a breach in the reflex arc e.g.
• Sensory nerve or root e.g. neuropathy, spondylosis
• Anterior horn cell e.g. MND, polio
• Motor nerve or root e.g. neuropathy, spondylosis
• Nerve endings e.g. myasthenia gravis
• Muscle e.g. myopathy

↑ reflex: Implies lack of higher control—an upper motor neurone lesion e.g. post-stroke

Infantile reflexes: 📖 p.816

Reinforcement: Method of accentuating reflexes. Use if a reflex seems absent. Ask the patient to clench his teeth (to reinforce upper limb reflexes) or clench his hands and pull in opposite directions (to accentuate lower limb reflexes). This effect only lasts ~1s., so ask the patient to perform the manoeuvre simultaneously with the tap from the tendon hammer.

Key tendon reflexes: Table 9.12 (📖 p.286). Record whether absent, present with reinforcement, normal, or brisk ± clonus.

Table 9.12 Tendon reflexes and nerve roots involved

Reflex	Test	Expected result	Nerve roots
Jaw	Ask the patient to let his mouth open slightly. Place a finger on the chin and tap the finger with a tendon hammer.	Contraction of the masseters and closure of the mouth	5th cranial nerve
Biceps	Tap a finger placed on the biceps tendon by letting the tendon hammer fall on it.	Contraction of the biceps + elbow flexion	C5, C6
Supinator	Tap the lower end of the radius just above the wrist with the tendon hammer.	Contraction of brachioradialis + elbow flexion	C5, C6
Triceps	Support elbow in flexion with 1 hand. Tap the triceps tendon with a tendon hammer held in the other hand.	Contraction of the triceps + elbow extension	C6, C7
Knee	Support the knees so relaxed and slightly bent. Let the tendon hammer fall onto the infrapatellar tendon.	Contraction of quadriceps + extension of the knee	L3, L4
Ankle	Externally rotate the thigh and flex the knee. Let the tendon hammer fall onto the Achilles tendon.	Contraction of the gastrocnemius + plantar flexion of the ankle	S1

Other reflexes

- **Gag reflex** (IXth/Xth cranial nerves): Touch the back of the patient's pharynx on each side with a spatula → contraction of the soft palate. If absent, ask the patient whether he can feel the spatula. If he can, then Xth nerve palsy.
- **Abdominal reflexes** (T7–12): Lightly stroke the abdominal wall diagonally towards the umbilicus in each of the 4 abdominal quadrants. Absent abdominal wall contractions can be normal or indicate UMN or LMN lesion.
- **Cremaster reflex** (L1): Male patients only. Pre-warn the patient. Stroke the superior and medial aspect of the thigh in a downwards direction → contraction of the cremasteric muscle → raising of scrotum and testis on the side stroked. Absent in UMN and LMN lesions.
- **Plantar reflex** (S1): Pre-warn the patient. Run a blunt object up the lateral side of the sole of the foot, curving medially before the MTP joints → flexion of the big toe (if >1y. old). Extension implies UMN lesion.
- **Anal reflex** (S4/S5): Scratch the perianal skin → reflex contraction of the external sphincter. Absent in UMN and LMN lesions.

Clonus: Rhythmic involuntary muscle contraction due to abrupt stretching of a tendon e.g. by dorsi flexing the ankle. Associated with UMN lesions.

Regurgitation: Gastric and oesophageal contents are brought back effortlessly into the mouth. Regurgitation is rarely preceded by nausea, and when due to gastro-oesophageal reflux, often associated with heartburn. *Causes:* Gastro-oesophageal reflux, oesophageal pouch.

❶ Very high GI obstructions (e.g. gastric volvulus) cause non-productive retching rather than true regurgitation.

Renal colic: 📖 p.684

Restless legs: 📖 p.624

Respiratory rate: Normal rate for an adult is 14 breaths/min. at rest. Higher in children:
- **Neonate:** 30–60 breaths/min.
- **Infant:** 20–40 breaths/min.
- **1–3y.:** 20–30 breaths/min.
- **4–10y.:** 15–25 breaths/min.
- **>10y.:** 15–20 breaths/min.

↑ **respiratory rate:** *Consider:*
- Lung disease e.g. pneumonia, asthma
- Heart disease e.g. LVF
- Metabolic disease e.g. ketoacidosis
- Drugs e.g. salicylate overdose
- Psychiatric causes e.g. hyperventilation

↓ **respiratory rate:** *Consider:*
- CNS disease e.g. CVA
- Drugs e.g. opiates
- Cheyne-Stokes respiration

Retention of urine: 📖 p.690

Rhinorrhoea: Runny nose. If clear discharge, then may be physiological (e.g. due to cold) or due to allergy (e.g. hayfever or viral URTI). If green, indicates active bacterial infection. A yellow discharge may indicate viral or bacterial infection or allergy.

Right iliac fossa pain: Treat the cause. *Common causes:*
Acute
- Gastroenteritis
- Ureteric colic
- UTI
- Appendicitis
- Torted ovarian cyst
- Salpingitis
- Ectopic
- Volvulus
- Pelvic abscess

Chronic/subacute
- Constipation
- Irritable bowel syndrome
- Colon cancer
- Inflammatory bowel disease
- Hip pathology

Right upper quadrant (hypochondrial) pain: Treat the cause.
Consider:
- Gallstones
- Hepatitis
- Appendicitis e.g. if pregnant
- Colonic cancer at the hepatic flexure
- Perinephric abscess
- Right kidney pathology e.g. renal colic; pyelonephritis
- Intrathoracic conditions e.g. pneumonia
- Subphrenic abscess

Rigors: Shaking episodes (sometimes violent) associated with sudden rise in fever.

Romberg's sign: Ask the patient to stand with feet together. Observe how steady he is. Then ask the patient to shut his eyes. Again, observe how steady he is. +ve if the patient requires vision to stand steadily.

Interpretation
- *Sensory ataxia:* Lack of proprioception → unsteadiness without visual feedback.
- *Cerebellar ataxia:* The patient is equally unsteady whether his eyes are open or closed.

Runny nose: Rhinorrhoea—📖 p.287

S

Scrotal lumps: *Causes:* Hydrocoele, epididymal cyst, testicular tumour, varicocoele. If you cannot get above the lump, consider inguinal hernia.

Sexual problems
- **Postcoital bleeding:** 📖 p.714
- **Dyspareunia:** 📖 p.726
- **Psychosexual problems:** 📖 p.746
- **Impotence/erectile dysfunction:** 📖 p.702

Short stature: 📖 p.885

Sinusitis: 📖 p.919

Skin discolouration
- **Hyperpigmentation:** 📖 p.656
- **Hypopigmentation:** 📖 p.656

Skin eruption: Clues come from:
- *Age and gender of patient*
- *History:* Time course, distribution, exposure to possible provoking factors, similar symptoms in others
- *PMH:* Atopy, similar symptoms, genetic conditions, drugs, alcohol
- *FH:* Atopy, similar symptoms, genetic conditions
- *Examination:* Distribution and characteristics of lesions (see skin lesions—see opposite), general examination
- *Investigation:* Often unnecessary—direct at confirming cause

Treat according to cause ([] p.631–75). *Differential diagnosis:*

- Psoriasis
- Eczema
- Urticaria
- Lichenoid eruptions
- Photodermatoses
- Heat rash

- Papulosquamous eruptions
- Erythroderma
- Vasculitis
- Blistering disorders

- Bacterial infection
- Viral infection
- Fungal infection
- Scabies
- Insect bites

Skin lesions

Blisters: [] p.652

Brown spots: *Consider:*

- Freckles
- Moles
- Lentigos—like freckles but darker and not affected by sunlight

- Melanoma
- BCC
- Café au lait spots— >5 associated with neurofibromatosis
- Seborrhoeic warts

- Senile keratoses
- Dermatofibroma
- Systemic disease— Addison's Acanthosis nigrans, Haemachromatosis

Linear lesions: *Consider:*

- Koebner phenomenon—psoriasis, eczema, lichen planus
- Linear urticaria
- Self-inflicted trauma—dermatitis artefacta
- Reaction to garden plants—psoralen-induced phytophotodermatitis
- Impetigo—may spread along scratch marks
- Herpes zoster—at the edge of a dermatome

Ring-shaped lesions: *Consider:*

- Psoriasis
- Fungal infection e.g. ringworm
- Granuloma annulare

- Discoid eczema
- Erythema multiforme
- BCC
- Urticaria

- Pityriasis rosea
- Lichen planus
- Burns (especially on a child—may be NAI)

Scaling

- Silvery scaling on the surface of red patches—psoriasis
- Fine scaling accompanied with rash—pityriasis
- Coarse, scaly skin with no rash—ichthyosis

Subcutaneous nodules: *Consider:*

- RA
- Xanthelasma

- Neurofibroma
- Granuloma annulare

- Sarcoid
- Polyarteritis

White patches: Consider all causes of patchy hypopigmentation:

- Vitiligo
- After inflammation—cryotherapy, eczema, psoriasis, morphoea
- Pityriasis alba—white post-inflammatory patch on a child's face; no treatment needed
- Following exposure to some chemicals—substituted phenols, hydroquinone
- Certain infections—pityriasis versicolor, leprosy, yaws
- Tuberous sclerosis
- Halo naevus (pale area around a mole)
- Piebaldism (from birth—associated with a white forelock)
- Extensive hyperpigmentation e.g. chloasma—the patches of normal skin may appear hypopigmented

White spots: *Consider:*
- Pustules/whiteheads e.g. due to acne, folliculitis, or rosacea
- Molluscum contagiosum—white, firm, raised spots with a pearl-like appearance
- Milia—small, white spots usually on upper arms/face of children; resolve spontaneously

Yellow crusting: Usually due to staphylococcal infection (impetigo).

Sleep apnoea: 📖 p.400

Sneezing: Often associated with rhinitis.

Snoring: 📖 p.400

Sore mouth: Treat the cause. *Consider:*
- Oral thrush
- Apthous ulcers
- HSV
- Dry mouth
- Trauma (e.g. burn)
- Side-effects of chemo- or radiotherapy
- Anaemia
- Hand, foot, and mouth disease (child)
- Gingivitis

Sore throat: 📖 p.914

Sore tongue: Tongue problems—📖 p.294

Speech problems
- **Dysarthria:** 📖 p.256
- **Dysphasia:** 📖 p.257
- **Stammer:** p.291

Spider naevi: Small red lesions in the distribution of the superior vena cava i.e. on the arms, neck, and chest wall. Consist of a large arteriole with numerous small vessels radiating from it giving the appearance of a spider—hence the name. Vary in size from barely visible to 0.5cm diameter. Pressure applied to the central arteriole (e.g. with a pointed object) causes blanching of the whole lesion. Presence of >2 spider naevi is abnormal. *Causes:*
- Cirrhosis—most frequently, alcoholic
- Oestrogen excess—usually in association with chronic liver disease; part of normal hepatic function is the inactivation of oestrogens
- Rheumatoid arthritis—rarely
- Viral hepatitis (transient)
- Pregnancy—usually appear during the 2nd–5th mo. and disappear in the final trimester

Splenomegaly: *Causes:*
- *Haematological:* Lymphoma; leukaemia; myeloproliferative disorders; sickle cell disease (children usually); thalassaemia
- *Inflammatory:* RA (Felty's syndrome); Sjogren's; sarcoid; amyloid
- *Infection:* Glandular fever; malaria; SBE; TB; leischmaniasis

Splinter haemorrhages: 📖 p.660

Sputum

- Smoking is the leading cause of excess sputum production (look for black specks of inhaled carbon).
- Yellow-green sputum is due to cell debris (bronchial epithelium, neutrophils, eosinophils) and is not always infected.
- Bronchiectasis causes copious greenish sputum.
- Blood-stained sputum (haemoptysis) always needs full investigation—📖 p.266.
- Pink froth suggests pulmonary oedema.
- Absolutely clear sputum is probably saliva.

Steatorrhoea: Excess fat in faeces. The stool is pale-coloured, foul smelling, and floats ('difficult to flush'). Usually due to malabsorption—📖 p.451.

Stammer: Disorder of rhythm and fluency of speech in which syllables, words, or phrases are repeated. ♂:♀≈4:1. Cause unknown. Can result in stress and embarrassment.
- *Younger children:* Often short-lived and, in most cases, resolves spontaneously
- *Older children/adults:* Refer to speech therapy

Strangury: Distressing desire to pass something *per urethra* that will not pass e.g. stone.

Stridor: 📖 p.916 and 1011

Sweating: Excess sweating—Hyperhydrosis 📖 p.659

Swelling of the ankles/legs: Occurs when the rate of capillary filtration > rate drainage. Capillary filtration ↑ occurs due to ↑ venous pressure, hypoalbuminaemia, or local inflammation. ↓ drainage occurs due to lymphatic obstruction. Consider whether the swelling is acute or chronic, symmetrical or asymetrical, localized or generalized. Ask about associated symptoms e.g. breathlessness. Treat according to cause. *Causes:*

Acute

- DVT
- Superficial thrombophlebitis
- Cellulitis
- Joint effusion/haemarthrosis
- Haematoma

- Baker's cyst
- Arthritis
- Fracture
- Acute arterial ischaemia
- Dermatitis

Chronic

- Gravitational oedema e.g. due to immobility—common in the elderly. Advise elevation of feet above waist level, support stockings (ideally apply stockings before getting out of bed), avoid standing still. Diuretics are not a long-term solution.
- Heart failure
- Hypoproteinaemia e.g. nephrotic syndrome
- Idiopathic oedema
- Reflex sympathetic dystrophy
- Lymphoedema—infection, tumour, trauma
- Post-thrombotic syndrome
- Chronic venous insufficiency/venous obstruction
- Lipodermatosclerosis
- Congenital vascular abnormalities.

Syncope: Loss of consciousness—📖 p.274

Micturition syncope: Occurs as an isolated symptom in middle-aged and elderly men—usually when they get up at night to urinate. Does not require further investigation. Advise patients to sit to urinate.

Cough syncope: May occur at any age after a prolonged bout of cough which impairs venous return.

T

Tall stature: 📖 p.885

Tachycardia: Heart rate >100bpm—📖 p.342

Tardive dyskinesia: Movement patterns (abnormal)—📖 p.276

Telangectasia: Visible dilation of distal venules or an arteriole (spider naevus). *Causes:*
- *Congenital* e.g. hereditary haemorrhagic telangectasia
- *Venous disease in the leg* e.g. venous stars
- *Rosacea*—facial
- *Excess oestrogen* e.g. liver disease; the COC pill; pregnancy
- *Skin atrophy* e.g. ageing skin; radiation dermatitis; topical steroids

Spider naevi: 📖 p.290

Tenesmus: This is a sensation, felt in the rectum, of incomplete emptying following defecation—as if there was something left behind which cannot be passed. It is very common in irritable bowel syndrome, but can be caused by a tumour.

Testicular pain: Treat the cause. *Causes:*
- Epididymo-orchitis
- Varicocoele
- Torsion of the testis
- Testicular tumour
- Trauma and haematoma formation

Testis
- **Absent testis:** 📖 p.248
- **Testicular lump:** 📖 p.698

Thought disorders: Consider disorders of:
Content
- *Ideas of reference:* The patient feels he is noticed by everyone around him/stands out from the crowd; media content e.g. television or radio, refers to himself; or that others are talking or thinking about him. Becomes a delusion of reference when insight is lost. Associated with schizophrenia, depressive states, and acute and chronic cognitive impairment.
- *Delusions:* 📖 p.255

- *Delusions of persecution:* Most common type of paranoid delusion. Belief that a person or organization is intentionally harassing or inflicting harm upon the patient. Associated with schizophrenia, depressive states, and acute and chronic cognitive impairment.
- *Delusions of grandeur:* Beliefs of possessing exaggerated power, importance, knowledge, or ability. Associated with manic depression.

Flow

- *Flight of ideas:* Leaps from idea to idea. There is always some association between ideas but may seem odd e.g. rhymes. Associated with manic illness.
- *Perseveration:* Persistence of a verbal or other behaviour beyond what is apparently intended, expected, or needed. Associated with dementia and brain damage e.g. cerebral palsy, CVA.
- *Loosening of association:* Series of thoughts appear only distantly (or loosely) related to one another or completely unrelated. Associated with schizophrenia.
- *Thought block:* Abrupt and complete interruption in the stream of thought, leaving a blank mind. Associated with schizophrenia.

Form

- *Preoccupation:* The patient thinks about a topic frequently but can terminate the thoughts voluntarily. Common symptom e.g. in anxiety states. Ask about preoccupation with suicide in depressed patients.
- *Obsession:* Thought or image repeated in spite of its inappropriateness or intrusiveness and associated discomfort. The thought and efforts to stop it can be disabling.

Possession

- *Thought insertion:* Thoughts do not belong to the patient but have been planted there by someone else. One of the 1st rank symptoms of schizophrenia.
- *Thought withdrawal:* Opposite of thought insertion. The patient perceives a thought is missing and has been removed by someone else. A 1st rank symptom of schizophrenia.
- *Thought broadcasting:* The patient believes his thoughts can be heard by other people—either directly or via the newspapers, radio, etc. Associated with schizophrenia.

Thrills: Palpable murmurs—always indicate pathology. Note whether systolic or diastolic and where felt strongest.

Systolic thrills

- *Felt most strongly at the apex:* VSD or mitral regurgitation
- *3rd/4th interspace:* VSD
- *Base of heart on the right:* Aortic stenosis, aortic aneurysm
- *Base of the heart on the left:* CHD e.g. pulmonary stenosis

Diastolic thrills

- *Apex:* Mitral stenosis

Tics: Movement patterns (abnormal)—p.276

Tinnitus: p.928

Tired all the time: 📖 p.582

Tongue problems
- *Blue tongue:* Central cyanosis—📖 p.254
- *Dry and furred:* Dehydration
- *Geographic tongue:* Irregular, smoother, redder patches on the dorsum of the tongue that change position over time. Due to papillae loss. May be asymptomatic or cause soreness. Rarely, due to vitamin B_2 deficiency.
- *Large tongue:* Consider acromegaly, amyloidosis, myxoedema.
- *Smooth tongue:* Iron, riboflavin, nicotinic acid, B_{12}, or folate deficiency; idiopathic—usually elderly; antibiotic use.
- *Sore tongue:* Glossitis of anaemia; Crohn's disease, coeliac disease, carcinoma of the tongue; psychogenic causes.
- *Strawberry tongue:* Yellowish-white tongue coating with the dark red papillae of the tongue projecting through. Associated with scarlet fever, though also present in Kawasaki's disease.
- *Ulcer:* Presume any non-healing ulcer is due to carcinoma of the tongue until proven otherwise. Refer to oral surgeon for biopsy. Treatment is with surgery or laser ablation ± radiotherapy.

Toothache: 📖 p.912

Tremor
- *Resting tremor:* Present at rest but abolished on voluntary movement. Most common cause—PD when tremor is rhythmic.
- *Intention tremor:* Irregular large-amplitude tremor worse on movement e.g. reaching for something. Typical of cerebellar disease.
- *Tremors on movement:* Thyrotoxicosis, anxiety, benign essential tremor (inherited), and drugs (e.g. β-agonists) cause a fine tremor abolished at rest. Alcohol and β-blockers may help.

U

Ulcer (leg): 📖 p.640

Unconscious patient: 📖 p.1032

Urgency: Dysuria and urgency—📖 p.259

Urticaria: 📖 p.642

V

Vaginal bleeding
- **Menorrhagia/heavy periods:** 📖 p.724
- **Intermenstrual bleeding:** 📖 p.714
- **Bleeding in early pregnancy:** 📖 p.736
- **Bleeding in later pregnancy:** 📖 p.792
- **Postcoital bleeding:** 📖 p.714
- **Post-menopausal bleeding:** 📖 p.713
- **Prolonged periods:** 📖 p.280

Vaginal discharge: 📖 p.740

Varicose veins: 📖 p.362

Vertigo: 📖 p.928

Visual disturbance: *Consider:*
- *Eye disease:* 📖 p.931–955.
- *Drugs*
- *CNS lesions*
  - History of visual field loss e.g. stroke
  - Double vision—MS, trauma, tumour, basilar artery insufficiency, chronic basilar meningitis
  - Flashing lights—migraine, seizure disorder
  - Visual hallucinations—seizure disorder, drugs
  - Transient blindness—vascular lesions, migraine

Visual field defects: Figure 9.2
- **Cortical blindness:** Normal eyes. Normal papillary responses but no conscious vision. Due to bilateral damage to the visual cortex.
- **Tunnel vision:** Loss of peripheral vision in all directions. *Consider:* migraine; glaucoma; optic atrophy; tertiary syphilis; papilloedema; retinal abnormalities e.g. retinitis pigmentosa; hysteria. Refer to ophthalmology.
- **Enlarged blind spot:** The blind spot is a small area lateral to the centre of the visual field where there is no vision perception. Due to interruption of the retina by the optic disc. Blind spot is enlarged if the optic disc is enlarged e.g. papilloedema.
- **Central scotoma:** Loss of central vision with normal vision around it. May be unilateral or bilateral. *Consider:*
  - Bilateral: methylated spirit ingestion, B_{12} deficiency, tobacco
  - Unilateral/bilateral: MS
  - Unilateral: glioma of the optic nerve, vascular lesion

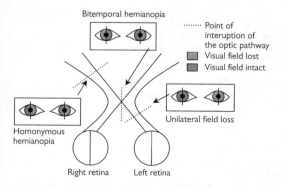

Figure 9.2 Visual pathways and visual field defects caused by interruption anterior to the optic chiasm, at the optic chiasm, and behind the optic chiasm

Loss of vision from one eye: Due to a lesion anterior to the optic chiasm (Figure 9.2) e.g. retinal artery occlusion, tumour.

- **Bitemporal hemianopia:** Due to interruption of the visual pathways at the optic chasm where fibres from the nasal half of the retina cross. Results in bilateral temporal field loss. If partial, may cause partial loss (i.e. quadrantinopia). *Consider:* pituitary tumours, craniopharyngioma, meningioma.

- **Homonymous hemianopia:** Due to interruption of the visual pathway after the optic chiasm. Results in loss of vision on the same side in both eyes i.e. left-hand sided lesions → nasal side visual loss in the left eye and temporal side visual loss in the right eye. Partial interruption results in quadrantinopia or macular sparing. *Causes include:* CVA, head injury, or brain tumour.

Visual loss
- **Sudden:** 🕮 p.942
- **Gradual:** 🕮 p.944

Voice disturbance
- **Dysarthria:** 🕮 p.256
- **Dysphasia:** 🕮 p.257
- **Stammer:** 🕮 p.291

Vomiting

In children: 🕮 p.857

In adults: Common symptom. *History:* duration, colour, and frequency, ability to retain food and fluids, nature of vomitus, presence of blood or 'coffee grounds', relationship to eating. *Examination:* abdomen (masses, tenderness, hepatomegaly), dehydration. Advise patients to drink small amounts of clear fluids regularly to maintain hydration. Treat according to cause. *Causes:*
- *GI:* food poisoning; gastroenteritis; GI obstruction; pyloric stenosis; 'acute abdomen'.
- *CNS:* ↑ICP; head injury; motion sickness; migraine; Ménière's disease; labyrinthitis; cerebellar disease.
- *Psychiatric:* anorexia; bulimia.
- *Metabolic:* pregnancy; uraemia; drugs (e.g. opiates); toxins.
- *Infection:* tonsillitis, OM—especially in children.
- *Carcinomatosis*

Vulval itching (Pruritus vulvae): Treat the cause. *Causes:*
- Infection (e.g. candida, herpes genitalis, genital warts, threadworms, pubic lice, scabies)
- Atrophic vulvitis
- Vulval dystrophy
- Vulval carcinoma
- Generalized causes of pruritus—🕮 p.281

Vulval lumps: Common and usually benign.

General causes
- Sebaceous cyst
- Varicose veins
- Haematoma
- Benign skin tumours (lipoma, papilloma, etc.)
- Malignant skin tumours (1° or 2°)

Specific causes
- Bartholin's gland cyst/abscess
- Urethral caruncle
- Endometriosis
- Carcinoma of the vulva
- Inguinal hernia
- Hydrocoele of the canal of Nuck.

W

Walking difficulty ('off legs'): Common amongst the elderly.
Causes:
- *Musculoskeletal:* Osteoarthritis or RA, osteoporotic fractures, frac-tured neck of femur, osteomalacia, Paget's disease, polymyalgia rheu-matica;
- *Psychological:* Depression, bereavement, fear of falling;
- *Neurological:* Stroke, Parkinson's disease, peripheral neuropathy;
- *Spinal cord compression*
- *Systemic:* Pneumonia, UTI, anaemia, hypothyroidism, renal failure, infection, hypothermia.

Management: Treat according to cause. Refer if inadequate support at home, cause warrants admission, or no cause is found.

Gait (abnormal): p.263

Watery eyes: p.939

Weight loss: Non-specific symptom. Treat the cause. *Causes:*
- *GI:* Malabsorption, malnutrition, dieting;
- *Chronic disease:* Hyperthyroidism, DM, heart failure, renal disease, degenerative neurological/muscle disease, chronic infection (e.g. TB, HIV) or infestation;
- *Malignancy*
- *Psychiatric:* Depression, dementia, anorexia.

Table 9.13 Fluorescence under Wood's light and its associations

Colour of fluorescence	Association
Golden yellow	Tinea versicolor
Pale green	Trichophyton schoenleini
Bright yellow-green	Microsporum canis
Greeny blue	Pseudomonas aeruginosa
Pinky orange	Porphyria cutanea tarda
Purple brown	Hyperpigmentation
Pale white	Hypopigmentation
Ash leaf-shaped spot	Tuberous sclerosis
Bright white or blue white	Depigmentation, vitiligo
Bright white	Albinism
Bluey white	Leprosy

Wood's light: Filtered UV rays (Wood's light) can be used as a diagnostic aid. Normal skin does not fluoresce or shine under ultraviolet light. Abnormal findings may indicate infection or depigmentation—Table 9.13, 📖 p.297.

Wheeze: Musical sound heard during expiration.
- *Polyphonic wheeze:* indicates narrowing of many small airways—typical of asthma or COPD.
- *Monophonic wheeze:* indicates single large airway obstruction e.g. due to foreign body or tumour.

X

Xanthomata: Localized collections of lipid-laden cells. Appear as yellowish coloured lumps. Often caused by ↑ lipids.
- **Plane xanthoma:** Yellow/orange macules/plaques in the skin—particularly skin creases. Palmar xanthoma are indicative of familial hypercholesterolaemia.
- **Tendon xanthoma:** Mobile nodules in tendons especially on the backs of the hands, fingers, elbows, knees, and heels. Associated with familial hypercholesterolaemia.
- **Eruptive xanthoma:** Crops of small yellowish brown papules surrounded by erythema on buttocks, posterior thighs, knees, and elbows. Associated with some types of lipoproteinaemia and uncontrolled DM.
- **Tuberous xanthoma:** Yellow/orange nodules in the skin over the elbow/knee. Associated with hyperlipoproteinaemia, myxoedema, and rarely, biliary cirrhosis.
- **Xanthelasma:** Collection of lipid-laden cells on the eyelid. Associated with ↑ lipids in ~ 50%. Also associated with cholestasis, myxoedema, and renal disease.

Laboratory tests

BIOCHEMISTRY

Alanine-amino transferase (ALT; SGPT): ↑ in liver disease—suggests hepatocyte damage.

Albumin
High albumin: *Causes:* dehydration; artefact (e.g. haemostasis).

Low albumin: Results in oedema. *Causes:*

- Malignancy
- Liver disease
- Nephrotic syndrome
- Burns
- Protein-losing enteropathy
- Malabsorption
- Malnutrition
- Late pregnancy
- Artefact (e.g. blood taken from arm with IVI)
- Posture (5g/L higher if upright)
- Genetic variations

Alkaline phosphatase: ↑ in liver disease—suggests cholestatsis; bone disease, especially Paget's; growing children; healing fractures; osteomalacia; metastases; hyperparathyroidism; and renal failure. The placenta makes its own isoenzyme in pregnancy.

Placental alkaline phosphatase (PLAP): ↑ in pregnancy, carcinoma of ovary, seminoma, and smokers.

Alpha-amylase: ↑ in acute pancreatitis; severe uraemia; diabetic ketoacidosis. Not ↑ in chronic pancreatitis.

ALT: Alanine amino transferase—see above.

Amylase: Alpha-amylase—see above.

Aspartate-amino transferase (AST; SGOT): ↑ in liver disease (suggesting hepatocyte damage); following MI; skeletal muscle damage; and haemolysis.

Calcium
- **Hypercalcaemia:** 📖 p.424
- **Hypocalcaemia:** 📖 p.424

Creatinine: Commonly ordered test to detect renal dysfunction (Table 9.14). Severity of renal impairment is measured in terms of glomerular filtration rate. Serum creatinine is a rough guide to glomerular filtration rate (GFR) when corrected for age, gender, and weight—↓ in GFR is associated with ↑ in serum creatinine,

$$ \text{GFR} = \frac{(140-\text{age (y.)}) \times \text{weight (kg)} \times 1.2 \ (\text{♂}) \ or \ 1.05 \ (\text{♀})}{\text{Serum creatinine}} $$

❶ Renal function ↓ with age. Many elderly patients have a GFR <50ml/min. which, because of ↓ muscle mass, may not be indicated by a ↑ serum creatinine.

Table 9.14 Causes of an abnormal serum creatinine

↑ creatinine (>150μmol/l)	↓ creatinine (<70μmol/l)
Renal disease/renal failure	Muscular dystrophy (late stage)
Drugs e.g. trimethoprim, probenecid, cimetidine, potassium sparing diuretics (e.g. amiloride)	Myasthenia gravis
Large muscle bulk	
Muscle breakdown e.g. muscular dystrophy	

Creatine kinase (CK): 📖 p.311

Gamma-glutamyl transpeptidase (GGT, γGT): ↑in liver disease—particularly alcohol-induced damage.

GGT: Gamma-glutamyl transpeptidase—see above.

Glucose
- **Blood glucose:** 📖 p.404
- **Glycosuria:** 📖 p.306

Lactate dehydrogenase (LDH): *Causes of ↑ LDH:*
- MI
- Liver disease—suggests hepatocyte damage
- Haemolysis
- PE
- Tumour necrosis

Potassium

Hyperkalaemia

⚠ Plasma potassium >6.5mmol/l *needs urgent treatment.*
- Check it is not an artefact e.g. due to haemolysis inside the bottle
- Admit for investigation of cause and treatment

ECG changes associated with hyperkalaemia: Tall tented T-waves; small P-wave; wide QRS complex becoming sinusoidal, VF.
Causes: Table 9.15. Treat the cause.

Hypokalaemia

⚠ Plasma potassium <2.5mmol/l *needs urgent treatment.*—admit.

Presentation: Muscle weakness, hypotonia, cardiac arrhythmias, cramps, and tetany.
ECG changes associated with hypokalaemia: Small or inverted T-waves; prominent u-wave (after T-wave); prolonged P-R interval; depressed ST segment.
Causes: Table 9.15

Treatment
- *If mild (>2.5mmol/l, no symptoms):* Give oral potassium supplement (at least 80mmol/24h. e.g. Sando-K 2 tabs bd). If the patient is taking a thiazide diuretic, hypokalaemia >3.0mmol/L rarely needs treating.
- *If severe (<2.5mmol/L, dangerous symptoms):* Admit to a general medical team

Table 9.15 Causes of altered serum potassium

↑ potassium (>5mmol/l)	↓ potassium (<3.5mmol/l)
Renal failure	Diuretics
Drugs, e.g. ACE inhibitors: excess K⁺ therapy; K⁺ sparing diuretics	Cushing's syndrome/steroids
Addison's disease	Vomiting and/or diarrhoea
Metabolic acidosis (DM)	Conn's syndrome
Artefact (haemolysed sample)	Villous adenoma of the rectum
	Purgative or liquorice abuse
	Intestinal fistulae
	Renal tubular failure
	Hypokalaemic periodic paralysis—interrmittent weakness lasting <72h

Renal function

- **Acute and chronic renal failure:** 📖 p.680
- **Creatinine:** 📖 p.299
- **Urea:** 📖 p.302

Table 9.16 Causes of altered serum sodium

↑ sodium (>145mmol/l)	↓ sodium (<135mmol/l)
Usually due to water loss > Na⁺ loss	*Renal loss of Na⁺*
• Fluid loss without water replacement (e.g. diarrhoea, vomit, burns)	• Diuretic excess—especially thiazides
• Diabetes insipidus—suspect if large urine volume	• Addison's disease
• Osmotic diuresis	• Renal failure
• Primary aldosteronism: suspect if ↑BP, ↓ K⁺, alkalosis (HCO₃↑)	• Loss of Na+ elsewhere
	• Diarrhoea
	• Vomiting
	• Fistula
	• Villous adenoma of the rectum
	• Small bowel obstruction
	• CF
	• Heat exposure
	Dilution with water
	• SIADH (📖 p.429)
	• Water overload (e.g. polydipsia in schizophrenia)
	• Severe hypothyroidism
	• Glucocorticoid deficiency
	• Nephrotic syndrome
	• Cardiac failure
	• Cirrhosis
	• Renal failure

Sodium

Hyponatraemia: Low serum sodium (<135mmol/l). Rarely symptomatic in general practice. May present with signs of water excess—confusion, fits, ↑BP, cardiac failure, oedema, anorexia, nausea, muscle weakness. *Causes:* Table 9.16. *Management:* Treat the cause. If unwell admit for investigation.

Hypernatraemia: Excess serum sodium (>145mmol/l). Rare in general practice. *Presentation:* Thirst, confusion, coma, fits, signs of dehydration; dry skin, ↓ skin turgor, postural hypotension, and oliguria if water deficient. *Causes:* Table 9.16. *Management:* Admit for further investigation.

Urea: Commonly ordered test to detect renal dysfunction. While ↓ in glomerular filtration rate (GFR) is associated with ↑ in serum urea, urea may alter independently of the GFR. Causes of abnormal serum urea—Table 9.17.

Table 9.17 Causes of an abnormal serum urea

↑ urea (>6.7mmol/l)	↓ urea (< 2.5mmol/l)
Renal failure	Liver disease (↓ urea production)
GI bleeding	Anabolic state
High-protein diet	High ADH levels (high GFR)
Drugs—high-dose steroids, tetracycline	Starvation or low-protein diet
Dehydration	Pregnancy

Uric acid/urate

Hyperuricaemia: *Causes:* ↑ turnover or ↓ excretion of urate.
- *Drugs:* Cytotoxics; thiazides; ethambutol
- ↑*cell turnover:* Lymphoma; leukaemia; psoriasis; haemolysis; muscle necrosis
- ↓ *excretion:* Primary gout; chronic renal failure; lead nephropathy; hyperparathyroidism

In addition: Associated with ↑ BP and hyperlipidaemia. Urate may be ↑ in disorders of purine synthesis (e.g. Lesch-Nyhan syndrome).

HAEMATOLOGY

Anaemia: 📖 p.522

B12: 📖 p.523

Basophils: ↑ in—viral infections; urticaria; myxoedema; post-splenectomy; CML; UC; malignancy; systemic mastocytosis (urticaria pigmentosa); haemolysis; polycythaemia rubra vera.

Coagulation tests: (sodium citrate tube; false results if under-filled).
- **Prothrombin time (PT):** Prolonged by coumarins (e.g. warfarin); vitamin K deficiency; liver disease
- **Thrombin time:** ↑ in heparin treatment, DIC, or afibrinogenaemia
- **INR:** Time the sample takes to clot as a ratio to a control sample—📖 p.366–7

Eosinophils: ↑ in:
- Parasitic infestations: e.g. ascaris, strongyloides
- Allergic disorders: e.g. hayfever, drug reactions
- Skin disorders: e.g. urticaria, pemphigus, eczema
- Pulmonary disorders: e.g. asthma, aspergillosis, PAN
- Malignant disorders: e.g. lymphoma, carcinoma, leukaemia
- Miscellaneous disorders: e.g. hypereosinophilic syndrome, sarcoidosis, hypoadrenalism, eosinophilic gastroenteritis.

Erythrocyte sedimentation rate (ESR): Rate of fall of red cells in a column of blood. A measure of the acute phase response—the pathological process may be infective, immunological, malignant, ischaemic, or traumatic. ESR ↑ with age; ♀>♂; ↑ in patients with severe anaemia.

Folate: 📖 p.523

INR: 📖 p.366–7

Lymphocytes: 1.3–3.5 x 10^9/l (20–45%).
↑ in
- Viral infections—EBV, CMV, rubella
- Toxoplasmosis
- Whooping cough
- Brucellosis
- Chronic lymphatic leukaemia.

❶ Large numbers of abnormal ('atypical') lymphocytes are characteristically seen with EBV infection.

↓ in
- Steroid therapy
- SLE
- Uraemia
- Legionnaire's disease
- AIDS
- Marrow infiltration
- Post chemotherapy or radiotherapy

Mean cell volume (MCV)

Low MCV (microcytic <75fl): *Most common cause:* Iron-deficiency anaemia. Confirm by showing that serum ferritin is ↓. *Rarer causes:* Thalassaemia (suspect if MCV is 'too low' for the level of anaemia); congenital sideroblastic anaemia (very rare).

High MCV (macrocytic >110fl): Vitamin B_{12} or folate deficiency; alcohol; liver disease; drugs (e.g. iron, azathioprine, zidovudine); haemolysis; pregnancy; hypothyroidism; marrow infiltration; myelodysplasia.

Monocytes: ↑ in—acute and chronic infections (e.g. TB; brucellosis; protozoa); malignant disease (including acute myeloid leukaemia and Hodgkin's disease); myelodyspalsia.

Neutrophils

↑↑ **in:** Leukaemia; disseminated malignancy; severe childhood infection.

↑ **in**

- Bacterial infection
- Trauma
- Surgery
- Burns
- Haemorrhage
- Inflammation
- Infarction
- Polymyalgia
- PAN
- Myeloproliferative disorders
- Drugs (e.g. steroids)

↓ **in**

- Viral infections
- Typhoid
- TB
- Septicaemia
- Drugs (e.g. carbimazole, sulfonamides)
- Hypersplenism
- Anti-neutrophil antibodies (e.g. in RA or SLE)
- B_{12} or folate deficiency—↓ manufacture
- Bone marrow failure

Pancytopoenia: *Causes:*

- Aplastic anaemia
- Megaloblastic anaemia
- Bone marrow infiltration or replacement (e.g. by lymphoma, leukaemia, myeloma, 2° carcinoma, myelofibrosis)
- Hypersplenism
- SLE
- Disseminated TB
- Paroxysmal nocturnal haemoglobinuria.

Platelets

↓ **platelets (thrombocytopoenia—<150x10⁹/l):** *Causes:*

- ↓ *production:* Marrow failure; megaloblastosis.
- ↓ *survival:* ITP; viruses; DIC; drugs; SLE; lymphoma; thrombotic thrombocytopenic purpura; hypersplenism; genetic disease.
- *Platelet aggregation:* Heparin (5% patients).

↑ **platelets (thrombocythaemia—>400x10⁹/l):** *Causes:* ~50% with unexplained thrombocytosis have a malignancy. *Other causes:* Kawasaki disease; myeloproliferative or inflammatory disease (e.g. RA); bleeding; splenectomy.

Polycythaemia: Increase in the number of circulating red cells. May be 1° (polycythaemia rubra vera) or 2°. 2° polycythaemia may be:

- *Appropriate*—high altitude, chronic lung disease (e.g. COPD), cardiovascular disease with a R → L shunt, heavy smoking, ↑ affinity for haemoglobin (familial polycythaemia) *or*
- *Inappropriate*—due to excess erythropoietin e.g. from renal tumour, hepatocellular tumour, or massive uterine fibroid.

❶ Hb may also appear ↑ if the patient is dehydrated—concentration effect.

Red cells

- **Polycythaemia:** See above
- **Anaemia:** 📖 p.522
- ↑ **MCV:** 📖 p.303

Thrombocytosis: ↑ platelet count >1000x10^9/l. *Causes:*
- Essential thrombocytosis: Rare
- Reactive (2°) throbocytosis: Due to infection, malignant disease, acute or chronic inflammatory disease, pregnancy, after splenectomy, iron deficiency, or following haemorrhage.

Thrombocytopoenia: Opposite and 📖 p.528

White cells
- **Neutrophils:** 📖 p.304
- **Lymphocytes:** 📖 p.303
- **Eosinophils:** 📖 p.303
- **Basophils:** 📖 p.302
- **Monocytes:** 📖 p.303

OTHER BLOOD TESTS

C-reactive protein (CRP): Acute phase protein which ↑ ≤6h. after an acute event. Follows clinical state more rapidly than ESR. Not ↑ by SLE, leukaemia, UC, pregnancy, OA, anaemia, polycythaemia, or heart failure. Highest levels are seen in bacterial infections (>10mg/L).

Plasma viscosity: Measure of the acute phase response—pathological process may be infective, immunological, malignant, ischaemic, or traumatic. ♂=♀; ↑ slightly with age; unaffected by the level of Hb.

Prostate specific antigen (PSA)
Causes of ↑ PSA: Prostate cancer, BPH, prostatitis, old age, acute urinary retention, prostate instrumentation (includes prostate biopsy, urinary catheterization, and rectal examination).

Screening for prostate cancer: There is no prostate screening programme in the UK but men can request a PSA test. Warn patients about the poor specificity of the test before performing the test, and provide information about the pros and cons of testing—📖 p.160.

Performing a PSA test^G: Do the PSA test before doing a digital rectal examination. If that's not possible, delay the test for 1wk. after the examination. Do NOT do a PSA test if the man has:
- A UTI
- Ejaculated within 48h.
- Exercised vigorously in the previous 48h.
- Had a prostate biopsy <6wk. ago

Referral^G: Table 9.18

Table 9.18 PSA cut-offs which should prompt referral

Age (y.)	Refer to urology if PSA (ng/ml) is
50–59	≥3.0
60–69	≥4.0
≥70	>5.0

Monitoring prostate cancer
- PSA >40: High chance of nodal or metastatic spread
- PSA >100: Metastatic spread is very likely

URINE

Creatinine clearance: A more accurate method of assessing GFR is to use 24h. collection of urine together with serum creatinine to measure creatinine clearance:

$$\text{Creatinine clearance (ml/min.)} = \frac{\text{Urinary creatinine (μmol/l) in 24h.} \times 0.7}{\text{Serum creatinine (μmol/l)}}$$

Glycosuria: *Causes:*

- DM
- Pregnancy
- Sepsis
- Renal tubular damage
- Low renal threshold

In all cases, check fasting blood glucose (+ glucose tolerance test if pregnant). Check immediate BM if other symptoms suggestive of DM.

Haematuria: 📖 p.265

Proteinuria: Normally discovered with urine dipstick If +ve, then repeat with another sample to exclude spurious results. Treat the cause where necessary.

If accurate estimation is needed, use 24h. urine collection. Normally, adults excrete <150mg protein/d. Protein:creatinine ratio in morning urine can be used for monitoring chronic proteinuria.

Causes
- UTI
- Vaginal mucus
- DM
- ↑ BP
- Glomerulonephritis
- Pyrexia
- CCF
- Pregnancy (and PET)
- Postural proteinuria—2–5% adolescents; rare >30y.
- Haemolytic-uraemic syndrome
- SLE
- Myeloma
- Drugs (e.g. gold, penicillamine)
- Amyloid

Microalbuminuria: Albuminuria in the range 30–200 mg/l. Not detectable with standard urine dipsticks. Special sticks are available for routine screening of high-risk groups e.g. diabetics. *Causes:*
- *DM:* Microalbuminuria precedes frank proteinuria. Treatment with antihypertensives slows progression in both type 1 and type 2 DM. In type 1 DM, patients should be started on an ACE inhibitor if they screen +ve for microalbuminuria, even if normotensive—📖 p.416.

- *Arteriopathy:* Microalbiminuria may be present in patients with CCF or ↑ BP. There is evidence from the HOPE study (Gerstein *et al.* (2001) *JAMA* 286: 421–6) that presence of microalbuminuria predicts ↑ risk of MI, CVA, CCF, and cardiovascular and all-cause mortality.
- *Other chronic illness:* Malignancy, COPD
- *Acute illness:* Inflammatory bowel disease, MI, acute pancreatitis, trauma, burns, meningitis

❶ Standard urine dipsticks do not detect Bence–Jones proteinuria.

Other relevant pages

Cardiology and vascular disease

Useful information
British Heart Foundation ☎0845 708 070 🖳 *http://www.bhf.org.uk.*
British Hypertension Society 🖳 *http://www.bhsoc.org*

Cardiac investigations

Electrocardiogram (ECG): Graphic recording of electric potentials generated by the heart. Many surgeries now have ECG machines that interpret and print out their findings. Analysis is easier, but it is still important to be able to understand significance of abnormalities and check computer analysis in the clinical context.

Interpreting ECGs: Many mistakes in ECG interpretation are errors of omission, so a systematic approach is best. *Check:*
- Standardization (calibration) and technical features (including lead placement and artefacts)
- Heart rate—usual speed (25mm/s). Each big square represents 0.2s (small square—0.04s.). Rate = $\frac{300}{\text{R-R interval}}$ (in larger squares)
- Rhythm—regular/irregular
- PR interval—normal if <0.2s
- QRS interval—abnormal if >0.12s
- QT interval—varies with rate; at 60bpm, normal if 0.35–0.43s
- P waves—present or absent; shape
- QRS voltages—height of complexes; see Table 10.1
- Mean QRS electrical axis—sum of all ventricular forces during ventricular depolarization. Normal axis: −30° to +120°
  - If more −ve is left axis deviation; if more +ve is right axis deviation
  - *Rule of thumb 1:* if the majority of the QRS complex is above the baseline (+ve) in leads I and II, the axis is normal
  - *Rule of thumb 2:* the axis lies at 90° to a QRS complex where the height above the baseline = height below the baseline
- Precordial R-wave progression
- Abnormal Q waves—>25% of the succeeding R-wave and/or >0.04s. wide
- ST segments—elevation/depression, shape
- T waves—height, inversion, shape
- U waves—small, rounded deflection (≤1mm), follows T wave and usually has the same polarity

Brief guide to common ECG changes: p.312

24h./ambulatory ECG: ECG monitoring equipment is worn for 24h. Continuous monitoring may detect intermittent arrythmias or ischaemia.

Exercise ECG: ECG testing whilst the patient undergoes graded exercise on a treadmill/exercise bicycle. Local referral criteria vary. Mortality ~1:10,000. Used for:
- Diagnosis of IHD—75% have a +ve test; false +ve rate of ~5%
- Assessment of exercise tolerance
- Response to treatment
- As a prognostic indicator
- Assessment of exercise-related arrhythmias

Contraindications: Recent MI (<7d.), unstable angina, electrolyte disturbance, aortic stenosis, severe heart failure, known left main coronary artery stenosis, LBBB (may not be possible to interpret the trace).

Cardiac enzymes: Biochemical blood assay of molecules released when the heart is damaged. Used in diagnosis of MI.

- **Troponins T and I:** Preferred markers as more sensitive/specific than CK, AST, or LDH. Together with CK, earliest to ↑ after MI.
- **Creatine kinase (CK):** ↑ in MI, muscle damage (e.g. prolonged running or seizures), after IM injection, and with dermatomyositis (e.g. due to statins). CK-MB assay may help clarify whether a cardiac event has occurred <48h. previously.
- **AST:** 2nd to ↑—📖 p.299   • **LDH:** Last to ↑—📖 p.300

Echocardiogram (Echo): Heart USS. Local referral procedures vary.

- **2-dimensional:** Produces a fan-shaped, cross-sectional, moving, real-time image of the heart. May be transthoracic or transoesophageal. Used to asses valvular abnormalities and prosthetic heart valves; aortic aneurysm/dissection; heart failure; pericardial effusion; masses within the heart; myocardial abnormalities (e.g. aneurysms, hypertrophy); IHD; congenital heart disease.
- **M-mode:** Plotted on a scrolling screen. Stationary structures appear as straight lines across the screen; moving structures appear as undulating lines. Usually displayed with an ECG trace to enable identification of phases of the cardiac cycle. Used to investigate movement of individual structural elements (e.g. valves, chamber walls).
- **Doppler:** Enables flow across valves and ASD/VSDs to be quantified.

Cardiac catheterization: Refer via 2° care. Involves passing a catheter, usually via the femoral or brachial artery, to the heart. Used to:

- Measure pressures within the heart and great vessels
- Assess oxygen saturation via blood samples
- Perform coronary angiography—contrast is injected into the coronary arteries to assess their anatomy and/or patency
- Perform intravascular ultrasound
- Perform other procedures (e.g. angioplasty, valvuloplasty, cardiac biopsy)

Complications: Arrhythmia (0.56%); MI (0.07%); stroke (0.07%); death (0.14%); haemorrhage at the site of insertion (0.56%); thromboembolism; trauma to heart and vessels; infection.

Radionucleotide imaging: Refer via 2° care. Involves iv administration of a γ-emitting radionucleotide and gamma camera monitoring.

- **Radionucleotide angiography:** Uses technetium^{99m}-labelled RBCs to calculate left ventricular ejection fraction and assess ventricular action.
- **Myocardial perfusion scintigraphy:** Uses thallium^{201} injected IV during exercise testing to demonstrate areas of poorly perfused myocardium.

Cardiac MRI/magnetic resonance angiography: Used increasingly in 2° care to provide detailed structural information about the heart and rapid angiographic images.

Further information

ABC of electrocardiography (2002) *BMJ* 📖 http://www.bmjjournals.com

Patient information

British Heart Foundation ☎0845 708 070 📖 http://www.bhf.org.uk

Brief guide to common ECG changes

❶ For detailed analysis of ECGs, refer to a specialist text e.g. Hampton (2003) *The ECG made easy*. Churchill Livingstone

Table 10.1 Common ECG abnormalities and their causes

ECG abnormality		Possible causes
Tachycardia	Rate >100bpm	Physiological, AF, atrial flutter, SVT, VT.
Bradycardia	Rate <60bpm	Physiological, drugs (e.g. β-blockers, digoxin), heart block (see 📖 p.346), sick sinus syndrome.
Irregular	Assess whether any pattern or not	AF (no pattern), sick sinus syndrome (no pattern), ventricular ectopics (normally no pattern), heart block (pattern).
P-R interval	Short P-R interval	Nodal rhythm, WPW syndrome** (📖 p.343)
	Prolonged >0.2s.	Heart block (📖 p.346); sick sinus syndrome, drugs (e.g. β-blockers, digoxin)
Left bundle branch block (LBBB)*	QRS >0.12s. wide. Last peak is below the isoelectric line in V1.	IHD, ↑BP, cardiomyopathy, aortic valve disease, SVT. Artificial pacemakers may produce a similar QRS complex.
Right bundle branch block (RBBB)	QRS >0.12s. wide. Last peak is above the isoelectric line in V1.	May be normal; congenital heart disease (e.g. ASD), valvular heart disease, IHD, pulmonary hypertension, during SVT.
Incomplete bundle branch block	QRS<0.12s with abnormal shaped QRS complex.	As for RBBB or LBBB
Q-T interval abnormalities	Prolonged Q-T interval	↓K⁺, drugs (e.g. TCAs, phenothiazines, amiodarone), SAH or CVA, hypothermia.
	Shortened Q-T interval	↑Ca²⁺, digoxin.
Abnormal P-waves	↑ P-wave amplitude (>2.5mm)	Right atrial overload—tricuspid stenosis, pulmonary hypertension, pulmonary stenosis.
	Biphasic P-wave in V1 ±broad (>0.12s) often notched P wave in ≥ 1 limb lead.	Left atrial abnormality—mitral stenosis, aortic stenosis, conduction abnormalities.

* No comment can be made about ST segment or T wave if LBBB.
** WPW = Wolff Parkinson White syndrome.

Table 10.1 (cont.)

ECG abnormality		Possible causes
Right ventricular hypertrophy (RVH)	Strain pattern—ST depression and T-wave inversion in leads V1-3. Dominant R in V1 with narrow QRS.	Pulmonary stenosis, mitral stenosis, pulmonary hypertension, ASD (±RBBB). Similar changes seen with inferior MI (T-wave upright); WPW syndrome.
Left ventricular hypertrophy (LVH)	Strain pattern—ST↓ and T-wave ↓ in leads V4-6. Large voltages of QRS complex—sum of S in V1 and R in V5 or V6 alone >35mm.	↑BP, aortic stenosis, coarctation of the aorta, HOCM.
Right axis deviation	📖 p.310	RVH/strain (e.g. following PE), cor pulmonale, pulmonary stenosis. Alone with normal QRS = left posterior hemiblock.
Left axis deviation	📖 p.310	LVH/strain (e.g. ↑BP, aortic stenosis, HOCM), VSD, ASD. If occurs alone with normal QRS = left anterior hemiblock.
Poor R-wave progression	Small or absent R waves in the R → midprecordial leads.	L or R ventricular enlargement, LBBB, left pneumothorax, dextrocardia, COPD.
	Reversed R-wave progression—↓in R-wave amplitude from V1 → mid/lateral pre-cordial leads.	Right ventricular enlargement.
Abnormal Q-waves	>25% of succeeding R-wave and/or >0.04s. wide.	Normal; left pneumothorax; dextrocardia; MI; myocarditis; hyperkalaemia; cardiomyopathy; amyloid; sarcoid; scleroderma; LVH; RVH; LBBB; WPW syndrome.
ST elevation	ST segment raised >1mm above baseline.	MI, prinzmetal angina, pericarditis, ventricular aneurysm.
ST depression	ST segment lowered >0.5mm below baseline.	Angina, ventricular strain, drugs (digoxin, verapamil), hyperkalaemia, myocarditis, cardiomyopathy, fibrosis, Lyme disease.
T-wave inversion	Abnormal if inverted in leads I, II, or V4-6.	MI (inverts <24h. after MI); ventricular strain (see above); PE (III); digoxin (V5-6).
U-waves	↑ amplitude > 1mm.	Drugs (e.g. quinidine, procainamide, disopyramide) or ↓K+.
Inversion in precordial leads		Subtle sign of ischaemia.

❶ Always compare with previous ECGs, if available.

Prevention of coronary heart disease

Coronary heart disease (CHD) is the most common cause of death in UK (1:4 deaths). Mortality is falling is but morbidity, rising.

Primary prevention: *Objective:* To stop heart disease developing in a population. *Strategies:*

• *Population strategy:* Influences the factors which ↑ risk of CHD in an entire population e.g. anti-smoking campaigns (📖 p.234). GPs can do this by displaying health education posters/literature where all patients have access (waiting room, practice leaflet).
• *High-risk strategy:* Identifies individuals at high risk and attempts to ↓ their risk. Selection of patients is based on overall risk which depends on the combination of risk factors a patient has and can be estimated using tables (📖 p.326–7). Only small benefit is gained by screening an entire population, and population screening is not cost-effective[R]. An opportunistic strategy targeting high-risk individuals is preferable.

Secondary prevention: *Objective:* To stop progression of symptomatic CHD. 46% people who die from MI are already known to have CHD. There is strong evidence that targeting patients with CHD for risk-factor modification is effective in ↓ risk of recurrent CHD[S].

The GP's role

• Identification of patients who would benefit from 1° prevention through opportunistic risk-factor screening or routine checks (e.g. new patient checks)
• Ensuring patients who have proven atherosclerotic disease have ongoing follow-up; disease registers; routine recall and follow-up by the practice, PCT, and/or 2° care services; and monitoring of drug prescriptions
• Promoting lifestyle modification in at-risk patients
• Ensuring current best care guidelines are followed and treatment regimes are updated as policies change
• Checking the process through audit

Aspirin in prevention of vascular disease: Antiplatelet therapy is effective in ↓ cardiovascular morbidity and mortality. Aspirin (75–300mg od for maintenance treatment; 150–300mg for acute stroke/MI) is the agent most widely used. For patients with contraindications to aspirin, clopidogrel (75mg od) is an alternative.

Cautions

• Risk of major GI bleed at doses of 75–300mg od is 1:500 patient-years. ↓ gastric intolerance by using 75mg od, using dispersible or enteric-coated preparations, PPIs, or H_2 receptor antagonists.
• Avoid concomitant use of warfarin, except on specialist advice, as it significantly ↑ risk of bleeding.

Indications

• *CHD*
  • Suspected acute MI or unstable angina (stat dose of 150–300mg).

- Previous MI, angina, coronary artery surgery, or angioplasty.
- 1° prevention—consider for 1° prevention of MI in adults with type 2 DM, type 1 DM with high or moderately high risk of arterial disease, and patients with 10y. CHD risk ≥ 15% or CVD risk ≥ 20%. 75mg od → 20% ↓ in non-fatal MI at a cost of a small ↑ in risk of bleeding. Benefit ↑ with ↑ absolute risk of CHD.
- **↑ BP:** 📖 p.316. Patients age ≥50y. with satisfactory BP control (<150/90mmHg) + target organ damage, DM, or 10y. CVD risk ≥ 20%.
- **Stroke:** 📖 p.606. Following ischaemic stroke/TIA or carotid endarterectomy. Warfarin is preferable for patients with AF (📖 p.344) or other causes of cardio-embolic stroke.
- **Peripheral arterial disease:** 📖 p.360. Patients with claudication, peripheral angioplasty, or arterial grafts.
- **AF:** 📖 p.344. AF but no additional risk factors. Aspirin 75–150mg od. If AF and ≥ 1 risk factor—consider treatment with warfarin in preference to aspirin. *Risk factors:* previous ischaemic stroke/TIA, >65y., ↑ BP, DM, cardiac failure, Echo showing LV dysfunction or mitral valve calcification.

Table 10.2 Risk factors for heart disease

Non-modifiable	Modifiable (proven benefit)	Modifiable (unproven benefit)
Age: ↑ with age	Smoking: 📖 p.234	Haemostatic factors: ↑ plasma fibrinogen
Sex: ♂>♀ in those <65y.	Hyperlipidaemia: 📖 p.322	
Ethnic origin: in the UK, people who originate from the Indian subcontinent have ↑ risk; Afro-Caribbeans have ↓ risk	Hypertension: 📖 p.316 DM: 📖 p.404 Diet: 📖 p.226 Obesity: 📖 p.230	Apolipoproteins: ↑ Lipoprotein(a) Homocysteine: ↑ blood homocysteine
Socio-economic position	Physical inactivity: 📖 p.232	Vitamin levels: ↓ blood folate, vitamin B_{12} and B_6
Personal history of CHD	Left ventricular dysfunction/heart failure (2° prevention): 📖 p.338	Depression
Family history of CHD: <55y. ♂; <65y. ♀		
Low birth weight (IUGR)	Coronary prone behaviour: competitiveness, aggression and feeling under time pressure (2° prevention)—behaviour modification is associated with ↓ risk.	

Further information

DoH National Service Framework: Coronary Heart Disease (2000) 🖥 http://www.dh.gov.uk
SIGN 🖥 http://www.sign.ac.uk
- Lipids and the 1° prevention of CHD (1999)
- 2° prevention of CHD following MI (2000)

Patient information

British Heart Foundation ☎0845 708 070 🖥 http://www.bhf.org.uk

Hypertension^G

Major risk factor for CHD and CVA. ↑BP is normally symptomless until it causes organ damage. ~50% age 65-74y. have ↑BP. Management aims to detect and treat ↑BP before damage occurs. Hypertension is under-diagnosed and under-treated in the UK.

Diagnosis of hypertension: BP is a continuous variable—the higher the BP, the greater the risk of CVA/CHD. There is no figure above which hypertension can be diagnosed definitively, although currently, treatment is considered at BP >140/90 (see management guidelines below).

Measurement of BP^G

• Regularly maintain and calibrate your sphygmomanometer.
• Use a cuff of correct width:
  • *Most adults*; 12 × 26cm bladder;
  • *Large adults with arm circumference >33cm*; use 12 × 40cm bladder;
  • *Thin adults and children with arm circumference ≤ 26cm*; use 10 × 18cm bladder size.
• Seat the patient with arm at the level of the heart.
• In patients with symptoms of postural hypotension (falls or dizziness), measure BP when standing. If drop in systolic BP of >20mmHg, consider specialist referral.
• Measure BP to nearest 2mmHg.
• Measure diastolic pressure when heart sounds completely disappear (K_5) (only use the pressure at which they suddenly muffle (K_4) when K_5 cannot be determined).
• BP varies throughout the day and can ↑ as a response to having BP checked ('white coat phenomenon'—prevalence 10%). Take ≥ 2 measurements on 2 occasions before classifying a patient as hypertensive.
• BP measurements should normally be made at monthly intervals, but should be done more frequently in severe hypertension.
• If BP is very variable, consider ambulatory BP monitoring (gives average BP over 24h.) or intermittent home BP monitoring. (NICE does not recommend the routine use of these methods at present due to lack of research evidence.)

Causes

• Unknown—95% (essential hypertension); alcohol (10%) or obesity may be contributory factors
• Renal disease—🕮 p.677–83
• Endocrine disease—Cushing's (both syndrome and 2° to steroids); Conn's syndrome; phaeochromocytoma; acromegaly; hyperparathyroidism; DM: (🕮 p.404–19)
• Pregnancy—🕮 p.786
• Coarctation of the aorta—🕮 p.356

Presentation

• Usually asymptomatic and found during routine BP screening or incidentally. Occasionally, headache or visual disturbance.
• May be symptoms of end-organ damage—LVH, TIAs, previous CVA/MI, angina, renal impairment, PVD.

Examination: Check BP, heart size, heart sounds, heart failure, examine fundi (📖 p.954).

Investigation
- **Blood:** FBC, U&E, creatinine, glucose, lipid profile, consider GGT if excess alcohol is a possibility
- **Urine:** RBCs, glucose, protein
- **ECG**
- **Echo:** Consider referral if left ventricular hypertrophy suspected

△ **Malignant hypertension:** Presents with headache, very elevated BP (diastolic >140mmHg), renal failure, fits, coma (encephalopathy), severe retinopathy. Life-threatening condition. If malignant hypertension is suspected, admit as an acute medical emergency.

Summary of hypertension management: (based on NICE and British Hypertension Society (BHS) Guidelines, 2004)
- **Provide lifestyle modifications** for all those with high, borderline, or high normal BP
- **Discuss the need to formally assess cardiovascular risk with patients**
- **Consider specialist referral** for patients with signs or symptoms of 2° hypertension
- **Initiate antihypertensive drug therapy** in those with sustained systolic BP of ≥160 and/or diastolic ≥100mmHg
- **Systolic BP 140–159 and/or diastolic BP 90–99mmHg:** Treat those with a history of cardiovascular disease (CVD), target organ damage or estimated risk of CVD of ≥ 20% (CHD of ≥15%) over 10y.
- **In those with DM:** Initiate antihypertensive drug therapy if systolic BP is sustained ≥ 140 mmHg or diastolic ≥ 90mmHg (BHS)
- **Optimal BP treatment goals (BHS):**
  - In non-diabetic: systolic BP <140mmHg, diastolic <85mmHg
  - In diabetics, chronic renal disease or established CVD: systolic <130mmHg, diastolic <80mmHg
- **Most patients with ↑BP require ≥2 BP lowering drugs** to achieve BP goals—see BHS AB/CD treatment algorithm (📖 p.320)
- **Use low-dose aspirin 75mg/d.** (unless contraindicated) for 2° prevention ischaemic CVD and for 1° prevention in >50y. with 10yr CVD risk ≥20% and BP controlled <150/<90mmHg (BHS)

Statin therapy is recommended (BHS) for all those with ↑BP complicated by CVD, irrespective of baseline cholesterol or LDL levels and for 1° prevention in patients >40y. with↑BP and 10y. CVD risk ≥20%

Essential reading
NICE (2004) Hypertension—Management of hypertension in adults in primary care
  🖥 http://www.nice.org.uk
BHS Guidelines for the management of hypertension (2004)
  🖥 http://www.bhsoc.org

Patient information
British Heart Foundation ☎0845 708 070 🖥 http://www.bhf.org.uk

Management of hypertension^G

Malignant hypertension: 📖 p.317

Education: Patients will not take tablets regularly, be motivated to change lifestyle, or turn up for regular checks if they don't understand why treating their ↑ BP is important or what side-effects of treatment they are likely to experience. On the other hand, some patients who were fit and well prior to their diagnosis, will assume a sick role unless it is explained that they are well and treatment is designed to stop illness developing. Reinforce management at follow-up and give opportunities for discussion.

Initial treatment

- Treat other modifiable risk factors for CHD (📖 p.315) and CVA (📖 p.608)
- Aim to ↓BP to <140/85 (diabetics <130/80)
- Benefits of treatment remain in patients up to 85y. of age—and probably beyond. Offer patients >80y. the same treatment as young patients, taking into account any comorbidity and existing drug use.

Non-drug treatment: Offer to all hypertensives and those with FH of ↑BP. Reinforce advice with written information.

- Offer smoking cessation advice and help (📖 p.234)
- ↓ weight to optimum for height (📖 p.230)
- Encourage regular exercise—dynamic is best e.g. walking, swimming, cycling (📖 p.232)
- ↓ alcohol to <21u/wk. for ♂ and <14u/wk. for ♀ (📖 p.236–9)
- ↓ dietary salt intake
- ↑ dietary fruit and vegetable intake—aim for 5 portions/d.
- ↓ excess coffee consumption and other caffeine-rich products
- Encourage relaxation and stress management
- *Don't* offer Ca^{2+}, Mg^{2+}, or K^+ supplements as a method to ↓BP

Drug treatment

- *BP lowering drugs:* 📖 p.320
- *Aspirin* (📖 p.314): Recommend 75mg od for hypertensive patients if:
  - Aged ≥50y.
  - Satisfactory control of BP (<150/90mmHg) *and*
  - Target organ damage, DM, or 10y. CHD risk ≥ 20%
- *Statin therapy* (📖 p.324): Prescribe:
  - If ↑BP complicated by CVD irrespective of baseline cholesterol or LDL levels *or*
  - For 1° prevention in patients >40y. with ↑BP and 10y. CVD risk ≥20%

❶ Side-effects of drug treatment for hypertension are common. 40–50% started on an antihypertensive drug discontinue, regardless of which class of drug is used. 80% of side-effects are seen in 1st year of treatment.

Follow-up: Regular review of patients with ↑BP is essential. Once ↑BP is controlled, routine review of BP can be undertaken by properly trained practice nurses, but annual review of medication should be undertaken by a GP and the GP must review if BP is not controlled.

Review interval: Depends on stability of BP:
- *After starting treatment:* Review after 1mo.
- *If BP is controlled:* Review after a further 3mo. and then every 3–6mo.
- *If BP is not controlled:*
  - Bring the patient back to repeat the BP reading. *Don't* alter medication on the strength of a single BP reading.
  - If ↑BP is sustained, alter medication—see AB/CD guidelines 📖 p.320. Most patients need >1 drug.
  - If ↑ dose causes ↑ side-effects without improvement in response, alter medication.
  - Review in the same way monthly until BP is controlled.

Format of the annual review
- Check BP
- Look for signs of end-organ failure, including annual urine test for proteinuria
- Discuss symptoms and medication
- Assess and treat other modifiable risk factors for CHD/CVA
- Reinforce non-drug treatment (see opposite)

Referral to cardiology/general medicine
E = Emergency admission; U = Urgent; S = Soon; R = routine
- Malignant hypertension—E
- Renal impairment—U/S/R
- Suspected 2° hypertension—S/R
- Patients <35y.—R
- Multiple risk factors—R
- BP difficult to treat—R
- Pregnancy—to obstetrician; urgency depends on stage of pregnancy and clinical features (📖 p.786)

Reducing or stopping treatment: ↓BP too far (<120/80) may ↑ mortality, especially in the elderly.
- *Don't* stop medication if high CVD risk or end-organ damage.
- If diastolic BP <80 and systolic BP <140 consistently, consider decreasing or stopping medication. 1–2y. after withdrawal of medication, 50% are normotensive and 40% stay off drug therapy permanently.
- Elderly people are prone to postural hypotension. Check for postural drop (sitting and standing BP). If present, ↓ dose of antihypertensive.
- Continue BP follow-up lifelong, even if off medication.

Essential reading
NICE (2004) Hypertension—management of hypertension in adults in primary care 🖥 http://www.nice.org.uk
BHS Guidelines for the management of hypertension (2004)
🖥 http://www.bhsoc.org

Patient information
British Heart Foundation ☎0845 708 070 🖥 http://www.bhf.org.uk

Drug treatment of hypertension[G]

At the time of writing, 2 major guideline-producing bodies in the UK have produced new guidelines for the treatment of hypertension in primary care. These do not concur. For more information, please obtain the original guidelines:
- *NICE:* Hypertension—Management of hypertension in adults in primary care (2004) 🖳 http://www.nice.org.uk
- *British Hypertension Society (BHS):* Guidelines for the management of hypertension (2004) 🖳 http://www.bhsoc.org

NICE (2004): Recommendations for drug treatment:
- Normally begin with a low-dose thiazide diuretic. If young (<55y.), consider starting with a β blocker.
- If necessary, as a 2nd line, add a β blocker *unless* the patient is at risk of new onset DM (strong FH, type 2 DM, impaired glucose tolerance, obese (BMI >30) or of South Asian or African-Caribbean origin).
- If the patient is at risk of new onset DM, add an ACE Inhibitor as 2nd line. Offer an angiotensin receptor blocker if ACE inhibitors are not tolerated due to cough.
- 3rd line—add a dihydropyridine calcium channel blocker. *Only* dihydropyridine calcium channel blockers should be used with a β blocker.
- 4th line—consider other drugs or refer.

General rules
- *If a drug is not tolerated:* Stop and move on to next line of therapy.
- *If a drug is tolerated but the BP target isn't met:* Add in the next line of therapy.

BHS (2004): The AB/CD algorithm is a guide to aid decision making when combining drugs. It operates on the theory that ↑BP can be broadly classified as 'high' or 'low renin'—Table 10.3.

Table 10.3 BHS guidance on combining BP lowering drugs

	The AB/CD rule	
	Younger (<55y.) and non-black	*Older (≥55y.) or black*
Step 1	A (or B*)	C or D
Step 2	A (or B*) + C or D	
Step 3	A (or B*) + C + D	
Step 4—resistant ↑BP	Add either an α blocker or spironolactone or other diuretic	

A: ACE inhibitor or angiotensin receptor blocker   B: β blocker
C: Calcium channel blocker   D: Diurectic
* Combination of B and D may induce more new onset DM compared to other combinations.

Reproduced with permission of the British Hypertension Society.

Table 10.4 First-line antihypertensive drugs

Class of 1st line drug	Reasons to choose the drug	Reasons to avoid the drug
α blockers BNF 2.5.4	Prostatism Dyslipidaemia	Urinary incontinence worsens Postural hypotension is common
ACE inhibitors BNF 2.5.5.1 ❶ Check U&E and Cr before starting and at first follow-up.	Heart failure or left ventricular dysfunction Post MI or established CVD Diabetic nephropathy 2° stroke prevention	⚠ Do not use: If known renovascular disease—can precipitate renal failure; or in pregnancy
Angiotensin receptor blocker BNF 2.5.5.2 ❶ Check U&E and Cr before starting and monitor K^+ at follow-up.	ACE inhibitor intolerance Diabetic nephropathy ↑BP + LVH Heart failure if ACE intolerant Post MI	Use with caution: If aortic or mitral valve stenosis and in obstructive hypertrophic cardiomyopathy
β blockers BNF 2.4 ❶ May accumulate in patients with renal failure—↓ dose.	MI and/or angina	Avoid in patients with: Asthma, COPD, heart block, heart failure, peripheral vascular disease, hyperlipidaemia. In patients with DM: May → small deterioration in glucose tolerance and ↓ awareness of hypoglycaemia.
Calcium channel blockers BNF 2.6.2 ❶ Different agents have different therapeutic effects.	Dihydropyridine agents: Of proven efficacy in the elderly and those with isolated systolic hypertension. Rate-limiting agents: Useful in those with angina or post MI.	Rate-limiting agents: Avoid in patients with heart block or heart failure. Do not combine with β blockers.
Thiazide diuretics BNF 2.2.1 ❶ Use the lowest dose. Higher doses don't have additional effect on BP.	More effective than β blockers in the elderly	Avoid in patients with gout. May adversely affect lipid profile.

❶ Most patients require >1 drug to control their BP
⚠ Avoid combination of β-blockers and rate-limiting calcium antagonists (verapamil, diltiazem) due to risk of bradycardia/asystole.

Hyperlipidaemia

Average cholesterol level in a population is a predictor of CHD risk and dependent on diet but, on an individual level, it is a much poorer predictor—only 42% who develop CHD have ↑ cholesterol. However, lowering cholesterol is of proven benefit in 1° and 2° prevention of CHD. Concern that low cholesterol is associated with ↑ risk of death from other causes (e.g. suicide, cancer) is unfounded.

Cholesterol: Fatty substance manufactured by the body (mainly liver) which plays a vital role in functioning of cell membranes. Total plasma cholesterol consists of:
- **LDL (low-density lipoprotein) cholesterol**—high levels associated with ↑ risk CHD
- **HDL (high-density lipoprotein) cholesterol**—low levels associated with ↑ risk CHD
- **Triglycerides (TGs)**—independent risk factor for CHD. If >5mmol/l refer for specialist opinion
- **Ratio of total cholesterol:HDL**—used to predict risk. No threshold; the higher the ratio, the greater the risk.

Testing for hyperlipidaemia: Blood cholesterol concentration is not steady over time. 1:4 ↑ cholesterols are normal on repeat testing. Check ≥ 2 samples at different times:
- **Before initiating treatment or if screening for familial dyslipidaemia**—take fasting samples checking triglycerides.
- **Screening and routine follow-up**—take non-fasting samples testing total blood cholesterol and total cholesterol:HDL ratio.

Screening
- **1° prevention:** Whole population screening + dietary advice has little effect on cholesterol levels and may ↓ impact of population strategies (less inclination to alter diet if cholesterol levels are known to be normal) and allow sufferers to assume a sick role. The alternative is opportunistic screening of those age 35–70y. with other risk factors or signs of ↑ cholesterol (corneal arcus <50y., xanthelasma, xanthomata).
- **2° prevention:** All those who have proven CHD—check cholesterol levels annually.
- **Familial hyperlipidaemia:** Screen 1st degree blood relatives >18y. old with fasting lipids if:
  - FH of familial hyperlipidaemia
  - FH of premature CHD (men <55y., women <65y.) or other atherosclerotic disease
  Screening interval has not been determined—5y. seems reasonable.

Familial hyperlipidaemia: There are many types of familial dyslipidaemia. If suspected, refer. Common forms include:
- **Polygenic hypercholesterolaemia**—most common form of familial dyslipidaemia. Presents with FH of premature CHD + ↑ total cholesterol
- **Familial combined hyperlipidaemia**—polygenic hyperlipidaemia affecting 0.5–1% of the population and ~15% of those suffering MI <60y.

Associated with obesity, insulin resistance/DM, ↑BP, xanthelasma, corneal arcus, and premature IHD. ↑ total cholesterol (6.5–10mmol/l); ↑ TGs (2.3–12mmol/l).

- *Familial hypercholesterolaemia* (type IIa)—autosomal dominant. Heterozygous form present in 1:500. Associated with tendon xanthomata and FH premature IHD. ↑ LDL (>4.9mmol/l); ↑ total cholesterol (>7.5mmol/l); normal TGs.
- *Familial hypertriglyceridaemia* (type IV/V)—autosomal dominant. Affects ~1% of the general population and ~5% having MI<60y. Associated with DM, obesity, gout, eruptive xanthomas, and pancreatitis. Normal (or slightly ↑) total cholesterol; ↑ TGs (2.3–>10mmol/l).

Secondary hyperlipidaemia: Conditions associated with 2° hyperlipidaemia include:

- Drugs
  - Steroids
  - β blockers
  - Thiazides
  - COC pill
  - Isotretinoin
- Obesity
- DM (📖 p.404)
- Excess alcohol
- Pregnancy
- ↓T₄*
- Renal failure
- Nephrotic syndrome
- Cholestasis
- Cushing's syndrome
- Porphyria
- Myeloma
- Lipodystrophies
- Glycogen storage disease

Management of hypercholesterolaemia: 📖 p.324.

Essential reading

British Hypertension Society (2004) Guidelines for the management of hypertension 🖥 http://www.hyp.ac.uk/bhs
SIGN 🖥 http://www.bhsoc.org
- Lipids and the 1° prevention of CHD (1999)
- 2° prevention of CHD following MI (2000)
Joint British recommendations on prevention of CHD in clinical practice: summary (2000) 🖥 http://www.bmj.com
NICE (in preparation) Hyperlipidaemia: identification and management of hyperlipidaemia as part of cardiovascular risk assessment in 1° care 🖥 http://www.nice.org.uk

Patient information

British Heart Foundation ☎0845 708 070 🖥 http://www.bhf.org.uk

---

* Patients with hypothyroidism should receive adequate thyroid replacement before assessing need for lipid-lowering treatment. Correction of hypothyroidism may resolve the lipid abnormality and untreated hypothyroidism ↑ risk of myositis with statins.

Management of hypercholesterolaemia[G]

Lowering LDL and raising HDL ↓ progression of coronary atherosclerosis—whatever the age of the patient.

Calculating cardiovascular disease (CVD) risk: Always consider ↑ cholesterol with other risk factors for CHD/CVD. Calculate risk using tables (📖 p.326–7) or a computer program e.g. Joint British Societies' Cardiac Risk Assessor (available free at *http://www.bhsoc.org*).

❶ Decisions on whether to treat ↑ cholesterol have been based in recent years on CHD risk, but there is a move to change this to CVD risk to reflect the importance of stroke as well as CHD prevention.

Non-drug therapy: Offer to all patients with ↑ cholesterol and those with DM or FH of CHD/CVD. Reinforce advice with written information.
• ↓ intake of saturated fats (<7% of total calories) and cholesterol (<200mg/d.). If cholesterol level >5mmol/l, low cholesterol diets → average ↓ in cholesterol of 8.5% at 3mo..
• Margarines and other foods enriched with plant sterol or stanol esters inhibit cholesterol absorption from the GI tract and can ↓ serum cholesterol in those on an average diet by 10%. Their effect on individuals already on a low-fat diet is less.
• Weight ↓—in patients with BMI ≥30kg/m², weight ↓ of 10kg → 7% ↓ in LDL and 13% ↑ in HDL.
• ↑ physical activity—enhances cholesterol-lowering effects of diet and weight ↓
• Give general advice about ↓ CHD/CVD risk (📖 p.315 and 608) e.g. smoking cessation.

Drug therapy with statins: Table 10.5

1° prevention
• Initiate statin therapy if 10y. CVD risk ≥30% (CHD risk ≥20%) and total cholesterol >5mmol/l. The long-term aim is to treat all patients with 10y. CVD risk ≥20% (CHD risk ≥15%)[G]. ↓ cholesterol → ↓ all cause mortality by 22% and ↓ CHD events by 31%.
• Treat all type 2 diabetics with a statin. This ↓ risk of MI/CVA by ~¼ regardless of initial cholesterol[R].

2° prevention: Although statin treatment is often only offered to patients with total cholesterol >5mmol/l at present, trial data suggest all patients with proven CHD benefit from ↓ in total cholesterol and LDL irrespective of initial cholesterol concentration[S]. ↓ in total cholesterol and LDL by 25–35% using statin therapy → ↓ CHD mortality by 25–35%[S]

Treatment target[G]: Aim to ↓ total cholesterol by 25% or to <4mmol/l—whichever is the lower value *or* to ↓ LDL cholesterol by 30% or to < 2.0mmol/l—whichever is the lower value.

Minimum audit standard[G]: Total cholesterol <5.0mmol/l or LDL cholesterol <3.0mmol/l or ↓ by 25% or 30%, respectively—whichever is the lower value. All type 2 diabetics offered a statin.

Routine referral to cardiology/general medicine for:
• Familial hypercholesterolaemia (± referral to genetics)
• High triglycerides
• Hypercholesterolaemia resistant to treatment or difficult to treat

Table 10.5 Notes on prescribing statins (*BNF 2.12*)

Contraindications	Pregnancy; breast-feeding; active liver disease.
Important interactions	↑ effect warfarin; ↑ risk myositis when taken with other lipid-lowering drugs, macrolide antibiotics (e.g. erythromycin), or ciclosporin.
Choice of statin	Evidence of efficacy in RCTs for simvastatin and pravastatin only. Others (e.g. fluvastatin, atorvastatin) may be cheaper.
Dose	Base either on doses used in trials (simvastatin 20mg/ pravastatin 40mg) or start at lowest dose and titrate upwards until effective.
Titration of dose	Measure cholesterol 4–6 wkly and adjust dose upwards until target levels are reached
Patient education	Statins are most effective taken in the evening. The most important adverse effect is myositis (<1:10,000). Ask to report any unexplained muscle pain/weakness. If this occurs, check CK—if >5x upper limit of normal, withdraw therapy.
Monitoring	Fasting sample for triglycerides and glucose pre-treatment.
	Measure total cholesterol (non-fasting) 4–6wk. after starting treatment or after any dose change. If stable; measure 6–12 monthly
	Measure liver function tests pre-treatment and after 1–3mo. Thereafter, measure each 6mo. for 1y. Discontinue if serum transaminase ↑ (and stays at) >3x normal.

Essential reading

BHS (2004) Guidelines for the management of hypertension 🖳 http://www.bhsoc.org
SIGN 🖳 http://www.sign.ac.uk
• Lipids and the 1° prevention of CHD (1999)
• 2° prevention of CHD following MI (2000)
Joint British recommendations on prevention of CHD in clinical practice: summary (2000) 🖳 http://www.bmj.com
MRC/BHF Heart Protection Study of cholesterol lowering with simvastatin of 5963 people with diabetes: a randomized placebo-controlled trial (2003) *Lancet* **362**: 2005–16
NICE Guidelines (due in 2005/6) 🖳 http://www.nice.org.uk

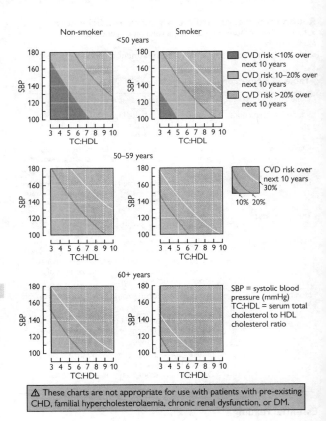

Figure 10.1 Cardiovascular risk chart for non-diabetic men. (Reproduced with permission of Manchester University.)

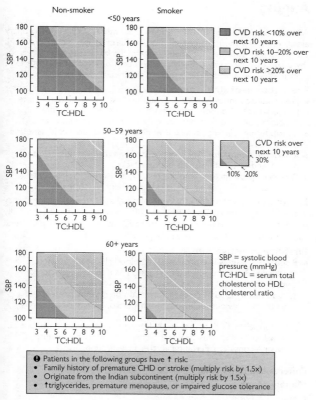

Figure 10.2 Cardiovascular risk chart for non-diabetic women. (Reproduced with permission of Manchester University.)

Angina^G

Affects ~2% population in UK. Incidence ↑ with age. ♂ > ♀. Coronary artery disease is the most common cause. Rarer causes include: HOCM, valve disease, hypoperfusion during arrhythmia, arteritis, anaemia, or thyrotoxicosis. Mortality (usually sudden death or after MI or acute LVF) is ~0.5–4%/y.—doubled if coexistent left ventricular dysfunction.

Presentation of stable angina: Diagnosis is usually made on history:
- *Pain:* Episodic central-crushing or band-like chest pain which may radiate → jaw/neck and/or 1 or both arms. Pain in the arms/neck may be the only symptom. Ask about frequency, severity, duration, and timing of attacks.
- *Precipitating/relieving factors:* Precipitated by exertion, cold, emotion, and/or heavy meals. Pain stops with rest or GTN spray.
- *Associated symptoms:* May be associated with palpitations, sweating, nausea, and/or breathlessness during attacks.
- *Presence of risk factors:* Smoking history; family history; history of other vascular disease e.g. CVA/TIA, peripheral vascular disease.

Examination: There are usually no physical signs, though anaemia may exacerbate symptoms. Check BMI and BP. Look for murmurs (especially ejection systolic murmur of aortic stenosis) and evidence of peripheral vascular disease and carotid bruits (especially in diabetics).

First-line investigations
- *Blood:* FBC, fasting lipid profile, fasting blood glucose. Consider checking ESR (to exclude arteritis) and TFTs if clinical suspicion of thyrotoxicosis.
- *12-lead resting ECG:* Provides information on rhythm, presence of heart block, previous MI, myocardial hypertrophy, and/or ischaemia.

❶ A Normal ECG does not exclude coronary artery disease, but an abnormal ECG identifies those at higher risk of cardiac events in the next year—consider referral for further investigation.

Differential diagnosis: Chest pain—📖 p.1046–7
Management
General advice
- *Driving:* Patients who drive should inform the DVLA and their insurance company of the diagnosis. Vocational drivers (📖 p.204).
- *Occupation:* Patients may not be able to undertake heavy work—give advice and support. Special rules apply to some occupations e.g. merchant seamen, airline pilots—advise patients to consult their occupational health department.

Non-drug treatment: Aimed at 2° prevention of CHD (📖 p.314).
- *Smoking cessation*—📖 p.234
- *Hypertension:* Check BP and treat if >140/90—📖 p.316
- *Diet:* Advise healthy diet (oily fish, low cholesterol, ↑ fruit and vegetables, ↓ salt) and, if obese, aim to ↓ weight until BMI <25
- *Alcohol:* ↓ excess consumption. Targets: <3u/d. ♂; <2u/d. ♀

- *Exercise:* ↑ aerobic exercise within the limits set by the disease state
- *Diabetes:* Treat any underlying DM—📖 p.404–19
- *Cardiac rehabilitation:* May be helpful for patients with severe angina and/or after surgery.

Drug treatment: 📖 p.330

Referral for exercise ECG: 📖 p.310. Refer all patients with angina, unless contraindicated, for an exercise tolerance test to allow risk stratification. If contraindicated, refer to cardiology. Advise patients to take their usual medication prior to going for the test.

Contraindications

- Symptoms uncontrolled by maximal medical treatment
- Uncertain diagnosis
- Proven or suspected aortic stenosis or cardiomyopathy or physically incapable of performing the test for reasons other than angina
- Results of stress testing would not affect management
- LBBB on ECG

Referral to cardiology: E = Admit; U = Urgent; S = Soon; R = Routine

- Unstable angina/rapidly progressive symptoms—E
- Aortic stenosis with angina—U
- Angina following MI—U/S
- Abnormal ECG at diagnosis—U/S
- Angina not controlled by medication—U/S/R
- If diagnosis is in doubt—S/R
- Exercise test contraindicated—R
- Strong family history—R
- Other factors e.g. occupation affected—R

Unstable angina: Pain on minimal or no exertion, pain at rest (may occur at night), or angina which is rapidly worsening in intensity, frequency, or duration. *Incidence:* 6/10,000/y.; 15% suffer MI in <1mo. **Management:** Urgent referral to cardiology. Admit if attacks are severe, occur at rest, or last >20min. even with GTN spray.

Bypass surgery (CABG) and coronary angioplasty: CABG ↓ mortality over 5y., 7y., and 10y. and ↓ symptoms in 80–90%. Angioplasty → improves symptoms in 70% though evidence of ↓ in mortality is lacking; coronary artery stenting improves symptom control and relapse rate.

Prinzmetal (variant) angina: Angina at rest due to coronary artery spasm. ECG shows ST elevation. *Management:* Refer to cardiology to exclude MI and atherosclerotic angina. GTN alleviates immediate episodes. Calcium channel blockers are used to prevent angina. (*After M. Prinzmetal (1908–87)—US cardiologist*)

Further information

SIGN (2001) Management of stable angina 🖥 http://www.sign.ac.uk
Cardiac rehabilitation 🖥 http://www.cardiacrehabilitation.org.uk

Patient information

British Heart Foundation ☎0845 708 070 🖥 http://www.bhf.org.uk

Drug treatment of angina

Symptom control: *(BNF 2.6)*

As required medication

- Glyceryl trinitrate (GTN) spray is used for 'as required' symptom relief for angina.
- If symptoms are infrequent (≤2 attacks/wk.), GTN may be used alone; if attacks are more frequent, add regular symptomatic treatment (below).
- Advise 1 or 2 puffs, as needed, in response to pain and before engaging in activities that bring on pain.
- If response to GTN spray is poor, consider a buccal preparation.

> ❶ Sublingual GTN tablets are an alternative to GTN spray but deteriorate after 8wk.

> ⚠ Warn patients to call for help (dial 999 or ring emergency GP) if chest pain lasts >20min. despite GTN spray.

Regular treatment

- If symptoms are severe or >2x/wk., prescribe regular symptomatic treatment—Table 10.6.
- Introduce medication in a stepwise manner according to response:
  - Start with a β blocker (e.g. atenolol 50–100mg od) unless contraindicated/intolerant.
  - Add a long-acting dihydropyridine calcium channel blocker (e.g. amlodipine 5mg od) as 2nd line.
  - Add a long-acting nitrate (e.g. isosorbide mononitrate 20mg bd/tds) as a 3rd line.
  - For patients without left ventricular dysfunction, and in whom β blockers are inappropriate, use diltiazem (60mg bd/tds) or vera-pamil (80–120mg tds) as 1st line treatment and add a long-acting nitrate if symptom control is not adequate.
  - For patients with left ventricular dysfunction, use a long-acting nitrate as 1st line treatment and add a long-acting dihydropyridine calcium channel blocker if symptom control is not adequate.
  - For those intolerant of standard treatment, or where standard treatment has failed, try nicorandil (5–10mg bd).
- Within any drug class, use the cheapest preparation that the patient can tolerate, will comply with, and which controls symptoms.

> ⚠ Avoid combination of β blockers and rate-limiting calcium channel blocker (verapamil, diltiazem) due to risk of bradycardia/asystole.

2° prevention

Aspirin: ↓ mortality by 34%. Unless contraindicated, give 75mg od to all patients with angina. Consider clopidogrel 75mg od if aspirin intolerant.

Statins: ↓ in total cholesterol and LDL by 25–35% using statin therapy → ↓ CHD mortality by 25–35%[S]. Trial data suggest all patients with proven CHD benefit from ↓ in total cholesterol and LDL irrespective of initial cholesterol concentration[S]—📖 p.324.

Table 10.6 Drug treatment of angina

Drug	Treatment notes
β blockers *(BNF 2.4)* ❶ May accumulate in patients with renal failure—↓ dose	Effective for symptom control and to prevent vascular events.
	Check fully β-blocked by monitoring heart rate—resting heart rate ≤65bpm; post-exercise (e.g. walking up 2 flights of stairs) heart rate ≤90bpm. Further increases in dose once adequately β-blocked are usually unhelpful.
	Warn patients not to stop suddenly or run out.
	If the patient needs to stop the drug, tail off over 4wk.
	Contraindications: asthma, left ventricular dysfunction, bradycardia.
Dihydropyridine calcium-channel blockers *(BNF 2.6.2)*	Amlodipine, felodipine, isradipine, lacidipine, lercanidipine, nicardipine, nifedipine, nimodipine, and nisoldipine.
	All equally effective in symptom control. No evidence of cardioprotective effect.
	Contraindications: vary. Don't use if aortic stenosis, <1mo. post MI or uncontrolled heart failure, except with specialist advice.
Rate-limiting calcium channel blockers *(BNF 2.6.2)*	Diltiazem and verapamil
	Contraindications: avoid in patients with heart block or heart failure. Do not combine with β blockers.
Long-acting nitrates *(BNF 2.6.1)* e.g. isosorbide mononitrate (ISMO)	Oral and patch preparations (dosages ≥10mg/24h.) are available.
	Start with a low dose and ↑ as tolerated. Side-effects are common.
	Side-effects: headache, postural hypotension and dizziness—wear off with use. Reflex tachycardia may ↓ coronary blood flow and worsen angina.
	Tolerance: many patients rapidly develop tolerance with ↓ therapeutic effect. To avoid this, allow a nitrate-free period of 4–8h./d. overnight by removing patches at night or giving the 2nd dose of ISMO at 4 p.m.
	Contraindications: HOCM, aortic stenosis, constrictive pericarditis, mitral stenosis, severe anaemia, closed-angle glaucoma.
Potassium channel activator *(BNF 2.6.3)*	Nicorandil
	Similar efficacy to other antianginal drugs in controlling symptoms.
	May produce additional symptomatic benefit in combination with other antianginal drugs (unlicensed).
	Headache is common—usually transitory.
	Contraindications: left ventricular failure; hypotension.

After myocardial infarction (MI)

Acute myocardial infarct: 📖 p.1048

Management post MI

Modification of risk factors: 2° prevention (📖 p.314).
- *Cholesterol:* Although statin treatment is often, at present, only offered to patients with total cholesterol >5mmol/l, trial data suggest *all* patients with proven CHD benefit from ↓ in total cholesterol and LDL irrespective of initial cholesterol concentration[5]. ↓ in total cholesterol and LDL by 25–35% using statin therapy → ↓ CHD mortality by 25–35%. Serum cholesterol levels ↓ after MI and remain ↓ for several weeks.
- *β blockers:* Unless contraindicated, start all patients on an oral β blocker (e.g. atenolol) soon after MI and continue indefinitely. Estimated to prevent 12 deaths/1000 treated/y.

ACE inhibitors: ↓ myocardial work and ↓ deaths within 1mo. post MI by 5/1000 treated. Survival advantage is sustained >1y. even if treatment is not continued long-term. Effects are greater for patients with heart failure at presentation. *Long-term ACE inhibitors:* Trials show ↓ mortality for all patients.

Aspirin: Starting aspirin <24h. after MI prevents 80 vascular events over the next 2y./1000 patients treated. Unless contraindicated, continue life long. There is some debate about optimal dose—usual practice is to give 150mg od for 1mo. after MI and then ↓ to 75mg od from then onwards. Occasionally (e.g. left ventricular aneurysm, AF), anticoagulation is indicated.

Exercise testing: Routine exercise testing identifies those likely to have angina post MI who might benefit from early angiography ± angioplasty or CABG.

Cardiac rehabilitation: ↓ risk of death by 20–25%. Provided by specialist multidisciplinary teams. *Components include:* Psychological support, information about CHD, modification of risk factors.

The role of the GP

Support after discharge
- *Physical activity*—advise gradual ↑ in activity. Ensure goals given match those given by local cardiac rehabilitation. *Guide:*
  - 2wk. after MI—stroll in garden or street
  - 4wk. after MI —walk ½ mile/d.
  - 4–6wk. after MI—↑ to 2 miles/d. by 6wk.
  - From 6wk.—↑ speed of walking; aim 2 miles in <30min.
- *Sexual activity*—resume after 6wk. A leaflet is available from the British Heart Foundation.
- *Return to work*—guide:
  - Sedentary workers—4–6wk. after uncomplicated MI
  - Light manual workers—6–8wk. after uncomplicated MI
  - Heavy manual workers—3mo. after uncomplicated MI

- *Psychological effects*—≈½ are depressed 1wk. after MI and 25% after 1y. Educate about CHD. Check for depression, counsel, and treat as needed.
- *Driving*—no driving for 1mo. after MI. Inform car insurance company but no need to inform DVLA. HGV and PSV licence holders must notify the DVLA. Driving may be allowed after assessment.
- *Flying*—most airlines will not carry passengers for 2wk. post MI and then only if able to climb 1 flight of stairs without difficulty.

Ongoing follow-up

- *Monitoring health*—'continue regular reviews at least annually' lifelong. Check for symptoms and signs of cardiac dysfunction (breathlessness, palpitations, angina); depression; carer stress.
- *Monitoring drug therapy*—ongoing prescription of drugs, monitoring of compliance and side-effects, changing medication if clinical circumstances or best practice alter.
- *2° prevention*
  - *Smoking cessation*—📖 p.234. ↓ risk of death by 50% over 15y.
  - *Hypertension*—Check BP and treat if >140/90 (📖 p.316)
  - *Diet*—Advise healthy diet (low cholesterol, ↑ fruit and vegetables, ↓ salt) and, if obese, aim to ↓ weight until BMI <25. Diets rich in omega-6 and omega-3 fatty acids (found in oily fish, vegetables, and nuts) ↓ CHD in 2° prevention but effect is through ↓ in risk of thrombosis and not associated with ↓ cholesterol.
  - *Alcohol*—↓ excess consumption. *Targets:* <3u/d. ♂; <2u/d. ♀
  - *Exercise*—↑ aerobic exercise within the limits set by the disease state.
  - *Diabetes*—Treat any underlying DM (📖 p.404).
  - *Reinforce information given during cardiac rehabilitation*

Dressler syndrome (post MI syndrome): Develops 2–10wk. after MI or heart surgery. Thought to be due to auto-antibodies to heart muscle. Presents with recurrent fever and chest pain ± pleural and/or pericardial effusion. *Management:* Refer urgently for cardiology/general medical advice. Treatment is with steroids and NSAIDs.
(W. Dressler (1890–1969)—U.S. physician)

Further information

DoH National Service Framework: Coronary heart disease (2000) 🖳 http://www.dh.gov.uk
Cardiac rehabilitation 🖳 http://www.cardiacrehabilitation.org.uk.

Patient information

British Heart Foundation ☎0845 708 070 🖳 http://www.bhf.org.uk

Chronic heart failure[G]

Chronic heart failure occurs when output of the heart is inadequate to meet the needs of the body. It is the end stage of all diseases of the heart. *Prevalence:* 3–20/1000 population (1–1.6%). Incidence ↑ with age.

Causes of chronic heart failure
- **High-output:** The heart is working at normal or ↑ rate but the needs of the body are ↑ beyond that which the heart can supply e.g. hyperthyroidism, anaemia, Paget's disease, A-V malformation.
- **Low-output:** ↓ heart function. *Causes:*
  - ↑ pre-load: e.g. mitral regurgitation, fluid overload.
  - *Pump failure:*
    — Cardiac muscle disease—IHD (46%), cardiomyopathy
    — ↓ expansion of heart and restricted filling—restrictive cardiomyopathy, constrictive pericarditis, tamponade
    — Inadequate heart rate—β blockers, heart block, post MI
    — Arrythmia—most common; AF ≈ 30% patients with heart failure
    — ↓ power—negatively ionotropic drugs e.g. verapamil, diltiazem
  - *Chronic excessive afterload:* ↑BP (70%—may be in combination with IHD), aortic stenosis.
- **Primary right heart failure:** e.g. pulmonary hypertension (📖 p.340), tricuspid incompetence.

Risk factors
- Smoking
- Alcohol (toxic effect on the heart) —cause of heart failure in 2–3%
- DM
- Obesity
- High total cholesterol: HDL ratio
- LVH on Echo

Presentation: Clinical diagnosis is difficult. 20–30% patients diagnosed by their GP as having heart failure do not have any demonstrable abnormality of cardiac function on Echo testing. Take a detailed history and do a clinical examination to exclude other disorders.

Algorithm for diagnosing heart failure: Figure 10.3 (📖 p.336)

Classification and symptoms
- **Left ventricular failure (LVF):** Failure of the left ventricle causing back pressure into pulmonary system and giving symptoms and signs within the respiratory system. *Symptoms include:*
  - Shortness of breath (on exertion, orthopnoea, PND)
  - ↓ exercise tolerance
  - Lethargy/fatigue
  - Nocturnal cough (may bring up pink froth or have haemoptysis)
  - Wheeze
- **Right ventricular failure (RVF):** Failure of the right ventricle causing back pressure into peripheral circulation resulting in symptoms /signs in the abdomen or limbs. *Symptoms include:*
  - Swelling of ankles
  - Abdominal discomfort due to liver distension
  - Nausea and anorexia
  - Fatigue and wasting
  - Often ↑ weight
- **Congestive cardiac failure (CCF):** Failure of both ventricles.

Signs:
- Cachexia and muscle wasting
- ↑ RR ± cyanosis
- ↑ pulse rate
- Cardiomegaly and displaced apex beat
- Right ventricular heave
- ↑ JVP
- Pulsus alternans
- 3rd heart sound
- Basal crepitations ± pleural effusions and/or wheeze
- Pitting oedema of the ankles
- Hepatomegaly
- Ascites

Other conditions that may present with similar symptoms
- Obesity
- Respiratory disease
- Venous insufficiency in lower limbs
- Drug-induced ankle swelling (e.g. calcium channel blockers) or fluid retention (e.g. NSAIDs)
- Hypoalbuminaemia
- Intrinsic renal or hepatic disease
- Pulmonary embolic disease
- Depression and/or anxiety
- Severe anaemia
- Thyroid disease
- Bilateral renal artery stenosis
- Intrinsic renal or hepatic disease
- Pulmonary embolic disease
- Depression and/or anxiety
- Severe anaemia or thyroid disease
- Bilateral renal artery stenosis.

Complications
- Arrythmias—especially AF and VT
- Stroke or peripheral embolus
- DVT/PE
- Malabsorption
- Hepatic congestion/dysfunction
- Muscle wasting

Management: 📖 p.338

Prognosis: Progressive deterioration to death. ~½ die suddenly—probably due to arrythmias. *Mortality:*
- Mild/moderate heart failure—20–30% 1y. mortality
- Severe heart failure—>50% 1y. mortality.

Acute heart failure: 📖 p.1056

Essential reading
NICE (2003) Chronic heart failure 🖥 www.nice.org.uk

Patient information
British Heart Foundation ☎0845 708 070 🖥 http://www.bhf.org.uk

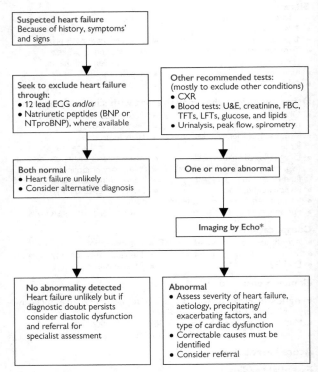

* Consider alternative methods of imaging if a poor image is produced
(e.g. transoesophageal Echo, radionuclide imaging, or cardiac MRI)

Figure 10.3 NICE algorithm for diagnosing heart failure. (Reproduced with permission of NICE from *Chronic heart failure: management of chronic heart failure in adults in primary and secondary care*, 2003.)

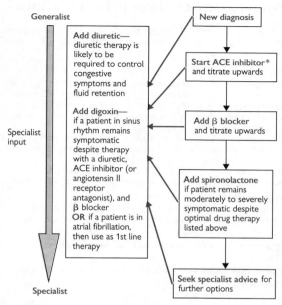

* If ACE inhibitor is not tolerated (e.g. due to severe cough), consider an angiotensin II receptor antagonist

Figure 10.4 NICE algorithm for pharmacological treatment of symptomatic heart failure due to left ventricular systolic dysfunction. (Reproduced with permission of NICE from *Chronic heart failure: management of chronic heart failure in adults in primary and secondary care*, 2003.)

Management of chronic heart failure

❶ Always look for the underlying cause and treat wherever possible. Review the basis for historical diagnoses and arrange Echo to confirm if diagnosis is in doubt.

Non-drug measures

- *Educate*—about the disease, current/expected symptoms' and need for treatment. Discuss prognosis. Support with written information.
- *Discuss ways to make life easier*—e.g. benefits, mobility aids, blue disability parking badge. Consider referral to social services for assessment for services such as home care.
- *Diet*—ensure adequate calories, ↓ salt, ↓ weight if obese, restrict alcohol.
- *Lifestyle measures*—smoking cessation (📖 p.234); regular exercise.
- *Restrict fluid intake*—if severe heart failure.
- *Vaccination*—influenza and pneumococcal vaccination.
- *Assess for depression*—common among patients with heart failure.

Drug treatment: Table10.7. *Aims to:*

- Improve symptoms—diuretics, digoxin, and ACE inhibitors *and*
- Improve survival—ACE inhibitors, β blockers, oral nitrates plus hydralazine, spironolactone.

Algorithm for drug treatment of heart failure: Figure 10.4 (📖 p.337).

Monitoring: Review every 6mo. or more often as required. *Check:*

- *Clinical state*—functional capacity, fluid status, cardiac rhythm, cognitive and nutritional status, mood.
- *Medication*—ensure drug record is up to date, review compliance and side-effects, change drugs if clinical circumstances/best practice alter.
- *Blood*—U&E and creatinine.

Referral to general medicine, cardiology, or elderly care

E = Emergency admission; U = Urgent; S = Soon; R = Routine
- Heart failure unable to be managed at home—E
- Severe heart failure—U/S
- Heart failure not controlled by medication—U/S/R
- Angina, AF, or other symptomatic arrhythmias—U/S/R
- If diagnosis is in doubt—S/R
- To initiate an ACE inhibitor or β blocker (see p.339)—S/R
- Heart failure due to valve disease or diastolic dysfunction—R
- Comorbidity that may impact on heart failure (COPD, renal dysfunction, anaemia, thyroid disease, peripheral vascular disease, urinary frequency, gout)—R
- Women with heart failure planning pregnancy—R

Essential reading
NICE (2003) Chronic heart failure 🖥 www.nice.org.uk

Patient information
British Heart Foundation ☎0845 708 070 🖥 http://www.bhf.org.uk

Table 10.7 Drugs used in the treatment of chronic heart failure

Drug class	Treatment notes
Diuretics (BNF 2.2)	*Loop diuretics* (e.g. furosemide) or *thiazides* (e.g. bendro-flumethiazide). Use the minimum effective dose to control congestive symptoms and fluid retention (e.g. furosemide 20mg od). Monitor for ↓ K⁺—co-treat with amiloride, ACE inhibitor, or K⁺ supplement as necessary.
ACE inhibitors (BNF 2.5.5.1) ❶ Check U&E and Cr before starting, at first follow-up, and after each ↑ dose. ⚠ Do not use: If renovascular disease, in pregnancy, if the patient has HOCM, or if significant valve disease.	Improve symptoms, ↑exercise capacity, ↓ progression of disease , ↓ hospital admissions, and ↑survival in symptomatic and asymptomatic patients. Start at low dose (e.g. ramipril 1.25mg od) and titrate upwards. Refer for specialist initiation if: • Age ≥70y. • Hypovolaemia • Hyponatraemia (Na⁺ <130mmol/l) • Renal impairment (creatinine >150μmol/l) • Receiving multiple or high-dose diuretic therapy (e.g. >80mg furosemide/d.) or high-dose vasodilator therapy • Severe or unstable heart failure • Hypotension—systolic BP <90mmHg If ACE inhibitors are not tolerated consider an angiotensin receptor blocker (ARB).
β blockers (BNF 2.4) ❶ Refer for specialist initiation if any contraindication, elderly, or severe heart failure.	Start a β blocker licensed for heart failure (e.g. bisoprolol 1.25mg mane) after diuretic and ACE inhibitor in all those with left ventricular dysfunction, regardless of whether symptoms persist. Use in a 'start low, go slow' manner with assessment of pulse, BP, and clinical status after each titration.
Digoxin (BNF 2.1.1)	Use when symptoms persist despite ACE inhibitor, β blocker, and diuretics, and for patients with AF + heart failure. 2 effects—antiarrhythmic and +ve inotrope. Improves symptoms, exercise tolerance, and → ↓ admissions to hospital. No improvement in overall survival.
Other drugs to consider depending on coexistent conditions	*Anticoagulation*—patients with heart failure and AF, PH thromboembolism, left ventricular aneurysm, or intra thoracic thrombus (🕮 p.366). *Aspirin*—75–150mg od if heart failure + atherosclerotic arterial disease (including CHD). *Statins*—only if other indications (🕮 p.324). *Amlodipine*—can be used for treatment of angina and ↑ BP in patients with heart failure. ❶ *Avoid verapamil, diltiazem, or short-acting dihydro-pyridine agents.*
Drugs initiated under specialist supervision only	*Amiodarone*—all patients require clinical review, LFTs, and TFTs every 6mo. *Spironolactone*—↑ survival if severe heart failure. Refer if moderate or severe symptoms despite optimal therapy. Dose 12.5–50mg od—monitor for ↑K⁺ and ↓ renal function. If ↑ K⁺, ½ the dose and recheck. *Isosorbide/hydralazine combination* *Inotropic agents*

Pulmonary hypertension and cor pulmonale

Pulmonary hypertension

Normal pulmonary arterial pressure is $<^1/_5$ of that in the systemic circulation. Pulmonary hypertension occurs by one of 3 mechanisms:
- High pulmonary blood flow (e.g. L → R shunt)
- ↑ pulmonary vascular resistance
- Chronic pulmonary venous hypertension

Causes

Lung disease
- Asthma
- Bronchiectasis
- Pulmonary fibrosis

Cardiac disease
- Mitral stenosis
- Congenital heart disease
- Severe LVF

Hypoventilation
- Sleep apnoea
- Enlarged adenoids in children
- CVA

Pulmonary vascular disease
- PE
- Sickle-cell disease

Neuromuscular disease
- MND
- Polio
- Myaesthenia gravis

Thoracic cage abnormalities
- Kyphosis
- Scoliosis

Consequences: With time, ↑ pressure in the pulmonary vascular tree → permanent damage to smaller pulmonary vessels and pulmonary hypertension becomes irreversible—even if the cause is removed. If a shunt is present, when pulmonary pressure > systemic pressure the shunt reverses and the patient becomes, cyanotic.

Diagnosis: Under-diagnosed—delay between onset of symptoms and diagnosis ≈ 2y.

Presentation: CCF ± infective bronchitis, chest pain, breathlessness, lethargy and fatigue, haemoptysis, syncope, nausea.

Examination: Check for cyanosis, peripheral oedema, ↑ JVP, 4th heart sound, diastolic murmur from pulmonary regurgitation, hepatomegaly ± ascites, crepitations at lung bases ± pleural effusion.

Investigations
- **CXR**—cardiomegaly + enlargement of proximal pulmonary arteries.
- **ECG**—right axis deviation, tall peaked P waves and dominant R wave in right precordial leads *or* RBBB.

Management: Refer to cardiologist or chest physician. Doppler Echo is used to assess ventricular function and pulmonary arterial pressure. In the UK, ongoing care is now organized into designated multidisciplinary pulmonary hypertension units.

Treatment
- Remove the underlying cause, if possible.
- Oxygen therapy for symptomatic relief.
- Epoprostenol analogues have now become the mainstay of treatment and ↑ exercise tolerance and survival. Bosentan is also used.

- Vasodilation with calcium channel blockers (in the 10–15% of patients who are responsive) can dramatically improve prognosis.
- Treat left ventricular failure with ACE inhibitors, β blockers, and diuretics.
- Anticoagulation.

Prognosis: If the cause is irreversible, a steady decline towards cor pulmonale and death is the likely outcome, and heart-lung transplantation the only option. However, newer drugs are improving prognosis.

Cor pulmonale: Right heart failure as a result of chronic hypoxia causing chronic pulmonary hypertension. Due to diseases of the lung, its vessels, or the thoracic cage.

Further information

British Heart Foundation (2003) *Factfile: pulmonary hypertension* 🖳 www.bhf.org.uk

Tachycardia/palpitations

Heart rate >100bpm. Palpitations are the sensation of rapid, irregular, or forceful heart beats. Common, and may be an incidental finding. History and examination can exclude significant problems in most patients.

History: Ask about:

- *Palpitations:* duration, frequency and pattern, rhythm (ask the patient to tap it out if not present when seen)
- *Precipitating/relieving factors*
- *Associated symptoms:* chest pain, collapse or funny turns, sweating, breathlessness or hyperventilation
- *Past history* e.g. previous episodes, heart disease, thyroid disease
- *Lifestyle:* drug history, caffeine/alcohol intake, smoking
- *Occupation:* arrythmias may affect driving (□ p.204) and/or work

> ⚠ **Red flag symptoms**
> - Pre-existing cardiovascular disease
> - FH of syncope, arrhythmia, or sudden death
> - Arrhythmia associated with falls and/or syncope

Examination

- *General examination:* for anaemia, thyrotoxicosis, anxiety, other systemic disease
- *Cardiovascular examination:* heart size, pulse rate and rhythm, JVP, BP, heart sounds and murmurs, evidence of left ventricular failure

Investigations

- *First-line:* resting ECG is all that is needed for many patients.
- *Further investigations:* consider if ECG is abnormal or other concerning features:
    - Ambulatory ECG or cardiac memo
    - Echo if <50y. or murmur/left ventricular failure detected
    - Exercise tolerance test if exercise-related
    - *Blood:* TFTs, FBC, ESR, U&E, fasting blood glucose, Ca^{2+}, albumin

Ventricular tachycardia (VT): Broad (>3 small squares) QRS complexes at a rate of >100bpm on ECG. Admit as 999 emergency. Meanwhile, give O_2 if available ± 100mg IV lidocaine. If no pulse, treat as VF cardiac arrest (□ p.1026)
Recurrent VT: May require surgery, insertion of a pacemaker or implantable cardioverter defibrillator.

Ventricular ectopic beats: Additional broad QRS complexes, without p-waves, superimposed on regular sinus rhythm. Common and usually of no clinical significance. Rarely, may be the presenting feature of viral myocarditis. *Management:*

- *Frequent ectopics (>100/h.) on ECG:* Refer urgently to cardiology
- *R on T phenomenon on ECG:* Rarely, ectopics can → VF particularly if they coincide with the T wave of a preceding beat ('R on T phenomenon'). If this occurs >10x/min. on *ECG,* then admit.
- *After MI:* Ventricular extrasystoles after MI are associated with ↑ mortality. Refer to cardiology.

- *No sinister features on ECG:* Explain the benign nature of the condition. Advise avoidance of caffeine, alcohol, smoking, and fatigue. β blockers can be helpful for patients unable to tolerate ectopics despite reassurance.

Paroxysmal supraventricular tachycardia (SVT): Narrow QRS complex tachycardia with a regular rate >100bpm on ECG.

Management
- *If seen during an attack:*
  - Get an ECG if possible.
  - Try carotid sinus massage (unless elderly, IHD, digoxin toxic, carotid bruit, history of TIAs), the Valsalva manoeuvre, and/or ice on the face (especially effective for children).
  - Admit as an emergency if the attack continues.
  - If the attack terminates, refer to cardiology for advice on further management enclosing a copy of the ECG trace during an attack, if available.
- *If diagnosed from history or ambulatory ECG trace, or if attack terminates rapidly:* Refer to cardiology for confirmation of diagnosis and initiation of treatment—urgent referral if chest pain, dizziness, or breathlessness during attacks. Enclose the ECG trace during an attack, if available.
- *Treatment options:* Sotalol, verapamil, or amiodarone.
- *Advice:* Advise patients to avoid caffeine, alcohol, and smoking.

Sinus tachycardia: Consider infection, pain, MI, shock, exercise, emotion (including anxiety), heart failure, thyrotoxicosis, drugs.

Atrial fibrillation/flutter: 📖 p.344

No tachycardia and no ECG abnormalities: Reassure. Explore the possibility of anxiety disorder (📖 p.960).

Wolff–Parkinson–White (WPW) syndrome: A congenital accessory conduction pathway is present between atrium and ventricle (bundle of Kent). *Clinical features:*
- Predisposes to SVT and AF
- *ECG:* short P-R interval followed by slurred upstroke ('delta wave') into the QRS complex.
- *Management:* Refer to cardiology. Treatment is with anti-arrythmics (SVT—verapamil; AF—amiodarone or DC shock) ± ablation of the accessory pathway.

(*L. Wolff (1898–1972) and P. D. White (1886–1973)—US physicians; J. Parkinson (1885–1976)—English physician*)

Further information
BMJ (2002) ABC of electrocardiography 🖳 http://www.bmjjournals.com
British Heart Foundation (2004) *Factfile: Palpitations: their significance and investigation* 🖳 http:www.bhf.org.uk
NICE: Guidance on the use of implantable cardioverter defibrillators for arrhythmias. 🖳 http://www.nice.org.uk

Atrial fibrillation (AF)^G

A common disturbance of cardiac rhythm which may be episodic (*paroxysmal*) or chronic. Characterized by rapid, irregular, narrow QRS complex tachycardia with absence of p-waves. Affects <1% <60y., >8% aged over 80y. Associated with 5x ↑ risk of stroke (📖 p.606).

Causes
- No cause (isolated AF) ~12%
- CHD
- Valvular heart disease (especially mitral valve disease)
- ↑BP (especially if left ventricular hypertrophy)
- Cardiomyopathy

Acute AF: May be precipitated by acute infection, high alcohol intake, surgery, electrocution, MI, pericarditis, PE, or hyperthyroidism.

Symptoms: Often asymptomatic but may cause palpitations, chest pain, dyspnoea, fatigue, lightheadedness, and/or syncope.

Examination
- *General examination:* Check for anaemia, thyrotoxicosis, anxiety, and other systemic disease.
- *Cardiovascular examination:* Check heart size, pulse rate and rhythm (apex rate > radial pulse rate when a patient is in AF), JVP, BP, heart sounds and murmurs, and for evidence of left ventricular failure.

Investigations
- *Routine investigations:* Resting ECG, CXR, *Blood:* TFTs, FBC, U&E.
- *Further investigations:* Ambulatory ECG or cardiac memo if paroxysmal AF; Echo if <50y. or murmur/left ventricular failure detected; consider exercise tolerance test if exercise-related.

Management: Figure 10.5. *Aims to:*
- Relieve symptoms e.g. palpitations, fatigue, dyspnoea
- Prevent thromboembolism and ↓ risk of stroke
- Maintain cardiac function

Referral to cardiology, general medicine, or elderly care
E = Emergency admission; U = Urgent; S = Soon; R = Routine
- Fast rate and patient compromised by arrhythmia (chest pain, ↓BP, or more than mild heart failure)—E
- Candidate for DC or chemical cardioversion—E/U
- Uncertainty about diagnosis or treatment—S/R
- Symptoms are uncontrolled by digoxin—S/R
- Paroxysmal AF for consideration of sotalol or amiodarone—S/R

Atrial flutter: ECG shows regular saw-tooth baseline at rate of 300bpm with a narrow QRS complex tachycardia superimposed at a rate of 150bpm or 100bpm. Manage in the same way as AF (though specialist drug treatment may differ).

Essential reading
ACC/AHA/ESC (2001) Guidelines for the management of patients with AF 🖥 http://www.acc.org

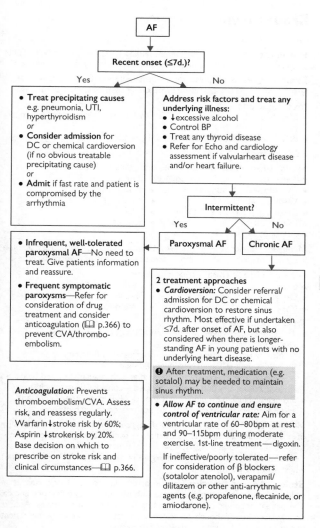

AF

Recent onset (≤7d.)?

Yes

- **Treat precipitating causes** e.g. pneumonia, UTI, hyperthyroidism
  or
- **Consider admission** for DC or chemical cardioversion (if no obvious treatable precipitating cause)
  or
- **Admit** if fast rate and patient is compromised by the arrhythmia

- **Infrequent, well-tolerated paroxysmal AF**—No need to treat. Give patients information and reassure.
- **Frequent symptomatic paroxysms**—Refer for consideration of drug treatment and consider anticoagulation (🕮 p.366) to prevent CVA/thrombo-embolism.

Anticoagulation: Prevents thromboembolism/CVA. Assess risk, and reassess regularly. Warfarin↓stroke risk by 60%; Aspirin ↓stroke risk by 20%. Base decision on which to prescribe on stroke risk and clinical circumstances—🕮 p.366.

No

Address risk factors and treat any underlying illness:
- ↓excessive alcohol
- Control BP
- Treat any thyroid disease
- Refer for Echo and cardiology assessment if valvular heart disease and/or heart failure.

Intermittent?

Yes — **Paroxysmal AF**

No — **Chronic AF**

2 treatment approaches
- *Cardioversion:* Consider referral/admission for DC or chemical cardioversion to restore sinus rhythm. Most effective if undertaken ≤7d. after onset of AF, but also considered when there is longer-standing AF in young patients with no underlying heart disease.

 ❶ After treatment, medication (e.g. sotalol) may be needed to maintain sinus rhythm.

- *Allow AF to continue and ensure control of ventricular rate:* Aim for a ventricular rate of 60–80bpm at rest and 90–115bpm during moderate exercise. 1st-line treatment—digoxin.

 If ineffective/poorly tolerated—refer for consideration of β blockers (sotalol or atenolol), verapamil/dilitazem or other anti-arrythmic agents (e.g. propafenone, flecainide, or amiodarone).

Figure 10.5 Management of AF in primary care

Bradycardia

Heart rate <60bpm.

Presentation: Often an incidental finding but may present with faints or blackouts, drop attacks, dizziness, breathlessness, or lack of energy.

Examination: Slow pulse rate; normal or low BP ± evidence of 2° heart failure. There may also be symptoms / signs of associated disease.

Investigations
- *ECG:* See below; ambulatory ECG may help with diagnosis of intermittent bradycardia (e.g. sick sinus syndrome).
- *Blood:* TFTs, FBC, ESR, U&E, LFTs, digoxin levels (if taking digoxin).

ECG changes

Sinus bradycardia: Constant bradycardia. P-waves present and P-R interval <0.2 sec. (1 large square). *Causes:*
- Physiological e.g. athletes
- Vasovagal attack
- Drugs e.g. β blockers, digoxin
- Inferior MI
- Sick sinus syndrome
- Hypothyroidism
- Hypothermia
- ↑ ICP
- Jaundice

Management: Admit acutely if symptomatic. Refer for cardiology opinion if asymptomatic but HR <40bpm despite treatment of reversible causes.

AV node block (heart block): *Causes:*
- IHD
- Drugs (digoxin, verapamil)
- Myocarditis
- Cardiomyopathy
- Fibrosis
- Lyme disease (rare)

Types of heart block
- *1st degree block*—fixed P-R interval >200ms (1 large square)
- *2nd degree block*
  - Mobitz type I (Wenckebach)—progressively lengthening P-R interval followed by a dropped beat
  - Mobitz type II—constant P-R interval with regular dropped beats (e.g. 2:1—every 2nd beat is dropped—consider drug toxicity)
- *3rd degree block* (complete heart block)—P-P intervals are constant and R-R intervals are constant but not related to each other.

Management: Untreated 2nd and 3rd degree heart block have a mortality of ≈ 35%. Refer all patients to cardiology even if asymptomatic. If symptomatic (↓BP <90mmHg systolic, left ventricular failure, heart rate <40bpm) admit as an emergency—give iv atropine and O₂ (if available) whilst awaiting admission.

Stokes–Adams attacks: Cardiac arrest due to AV block. Results in sudden loss of consciousness ± some limb twitching due to cerebral anoxia. The patient becomes pale and pulseless but respiration continues. Attacks usually last ~30sec., though occasionally are fatal. On recovery the patient becomes flushed. Refer to cardiology if suspected.
(W. Stokes (1804–1878)—Irish physician and R. Adams (1791–1875)—Irish surgeon)

Sick sinus syndrome: Due to sinus node dysfunction causing bradycardia ± asystole, sinoatrial block (complete heart block), AF, or SVT alternating with bradycarida (tachy/brady syndrome). Common amongst elderly patients. If symptomatic, heart rate <40bpm, or pauses >3sec. on ECG, refer to cardiology for pacemaker insertion.

Pacemakers: Electrically stimulate the heart to beat. *Indications:*
• Symptomatic bradycardia
• 2nd or 3rd degree heart block
• Suppression of resistant tachycardia

Insertion: Pacemaker box is attached under the skin of the chest—usually medial to the left axilla under LA. Wires are fed into the great veins of the chest and thus to the heart under X-ray and/or US guidance.

Types: Classified according to,
• Chamber paced—atrium, ventricle, or both ('dual')
• Chamber sensed—atrium, ventricle, or both ('dual')
• Mode of response to sensing—inhibited output, triggered, inhibited and triggered ('dual').

Thus, a V V I pacemaker both paces and senses the ventricle in inhibited mode—i.e. if the ventricle beats spontaneously, the pacemaker will not fire.

ECG changes with a pacemaker: If the pacemaker is in operation, a pacing 'spike' (vertical line) is seen on ECG.

❶ In devices pacing on demand, a spike will not be seen if the natural rate is in excess of the rate set on the pacemaker.

Lifespan: Pacemakers last 7–15y. Regular checks are made by pacemaker clinics to ensure the pacemaker remains operational. Reprogramming through the skin is possible. Batteries can be changed via a small surgical procedure under local anaesthetic.

Driving with a pacemaker: Inform DVLA and insurance company (📖 p.203). Stop driving for 1mo. after insertion.

⚠ Pacemakers must be removed after death, before cremation can occur. A fee is payable.

Further information
BMJ (2002) ABC of electrocardiography ▣ http://www.bmjjournals.com
NICE (2004) Dual-chamber pacemakers for symptomatic bradycardia due to sick sinus syndrome and/or atrioventricular block ▣ http://www.nice.org.uk

Infective endocarditis

⚠ New murmur + fever = endocarditis, until proven otherwise

Infective endocarditis occurs when there is Infection of a heart valve. The valve may be normal (50%—may be associated with iv drug abuse), rheumatic, degenerative, congenitally abnormal, or prosthetic (Table 10.8). Uncommon, but consequences may be disastrous and often detected late.

Causes
- **Common organisms:** Strep. viridans (35–50%); Staph. aureus (20%)
- **Non-bacterial causes:** SLE, malignancy.

Presentation: May be acute (acute heart failure) or subacute (course worsening over days/weeks). *Symptoms/signs:*
- *Infective:* fever, weight ↓, night sweats, malaise, lethargy, clubbing, splenomegaly, anaemia, mycotic aneurysms
- **Heart murmurs ± heart failure**
- *Embolic:* stroke, lung abscesses (right heart endocarditis)
- *Vasculitic:* microscopic haematuria, splinter haemorrhages, Osler's nodes (painful lesions on finger pulps), Janeway lesions (palmar macules), Roth's spots (retinal vasculitis), renal failure.

Management: Have a high index of suspicion for patients at ↑ risk i.e. with valve lesions or prosthetic valves. Admit as an emergency if suspected. Avoid starting antibiotics prior to admission as this might cause delay in diagnosis by rendering the blood cultures sterile. Hospital treatment is with prolonged iv broad spectrum antibiotics (≥2wk.).

Prognosis: 20–25% of those admitted with a diagnosis of infective endocarditis die; 80% have major complications during admission e.g. heart failure. Valve replacement may be required—especially if endocarditis is on a prosthetic valve.

Table 10.8 Risk of developing infective endocarditis

Risk	Condition	Antibiotic prophylaxis
High	Prosthetic heart valve Past history of infective endocarditis Complex cyanotic congenital heart disease	Required
Moderate	Mitral valve prolapse Valvular dysfunction (e.g. following rheumatic heart disease) Ventricular septal defects Primum atrial septal defects HOCM Past history of rheumatic fever	Required
Low	Murmurs not due to valve disease (e.g. flow murmurs in pregnancy)	Not required

Prevention: Those at high/moderate risk of infective endocarditis (Table 10.8) should take prophylactic antibiotics prior to any procedure that might cause a transient bacteraemia (Tables 10.9 and 10.10). Good dental hygiene is also important including regular dentist check-ups.

Table 10.9 Requirements for antibiotic prophylaxis

Procedures requiring prophylaxis		Procedures not requiring prophylaxis
High and moderate-risk patients	*High-risk patients only*	
• Dental procedures which can → gum bleeding (i.e. virtually all dental procedures) • Surgery (excluding skin surgery)—warn consultant in referral letter) • Lower GI or GU endoscopy	• All endoscopic procedures including proctoscopy and sigmoidoscopy • Normal obstetric delivery • Insertion of IUCD • Insertion of a urethral catheter in a patient with infected urine (ensure infecting organism is sensitive to prophylactic antibiotics)	• Routine phlebotomy • Cervical smear • Insertion of IV cannula (though should be changed frequently)

⚠ If in doubt, ask advice from the cardiologist in charge of the patient's care or a specialist in infectious diseases.

Table 10.10 Antibiotic regimes for use in primary care (*BNF 5.1*)

Patients	Antibiotics
All patients *except* • those with a past history of endocarditis • those who are penicillin-allergic • those who have had >1 dose of penicillin in the previous month	Amoxycillin 3g po 1h. before the procedure (Child <5y.—¼ adult dose; child 5–10y.—½ adult dose)
Patients allergic to penicillin *or* Patients who have received >1 dose of penicillin in the previous month	Clindamycin 600mg po 1h. before the procedure (Child <5y.—¼ adult dose; child 5–10y.—½ adult dose)
Patients with a past history of endocarditis	The procedure should be carried out in hospital with iv gentamicin 120mg prior to the procedure, then amoxycillin 500mg 6h. after the procedure

Further information

British Heart Foundation (2003/2004) *Factfiles: Infective endocarditis* 🖳 www.bhf.org.uk

Rheumatic fever, myocarditis, and pericarditis

Rheumatic fever: There has been a dramatic ↓ in incidence of rheumatic fever in industrialized countries since 1950s, but recently numbers of cases have ↑. Rheumatic fever is still an endemic disease in developing countries. *Peak incidence:* age 5–15y.

Cause: Rheumatic fever is due to an abnormal immunological response to β-haemolytic streptococcal infection (e.g. 2–4wk. after sore throat). Its importance lies in the permanent damage caused to heart valves in some of those affected and subsequent risk of endocarditis.

Diagnosis: Can be made if revised Jones criteria are met (Table 10.11)

Management: If suspected, refer for specialist care. Specialist management includes evaluation of heart lesions with Echo; bed rest; penicillin, and symptom control (e.g. analgesia, sedatives for chorea). Anti-inflammatory agents such as corticosteroids and aspirin may be used to try to ↓ complications of carditis but their use is controversial.

Prognosis
- 60% develop chronic rheumatic heart disease (70% mitral valve; 40% aortic; 10% tricuspid; 2% pulmonary). Likelihood correlates with severity of initial disease.
- Recurrence may occur after further streptococcal infection or be precipitated by pregnancy or the COC pill.

Table 10.11 Revised Jones criteria for diagnosis of rheumatic fever

Evidence of previous streptococcal infection (scarlet fever, +ve throat swab, and/or ↑ ASO titre >200U/ml)

and

2 major criteria

or

1 major + 2 minor criteria

Major criteria	Minor criteria
Carditis (45–70%)—arrhythmia, new murmur, pericardial rub, heart failure, conduction defects	Prolonged P-R interval on ECG (but not if carditis is one of the major criteria)
Migratory polyarthritis ('flitting'—75%) red, tender joints	Arthralgia (but not if arthritis is one of the major criteria)
Sydenham's chorea (St. Vitus' dance—10%)	Fever
Subcutaneous nodules (2–20%)	↑ESR or ↑CRP
Erythema marginatum (2–10%)	History of rheumatic heart disease or rheumatic fever

2° prevention

- Penicillin 250mg bd po or sulfadiazine 1g od (500mg od for patients <30kg) for ≥5y. to prevent recurrence. Duration of prophylaxis is dependent on whether there was carditis in the initial attack (no carditis—continued for 5y.; if cardiac involvement—continued until age 25y. or longer).
- Once regular prophylaxis has stopped, patients should continue to have prophylactic antibiotics for dental and other operative procedures for life (Tables 10.9 and 10.10—📖 p.349).

Acute myocarditis: Inflammation of the myocardium. May present in a similar way to MI or with palpitations. *Causes:* Viral infection (e.g. Coxsackie virus; diptheria; rheumatic fever; drugs).

Management: Admit for specialist cardiologist care. Treatment is supportive. Some recover spontaneously, others progress to intractable heart failure requiring transplantation.

Pericarditis: Sharp, constant sternal pain relieved by sitting forwards. May radiate to left shoulder ± arm or into the abdomen. Worse lying on the left side and on inspiration, swallowing, and coughing. A pericardial rub may be present at the left sternal edge on auscultation. *Causes:*

- Infection (e.g. Coxsackie virus, TB)
- Malignancy
- Uraemia
- MI (Dressler's syndrome—📖 p.333)
- Trauma
- Radiotherapy
- Connective tissue disease
- Hypothyroidism

Investigations: ECG—concave (saddle-shaped) ST elevation in all leads.

Management: Refer to cardiology; treat the cause (if possible); symptomatic treatment with NSAID for pain; steroids in resistant cases.

Complications

- *Pericardial effusion:* Fluid in the pericardial sac. *Presentation:* left or right heart failure, cardiac tamponade (inability of the heart to dilate in diastole resulting in tachycardia, ↓ BP, ↑ JVP). CXR—large, globular heart. Echo is diagnostic. *Management:* admit for urgent cardiology assessment.
- *Constrictive pericarditis:* Pericardium becomes fibrosed and non-expansile. Most common cause is TB. *Presentation:* right heart failure, hepatosplenomegaly, ascites, ↓ BP, ↑ JVP. *Management:* refer to cardiologist for confirmation of diagnosis. Treatment involves surgical release of the pericardium.

Cardiomyopathy and heart transplant

Cardiomyopathy: Primary disease of the heart muscle.

Dilated (congestive) cardiomyopathy: Prevalence ≈ 35/100,000 population. ♂>♀. Dilation of left ± right ventricle and ↓ contractility. Presents with heart failure. ECG shows non-specific S-T abnormalities. CXR shows cardiac enlargement and pulmonary venous hypertension. Echo is diagnostic. *Causes:*

- Idiopathic
- Familial (20%)
- Cardiovascular—IHD, ↑ BP, congenital heart disease, rheumatic heart disease
- Alcohol
- Infection (Coxsackie virus)
- Endocrine disease—myxoedema, thyrotoxicosis, acromegaly
- Cardiotoxic drugs
- Pregnancy
- Connective tissue disease (SLE, PAN, systemic sclerosis)
- Sarcoidosis
- Amyloidosis
- Haemachromatosis
- Malignancy
- Muscular dystrophy

Management and prognosis: Advise patients to stop drinking alcohol as may make the cardiomyopathy worse. Specialist management is needed in all cases and involves treatment of heart failure and arrythmias. Most patients require long-term anticoagulation. Surgical options include cardiomyoplasty and/or heart transplantation. *Mortality:* 40% in 2y. (sudden death, cardiogenic shock).

Hypertrophic cardiomyopathy: Familial inheritance (autosomal dominant) though 1:2 cases are sporadic. In its most common form causes asymetrical septal hypertrophy ± aortic outflow obstruction (obstructive hypertrophic cardiomyopathy).

Presentation: Many cases are detected through screening of asymptomatic patients with a FH using echocardiography. *Symptoms/signs:*

- Palpitations—associated with arrythmias; 5% have AF
- Breathlessness on exertion
- Chest pain—may be angina or atypical pain
- Murmur—may be due to outflow obstruction and/or mitral valve dysfunction
- Faints/collapses

Investigations

- *ECG*—left ventricular hypertrophy and ischaemic changes (e.g. T wave invesion)
- *CXR*—normal until disease is in its late stages
- *Echo*—diagnostic; refer if suspicious symptoms or FH.

Management and prognosis: Patients require antibiotic prophylaxis for dental and other operative procedures (Tables 10.9 and 10.10—□ p.349). Specialist management is needed in all cases and involves symptomatic treatment e.g. β blockers for chest pain, amiodarone for arrythmias (digoxin is contraindicated). Surgical options include myotomy and myectomy. *Mortality:* The major cause of mortality is sudden death which is unrelated to severity of symptoms. Though ultimately fatal in the majority, interval between diagnosis and death is often decades.

Restrictive cardiomyopathy: Stiff ventricle which limits filling. Presents with heart failure. Echo is diagnostic. *Causes:* amyloid, sarcoidosis, haemachromatosis. *Management:* specialist management is required. Treatment is symptomatic.

Obliterative cardiomyopathy: Rare in Western countries. Idiopathic fibrosis of inflow tract prevents filling and eventually leads to cavity obliteration.

Heart transplantation: Considered in patients with estimated 1y. survival <50%. *Indications/contraindications:* Table 10.2.

Assessment: Each eligible patient is assessed for psychosocial factors and physical factors (e.g. renal failure, obesity, age, peripheral vascular disease) which affect prognosis before a decision whether to place the patient on the transplant list is made.

Post-operative: Patients require lifelong immunosuppression—usually with ciclosporin. Follow-up is undertaken in specialist clinics.

Prognosis: 1:4 patients die on the transplant list; 60% receive transplant in <2y.; perioperative mortality <10%; 1y. survival 92%; 5y. survival 75%; 10y. survival 60%. Patients have accelerated graft atherosclerosis for reasons that are not clear. Complications of immunosuppression include ↑ risks of infection and cancer.

Table 10.12 Indications and contraindications for heart transplant

Indications	Contraindications
All patients must have end-stage heart disease. Causes:	Systemic disease likely to affect life expectancy (e.g. malignancy)
• IHD (50%)	Active infection (HIV, hepatitis B or C)
• Cardiomyopathy (40%)	Significant pulmonary vascular disease
• Valvular and congenital heart defects (5%)	Continued excess alcohol consumption
	Significant cerebral/systemic vascular disease
	Upper age limit is generally taken at ~60y.

Patient information and support
Cardiomyopathy Association. ☎01923 249 977 🖳 http://www.cardiomyopathy.org
Transplant Support Network ☎01535 210101
　🖳 http://www.transplantsupportnetwork.org.uk
Society of cardiothoracic surgeons of Great Britian and Ireland. Patient information
　🖳 http://www.scts.org

Valve disease

Heart murmurs: 📖 p.267

> ⚠ All patients with newly detected valve disease, except those with mitral valve prolapse or aortic sclerosis, require cardiology referral.
> - Admit if suspected endocarditis
> - Refer urgently/admit if symptomatic valve disease or if valve disease underlies the presenting condition e.g. heart failure caused by aortic stenosis, AF caused by mitral valve disease.

Mitral stenosis: Usually due to rheumatic fever.

Presentation

- *Symptoms:* Breathlessness, palpitations, fatigue. May → pulmonary hypertension which presents with right heart failure, haemoptysis, and/or recurrent bronchitis.
- *Signs:* Peripheral cyanosis ('malar flush' on cheeks), left parasternal heave, tapping apex beat, AF, rumbling mid-diastolic murmur at the apex.

Management: Confirm with Echo. Refer to cardiology. Treatment is medical (digoxin, diuretics, anticoagulation) ± surgical (valvotomy, balloon valvoplasty, valve replacement). Give antibiotic prophylaxis—📖 p.349.

Mitral regurgitation (incompetence): *Causes:*

- Congenital
- Rheumatic fever
- Mitral valve prolapse
- Ventricular dilatation
- Endocarditis
- Cardiomyopathy
- Ruptured papillary muscle /chordae tendinae following MI
- RA

Presentation

- *Symptoms:* Dyspnoea, fatigue.
- *Signs:* Displaced apex (→ left axilla), pansystolic murmur at the apex radiating to axilla, AF, left ventricular failure.

Management: Confirm with Echo. Refer to cardiology. Treatment is medical (digoxin and anticoagulation for AF, diuretics) ± surgical (valve replacement). Give antibiotic prophylaxis —📖 p.349.

Mitral valve prolapse: Prevalence ~1:20.

Presentation

- *Symptoms:* Usually none. Rarely, atypical chest pain, palpitations, syncope, postural hypotension, emboli.
- *Signs:* Late systolic murmur over apex.

Management: Confirm with Echo. Antibiotic prophylaxis for dental or surgical procedures if regurgitation or thickened (myxomatous) mitral valve leaflets (📖 p.349). If syncope or palpitations, refer to cardiology—a rare complication is ventricular arrhythmia.

Aortic sclerosis: Senile thickening and stiffening of the aortic valve not associated with outflow obstruction. Clinically, an ejection systolic murmur is present but no other symptoms or signs. CXR may show a calcified valve. No treatment is required.

Aortic stenosis: *Causes:*
- Congenital
- Rheumatic fever
- Bicuspid valve
- Degenerative calcification
- Hypertrophic cardiomyopathy

Presentation
- *Symptoms:* Angina, breathlessness, syncope or 'funny turns', dizziness, sudden death.
- *Signs:* Small volume pulse, low pulse pressure (difference between systolic and diastolic BP), ejection systolic murmur loudest in the aortic area which radiates to carotids and apex.

Management: Echo is diagnostic and gives an estimate of the gradient across the valve and thus severity of the condition. Refer to cardiology. Surgery (valve replacement or transcutaneous vulvoplasty) is considered for those with syncope or if systolic gradient across the valve is >50mmHg. Avoid treatment with ACE inhibitors. Give antibiotic prophylaxis—📖 p.349.

Aortic regurgitation *Causes:*
- Congenital e.g. VSD
- Bicuspid aortic valve
- Rheumatic fever
- Aortic dissection
- Endocarditis
- Cardiomyopathy
- Syphilis
- Marfan's or Ehlers Danlos syndrome

Presentation
- *Symptoms:* Dyspnoea, palipitations (extrasystoles).
- *Signs:* Prominent pulse ('water-hammer'), wide pulse pressure, visible neck pulsation (Corrigan's sign), head nodding in time with pulse (De Musset's sign), visible capillary pulsations (e.g. in nail bed—Quincke's sign), displaced apex beat, high-pitched early diastolic murmur (easily missed).

Management: Confirm with Echo. Refer to cardiology for consideration of surgery. Give antibiotic prophylaxis—📖 p.349.

Right heart valve disease: Echo is diagnostic. Always requires specialist management. Give antibiotic prophylaxis (📖 p.349).
- *Tricuspid stenosis:* Mitral valve disease always coexists. *Cause:* rheumatic fever. *Murmur:* early diastolic (left sternal edge in inspiration). *Treatment:* diuretics ± surgery (valvotomy or replacement).
- *Tricuspid regurgitation: Causes:* RV enlargement, endocarditis (iv drug abusers), carcinoid, rheumatic fever, congenital. *Presents* with oedema, breathlessness, pulsatile hepatomegaly (± jaundice), ascites, pansystolic murmur loudest at left sternal edge. *Treatment:* diuretics, vasodilators ± surgery (valve replacement or annuloplasty).
- *Pulmonary stenosis: Causes:* congenital (Fallot's tetralogy), rheumatic, carcinoid. *Murmur:* ejection systolic murmur (loudest to left of upper sternum, radiating to left shoulder). *ECG:* RVH. *CXR*—dilated pulmonary artery. *Treatments:* (if required) is with pulmonary valvotomy.
- *Pulmonary regurgitation: Causes:* pulmonary hypertension (📖 p.340). *Murmur:* decrescendo early diastolic murmur at left sternal edge.

⚠ Women planning pregnancy who have known valve disease require review for specialist advice.

Other structural abnormalities of the heart

Coarctation of the aorta: Localized narrowing of the descending aorta usually distal to the origin of the left subclavian artery.

Presentation: Heart failure, ↑BP, murmur heard incidentally (ejection systolic murmur over the left side of the chest radiating to the back), lack of femoral pulses. Rarely presentation is with a complication e.g. subarachnoid haemorrhage or endocarditis. *CXR*—prominent left ventricle. *ECG*—left ventricular hypertrophy.

Management: Refer to cardiology—surgery to remove the narrowed portion of the aorta is usually indicated.

Atrial septal defect (ASD): A hole connects the 2 atria. Holes high in the septum (ostium secundum) are most common; holes lower in the septum (ostium primum) are associated with AV valve abnormalities. Blood flows from L → R through the shunt and the right heart takes the burden.

Presentation
- *Ostium secundum defects:* Symptoms are rare in infancy and uncommon in childhood. If detected in these groups, presents as a murmur (systolic—loudest in the 2nd left interspace) which is found incidentally, with breathlessness or tiredness on exertion or recurrent chest infections. Presentation is usually in the 3rd or 4th decade with heart failure, pulmonary hypertension, or atrial arrythmias.
- *Ostium primum defects:* Heart failure commonly develops in infancy/childhood ± severe pulmonary hypertension. In addition to the ASD murmur, there may be a pansystolic murmur signifying mitral or tricuspid valve regurgitation.

Investigation
- *CXR:* Cardiomegaly with a prominent right atrium ± pulmonary artery ± pulmonary plethora.
- *ECG:* Right axis deviation (ostium secundum defect) or left axis deviation (ostium primum defect), RVH ± RBBB.
- *Echo:* Diagnostic.

Management: Refer to cardiology. Cardiac surgery to close the defect is usually indicated. All patients with ostium primum defects require prophylactic antibiotics (☐ p.349).

Ventricular septal defect (VSD): A hole connects the 2 ventricles. Blood flows initially from L → R through the hole. All patients with VSD require prophylactic antibiotics (☐ p.349). May be congenital or acquired (usually septal rupture post MI).

Congenital VSD
Small VSD ('maladie de Roger'): Normally asymptomatic.
- *Examination:* Thrill palpable at lower left sternal border; harsh pansystolic murmur—small holes give loud murmurs.

- *Investigations:* CXR and ECG are normal. Diagnosis is confirmed on Echo.
- *Management:* Refer to cardiology. Usually surgery is not indicated.

Moderate VSD: Symptoms usually appear in infancy—breathlessness on feeding/crying, failure to thrive, recurrent chest infections. As the child gets older, symptoms improve (relative size of the defect ↓).
- *Examination:* Cardiomegaly, thrill palpable at left sternal edge, pansystolic murmur.
- *Investigations:* Cardiomegaly ± prominent pulmonary arteries ± pulmonary plethora. Diagnosis is confirmed on Echo.
- *Management:* Refer to cardiology. Surgery is indicated if the child is not improving or there is evidence of pulmonary hypertension.

Large VSD: Presents with heart failure at ~3mo. of age, though there may be symptoms of breathlessness on feeding/crying prior to this.
- *Examination:* Baby is obviously unwell—underweight, breathless, pulmonary oedema ± cyanosis, large heart, thrill over left sternal edge ± parasternal heave, murmur—often not pansystolic due to high right ventricular pressures.
- *Management:* Admit to paediatrics. Medical treatment ± surgery is always needed.

Acquired VSD: Suspect if new pansystolic murmur ± heart failure develop after MI. Investigate as for congenital VSD. Refer to cardiology (speed of referral will depend on state of the patient) for advice on further management.

Marfan syndrome: Autosomal dominant connective tissue disease causing abnormalities of fibrillin (a glycoprotein in elastic fibres). *Features include:*
- Arachnodactyly (long spidery fingers)
- High-arched palate
- Arm span > height
- Lens dislocation ± unstable iris
- Aortic dilatation (β blockers appear to slow this)
- Aortic incompetence may occur e.g. in pregnancy
- Aortic dissection may cause sudden death—Echo screening may be helpful for affected individuals.

If suspected, refer to cardiology ± genetics.
(*E.J.A. Marfan (1858–1942)—French paediatrician*)

Other congenital heart disease: 📖 p.842

Aneurysms

An arterial aneurysm forms when there is a 50% ↑ in normal diameter of the vessel. Aneurysms may affect any medium/large artery—aorta/iliac arteries>popliteal>femoral>carotid. FH of aneurysm is a risk factor.

Causes: Atheroma (most common); injury; infection (e.g. endocarditis, syphilis—mycotic aneurysms).

Abdominal aortic aneurysm (AAA): Prevalence 5% and increasing. The typical patient with an AAA is a ♂ smoker >65y. Risk ↑ x4–10 if there is an affected 1st degree relative.

Presentation: Often discovered as an incidental finding on abdominal examination, X-ray (calcification of aneurysm wall in 50% cases), or USS (¾ asymptomatic at diagnosis). Otherwise presents with:
- *Local symptoms:* vague abdominal or back pain.
- *Distant symptoms:* embolization/acute ischaemia of a limb. Multiple small infarcts (e.g. of toes) with good peripheral pulses suggests an aneurysm proximally.
- *Collapse due to rupture:* hypovolaemic shock ± pulsatile abdominal mass ± abdominal or back pain—📖 p.1042.

Investigation: USS confirms diagnosis and gives an estimate of diameter, site, and extent.

Factors predisposing to rupture of AAA

- Diameter (risk ↑ with diameter)
- COPD
- Smoking
- ↑ diastolic BP
- FH
- Fast rate of expansion
- Inflammation within the aneurysm wall
- Thrombus-free surface area of aneurysm sac

Screening: Acute rupture of AAA in the community has ~90% mortality rate. Elective surgical repair has ~5–7 % mortality. Single abdominal USS in men age 65y. would exclude 90% of the population from future AAA rupture. A large RCT of population screening in the UK showed 44% ↓ in death due to AAA in the screened group over 4y. Trials evaluating cost-effectiveness of screening have suggested that screening smoking ♂ at 65y. may be more cost-effective. Decisions on population screening are awaited. In the meantime, consider screening men with CHD and ↑ BP.

Problems: Identifies small aneurysms not requiring repair but just surveillance. This may cause morbidity in low-risk, healthy individuals.

Management of AAA
- *Acute rupture:* 📖 p.1042.
- *Referral for elective surgery:* Refer if risk of rupture>risk elective repair. The greater the diameter, the more the risk (5.5cm diameter ≈10% 1y. rupture rate; 10cm diameter >75% 1y. rupture rate). AAAs >5.5cm are routinely repaired unless the patient has other factors that ↑ risk of surgery substantially. There is no survival benefit from treating

smaller aneurysms. Symptomatic aneurysms are urgent cases as symptoms may indicate stretching of the aneurysm sac (through rapid expansion) or inflammation—both risk factors for rupture.

- *USS surveillance:* Usually annual—patients with AAAs <5.5cm diameter. Routine repair takes place when and if the aneurysm expands to >5.5cm. 3:5 eventually warrant surgery.

Inflammatory aneurysms: Characterized by inflammatory infiltrate in the aneurysm wall. May be adherent to surrounding structures. *Presentation:* fever, malaise, and abdominal pain. Associated with ↑ mortality at operation.

Thoracoabdominal aneurysm: Involves thoracic and abdominal aorta—including the origins of the visceral and renal arteries. Surgery is more complex and carries higher mortality.

Dissecting thoracic aortic aneurysm: 📖 p.1042

Popliteal aneurysms: 80% peripheral aneurysms. Most are >2cm diameter; 50% are bilateral. Associated with AAA (40%).

Presentation: Acute below knee ischaemia 2° aneurysm thrombosis or embolization. Popliteal pulses are pronounced. Diagnosis is confirmed on USS.

Management
- Acute ischaemia—📖 p.1084
- Elective surgery (popliteal bypass)—when aneurysm >2.5cm diameter

Femoral artery aneurysms: *Presentation:* local pressure symptoms, thrombosis, or distal embolisation. *Surgical treatment:* bypass surgery.

Cerebral artery aneurysms: 📖 p.604

Further information
British Heart Foundation (2003) *Factfiles: Abdominal aortic aneurysms* 🖥 http://www.bhf.org.uk

Patient information and support
British Vascular Foundation 🖥 http://www.bvf.org.uk
Vascular Society of GB & Ireland 🖥 http://www.vascularsociety.org.uk

Chronic peripheral ischaemia

Peripheral vascular disease (normally atherosclerotic) commonly affects arteries supplying the legs. *Incidence:* 10% patients age 60–70y., 20% >70y.

Natural history: Most remain stable. A few (2% over 10y.) progress from intermittent claudication to critical limb ischaemia. Management of cardiovascular risk factors is essential.

Intermittent claudication: Restriction of blood flow causes pain on walking. *Risk factors:*

- ♂>♀
- Smoking
- Obesity
- ↑BP
- Hyperlipidaemia
- DM
- Physical inactivity
- Hypercoagulable states
- Postmenopausal

Presentation: Presents with muscular, cramp-like pain in the calf, thigh, or buttock on walking that is rapidly relieved on resting. The leg is cool and white with atrophic skin changes and absent pulses (Table 10.13):

- *Disease in the superficial femoral artery*—absent popliteal and foot pulses. Causes calf claudication.
- *Disease of the aorta or iliac artery*—weak or absent femoral pulse ± femoral bruit. Causes calf, thigh, or buttock claudication.

Differential diagnosis: Nerve root compression e.g. sciatica; spinal stenosis—usually bilateral pain which may occur after prolonged standing as well as exercise—not rapidly relieved by rest.

Investigation

- *Blood*—FBC, U&E, Cr (peripheral vascular disease is associated with renal artery stenosis—📖 p.683), glucose, lipids.
- *Ankle: brachial systolic pressure index (ABI)*—
  - Good history + ABI<0.95 confirms diagnosis
  - If good history but normal ABI (=1), consider exercise testing*
- *Duplex USS*—used to determine site of disease*

Management

- ↓ *risk factors* (📖 p.314): Patients with claudication have a 3x ↑ risk of death from MI/stroke. Advise to stop smoking, and lose weight. Ensure optimum treatment of ↑BP, lipids, and DM.
- *Foot care:* Regular chiropody.
- *Drugs*
  - *Aspirin* (75–300mg od)—↓ risk of cardiovascular events. Alternatives are dipyridamole (200 mg bd) or clopidogrel (75mg od).
  - *Naftidrofuryl*—may ↑ walking distance; unclear whether influences outcome. Reassess after 3–6mo. Discontinue if no improvement.
  - *Cilostazol*—↑ walking distance in those with ongoing symptoms despite risk factor management.
- *Exercise:* Training for ≥6mo. by regularly walking as far as possible before being stopped by pain, ↑ pain-free and maximum walking distances. Effect is greater than the effect of angioplasty.

*May only be available via 2° care referral

Table 10.13 Location of the pulses of the lower limbs

Pulse	Location
Femoral	Below inguinal ligament; $^1/_3$ of the way up from pubic tubercle
Popliteal	With knee flexed at right angles, palpate deep in the midline
Posterior tibial	1cm behind medial malleolus
Dorsalis pedis	Variable—on the dorsum of the foot just lateral to the tendons to the big toe. ❶ Many healthy people have only 1 foot pulse.

Referral to vascular surgery

E = Emergency admission; U = Urgent; S = Soon; R = Routine
- Critical limb ischaemia—E/U
- Severe symptoms—S
- Job affected—S/R
- Uncertainty about diagnosis—R
- No better after exercise training—R

The diabetic foot: 📖 p.418

Critical limb ischaemia

Presentation: Deteriorating claudication and nocturnal rest pain (usually just after fallen asleep—hanging the foot out of bed improves the pain). Ulceration or gangrene results from minor trauma.

Examination: Look for:
- Atrophic skin changes—pallor, cool to the touch, hairless, shiny
- On lowering the leg—turns a dusky blue-red colour; on elevation, pallor and venous guttering
- Ulceration—check under the heel and between the toes
- Swelling suggests the patient is sleeping in a chair to avoid rest pain or, rarely, pain from deep infection
- Absent foot pulses—if present, consider alternative diagnosis
- ABI<0.5—❶ arterial calcification can result in falsely high readings.

Management: Analgesia (often requires opiate); refer for urgent vascular surgical assessment.

Specialist management
- *Angiography:* to assess extent and position of disease.
- *Percutaneous transluminal angioplasty ± stenting:* most suitable for short occlusions/stenoses of the iliac and superficial femoral vessels. 1y. patency rate 80-90%.
- *Surgery:* most suitable for longer occlusions/multiple stenoses—aortobifemoral bypass grafts have 5y. patency rates >90%; femoro-popliteal bypass grafting gives 5y. patency rates of <70% of re-occlusion. Amputation is a last option.

Acute limb ischaemia: 📖 p.1084

Further information
British Heart Foundation (2001) *Factfiles: peripheral vascular disease* 🖥 www.bhf.org.uk

Patient information and support
British Vascular Foundation 🖥 http://www.bvf.org.uk

Varicose veins and thrombophlebitis

Tortuous, twisted, or lengthened veins. *Prevalence:* 17–31%. ♂ > ♀ (≈5:4). The vein wall is inherently weak → dilatation and separation of valve cusps so they become incompetent. Blood flows backwards from the deep to superficial venous system, causing back pressure and further dilatation.

Most varicose veins are primary. *Risk factors:* age, parity, occupations requiring a lot of standing, obesity (women only). 2° *causes:* DVT, pelvic tumour, pregnancy, or A-V fistula.

Types
- **Trunk:** Varicosities of the long or short saphenous vein or their branches. May be symptomatic.
- **Reticular:** Usually asymptomatic. Dilated tortuous subcutaneous veins not belonging to the main branches of the long or short saphenous vein.
- **Telangectasia:** Spider veins, star bursts, thread veins, or matted veins. Intradermal venules <1mm. Unsightly but otherwise asymptomatic.

Presentation: *Consider:*
- **Why is the patient consulting now?** Patients are often worried about appearance of varicose veins or prognosis if left untreated, but have no other symptoms attributable to the veins (1:3 consultations).
- **Symptoms:** Heaviness, tension, aching (worse on standing and in the evening; improved by elevating the leg and support stockings), itching.
- **Complications:** See opposite.
- **PMH:** Previous surgery or injection for varicose veins; pregnancy; past history of DVT or thrombophlebitis; COC pill or HRT.
- **FH:** Varicose veins or DVT.

Examination
- **Abdominal examination:** To exclude 2° causes.
- **Veins:** With the patient standing, inspect distribution of the veins and any 2° skin changes. Patterns of distribution:
  - *Long saphenous distribution*—thigh and medial aspect of the calf.
  - *Short saphenous distribution*—below the knee on the posterior and lateral aspects of the calf.

Management: Reassurance is often all that's needed.
- **If symptoms are troublesome:** Advise support stockings; avoid standing for prolonged periods and if standing, don't stand still; walk regularly; ↓ weight (if obese).
- **If any complications or severe symptoms:** Refer for surgical assessment. In general, patients with purely cosmetic problems are not treated under the NHS.

Bleeding varicose veins: Bleeding can be stemmed by raising the foot above the level of the heart and applying compression. If the patient is fit for surgery, refer for surgical assessment. Once recovered from the bleed, advise compression hosiery.

Complications

- Haemorrhage
- Varicose eczema
- Skin pigmentation
- Thrombophlebitis
- Lipodermatosclerosis—fibrosis of the dermis and subcutis around the ankle → firm induration
- Oedema
- Venous ulceration—40% don't have visible varicose veins
- Atrophie blanche— white, lacy scars

COC pill and HRT: Women with varicose veins taking the COC pill or HRT are not at ↑ risk of DVT but are at ↑ risk of thrombophlebitis.

Saphena varix: Dilatation of the saphenous vein at its confluence with the femoral vein which transmits a cough impulse. May have bluish tinge and disappears on lying down. A cause of a lump in the groin. Action only needed if symptomatic.

Thrombophlebitis: Presents as severe pain, erythema, pigmentation over, and hardening of the vein. Thrombophlebitis in varicose veins results from stasis. Consider underlying malignancy or thrombophilia if thrombophlebitis occurs in normal veins; there is recurrent thrombophlebitis in varicose veins.

Management: There is no indication for antibiotics.
- Crepe bandaging to compress vein and minimize propogation of thrombus
- Analgesia—preferably NSAID
- Ice packs and elevation
- Low-dose aspirin—75–150mg od

⚠ If phlebitis extends up the long saphenous vein towards the saphenofemoral junction, refer for urgent duplex scanning—saphenofemoral ligation may be indicated if thrombus extends into the femoral vein.

Follow-up: If the patient is fit for surgery, refer for surgical assessment as thrombophlebitis tends to recur if the underlying venous abnormality is not corrected.

❶ History of thrombophlebitis is a contraindication to the COC pill and a reason to stop for current users. Evidence regarding HRT is less clear.

Thrombophlebitis migrans: Recurrent tender nodules affecting veins throughout the body. Associated with carcinoma of the pancreas.

Patient information
British Vascular Foundation ▣ http://www.bvf.org.uk

Deep vein thrombosis (DVT)

Deep vein thrombosis may be proximal (involving veins above the knee) or isolated to the calf veins. May also occur in the cerebral sinus, and veins of the arms retina and mesentery. *Incidence:* 1 in 1000 people/y. in developed countries.

Risk factors

- Age >40y.
- Smoking
- Obesity
- Immobility
- Recent long-distance travel
- Pregnancy
- Puerperium
- COC pill/HRT use
- Surgery
- Recent trauma
- Malignancy
- Heart failure
- Nephrotic syndrome
- Inflammatory bowel disease
- PMH of venous thromboembolism
- Inherited thrombophilic clotting disorders
- Other chronic illness

Presentation: Unilateral leg pain, swelling and/or tenderness ± mild fever, pitting oedema, warmth, and distended collateral superficial veins.

Differential diagnosis

- Cellulitis
- Haematoma
- Ruptured Baker's cyst
- Superficial thrombophlebitis
- Chronic venous insufficiency
- Venous obstruction
- Post-thrombotic syndrome
- Acute arterial ischaemia
- Lymphoedema
- Fracture
- Hypoproteinaemia

Immediate action: Clinical diagnosis is unreliable. <50% with clinically suspected DVT have diagnosis confirmed on diagnostic imaging. Refer all suspected DVTs for further assessment. *Specialist assessment:* Clinical probability scores are used to decide whether patients fall into high or low probability groups for DVT.

- *If low probability:* A blood D-dimer test is done (detects a degradation product of fresh venous thrombus). If the D-dimer test is –ve, DVT is excluded. If +ve, the patient is assessed as if medium/high probability.
- *If medium/high probability:* USS assessment is undertaken. If USS is –ve and low probability or –ve D-dimer, DVT is excluded. If USS is +ve, diagnosis of DVT is confirmed. If USS is –ve and medium/high probability or +ve D-dimer, USS is repeated after 1wk. or the patient is assessed with venography, CT, or MRI.

Management of patients with confirmed DVT

- Initial anticoagulation is with low molecular weight heparin (LMWH) followed by oral anticoagulation (warfarin)—usually as an out-patient.
- LMWH should be continued for at least 4d. and until INR is in therapeutic range for ≥2d. Target INR 2.5 (range 2–3).
- Oral anticoagulants ↓ risk of further thromboembolism and should be continued for 3–6mo. after a single DVT (📖 p.366).
- Graduated elastic compression stockings should be worn for >2y. as they ↓ risk post-thrombotic leg syndrome by 12–50%.

Management during pregnancy: 📖 p.785

Isolated calf DVT: There is some debate whether anticoagulation is necessary. Untreated 40–50% extend to proximal DVT and anticoagulation ↓ risk extension. Some specialists prefer to treat with compression stockings and follow with serial USS.

Complications of DVT

- *Pulmonary embolus:* Without treatment, 20% with proximal DVT develop PE (📖 p.1054).
- *Post-thrombotic syndrome:* Occurs after DVT. Results in chronic venous hypertension causing limb pain, swelling, hyperpigmentation, dermatitis, ulcers, venous gangrene, and lipodermatosclerosis.
- *Recurrent venous thromboembolism:* Patients with history of DVT or PE have ↑ risk of recurrence in high-risk situations (trauma, surgery, immobility, pregnancy) and should receive prophylaxis with heparin/oral anticoagulants in such situations.

Table 10.14 Dose regime for starting warfarin in the community

INR on day 5	Dose days 5–7	INR on day 8	Dose from day 8	Instructions:
≤1.7	5mg	≤1.7	6mg	• Give warfarin 5mg od for 4d. then check INR
		1.8–2.4	5mg	• Adjust dose as in Table 10.4
		2.5–3	4mg	
		>3	3mg for 4d.	
1.8–2.2	4mg	≤1.7	5mg	• Recheck INR on day 8 and adjust dose as in table 10.4
		1.8–2.4	4mg	• Thereafter, check INR weekly (unless 4d. interval stated) and adjust dose accordingly until dose is stable in the target range
		2.5–3	3.5mg	
		3.1–3.5	3mg for 4d.	
		>3.5	2.5mg for 4d.	
2.3–2.7	3mg	≤1.7	4mg	
		1.8–2.4	3.5mg	
		2.5–3	3mg	
		3.1–3.5	2.5mg for 4d.	
		>3.5	2mg for 4d.	
2.8–3.2	2mg	≤1.7	3mg	⚠ **High INR**
		1.8–2.4	2.5mg	
		2.5–3	2mg	INR ≥ 8 (lower if other risk factors for bleeding)—admit to hospital even if not, bleeding.
		3.1–3.5	1.5mg for 4d.	
		>3.5	1mg for 4d.	
3.3–3.7	1mg	≤1.7	2mg	
		1.8–2.4	1.5mg	INR >3.7 and <8—omit warfarin 1–2d. and recheck INR. Restart when INR <5 and re-titrate dose.
		2.5–3	1mg	
		3.1–3.5	0.5mg for 4d.	
		>3.5	omit for 4d.	
>3.7	0mg	<2	1.5mg for 4d.	
		2–2.9	1mg for 4d.	
		3–3.5	0.5mg for 4d.	

Reproduced with permission from *British Journal of Clinical Pharmacology* (1998) **46**: 157–61.

Anticoagulation

Heparin in the community: Only use on specialist advice. Usually s/cut low molecular weight (LMW) heparin used as it does not need daily monitoring.

Table 10.15 Indications for oral anticoagulation and target INR

Indication	Target INR (target range)	Duration of treatment
Cardiac		
Mechanical prosthetic heart valves		
1st generation	3.5 (3.0–4.0)	Long term
2nd generation	3.0 (2.5–3.5)	
Rheumatic mitral valve disease	2.5 (2.0–3.0)	Long term
Valvular AF and AF due to congenital heart disease or thyrotoxicosis	2.5 (2.0–3.0)	Long term
Non-valvular AF and medium/high risk of stroke (📖 p.607)	2.5 (2.0–3.0)	Long term
Dilated cardiomyopathy	2.5 (2.0–3.0)	Long term
Mural thrombus post MI	2.5 (2.0–3.0)	3mo.
Cardioversion	2.5 (2.0–3.0)	3wk before procedure and for 4wk. after procedure
Venous thromboembolism		
1st PE/proximal vein thrombosis and no persistent risk factors	2.5 (2.0–3.0)	6mo.
1st calf vein thrombosis and no persistent risk factors	2.5 (2.0–3.0)	3 mo.
Prophylaxis of recurrent DVT/PE		
Occurring on warfarin	3.5 (3.0–4.0)	Long term
Occurring off warfarin	2.5 (2.0–3.0)	
Other disorders		
Inherited thrombophilia with no previous thrombosis	2.5 (2.0–3.0)	Anticoagulate for high-risk activities e.g. surgery
Inherited thrombophilia with previous episode of thrombosis	2.5 (2.0–3.0)	Long term
Antiphospholipid syndrome	2.5–3.5	Long term

Warfarin: Acts by antagonizing the effects of vitamin K and thus ↓ clotting tendency. It takes 48–72h. for anticoagulant effect to develop, fully, so not used initially when acute effect is required. Indications and target INRs—Table 10.15.

Initiation of warfarin
- *Acute anticoagulation (e.g. PE)*—admit to hospital for heparinization, then warfarinization with heparin cover.
- *For DVT*—anticoagulation is often started in the community with heparin, and then warfarin under specialist direction.
- *If no urgency (e.g. chronic AF)*—warfarin can be started in the community. Check baseline blood sample for FBC, clotting screen, urea and liver function tests. Complete a DoH oral anticoagulant booklet for the patient to carry. Take patients (or carers) through the educational dos and don'ts in the booklet. Advise that the daily dose of warfarin should be taken at a fixed time.

Dose regime for starting warfarin in the community: Table 10.14 (📖 p.365).

Monitoring: Table 10.16. If there is a change in clinical state, monitor more frequently until steady state is re-established. Have an explicit system for handling results promptly, making informed decisions on further treatment and testing, and communicating results to patients. Monitor the process with regular audit.

Table 10.16 Warfarin therapy: recall periods during maintenance therapy

INR	Recall interval and action
1 INR high ⚠ If INR >8—admit	Recall 7–14d. Stop treatment for 1–3d. (max 1wk. in prosthetic valve patients) and restart at a lower dose.
1 INR low	↑ dose and recall in 7–14d.
1 therapeutic INR	Recall 4wk.
2 therapeutic INRs	Recall 6wk. (maximum interval if prosthetic heart valve)
3 therapeutic INRs	Recall 8wk.*
4 therapeutic INRs	Recall 10wk.*
5 therapeutic INRs	Recall 12wk.*

*Except prosthetic heart valves, where maximum recall interval is 6wk.

Recurrent arterial thrombosis/embolism on anticoagulants
Seek specialist advice. *Consider:*
- Compliance
- Modifiable risk factors—smoking, ↑BP, lipids
- Cardiac sources of emboli (Echo)
- Thrombophilias— 📖 p.529
- Arteritis e.g. collagen disorders, syphilis
- Malignant disease

Further information
SIGN (1999) Antithrombotic therapy 🖳 http://www.sign.ac.uk
B J Haematology (1999) Guidelines on oral anticoagulation, (3rd edition) **101**: 374–87
🖳 http://www.bcshguidelines.com

Respiratory medicine

Bronchodilators and steroids

Bronchodilators: Cause relaxation of bronchial smooth muscle.

Short-acting β_2 agonists: e.g. salbutamol, terbutaline. Safest, most effective β_2 agonists for use as quick relievers in asthma and COPD.

- Duration of action: ~3–5h. Oral preparations are less effective than inhaled preparations. Prescribe as 1 or 2 puffs prn.
- Warn patients to seek medical advice if usual dose does not relieve symptoms or relieves symptoms for <3h.
- Consider using a nebuliser if high doses are needed.
- Regular treatment with bronchodilators alone may be linked with worsening of asthma and asthma deaths. If asthmatic and using >1x/d., consider starting prophylaxis—📖 p.380.

Longer-acting β_2 agonists: e.g. salmeterol, formoterol

- *Asthma:* e.g. salmeterol 50–100mcg bd—use as an adjunct to existing corticosteroid treatment (📖 p.380). Particularly useful for night-time asthma. Usual duration of action is ~12h. Do not use for relief of acute attacks.
- *COPD:* 📖 p.385.

Steroids: Short- and long-term treatment of inflammatory conditions.

Side-effects

- ↑BP
- Osteoporosis ± fracture (📖 p.568)
- Proximal muscle wasting
- Euphoria
- Paranoid states or depression— especially if past history of psychiatric disorder
- Peptic ulceration—soluble or EC versions may ↓ risk
- Suppression of clinical signs— may allow diseases (e.g. septicae- mia), to reach advanced stage before being recognized
- Spread of infection (e.g. chickenpox)
- DM and worsening of diabetic control in diabetic patients
- Cushing's syndrome—moon face, striae, and acne (📖 p.426)
- Adrenal atrophy—can persist for years after stopping long-term steroids; illness or surgical emergencies may require steroid supplements
- Growth suppression in children
- Na^+ and water retention; K^+ loss

Administration: Often started at high dose to suppress disease process and stepped down with improvement. Use the minimum dose that controls disease as maintenance therapy.

- *Oral steroids:* Prescribe as a single dose in the morning to ↓ circadian rhythm disturbance. Supply with a 'steroid card'.
- *Inhaled steroids:* Use regularly to obtain maximum benefit. Alleviation of symptoms occurs 3–7d. after initiation. Supply patients using high-dose inhalers with a 'steroid card'.
  - If the inhaled corticosteroid causes coughing, a short-acting β_2 agonist before use might help.
  - Common unwanted effects are oral candidiasis (5%) and hoarseness—↓ by use of a large-volume spacer or mouth washing after use.

Steroid cards: Should be carried at all times by patients on oral or high doses of inhaled steroids. The card:
• Informs other practitioners your patient is on steroids *and*
• Gives the patient advice on use of steroids and risk of infection

Obtaining steroid cards
• England and Wales: Department of Health ☎08701 555 455
• Scotland: Banner Business Supplies: ☎01506 448 440

Withdrawal of steroids: Stop abruptly if disease is unlikely to relapse, the patient has received treatment for ≤3wk., and is not included in the patient groups described below. Withdraw gradually if disease is unlikely to relapse and the patient has:
• Recently had repeated steroid courses (particularly if taken for >3wk.)
• Taken a short course <1y. after stopping long-term therapy
• Other possible causes of adrenal suppression
• Received >40mg od of prednisolone (or equivalent)
• Been given repeat doses in the evening
• Received treatment with steroids for >3wk.

During corticosteroid withdrawal, ↓ dose rapidly to physiological levels (~ prednisolone 7.5mg od); thereafter ↓ more slowly. Assess the disease during withdrawal to ensure relapse doesn't occur.

Home nebuliser therapy: In England and Wales, nebulisers are not available via the NHS (but are free of VAT). Some nebulisers are available in Scotland on form GP10A. Nebulisers convert a solution of drug into an aerosol for inhalation. They are used to deliver a higher dosage of drug than is usual with inhalers over a short period of time (5–10min.). *List of available devices—BNF 3.1.5.*

Indications
• Acute exacerbations ± regular treatment of asthma/COPD
• Antibiotic treatment—for patients with chronic purulent infection e.g. CF, bronchiectasis; prophylaxis and treatment of pneumocystis pneumonia with pentamidine in patients with AIDS
• Palliative care—palliation of breathlessness and cough e.g. bronchodilators, lignocaine, or bupivacaine for dry, persistent cough.

Use in asthma/COPD: Before suggesting long-term use:
• Review diagnosis
• Review technique using hand-held device ± spacer and device
• Review compliance with medication
• Try ↑ dose of bronchodilator via a hand-held device for at least 2wk.
• Perform a 2wk. trial of nebuliser therapy and monitor therapeutic effect (e.g. with PEFR in asthma or dyspnoea score with COPD)

Provide clear instructions on the use of the nebuliser, monitoring, and when to seek help. All patients with home nebulisers should be followed up regularly.

Essential reading
British Thoracic Society (1997) Current best practice for nebuliser treatment *Thorax* 52 (Suppl 2): S4–24 🖳 http://www.brit-thoracic.org.uk

Measuring lung function in the surgery

Peak flow: A simple and cheap test. Peak flow is not a good measure of airflow limitation as it tends to overestimate lung function. It is best used to monitor progress of disease and affects of treatment for patients with asthma. Link with self-management plan (📖 p.378). Peak flow meters are available on NHS prescription. Since 2004, EN 13826/EU standard peak flow meters are supplied. Peak flow charts are available from NHS supplies (Form FP1010) and drug companies.

Measuring peak expiratory flow rate (PEFR)

- Ask the patient to stand up (if possible) and hold the peak flow meter horizontally. Check the indicator is at zero and the track clear.
- Ask the patient to take a deep breath and blow out forcefully into the peak flow meter ensuring lips are sealed firmly around the mouthpiece.
- Read the PEFR off the meter. The best of 3 attempts is recorded.
- Consider using a low-range meter if predicted or best PEFR is <250L/min.
- Normal values—see Table 11.2 (📖 p.374).

Spirometry: Measures the volume of air the patient is able to expel from the lungs after a maximal inspiration.
- **FEV_1:** Volume of air the patient is able to exhale in the first second of forced expiration.
- **FVC:** Total volume of air the patient can forcibly exhale in 1 breath.
- **FEV_1/FVC:** Ratio of FEV_1 to FVC expressed as a %.

Measuring FEV_1 and FVC

- Sit the patient comfortably
- Ask the patient to take a deep breath in
- Ask the patient to blow the whole breath out as hard as possible until there is no breath left to expel and ensuring lips are sealed firmly around the mouthpiece
- Encourage the patient to keep breathing out
- Repeat the procedure x 2 (i.e. 3 attempts in all)
- At least 2 readings should be within 100ml or 5% of each other
- Normal values—see Table 11.3 (📖 p.375)

Table 11.1 Interpretation of spirometry results

	Restrictive lung disease (e.g. fibrosing alveolitis)	Obstructive lung disease (e.g. COPD)
FEV_1 (% of predicted normal)	↓ (<80%)	↓ (<80%)
FVC (% of predicted normal)	↓ (<80%)	Normal or ↓
FEV_1/FVC	Normal (>70%)	↓ (<70%)

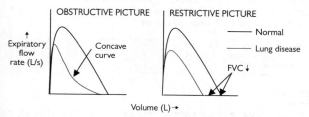

Figure 11.1 Flow volume curves for patients with restrictive and obstructive lung disease

Flow volume measurement: Available with some spirometers. Shape of the flow-volume curve may suggest an obstructive picture—see Figure 11.1.

The Revised Jones Morbidity Index: Useful tool to identify patients with poor asthma control in general practice and monitor effect of changes of treatment. Morbidity categories correlate with lung function. Not designed for use during an acute attack.

During the last 4 weeks
- Have you been in a wheezy or asthmatic condition at least once a week?
- Have you had time off work or school because of your asthma?*
- Have you suffered from attacks of wheezing during the night?

NO to all questions = low morbidity
1 x YES answer = medium morbidity
2 or 3 x YES answer = high morbidity

Further information

British Thoracic Society *Spirometry in practice: A practical guide to using spirometry in primary care.* Available from 🖳 http://www.brit-thoracic.org.uk
ARTP/BTS Certificate in Spirometry. Further details and list of approved training centres is available from ☎0121 697 8339

---

* If the patient does not work/go to school count as a NO answer.

Table 11.2 Predicted PEFR measurements in L/min (EU scale)[*]
Children: Height is the only determinant of PEFR in children. With ↑ age, the pattern of adult values takes over.

Height: ft	3'	3'4"	3'8"	4'	4'4"	4'8"	5'	5'4"	5'8"	6'
m	90cm	1	1.1	1.2	1.3	1.4	1.5	1.6	1.7	1.8
PEFR l/min.	88	105	136	172	220	265	313	371	427	487

Women
Height →

ft	4'10"	4'11"	5'	5'1"	5'2"	5'3"	5'4"	5'5"	5'6"	5'7"	5'8"	5'9"	5'10"
m	1.47	1.5	1.52	1.55	1.57	1.6	1.62	1.65	1.67	1.7	1.72	1.75	1.77
Age													
15y.	379	382	385	389	391	394	397	400	402	405	407	411	413
20y.	402	406	409	413	416	419	422	425	428	431	434	437	439
25y.	415	419	422	426	429	433	435	439	441	445	447	451	453
30y.	419	424	427	431	433	437	440	444	446	450	452	456	458
35y.	418	423	425	430	432	436	439	443	445	449	451	454	457
40y.	413	417	420	424	427	431	433	437	439	443	445	449	451
45y.	405	409	412	416	418	422	425	428	431	434	436	440	442
50y.	394	399	401	405	407	411	414	417	419	423	425	428	430
55y.	383	387	389	393	395	399	401	404	407	410	412	415	417
60y.	370	373	376	379	382	385	387	391	393	396	398	401	403
65y.	356	360	362	366	368	371	373	376	378	381	383	386	388
70y.	343	346	348	351	353	356	358	361	363	366	368	371	372

Men
Height →

ft	5'2"	5'3"	5'4"	5'5"	5'6"	5'7"	5'8"	5'9"	5'10"	5'11"	6'	6'1"	6'2"
m	1.57	1.6	1.62	1.65	1.67	1.7	1.72	1.75	1.77	1.8	1.82	1.85	1.87
Age													
15y.	479	485	489	494	498	503	506	511	515	520	523	528	531
20y.	534	540	545	551	555	561	565	571	575	580	584	589	593
25y.	568	575	580	587	591	598	602	608	612	618	622	628	632
30y.	587	594	599	606	611	617	622	628	633	639	643	649	653
35y.	594	601	606	613	618	625	629	636	640	646	650	657	661
40y.	592	599	604	611	615	622	627	633	637	644	648	654	658
45y.	582	590	594	601	606	612	617	623	627	634	638	644	647
50y.	568	575	580	586	591	597	601	608	612	618	622	627	631
55y.	550	557	561	568	572	578	582	588	592	598	602	607	611
60y.	529	536	540	546	550	556	560	566	570	575	579	584	588
65y.	507	513	517	523	527	533	536	542	545	551	554	559	562
70y.	484	490	493	499	503	508	511	517	520	525	528	533	536

❶ For normal values in age groups/heights not represented on these charts or for conversion from the old Wright scale peak flow meters, see 🖥 http://www.peakflow.com

[*] Based on values from Gregg I and Nunn AJ (1989) *BMJ* **298**:1068–70, and from Godfrey S et al. (1970) *Brit J Dis Chest* **64**:15
Spirometry normal values reproduced with permission of the British Thoracic Society

Table 11.3 Predicted FEV1 and FVC measurements (in L)

❶ These values apply for Caucasians. ↓ values by 7% for Asians and 13% for people of Afro-Caribbean origin.

Women

Height	ft	4'11"	5'1"	5'3"	5'5"	5'7"	5'9"	5'11"
	m	1.5	1.55	1.6	1.65	1.7	1.75	1.8
Age								
38–41y.	FEV_1	2.3	2.5	2.7	2.89	3.09	3.29	3.49
	FVC	2.69	2.91	3.13	3.35	3.58	3.80	4.02
42–45y.	FEV_1	2.2	2.4	2.6	2.79	2.99	3.19	3.39
	FVC	2.59	2.81	3.03	3.25	3.47	3.69	3.91
46–49y.	FEV_1	2.1	2.3	2.5	2.69	2.89	3.09	3.29
	FVC	2.48	2.7	2.92	3.15	3.37	3.59	3.81
50–53y.	FEV_1	2	2.2	2.4	2.59	2.79	2.99	3.19
	FVC	2.38	2.6	2.82	3.04	3.26	3.48	3.71
54–57y.	FEV_1	1.9	2.1	2.3	2.49	2.69	2.89	3.09
	FVC	2.27	2.49	2.72	2.94	3.16	3.38	3.6
58–61y.	FEV_1	1.8	2	2.2	2.39	2.59	2.79	2.99
	FVC	2.17	2.39	2.61	2.83	3.06	3.28	3.5
62–65y.	FEV_1	1.7	1.9	2.1	2.29	2.49	2.69	2.89
	FVC	2.07	2.29	2.51	2.73	2.95	3.17	3.39
66–69y.	FEV_1	1.6	1.8	2	2.19	2.39	2.59	2.79
	FVC	1.96	2.18	2.4	2.63	2.85	3.07	3.29

For women ≥70y, use the formulae:
- $FEV_1 = (0.0395 \times \text{height in m.} \times 100) - (0.025 \times \text{age in y.}) - 2.6$
- $FVC = (0.0443 \times \text{height in m.} \times 100) - (0.026 \times \text{age in y.}) - 2.89$

Men

Height	ft	5'3"	5'5"	5'7"	5'9"	5'11"	6'1"	6'3"
	m	1.6	1.65	1.7	1.75	1.8	1.85	1.9
Age								
38–41y.	FEV_1	3.2	3.42	3.63	3.85	4.06	4.28	4.49
	FVC	3.81	4.1	4.39	4.67	4.96	5.25	5.54
42–45y.	FEV_1	3.09	3.3	3.52	3.73	3.95	4.16	4.38
	FVC	3.71	3.99	4.28	4.57	4.86	5.15	5.43
46–49y.	FEV_1	2.97	3.18	3.4	3.61	3.83	4.04	4.26
	FVC	3.6	3.89	4.18	4.47	4.75	5.04	5.33
50–53y.	FEV_1	2.85	3.07	3.28	3.5	3.71	3.93	4.14
	FVC	3.5	3.79	4.07	4.36	4.65	4.94	5.23
54–57y.	FEV_1	2.74	2.95	3.17	3.38	3.6	3.81	4.03
	FVC	3.39	3.68	3.97	4.26	4.55	4.83	5.12
58–61y.	FEV_1	2.62	2.84	3.05	3.27	3.48	3.7	3.91
	FVC	3.29	3.58	3.87	4.15	4.44	4.73	5.02
62–65y.	FEV_1	2.51	2.72	2.94	3.15	3.37	3.58	3.8
	FVC	3.19	3.47	3.76	4.05	4.34	4.63	4.91
66–69y.	FEV_1	2.39	2.6	2.82	3.03	3.25	3.46	3.68
	FVC	3.08	3.37	3.66	3.95	4.23	4.52	4.81

For men ≥70y. use the formulae:
- $FEV_1 = (0.043 \times \text{height in m.} \times 100) - (0.029 \times \text{age in y.}) - 2.49$
- $FVC = (0.0576 \times \text{height in m.} \times 100) - (0.026 \times \text{age in y.}) - 4.34$

Asthma

Symptoms/signs of a severe asthma attack

- Unable to talk in sentences without stopping for breath
- Intercostal recession
- PEFR <50% best
- Tachypnoea (respiratory rate >25 breaths/min.)
- Tachycardia (heart rate >110bpm)

Life-threatening signs

- Central cyanosis
- Silent chest (inaudible wheeze)
- Confusion or exhaustion
- PEFR <33% predicted or best
- Hypotension
- Bradycardia

Management of an acute asthma attack: 📖 p.1058

Asthma is a condition of paroxysmal, reversible airways obstruction and has 3 characteristic features:
- Airflow limitation which is usually reversible spontaneously or with treatment
- Airway hyper-responsiveness to a wide range of stimuli
- Inflammation of the bronchi

Personal or family history of asthma or other atopic conditions (e.g. eczema or hayfever), makes diagnosis of asthma more likely.

Classification

- *Intrinsic:* no specific triggers—typically starts in middle age
- *Extrinsic:* identifiable triggers—typically affects children and young people.

Prevalence: Estimates of prevalence vary widely dependant on criteria used. European Respiratory Health Survey figures:
- 25% adults aged 20–44y. suffer from wheeze
- 15% suffer from wheeze with breathlessness
- 7% have doctor-diagnosed asthma

There is marked geographical variation. Occupational asthma accounts for 1–2% of adult asthma (📖 p.399).

Asthma in special groups

- *Children:* 📖 p.860
- *Occupational asthma:* 📖 p.399
- *Pregnancy:* 📖 p.780

Asthma in adults: Diagnosis can be difficult as people who have asthma suffer from a variety of symptoms—none of which are specific for asthma.

Symptoms

- wheeze
- shortness of breath
- chest tightness
- cough

Typically, symptoms are: variable, intermittent, worse at night and in the early morning (when PEFR dips) and/or provoked by triggers e.g. exercise, pollen.

Signs

- **None:** common if patient is well
- **Wheeze:** bilateral, diffuse, polyphonic, expiratory>inspiratory— document in notes if heard
- **'Barrel chest':** signs of hyperinflation ± wheeze in a patient with chronic asthma.

Tests: Objective tests should be used to confirm diagnosis of asthma before long-term treatment is started. In general practice, this involves PEFR measurement ± spirometry (📖 p.372).

- **PEFR**
  - Normal PEFR in the presence of symptoms suggests diagnosis is NOT asthma
  - Variability of PEFR over time (either spontaneous or in response to medication) is a characteristic feature of asthma (Table 11.4)
- **Spirometry:** Use to exclude other forms of lung disease e.g. COPD. Can also be used instead of PEFR to demonstrate variability (≥15% variation in FEV_1 with a minimum change in FEV_1 ≥200l/min. suggests asthma).
- **CXR:** Consider for any patient with atypical/additional symptoms

Table 11.4 Objective tests to confirm asthma

Test	Positive outcome[*]
Serial PEFR measurements	Demonstrate variability on ≥3d./wk.
Trial of β-agonists	Inhaled salbutamol (2.5mcg via nebuliser or 400mcg via MDi with spacer) → ↑ PEFR
Trial of steroids	Prednisolone 30mg od for 14d. → ↑ PEFR
Exercise test	6min. exercise (e.g. running) → ↓ PEFR

[*] >20% variability from the best or baseline reading, with a minimum change in PEFR of ≥60l/min. is highly suggestive of a diagnosis of asthma.

Common precipitating/exacerbating factors

- Exercise
- Emotion
- Weather (fog, cold air, thunder-storms)
- Air pollutants (smoke and dust)
- Household allergens (e.g. house dust mite, animal fur, feathers)
- Smoking
- Occupational exposure to animal products, wood dusts, grain dusts, chemicals (e.g. isocyanates)
- Infection (commonly viral URTI and chest infections)
- Drugs (NSAIDs, β blockers)
- Gastro-oesophageal reflux

Cough variant asthma: Asthma in which cough without wheeze is the predominant feature

Differential diagnosis

- **Localized obstruction of the airways:** cancer (lung, trachea, larynx), foreign body, post tracheostomy stenosis
- **Generalized obstruction of the airways:** COPD (predominantly irreversible), cardiac disease, PE, interstitial lung disease, aspiration, bronchiectasis, CF.

Asthma management in practice

Aims of treatment
- To minimize symptoms and impact on lifestyle (e.g. absence from work/school; limitations to physical ability)
- To minimize the need for reliever medication
- To prevent severe attacks/exacerbations

GP services: Ideally, routine asthma care should be carried out in a specialized clinic. Doctors and nurses involved in asthma clinics need appropriate training with regular updates. Practices should keep an asthma register of affected patients to ensure adequate follow-up and allow audit. High quality asthma care is rewarded in the quality and outcomes framework.

Reviews and monitoring Frequency depends on needs. Aim to review all patients with asthma at least annually.
- Check symptoms since last seen. Use objective measures e.g. Revised Jones Morbidity Index (📖 p.373)
- Record smoking status and advise smokers to stop
- Record any exacerbations/acute attacks since last seen
- Check medication—use, concordance (prescription count—📖 p.124), inhaler technique, problems, side-effects
- Check influenza/pneumococcal vaccination received
- Review objective measures of lung function e.g. home PEFR chart, PEFR at review
- Address any problems or queries and educate about asthma
- Agree management goals and date for further review

Self-management: All patients should receive—
- *Self-management education:* Brief, simple education linked to patient goals is most likely to be successful. Include information about: nature of disease, nature of the treatment and how to use it, self-monitoring/self-assessment, recognition of acute exacerbations, allergen/trigger avoidance, patients own goals of treatment.
- *Written action plan:* Focus on individual needs. Include information about features which indicate when asthma is worsening and what to do under those circumstances. Action plans ↓ morbidity and health costs from asthma[S].
- *PEFR monitoring:* Record PEFR at asthma review and if acute exacerbation. Home monitoring in combination with an action plan can be useful, especially for patients with severe asthma, brittle asthma (i.e. rapid development of acute asthma attacks), and for those who are poor perceivers of their symptoms.

Management of acute asthma: 📖 p.1058

Non-pharmacological measures
- *Smoking:* Smoking may ↑ symptoms of asthma—advise to stop[G].
- *Weight:* There is some evidence that weight ↓ in obese patients with asthma results in ↑ asthma control[R].

- *Allergen avoidance*
  - *House dust mite:* There is little evidence that ↓ house dust mite results in clinical improvement[C]. In commited families advise: complete barrier bed coverings; removal of carpets; removal of soft toys from bed; high temperature washing of bed linen; acaricides to soft furnishings; dehumidification. There is no evidence that air ionizers have any beneficial effect.
  - *Pets:* There is no evidence that removing pets from a home results in improved symptoms but many experts still advise removal of the pet for patients with asthma who also have an allergy to the pet.

Drug therapy: 🕮 p.380

Complementary and alternative therapy: Table 11.5

Evidence	Therapy	
Inconclusive but some evidence of benefit	• Hypnosis[S] • Acupuncture[C] • Physical training[C] • Immunotherapy[C]—only in specialized clinic	• Magnesium supplements[R] • Breathing exercises[C] • Herbal medicine[S]
Insufficient evidence	Massage[C]	Homeopathy[C]
No benefit	Chiropractic[C]	Fish oil supplements[C]

Psychosocial factors: Depression, anxiety, and denial of disease are associated strongly with asthma deaths. Other associations with asthma severity include: life crises, family conflict, social isolation, shame, anger, and high-risk lifestyles e.g. smoking and alcohol abuse. When asthma proves difficult to control on usually effective therapy, find out about any family, psychological, or social problems which may be interfering with effective management

Referral: Consider referral if:
- Diagnostic confusion e.g. unexpected clinical findings (e.g. clubbing, cyanosis); spirometry or PEFR does not fit the clinical picture
- Suspected occupational asthma
- Persistent shortness of breath

- Unilateral or fixed wheeze
- Stridor
- Chest pain
- Weight loss
- Persistent cough ± sputum production
- Non-resolving pneumonia

Essential reading
British Thoracic Society/SIGN British guidelines on the management of asthma (revised 2004) 🖳 http://www.sign.ac.uk

Patient information and support
Asthma UK ☎08457 01 02 03 🖳 http://www.asthma.org.uk

Drug treatment of asthma

Management of acute asthma: 📖 p.1058

Asthma in pregnancy: 📖 p.780

Use a stepwise approach: Figure 11.2. Start at the step most appropriate to the initial severity of symptoms. The aim is to achieve early control of the condition and then to ↓ treatment by stepping down.

Exacerbations: Treat exacerbations early. A rescue course of prednisolone 30–40mg od for 1–2wk. may be needed at any step and any time.

Selection of inhaler device: If possible, use a metred dose inhaler. Inadequate technique may be mistaken for drug failure. Emphasize patients must inhale slowly and hold their breath for 10s. after inhalation. Demonstrate inhaler technique before prescribing and check at follow-ups. Spacers or breath-activated devices are useful for patients who find activation difficult. Dry powder inhalers are an alternative.

Short-acting β_2 agonists: 📖 p.370 (e.g. salbutamol). Work more quickly and/or with fewer side-effects than alternatives. Use prn unless shown to benefit from regular dosing. Using ≥1 canister/mo. or >10–12puffs/d. is a marker of poorly controlled asthma.

Inhaled corticosteroids: 📖 p.370. Most effective preventer for achieving overall treatment goals. May be beneficial even for patients with mild asthma. Consider if:
• Exacerbations of asthma in the last 2y.
• Using inhaled β_2 agonists >3x/wk.
• Symptomatic ≥3x/wk. or ≥1night /wk.

Oral steroids: 📖 p.370

Add on therapy: Before initiating a new drug, check compliance and inhaler technique and eliminate trigger factors.
• *Long-acting β_2 agonists (LABA):* 📖 p.370—inhaled preparations (e.g. salmeterol) improve lung function/symptoms. Slow-release tablets have similar effect but side-effects are greater. Do not use without inhaled steroids. Only continue if demonstrable benefit.
• *Theophylline:* Improves lung function/symptoms. Side-effects common.
• *Leukotriene receptor antagonists:* e.g. montelukast. Provide improvement in symptoms and lung function and ↓ exacerbations.
• *Sodium cromoglycate and nedocromil sodium:* Some evidence of benefit in adults (nedocromil sodium > sodium cromoglycate).

Stepping down: Review and consider stepping down at intervals ≥3mo. Maintain on the lowest dose of inhaled steroid controlling symptoms. When reducing steroids, cut dose by 25–50% each time.

Further information

British Thoracic Society/SIGN: British guidelines on the management of asthma (revised 2004).
    📖 http://www.sign.ac.uk
BNF Section 3 📖 http://www.bnf.org

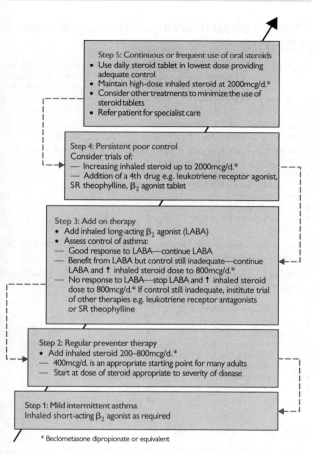

Step 5: Continuous or frequent use of oral steroids
- Use daily steroid tablet in lowest dose providing adequate control
- Maintain high-dose inhaled steroid at 2000mcg/d.*
- Consider other treatments to minimize the use of steroid tablets
- Refer patient for specialist care

Step 4: Persistent poor control
Consider trials of:
— Increasing inhaled steroid up to 2000mcg/d.*
— Addition of a 4th drug e.g. leukotriene receptor agonist, SR theophylline, β_2 agonist tablet

Step 3: Add on therapy
- Add inhaled long-acting β_2 agonist (LABA)
- Assess control of asthma:
— Good response to LABA—continue LABA
— Benefit from LABA but control still inadequate—continue LABA and ↑ inhaled steroid dose to 800mcg/d.*
— No response to LABA—stop LABA and ↑ inhaled steroid dose to 800mcg/d.* If control still inadequate, institute trial of other therapies e.g. leukotriene receptor antagonists or SR theophylline

Step 2: Regular preventer therapy
- Add inhaled steroid 200–800mcg/d.*
— 400mcg/d. is an appropriate starting point for many adults
— Start at dose of steroid appropriate to severity of disease

Step 1: Mild intermittent asthma
Inhaled short-acting β_2 agonist as required

* Beclometasone dipropionate or equivalent

Figure 11.2 Summary of stepwise management in adults

All doses given refer to beclometasone dipropionate (BDP) administered via metred dose inhaler. For other drugs/formulations, adjust dose accordingly (see BNF Section 3).

Reproduced with permission of the British Thoracic Society and SIGN

Chronic obstructive pulmonary disease (COPD)

Slowly progressive disorder characterized by airflow obstruction. Affects ~16% of the population in the 40–68y. age group (♂>♀) and is responsible for ~5% of deaths. *Causes:* cigarette smoking; genetic (bronchial hyperresponsiveness; α_1-antitrypsin deficiency); race (Chinese and Afro-Caribbean's have ↓ susceptibility); diet (poor diet and low birthweight).

Presentation: Affects different patients in different ways. Diagnosis is suggested by a combination of history, signs, and baseline spirometry.

History: Consider diagnosis in any patient >35y. with a risk factor for COPD (generally smoking) and ≥1 of:
• Shortness of breath on exertion—use an objective measure e.g. MRC dyspnoea scale (Table 11.6) to grade breathlessness
• Chronic cough
• Regular sputum production
• Frequent winter 'bronchitis'
• Wheeze

If diagnosis is suspected, also ask about: weight ↓, effort intolerance, waking at night, ankle swelling, fatigue, and occupational hazards.

⚠ Chest pain or haemoptysis are uncommon in COPD—if present, consider an alternative diagnosis.

Signs: May be none. Possible signs:
• Hyperinflated chest ± poor chest expansion on inspiration
• ↓ crico-sternal distance
• Hyper-resonant chest with ↓ cardiac dullness on percussion
• Use of accessory muscles
• Paradoxical movement of lower ribs
• Tachypnoea
• Wheeze or quiet breath sounds
• Pursing of lips on expiration (purse lip breathing)
• Peripheral oedema
• Cyanosis
• ↑ JVP
• Cachexia

Table 11.6 MRC dyspnoea scale

Grade	Degree of breathlessness related to physical activity
1	Not troubled by breathlessness except on strenuous exercise
2	Short of breath when hurrying or walking up a slight hill
3	Walks slower than contemporaries on level ground because of breathlessness or has to stop for breath when walking at own pace
4	Stops for breath after walking about 100m or after a few minutes on level ground
5	Too breathless to leave the house or breathless on dressing/undressing

Table 11.7 Comparison of COPD and asthma

	COPD	Asthma
Symptoms <35y.	Rare	Common
Smoking history	Nearly all	Maybe
Breathlessness	Persistent and progressive. Poor response to inhaled therapy—if good, recon-sider diagnosis.	Variable throughout the day and from day to day. Good response to inhaled therapy typical.
Chronic productive cough	Common	Uncommon
Waking at night with cough/wheeze	Uncommon	Common

Tests

- *Spirometry:* ☐ p.372. Predicts prognosis but not disability/quality of life. A diagnosis of airflow obstruction can be made if:
  - $FEV_1/FVC < 0.7$ (<70%) *and*
  - $FEV_1 < 80\%$ predicted
  Reversibility testing may be confusing. Consider if diagnostic doubt:
  - >400ml ↑ in FEV_1 following trial of bronchodilator or prednisolone (30mg od for 2wk.) suggests asthma.
  - Clinically significant COPD is *not* present if FEV_1 and FEV_1/FVC return to normal after drug therapy.
- *PEFR:* ☐ p.372. Patients with COPD have little variability in PEFR. Serial home PEFR measurements can help distinguish between asthma and COPD. PEFR may underestimate severity of airflow limitation and a normal PEFR does not exclude airflow obstruction.
- *CXR:* Indicated to exclude other diagnoses e.g. lung cancer
- *FBC:* To identify polycythaemia or anaemia
- *BMI*
- *Other investigations :* Only if indicated clinically:
  - α_1-antitrypsin—if early onset COPD or family history
  - ECG/Echo—if cor pulmonale suspected
  - Sputum culture—if persistent purulent sputum

Differential diagnosis: Asthma, bronchiectasis, CCF, lung cancer.

Table 11.8 Severity of COPD and expected clinical picture

Severity	Clinical state	Spirometry
Mild	Cough but little or no breathlessness. No abnormal signs. No ↑ use of services.	FEV_1 50–80% predicted
Moderate	Breathlessness, wheeze on exertion, cough ± sputum, and some abnormal signs. Usually known to GP—intermittent complaints.	FEV_1 30–49% predicted
Severe	SOBOE. Marked wheeze and cough. Usually other signs too. Likely to be known to GP and hospital consultant with frequent problems/admissions.	FEV_1 <30% predicted

Management of COPD

Record values of spirometric tests performed at diagnosis and review. At each review, record current symptoms, problems since last seen, exercise tolerance, and smoking status. Educate the patient and family about the disease, medication, and self-help strategies.

Non-drug therapy

- *Smoking cessation:* Most important way to improve outcome.
- *Vaccination:* All patients with COPD should have influenza and pneumococcal vaccination.
- *Exercise:* Lack of exercise ↓ FEV_1. Pulmonary rehabilitation is of proven benefit—refer via respiratory physicians, if available locally.
- *Nutrition:* Weight ↓ in obese patients improves exercise tolerance.

Drug therapy: Document effects of each drug treatment on symptoms, quality of life, and lung function, as tried—Figure 11.3.

Management of acute exacerbations: 📖 p.386

Referral for specialist care

- Uncertain diagnosis
- Age <40y.
- Severe COPD
- Rapid decline in FEV_1
- Cor pulmonale
- Frequent infections
- Haemoptysis
- α_1 antitrypsin deficiency

- Assessment for:
  - LTOT (see below)
  - Long-term oral steroids
  - Withdrawal of long-term steroids
  - Long-term nebuliser therapy
  - Pulmonary rehabilitation
  - Surgery e.g. lung transplant

Long-term oxygen therapy (LTOT): *Only* prescribe after evaluation by a respiratory physician. Refer patients with:

- Severe airflow obstruction (FEV_1<30%—consider if 30–49%)
- Cyanosis
- Polycythaemia

- Peripheral oedema
- ↑JVP
- Hypoxaemia (oxygen saturation ≤92% breathing air)

Treatment for >15h./d ↑ survival and quality of life. Ambulatory oxygen therapy can ↑ exercise tolerance in some patients. Always warn patients about the fire risks of having pure oxygen in their home.

O_2 cylinders and associated equipment: A list of pharmacies supplying O_2 is available via local PCOs. O_2 concentrators are more economical for LTOT. Prescribe on FP10. Specify amount of O_2 required (h./d.) and flow rate. Arrangements for supply vary—see BNF section 3.6. Supply back-up cylinders in case of breakdown or power cut.

Essential reading

RCP/NICE: National clinical guidelines on management of chronic obstructive pulmonary disease in adults in primary and secondary care (2004). *Thorax* **59** (Suppl.1): 1–232.

Patient support

British Lung Foundation ☎020 7688 5555 🖥 http://www.britishlungfoundation.org

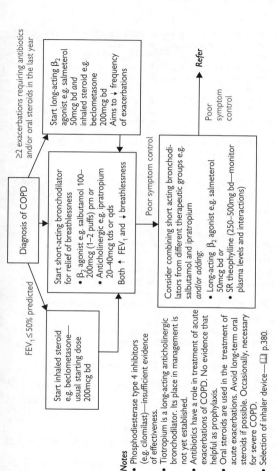

Figure 11.3 Drug management of COPD

The figure contains the following text elements:

Diagnosis of COPD

FEV$_1$ ≤ 50% predicted

≥2 exacerbations requiring antibiotics and/or oral steroids in the last year

Start inhaled steroid e.g. beclometasone—usual starting dose 200mcg bd

Start short-acting bronchodilator for relief of breathlessness
• β$_2$ agonist e.g. salbutamol 100–200mcg (1–2 puffs) prn or
• Anticholinergic e.g. ipratropium 20–40mcg tds or qds
Both ↑ FEV$_1$ and ↓ breathlessness

Start long-acting β$_2$ agonist e.g. salmeterol 50mcg bd and inhaled steroid e.g. beclometasone 200mcg bd
Aims to ↓ frequency of exacerbations

Poor symptom control

Consider combining short acting bronchodilators from different therapeutic groups e.g. salbutamol and ipratropium and/or adding:
• Long-acting β$_2$ agonist e.g. salmeterol 50mcg bd or
• SR theophylline (250–500mg bd—monitor plasma levels and interactions)

Poor symptom control

Refer

Notes
• Phosphodiesterase type 4 inhibitors (e.g. cilomilast)—insufficient evidence of effectiveness.
• Tiotropium is a long-acting anticholinergic bronchodilator. Its place in management is not yet established.
• Antibiotics have a role in treatment of acute exacerbations of COPD. No evidence that helpful as prophylaxis.
• Oral steroids are used in the treatment of acute exacerbations. Avoid long-term oral steroids if possible. Occasionally, necessary for severe COPD.
• Selection of inhaler device—🕮 p.380.

Management of acute exacerbations of COPD

Presentation: Worsening of previous stable condition. Features: ≥1 of

- ↑ dyspnoea—marked dyspnoea, tachypnoea (>25breaths/min), use of accessory muscles at rest and purse lip breathing are signs of severe exacerbation
- ↓ exercise tolerance—marked ↓ in activities of daily living is a sign of severe exacerbation
- ↑ fatigue
- ↑ fluid retention—new onset oedema is a sign of severe exacerbation

- ↑ wheeze
- Chest tightness
- ↑ cough
- ↑ sputum purulence
- ↑ sputum volume
- Upper airways symptoms e.g. colds, sore throats
- New onset cyanosis—severe exacerbation
- Acute confusion—severe exacerbation

❶ Fever and chest pain are uncommon presenting features—consider alternative diagnosis

Causes of exacerbations: 30% have no identifiable cause.
- *Infections:* Viral upper and lower respiratory tract infections e.g. common cold, influenza, bacterial lower respiratory tract infections.
- *Pollutants* e.g. nitrous oxide, sulphur dioxide, ozone.

Differential diagnosis

- Pneumonia
- LVF/pulmonary oedema
- Lung cancer
- Pleural effusion

- Recurrent aspiration
- Pneumothorax
- PE
- Upper airway obstruction

Investigations

- *Pulse oximetry:* If available, can be used as a measure of severity (saturation ≤92% breathing air suggests hypoxaemia—consider admission) and to monitor progress.
- *CXR:* Consider if diagnostic doubt and/or to exclude other causes of symptoms.
- *Sputum culture:* Not recommended routinely in the community[G].

Management: Decide whether to treat at home or admit to hospital—Table 11.9.

Home treatment of acute exacerbations

- *Add or ↑ bronchodilators:* Consider if inhaler device and technique are appropriate.
- *Start antibiotics:* Use broad spectrum antibiotic e.g. erythromycin 250–500mg qds if sputum becomes more purulent *or* clinical signs of pneumonia *or* consolidation on CXR.
- *Oral corticosteroids:* Start early in the course of the exacerbation if ↑ breathlessness which interferes with daily activities. Dosage: 30mg/d. of prednisolone for 1–2wk. Consider osteoporosis prophylaxis with a bisphosphonate if frequent courses are required (📖 p.568).

Table 11.9 Deciding whether to treat acute exacerbations at home or in hospital. (The more features in the 'treat in hospital' column, the more likely the need for admission.)

	Treat at home	Treat in hospital*
Ability to cope at home	Yes	No
Breathlessness	Mild	Severe
General condition	Good	Poor—deteriorating
Level of activity	Good	Poor/confined to bed
Cyanosis	No	Yes
Worsening peripheral oedema	No	Yes
Level of consciousness	Normal	Impaired
Already receiving LTOT	No	Yes
Social circumstances	Good	Living alone/not coping
Acute confusion	No	Yes
Rapid rate of onset	No	Yes
Significant comorbidity (e.g. cardiac disease, IDDM)	No	Yes
Changes on CXR (if available)	No	Present

* Hospital-at-home schemes and assisted discharge schemes are a suitable alternative.
Reproduced with permission of BMJ Journals.

Follow-up

- Reassess as necessary. If the patient deteriorates, reconsider the need for hospital admission (above). If not fully improved within 2wk., consider CXR and hospital referral.
- Reassess patients who have been admitted 4–6wk. after discharge. Assess their ability to cope at home. ~1:3 are readmitted within 3mo.
- Reassess inhaler technique and understanding of treatment regime.
- In severe cases, reassess the need for LTOT and/or home nebuliser.
- Check FEV_1.
- Emphasize the potential benefit of lifestyle modification—smoking cessation, exercise, weight loss if obese.
- Arrange ongoing regular follow-up.

Essential reading

RCP/NICE: National clinical guidelines on management of chronic obstructive pulmonary disease in adults in primary and secondary care (2004). *Thorax* **59** (Suppl.1): 1–232.

Lung cancer

Most common cancer (37,000cases/y.) and 3rd most common cause of death in the UK. Small cell lung cancer accounts for ~¼ all cases—the remainder are mainly adenocarcinoma or squamous cell carcinoma. Incidence ↑ with age—85% are aged >65y. and 1% <40y. at presentation.

Screening: A 2003 Cochrane review concluded that current evidence does not support screening for lung cancer with chest radiography or sputum cytology. Frequent CXR screening might be harmful. Results of trials of screening with CT scanning are awaited from the US but preliminary results do not suggest this will be an effective screening strategy.

Prevention
- *Smoking cessation* (📖 p.234)—90% of lung cancer patients are smokers or ex-smokers.
- *Diet*—↑ consumption of fruit, carrots, and green vegetables may ↓ incidence but there is no evidence that vitamin supplements are beneficial, and they might be harmful[C].

Presentation: >90% have symptoms at the time of diagnosis. Common presenting features:
- Cough (56%)
- Chest / shoulder pain (37%)
- Haemoptysis (7%)
- Dyspnoea
- Hoarseness
- Weight ↓
- Finger clubbing
- General malaise
- Distant metastases
- Incidental finding on CXR

Guidelines for urgent referral if suspected lung cancer

Referral for urgent CXR
- Haemoptysis
- Unexplained and persistent
  - Cough (>3wk.)
  - Chest/shoulder pain
  - Dyspnoea
- Unexplained weight ↓
- Features suggestive of metastases e.g. hepatomegaly
- Persistent
  - Hoarseness (>3wk.— 📖 p.916)
  - Chest signs e.g. infection slow to clear on antibiotics
  - Cervical/supraclavicular LNs
- Finger clubbing

Urgent referral to a chest physician
- Suspicious CXR
- Persistent haemoptysis in smokers/ex-smokers >40y. of age
- SVC obstruction (📖 p.1012)
- Stridor (acute admission)

Management: Once the diagnosis has been confirmed, liaise with the chest physician, specialist lung cancer team, primary health care team, and specialist palliative care services (e.g. Macmillan Nurses). Follow-up regularly. 80% die in <1y.

Palliative care: 📖 p.999–1015.

Pancoast syndrome: Apical lung cancer + ipsilateral Horner's syndrome. *Cause:* invasion of the cervical sympathetic plexus. *Other features:* shoulder and arm pain (brachial plexus invasion C8-T2) ± hoarse voice/bovine cough (unilateral recurrent laryngeal nerve palsy and vocal cord paralysis). *(H.K. Pancoast (1875–1939)—US radiologist).*

Further information

DoH: Guidelines for urgent referral of patients with suspected cancer (2000)
  ⟐ *http://www.dh.gov.uk*
SIGN: Management of lung cancer (1998) ⟐ *http://www.sign.ac.uk*

Patient support/information

Lung Cancer Resources Directory ⟐ *http://www.cancerindex.org*
The Roy Castle Lung Cancer Foundation ☎0800 358 7200
  ⟐ *http://www.roycastle.org*

Pneumonia

Common condition with annual incidence of ~8 cases/1000 adult population. Incidence ↑ with age and peaks in the winter. Mortality for those managed in the community is <1%, but 1 in 4 patients with pneumonia are admitted to hospital and mortality for those admitted is ~9%.

Presentation: Acute illness characterized by:
- Symptoms of an acute lower respiratory tract illness (cough + ≥ 1 other lower respiratory tract symptom e.g. purulent sputum, pleurisy)
- New focal chest signs on examination (consolidation or ↓ air entry, coarse crackles, and/or pleural rub)
- ≥1 systemic feature
  - Sweating, fevers, shivers, aches and pains *and/or*
  - Temperature ≥38°C
- No other explanation for the illness

❶ The elderly may present atypically e.g. 'off legs' or acute confusion.

Common causative organisms
- S. pneumoniae (36%)
- H. influenzae (10%): More common amongst the elderly
- Influenza A&B (8%): Annual epidemics during the winter months—~3% develop pneumonia
- Mycoplasma oneumoniae (1.3%): Less common in the elderly; epidemics occur every 4y. in the UK
- Gram –ve enteric bacteria (1.3%)
- C. psittaci (1.3%): ~20% have history of bird contact
- S. aureus (0.8%): More common in the winter months—may be associated with viral infection e.g. flu
- Legionella spp. (0.4%): Most common in September/October—>50% related to travel

TB: 📖 p.488   **Immunocompromised patients:** 📖 p.504

Prevention
- Influenza vaccination: 📖 p.481
- Pneumococcal vaccination: 📖 p.481

Differential diagnosis
- Pneumonitis e.g. 2° to radiotherapy, chemical inhalation
- Pulmonary oedema (may coexist in the elderly)
- PE

Investigations: Often unnecessary in general practice. Consider:
- *Pulse oximetry* (if available): Use to assess severity. If oxygen saturation ≤92% in air, the patient is hypoxic and requires admission.
- *CXR:* If diagnostic uncertainty or symptoms not resolving. CXR changes may lag behind clinical signs but should return to normal <6wk. after recovery. Persistent changes on CXR >6wk. after recovery require further investigation.
- *Sputum culture:* If not responding to treatment. If weight ↓, malaise, night sweats, or risk factors for TB (ethnic origin, history of TB exposure, social deprivation, or elderly), request mycobacterium culture.
- *Blood: FBC:* ↑ WCC; ESR ↑; acute and convalescent titres to confirm 'atypical' pneumonia (Legionella, C. psittaci, M. pneumonia).

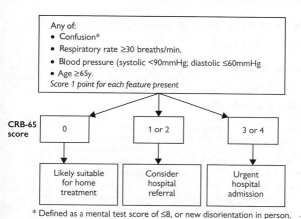

Any of:
- Confusion*
- Respiratory rate ≥30 breaths/min.
- Blood pressure (systolic <90mmHg; diastolic ≤60mmHg
- Age ≥65y.

Score 1 point for each feature present

CRB-65 score

| 0 | 1 or 2 | 3 or 4 |

| Likely suitable for home treatment | Consider hospital referral | Urgent hospital admission |

* Defined as a mental test score of ≤8, or new disorientation in person, place or time

Figure 11.4 Assessment of severity and management of pneumonia

Management

- *Consider the need for admission:* See Figure 11.4. Have a low threshold for admission if ill but apyrexial, concomitant illness (e.g. CCF, chronic lung, renal or liver disease, DM, cancer) or poor social situation. If life-threatening infection or considerable delay (>2h.), consider administering antibiotics before admission.
- *If a decision is made to treat at home:*
  - Advise not to smoke, to rest, and drink plenty of fluids.
  - Start antibiotics e.g. amoxicillin 500mg–1g tds, erythromycin 500mg tds, or clarithromycin 500mg bd.
  - Treat pleuritic pain with simple analgesia e.g. paracetamol 1g qds.
  - Review within 48h. Reassess clinical state. If deteriorating or not improving, consider CXR or admission.

Complications: Require specialist management—refer.
- Pleural effusion (may be reactive or empyema—pus in the lung cavity)
- Lung abscess (presents with swinging fever and worsening pneumonia)
- Septicaemia
- Metastatic infections
- Respiratory failure
- Jaundice

Essential Reading

British Thoracic Society: Guidelines for the management of community acquired pneumonia in adults (2001) and Update (2004). 🖳 www.brit-thoracic.org.uk

Pleural effusion, pneumothorax, and bronchiectasis

Pleural effusion: Fluid in the pleural cavity. Simple effusions may be transudates (<30g/L protein) or exudates (>30g/L protein). Alternatively, effusions can be made of blood, lymph, or pus (empyema).

Causes of simple effusion

- Malignancy (lung cancer, mesothelioma, Meig's syndrome, lymphangitis, lymphoma, metastatic cancer)
- Infection (e.g pneumonia, TB)
- Heart failure
- Inflammation (SLE, RA, pancreatitis, asbestos exposure)
- Infarction (PE)
- Constrictive pericarditis
- Hypoproteinaemia
- Hypothyroidism

Presentation

- *Symptoms:* Dyspnoea, pleuritic pain, symptoms of underlying cause. May be incidental finding on CXR.
- *Signs:* Absent breath sounds, dullness to percussion, ↓ tactile vocal fremitus, ↓ vocal resonance. Above the effusion there is usually a zone of bronchial breathing. Early on there may be a pleural rub. Large effusions shift the mediastinum away from the affected side and there may be ↓ chest wall movement.

Investigations: Confirmed on CXR. If cause is not immediately apparent, refer for diagnostic tap (should be done where X-ray facilities are available).

Management: Treat the underlying cause. Refer for drainage if symptomatic. Repeated drainage ± pleurodesis may be necessary.

Further information

British Thoracic Society: guidelines for the management of pleural effusion (2003)
🖳 http://www.brit-thoracic.org.uk

Pneumothorax: Air in the pleural cavity. > ½ cases are due to trauma of some kind—the rest are spontaneous. 2 peaks in incidence are seen—3rd–4th decade and 8th–9th decade.

⚠ Tension pneumothorax can be rapidly fatal. Suspect if unwell (distressed, sweating, tachycardic), signs of pneumothorax, and mediastinal, shift away from the pneumothorax—📖 p.1055

Spontaneous pneumothorax: *Risk factors:* Previous pneumothorax, smoking, ascent in an aeroplane, diving. *Cause:*

- *In patients <40y.:* usually due to rupture of a pleural bleb. Typical patient is tall, thin, and male (♂:♀ ≈ 6:1).
- *Patients >40y.:* Usually due to COPD (70–80%).
- *Rarer causes:* Asthma, pneumonia, TB, lung cancer, pulmonary fibrosis.

Presentation

- Sudden onset of pleuritic chest pain or ↑ breathlessness ± pallor and tachycardia.

- *Examination:* Look for resonant percussion note, ↓ or absent breath sounds—signs may be absent if the pneumothorax is small.

Management
- Refer for CXR.
- If pneumothorax is confirmed, seek specialist advice about further management.
- Small pneumothoraces usually resolve spontaneously (50% collapse takes ~40d. to resorb)—monitor until completely resolved.
- Larger pneumothoraces may require admission for aspiration or a chest drain.
- Smoking cessation ↓ risk of recurrence.

Traumatic pneumothorax: Trauma may not initially be obvious— ask about injections around the chest area e.g. acupuncture (to neck and shoulders as well as chest); aspiration of breast lump; etc. Presentation and management: As for spontaneous pneumothorax (above).

Further information
British Thoracic Society: Guidelines for the management of spontaneous pneumothorax (2003) 🖳 http://www.brit-thoracic.org.uk

Bronchiectasis: Consider in any patient with persistent or recurrent chest infections. Permanently dilated bronchi act as sumps for infected mucus. *Causes:*
- *Congenital*—CF, Kartagener syndrome;
- *Post-infection*—TB, pertussis, measles, pneumonia;
- *Other*—bronchial obstruction, aspergillosis (📖 p.502), hypogamma-globulinaemia (📖 p.537), gastric aspiration.

Presentation
- *Mild cases*—asymptomatic with winter exacerbations consisting of fever, cough, purulent sputum, pleuritic chest pain, dyspnoea;
- *More severe cases*—persistent cough and sputum, haemoptysis, club-bing, low-pitched inspiratory and expiratory crackles and wheeze.

Investigations
- CXR;
- Sputum—M,C&S;
- Spirometry—reversible airways obstruction is common.

Management: Refer to a respiratory physician. Treatment includes physiotherapy, antibiotics, bronchodilators, and (rarely) surgery.

Kartagener syndrome (immotile cilia syndrome): Combination of bronchiectasis, chronic sinusitis, and male infertility plus situs inversus (transposed heart and abdominal organs). Due to defect in cilia function. Otitis media and salpingitis are frequent. (*M. Kartagener (1897–1975)— Swiss physician*)

Cystic fibrosis

Cystic fibrosis (CF) is the most common inherited disorder in the UK (prevalence: 1:2500). Median survival has ↑ dramatically and is now >40y. But of the 7500 CF patients in the UK, 6000 are <25y. old.

Genetics

- Results from mutation of a single gene (cystic fibrosis transmembrane conductance regulator) essential for salt and water movement across cell membranes → thickened secretions.
- Autosomal recessive inheritance—1:4 chance of having a child with CF if both parents are carriers.
- ~1:25 adults in the UK carry the CF gene (~2.3 million adults).
- Most common in Caucasians—rare in people of Afro-Caribbean origin.

Screening: Several possibilities:
- **Preconceptual screening:** Buccal smears to karyotype prospective parents.
- **Antenatal screening:** CVS at ~10wk.—for parents with an affected child already or where both parents are +ve on karyotyping.
- **Neonatal screening:** A national neonatal screening policy using the Guthrie bloodspot card will be introduced in the UK shortly.

Presentation: Wide range of clinical presentation and severity:
- Neonatal (meconium ileus): 10%
- Infancy
  - GI symptoms alone (failure to thrive; steatorrhoea)—30%
  - Recurrent respiratory infections—25%
  - Combination of GI and respiratory symptoms—15%
- >16y.: Variety of presentations (e.g. malabsorption)—10%
- +ve family history or screening—10%.

Diagnosis: Refer to paediatrics (or general medicine if >16y.). A +ve sweat test (Na^+ >70mmol/l; Cl^- >60mmol/l on 2 occasions) is diagnostic.

Common problems
Lung disease

- **↑viscosity of secretions:** Treated with physiotherapy ± postural drainage ± dornase alpha (nebulised mucolytic enzyme).
- **Bronchiectasis and infection:** Responsible for most morbidity and >90% mortality. *Infecting organisms:* Small children—*S. aureus* and *H. influenzae.*; older children/adults—Pseudomonas infection is common. Prevention and control of chronic Pseudomonas infection minimizes ↓ in lung function and ↑ survival.
- **Airways inflammation and bronchoconstriction:** Managed with inhaled bronchodilators and anti-inflammatories.
- **Pneumothorax:** 📖 p.392.
- **Aspergillus fumigatus and allergic bronchopulmonary aspergillosis:** ~20%. Recurrent episodes of eosinophilic pneumonia.
- **Cor pulmonale and/or respiratory failure:** Major cause of death. Cadaveric heart-lung transplantation (50% 5y. survival) or partial lung transplant from a related donor is a last resort.

GI disease

- *Failure to thrive:* Affects ~50% of children with CF—📖 p.884
- *Pancreatic disease:* 85% of CF patients have pancreatic insufficiency → malabsorption. Patients require pre-meal oral pancreatic enzymes (e.g. Creon) and a high-calorie diet supplemented with fat-soluble vitamins (A, D, and E)—advice from a dietician is essential. *Other problems:* Acute pancreatitis—📖 p.448; IDDM—📖 p.404.
- *Liver disease:* Abnormal bile → intrahepatic biliary stasis and gallstone formation → chronic liver disease, biliary colic, cholecystitis, and biliary stricture.
- *Bowel disease:* Meconium ileus (📖 p.816); distal ileus obstruction syndrome (meconium ileus equivalent); intussusception; rectal prolapse due to bulky stools.

Other problems

- *Nasal polyps*
- *Infertility:* ♂ infertility and ♀ subfertility. Have a low threshold for referral.
- *Vasculitis*
- *Musculoskeletal problems:* Osteoporosis (1:3 adults with CF); hypertrophic pulmonary arthropathy; CF arthropathy.
- *Behavioural and psychological problems:* Common.

Management: CF is a multisystem disease requiring a holistic approach to care which aims to maintain patients' independence, improve quality of life, *and* extend life expectancy through:
- Preventing chronic infection as long as possible and later stabilizing respiratory infection *and*
- Maintaining good nutritional state.

A multidisciplinary team in a specialist CF centre is best placed to achieve this. Patients usually have direct access.

Role of the GP

- Communication and ongoing support
- Prescribing routine treatment, including O_2, as directed by the CF team
- Providing routine childhood immunizations, pneumococcal vaccination, and annual influenza vaccination
- Managing unrelated illness e.g. URTI
- Referral for specialist care e.g. for infertility or genetic counselling
- Certification of illness
- Support of carers
- Terminal care

Further information

CF Trust Standards for the clinical care of children and adults with CF in the UK (2001) 🖳 http://www.cftrust.org.uk

Patient support

Cystic Fibrosis Trust 🖳 http://www.cftrust.org.uk
Association of Cystic Fibrosis Adults 🖳 http://www.acfa.org.uk

Diffuse parenchymal lung diseases

Comprise a variety of conditions in which inflammation affects the alveolar wall, leading to fluid in the alveolar air spaces. CXR generally shows diffuse shadowing. Careful history of occupational and environmental exposure to allergens and drug history is important.

Sarcoidosis: Characterized by non-caseating granulomata. May affect any organ and patients of any age but typical presentation is with lung granulomata in a young adult.

Presentation
- *Acute sarcoidosis (Löfgren's syndrome):* Erythema nodosum, bilateral hilar lymphadenopathy on CXR, swinging fever, polyarthralgia.
- *Insidious onset:* Hilar lymphadenopathy may be an incidental finding on CXR. *Symptoms/signs:* Gradual onset of exertional dyspnoea, dry cough, malaise, tiredness, and weight loss.
- *Extrathoracic sarcoidosis:* Erythema nodosum, lupus pernio, scar infiltration, enlarged lacrimal glands, hypopyon, uveitis, arthralgia, arrythmias, heart failure, pericardial effusion, cranial and peripheral nerve palsies, seizures, hypercalcaemia, renal stones, lymphadenopathy, hepatosplenomegaly, fever, and malaise.

Management: Refer any patient with bilateral hilar lymphadenopathy for further investigation. Steroids are widely used to treat sarcoidosis (± azathioprine, methotrexate, or chloroquine)—relapse is common following withdrawal. Remits without treatment in 2 out of 3 cases. Mortality is <3% (usually die due to CCF and/or cor pulmonale).

Fibrosing alveolitis: Incidence ↑ with age. May be:
- *Associated with other diseases:* Connective tissue disease (33%); chronic active hepatitis; renal tubular acidosis; autoimmune thyroid disease; ulcerative colitis.
- *Associated with drug use*
  - Cytotoxics e.g. busulphan, bleomycin, methotrexate
  - Cardiac drugs e.g. amiodarone
  - Antibiotics e.g. nitrofurantoin
  - Analgesics e.g. diamorphine
  - Rheumatological drugs e.g. gold, penicillamine
  - Poisons e.g. paraquat
- *Idiopathic ('cryptogenic fibrosing alveolitis'):* occupational exposure to wood or metal dust may be implicated.

Presentation: Progressive exertional dyspnoea and dry cough; clubbing (>50%); fine end inspiratory crepitations; malaise; weight ↓. *In advanced state:* Central cyanosis and right heart failure. *CXR:* Diffuse shadowing. *Lung function tests:* Restrictive picture.

Differential diagnosis: LVF; COPD; other causes of lung fibrosis—dust exposure (coal, asbestos, silica, farmer's lung, bird fancier's lung); inhalant exposure (O_2, NO_2); drugs; radiation.

Management: Refer to a respiratory physician—if due to industrial exposure may be classified as an industrial disease and qualify for compensation (📖 p.115) Treatment is with oral steroids ± immunosuppressants. Lung transplant is a last option. 5y. survival is <50% but can be very variable (range 1–20y.).

Extrinsic allergic alveolitis: *(farmer's lung; bird fancier's lung)* Inhaled particles (e.g. fungal spores or avian proteins) provoke an allergic reaction in the lungs of hypersensitive individuals.

Presentation: Both may occur together:
• *Acute reaction:* 2–4h. post exposure. Fever, malaise, dry cough, shortness of breath.
• *Chronic reaction:* Malaise, weight ↓, exertional dyspnoea, fine crepitations in both lung fields.

Investigations
• *FBC:* ↑ neutrophils (acute reaction)
• *ESR* ↑ (acute reaction)
• *CXR* may be normal or show typical changes (shadowing, widespread small nodules, or ground glass appearance)
• Diagnosis is confirmed by demonstrating serum precipitins to the provoking factor

Management: Both acute and chronic disease are treated with prednisolone. For acute attacks use 40mg od reducing the dose and stopping as soon as symptoms disappear. Refer for advice on chronic management.

Further information
British Thoracic Society (1999) The diagnosis, assessment and treatment of diffuse parenchymal lung disease in adults. *Thorax*, **54**: Suppl 1.🖳 http://www.brit-thoracic.org.uk

Patient support
British Lung Foundation ☎020 7688 5555 🖳 http://www.britishlungfoundation.org

Occupational lung disease

Exposure to gases, vapours, and dusts at work can lead to lung disease.

Coal-worker's pneumoconiosis: 90% of all compensated industrial lung disease in the UK. 'Pneumoconiosis' means accumulation of dust in the lungs and tissue reaction to its presence. Incidence is related to total dust exposure. Divides into:

- **Simple pneumoconiosis:** Deposition of coal dust in the lung. Graded on CXR appearance. Grading determines whether disability benefit is payable in the UK. Effect on lung function is debated. Predisposes to progressive massive fibrosis (below).
- **Progressive massive fibrosis:** Round fibrotic masses several cm diameter form in the upper lobes. Presents with exertional dyspnoea, cough, black sputum, and, eventually, respiratory failure. Symptoms progress (or may even start) after exposure to coal dust has ceased. Lung function tests show a mixed restrictive and obstructive picture with loss of lung volume, irreversible airflow limitation, and ↓ gas transfer.

Asbestosis: Before legislation banning its use, exposure was widespread and occurred particularly in naval shipyards and power stations. *Effects:*

- **Pleural plaques:** Patches of pleural thickening ± calcification. Usually follows light exposure to asbestos. *Symptoms:* rare—occasional mild exertional dyspnoea. *Lung function tests:* mild restrictive picture.
- **Benign pleural effusion:** Usually occurs <20y. after exposure. *Symptoms:* increasing dyspnoea ± pleuritic pain. *Management:* refer for drainage. May be recurrent and require pleurodesis.
- **Bilateral diffuse pleural thickening :** Defined as pleural thickening >5mm thick, covering >¼ of the chest wall. Follows light or moderate exposure to asbestos. *Symptoms:* exertional dyspnoea. May progress even in the absence of further exposure. *Lung function tests:* restrictive pattern.
- **Mesothelioma***: Can follow even light exposure to asbestos. 20–40y. time lag between exposure and appearance of disease. Presents with increasing shortness of breath ± pleuritic pain. Examination and CXR show unilateral effusion (rarely bilateral). *Median survival:* 2y. from diagnosis.
- **Asbestosis*:** Follows heavy exposure after a 5–10y. interval. Presents with progressive dyspnoea, finger clubbing, basal end-expiratory crackles. *CXR:* 'honeycomb lung'—diffuse streaky shadowing. *Lung function tests:* severe restrictive defect and ↓ gas transfer.
- **Asbestosis-related lung cancer*:** Patients exposed to asbestos who have evidence of that exposure (pleural plaques, bilateral pleural thickening, or asbestosis) have an ↑ risk of bronchial carcinoma (usually adenocarcinoma). Smokers exposed to asbestos have a 5x ↑ risk compared to non-smokers exposed to asbestos.

There is no effective treatment for any of these conditions—management is symptomatic.

---

* Eligible for Industrial Injuries Benefit in the UK.

Occupational asthma: >200 industrial materials are known to cause occupational asthma. The important causes are recognized occupational diseases in the UK—patients may be eligible for statutory compensation provided they apply <10y. after leaving the occupation in which the asthma developed. Suspect if the patient has symptoms which improve on days away from work or on holiday. Always refer to a respiratory physician.

Extrinsic allergic alveolitis ('Farmer's lung'): p.397.

Silicosis: Uncommon. Affects stonemasons, pottery workers, workers exposed to sand-blasting, and fettlers (remove sand from metal casts). Caused by inhalation of silica. CXR appearance is distinctive. Presents with exertional dyspnoea ± cough. *Lung function tests:* as for progressive massive fibrosis (opposite).

Byssinosis: Affects workers in cotton mills. Symptoms (tightness in the chest, cough, and breathlessness) start on the 1st day back at work after a break (Monday sickness) with improvement as the week progresses. CXR is normal.

Berylliosis: Rare. Affects workers in the aerospace, nuclear power, and electrical industries. Presents similarly to sarcoidosis (p.396).

Iron (siderosis), barium (baritosis), and tin (stannosis) dust inhalation: Results in dramatic dense nodular shadowing on the CXR but effects on lung function and symptoms are often minimal.

Benefits: p.98–115.

Notification and compensation: p.114–115

Patient support
British Lung Foundation ☎020 7688 5555 🖳 http://www.britishlungfoundation.org

Snoring and obstructive sleep apnoea

Snoring: During sleep, the pharyngeal airway narrows due to ↓ dilator muscle tone. Snoring is vibratory noise generated from the pharynx and soft palate as the air passes through this narrowed space. Further narrowing produces louder snoring, laboured inspiration, and, eventually, apnoeic episodes (see below). Social consequences are the usual reason for the patient to seek help. They can be distressing: banishment from the bedroom, marital disharmony, no holidays, fear of travelling or falling asleep in a public place, etc.

> **❶** Snoring may be used by the spouse as an excuse to leave the marital bed and may actually be trivial/absent. If suspected, ask the patient to bring a recording of the offending noise.

Obstructive sleep apnoea: Occurs when the pharyngeal airway completely closes during sleep resulting in apnoeic episodes. ↑ inspiratory effort is sensed by the brain and a transient arousal provoked. A few of these arousals don't matter—but many (sometimes hundreds) per night → fragmented sleep and consequent daytime sleepiness.

Clinical features

- **Dominant features:** Excessive daytime sleepiness (not tiredness—Epworth Sleepiness Scale is a useful assessment tool), impaired concentration, snoring,
- **Other features:** Unrefreshing sleep, choking episodes during sleep, witnessed apnoeic episodes, restless sleep, irritability/personality change, nocturia, ↓ libido.

Causes of snoring and sleep apnoea: Overweight (neck circumference >16"), nasal congestion, evening alcohol/sedatives, large tonsils, receding lower jaw, smoking, hypothyroidism, menopause.

Management

Snoring without sleep apnoea

- **Initial approaches:** Suggest changing sleeping position (discourage from sleeping on back); elevate head of the bed (e.g. prop up on bricks—can ↓ nasal congestion); limit number of pillows to 1thick/2thin pillows to maximize pharyngeal size; ↓ weight if obese; ↓ or stop evening alcohol/sleeping tablets; suggest partner tries ear plugs (purchase from chemist—takes several nights to get used to wearing them).
- **If clinically indicated**
  - Nasal congestion—start beclometasone nasal spray (applied head downwards) 2puffs bd ± ipratropium bromide nasal spray 2 puffs nocte
  - Check TFTs to exclude hypothyroidism
  - Discuss the use of HRT in menopausal women (📖 p.734)
- **If simple measures fail:** Refer to:
  - Dentist or ENT for a mandibular advancement device
  - ENT for surgery—septal straightening, polypectomy, turbinate reduction, tonsillectomy, or uvulopalatopharyngoplasty

Sleep apnoea

- Advise patients to: ↓ weight if obese; ↓ or stop evening alcohol/sleeping tablets *and*
- Refer to a sleep unit or physician with a special interest in sleep problems. If diagnosis is proven and causing significant daytime sleepiness, usual treatment is with CPAP therapy at night. Mandibular advancement devices are alternatives for patients who cannot tolerate CPAP or have very mild symptoms with no daytime sleepiness. Occasionally, if large tonsils, referral to ENT for surgery is warranted.

⚠ **Driving:** Warn patients NOT to drive if sleepy. Once diagnosis is confirmed, they must inform the DVLA and their insurance company (💷 p.205).

Sleep apnoea in children: Common in children aged 2–7y. in association with tonsil enlargement during URTI. Sleep disruption can cause daytime sleepiness, hyperactivity, poor attention span, and bad behaviour. If tonsils are big enough to produce sleep apnoea in the absence of current infection, refer to ENT for consideration of tonsillectomy.

The Epworth Sleepiness Scale: How likely are you to doze off or fall asleep in the following situations, in contrast to feeling just tired?

This refers to your usual way of life in recent times. Even if you have not done some of these things recently, try to work out how they would have affected you.

Situation	Chance of dozing
Sitting and reading	☐
Watching TV	☐
Sitting inactive in a public place (e.g. a theatre or a meeting)	☐
As a passenger in a car for an hour without a break	☐
Lying down to rest in the afternoon when circumstances permit	☐
Sitting and talking to someone	☐
Sitting quietly after a lunch without alcohol	☐
In a car, while stopped for a few minutes in traffic	☐

0 = no chance of dozing　　*2 = moderate chance of dozing*
1 = slight chance of dozing　　*3 = high chance of dozing*

Score >10—consider sleep apnoea

Further information

SIGN/British Thoracic Society (2003) Management of obstructive sleep apnoea/hypopnoea syndrome in adults 🖥 http://www.sign.ac.uk

Patient support

The Sleep Apnoea Trust (SATA) ☎01494 527772 🖥 http://www.sleep-apnoea-trust.org

Endocrinology

Diabetes

Diabetes mellitus (DM) is a common syndrome affecting 3% of the population of the UK and caused by lack or ↓ effectiveness of endogenous insulin. It is characterized by ↑ blood sugars and abnormalities of carbohydrate and lipid metabolism.

Presentation

- *Acute:* Ketoacidosis or hyperosmolar non-ketotic coma (📖 p.1070).
- *Sub-acute:* Weight ↓, polydipsia, polyuria, lethargy, irritability, infections (candidiasis, skin infection, recurrent infections slow to clear), genital itching, blurred vision, tingling in hands/feet.
- *With complications:* Presentation with skin changes, neuropathy, nephropathy, arterial or eye disease (📖 p.414–419).
- *Asymptomatic:* DM may be detected on routine screening during well man/woman checks or opportunistic urine screening for glucose. A national screening programme is under consideration.

Diagnosis

If symptomatic: ↑ venous plasma glucose—random ≥11.1mmol/l; fasting ≥7.0mmol/l. If child, suspected ketoacidosis or unwell, don't delay to get a laboratory sample, admit, or refer for same-day specialist assessment on BM alone. Otherwise, only make diagnosis based on laboratory sample.

If asymptomatic: ↑ venous plasma glucose on two separate measurements on different days—random ≥11.1mmol/l; fasting ≥7.0mmol/l.

Impaired fasting glycaemia: Fasting plasma glucose ≥6.1mmol/l and <7mmol/l. Do a glucose tolerance test to clarify diagnosis.

Glucose tolerance test: Performed if impaired fasting glycaemia, borderline random plasma glucose, or if inconsistent results on repeat testing of fasting blood glucose. Ask the patient to fast overnight. Give 75g of glucose (350ml Lucozade). Check plasma glucose after 2h.
- If ≥11.1mmol/l, the patient is diabetic
- If ≥7.8 and <11.1mmol/l, the patient has *impaired glucose tolerance*
- If <7.8mmol/l, the patient is not diabetic

> ❶ Both impaired glucose tolerance and impaired fasting glucose are risk factors for DM and cardiovascular disease. Follow-up with annual fasting blood glucose—4%/y. develop DM. Treat cardiovascular risk factors aggressively.

> ⚠ Blood glucose may be temporarily ↑ during acute illness, after trauma or surgery, or during short courses of blood glucose raising drugs (see 2° causes). If HbA$_{1c}$ >7%, DM is likely.

Classification of primary diabetes

Type 1 (insulin-dependent (IDDM), juvenile onset)

- May occur at any age but more common in patients <30y.
- Autoimmune disease. Islet cell antibodies may initially be present. Associated with other autoimmune disease and certain genotypes (HLA DR3/4—though identical twin concordance ≈30%.).

- Patients are prone to profound weight ↓ and ketoacidosis.
- Insulin is needed from diagnosis.

Type 2 (non-insulin dependent (NIDDM), maturity onset)

- 80–90% patients with DM. ♂:♀≈3:2.
- Prevalence is ↑ing. Lifetime risk of developing type 2 DM is >10% and it is estimated ~½ remain undiagnosed.
- *Risk factors*
  - Age > 65y.
  - Obesity
  - FH of DM (identical twin concordance ≈100%)
  - Impaired glucose tolerance
  - Ethnic group (South Asians, Afro-Caribbean, Hispanics have 5–10x ↑ risk)
  - PMH of gestational diabetes or a baby >4kg at birth
- Due to impaired insulin secretion *and* insulin resistance in the liver, adipose tissue, and skeletal muscle.
- Type 2 diabetes is a 'silent killing disease' in which life expectancy is ↓ by 30–40% in the age range 40–70y.—a loss of 8–10y. of life.
- Onset tends to be insidious.
- Treatment is usually with diet ± tablets. Type 2 DM is progressive and many patients eventually require insulin treatment (though the patient is *still* a type 2 diabetic).
- ½ have complications at diagnosis.

Diabetes in pregnancy: 📖 p.781 and 784.

2° causes of DM

- *Drugs* (steroids, thiazides)
- *Pancreatic disease* (pancreatitis, surgery, cancer, haemochromatosis, cystic fibrosis)
- *Endocrine disease* (Cushing's disease, acromegaly, thyrotoxicosis, phaeochromocytoma)
- *Others* (glycogen storage diseases, insulin receptor antibodies)

Metabolic syndrome: Insulin resistance syndrome or syndrome X. Consists of impaired glucose tolerance or diabetes, insulin resistance + other metabolic disorders of ↑ cardiovascular risk including:

- Truncal obesity: waist circumference >0.9m (♀); >1.0m (♂)—use 0.1m lower figures for people of South Asian extraction
- ↑BP: >135/80
- Dyslipidaemia: serum HDL < 1.2mmol/l (♀) or <1.0mmol/l (♂); fasting serum triglycerides > 1.8mmol/l

Patients have a very high risk of cardiovascular disease and all risk factors should be treated aggressively.

❶ In patients on insulin, insulin resistance is suggested by high insulin doses (>1unit/kg/d.)

Further information

WHO (2000) Definition, diagnosis and classification of diabetes mellitus and its complications 🖥 http://www.diabetes.org.uk

Patient advice and support

Diabetes UK ☎ 0845 120 2960 🖥 http://www.diabetes.org.uk

Organization and monitoring of diabetic care

Aims of diabetic care

- Alleviation of symptoms
- Minimization of complications
- Reduction of early mortality
- Quality of life enhancement
- Education of the patient and family

GP diabetic clinics can be as effective as hospital clinics in achieving diabetic control. High-quality diabetic care is rewarded within the quality and outcomes framework.

Features of well organized care

- Use of a register and structured records (usually available as part of in-house computer software)
- Regular review, with follow-up of defaulters, following a protocol for care
- Thorough annual review (see below) with recall system
- Provision of protected time for the clinic
- Availability of good quality written information for patients
- Open access for patients to receive advice
- Multidisciplinary team covering all aspects of diabetes care—GPs, diabetes nurse specialists/assistants, and educators
- Access to dieticians and podiatrists
- Quality monitoring through audit and patient feedback
- Continuing education for professional staff

Routine diabetic review: Each diabetic patient requires 6 monthly review (or more frequent as necessary). This should include a thorough annual review of all aspects of disease and care. Reviews should cover:

- **Problems:** Recent life events; new symptoms; difficulties with management since last visit.
- **Review of:**
  - Indices of control e.g. HbA_{1c}
  - Self-monitored results and discussion of their meaning
  - Dietary behaviours
  - Physical activity
  - Smoking
  - Diabetes education
  - Skills e.g. injection technique
  - Foot care
  - Blood glucose, lipid, and BP therapy and results
  - Other medical conditions and therapy affecting DM
- **Review of complications:** Annual review—more frequent if established complications. Cardiovascular disease; nephropathy; neuropathy; eye disease; foot problems—📖 p.414–19; erectile dysfunction—📖 p.702.
- **Review of services:** Annual review—more frequent if problems.
- **Analysis and planning:** Agreement on the main points covered, targets for coming months, changes in therapy, interval to next consultation.
- **Recording:** Completion of structured record ± patient-held record.

❶ 7–10% of patients in long-term residential care have DM and they tend to be neglected. Agree a diabetes care plan for each affected resident and ensure at least annual diabetic review.

Monitoring blood glucose: All patients *can* achieve good levels of control (Table 12.1). Poorer control is acceptable in the elderly or others with limited life expectancy, as long as they are symptom free.

- **Urine monitoring:** Adequate for those who do not require tight control or for those who cannot cope with more complex techniques of monitoring or their interpretation.
- **Blood monitoring:** Essential for all patients using insulin and desirable for many on oral medication.
  - Explain the range of suitable monitoring devices available (BNF 6.1.6) and train in the use of the selected method.
  - Frequency of self-monitoring varies according to need.
  - Set targets for pre-prandial glucose levels.
  - Assess skills (and meters if used) yearly or if problems with self-monitoring.
  - Evaluate reliability of results by comparison with HbA$_{1c}$ results and results obtained at review.
- **Glycosylated haemoglobin (HbA$_{1c}$):** Measure at least 2x/y. Represents an average of blood sugar control over the previous 6–8wk..

Table 12.1 Indices of control

Measure	Target
Fasting blood glucose (mmol/l)	4–7mmol/l (post-prandial <9)—adults 4–8mmol/l (post-prandial <10)—children
Urine	–ve (post-prandial sugars <0.5%)
HbA$_{1c}$ (normal 4.0–6.0%)—measure every 2–6mo. depending on control	<7.5 (≤6.5 if ↑ risk of arterial disease)
Serum cholesterol (mmol/l)—2° prevention, type 2 DM or type 1 DM with risk factors for CVD, metabolic syndrome, or microalbuminuria	↓ total cholesterol by 25% or to <4mmol/l—whichever is the lower value or ↓ LDL cholesterol by 30% or to <2.0mmol/l—whichever is the lower value
BMI (kg/m^2)	25–30
BP—without macrovascular disease	<135/85
BP—with macrovascular disease	<130/80

❶ Reference values may vary between laboratories. Aim for glycosylated Hb to be within 1% of the upper limit of normal range.

Further information

Diabetes UK (1999) Guidelines of practice for residents with diabetes in care homes 🖳 http://www.diabetes.org.uk

Management of diabetes: education

Education is an essential aspect of diabetic care. Diabetes is a chronic condition, and however well it is managed in the clinic, the patient has to manage his or her own disease the rest of the time. Education enables patients and their carers to become equal partners in the management of their disease.

Topics to cover

General knowledge: Information about:
- DM—its progressive nature and complications
- Aims of management
- Structure of diabetic services and ways to access them
- Equipment required and usage instructions—syringes, needles, blood testing equipment, etc.
- Free prescriptions for patients requiring drugs or insulin to control their diabetes
- Problems of pregnancy (women of childbearing age only)
- Alert bracelets—Medic-Alert (☎ 020 7833 3034) provides stainless steel bracelets or necklets, and identity tags are also available from Medi-Tag (☎ 0121 200 1616)

Diet: Patients do *not* need a separate diet from the rest of the family or expensive 'diabetic' food products. A diabetic diet is a healthy diet.
- ≥50% of calorie intake should be from fibre-rich carbohydrate, with a minimum of fat (especially saturated fat), refined carbohydrate, and alcohol.
- Adjust total calorie intake according to desired BMI.
- Recommend at least 5 portions of fresh fruit or vegetables/d.
- Spread food intake evenly across the day for patients controlled with tablets or diet.
- Diet sheets are available from Diabetes UK and should be provided.
- Ready-made meals, processed foods, and alcohol are often sources of hidden sugar.

Immunizations: Offer influenza and pneumococcal vaccine to all diabetics.

Psychological problems: Discuss concerns underlying the diagnosis of DM or development of complications. Arrange counselling/refer to self-help resources as needed. Teenagers with diabetes can be a particularly difficult group to manage. Often control is poor due to a combination of rapid bodily changes and rebellion against the diagnosis of DM. Support information and advice given in specialist clinics.

Exercise: Encourage regular exercise.
- Review activity at work, and in getting to and from the workplace, hobbies, and physical activity in the home.
- Advise physical activity can ↑ insulin sensitivity, ↓ BP, and improve blood lipid control.
- If appropriate, suggest regular physical activity tailored to individual ability (e.g. brisk walking for 30min/d.; exercise prescription).

Smoking: Advice on and assistance with smoking cessation.

Driving: Advise all drivers they must notify their car insurance company and the DVLA, unless their diabetes is controlled by diet alone. Be aware of insurers who cater for diabetic drivers.

Foot care: 📖 p.418

Employment: Advise those on insulin that certain jobs are no longer possible:
• Working on scaffolding or with dangerous machinery
• Joining the Police or the Armed Services
• Driving a heavy goods or public service vehicle.

Jobs without these hazards should pose no problems, though the patient might wish to tell his/her employer. Special advice may be needed for shift work.

Travel: Give advice on:
• Management of change in time zones (📖 p.209)
• Transport of insulin
• Keeping monitoring and injection equipment in hand luggage
• Differences in insulin types and concentrations between countries
• Travel-related illness (especially gastroenteritis)
• Need for immunization and travel insurance.

Be aware of insurers who cater for diabetic travellers.

Further information
DoH: National Service Framework for Diabetes (2001) 🖥 *http://www.dh.gov.uk*

Patient advice and support
Diabetes UK ☎ 0845 120 2960 🖥 *http://www.diabetes.org.uk*

Treatment of type 2 diabetes

Tight control of type 2 DM ↓ retinopathy and development of micro-albuminuria by ¼ . Optimal results are obtained if HbA_{1c} is maintained at <7%. Benefits are only evident after a decade of good control[R].

⚠ *Always* combine treatment of hyperglycaemia with modification of other risk factors for vascular complications—📖 p.414.

Healthy eating and exercise: Diet is the cornerstone of diabetic treatment. In type 2 DM, try for at least 3mo. before medication is considered. Diet sheets are available from Diabetes UK. Increasing physical activity is also beneficial (↓ weight, ↓ lipids, and ↑ insulin sensitivity), though not always possible.

First-line oral hypoglycaemic agents: Figure 12.1 and *BNF 6.1.2*

Sulphonylureas: e.g. gliclazide 40–80mg od
- Act by augmenting insulin secretion. Effective only if there is some residual endogenous insulin production. All are equally effective. If one sulphonylurea does not work, another is not likely to either.
- Sulphonylureas should be taken before meals—warn patients about possible hypoglycaemia if meals are omitted. Start at the minimum dose and ↑ until either blood sugar is controlled or the maximum dose is reached. Wait ≥1mo. between adjustments.
- Main side-effect is weight gain.

Biguanides: e.g. metformin 500mg od qds
- 1st line oral treatment for obese patients (BMI>25). Acts by ↓ gluconeogenesis and ↑ peripheral utilization of glucose. Only effective if some endogenous insulin production.
- Avoid in very elderly patients, those with serious heart disease, liver, or renal failure (even mild) or high alcohol intake as ↑ risk of lactic acidosis. Hypoglycaemia is not a problem.
- Start with the minimum dose and ↑ monthly until control is achieved or maximum dose reached.

Other oral hypoglycaemic agents: *BNF 6.1.2*

Glitazones: e.g. rosiglitazone 4mg od. Cause ↑ insulin secretion, ↑ insulin sensitivity, and have beneficial effect on blood lipid profile.
- Use only in combination with metformin or a sulphonyl urea and *only* if combination of metformin and a sulphonyl urea is impossible due to contraindications or side-effects[N].
- Do not use in combination with insulin.
- Check liver function tests before starting treatment and every 2mo. in the 1st year of treatment, then 6–12 monthly thereafter.

Nateglinide and repaglinide: Stimulate insulin release. Rapid onset of action and short duration of activity. Both drugs can be given in combination with metformin. Repaglinide is also licensed as monotherapy.

Acarbose: Inhibitor of intestinal alpha glucosidase. Delays digestion and absorption of starch and sucrose. Lowers blood glucose alone or in combination with metformin *or* a sulphonyl urea. Unacceptable to many patients as it causes severe flatulence, though this side-effect ↓ with time.

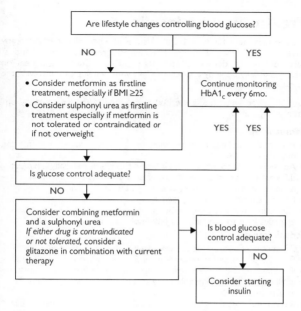

Figure 12.1 Using oral hypoglycaemic agents in type 2 DM

Indications to start insulin*: 📖 p.412
- Continuing weight loss and/or persistent symptoms.
- Non-obese patients who are on maximum oral therapy but still have poor diabetic control. Obese patients on maximal oral therapy but with poor control may benefit from insulin, though insulin causes weight gain. A concerted effort to lose weight is preferable, but not always achievable.
- Patients planning pregnancy.

Drug treatment of obesity: Anti-obesity drugs should only be prescribed for patients with type 2 DM if they have BMI ≥27kg/m² (sibutramine) or ≥28kg/m² (orlistat) and they have previously made serious attempts to lose weight by diet and exercise[N].

Essential reading
NICE 🖳 http://www.nice.org.uk
- Management of type 2 diabetes: blood glucose (2002)
- Diabetes (type 2)—glitazones (review) (No. 63) (2003)
- Obesity—orlistat (No. 22) and sibutramine (No. 31) (2004)
UKPDS 33 (1998) Lancet **352**: 837–53

*Continue metformin except if planning pregnancy; discontinue sulphonyl urea and/or glitazone.

Treatment with insulin

1st line treatment for type 1 DM. Also used when diet ± oral therapy have failed for type 2 DM. Local guidelines agreed between 1° and 2° care govern who does what and targets of care. Starting a patient on insulin is usually done by a specialist clinic with ongoing care involving the primary care team.

⚠ All drivers must notify the DVLA and their insurance company on starting insulin.

Monitoring

- Ask patients to keep a written diary of blood sugar values and time and date they are taken.
- Advise patients to measure their blood sugar pre-prandially ≥1x/d. at different times of the day—more often if using multiple injection regimes, after dose changes, or during intercurrent illness.
- Record episodes of hypoglycaemia.
- *Target:* blood glucose 4–7mmol/l pre-meals with hypoglycaemic episodes kept to a minimum. (4–8mmol/l pre-meals if <18y. old)

Administration

- Deep sc injection into upper arm, thigh, buttock, or abdomen.
- Fat hypertrophy and scarring are minimized by rotation of injection sites.
- 'Pen' devices and conventional syringe and needle are equally effective. In all cases, prime the needle using an 'air shot' (an empty needle ↓ insulin dose by ~2u).
- Rock 'pens' containing pre-mixed insulins to mix contents before use.

Common injection regimes

- Intermediate ± short-acting insulin od (type 2 only);
- Short + intermediate-acting insulin bd (pre-main and evening meal);
- Short + intermediate-acting insulin (pre-main meal), short-acting or rapid-acting* insulin (before evening meal), and intermediate-acting insulin (before bed);
- Short-acting or rapid-acting* insulin tds (pre-meals) and intermediate-acting insulin (before bed);
- Combinations of oral therapy and od or bd and long or intermediate-acting insulin.

Exercise: ↓ insulin dose acting at the time of exercise *or* take 1 or 2 glucose tablets before exercise, then check blood glucose afterwards. Adjust alterations/glucose dose with experience of effects of exercise. ↑ absorption of insulin from a limb site occurs if the limb is used in strenuous exercise following injection.

Intercurrent illness

- Continue insulin in usual dose.
- Keep a regular check (≥qds) of blood sugar.

---

* Rapid-acting insulin should be used as an alternative to meal-time soluble insulin where nocturnal or late inter-prandial hypoglycaemia is a problem or to eliminate the need for snacks between meals.

- If >13mmol/l, ↑ insulin by 2u./d. until control is achieved or use top-up injections of short-acting insulin qds prn.
- Maintain glucose intake even if not eating (with e.g. Lucozade or milk).
- Admit to hospital if: condition warrants admission; unable to take glucose; persistent vomiting; dehydration; ketotic (check urine if blood sugar >13mmol/l).

Poor control

- Exclude intercurrent illness
- Consider diet and/or gastroparesis
- Check insulin is being used as directed and injection sites are not scarred or hypertrophic
- Consider psychosocial factors which might be upsetting control
- Consider changing insulin dose—ask the patient to record a glucose profile (blood sugar pre-meals and before bed)
- If using >1 insulin, adjust 1 at a time
- Alter by ≤10% each time; allow ≥48h. between dose adjustments; alter dose of insulin acting at the time the blood sugar is most out of control
- If blood sugar is too high, ↑ insulin dose and vice versa

Hypoglycaemia

Emergency management: 📖 p.1070

Advice for patients

- Check blood sugar before driving and every 2h. during a long journey
- Carry glucose everywhere and sandwiches on long journeys
- If hypoglycaemia occurs, stop hazardous activities and take evasive action
- Wait until fully recovered before resuming activities

In case of severe hypoglycaemia: Supply a responsible member of the family with glucose gel (e.g. Hypostop) and glucagon injection. Teach him/her to use it. Response is short-lived—give oral glucose (e.g. Lucozade, glucose tablets, milk) as soon as the patient is conscious.

Recurrent hypoglycaemia

- If hypoglycaemia occurs in a regular pattern, check pattern of meals and activity and alter insulin to match needs
- If erratic, consider erratic lifestyle, alcohol, problems with absorption, errors in administration, gastroparesis
- If no obvious cause, consider change in underlying insulin sensitivity (e.g. age, renal impairment)

Hypoglycaemia unawareness: Associated with human insulins (but can occur with any). To restore warning signs, adjust insulin and food intake to stop glucose levels dropping to <4mmol/l.. Consider undetected night-time hypoglycaemia if HbA$_{1c}$ < expected from blood sugar diary. Driving is not permitted when hypoglycaemic awareness has been lost.

Essential reading

NICE (2004) Type 1 diabetes: diagnosis and management 🖥 http://www.nice.org.uk

Diabetic complications: cardiovascular disease and eye disease

Cardiovascular disease: Diabetics are at ↑ risk of MI (2–5x), stroke (2–3x), and peripheral vascular disease. Protective effect of female sex is lost. Atherosclerotic disease accounts for most of the excess mortality due to DM. Check arterial risk factors annually:

- Albumin excretion rate
- Blood glucose control
- BP
- Age
- Smoking—give advice on smoking cessation at every available opportunity. Help patients who want to give up with advice, medication, and smoking cessation support.
- Lipid profile (LDL, HDL cholesterol, and triglycerides)
- Family history of arterial disease
- Abdominal adiposity

> ⚠ **Don't use arterial risk tables for adults with DM.**

High risk for CVD
- Pre-existing CVD
- All type 2 diabetics >50y. or who have had DM for ≥10y.
- Adults with type 1 DM and *either* microalbuminuria/proteinuria *or* ≥2 features of the metabolic syndrome (📖 p.405)

Medium risk of CVD
- Adults with type 1 DM who do *not* have microalbuminuria/proteinuria or ≥2 features of the metabolic syndrome (📖 p.405) but *do* have other risk factors—age >35y., FH premature heart disease, of an ethnic group with higher risk of arterial disease, with abnormal lipids or BP

Aspirin: Give 75mg od to all type 2 diabetics aged >50y. (or if DM for ≥ 10y.) and type 1 diabetics with high/moderately high risk of arterial disease. Control systolic BP to ≤145mmHg before starting treatment.

Statin: Give to all type 2 diabetics[R] and type 1 diabetics in high-risk and moderately high-risk groups for arterial disease. Aim to ↓ total cholesterol by 25% or to <4mmol/l—whichever is the lower value *or* ↓ LDL cholesterol by 30% or to <2.0mmol/l—whichever is the lower value.

Blood glucose: Aim HbA$_{1c}$ <7.5%. If type 1 DM and high or moderately high risk of arterial disease, aim HbA$_{1c}$ ≤6.5%.

BP: Any ↓ in average BP ↓ risk of cardiovascular complications.
- *Type 1 DM[N]:* Treat if systolic BP >135 or diastolic BP >85mmHg *unless* microalbuminuria/proteinuria or ≥ 2 features of the metabolic syndrome (📖 p.404) when treat if systolic BP >130 or diastolic BP >80mmHg.
- *Type 2 DM[G]:* Treat if systolic BP ≥140 or diastolic BP ≥90mmHg regardless of absolute risk of CVD. Aim to ↓ BP to <130/80mmHg (or <125/75mmHg if proteinuria is present).

Thiazide diuretics (e.g. bendrofluazide 2.5mg od) are the drugs of choice as first-line treatment of ↑ BP unless albuminuria[R]. If albuminuria is present, an ACE inhibitor should be used as first-line agent.

❶ Most diabetics will need combination therapy to achieve adequate control. Other suitable agents for use alone or in combination include β-blockers and alpha 2 receptor antagonists. Only use calcium channel blockers as second-line or in combination therapy.

Eye disease

Blurred vision: May occur if control is poor. Caused by osmotic changes in the lens. Corrects with normalization of blood sugar. Wait before changing glasses.

Cataract: Juvenile 'snowflake' cataracts are more common and senile cataracts occur earlier.

Glaucoma: DM is a risk factor for developing glaucoma.

Retinopathy
* Most common cause of blindness in people of working age in industrialized countries (risk is ×20 non-diabetics).
* 20–40% type 2 diabetics have retinopathy at diagnosis.
* 20y. after diagnosis, all type 1 diabetics and 60% type 2 diabetics have retinopathy—sight-threatening is 5–10%.
* Small retinal blood vessels become blocked, swollen, or leaky causing exudate formation, oedema, or new vessels. Laser treatment (photo-coagulation) halts progression but does not restore vision.
* Monitor and treat associated risk factors—BP, lipids (hard exudates), smoking.
* Measure visual acuity (with glasses or pinhole) annually. Digital retinal photography is available throughout the UK. Screening (at least annually) to detect retinopathy before visual loss occurs is essential.

Classification of diabetic retinopathy: 📖 p.954.

Refer to ophthalmologist if:
* Sudden loss of vision—E
* Rubeosis iridis—E
* Pre-retinal or vitreous haemorrhage—E
* Retinal detachment—E
* New vessel formation—U
* Maculopathy—R
* Pre-proliferative retinopathy—R
* Cataract affecting visual acuity—R
* Unexplained drop in visual acuity—R

E = Emergency; U = urgent; R = routine

Essential reading
NICE 🖥 http://www.nice.org.uk
* Type 1 diabetes: diagnosis and management (2004)
* Management of type 2 diabetes: BP and lipids (2002)
* Management of type 2 diabetes: retinopathy (2002)
BHS Guidelines for the management of hypertension (2004)
🖥 http://www.hyp.ac.uk/bhs/home.htm

Further information
MRC/BHF (2003) Heart Protection Study of simvastatin in diabetic patients *Lancet* **362**: 2005–16
ALLHAT (2002) Major outcomes in high-risk hypertensive patients randomized to ACE inhibitor or calcium channel blocker vs. diuretic *JAMA* **288**: 2981–97

Diabetic complications: renal disease, neuropathy, and skin changes

Renal disease

Urinary tract infections: More common in patients with poorly controlled DM. May exacerbate renal failure and → renal scarring. Consider papillary necrosis if recurrent (more common in DM).

Nephropathy

- Most common cause of end-stage renal failure in adults starting dialysis in the UK. 25% diabetics have renal damage—more common if of Asian or African ethnic origin.
- Nephropathy is characterized by proteinuria (albumin:creatinine ratio ≥30mg/mmol or albumin concentration ≥200mg/l), ↑BP, and progressive ↓ in renal function.
- Before overt nephropathy occurs there is a phase (microalbuminuria or incipient nephropathy) in which the urine contains traces of protein not detected by standard protein dipstick. Microalbuminuria is defined as albumin:creatinine ratio ≥2.5mg/mmol (♂) or ≥3.5mg/mmol (♀) or albumin concentration ≥20mg/l.
- Presence of ↑ urine albumin levels and/or ↑ serum creatinine is associated with ↑ risk of premature cardiovascular events and renal failure.
- Check renal function annually (first pass urine specimen for albumin:creatinine ratio, serum creatinine, microalbuminuria dipstick). If abnormal, repeat more frequently (every 3–6mo.).
- Diabetic nephropathy is nearly always associated with retinopathy. If ↑ urine albumin *without* retinopathy, look for non-diabetic causes of renal disease (📖 p.678).

Management of nephropathy

- Optimize blood glucose control.
- Monitor and treat ↑BP (target BP <130/80mmHg or <135/75 or ≤ 125/75 depending on guidelines used—may require combination of antihypertensive agents) and treat other arterial risk factors aggressively.
- Modify diet (↓ salt intake, ↓ protein intake with target of 0.8g/kg).
- ACE inhibitors are protective of renal function and ↓ proteinuria whether or not the patient is hypertensive.
- Refer to a nephrologist if overt proteinuria (UTI excluded) or ↑ creatinine >150μmol/l.

Neuropathy: Enquire annually about painful and other symptomatic neuropathy, impotence in men, and manifestations of autonomic neuropathy, especially if renal complications or erratic blood glucose control. Optimize blood sugar control.

Symmetrical sensory progressive polyneuropathy: 40–50% patients with DM. Starts distally, feet>hands. Glove and stocking distribution. May be asymptomatic or cause numbness, tingling, or neuropathic pain. Pain can be depressing and disabling. Be supportive. If simple analgesia with paracetamol or NSAID is ineffective, try neuropathic painkillers—TCAs (e.g. amitriptyline 25–75mg nocte), carbamazepine (100–400mg bd), gabapentin, or counter-irritants (e.g. capsaicin 0.075%).

Mononeuropathies/mononeuritis multiplex: Especially cranial nerves III and VI (📖 p.590).

Amyotrophy: Painful wasting of quadriceps muscles. Reversible with improved blood sugar control.

Autonomic neuropathy

- *Postural ↓ BP:* Common, especially in the elderly. Increasing dietary salt intake may help. Other treatments are all unlicensed. They include fludrocortisone 100–400mcg od (uncomfortable oedema is a common side-effect) ± flurbiprofen or ephedrine hydrochloride (30–60mg tds to relieve oedema), and midodrine (alpha agonist).
- *Urinary retention:* 📖 p.690
- *Diabetic diarrhoea:* Exclude other causes of change in bowel habit— 📖 p.251. Diabetic diarrhoea can be treated with 2 or 3 doses of tetracycline (250mg—unlicensed). Otherwise treat with codeine phosphate 30mg tds/qds prn.
- *Erectile dysfunction:* 📖 p.702
- *Gastric paresis:* Treat with an antiemetic which promotes gastric transit e.g. domperidone 30mg tds. When this fails, erythromycin may be used, but evidence of effectiveness is lacking.
- *Gustatory sweating:* Can be treated with an antimuscarinic such as propantheline bromide but side-effects are common. Hyperhidrosis— 📖 p.659

Skin changes associated with DM: Numerous skin problems are associated with DM. These include:
- Predisposition to infection e.g. candidiasis, staphylococcal infection (e.g. folliculitis, boils).
- Pruritus.
- Xanthomas.
- Vitiligo (type 1 DM).
- Neuropathic and/or ischaemic ulcers—see the diabetic foot (📖 p.418).
- Fat atrophy/hypertrophy at insulin injection sites.
- Necrobiosis lipoidica—50% associated with DM. Small, dusky red nodules with well circumscribed borders. Can be single or multiple. Usually on outside of shin. Enlarge slowly becoming brownish yellow, irregular, and flattened/depressed. Longstanding lesions may ulcerate. No effective treatment.
- Diabetic dermopathy—pigmented scars over shins.
- Granuloma annulare ✐—asymptomatic dermal nodules. Association with DM is controversial.
- Diabetic cheiroarthropathy—waxy skin-thickening over the dorsum of the hand, with restricted mobility.

Essential reading

NICE 🖥 http://www.nice.org.uk
- Type 1 diabetes: diagnosis and management (2004)
- Management of type 2 diabetes: renal disease (2002)

The diabetic foot

Foot problems are common amongst diabetics. 5% develop a foot ulcer in any year and amputation rates are 0.5%/y. Foot problems are due to:
- Peripheral neuropathy (affects 20–40% diabetic patients) → ↓ foot sensation *and*
- Peripheral vascular disease (affects 20–40% diabetic patients) → pain and predisposition to ulceration

Information about foot care
- Self-care and self-monitoring:
  - Daily examination of the feet for problems—colour change; swelling; breaks in the skin; numbness
  - Footwear—importance of well-fitting shoes and hosiery
  - Hygiene (daily washing and careful drying) and nail care
  - Dangers associated with procedures such as corn or verruca removal
  - Methods to help self-monitoring e.g. mirrors if ↓ mobility
- When to seek advice from a health professional—if any colour change; swelling; breaks in the skin; numbness; or if self-monitoring is not possible (e.g. due to mobility problems).
- For patients at increased or high risk or with ulcers, additionally advise no barefoot walking and that, due to ↓ sensation, extra care and attention is needed.
- If skin lesions, advise patients to seek help if any change in the lesion, if ↑ swelling, pain, odour, colour change, or systemic symptoms.

Risk factors
- Neuropathy
- Peripheral vascular disease
- Previous ulceration or amputation
- Age >70y.
- Plantar callus
- Foot deformities
- Poor footwear
- Long duration of DM
- Social deprivation and isolation
- Poor vision
- Smoking

The foot check: Check the feet as part of the annual review.

History
- Foot problems since last review
- Visual or mobility problems affecting self-care of feet
- Self-care behaviours and knowledge of foot care
- History of numbness, tingling, or burning—may be worse at night.

Table 12.2 Classification of foot risk

Foot risk	Features
Low current risk	Normal sensation, palpable pulses
Increased risk	Neuropathy, absent pulses, or other risk factors
High risk	Neuropathy or absent pulses + deformity or skin changes or previous ulcer
Ulcerated foot	Foot ulcer on examination

Examination
- Foot shape, deformity, joint rigidity, and shoes
- Foot skin condition—fragility, cracking, oedema, callus, ulceration, sweating, presence of hair
- Foot and ankle pulses
- Sensitivity to 10g monofilament or vibration

Management

General points
- Optimize diabetic control and risk factors for vascular disease (including smoking cessation).
- Review drug therapy—stop β-blockers if evidence of peripheral vascular disease
- Educate about foot care

Specific management: Classification—Table 12.1
- *Low risk:* Foot care education.
- *Increased risk:* Foot care education. Refer to the foot protection team. Check feet every 3–6mo. Consider referral for vascular assessment. Consider regular podiatry if poor vision, immobility, or poor social conditions/foot hygiene. If previous foot ulcer, deformity, or skin changes—manage as high risk.
- *High risk:* Stress importance of foot care. Refer to the foot protection team for specialist podiatry. Inspect feet every 3–6mo. Review need for vascular assessment. Treat fungal infection.
- *Foot ulcer:* Refer to the multidisciplinary specialist foot care team urgently. Assess ischaemia using Dopplers. Consider referral for angiography. Treat infection. If new ulceration, cellulites, or discolouration, refer to a specialized podiatry/foot care team within 24h.

Table 12.3 Clinical features of neuropathic and vascular foot ulcers

Neuropathic	Vascular
Warm foot	Cool foot
Bounding pulses, normal ABI	Absent pulses, ↓ ABI
Located at pressure points	Located at extremities (e.g. between toes)
Painless	Painful
Clearly defined or 'punched out' Surrounded by callus	Less clearly delineated

❶ Diabetics may have coexisting peripheral neuropathy and peripheral vascular disease. ABI may be artificially ↑ due to calcification of vessels.

Charcot osteoarthropathy (Charcot's joint): Neuropathic foot damaged because of trauma 2° to loss of pain sensation. If suspected, refer immediately to the multidisciplinary foot care team for immobilization and long-term management.

Essential reading
NICE 🖳 http://www.nice.org.uk
  Type 1 diabetes: diagnosis and management (2004)
  Type 2 diabetes: prevention and management of foot problems (2004)

Lumps in the thyroid gland and goitres

Faced with a lump in the pre-tracheal region of the neck, ask:
• Is it in the thyroid (moves up and down on swallowing)?
• Is it a solitary lump or more generalized (a goitre)?
• Is the patient thyrotoxic, euthyroid, or hypothyroid?
• Is the trachea being compressed (patient is breathless)?

Solitary thyroid nodules: Investigate *all* solitary nodules. Check
TFTs and refer for thyroid USS. Refer to a thyroid surgeon urgently
Differential diagnosis:
• *Benign* (~90%): cyst, adenoma, discrete nodule in a nodular goitre.
• *Malignant* (~10%):
    • *Primary*—thyroid adenocarcinoma, lymphoma, medullary carcinoma
    • *Secondary*—direct spread from local tumour, metastatic spread
      from breast, colon/rectum, kidney, lung, lymphoma.

Thyroid cyst: Usually a degenerative part of a nodular goitre, though
true cysts do occur. There may be haemorrhage into a cyst in which case
there is rapid enlargement and the lump may be painful. Refer for confirmation of diagnosis.

Thyroid adenoma: 4 types, classified according to histological appearance—papillary, follicular, embryonal, hurtle cell. A minority of adenoma
produce thyroxine and cause thyrotoxicosis. Haemorrhage into an adenoma is rare and results in rapid ↑ in size. Refer for confirmation of diagnosis
± surgery.

Goitre: There are 4 main types of goitre—see Table 12.4.

Carcinoma of the thyroid: *Primary tumours:*
• **Papillary adenocarcinoma** (60%): Typical age range: 10–40y. ♀ > ♂.
  Low-grade malignancy which is rarely fatal. Spread occurs to local
  LNs and/or lung. The tumour is sensitive to TSH, so following
  thyroidectomy, treatment with thyroxine continues lifelong.
• **Follicular carcinoma** (25%): Typical age range: 40–60y. ♀ > ♂. May
  arise in a pre-existing multinodular goitre. Metastasizes via the
  bloodstream and boney secondaries are common. Treatment is with
  surgery and thyroxine suppression therapy and/or radioactive iodine.
• **Anaplastic carcinoma** (rare): Typical age range: 50–60y. ♀ > ♂.
  Aggressive tumour which grows rapidly and infiltrates the tissues of the
  neck. Compression of the trachea is common. Metastasizes locally to
  LNs and via lymphatics. Poor response to treatment.
• **Medullary carcinoma** (rare): Occurs at any age. ♀ = ♂. Familial
  incidence; associated with adenomas elsewhere. Often secretes
  calcitonin which is used as a tumour marker. Spreads to local LNs.
  Treated by excision then chemotherapy ± radiotherapy.
• **Lymphoma** (5%): Occurs at any age. May be primary or secondary. May
  be associated with Hashimoto's thyroiditis. Staged and treated as for
  lymphomas elsewhere (📖 p.534). Prognosis is good.

Table 12.4 Types of goitre—presentation and management

Type of goitre	Features	Management
Physiological	Occurs at puberty, during pregnancy, and in conditions of iodine deficiency	Usually requires no treatment. If iodine-deficient, treat with iodine supplements
Nodular	Benign enlargement of the thyroid gland with areas of hyperplasia and involution	No treatment is necessary unless: • Thyrotoxic • Compression of the neck structures → dyspnoea or dysphagia • Worried by cosmetic appearance • Focal ↑ in size or recurrent laryngeal nerve palsy (hoarseness)—suggest malignant change If treatment is needed, refer to surgery or endocrinology depending on symptoms.
Toxic	Grave's disease—smooth enlargement of the thyroid and thyrotoxicosis	See 📖 p.422
Inflammatory	*Hashimoto's thyroiditis:* • ♀ > ♂ • Antibodies to thyroid tissue are produced • Initially, goitre and thyrotoxicosis • Later myxoedema (H. Hashimoto (1881–1934)—Japanese surgeon) *De Quervain's thyroiditis:* • Inflammation due to viral infection—usually Coxsackie virus • Acutely swollen, tender thyroid gland and transient thyrotoxicosis often preceded by sore throat/malaise • Settles spontaneously (F. de Quervain (1868–1940)—Swiss surgeon) *Riedel's thyroiditis:* Rare. Thyroid becomes infiltrated by scar tissue → hypothyroidism ± recurrent laryngeal nerve palsy ± stridor. (B. Riedel (1846–1916)—German surgeon)	In all cases refer to endocrinology for confirmation of diagnosis and management guidance.

Thyroid disease

Hyperthyroidism: Affects 2% ♀ and 0.2% ♂. *Peak age: 20–49y. Causes:*
- Graves disease (see below)
- Toxic nodular goitre—older women with past history of goitre
- Thyroiditis
- Amiodarone
- Kelp ingestion

Presentation
- Weight loss
- Tremor
- Palpitations
- Hyperactivity
- AF
- Eye changes (opposite)
- Infertility

❶ In elderly patients, symptoms may be less obvious and include confusion, dementia, apathy, and depression.

Management: Refer to endocrinology at presentation. *Treatment:*
- *β-blockers:* e.g. propranolol, atenolol. Useful for symptom control until antithyroid drug therapy takes effect.
- *Carbimazole:* Inhibits synthesis of thyroid hormones. Ineffective for treatment of thyroiditis. May be given short term to render a patient euthyroid prior to surgery/treatment with radioactive iodine or long term (12–18mo.) in an attempt to induce remission (but >50% relapse). 3/1000 patients have serious adverse effects—agranulocytosis, hepatitis, aplastic anaemia, or lupus-like syndromes.
- *Radioactive iodine (^{131}I):* Effects take 3–4mo. to become apparent. Withdraw carbimazole >4d. prior to treatment and do not restart until >3d. after. Advise women of childbearing age to avoid pregnancy for 4mo. Most become hypothyroid at some point (sometimes years) after treatment. Continue monitoring TFTs long term. Associated with small ↑ risk of thyroid malignancy.
- *Surgery:* Partial or total thyroidectomy—reserved for patients with large goitres or who decline radioactive iodine. Carries risk of damage to recurrent laryngeal nerve or parathyroids.

⚠ Warn *all* patients starting carbimazole to stop the drug and seek urgent medical attention if they develop sore throat or other infection.

Thyrotoxic crisis/storm: p.1071.

Graves disease: Most common cause of hyperthyroidism. ♀:♂ ≈ 5:1 Peak age: 30–50y. Associated with smoking and stressful life events Autoimmune disease in which antibodies to the TSH receptor are produced. *(R.J. Graves (1797–1853)—Irish physician)*

Clinical features
- Hyperthyroidism
- Diffuse goitre ± thyroid bruit due to ↑ vascularity
- Extrathyroid features:
  - Eye disease—40% (see opposite page)
  - Pretibial myxoedema—5%
  - Thyroid acropachy—rare; clubbing, finger swelling
  - Onycholysis—rare

Management: As for hyperthyroidism.

Table12.5 Interpretation of thyroid function test results

Results of TFTs	Interpretation	Notes
TSH$\downarrow$, T$_4\uparrow$	Thyrotoxic	Occasionally T$_4$ is normal but T$_3$ $\uparrow$
TSH$\uparrow$, T$_4\downarrow$	Hypothyroid	TSH $\downarrow$ if hypothyroidism is 2° to pituitary failure (rare)
TSH$\uparrow$, T$_4\leftrightarrow$	Subclinical hypothyroidism	If any symptoms (including depression and non-specific symptoms or hypercholesterolaemia), consider a trial of treatment. If no symptoms, monitor annually.

Thyroid eye disease: Presents with:
- Double vision
- Eye discomfort ± protrusion (exopthalmos and proptosis)
- Lid lag
- Ophthalmoplegia (especially of upward gaze)
- TFTs can be $\uparrow$ or normal

Management: Refer to ophthamologist. If $\downarrow$ acuity or loss of colour vision, refer urgently, as there may be optic nerve compression.

Hypothyroidism (myxoedema): Common—10% $\female$ > 60y. $\female$:$\male$ ≈ 8:1.

Causes: Chronic autoimmune thyroiditis; post radioactive iodine; thyroidectomy.

Presentation
- Onset tends to be insidious and may go undiagnosed for years.
- *Always* consider hypothyroidism when a patient has non-specific symptoms, depression, fatigue, lethargy, or general malaise.
- Other symptoms—weight $\uparrow$, constipation, hoarse voice, or dry skin/hair.
- Signs are often absent—there may be a goitre, slow-relaxing reflexes, or non-pitting oedema of the hands, feet, or eyelids.

Screening: Check TFTs in patients:
- With persistent symptoms of tiredness/lethargy without clear cause.
- On amiodarone or with a history of ^{131}I administration.
- With hypercholesterolaemia, infertility, depression, dementia, obesity, other autoimmune disease, Turner's syndrome, or congenital hypothyroidism.

Management: Patients taking thyroxine replacement are entitled to apply for free prescriptions.
- *<65y. and healthy:* 150mcg od thyroxine. Re-check TFTs after 12wk. Adjust dose to keep TSH in normal range. Once dose is stable and TSH is within normal range, monitor annually and if symptomatic or worries about compliance.
- *If elderly or pre-existing heart disease:* Start 25mcg od thyroxine and $\uparrow$ dose every 4wk. according to TFTs. Consider adding propranolol if history of IHD as thyroxine can provoke angina.

Withdrawal of thyroxine: Usually patients requiring thyroxine are on it lifelong. If diagnosis is in doubt, stop thyroxine and re-measure TFTs after 4–6wk.

Hypothyroid coma: p.1071.

Hyper- and hypocalcaemia

Checking Ca^{2+}: Check calcium level on an *uncuffed* sample (to avoid falsely high readings) and correct for serum albumin—for every mmol/l less than 40, a correction of 0.02mmol/l should be added to the serum calcium concentration measured. For example:

Calcium 2.40   Corrected calcium = $(40 - 24) \times 0.02 + 2.4$
Albumin 24   = $0.32 + 2.4 = 2.72$

Hypocalcaemia: *Causes:*
- *If phosphate ↑:* CRF, hypoparathyroidism (may be 2° to thyroid or parathyroid surgery), pseudohypoparathyroidism (insensitivity to parathyroid hormone)
- *If phosphate normal or ↓:* Osteomalacia, overhydration, pancreatitis

Presentation
- Tetany
- Depression
- Perioral paraestheia
- Carpo-pedal spasm (wrist flexion and fingers drawn together)
- Neuromuscular excitability (tapping over parotid causes facial muscles to contract—Chvostek's sign)

❶ Apparent hypocalcaemia may be an artefact of hypoalbuminaemia.

Management: Supplement with calcium. Secondary care referral is usually needed to investigate and treat the underlying cause.

Hypercalcaemia: Presence of ↑ level of serum calcium (>2.6mmol/l). *Prevalence* ≈ 1:1000; ♂:♀ ≈ 1:3. Rare <age 50y.

Causes

Common
- Primary hyperparathyroidism
- Malignancy (10% tumours—usually myeloma, breast, lung, kidney, thyroid, prostate, ovary or colon)
- Chronic renal failure

Uncommon
- Familial benign hypercalcaemia
- Sarcoidosis
- Thyrotoxicosis
- Milk alkali syndrome
- Vitamin D treatment

Presentation: Often very non-specific but if increasing serum Ca^{2+} is left untreated, it can be fatal. May be an incidental finding. Other symptoms: *'bones, stones, groans, and abdominal moans'*.
- Tiredness
- Lethargy
- Weakness
- Mild aches and pains
- Anorexia
- Weight loss
- Low mood
- Stone formation
- Nausea/vomiting (often intractable)
- Polyuria and polydipsia
- Abdominal pain
- Constipation
- Confusion
- Corneal calcification

Management
- Treat according to cause (Figure 12.2)—malignancy (📖 p.1008)
- If diagnosis is unclear, refer to endocrinology. Urgency depends on serum Ca^{2+} and severity of symptoms.

- If Ca^{2+}>3.5mmol/l or severe symptoms, admit for lowering of Ca^{2+} with forced diuresis and IV pamidronate.

Familial benign hypercalcaemia: Asymptomatic. Inherited condition in which serum calcium concentrations are mildly ↑ throughout life. Confirm (if possible) by demonstrating ↑ Ca^{2+} in other family members. No adverse consequences and no treatment needed.

Milk alkali syndrome: Usually due to high ingestion of OTC indigestion remedies (e.g. Rennies). Ca^{2+} levels revert to normal on stopping. Investigate why the patient is taking these remedies (? peptic ulcer).

Hyperparathyroidism: ↑ secretion of parathyroid hormone (PTH).
- **1°hyperparathyroidism:** Incidence 0.5/1000. Peak age 40–60y. ♀:♂≈2:1. Circulating level of PTH is inappropriately high. Most patients are hypercalcaemic (but may be normocalcaemic if co-existent vitamin D deficiency). Due to ↑ secretion of PTH from one or both of the parathyroid glands. Refer. Treatment is usually surgical.
- **2°hyperparathyroidism:** ↑ PTH in response to chronic hypocalcaemia or hyperphosphataemia. Treat cause.
- **3°hyperparathyroidism:** Inappropriately ↑PTH → ↑Ca^{2+}. Follows prolonged 2° hyperparathyroidism. Most common in patients with chronic renal failure (especially if on dialysis) or chronic malabsorption. Treatment is usually surgical.

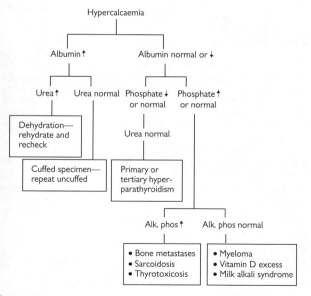

Figure 12.2 Guide to the diagnosis of cause of hypercalcaemia (must be taken in clinical context)

Adrenal disorders

Disorders of the adrenal cortex: The adrenal cortex produces 3 classes of steroids:

- Glucocorticoids e.g. cortisol
- Mineralocorticoids e.g. aldosterone
- Sex hormones e.g. androstenedione, testosterone, and oestrogen.

Disorders result from disturbance in production of these steroids.

Cushing's syndrome: In the majority of cases, Cushing's syndrome is iatrogenic—caused by exogenous administration of prednisolone or other corticosteroids. Non-iatrogenic Cushing's syndrome is much rarer, with annual incidence of 1–2/million (♀:♂ ≈ 3:1).

- 80% have a pituitary adenoma which secretes adrenocorticotrophic hormone (ACTH) causing hypersecretion of glucocorticoids and sex hormones (Cushing's disease).
- 20% are due to ectopic ACTH secretion by other tumours (e.g. small cell lung cancer) or hypersecreting tumours of the adrenal cortex.

(H.W. Cushing (1869–1939)—US neurosurgeon)

Presentation: Cushing's syndrome has high morbidity and mortality. Clinical features include:

- Moon face (90%)
- Truncal obesity (85%)
- Hypertension (80%)
- Menstrual disturbance (80%)
- Striae and bruising (60%)
- Osteoporosis (60%)
- Lethargy/depression (60%)
- Hirsuitism
- Acne
- Pigmentation
- Feminization in men
- Polyuria and polydipsia
- Psychosis

Investigation of non-iatrogenic Cushing's syndrome: Dexamethasone suppression test—dexamethasone 1mg po at midnight, then serum cortisol measured at 9 a.m. If <50mmol/l—excludes diagnosis, unless cortisol secretion is episodic. False positives are common. Expert advice is needed before proceeding with further tests.

Management
- Stop/minimize exogenous steroids.
- If no exogenous steroids and Cushing's syndrome is suspected, refer to endocrinology. Usually treated surgically.

Addison's disease: Primary adrenocortical insufficiency. In the UK most cases are due to autoimmune disease, surgery, or cessation of therapeutic steroids (or failure to ↑ dose to cover stress). Worldwide, TB is a major cause. Prevalence 50/million (♀:♂ ≈ 3:1).

(T. Addison (1795–1860)—English physician)

Clinical features
- Tiredness (95%)
- Weakness (95%)
- Anorexia (95%)
- Weight loss (90%)
- Pigmentation (buccal, palmar creases, new scars—90%)
- Abdominal pain (30%)
- Myalgia (20%)
- Postural hypotension and fainting (15%)
- Nausea
- Arthralgia

Presentation
- Can be dramatic with coma and severe hypoglycaemia or insidious with vague symptoms of malaise and lassitude.
- 50% patients with autoimmune Addison's disease have or will develop another autoimmune disease (e.g. Graves disease, pernicious anaemia) and 5% of women develop premature ovarian failure, so review regularly with these possibilities in mind.

Investigation
- Biochemical abnormalities—↓K$^+$, ↓Na$^+$, ↓ glucose (may not be symptomatic), uraemia, ↑Ca^{2+}, abnormal LFTs.
- FBC—neutropoenia, lymphocytosis.

Management
- Refer to endocrinology. Patients have a normal lifespan if treated.
- Treatment usually involves replacing deficient steroids with hydrocortisone and fludrocortisone. Adjust doses carefully.
- Warn patients not to stop steroids abruptly and to tell any doctor treating them about their condition (and wear warning bracelet in case of emergency).
- Double dose of hydrocortisone prior to dental treatment or if intercurrent illness (e.g. URTI). If vomiting, replace hydrocortisone po with im hydrocortisone.

Hyperaldosteronism (Conn's syndrome): Suggested by presence of ↑BP with ↓K$^+$—but normokalaemic cases are also described. $^2/_3$ have an aldosterone-secreting adenoma. Referral for endocrine assessment is important as adenomas can be removed surgically. Spironolactone is an effective alternative treatment.

Congenital adrenal hyperplasia: 📖 p.882

Disorders of the adrenal medulla

Phaechromocytoma: Rare but serious disorder affecting 0.1% hypertensive patients. Usually caused by catecholamine-secreting tumours—10% are bilateral; 10% extra-adrenal; 10% occur in children; 10% are malignant.

Presentation: May present with a huge array of symptoms and signs. ↑BP may be sporadic or sustained. Suspect in young patients with ↑BP, patients with very labile BP, or if associated headaches, sweating, and/or palpitations. May be associated with other conditions (e.g. neurofibromatosis).

Investigation: Urine catecholamine/metabolite levels.

Management: Consult local guidelines. Refer for specialist opinion if suspected. Treatment is usually surgical.

Patient advice and support
The Pituitary Foundation ☎ 0845 450 0375 🖥 http://www.pituitary.org.uk (booklet on Cushing's disease and GP Factfile)
Addison's Disease Self Help Group 🖥 http://www.adshg.org.uk

Pituitary problems

Hypopituitarism: ↓ production of all pituitary hormones (ACTH, growth hormone, FSH, LH, TSH, and prolactin). *Causes:*
- Surgery
- Irradiation
- Tumour (may be non-secreting or secrete one pituitary hormone with ↓ secretion of the others)
- Infection—TB
- Sheehan's syndrome—pituitary necrosis after post-partum haemorrhage (*H.L. Sheehan (b. 1900)—English pathologist*)

Presentation
- Hypothyroidism
- Hypogonadism
- Anorexia
- Headache
- Depression
- Hair loss
- Hypotension
- Visual field defect

Management: If suspected, refer to neurology or endocrinology for further investigation and advice on treatment.

Pituitary tumours: 10% intracranial tumours. Almost all are benign. Classified by histological type (chromophobic, acidophilic, or basophilic) or by the hormone secreted:
- No hormone (30%)
- Prolactin (35%)
- Growth hormone (20%)
- ACTH (7%)
- Prolactin and growth hormone (7%)
- LH, FSH, and TSH (1%)

Presentation: Present with symptoms caused by:
- Local pressure—bilateral hemianopia, cranial nerve palsies, headache
- Hormone secretion and/or
- Hypopituitarism (see above)

Management: Refer for further investigation and treatment if suspected.

Pituitary apoplexy: Rapid expansion of a pituitary tumour due to infarction or haemorrhage. Suspect if sudden onset of headache in a patient with a known pituitary tumour. Admit as a medical/neurosurgical emergency.

Craniopharyngioma: Tumour originating from Rathke's pouch. 50% present with local pressure effects in children (see 'pituitary tumours' above). Refer as for pituitary tumours.

Hyperprolactinaemia: The most common pituitary disorder. Due to pituitary adenoma.

Presentation: Tends to present earlier in women than men. Symptoms are due to pressure effects or ↑ prolactin. Symptoms of ↑ prolactin:
- ♀: Loss of libido, weight gain, apathy, vaginal dryness, menstrual disturbance, infertility, galactorrhoea
- ♂: Impotence, ↓ facial hair

Investigation: Check basal plasma prolactin (ask the lab for conditions under which they would like the sample taken).

Management: If suspected, refer for specialist opinion.

Other causes of ↑ prolactin
- Pregnancy
- Breast-feeding
- Stress
- Sleep
- Hypothyroidism
- Drugs—phenothiazines, metoclopramide, α-methyldopa, oestrogens
- Chronic renal failure
- Sarcoidosis

Acromegaly: Rare condition due to a growth hormone secreting pituitary tumour. Typical age at presentation: 30–50y.

Presentation
- Local pressure symptoms
- Changes in appearance—coarse oily skin, coarsening of facial features, ↑ foot size, ↑ teeth spacing
- Other effects—deepening of voice, sweating, paraesthesiae, proximal muscle weakness, progressive heart failure, goitre.
- *Complications*—DM, ↑BP, cardiomyopathy, large bowel tumours

Investigation and management: Refer to endocrinology.

Diabetes insipidus (DI): Caused by impaired water resorption by the kidney. 2 mechanisms:
- *Cranial DI:* ↓ ADH secretion from the posterior pituitary. 50% idiopathic. *Other causes:* head injury, tumour, infection, sarcoidosis, vascular, inherited.
- *Nephrogenic DI:* Impaired response of the kidney to ADH. *Causes:* drugs (e.g. lithium), hypercalcaemia, pyelonephritis, hydronephrosis, pregnancy (rare).

Presentation: Polydipsia, polyuria, dilute urine, dehydration.

Investigations: U&E (Na^+ ↑), Ca^{2+}, plasma and urine osmolality (plasma ↑, urine ↓). Specialist investigations (e.g. water deprivation test) confirm diagnosis.

Management: Treat the cause.
- Cranial DI may be treated with intranasal desmopressin or surgery.
- Nephrogenic DI may be treated with dietary restriction of protein and salt and/or bendrofluazide.

Syndrome of inappropriate ADH (SIADH): Important cause of hyponatraemia. Diagnosis is made by finding a concentrated urine (sodium >20mmol/l) in the presence of hyponatraemia (<125mmol/l) or low plasma osmolality (<260mmol/kg), and absence of hypovolaemia, oedema, or diuretics. Always requires specialist management. *Causes:*
- *Malignancy* e.g. small-cell lung cancer; pancreas; lymphoma.
- *CNS disorders* e.g. stroke; subdural haemorrhage; vasculitis (SLE).

Patient advice and support
The Pituitary Foundation ☎ 0845 450 0375 🖳 http://www.pituitary.org.uk (also GP Factfile)

Other relevant pages

Gastrointestinal medicine

Dyspepsia

In any year, up to 40% of the adult population suffer from dyspepsia. 1:10 seek their GP's advice and ~10% of these are referred. **Causes:**

- Gastro-oesophageal reflux disease (GORD)—15–25% (📖 p.436)
- Peptic ulcer (PU)—15–25% (📖 p.438)
- Stomach cancer—2% (📖 p.440)
- The remaining 60% are classified as *non-ulcer dyspepsia* (NUD, 'functional' dyspepsia)—manage as for uninvestigated dyspepsia
- *Rare causes*—oesophagitis from swallowed corrosives; oesophageal infection (especially in the immunocompromised)

Differential diagnosis: Cardiac pain (difficult to distinguish), gallstone pain, pancreatitis, bile reflux.

Presentation: Common symptoms include retrosternal or epigastric pain, fullness, bloating, wind, heartburn, nausea and vomiting. Examination is usually normal though there may be epigastric tenderness. Check for clinical anaemia, epigastric mass/hepatomegaly, and LNs in the neck.

Management: Figure 13.1

Helicobacter pylori: Infection is associated with:
- **GI disease**—peptic ulcer disease; gastric cancer; non-ulcer dyspepsia; oesophagitis
- **Non-GI disease**—ranging from cardiovascular disease and haematological malignancy to cot death

Testing for H. pylori [N]: 'Test and treat' all patients with dyspepsia who do not meet referral criteria (Figure 13.1). In practice, choice of test is limited by availability, ease of access, and cost. Options in the community are: serology, urea breath test, and faecal antigen test. A 2wk. washout period following PPI use is necessary before testing for *H. pylori* with a breath test or a stool antigen test.

Eradication [N]: Clears 80–85% *H. pylori* infections. Options:
- **PAC$_{500}$ regimen:** Full-dose PPI (e.g. omeprazole 20mg bd) + amoxycillin 1g bd + clarithromycin 500mg bd for 1wk. *or*
- **PMC$_{250}$ regimen:** Full-dose PPI (e.g. omeprazole 20mg bd) + metronidazole 400mg bd + clarithromycin 500mg bd for 1wk.

❶ Do not re-test, even if dyspepsia remains, unless there is a strong clinical need. Re-test using a urea breath test.

Lifestyle advice: Give advice on healthy eating, weight ↓, and smoking cessation. Advise patients to avoid precipitating factors e.g. coffee, chocolate, fatty foods. Raising the head of the bed and having a main meal well before going to bed may help some people. Promote continued use of antacids/alginates.

Essential reading
NICE (2004) Management of dyspepsia in adults in primary care 🖳 http://www.nice.org.uk

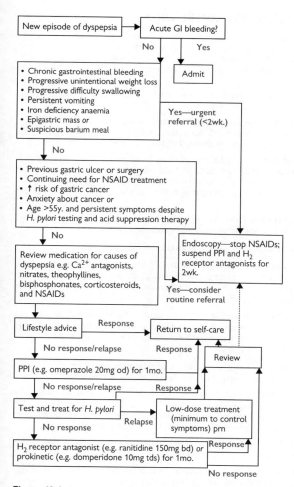

Figure 13.1 Algorithm for management of uninvestigated dyspepsia in general practice

Oesophageal conditions

Oesophagitis: Common condition. Reflux of acid from the stomach to the oesophagus causes mucosal damage resulting in inflammation and ulceration. *Other causes:* drugs (e.g. NSAIDs); infection (e.g. CMV, HSV, candida—especially in the immunocompromised); ingestion of caustic substances.

Management: Treat reflux-induced oesophagitis as for GORD (📖 p.436). Otherwise treat the cause.

Chronic benign stricture: Recurrent oesophagitis (e.g. 2° to GORD, NSAIDs, K^+ preparations) scars the oesophagus resulting in stricture formation. Most common amongst elderly women.

Presentation: Long history of reflux with more recent dysphagia. If obstruction is severe, undigested food may be regurgitated immediately after swallowing. May be associated with night-time coughing paroxysms due to aspiration of gastric contents into the chest. Examination is usually normal.

Management: Refer for urgent endoscopy to confirm diagnosis and exclude carcinoma. Treatment is by endoscopic dilatation of the stricture.

Carcinoma of the oesophagus: 📖 p.440

Presbyoesophagus: Common among the elderly. Intermittent sensation that food is getting stuck—usually at the back of the throat. Examination is normal, as is endoscopy. Barium swallow may reveal oesophageal spasm. Reassure.

Globus hystericus: Sensation of a lump in the throat without difficulty swallowing is common. It may indicate anxiety. Reassure if no organic signs and treat any dyspepsia. If not responding, refer to ENT for exclusion of an organic cause.

Oesophageal achalasia: Failure of relaxation of the circular muscles at the distal oesophagus. Peak incidence: 30–40y. ♀ slightly >♂.

Presentation: Gradual onset of dysphagia over years accompanied by regurgitation of stagnant food and foul belching. Night-time coughing fits are due to aspiration which can result in recurrent chest infections. Examination is usually normal, though may be signs of aspiration pneumonia.

Management: CXR to exclude aspiration pneumonia; endoscopy confirms diagnosis. Refer for surgery.

Plummer–Vinson syndrome: Iron deficiency anaemia + dysphagia due to a post-cricoid web in the oesophagus. ♀ > ♂. Peak incidence: 40–50y. Presents with high dysphagia with food sticking in the back of the throat ± retching/choking sensation. This is a pre-malignant condition so refer for biopsy and dilatation of pharyngeal web; replace iron. *(H.S. Plummer (1874–1936) and P.P. Vinson (1890–1959)—US physicians)*

Phanryngeal pouch: Pulsion diverticulum of the pharyngeal mucosa through Killian's dehiscence (area of weakness between the 2 parts of the inferior pharyngeal constrictor). ♂>♀; ↑ with age. Usually develops posteriorly, then protrudes to 1 side (L>R). As the pouch gets larger, the oesophagus is displaced laterally.

Presentation: Dysphagia—the first mouthful is swallowed easily, then fills the pouch, which makes further swallowing difficult. Accompanied by regurgitation of food from the pouch ± symptoms of aspiration (night-time coughing, recurrent chest infection). A swelling is palpable in the neck in $^2/_3$ of cases.

Management: Refer for further investigation. Diagnosis is confirmed with barium swallow. Treatment is surgical.

Oesophageal varices: Result from portal hypertension (📖 p.445) and can bleed massively. Admit as a 'bluelight' emergency.

Impacted oesophageal foreign body: Usually the patient notices something has stuck, resulting in pain, difficulty swallowing ± retching. If suspected, refer immediately to A&E for further investigation ± removal of the foreign body.

Oesophageal perforation: Rare—usually a complication of endoscopy. Less commonly due to violent vomiting. The patient becomes very distressed with pain relating to the site of perforation which is worse on swallowing. Examination reveals tachycardia, shock ± pyrexia ± breathlessness ± surgical emphysema in neck. Admit as a surgical emergency.

Gastro-oesophageal reflux disease and gastritis

Gastro-oesophageal reflux disease (GORD): Caused by retrograde flow of gastric contents through an incompetent gastro-oesophageal junction. It affects ~5% of the adult population.

Risk factors

- Smoking
- Alcohol
- Coffee
- Fatty food
- Big meals
- Obesity
- Hiatus hernia
- Tight clothes
- Pregnancy
- Drugs (TCAs, anticholinergics, nitrates, alendronate)
- Systemic sclerosis
- Surgery for achalasia

Conditions caused by GORD

- Oesophagitis (defined by mucosal breaks) ± oesophageal ulcer
- Benign oesophageal stricture (📖 p.434)
- Intestinal metaplasia: Barrett's oesophagus (see p.437)
- Oesophageal haemorrhage
- Anaemia

Presentation

- *Heartburn:* Most common symptom. Burning retrosternal or epigastric pain which worsens on bending, stooping, or lying, and with hot drinks. Relieved by antacids.
- *Other symptoms:*
  - Waterbrash—mouth fills with saliva
  - Reflux of acid into the mouth—especially on lying flat
  - Nausea and vomiting
  - Nocturnal cough/wheeze due to aspiration of refluxed stomach contents.
- *Examination:* Usually normal. Check for clinical anaemia, epigastric mass/hepatomegaly, and LNs in the neck.

Investigation: Endoscopy if indicated—see Figure 13.1, 📖 p.433

> ❶ Symptoms are poorly correlated with endoscopic findings. Reflux may remain silent in patients with Barrett's oesophagus but heartburn can severely affect quality of life of patients with –ve endoscopy results.

Initial management[N]

- In all cases, give lifestyle advice (📖 p.432).
- If diagnosis is clinical (i.e. patient presents with 'reflux-like' symptoms), treat as for uninvestigated dyspepsia (Figure 13.1, 📖 p.433).
- For patients with reflux confirmed on endoscopy or barium swallow, offer treatment with a PPI (e.g. omeprazole 20mg od) for 1–2mo. If oesophagitis at endoscopy and the patient remains symptomatic, double the dose of PPI for a further 1mo.
- If inadequate response to PPI, try an H_2 receptor antagonist (e.g. ranitidine 150mg bd) or prokinetic (e.g. domperidone 10mg tds) for 1mo.

Long-term management of endoscopically or barium confirmed GORD[N]

- Patients who have had dilatation of an oesophageal stricture should remain on long-term full-dose PPI therapy.
- For all other patients, if symptoms recur following initial treatment, offer a PPI at the lowest dose possible to control symptoms, with a limited number of repeat prescriptions. Discuss using the treatment on an as-required basis with patients to manage their own symptoms.
- Refer for consideration of surgery if quality of life remains significantly impaired despite optimal treatment. Surgery of any type is >90% successful, though results may deteriorate with time.

Hiatus hernia: Common (30% of over 50s). 50% have GORD. Obesity is a risk factor. The proximal stomach herniates through the diaphragmatic hiatus into the thorax.

- 80% have a 'sliding' hiatus hernia where the gastro-oesophageal junction slides into the chest.
- 20% have 'rolling' hernias where a bulge of stomach herniates into the chest alongside the oesophagus. The gastro-oesophageal junction remains in the abdomen.

Management: Treat as for GORD.

Barrett's oesophagus: Usually found incidentally at endoscopy for symptoms of GORD, and caused by chronic GORD. The squamous mucosa of the oesophagus undergoes metaplastic change and the squamo-columnar junction appears to migrate away from the stomach. The length affected varies. It carries a x40 ↑ risk of adenocarcinoma of the oesophagus, so regular endoscopy is essential. Treatment is with long-term PPIs (e.g omeprazole 20–40mg od) ± laser therapy ± resection.
(N.R. Barrett (1903–1979)—British surgeon)

Acute gastritis: Mucosal inflammation of the stomach with no ulcer.

- *Type A:* Affects the entire stomach; associated with pernicious anaemia; pre-malignant.
- *Type B:* Affects antrum ± duodenum; associated with H. pylori.
- *Type C:* Due to irritants e.g. NSAIDs, alcohol, bile reflux.

Presentation and investigation: Dyspepsia—□ p.432

Management

- Treat the cause where possible (e.g. vitamin B_{12} injections; H. pylori eradication; avoidance of alcohol)
- Acid suppression—H_2 receptor antagonist (e.g. cimetidine, nizatidine) or PPI for 4–8wk.
- Re-endoscope to confirm healing.

Complications: Haemorrhage; gastric atrophy ± gastric cancer (type A only).

Essential reading

NICE (2004) Management of dyspepsia in adults in primary care
⌨ http://www.nice.org.uk

Peptic ulceration

Peptic ulceration (PU) is a term which includes both gastric and duodenal ulceration (Table 13.1). Presents with dyspepsia (📖 p.432).

Table 13.1 Features of gastric and duodenal ulcers

	Gastric ulcer (GU)	Duodenal ulcer (DU)
Population	Typically affects middle aged/elderly ♂'s.	Typically affects young/middle-aged ♂'s, though can affect any adult. ♂>♀
Risk factors	• H. pylori (70–90% of gastric ulcer patients) • NSAID use (↑ risk 3–4x) • Delayed gastric emptying • Reflux from the duodenum (↑ by smoking)	• H. pylori (>90%) • NSAID use • Gastric hyperacidity • Rapid gastric emptying • Smoking • Stress (controversial)
Presentation	• May be asymptomatic • Epigastric pain worsened by food and helped by antacids or lying flat ± weight loss • With complications (see below)	• May be asymptomatic or spontaneously relapse and remit • Epigastric pain typically relieved by food and worse at night ± weight ↑ ± water brash (saliva fills the mouth) • With complications (see below)
Examination	In uncomplicated gastric ulceration, examination is usually normal, though there may be epigastric/left upper quadrant tenderness	In uncomplicated duodenal ulceration, examination is usually normal, though there may be epigastric tenderness
Investigation	As for dyspepsia (📖 p.432)	
Complications	• *Bleeding:* Acute GI bleeding (📖 p.1040); iron deficiency anaemia (📖 p.524) • *Perforated peptic ulcer:* DU>GU; GUs may perforate posteriorly into the lesser sac; DUs usually perforate anteriorly into the peritoneal cavity. There may not be a past history of indigestion. Presents with sudden onset severe epigastric pain which rapidly becomes generalized. When a GU perforates into the lesser sac, symptoms may remain localized or be confined to the right side of the abdomen. *Examination:* generalized peritonism with 'board-like rigidity'. *Management:* acute surgical admission. • *Pyloric stenosis in adults:* duodenal stenosis 2° to scarring from a chronic DU. Characterized by copious vomiting of food 1–2d. old. There may not be a past history of indigestion. *Examination:* if prolonged vomiting, may be evidence of dehydration ± weight ↓. Succussion splash may be audible. *Management:* surgical referral for confirmation of diagnosis and surgical relief.	

Management of peptic ulceration

For patients not taking NSAIDs

- *Eradicate* H. pylori *if present:* 📖 p.432—speeds ulcer healing and ↓ relapse. Confirm eradication has been achieved with a urea breath test (duodenal ulcer) or repeat endoscopy (gastric ulcer), and retreat if still present.
- *If* H. pylori *–ve:* Treat with full-dose PPI (e.g omeprazole 20mg od) for 1–2mo. For gastric ulcers, re-endoscope to check ulcer is healed.

For patients using NSAIDs

- Stop NSAIDs where possible. If not possible, consider changing to safer alternative (e.g. paracetamol, lowering dose of NSAID, COX2 selective NSAID) and/or adding gastric protection with a PPI or misoprostol.
- Offer full-dose PPI or H_2 receptor antagonist (H_2RA) therapy for 2mo. and, if *H. pylori* is present, subsequently offer eradication therapy.
- Check eradication with repeat endoscopy (gastric ulcer) or urea breath test (duodenal ulcer).

For all patients

- Lifestyle measures: Avoid foods (or alcohol) which exacerbate symptoms; eat little and often; and avoid eating for 3h. before bed. Stop smoking.
- If symptoms recur following initial treatment, offer a PPI at lowest dose to control symptoms, with a limited number of repeat prescriptions. Discuss using the treatment on a prn basis.
- Offer H_2RA therapy if there is an inadequate response to a PPI.
- In patients with unhealed ulcer or continuing symptoms despite adequate treatment, exclude non-adherence, malignancy, failure to detect *H. pylori*, inadvertent NSAID use, other ulcer-inducing medication, and rare causes such as Zollinger-Ellison syndrome or Crohn's disease.
- Once symptoms are controlled, review at least annually to discuss symptom control, lifestyle advice, and medication.
- Refer if gastric ulcer fails to heal or if symptoms do not respond to medical treatment. Possible surgical procedures include: gastrectomy, vagotomy and drainage procedure; highly selective vagotomy.

Zollinger–Ellison syndrome: Association of peptic ulcer with a gastrin-secreting pancreatic (rarely gastric or duodenal) adenoma— 50–60% are malignant, 10% are multiple, and 30% are associated with multiple endocrine adenomatosis (type 1). *Incidence:* 0.1% of patients with duodenal ulcer disease. Suspect in those with multiple peptic ulcers resistant to drugs, particularly if associated with diarrhoea ± steatorrhoea or a family history of peptic ulcers (or islet cell, pituitary, or parathyroid adenomas). Refer for further investigation. Treatment is with PPIs (e.g omeprazole 10–60mg bd) ± surgery. (*R.M. Zollinger (1903–1992) and E.H. Ellison (1918–1970)—US surgeons*)

Essential reading

NICE (2004) Management of dyspepsia in adults in primary care 🖥 http://www.nice.org.uk

Gastro-oesophageal malignancy

Carcinoma of the oesophagus: 99% squamous cell carcinoma; 1% adenocarcinoma (lower 1/3 of oesophagus). Most common in patients >60y. ♂ ≈ ♀. Spreads locally to adjacent structures and to the lymph system. Usually presents late, when prognosis is poor. Causes ~7000 deaths/y. in the UK.

Risk factors

- Smoking
- Alcohol
- Achalasia
- Barrett's oesophagus (📖 p.437)
- Plummer–Vinson syndrome (📖 p.434)
- Tylosis—rare, inherited disorder with hyperkeratosis of the palms; 40% develop oesophageal cancer

Presentation

- Usually presents with a short history of rapidly progressive dysphagia affecting solids initially, then solids and liquids, ± weight loss ± regurgitation of food and fluids (may be bloodstained). Retrosternal pain is a late feature.
- Examination may be normal. Look for evidence of recent weight loss, hepatomegaly, and cervical lymphadenopathy.

Management: Refer for urgent endoscopy if the diagnosis is suspected. Specialist management involves resection, radiotherapy, and/or palliation with a stenting tube e.g. Celestin tube. Tubes commonly become blocked. Palliative care (📖 p.999–1015).

Stomach cancer: Fairly common cancer in the UK causing ~7500 deaths/y. Disease affecting older people with 80% diagnosed >65y.—though peak age of diagnosis of early stage cancer is ~55y. ♂>♀ (3:1). Other risk factors include:

- Geography—common in Japan
- Blood group A
- *H. pylori* infection (though it is not clear if eradication ↓ risk)
- Atrophic gastritis
- Pernicious anaemia
- Smoking
- Adenomatous polyps
- Social class
- Previous partial gastrectomy

Presentation

- *History:* Often non-specific. Presents with dyspepsia (📖 p.432); weight ↓; anorexia; vomiting; dysphagia; anaemia; and/or GI bleeding. Have a high index of suspicion in any patient >55y. with recent onset dyspepsia (within 1y.) and/or other risk factors.
- *Examination:* Usually normal until incurable. Look for epigastric mass; hepatomegaly; jaundice; ascites; palpable, enlarged supraclavicular LN (Virchow's node); acanthosis nigricans.

Management: If suspected, refer for urgent endoscopy. In the early stages, total or partial gastrectomy may be curative. Most present at a later stage when 5y. survival <10%. Palliative care (📖 p.999–1015).

Post-gastrectomy syndromes

Abdominal fullness: A feeling of early satiety ± weight loss. Advise to take small, frequent meals.

Bilious vomiting: Vomiting of pure bile. Affects ~10% patients post-gastrectomy. Presents with intermittent sudden attacks of bilious vomiting 15–30min. after eating ± epigastric cramping pain relieved by vomiting.

Management: Usually settles spontaneously. Metoclopramide or domperidone may be helpful in the interim. If symptoms are severe or fail to settle, request surgical review. Surgical bile diversion or stomach reconstruction may alleviate symptoms.

Dumping: Abdominal distension, colic, and vasomotor disturbance (e.g. sweating, fainting) after meals. Affects 1–2% of gastrectomy patients (more common early after surgery—most settle within 6mo.). 2 types:
- *Early dumping:* Due to rapid gastric emptying. Starts immediately after a meal. Consists of sweating, flushing, tachycardia, palpitations, epigastric fullness, nausea. Occasionally, there may be vomiting, diarrhoea ± colicky abdominal pain. *Advise:* small, dry meals with restricted carbohydrate. Take drinks between meals. In severe cases, re-refer for surgery.
- *Late dumping:* Due to rapid gastric emptying → hyperglycaemia. The resultant hyperinsulinaemia causes a rebound hypoglycaemia. Starts 1–2h. after meals. Consists of faintness, sweating, tremor, and nausea. Advise patients to ↓ the sugar content of meals, rest for 1h. after each meal, and take glucose if symptoms occur. In severe cases, re-refer for surgery.

Diarrhoea post-gastrectomy: 50% of patients who have had a truncal vagotomy or gastrectomy suffer some frequency of defaecation; 5% require treatment. The diarrhoea is typically episodic and unpredictable. The exact mechanism is not clear. Treatment is with codeine phosphate or loperamide prn. Antibiotic treatment is occasionally successful—seek expert advice. Surgical measures are rarely necessary.

Anaemia: Gastrectomy can result in both vitamin B_{12} deficiency and iron deficiency anaemia. Prophylactic B_{12} injections may be advised by the operating surgeon. Many advise iron supplements for life. An annual FBC to monitor for anaemia is advisable. Treat with iron/B_{12} supplements.

Stomach cancer: Risk of stomach cancer is ↑ after partial gastrectomy (2x after 20y. and 7x after 45y.)

Further information
British Society of Gastroenterology (2002) Guidelines for the management of oesophageal and gastric cancer ◻ http://www.bsg.org.uk

Patient advice and support
British Association of Cancer United Patients (BACUP) ☎0800 800 1234
◻ http://www.bacup.org.uk

Liver disease

'Jaundice is the disease that your friends diagnose'
Aphorisms, Sir William Osler (1849–1920)

Acute liver failure: Presents with sudden onset of severe illness.

Major problems
- Jaundice
- Hypoglycaemia
- Hepatic encephalopathy—ranges from mild confusion and irritability through drowsiness and increasing confusion to coma
- Haemorrhage—due to deranged clotting factors
- Ascites—hepato-splenomegaly and ascites are not usually prominent
- Infection

Other symptoms/signs: Nausea ± vomiting; ↑ BP; foetor hepaticus (sweet smell on the breath).

Causes

In previously healthy patients

- Viral hepatitis
- Weil's disease
- Paracetamol overdose
- Halothane
- Idiosyncratic drug reactions
- Fungal/plant toxins
- Malignant infiltration

- Chemical exposure (e.g. carbon tetrachloride)
- Heatstroke
- Budd-Chiari syndrome
- Pregnancy (acute fatty liver—🕮 p.785)
- Wilson's disease
- Reye's syndrome

In patients with chronic liver disease

- Infection
- GI bleeding
- Sedation

- Diuretics and/or electrolyte imbalance
- Alcohol binges
- Constipation

Management: Admit as emergency to a hepatologist/gastroenterologist unless an expected terminal event. Prognosis is poor (<60% survive).

Gilbert syndrome: Inherited metabolic disorder causing unconjugated hyperbilirubinaemia. *Prevalence:* ~1–2%. Onset is shortly after birth, but the condition may go unnoticed for years. Jaundice occurs during intercurrent illness. ↑ bilirubin on fasting can confirm the diagnosis. Liver biopsy is normal. No treatment is required and prognosis is excellent. (*A. Gilbert (1858–1927)—French physician*)

Acute hepatitis: May be asymptomatic or present with fatigue, flu-like symptoms, fever, light stools, dark urine, and/or jaundice. *Causes:*
- Viral hepatitis (🕮 p.496)
- Alcohol
- Drugs (e.g. diclofenac, co-amoxiclav)
- Toxins

- Obstructive jaundice
- Other infections—malaria, Q fever, leptospirosis, yellow fever

Management: *Investigation:* LFTs; FBC; U&E; hepatitis serology. Treat according to cause. Admit acutely if condition is poor or rapidly deteriorating; refer for investigation if cause is unclear.

Complications: Chronic hepatitis, acute liver failure.

Chronic hepatitis: Hepatitis lasting >6mo. *Causes:*

- Viral hepatitis (B,C, and D—📖 p.496)
- Alcohol
- Drugs (e.g. nitrofurantoin, methyldopa, isoniazid)
- Chronic autoimmune hepatitis
- Primary biliary cirrhosis
- Sarcoidosis
- Wilson's disease
- Haemochromatosis
- α_1-antitrypsin deficiency

Presentation: May be asymptomatic or present with:

- Fatigue
- Right upper quadrant (RUQ) pain
- Jaundice
- Arthralgia
- Signs of chronic liver disease (gynaecomastia, testicular atrophy, clubbing, palmar erythema, leuconychia, peripheral oedema, spider naevi, portal hypertension, recurrent infection)
- Complications (acute liver failure, cirrhosis, hepatocellular carcinoma).

Management: Investigations: LFTs; FBC; U&E; hepatitis serology. Refer for specialist care.

Chronic autoimmune hepatitis: Typically presents in a young woman with chronic hepatitis. Associated with personal or family history of autoimmune disease (e.g. RA, vitiligo). Diagnosis is confirmed with liver biopsy and autoimmune markers. Long-term specialist management is required. Treatment is with steroids.

Hepatic tumours

Benign tumours: Hepatomegaly ± RUQ or an incidental finding. *Common types:* hepatic adenoma, fibroma, leiomyoma, lipoma, haemangioma, focal nodular hyperplasia (e.g. with cirrhosis). *Management:* refer to gastroenterology.

Primary malignant tumours: All are rare in the UK.

- *Hepatocellular carcinoma: Risk factors:* chronic hepatitis B; cirrhosis; UC; parasites (e.g. *Clonorchis sinensis*); COC pill (>8y. use ↑ risk ×4). *Presentation:* malaise, weight loss, anorexia, RUQ pain, jaundice (late). *Examination:* hepatomegaly ± RUQ tenderness. *Management:* USS liver. Refer to gastroenterologist. *Prognosis:* death in <6mo.
- *Cholangiocarcinoma:* Develops from the intra- or extra-hepatic tree. <10% hepatic malignancy. *Peak age:* 50–70y. *Risk factors:* UC, parasites (e.g. *Clonorchis sinensis*), congenital biliary tract disease. *Presentation:* painless jaundice (early), cachexia, abdominal pain (late). *Management:* investigate and refer as for jaundice (📖 p.270). *Prognosis:* death in 4–6mo.

2° tumours: Most common type of liver tumour, usually signalling late disease. *Presentation:* hard, enlarged, knobbly liver ± RUQ pain ± jaundice (late).

1° tumours commonly metastasizing to the liver: Lung, breast, large bowel, stomach, uterus, pancreas, carcinoid, lympoma, leukaemia.

Patient advice and support

British Liver Trust ☎01425 463080 🖳 *http://www.britishlivertrust.org.uk*

Cirrhosis and portal hypertension

Cirrhosis: The liver is replaced by fibrotic tissue and regenerating nodules of hepatocytes. *Causes:*

- Unknown (30%)
- Alcohol (25%)
- Viral hepatitis
- Primary biliary cirrhosis
- Haemachromatosis
- Wilson disease
- Budd-Chiari syndrome
- Chronic active hepatitis
- α_1-antitrypsin deficiency (autosomal recessive condition causing lung and liver disease)

Presentation: Variable. May be an incidental finding.
Symptoms/signs:

- Hepatomegaly (though liver becomes small and hard in late stages)
- Spider naevi
- Dupytrens contracture
- Palmar erythema
- Gynaecomastia
- Testicular atrophy
- Clubbing
- Xantholasma/xanthomata
- Portal hypertension
- Splenomegaly.

Late signs: Occur when the liver can no longer compensate for the damage to it—jaundice, hepatic encephalopathy, leuconychia, and oedema (due to hypoalbuminaemia).

Investigation

- *Blood:* FBC, LFTs (may be normal until late stages), γGT, U&E, Cr
- *Liver* USS

Management

- Refer to gastroenterology for expert advice
- Treat the cause where possible
- Avoid alcohol and refer to dietician for advice on nutrition
- Pruritus 2° to jaundice may respond to cholestyramine
- Give flu and pneumococcal vaccination

Complications

- Portal hypertension (± bleeding oesophageal varices)
- Encephalopathy
- Hepatocellular carcinoma
- Ascites (bacterial peritonitis complicates 1:4 cases—consider prophylaxis with ciprofloxacin)
- Renal failure

Prognosis: Very variable. ½ survive 5y.

Haemochromatosis: May be 1° or 2°.

Primary haemochromatosis: Autosomal recessive condition of excess gut absorption of iron → iron deposition in and damage to heart, liver, pancreas, joints, and pituitary. ~1:400 people are homozygous for the condition but expression of disease is highly variable. ♂>♀ (and women tend to present ~10y. later). Often an incidental finding in an asymptomatic patient or found by screening relatives of affected individuals (genetic testing or serum ferritin).
Symptoms/signs:

- Tiredness
- Arthralgia/arthritis
- Impotence and testicular atrophy
- Hepatomegaly ± signs of cirrhosis
- DM
- Cardiomyopathy
- Skin pigmentation

Investigation: Serum ferritin ↑; serum iron ↑; transferrin saturation >70%; total iron binding capacity ↓.

Management: Refer for specialist care. Diagnosis is confirmed with liver biopsy. Venesection returns life expectancy to normal.

Secondary haemochromatosis: Iron overload from frequent transfusions e.g. for haemolysis. Specialist management with desferrioxamine infusions to ↑ iron excretion is required.

Wilson disease (hepatolenticular degeneration): Rare, autosomal recessive (gene located on chromosome 13), inborn error of metabolism characterized by defective biliary copper excretion → accumulation of toxic amounts of copper in the liver, brain, kidney, and cornea. Treatment is with penicillamine. Liver transplantation is the only treatment in patients who present with acute liver failure. (*S.A.K. Wilson (1877–1937)—Scottish neurologist*)

Primary biliary cirrhosis: Slow progressive cholangio-hepatitis eventually → cirrhosis. ♀:♂ ≈ 9:1. Peak age at presentation: 45y. *Cause:* probably autoimmune. *Associations:*

- Thyroid disease
- Sjögren's syndrome
- CREST syndrome
- Coeliac disease
- Hepatic and extra-hepatic malignancy
- Pancreatic hyposecretion

Presentation: 50% are asymptomatic at presentation.

Symptoms/signs:

- Fatigue
- Pruritus
- Arthralgia
- Osteoporosis/osteomalacia
- Hirsutism
- Obstructive jaundice (late)
- Symptoms/signs of cirrhosis (above) or liver failure (📖 p.442)

Investigation: LFTs (↑Alk. Phos.; ↑ALT; ↑γGT). Liver biopsy confirms diagnosis.

Management and prognosis: Refer for specialist care. If asymptomatic, 1:3 remain symptom free over many years; the rest develop symptoms in 2–4y. Median survival is 7–10y. Liver transplant is an option. Recurrence may occur in the transplanted liver but prognosis following transplant is good.

Portal hypertension: Portal venous pressure is raised due to obstruction of the portal system before, within or after the liver. In Western countries, the most common cause is cirrhosis.

- Elevated portal venous pressure → collaterals between the portal and systemic circulation (including oesophageal varices). Usually presents with haematemesis and/or melaena from bleeding varices.
- Ascites develops if there is coexistent liver failure with hypoproteinaemia and hyperaldosteronism.
- Splenomegaly is common → thrombocytopoenia and leucopoenia.
- *Signs:* splenomegaly (80–90%), ascites, dilated veins around the umbilicus (rare), purpura, signs of chronic liver disease (jaundice, clubbing, spider naevi, palmar erythema, gynaecomastia, testicular atrophy), encephalopathy.
- Refer to gastroenterology. Specialist management is essential.

Gallbladder disease

Gallstones: Gallstones are increasingly common. 9% of 60y.-olds have them, and prevalence ↑ with age.

Other risk factors
- Gender (♀>♂)
- Body weight—prevalence ↑ with weight; also associated with rapid weight ↓
- Race—in the USA, native American > hispanic > white > black
- Affluency
- Pregnancy (and possibly HRT but not COC pill)
- Alcohol is protective
- Diet—vegetarian diet is protective.

Associated conditions
- Haemolysis
- DM
- Hypertriglyceridaemia
- Cirrhosis
- Crohn's disease
- Partial gastrectomy

Drugs which cause gallstones: Clofibrate (and other fibric acid derivatives); octreotide (somatostatin analogue).

Presentation: Gallstones are blamed for many digestive symptoms—they are probably innocent in most cases. 70% of stones in the gallbladder do not cause symptoms. Common presentations—Table 13.2.

Management of gallstones
- Advise the patient to stick to a low-fat diet.
- Refer for surgical review ± further evaluation (e.g. ERCP—endoscopic retrograde cholangiopancreatography).
- Gallstones can be removed by cholecystectomy (laparoscopic or open) or ERCP or may be dissolved with ursodeoxycholic acid (stones <5mm diameter—40% recur in <5y.) or shattered with lithotripsy (1:3 develop biliary colic afterwards).
- Persistent digestive symptoms after surgery are common (50% after cholecystectomy) and difficult to treat.

Primary cancer of the gallbladder: Rare. Usually seen in patients with a non-functioning gallbladder containing stones. Carries poor prognosis.

Patient advice and support
British Liver Trust ☎01425 463080 💻 http://www.britishlivertrust.org.uk

Table 13.2 Presentation and management of gallstone disease

	Presentation	Management
Biliary colic	Clear cut attacks of severe upper abdominal pain which may radiate → back/shoulder tip, lasting ≥ ½ h. and causing restlessness ± jaundice ± nausea or vomiting. *Examination:* Tenderness ± guarding in the right upper quadrant (↑ on deep inspiration—Murphy's sign).	*Treat* acute attacks with pethidine (50mg im/po) or diclofenac (50–100mg im/po/pr) + prochlorperazine 12.5mg im for nausea. *Admit if:* Uncertain of diagnosis, inadequate social support, persistent symptoms despite analgesia, suspicion of complications, and/or concomitant medical problems (e.g. dehydration, pregnant, DM, Addison's). *Investigate* for gallstones with abdominal USS to prove diagnosis when the episode has settled. *Differential diagnosis:* see acute abdomen (☐ p.1066). *Treat* gallstones to prevent recurrence.
Acute cholecystitis/ cholangitis	Pain and tenderness in the right upper quadrant/epigatrium ± vomiting. *Examination:* tenderness ± guarding in the right upper quadrant ± fever ± jaundice.	*Treatment:* broad spectrum antibiotic (e.g. ciprofloxacin) and analgesia as for biliary colic. *Admit if:* generalized peritonism, diagnosis uncertain, very toxic, concomitant medical problems (e.g. dehydration, DM, Addison's, pregnancy), inadequate social support, or not responding to medication *Empyema* occurs when the obstructed gallbladder fills with pus. Presents with persistent swinging fever and pain. Usually requires cholecystectomy ± surgical drainage. *Investigate* and follow-up to prevent recurrence, as for biliary colic.
Pancreatitis	☐ p.448	☐ p.448
Gallstone ileus	Occurs usually after an attack of cholecystitis. A stone from the gallbladder perforates the duodenum and impacts in the terminal ileum causing bowel obstruction.	☐ p.466
Chronic cholecystitis	Vague, intermittent, abdominal discomfort, nausea, flatulence, and intolerance of fats.	*Investigate* for gallstones with abdominal USS to prove the diagnosis. *Differential diagnosis:* reflux, IBS, upper GI tumour, PU. Refer for treatment of gallstones
Jaundice	Obstructive jaundice (☐ p.270) ± right upper quadrant pain.	☐ p.270

Pancreatic disease

Acute pancreatitis: Premature activation of pancreatic enzymes results in autodigestion and tissue damage. Most episodes are mild and self-limiting but 1:5 patients have a severe attack. Overall mortality ≈ 5–10%. May be recurrent.

Causes: In 10% patients no cause is identified.
- *Common causes (80%):* Gallstones, alcohol.
- *Rarer causes*
  - Drugs (e.g. azathioprine)
  - Trauma
  - Pancreatic tumours
  - Post-ERCP
  - Viral infection (mumps, HIV, Coxsackie B)
  - Mycoplasma infection
  - Hypercalcaemia
  - Hyperlipidaemia
  - Pancreas divisum (normal variant in 7–8% of the white population)
  - Familial pancreatitis
  - Vasculitis
  - Ischaemia or embolism
  - Pregnancy
  - End-stage renal failure

Presentation
- Poorly localized, continuous, boring epigastric pain which ↑ over ~1h.— often worse lying down ± radiation to the back (50%)
- Nausea ± vomiting

Examination
- *General:* Tachycardia, fever, shock, jaundice
- *Abdominal:* Localized epigastric tenderness or generalized abdominal tenderness; abdominal distension ± ↓ bowel sounds; evidence of retroperitoneal haemorrhage (periumbilical and flank bruising—rare)

Management: Admit as an acute surgical emergency. Prior to transfer, give analgesia with pethidine (morphine may induce spasm of the sphincter of Oddi).

Complications: Delayed complications may present in general practice— suspect if persistent pain or failure to regain weight or appetite. Complications include pancreatic necrosis; pseudocyst (localized collection of pancreatic secretions); fistula/abscess formation; bleeding, or thrombosis.

Prevention of further attacks
- Avoid factors that may have caused pancreatitis e.g. alcohol, drugs
- Advise patients to follow a low-fat diet
- Treat reversible causes e.g. hyperlipidaemia, gallstones

Chronic pancreatitis: Chronic inflammation of the pancreas results in gradual destruction and fibrosis of the gland ± loss of pancreatic function → malabsorption and DM.

Cause: Alcohol is responsible for most cases. *More rarely:* familial; CF; haemochromatosis; pancreatic duct obstruction (gallstones/pancreatic cancer); hyperparathyroidism.

Presentation

- Constant or episodic epigastric pain radiating to the back and relieved by sitting forwards
- Vomiting
- Weakness
- Jaundice
- Steatorrhoea
- Weight ↓
- DM
- Chronic poor health

Management: Refer to gastroenterology. *Treatment:*

- *Diet:* Low-fat, high-protein, high-calorie diet with fat-soluble vitamin supplements. Refer to dietician.
- *Pancreatic enzyme supplementation:* e.g. Creon capsules, pre-meals. May improve diarrhoea.
- *Alcohol abstinence.*
- *Pain control:* Provide analgesia—beware of opiate abuse. Consider referral for coeliac plexus block.
- *Surgery:* Pancreatectomy or pancreaticojejunostomy for pancreatic duct stricture, obstructive jaundice, unremitting pain, or weight loss.
- *Diabetes management:* 📖 p.404–19.

Pancreatic cancer: 1–2% of all malignancies accounting for 6500 deaths/y. in the UK. *Peak age:* 50–70y. Most cancers are adenocarcinomas. Rarely, tumours arise from exocrine or endocrine cells—these have better prognosis. $^2/_3$ pancreatic cancers occur in the head of the pancreas and compress the common bile duct → jaundice. Those in the body/tail of the gland present late. Most patients have disseminated disease at presentation.

Presentation

- Non-specific with gradual deterioration in health
- Weight ↓
- Pain—epigastric ± radiation → back—may be relieved by sitting forward
- Spontaneous venous thrombosis (thrombophlebitis migrans—📖 p.363)
- Pancreatitis
- Vomiting due to gastric outlet obstruction
- Dyspepsia

Examination: Check for weight ↓, epigastric or LUQ mass, hepatomegaly, jaundice. If jaundice is present, the gallbladder may be palpable as a small, rounded mass beneath the liver.

Management: Refer for urgent surgical assessment. Diagnosis is confirmed using a combination of USS, CT, and/or ERCP. Depending on stage at presentation, laparotomy ± resection may be attempted or palliative bypass of obstructed common bile duct. Radiotherapy and chemotherapy are not helpful. *Prognosis:* median survival after surgery is 24wk. (40wk. after Whipples procedure). Palliative care—📖 p.999–1015.

Patient advice and support

British Association of Cancer United Patients (BACUP) ☎0800 800 1234
🖥 *http://www.bacup.org.uk*

Chronic diarrhoea, malabsorption, and faecal incontinence

Chronic diarrhoea[G]: Patients' perceptions of diarrhoea vary widely. When a patient reports diarrhoea, clarify what is meant. Diarrhoea is the abnormal passage of loose or liquid stools >3x/d. When it lasts >4wk. it is 'chronic'. Chronic diarrhoea affects ~4–5% of adults in the UK. There are many causes (Table 13.3) and all patients require investigation.

Assessment: Careful history is vital. Ask about:

- *Symptoms suggestive of organic disease:* History of <3mo. duration; predominantly nocturnal or continuous (as opposed to intermittent) diarrhoea; significant weight ↓; liquid stools with blood and/or mucus.
- *Symptoms suggestive of malabsorption:* Pale and/or offensive stools/steatorrhoea.
- *Family history:* Neoplastic disease, inflammatory bowel disease, and coeliac disease.
- *Past history:* Previous surgery (especially ileal resection which can cause short bowel syndrome and cholecystectomy); pancreatic disease; systemic disease (e.g. thyrotoxicosis, DM).
- *Drugs and alcohol history:* Recent antibiotics; alcoholism; regular medications (cause 4% chronic diarrhoea).
- *Travel*

Examination: Full examination. Look for signs of systemic disease and examine abdomen for scars and masses.

Investigations
- *Blood:* FBC, ESR, Ca^{2+}, LFTs, haematinics, thyroid function tests, and coeliac serology (if available in the community).
- *Stool:* M,C&S.

Management
- If obvious identifiable cause (e.g. GI infection, constipation, drug side-effect), then treat and review. Refer to gastroenterology if treatment does not relieve symptoms.
- If symptoms suggestive of functional bowel disease and <45y. with normal investigations, irritable bowel syndrome is likely. Reassure, offer advice, and review as necessary. Refer to gastroenterology if atypical symptoms appear or the patient is unhappy with the diagnosis.
- Otherwise refer to gastroenterology for assessment. Speed of referral depends on age and severity of symptoms.

Further information
British Society of Gastroenterology (2002) Guidelines for the investigation of chronic diarrhoea (2nd edition) ▣ http://www.bsg.org.uk

Factitious diarrhoea: Responsible for 4% referrals to gastroenterology departments and 20% of tertiary referrals. Due to laxative abuse or adding of water or urine to stool samples. Difficult to spot—have a high index of suspicion, especially in patients with history of eating disorder or somatization.

Table 13.3 Causes of chronic diarrhoea

Colonic	Small bowel	Pancreatic
Colonic cancer	Crohn's disease	Pancreatic cancer
Ulcerative colitis	Coeliac disease	Chronic pancreatitis
Crohn's disease	Other enteropathies e.g. Whipple's disease	CF
Constipation with overflow diarrhoea	Bile acid malabsorption	**Other causes**
Endocrine	Ischaemia	Bowel resection
		Intestinal fistula
DM (autonomic neuropathy)	Enzyme deficiencies e.g. lactase deficiency	Drugs
Hyperthyroidism	Radiation damage	Alcohol
Hypoparathyroidism	Bacterial overgrowth	Autonomic neuropathy
Addison's disease	Lymphoma	'Factitious' diarrhoea
Hormone-secreting tumours e.g. carcinoid	Infection e.g. giardiasis, cryptosporidium	
	Irritable bowel syndrome	

Malabsorption: Presents with chronic diarrhoea, ↓ in weight, steatorrhoea, vitamin/iron deficiencies, and/or oedema due to protein deficiency. In all cases, refer to gastroenterology for investigation and treatment of the cause.

Usual causes: Coeliac disease, chronic pancreatitis, Crohn's disease.

Rarer causes: CF, pancreatic cancer, Whipple's disease, biliary insufficiency, bacterial overgrowth, chronic infection (e.g. giardiasis, tropical sprue), following gastric surgery.

Faecal incontinence: Affects ~2% of all ages, causing great personal disability. It is a common reason for carers to request placement in a nursing home. *Causes:*

- Age
- Constipation (overflow incontinence)
- Childbirth
- Anal surgery
- Rectal prolapse
- Haemorrhoids
- Inflammatory bowel disease
- After radiotherapy
- Systemic sclerosis
- Neurological disorders
- Cognitive deficit
- Congenital disorders (e.g. anal atresia, Hirschsprung's disease)
- Emotional problems (encoparesis in children—📖 p.895)

Management

- Clear any constipation.
- If symptoms are mild or infrequent, treat with loperamide or codeine phosphate, prn or continuously.
- If unsuccessful, daily enemas to empty the distal bowel together with loperamide to prevent soiling are useful.
- If symptoms are not controlled with simple measures, refer to surgeon or DN (for advice re skin care and hygiene) as appropriate. Devices such as anal plugs and faecal collectors can be useful in some situations.

Gastroenteritis/food poisoningND

Ingestion of viruses, bacteria, or their toxins commonly cause diarrhoea and/or vomiting. Affects 1:5 of the UK population each year, costing £¾ billion. Source of infection may not be clear; might be traced back to contaminated food or water or infection may spread from person-person contact (especially if personal hygiene is poor).

Prevention: Handwashing after using the toilet; longer cooking and rewarming times; prompter consumption.

Presentation
- *History:* Severity and duration of symptoms, food eaten and water drunk, time relationship between ingestion and symptoms, other affected contacts.
- *Examination:* Usually normal. Dehydration may prompt admission.

Investigation: Stool sample if:
- Diarrhoea >1wk.
- Recent return from abroad
- Food worker
- Patient lives or works in an institution e.g. residential care home
- An outbreak is suspected

Management: See diarrhoea (📖 p.255). Advise small amounts of clear fluids frequently. Only give antibiotics if recommended following stool culture (exception is giardia diarrhoea—📖 p.509). Consider admission if becoming dehydrated. Refer to gastroenterology/paediatrics if lasts >3wk. and –ve stool culture or blood in stool.

Vomiting: 📖 p.296

Traveller's diarrhoea: 📖 p.509

Further information
Health Protection Agency (HPA) Infections: Topics A-Z:—gastrointestinal disease
🖥 http://www.hpa.org.uk

Table 13.4 Common causes of gastroenteritis in the UK

Organism/ source	Incubation	Symptoms					Food
		D	**V**	**P**	**F**	**O**	
Staph. Aureus	1–6h.	✓	✓	✓		↓BP	Meat
B. cereus	1–5h.	✓	✓				Rice
C. perfringens	6–24h.	✓		✓			Meat
C. botulinum	12–36h.		✓			Paralysis	Canned food
Salmonella species	12–48h.	✓	✓	✓	✓		Meat, eggs, poultry
Shigella	48–72h.	✓		✓	✓	Blood in stool	Any food
Campylobacter	48h.–5d.	✓		✓	✓	Blood in stool	Milk, water
E. coli	12–72h.	✓		✓	✓	Blood in stool	Food, water
Y. enterocolitica	24–36h.	✓		✓	✓		Milk, water
Giardia lamblia	1–4wk.	✓					Water
Cryptosporidium	4–12d.	✓		✓	✓		Water
Listeria (Pregnant women— 📖 p.790)						Flu-like illness, pneumonia	Milk products, pâtés, raw vegetables
V. para- haemolyticus	12–24h.	✓	✓	✓			Fish
Rotavirus	1–7d.	✓	✓		✓	Malaise	Food, water
Small viruses	36–72h.	✓	✓		✓	Malaise	Any food
Entamoeba histolytica	1–4wk.	✓		✓	✓	Blood in stool	Food, water
Mushrooms	15min.–24h.	✓	✓	✓		Fits, coma, renal/liver failure	
Scrombrotoxin	10–60min.	✓				Flushes, erythema	Fish
Heavy metals e.g. zinc	5min.–2h.		✓	✓			
Red beans	1–3h.	✓	✓				

D = diarrhoea; V = vomiting; P = abdominal pain; F = fever; O = other
❶ All cases of food poisoning are notifiable diseases in the UK—📖 p.481

Coeliac disease^G

Common disorder (UK prevalence 1:300), though only a minority have clinically recognized disease. Inflammatory disease of the upper small intestine resulting from gluten ingestion. Inflammation → malabsorption. It can occur at any age but the majority are diagnosed in adulthood (peak incidence—5th decade). ♀:♂ ≈ 3:1. In children, peak incidence is ≈ 4y.
Predisposing factors:
- Genetic—1:10 chance if a 1st degree relative is affected
- Environmental—60–70% concordance in twin studies so other factors (e.g. infection, hormonal status) must intervene.

Presentation: Many patients (especially adults) have minimal or atypical symptoms. Common presentations are listed in Table 13.5. Check FBC, ESR, LFTs, and Ca^{2+} in all cases. If presenting with diarrhoea, check stool sample to exclude infective causes.

Table 13.5 Presentation of coeliac disease

Children	Adults	Associated disorders
<2y.	General lassitude (80–90%)	Dermatitis herpetiformis
Chronic diarrhoea	Anaemia (85%)	(📖 p.653)
Failure to thrive	Diarrhoea (75–80%)	Type 1 DM (📖 p.404)
Abdominal distension	Weight loss	Autoimmune thyroid
Vomiting	Constipation	disease (📖 p.422)
Typically pale and	Apthous mouth ulcers	Primary biliary cirrhosis
miserable	Sore tongue and mouth	Sjögren's syndrome
Hair thinning	Dyspepsia	IgA deficiency
	Abdominal pain/bloating	Osteoporosis
>2y.	Anxiety or depression	Epilepsy
Loss of appetite	Bone pain due to	
Diarrhoea	osteoporosis	
Constipation	Muscle wasting	
Anaemia	Neuropathies	
Short stature	Infertility	

Management

Initial management: Refer all suspected cases for specialist investigation to confirm the diagnosis.
- Endomysial antibodies—sensitivity >86% and 100% specificity in the right clinical setting. ❶ available in the community in some areas
- Small intestinal biopsy—shows villous atrophy.

Diet
- Permanent withdrawal of gluten from the diet → complete remission with symptom resolution within weeks. Explain that a gluten-free diet will be needed for life.

- Refer to a dietician for specialist dietary advice. The Coeliac Society also publishes recipes and guidelines.
- Advise patients to exclude wheat, barley, and rye cereal products. Moderate amounts of oats can be consumed, but emphasize oats must be free of other contaminating cereals.
- Prescribe adequate amounts of gluten-free products, marking the prescription 'ACBS'.
- Add supplements of deficient nutrients e.g. iron, folic acid, calcium until well established on a gluten-free diet.
- Women with coeliac disease contemplating pregnancy should take folic acid 5mg od until 12wk. gestation.

Pneumococcal vaccination: All patients with coeliac disease have a degree of hyposplenism and are more prone to pneumococcal infection. Advise patients to have pneumococcal vaccination.

Follow-up: Patients should be followed-up every 6–12mo. in a specialist clinic or by a GP under a shared care arrangement. Routine checks include: symptoms; weight; blood—Hb, B_{12}, folate, iron, albumin, Ca^{2+}, antigliadin or antiendomysial antibodies. Consider bone densitometry to exclude osteoporosis.

Failure to respond to diet: The most common reason is continued ingestion of gluten (intentional or inadvertent). Re-refer to dietician. If symptoms recur after a period of remission, re-refer to a specialist for reassessment of the diagnosis.

Complications: Osteoporosis and malignancy (lymphoma or carcinoma of the small intestine). Both are virtually eliminated by adherence to a strict gluten-free diet, but remain vigilant and refer if suspected.

Essential reading
British Society of Gastroenterology (2002) Interim guidelines for the management of patients with coeliac disease ◱ http://www.bsg.org.uk

Patient advice and support
Coeliac UK ☎0870 444 8804 ◱ http://www.coeliac.co.uk

Inflammatory bowel disease[G]

Ulcerative colitis (UC) and Crohn's disease (B.B. Crohn (1884–1983)—US gastroenterologist) are collectively termed inflammatory bowel disease.

Both are chronic, relapsing-remitting diseases characterized by acute, non-infectious inflammation of the gut. In the case of UC, inflammation is limited to the colorectal mucosa. Extent varies from disease limited to the rectum (proctitis) to disease affecting the whole colon (pancolitis). In the case of Crohn's, any part of the gut from mouth to anus can be affected with normal bowel between affected areas (skip lesions).

Cause: Cause is unknown. It is thought both diseases are the result of effects of an environmental trigger on genetically susceptible individuals Factors implicated (none proven) include: gut flora, food constituents, infections e.g. measles, mycobacterium paratuberculosis.

Presentation and investigation: Tables 13.6, 13.7, and 13.8

Differential diagnosis

- Irritable bowel syndrome
- Coeliac disease
- Anal fissure
- Gut Infection e.g. giardiasis
- Diverticulitis
- Colonic tumour
- Food-sensitive colitis (infants)
- Pseudomembranous colitis
- Ischaemic colitis
- Microscopic colitis

Table 13.6 Assessing the severity of ulcerative colitis

Severity	Symptoms
Mild	<4 liquid stools/d. Little/no rectal bleeding No signs systemic disturbance
Moderate	4–6 liquid stools/d. Moderate rectal bleeding Some signs of systemic disturbance Mild disease that does not respond to treatment
Severe	>6 liquid stools/d. Severe rectal bleeding Systemic disturbance (↑ pulse rate, pyrexia, ↑ ESR, ↑WCC, ↓Hb) Signs of malnutrition (e.g. hypoalbuminaemia) Weight loss >10%

Management: 📖 p.458

Essential reading

British Society of Gastroenterology (2004) Guidelines for the management of inflammatory bowel disease in adults 🖥 http://www.bsg.org.uk

Patient advice and support

National Association for Colitis and Crohn's disease (NACC) ☎0845 130 2233 (info); 0845 130 3344 (support) 🖥 http://www.nacc.org.uk

Table 13.7 Epidemiology of inflammatory bowel disease

	UC	Crohn's disease
Incidence	10–20/100,000/y.	5–10/100,000/y. and increasing
Prevalence	100–200/100,000	50–100/100,000
Peak age of incidence	40–60y. (85% <60y.)	
Gender	♂=♀	
Risk factors	Smoking is protective	Smoking is a risk factor

Table 13.8 Features of inflammatory bowel disease

	UC	Crohn's disease
GI symptoms	Diarrhoea + blood/mucus (stool may be solid if rectal disease only) Faecal urgency/incontinence Tenesmus Lower abdominal pain	Diarrhoea ± blood/mucus Malabsorption Abdominal pain (cramp) Mouth ulcers Bowel obstruction due to strictures Fistulae (often perianal) Abscesses (perianal and intra-abdominal)
Systemic symptoms	Tiredness and/or malaise Weight ↓ or failure to thrive/grow (children) Fever	
Associated conditions	*Joint disease*—arthritis, sacroileitis, ankylosing spondylitis—(🕮 p.576) *Eye disease*—iritis or uveitis *Skin changes*—erythema nodosum, pyoderma gangrenosum (UC>>Crohn's) *Liver disease*—autoimmune hepatitis (UC), gallstones (Crohn's), sclerosing cholangitis (UC>>Crohn's) *Miscellaneous*—thromboembolism, osteoporosis (Crohn's), amyloidosis (Crohn's)	
Examination	*Abdominal + rectal examination*—abdominal tenderness. Anal and perianal lesions (pendulous skin tags, abscesses, fistulae) and/or mass in the right iliac fossa are characteristic of Crohn's disease. *General examination*—clubbing, apthous ulcers in the mouth (Crohn's), signs of weight loss, anaemia or hypoproteinaemia.	
Investigation	*Blood*—FBC (anaemia, ↑WCC), ESR (↑ when disease is active), U&E,Cr, LFTs (including serum albumin) *Stool*—M,C&S (including *Cl. difficile*) to exclude infection *AXR*—consider to clarify extent of disease, exclude toxic megacolon or bowel obstruction, and/or identify proximal constipation *Proctoscopy*—inflammation and shallow ulceration extending proximally from the anal margin suggests UC	

Management of inflammatory bowel disease[G]

❶ A multidisciplinary approach, coordinating care in general practice with specialist gastroenterology and surgery services, is essential

Suspected diagnosis: Refer to gastroenterology for further investigation if persistent, unexplained diarrhoea lasting >4wk. with −ve stool cultures and/or persistent abdominal pain.

Ulcerative colitis: *BNF 1.5*

Active disease

- Mesalazine 2–4g daily. Topical 5-ASA derivatives are a useful adjunct if troublesome rectal symptoms.
- Add steroids (prednisolone 40mg od po + rectal preparation) if prompt response is needed or mesalazine is unsuccessful. Review frequently and ↓ dose over 8wk. Rapid withdrawal ↑ risk of relapse.
- Azathioprine is substituted if steroids are not effective, frequent steroids (≥2courses/y.), disease relapses as dose of steroid is ↓, or relapse <6wk. after stopping steroids. Requires consultant supervision. Monitoring (📖 p.575).
- Ciclosporin (consultant supervision) may be effective for severe, steroid refractory disease.

⚠ **Admit acutely if:**
- Severe abdominal pain (especially if associated with tenderness)
- Severe diarrhoea (>8x/d.) ± bleeding
- Dramatic weight loss
- Fever or other signs of systemic disease.

Maintenance treatment: Follow-up in 2° care is routine. Most patients require lifelong therapy.
- Mainstays of treatment are 5-ASA derivatives (e.g. mesalazine 1–2g/d. or balsalazide 1.5g/d.). Use a rectal formulation (e.g mesalazine 1g daily pr) if disease is confined to the rectum or descending colon. Long-term treatment ↓ risk of colonic cancer by 75%. 10% are intolerant to 5-ASA derivatives—the alternative is azathioprine (see above).
- Treat proximal constipation with stool-bulking agents or laxatives.
- NSAIDs can precipitate relapse, so avoid.

Surgery: Last resort. 20–30% of patients with pancolitis require colectomy—1:3 develop pouchitis (non-specific inflammation of the ileal reservoir) within 5y. of surgery.

Prognosis: At any time, 50% are asymptomatic, 30% have mild symptoms, and 20% have moderate/severe symptoms. <5% are free from relapse after 10y. Relapses usually affect the same part of the colon.

Crohn's disease

Active ileal and/or colonic disease
- Treat with mesalazine 4g daily.

- Add steroids (prednisolone 40mg od po or budesonide 3mg tds) if unresponsive to mesalazine. Review frequently and ↓ dose over 8wk. Rapid withdrawal ↑ risk of relapse.
- Elemental or polymeric diets for 4–6wk. can be a useful adjunct or alternative to steroid treatment—take consultant advice.
- Other medical treatments used with consultant supervision include metronidazole, azathioprine, and antitumour necrosis factor (infliximab).
- Surgery is an option if medical treatment has failed. 50% need surgery within 10y. of onset. Surgery is not curative and 50% will require a further operation at a later stage. After ileal resection, check B_{12} levels annually.

⚠ Admit acutely if:

- Severe abdominal pain (especially if associated with tenderness)
- Severe diarrhoea (>8x/d.) ± bleeding
- Dramatic weight loss
- Bowel obstruction
- Fever/other signs of systemic disease.

❶ For disease elsewhere, take specialist advice

Maintenance treatment: Follow-up in 2° care is routine. Treatment is aimed at minimizing impact of the disease.
- The most effective measure is to stop smoking.
- Mesalazine has limited benefit. It is ineffective at doses <2g daily.
- Other agents used include azathioprine, methotrexate, and intermittent courses of infliximab. All require consultant supervision.
- Treat diarrhoea symptomatically with codeine phosphate or loperamide. Cholestyramine (4g 1–3x/d.) ↓ diarrhoea due to terminal ileal disease/resection.
- NSAIDs can precipitate relapse so avoid.

Prognosis: 75% are back to work after the first year but 15% remain unable to work long term. Complications—Table 13.9.

Table 13.9 Complications of inflammatory bowel disease

UC	Crohn's
Toxic megacolon—colon distends and may perforate.	*Intra-abdominal abscess*
	Intestinal stricture—common; may require surgery
Colonic cancer—risk ↑ if disease >8y., onset in childhood/adolescence, age >45y., FH of colon cancer, extensive colitis, sclerosing cholangitis. *Prevention:* screening with colonoscopy. Frequency depends on severity of the disease and duration of symptoms.	*Toxic megacolon*—rare (see UC)
	Bowel obstruction
	Fistula formation
	Perianal disease
Sclerosing cholangitis—fibrosis and stricture of intra- and extra-hepatic bile ducts. Presents with obstructive jaundice.	*Malignancy*—large and small bowel cancer—5% 10y. after diagnosis
	Osteoporosis

❶ *psychological effects*—Both UC and Crohn's are chronic lifelong conditions which have major impact on work and domestic life. Self-help groups can be useful.

Irritable bowel syndrome

Relapsing and remitting condition of unknown cause. It is a diagnosis of exclusion, with no confirmatory test and no cure. Extremely common. Lifetime prevalence ≥ 20%, though ~75% never consult a GP. ♀>♂ (2.5:1). Symptoms can appear at any age.

Diagnosis of irritable bowel syndrome (IBS): Consistent features are abdominal pain and some form of change in bowel habit (either constipation or diarrhoea). Other bowel, urinary, and gynaecological symptoms are also common. Symptoms are often precipitated by stressful events, dietary indiscretion or GI infection. Examination is normal or there may be some abdominal distension ± tenderness, though never any guarding or rebound tenderness.

❶ The more of the following criteria present—the *less* likely there is to be organic disease:

- Abdominal distention
- Relief of pain with bowel movement
- Looser motions with the onset of pain
- Mucus
- More frequent motions with the onset of pain
- A feeling of incomplete evacuation of the rectum

Differential diagnosis

- Colonic carcinoma
- Coeliac disease
- Inflammatory bowel disease (Crohn's disease or UC)
- Pelvic inflammatory disease
- Endometriosis
- GI infection
- Thyrotoxicosis

Investigation A diagnosis of exclusion. How far to investigate is a clinical judgement weighing risks of investigation against possibility of serious disease. Judgement is based on age of the patient, family history, length of history, and symptom cluster.

- *Patients <40y.:* Investigation may be unnecessary. Consider—FBC, ESR, faecal occult blood ± sigmoidoscopy if symptoms are severe/persistent.
- *Patients >40y.:* Colonic cancer must be excluded for any patient with a change in bowel habit (🕮 p.251).
- *Other investigations to consider*
  - Thyroid function tests if other symptoms/signs of thyroid disease
  - Stool samples to exclude GI infection if diarrhoea
  - Endocervical swabs for *Chlamydia*
  - Colonoscopy to exclude inflammatory bowel disease
  - Laparoscopy to exclude endometriosis
  - Antibody testing to exclude coeliac disease.

Referral: Gastroenterology/general surgery if:

- >40y. with symptoms of recent onset—U
- Passing blood (except if from an anal fissure or haemorrhoids)—U
- Change in symptoms, especially if >40y.—U/S
- Weight loss—U/S
- Atypical features (i.e. not those listed above)—U/S/R
- Patient is unhappy to accept a diagnosis of IBS despite explanation—R

U=urgent; S=soon; R=routine.

Treatment: Reassure. Information leaflets are helpful.

Specific measures

Fibre/bulking agents: Constipation-predominant IBS. Bran can make some patients worse. Ispaghula husk is better tolerated. Lactulose is an alternative but worsens bloating.

Antispasmodics: e.g. mebeverine, peppermint oil. All equally effective. If no response in a few days, switch to another—different agents suit different individuals. Once symptoms are controlled, use prn dosing.

Antidiarrhoeal preparations: e.g. loperamide, co-phenotrope. Codeine phosphate may cause dependence. Use prn for patients with diarrhoea—predominant disease. Use pre-emptive doses to cover difficult situations (e.g. air travel).

Antidepressants: No evidence of benefit in IBS unless the patient is overtly depressed. Withdraw if no response after 4–6wk.

Dietary manipulation: Exclusion diets can be helpful in up to 50% patients (especially patients with diarrhoea—predominant disease). If a patient keeps a diary, it may be possible to identify foods which provoke symptoms. Common candidates are dairy products, citrus fruits, caffeine, alcohol, tomatoes, gluten, eggs.

Psychotherapy and hypnosis: Some effect in trials. Reserve for cases which have failed to respond to more conventional treatment.

Failure to respond to treatment: Consider another diagnosis might have been missed. Review history and examination ± refer for further investigation.

Prognosis: >50% still have symptoms after 5y.

Further information

British Society of Gastroenterologists (2000) Guidelines for the management of irritable bowel syndrome ☐ http://www.bsg.org

Patient advice and support

IBS Network ☎01543 492 192 (6–8 p.m. weekdays and 9 a.m.–12 noon on Saturdays) ☐ http://www.ibsnetwork.org.uk

Hernias

Differential diagnosis of groin lumps: Groin lumps—📖 p.265

> **Irreducible hernia**
> - Most types of hernia may become irreducible.
> - It may be the 1st presentation of a hernia or a complication of a longstanding hernia.
> - If obstructed (incarcerated) or strangluated (blood supply to bowel contained within the hernia sac is compromised), the hernia is tender and there are symptoms/signs of small bowel obstruction.
> △ In all cases, if you are unable to reduce a hernia, admit urgently for surgical assessment.

Inguinal hernia: Protruberance of peritoneal contents through the abdominal wall where it is weakened by the presence of the inguinal canal. Common condition (♂>♀) which can occur at any age.

Presentation: Presents with a lump in the groin ± discomfort or straining or standing for any length of time. There may be a distinct precipitating event (e.g. heavy lifting). *Risk factors:* chronic cough (e.g. COPD); constipation; urinary obstruction; heavy lifting; ascites; previous abdominal surgery. *2 types:*
- *Indirect (80%):* Follow the course of the spermatic cord or round ligament down the inguinal canal through the internal inguinal ring (located at the mid-point of the inguinal ligament, 1.5cm above the femoral pulse) and sometimes out through the external inguinal ring into the scrotum/vulva.
- *Direct (20%):* Pass through a defect in the abdominal wall into the inguinal canal. Rare in children and more common in the elderly.

Examination: Examine the patient standing up. Look for a bulge in the groin above the line of the inguinal ligament. Unless incarcerated, the lump should have a cough impulse. Check you are able to reduce it (sometimes it is easier the patient lies down; ask the patient to do it if you can't).

Management
- *Conservative:* Small hernias often require no treatment other than reassurance. Trusses can be useful for symptomatic hernias in elderly patients, those unfit for surgery, or whilst awaiting surgery (may be prescribed on FP10).
- *Referral:* For surgical repair. Various methods are used—all have a high level of success (<2% recurrence rate).

Femoral hernia: Less common than inguinal hernias. ♀>♂. The patient is usually elderly, though a femoral hernia can occur at any age. The peritoneal contents protrude down the femoral canal. Risk of strangulation is high.

Presentation: Presents as a painful lump in the groin and/or small bowel obstruction.

Examination: There is a rounded swelling medially in the groin and lateral to the pubic tubercle. If reducible, a soft palpable lump remains after reduction.

Management: Always refer for urgent surgical repair. Admit as surgical emergency if obstructed or irreducible.

Incisional hernia: Breakdown of the muscle closure in an abdominal wound some time after surgery. There may be a history of wound sepsis, haematoma, or breakdown.

Presentation: Presents with a bulge at the site of the operation scar ± discomfort.

Examination: The hernia is usually visible when the patient stands—it can be made more obvious by asking the patient to cough or raise straight leg whilst lying flat. The margins of the muscular defect are palpable under the skin. Note whether fully reducible or not.

Management: Often reassurance suffices. If obstructed/strangulated or causing discomfort refer for surgical assessment.

Umbilical hernia: Most common in infants (📖 p.840). In adults, para-umbilical hernias, presenting as a bulge adjacent to the umbilicus, may occur due to weakness in the linea alba. ♀>♂.

Management: Refer for surgical assessment. Usually repaired, as risk of strangulation is high. Admit as a surgical emergency if obstructed or irreducible.

Epigastric hernia: Midline hernia through a defect in the linea alba above the umbilicus. Never contains bowel. Usually symptomless, though occasionally causes epigastric pain ± vomiting. *Examination:* epigastric mass with cough impulse.

Management: Refer for surgical repair.

Spigelian hernia: A hernial sac protrudes lateral to the rectus sheath midway between umbilicus and pubic bone. Presents with discomfort ± vomiting. Refer for surgical repair.

Obturator hernia: Hernia protrudes out from the pelvis through the obturator canal. Usually presents with strangulation ± pain referred to the knee. Admit for surgery.

Richter hernia: A knuckle of the side wall of the gut gets caught in a hernia sac and becomes strangulated, but the bowel is not obstructed. Presents with abdominal pain which rapidly becomes worse ± shock. *(A.G Richter (1742–1812)—German surgeon)*

Conditions affecting the small bowel

Acute appendicitis: Most common surgical emergency in the UK—lifetime incidence ≈ 6%. Peak age: 10–30y.

Presentation
- Central abdominal colic progresses and localizes in the RIF, becoming worse on movement (especially coughing, laughing)
- Anorexia
- Dysuria
- Nausea ± vomiting
- Rarely, diarrhoea.

Examination
- Discomfort on walking (tend to walk stooped)
- Discomfort on coughing
- Flushed and unwell
- Pyrexia (~37.5°C)
- Furred tongue and/or foetor oris
- Tenderness and guarding in the right iliac fossa (especially over McBurney's point—2/3 of the distance between the umbilicus and anterior superior iliac spine)
- Pain in the right iliac fossa on palpation of the left iliac fossa (Rovsing's sign)
- Rectal examination—tender high on the right
- Vaginal examination—no cervical excitation but may be tender on the right.

Investigation: Urinalysis—NAD or trace of blood.

Differential diagnosis
- UTI
- Diverticulitis
- Food poisoning
- Mesenteric adenitis
- Ectopic pregnancy
- Salpingitis
- Torsion of the right ovary
- Cholecystitis
- Perforated peptic ulcer
- Crohn's disease.

Management: Admit as a surgical emergency—expect to be wrong ~½ the time.

Complications
- Generalized peritonitis 2° to perforation
- Appendix abscess
- Appendix mass
- Female infertility

⚠ Symptoms and signs may be atypical—especially if the patient is very young or very old. In pregnancy, pain is typically higher (📖 p.796). If unsure of diagnosis and the patient is well, either arrange to review a few hours later or ask the patient/carer to contact you if any deterioration or change in symptoms occurs.

Meckel's diverticulum: Remnant of the attachment of the small bowel to the embryological yolk sac. It is 2 inches long, ~2 foot (100cm) proximal to the appendix, and present in 2% of the population. A Meckel's diverticulum may not cause any problems or cause an appendicitis-like picture, acute intestinal obstruction, or GI bleeding. Symptoms can occur at any age but are most common in children. (J.F. Meckel (1781–1833)—German anatomist)

Intussusception: 📖 p.858

Crohn's disease: 📖 p.456

Coeliac disease: 📖 p.454

Intestinal obstruction and ischaemia: 📖 p.466

Whipple's disease: A cause of malabsorption which usually occurs in ♂>50y. *Other features:* arthralgia, pigmentation, weight ↓, lymphadenopathy, ± cerebellar or cardiac signs. *Cause: Tropheryma whippelii. Management:* refer for gastroenterological assessment. Jejunal biopsy is characteristic. *Treatment:* co-trimoxazole or prolonged tetracycline may bring a remission. (G.H. Whipple (1878–1976)—US pathologist)

Peutz–Jeghers syndrome: Autosomal dominant disorder. Benign intestinal (usually small intestine) polyps in association with dark freckles on lips, oral mucosa, face, palm, and soles. May cause GI obstruction or GI bleeding. Malignant change occurs in ≈3%. (J.L.A. Peutz (1886–1957)—Dutch physician; H. Jeghers (1904–90)—US physician)

Adhesions: Adhesions arise as a result of intra-abdominal inflammation. Bowel loops become adherent to each other, omentum, mesentery and abdominal wall. Fibrous bands may form, connecting adjacent structures. *Causes:* surgery; intra-abdominal sepsis (e.g. appendicitis, cholecystitis, salpingitis); inflammatory bowel disease; endometriosis.

Presentation: Variable—abdominal pain; bowel obstruction.

Management: Refer to a surgeon. Treatment is difficult as any surgery will result in new adhesions; conservative management with analgesia and stool softeners is preferred. Open or laparoscopic division of adhesions is occasionally necessary.

Carcinoid syndrome: Carcinoid tumours are normally in the small bowel—rarely in the bronchus, testis, or ovary. Carcinoid tumours cause release of hormones (serotonin, kinins, prostaglandin, and histamine) resulting in:
- Flushing attacks—often precipitated by alcohol
- Diarrhoea
- Episodic bronchospasm
- Pulmonary stenosis ± tricuspid incompetence ± CCF.

❶ Symptoms normally appear only after hepatic metastasis.

Management: Refer for specialist care (gastroenterology). Admit immediately if any sudden worsening of symptoms as carcinoid crisis is life-threatening. *Median survival:* 5–8y. from diagnosis (though may be much longer).

Conditions affecting the large bowel

Intestinal obstruction: Blockage of the bowel due to either mechanical obstruction or failure of peristalsis (ileus).
Causes:
- *Obstruction from outside the bowel:* Adhesions or bands; volvulus; invasion by neighbouring malignancy (e.g. bladder, ovary); obstructed hernia (📖 p.462).
- *Obstruction from within the bowel wall:* Tumour; infarction; congenital atresia; Hirschsprung's disease (📖 p.841); inflammatory bowel disease (📖 p.456); diverticulitis.
- *Obstruction in the lumen:* Impacted faeces/constipation (📖 p.472); bolus obstruction (e.g. swallowed foreign body); gallstone ileus; intussusception (📖 p.858); large polyps.
- *Ileus/functional obstruction:* Post-op; electrolyte disturbance; uraemia; DM; back pain; anticholinergic drugs.

Presentation
- Anorexia; nausea; vomiting (may be faeculent) gives relief; colicky central abdominal pain and distension; absolute constipation for stool and gas (though if high obstruction, constipation may not be absolute).
- *Examination:* Uncomfortable and restless; abdominal distension ± tenderness (though no guarding/rebound); active tinkling bowel sounds or quiet/absent bowel sounds (later).

Management: Admit as surgical emergency.

Ischaemic bowel: Interruption of the blood supply of the bowel.
- *1° ischaemia:* Usually due to either mesenteric embolus from the right side of the heart or venous thrombosis and typically occurs in elderly patients who might have pre-existing heart or vascular disease.
- *2° ischaemia:* Usually due to intestinal obstruction (e.g. strangulated hernia, volvulus, intussusception).

Presentation: Sudden onset of abdominal pain which rapidly becomes severe. There may be a history of pain worse after meals prior to this event (mesenteric angina). *Examination:* Very unwell; shocked; may be in AF; generalized tenderness but normally no guarding/rebound. Often signs are out of proportion to symptoms.

Management: Give opiate analgesia. Admit as surgical emergency.

Sigmoid volvulus: Occurs in people who have redundant colon on a long mesentery with a narrow base. The sigmoid loop twists causing intestinal obstruction. The loop may become ischaemic. Risk factors: constipation, laxatives, tranquillisers.

Presentation: Acute onset of abdominal distension and colicky abdominal pain with complete constipation and absence of flatus. There may be a history of repeated attacks.

Management: Admit acutely to hospital. Treatment is release by passing a flatus tube and/or surgery. Once the condition has been treated, ↓ recurrences by preventing constipation and stopping tranquillisers if possible.

Carcinoma of the colon: 📖 p.468
Inflammatory bowel disease: 📖 p.456
Diverticulitis: Common condition of the colon associated with muscle hypertrophy and ↑ intraluminal pressure. Mucosa-lined pouches are pushed out through the colonic wall, usually at the entry points of vessels. These pouches are the diverticula. 95% are in the sigmoid colon, though they may occur anywhere in the bowel. They are present in >$\frac{1}{3}$ of people >60y. in the UK. *Risk factors:* include low-roughage diet and age. Diverticular disease implies the diverticula are symptomatic—Table 13.10.

Table 13.10 Presentation and management of diverticular disease

	Presentation	Management
Chronic diverticulitis (painful diverticular disease)	Presents with altered bowel habit, abdominal pain (often colicky and left sided), nausea, and flatulence. Symptoms are often improved by defaecation.	Investigate for change in bowel habit (📖 p.251). Once diverticular disease is confirmed, treat with high-fibre diet ± antispasmodics (e.g. mebeverine 135mg tds). Refer if severe symptoms.
Acute diverticulitis	Presents with: <ul><li>Altered bowel habit</li><li>Colicky left-sided abdominal pain—may become continuous and cause guarding/peritonism in the left iliac fossa</li><li>Fever</li><li>Malaise ± nausea</li><li>Flatulence</li></ul> ❶ There may be few abdominal signs in the elderly	Treat with oral antibiotics (e.g. co-amoxiclav 250mg tds or cefaclor 250–500mg tds and metronidazole 400mg bd or ciprofloxacin 500–750mg bd). There may also be some benefit from a low-residue diet. If severe symptoms, uncertain diagnosis, or not settling, admit as an acute surgical emergency.
Diverticular abscess	Presents with swinging fever, general malaise ± other localizing symptoms e.g. pelvic pain.	Refer for urgent surgical assessment/admit as a surgical emergency.
Perforated diverticulum	Presents with ileus, peritonitis, and shock.	Admit as an acute surgical emergency.
Fistula formation	A fistula may form if a diverticulum perforates into bladder, vagina, or small bowel (📖 p.196).	Refer for surgical assessment. Treatment is usually with surgery.
Haemorrhage from a diverticulum	Common cause of rectal bleeding—usually sudden and painless.	Gain IV access. Admit as an acute surgical emergency (📖 p.1040).
Post-infective stricture	Fibrous tissue formation following infection can cause narrowing of the colon → sub-acute obstruction (📖 p.466).	Keep stool soft. If recurrent problems, refer for surgery.

Anal conditions: 📖 p.474

Colorectal cancer

Lifetime risk: 1:25. Incidence ↑ with age—99% occur in people >40y. and 85% in people >60y.

Risk factors: FH (if 1x 1st degree relative, risk ↑ x2–3); UC; Crohn's disease; previous colorectal cancer (at risk of 2nd primary).

Screening: Patients presenting with tumour confined to the bowel wall have >90% long-term survival. If tumour is detected when invasion through the bowel wall to the local LNs has occurred, <10% survive long term. However, most tumours are detected at advanced stages and overall 5y. survival ≈40%. Screening with faecal occult blood testing to detect cases earlier ↑ survival rates[R], and a screening programme is likely in the next few years (📖 p.161).

⚠ **Red flag symptoms/signs:** Refer all suspected cases for *urgent* surgical assessment:
- **All ages:** Refer if:
  - Definite, palpable right-sided mass
  - Definite, palpable rectal (not pelvic) mass
  - Rectal bleeding with change in bowel habit to more frequent defaecation or looser stools (or both) persistent over ≥6wk.
  - Iron deficiency anaemia (Hb <110g/l in men; <100g/l in post-menopausal women) without obvious cause.
- **>50y. or younger patients with FH of ≥1 1st degree relative who had colorectal cancer age <55y. or 2 1st degree relatives with the disease at any age:** Refer if:
  - Rectal bleeding persistently without anal symptoms
  - Change in bowel habit to more frequent defaecation or looser stools (or both) without rectal bleeding and present ≥6wk.
- **Younger patients:** If no FH and normal examination, treat rectal bleeding without anal symptoms and/or change in bowel habit symptomatically but refer if symptoms persist.

2° care management: Treatment is usually surgical—procedure depends on the site of the lesion. Once successfully treated, younger patients are followed-up with 5-yearly colonoscopy until aged 70y.

1° care management: Once diagnosis has been made offer:
- *Support and advice*—explanation of the condition and reinforcement of information; advice on benefits, self-help groups; need for relatives to have genetic advice/screening; provision of stoma products if needed.
- *Active treatment*—much chemotherapy for colorectal cancer is given on an out-patient basis. The PHCT may become involved if there are problems with side-effects or delivery of the chemotherapy. Liaise with hospital services as needed.
- *Palliative care*—📖 p.999–1015
- *Monitoring for recurrence*—mostly done in 2° care but there is evidence that effective monitoring can be undertaken in 1° care with suitable training. Even if 2° care monitoring is in progress, remain vigilant for recurrences and re-refer urgently if suspected.

- *Referral of relatives for screening*
  - If FH of familial adenomatous polyposis, juvenile polyposis, Peutz-Jehger's syndrome, hereditary non-polyposis colorectal cancer, >2 1st degree relatives with history of colorectal cancer, or family history of the MMR oncogene. Refer for specialist follow-up and genetic counselling.
  - If 2 1st degree relatives with a history of colorectal cancer or a 1st degree relative with a history of colorectal cancer aged <45y.— refer for colonoscopy at presentation or aged 35–40y., whichever is later. Repeat colonoscopy aged 55y.

Adenomatous polyps: Bowel cancers arise from these polyps over many years. All polyps are removed due to risk of malignant change. Follow-up surveillance with repeated colonoscopy may be necessary depending on the number of polyps and their size (>1cm diameter polyps are associated with higher risk of malignant change).

Familial colorectal cancer

Familial adenomatous polyposis (FAP): 0.5% of all colorectal cancers. Lifetime risk of death from colorectal cancer is 1:2.5 if untreated. Patients usually develop cancer <40y. of age, so all affected patients require annual sigmoidoscopy from puberty ± prophylactic total colectomy if polyps develop. Refer for long-term specialist surgical follow-up. Refer relatives for genetic counselling.

Juvenile polyposis: Lifetime risk of death from colorectal cancer is 1:3. All affected patients require annual sigmoidoscopy from puberty ± prophylactic total colectomy. Refer for long-term specialist surgical follow-up. Refer relatives for genetic counselling.

Hereditary non-polyposis colorectal cancer (HNPCC): Patients with ≥3 family members with colorectal cancer where ≥2 generations have been affected and ≥1 affected family member developed the disease <50y. of age, have a 40% lifetime risk of colorectal cancer. Refer for specialist surgical follow-up with regular colonoscopy. Refer high-risk relatives for genetic counselling.

Further information

DoH (1997 + updates) Manual of colorectal cancer ▣ www.dh.gov.uk
British Society of Gastroenterology (2002) Summary of recommendations for colorectal cancer screening and surveillance in high risk groups ▣ http://www.bsg.org.uk
SIGN (2003) Management of colorectal cancer ▣ http://www.sign.ac.uk

Patient advice and support

British Association of Cancer United Patients (BACUP) ☎0800 800 1234 ▣ http://www.bacup.org.uk
British Colostomy Association ☎0800 328 4257 ▣ http://www.bcass.org.uk

Patients with ostomies

The first iatrogenic stoma was constructed in France in 1776 for an obstructing rectal cancer. Stomas (from the Greek meaning 'mouth') may be temporary or permanent.

Table 13.11 The 3 main types of stoma

Colostomy	Ileostomy	Urostomy
Age: Most >50y.	*Peak age range:* 10–50y.	*Age:* Most >50y.
Output: Depends on site: • transverse colostomy—soft stool • descending/sigmoid colostomy—formed stool	*Output:* Soft/fluid stool	*Output:* Urine—continent procedures using bowel to fashion a bladder which is then drained with a catheter through the stoma are becoming common
Reasons for colostomy Carcinoma Diverticular disease Trauma Radiation enteritis Bowel ischaemia Hischprung's disease Congenital abnormalities Obstruction Crohn's disease Faecal incontinence	*Reasons for ileostomy:* Ulcerative colitis Crohn's disease Familial polyposis coli Obstruction Radiation enteritis Trauma Bowel ischaemia Meconium ileus Carcinoma	*Reasons for urostomy:* Carcinoma Urinary incontinence Fistulas Spinal column disorders

Common problems

Psycho-social problems: Self-help groups provide information and tips on lifestyle and stoma care; specialist stoma nurses can provide support and counselling.

Stoma retraction: Can → leakage and severe skin problems. Most common reason for re-operation. Refer for specialist advice.

Prolapse: Seen most frequently with loop colostomy. If persists and disrupts pouching, refer for consideration of revision.

Peristomal hernia: Common complication. Symptomatic cases require referral for repair.

Stenosis: Narrowing of the stoma may result in difficulty or pain passing stool and/or obstruction. If problematic refer for revision.

Skin complications: Skin irritation can be due to:
• leakage onto the skin
• allergic reactions to the adhesive material in a skin barrier
• fungal infection
• inadequate hygiene.

Prevention of skin complications
- Advise patients to clean, rinse, and pat the skin dry between pouch changes
- Avoid using an oily soap, which can leave a film that interferes with proper adhesion of the skin barrier
- Ensure the pouch system fits
- Treat any infection with oral antibiotics and/or oral or topical antifungals
- Apply skin barrier cream
- If the skin is uneven (e.g. due to scarring), fill irregularities with stoma paste to give a better fit
- Consider the use of convex discs or stoma belts (refer to specialist stoma nurse for advice).

Drugs: Enteric-coated and modified-release preparations are unsuitable for people with bowel stomas—particularly for patients with ileostomy.

Diet
- Avoid foods that cause intestinal upset or diarrhoea.
- In the case of descending/sigmoid colostomy, avoid foods that cause constipation. If constipation does occur, ↑ fluid intake and/or dietary fibre.
- Certain foods (e.g. beans, cucumbers, and carbonated drinks) can cause gas, along with certain habits such as talking or swallowing air while eating, using a straw, breathing through the mouth, and even chewing gum.
- A daily portion of apple sauce, cranberry juice, yogurt, or buttermilk can help control odour. If odour is strong and persistent, consider use of charcoal filters.

Activities: Advise patients to avoid rough contact sports and heavy lifting as these might → herniation around the stoma. Patients with stomas may swim. Water will not enter a stoma due to peristalsis, so stomas do not need to be covered when bathing.

Travel: Advise patients to pack sufficient supplies of their stoma products and carry supplies with them in case baggage is misplaced. Avoid storing supplies in a very hot environment as heat may damage pouches.

❶ In all cases, liaise with a specialist stoma nurse if possible.

Patient advice and support
British Colostomy Association ☎0800 328 4257 ▣ *http://www.bcass.org.uk*

Constipation

3 million GP consultations/y. are due to constipation and 1:5 people believe they are constipated.

Definition: 2 or more of the following for ≥3mo.:

- Straining at defaecation ≥ ¼ of the time
- A sensation of incomplete evacuation ≥¼ of the time
- ≤2 bowel movements/wk.
- Lumpy and/or hard stools ≥¼ of the time

❶ Most patients consulting in general practice do not meet these criteria.

Young patients with lone constipation: ♀:♂≈9:1.

Assessment

- Establish symptoms—constipation is usually longstanding in this group
- Include drug history
- Ask about health beliefs—80% believe their bowels should open daily
- Explore concerns about underlying disease
- If longstanding, ask why the patient is consulting now
- Examine the abdomen
- Only investigate if symptoms/signs suggestive of organic disease (Table 13.12).

Management: Treat organic causes. Otherwise:

- *Mild symptoms:* Reassure.
- *More severe symptoms*
  - Lifestyle advice—↑ fluid intake, exercise regularly, add fibre to diet (helps 50%) e.g. add 3 tablespoons of coarse bran to food daily.
  - If lifestyle advice alone fails, start an osmotic laxative e.g. magnesium hydroxide 15mls bd.
  - If an osmotic laxative fails, try a short course of stimulant laxative e.g. senna 1–2 tablets at 5p.m. Long-term use of some stimulant laxatives is reported to cause cathartic atonic colon. Although there is no evidence senna causes this, in young, fit patients only use short courses or use intermittently e.g twice weekly.
  - If still constipated, specialist referral is warranted.

Irritable bowel syndrome with constipation: 20% develop symptoms of irritable bowel syndrome (IBS) in their lifetime (📖 p.460). Constipation is the predominant symptom in 30%. Other symptoms are usually present.

Assessment

- Establish symptoms
- Examine the abdomen
- Investigation is usually unnecessary, unless atypical features

Management: If <40y., examination is normal, and constipation is associated with abdominal pain that is relieved by opening bowels, IBS can be diagnosed. Manage as for young patients with lone constipation but avoid osmotic laxatives as they make bloating worse.

Table 13.12 Organic causes of constipation

Colonic disease	Carcinoma	Stricture
	Diverticular disease	Intussusception
	Crohn's disease	Volvulus
Anorectal disease	Anterior mucosal prolapse	Anal fissure
	Distal proctitis	Perianal abscess
Pelvic disease	Ovarian tumour	Endometriosis
	Uterine tumour	
Endocrine/metabolic disorders	Hypercalcaemia	DM with sutonomic neuropathy
	Hypothyroidism	
Drugs	Opioids	Antiparkinsonian drugs
	Antacids containing calcium or aluminium	Anticholinergics
	Antidepressants	Anticonvulsants
		Antihistamines
	Iron	Calcium antagonists
Other	Pregnancy	Poor fluid intake
	Immobility	

Constipation in the over 40s: Any change in bowel habit should always be taken seriously and investigated, if appropriate.

Assessment
- Establish symptoms and onset. Specifically, ask about tenesmus, blood in stool, abdominal pain, and diarrhoea.
- Check current medication.
- Examine the abdomen for masses and hepatomegaly. Rectal examination is essential to exclude low rectal or anal carcinoma and detect faecal impaction.
- Check FBC, ESR, renal function tests, LFTs, TFTs, and serum glucose.
- Image the lower bowel by colonoscopy or barium enema.

> ❶ Occult presentations of constipation are common in the very elderly and include confusion, urinary retention, abdominal pain, overflow diarrhoea, loss of appetite, and nausea.

Management: Treat any reversible, underlying organic cause—Table 13.12. Treat symptomatically if no cause is found or the underlying cause is untreatable:
- *Constipation:* Treatment with stimulant laxatives in combination with bulking agents e.g. Fybogel is more effective at increasing stool frequency than osmotic laxatives, and at lower cost. Long-term use of stimulant laxatives including co-danthrusate is acceptable in the very elderly. Otherwise, use prn or intermittently.
- *Faecal impaction:* Treat with glycerol suppositories if the mass is hard, followed by phosphate or bisocodyl enemas.

Anal conditions

Anal fissure: The anal mucosa is torn—usually on the posterior aspect of the anal canal. May occur at any age.

Presentation: Pain on defaecation ± constipation ± fresh rectal bleeding ('blood on toilet paper'). The fissure is often visible as is a 'sentinel pile' (bunched up mucosa at the base of the tear). Rectal examination is extremely tender due to muscle spasm.

Management: Soften stool (e.g. bran, Fybogel); analgesic suppositories (e.g. 5% lignocaine ointment; OTC haemorrhoid preparations). If unsuccessful, add glyceryl trinitrate ointment (0.2–0.3%) which relieves pain and spasm but may cause headache. If interventions fail, refer to surgeon.

Haemorrhoids ('piles'): Common in all age groups from mid-teens onwards. Represent distention of the submuscosal plexus of veins in the anus. 3 main groups situated at 3, 7, and 11 o'clock positions (relative to the patient viewed in lithotomy position). *Risk factors:* constipation; FH; varicose veins; pregnancy; ↑ anal tone (cause not understood); pelvic tumour; portal hypertension. *Classification:*
- *1st degree:* piles remain within the anal canal.
- *2nd degree:* prolapse out of anal verge but spontaneously reduce.
- *3rd degree:* prolapse out of anus and require digital reduction.
- *4th degree:* permanently prolapsed.

Presentation: Discomfort or discharge ± fresh red rectal bleeding (blood on toilet paper, coating stool, or dripping into pan after defaecation); feeling of incomplete emptying of the rectum; mucus discharge; pruritus ani. *Rectal examination:* prolapsing piles are obvious; 1st degree piles are not visible or palpable.

Management: If piles are not obvious on examination, arrange proctoscopy ± sigmoidoscopy for all patients >40y.. *Treatment:* soften stool (bran, Fybogel) and recommend topical analgesia (e.g. lignocaine 5% ointment or OTC preparation). If not responding to treatment, uncertainty over diagnosis, or severe symptoms (e.g. soiling of underwear), refer for surgical assessment.

Complications
- *Strangulation:* circulation to the pile is obstructed by the anal sphincter. Results in intense pain and anal sphincter spasm. Treat with analgesia. If severe pain or symptoms not settling, may require admission.
- *Thrombosis:* pain and anal sphincter spasm. Treat with analgesia, ice packs, and bed rest—consider referral for surgery to prevent recurrence.

Perianal haematoma (thrombosed external pile): Due to a ruptured superficial perianal vein → a subcutaneous haematoma. Presents with sudden onset of severe perianal pain. A tender, 2–4mm 'dark blue berry' under the skin adjacent to the anus is visible. Treat with analgesia. Settles spontaneously over ~1wk. If <1d. old can be evacuated via a small incision under LA.

Rectal prolapse: Occurs in 2 age groups—the very young (📖 p.856) and those >60y. In adults there are 2 types:

• *Mucosal:* Bowel musculature remains in position but redundant mucosa prolapses out of the anal canal. Occurs in adults with 3rd degree piles.
• *Complete:* Descent of the upper rectum into the lower anal canal. Usually due to weak pelvic floor from childbirth. The whole bowel wall is inverted and passed out through the anus. There may be associated uterine prolapse.

Presentation: Often presents late with a mass coming down through the anus ± anal discharge.

Management: Refer for surgery. For patients unfit for surgery, a supporting ring is occasionally used.

Perianal abscess: Usually caused by infection arising in a perianal gland. Tends to lie between the internal and external sphincters and points towards the skin at the anal margin. May affect patients of any age and presents with gradual onset of perianal pain which becomes throbbing and severe; defaecation and sitting are painful—characteristically patients sit with one buttock raised off the chair. Examination may reveal the abscess in the skin next to the anus. Refer for as an acute surgical emergency for drainage.

Perianal fistula: Abnormal connection between the lumen of the anus (or rectum) and skin. Usually develops from perianal abscess. Fistulas are either 'high' (open into the bowel above the deep external anal sphincter) or 'low' (open into the bowel below this point). High fistulae are rare and usually due to UC, Crohn's disease, or tumour—they are more complex to repair. Presents with persistent perianal discharge and/or recurrent abscesses. The external opening is usually visible lateral to the anus; the internal opening may be palpable on rectal examination. Refer for surgical repair.

Pilonidal sinus: Obstruction of a hair follicle in the natal cleft. The ingrowing hair triggers a foreign body reaction → pain, swelling, abscess, and/or fistula formation ± foul smelling discharge. *Management:* refer for surgery.

Anal ulcers: Rare. Consider Crohn's disease, syphilis, tumour.

Anal cancer: Squamous cell cancer. *Risk factors:* anal sex, syphilis, anal warts. *Presentation:* bleeding, pain, anal mass or ulcer, pruritus, stricture, change in bowel habit. *Management:* refer for urgent surgical review and confirmation of diagnosis. Treatment is usually with a combination of radiotherapy ± chemotherapy.

Other relevant pages

Infectious disease

⚠Throughout this chapter ND indicates notifiable disease

Immunization

> 'It is every child's right to be protected against infectious diseases. No child should be denied immunization without serious thought as to the consequences, both for the individual child and for the community.'
> Department of Health *Immunization against infectious disease*, 1996

Immunity can be induced in 2 ways

- *Active immunity:* Induced using inactivated or attenuated live organisms or their products. Act by inducing cell-mediated immunity and serum antibodies. Generally long-lasting.
- *Passive immunity:* Results from injection of human immunoglobulin. The protection afforded is immediate but lasts only a few weeks.

Storage of vaccines: Manufacturers' recommendations for storage must be observed. Do not store vaccines in the door of a vaccine fridge and make sure there is a maximum and minimum thermometer in the fridge. Record readings regularly and discard vaccines if not stored at the correct temperature.

Giving immunizations: Only GPs and nursing staff suitably trained should give immunizations.

- Check immunization is necessary
- Check the patient is fit and well
- Check that consent has been obtained (prior written consent from parents is usually obtained for childhood vaccinations but this only consents for the child to be included in the vaccination programme—check verbally at the time that patient/parents are aware of the nature of the vaccination and consent to its administration)
- Check that immunizations are the correct ones and in date
- Ensure resuscitation facilities are available
- Record vaccine expiry date and batch number
- Reconstitute the vaccine (if necessary) and give according to manufacturer's instructions
- Record date of vaccination and site in medical notes

Contraindications

- *Acute illness:* Delay until fully recovered. Minor ailments without fever or systemic upset are not reasons to postpone immunization.
- *Severe local reaction to a previous dose:* Extensive area of redness and swelling which becomes indurated and involves much of the antero-lateral surface of the thigh or a major part of the circumference of the upper arm.
- *Severe generalized reaction to a previous dose:*
  - Fever $\geq 39.5°C$ <48h. after vaccination
  - Anaphylaxis, bronchospasm, laryngeal oedema, and/or generalized collapse
  - Prolonged unresponsiveness
  - Prolonged high-pitched or inconsolable screaming for >4h.
  - Convulsions or encephalopathy <72h. after vaccination

Contraindications to live vaccines: BCG; measles; mumps; oral typhoid; polio; rubella; yellow fever. *Do not* give live vaccines:
• To pregnant women
• To immunocompromised patients:
  • Patients on high-dose steroids for >1wk. (e.g. >1mg/kg/d. prednisolone for children or ≥40mg/d. prednisolone for adults)
  • Haematological malignancy
  • Radiotherapy or chemotherapy in the last 6mo.
  • Another immunodeficiency syndrome
• If <3wk. after another live vaccine (but 2 live vaccines may be given together at different sites).
• With immunoglobulin (from 3wk. before to 3mo. after immunoglobulin).

❶ Patients with HIV infection may receive live vaccines except BCG and yellow fever.

Specific contraindications: See individual vaccinations listed in the 'Green' book.

Vaccine damage payments: Only payable if a patient is >80% impaired by a vaccination given within the NHS. Apply to the Vaccine Damage Payments Unit, Palatine House, Lancaster Road, Preston. PR1 1HB. ☎01772 899944 🖳 *http://www.dwp.gov.uk* Recipients receive a lump sum.

Essential reading
DoH: The Green book: immunization against infectious disease.
🖳 *http://www.dh.gov.uk*

Further information
Health Protection Agency (HPA) Information on vaccines and vaccination schedules and on notifications of infectious diseases.
🖳 *http://www.hpa.org.uk*

Patient information
Immunization: NHS website for patients.
🖳 *http://www.immunisation.org.uk*

Immunization schedule and notification of infectious diseases

Table 14.1 UK schedule of childhood immunization

Disease (vaccine)	Age	Comment
Diphtheria/tetanus/pertussis/ haemophilus influenzae type b/ inactivated polio (DTaP/IPV/Hib) Meningococcus type C (men C)	2, 3, and 4 mo.	Primary course (3 doses, a month between each dose) 2 injections
Measles/mumps/rubella (MMR)	12 to 15mo. (can be given at any age >12mo.)	1st dose, 1 injection
Diphtheria/tetanus/acellular pertussis/inactivated polio (DTaP/IPV)	3y.4mo.–5y. (3y. after completion of the 1° course)	Booster dose 1 injection
Measles/mumps/rubella (MMR)	3y.4mo.–5y.	2nd dose, 1 injection
Tuberculosis (BCG)	10–14y. and neonates at high risk	Skin test; then, if needed, 1 injection
Tetanus/low-dose diphtheria (Td/IPV)/inactivated polio	13–18y.	Booster dose 1 injection

❶ Pneumococcal vaccination is due to be added to this schedule in 2006/7.

Childhood immunization: In the UK, routine vaccinations for the under 5s are usually done in the GP surgery. Routine vaccinations for older children are normally done through the school health service. Schedule for childhood immunizations—Table 14.1.

Payment: Payment can be made:

- *Through the global sum:* All routine vaccinations for the under 5s and vaccinations for older children missed by the school vaccination programme can be provided as an additional service. Opting out of giving vaccinations to the under 5s results in a 1% ↓ in global sum.
- *As a directed enhanced service:* This continues the target payment scheme for routine childhood vaccination for pre-school children that existed under the terms of the 'Red book'.

Target payments: There are 2 payments available—one for children aged 2 and another for children aged 5. These are paid quarterly, in arrears, when children complete their vaccinations.

- *For children aged 2 this includes:*
  - Group 1—Diphtheria, tetanus, and poliomyelitis
  - Group 2—Pertussis
  - Group 3—MMR
  - Group 4—Hib

❶ Although meningitis C vaccination is now routinely given at 2, 3, and 4mo., it is not currently included for target calculation purposes.

● *For children aged 5 this includes:* A single booster dose of diphtheria, tetanus, and polio.

Within each age group and subgroup there are 2 levels of payment—the lower payment is achieved when ≥70% of the eligible children have been vaccinated; the higher figure when this proportion is ≥90%.

Adult immunization

Influenza and pneumococcal vaccination: Available as a directed enhanced service—existing practices do not have preferred provider status, so may be provided through an outside agency, depending on local arrangements. Additional payments are available through the quality and outcomes framework for ensuring at-risk patients receive vaccination.

Other necessary vaccinations: Can be provided as an additional service. Opting out incurs a 2% global sum reduction. A list of eligible vaccinations and terms and conditions of eligibility is available on the BMA website (⌨ *http://www.bma.org.uk*). Travel vaccinations which do not fall into these criteria can be administered as a private service and the patient must then pay a fee.

Notifiable diseases (^ND): Notification of certain diseases is required under the Public Health (Control of Disease) Act 1984 and Public Health (Infectious Disease) Regulations 1988. Notification is made to the local authority's Medical Officer for Environmental Health (who also provides forms for notification purposes). A fee is payable to the notifying doctor.

Diseases included

- Acute encephalitis
- Acute poliomyelitis
- Anthrax
- Cholera
- Diphtheria
- Dysentery
- Food poisoning
- Leprosy
- Leptospirosis
- Malaria
- Measles
- Meningitis (all types)

- Meningococcal septicaemia (without meningitis)
- Mumps
- Ophthalmia neonatorum
- Paratyphoid fever
- Plague
- Rabies
- Relapsing fever
- Rubella
- Scarlet fever

- Smallpox
- Tetanus
- Tuberculosis
- Typhoid fever
- Typhus fever
- Viral haemorrhagic fever
- Viral hepatitis (all types)
- Whooping cough
- Yellow fever

Essential reading

DoH: The Green book: immunization against infectious disease.
⌨ *http://www.dh.gov.uk*

Further information

Health Protection Agency (HPA) Information on vaccines and vaccination schedules and on notifications of infectious diseases ⌨ *http://www.hpa.org.uk*

Patient information

Immunization ⌨ *http://www.immunisation.org.uk*

Bacterial infection: streptococcal and staphylococcal infections

Streptococcal infection: Several groups are pathogenic to man—A, B, C, G, D, and Viridans streptococci.

Presentation

- Pharyngitis
- Tonsillitis
- Wound/skin infections
- Septicemia
- Scarlet fever
- Pneumonia
- Rheumatic fever
- Glomerulonephritis
- Neonatal sepsis
- Postpartum sepsis
- Endocarditis
- Septic arthritis
- Pneumonia
- UTI
- Dental caries

Investigation: Diagnosis is usually clinical. Evidence of infection can be obtained by measuring changing antibody response to infection (ASO titres). ASO titres ↑ in ~80% infections. Wound swabs are +ve if infection is on the skin and throat swabs may be +ve in pharyngitis/tonsillitis.

Treatment: Most streptococci are sensitive to penicillin (e.g. penicillin V 250–500mg qds for 7–10d.), though resistance is increasingly common.

Pneumococcal infection: There are >85 types of S. Pneumoniae. Pneumococci are carried in the noses and throats of ½ the population. In most people, they are harmless. Spread is by droplet infection.

Presentation

- Pneumonia
- Acute otitis media
- Sinusitis
- Meningitis
- Endocarditis
- Septic arthritis (rare)
- Peritonitis (rare)

Treatment: Amoxicillin 250–500mg tds for 7d. (erythromycin in allergic individuals). Resistance to penicillin in the community is still low.

Vaccination: Routine vaccination will be offered as part of the childhood immunization schedule in the near future. Meanwhile, offer to high-risk patients (see box). Ineffective in children <2mo.. In children aged 2mo.–5y., give conjugate vaccine initially and then polysaccharide vaccine after 2y. Booster doses are not needed except for patients with asplenia or nephrotic syndrome (when give a booster after 5–10y.).

High-risk patients for pneumococcal infection

- ≥65y. of age
- Asplenia or functional asplenia (📖 p.505) e.g. splenectomy, sickle cell
- Chronic renal disease or nephrotic syndrome
- Immunodeficiency or immunosuppression e.g. lymphoma, Hodgkin's disease, multiple myeloma, HIV, chemotherapy
- Chronic heart disease, lung disease e.g. asthma or COPD, or liver disease
- Coeliac disease
- Cochlear implant
- DM
- CSF shunts
- Children <5y. who have had previous invasive pneumococcal disease

---

Scarlet fever: Gp.A haemolytic streptococcus infection.
- *Incubation:* 2–4d.
- *Presentation:* Fever, malaise, headache, tonsillitis, rash (fine punctate erythema sparing face), 'scarlet' facial flushing, strawberry tongue (initially white turning red by 3rd/4th d.)
- *Treatment:* Penicillin V 250–500mg qds for 10d.
- *Complications:* Rheumatic fever (📖 p.350); acute glomerulonephritis

Staphylococcal infection: Usually *Staph. aureus*—occasionally *Staph. epidermidis*. Carried in the nose of ~30% of healthy adults. Antibiotic-resistant strains are common.

Presentation

- Neonatal infections: usually appear <6wk. after birth—pustular or bullous skin lesions on neck, axilla, or groin
- Breast abscess/ mastitis
- Abscesses/ faruncles/ carbuncles
- Septicaemia
- Endocarditis
- Wound infection
- Pneumonia: especially patients with COPD, influenza, or those receiving corticosteroids or immuno-suppressive therapy
- Osteomyelitis/septic arthritis

Management: Antibiotics (usually flucloxacillin or erythromycin 250–500mg qds for 7–10d.), abscess drainage (where appropriate), and general supportive measures. Where possible, obtain specimens for culture before instituting or altering antibiotic regimens.

Methicillin-resistant *Staph. aureus* (MRSA): MRSA acts in exactly the same way as any other *Staph. aureus*—it is carried harmlessly in most but occasionally causes a range of infections. It is only different due to its multiple resistance to antibiotics. Often contracted in hospital.
- ↓ tendency for multiple resistance by prudent use of antibiotics[N].
- Wash hands thoroughly with an appropriate antibacterial preparation if they appear soiled[N].
- If hands appear clean, wash with an alcoholic rub between each and every patient contact[N].
- Follow local policies for management of patients who are known to be infected with or carry MRSA.

Toxic shock syndrome: Caused by staphylococcal exotoxin.
- *Risk factors:* Tampon use, postpartum, staphylococcal wound infection, influenza, osteomyelitis, cellulitis.
- *Presentation:* Sudden onset high fever, vomiting, diarrhoea, confusion, and skin rash. May progress to shock ± death.
- *Management:* Admit as a medical emergency—mortality 8–15%.

Further information

DoH (2004) Winning ways: reducing healthcare associated infection in England 🖥 http://www.dh.gov.uk

NICE (2003) Infection control, prevention of healthcare-associated infection in primary and community care 🖥 http://www.nice.org.uk

Health Protection Agency (HPA) Topics A–Z: streptococcal infections, staphylococcus aureus 🖥 http://www.hpa.org.uk

Bacterial infection: other gram-positive infections

Clostridium infections: Anaerobic, spore-forming bacilli found in dust, soil, vegetation, and GI tracts of humans and animals. 25–30 species cause disease in humans.

Presentations

- Food poisoning—*C. perfringens*
- Pseudo-membranous colitis—overgrowth of *C. difficile* following antibiotic therapy. Presents with bloody diarrhoea. Treated with vancomycin or metronidazole if toxin is isolated from stool.
- Botulism—caused by a toxin released by *C. botulinum* which is ingested in contaminated food. Presents with neurological symptoms and warrants immediate admission for antitoxin.
- Wound infections—*C. perfringens* causes cellulitis which may → gas gangrene, septicaemia, ± death. Admit for iv antibiotics.
- Tetanus—see below

Tetanus (Lockjaw)[ND]: 50 cases/y. in the UK.

- *Incubation:* 2–50d.
- *Presentation: C. tetani* infects contaminated wounds (which may be trivial), the uterus postpartum (maternal tetanus), or newborn umbilicus (tetanus neonatorum). Tetanus toxin → generalized or localized tonic spasticity ± tonic convulsions. Suspect in any patient who has not been immunized who develops muscle stiffness or spasm several days after incurring a skin wound or burn.
- *Management:* If suspected, admit for specialist care. Treatment is with antitoxin, wound debridement, and general support. Effects may last several weeks. Mortality—40%.

Tetanus-prone injuries

- Any burn or wound sustained >6h. before surgical treatment of that wound
- Any burn or wound that:
  - Has a significant amount of dead tissue within it
  - Is a puncture-type wound
  - Has been in contact with soil or manure likely to harbour tetanus organisms
  - Is clinically infected

Prevention: Tetanus vaccine:

- *Primary immunization:* 3 doses of vaccine each 1mo. apart. If the schedule is disrupted, the course should be resumed from where it was stopped as soon as possible.
- *Booster doses in children:* 1 dose >3y. after the 1° course of immunization (usually given pre-school) and another 10y. later (usually given on leaving school).
- *Booster doses in adults:* 10y. after the primary course and again 10y. later. Probably gives lifelong protection. If an adult has received >5 doses in total, further routine boosters are not recommended.

- *Open wounds:* Last dose <10y. before—no vaccination required; last dose >10y. before—booster dose of tetanus vaccine + human tetanus immunoglobulin if tetanus-prone wound (see p.484). If no previous vaccination—1° course of vaccination + human tetanus immunoglobulin if tetanus-prone wound.

Diphtheria[ND]**:** Caused by *Corynebacterium diphtheriae*. Rare in the UK since routine immunization.
- *Spread:* Droplet infection, contact with articles soiled by an infected person.
- *Incubation:* 2–5d.
- *Presentation:* In countries where hygiene is poor, cutaneous diptheria is the predominant form. Elsewhere, characterized by an inflammatory exudate which forms a greyish membrane in the respiratory tract (may cause respiratory obstruction). *C. diphtheriae* secretes a toxin which affects myocardium, nervous and adrenal tissues.
- *Management:* Admit for antitoxin and iv erythromycin. Patients may be infectious for up to 4wk., but carriers shed *C. diphtheriae* for longer.

Prevention: Vaccination—part of the routine childhood vaccination programme in the UK (📖 p.480). In addition, give booster dose to people in contact with a patient with diphtheria or carrier, or before travel to epidemic or endemic areas.

Further information
Health Protection Agency (HPA) Topics A-Z: clostridium, tetanus, diphtheria
📖 http://www.hpa.org.uk

Bacterial infection: gram-negative infections

Enterobacteria: Examples include:

- Salmonella (📖 p.453)
- Shigella (📖 p.453)
- Escherichia
- Klebsiella
- Enterobacter
- Proteus
- Morganella
- Providencia
- Yersinia

Some are normal gut commensals. Others are pathogenic causing:

- Diarrhoea
- UTI—frequently *E.coli*; *Proteus* species are associated with bladder stones
- Intra-abdominal infections including peritonitis and hepatobiliary infection
- Septicaemia
- Meningitis—*E.coli* is the most common cause in neonates
- Chest infection—*Klebsiella* may cause a severe form of pneumonia
- Endocarditis—rare

Organisms are usually sensitive to co-amoxiclav and/or trimethoprim. Severe infection requires admission to hospital for iv antibiotics.

Pertussis (whooping cough)ND: Caused by *Bordetella pertussis*.

- *Incubation:* 7d.
- *Symptoms:*
    - Catarrhal stage—symptoms and signs of URTI; lasts 1–2wk.
    - Coughing stage—increasingly severe and paroxysmal cough with spasms of coughing followed by a 'whoop'; associated with vomiting, cyanosis during coughing spasms, and exhaustion. Lasts 4–6wk., then cough improves over 2–3wk.
- *Examination:* Chest is clear between coughing bouts.
- *Investigation:* Microscopy and culture of pernasal swabs (special swab and culture medium available from the lab); FBC—lymphocytosis.
- *Management:* Erythromycin in the catarrhal stage. Once coughing stage has started, treatment is symptomatic.
- *Complications:* Pneumonia, bronchiectasis, convulsions, subconjunctival haemorrhages, and facial petechiae.

Prevention

- *Proven contacts:* Treat with erythromycin.
- *Vaccination:* Routinely given in childhood (📖 p.480). Children with a personal or family history of febrile convulsion, FH of epilepsy, and children with well-controlled epilepsy can be vaccinated—give advice on fever prevention. Defer vaccination for children with any undiagnosed or evolving neurological condition or poorly controlled epilepsy until the condition is stable. If in doubt, refer to paediatrics.

Haemophilus influenzae: 99% of infections are due to type b. Rare <3mo. then incidence rises, reaching peak incidence at 10–11mo. Thereafter, incidence declines until the age of 4y. after which infection is rare.

Presentation:

- Meningitis—(60%); 8–11% have permanent neurological sequelae; mortality—(5%)
- Epiglottitis—(15%)
- Septicaemia—(10%)
- Osteomyelitis
- Septic arthritis
- Cellulitis
- Pneumonia
- Pericarditis

Management: Admit patients with severe infections. Organisms are often penicillin-resistant and treatment is usually with iv cefotaxime.

Prevention: Vaccination is routinely offered to all children (📖 p.480). In addition, offer a one-off vaccination to all unimmunized asplenic patients (preferably 2wk. prior to splenectomy) and HIV +ve patients.

Pseudomonas aeruginosa: Common and serious pathogen.

- In immunocompetent patients may cause UTI, wound infections (particularly leg ulcers—gives a characteristic greenish colouring), osteomyelitis, and skin infections (e.g. otitis externa).
- In immunocompromised patients and patients with CF, a common cause of pneumonia and septicaemia.
- Treatment is difficult due to multiple antibiotic resistance. Always send a specimen for culture and sensitivity if suspected.

Mycoplasma: *Mycoplasma pneumoniae* causes epidemics of lower respiratory tract infection every 3–4y. Spread by droplet infection.

- *Incubation:* 12–14d.
- *Presentation:* Dry, persistent cough ± arthralgia. CXR shows bilateral, patchy consolidation. Infection is confirmed with serology.
- *Management:* Erythromycin 500mg qds for 2wk. (alternative is tetracycline). Relapse is common. Severe infections may require hospital admission.

Chlamydial infection: 3 species:

- *C. trachomatis:* Includes 15 serotypes. Causes trachoma and inclusion conjunctivitis; sexually transmitted diseases (📖 p.743); pharyngitis.
- *C. pneumoniae:* Responsible for 6–19% of community-acquired pneumonia, especially in children and young adults. May be clinically indistinguishable from pneumonia caused by Mycoplasma (see above). Treat with tetracycline or erythromycin po for 2wk. or azithromycin 500mg od for 3d.
- *C. psittaci:* Infects many animals, but human infection is closely related to contact with birds. Treat as for *C. pneumoniae* (above).

Cholera: 📖 p.509   **Campylobacter:** 📖 p.453

Meningococcal meningitis: 📖 p.1044 **Gonorrhoea:** 📖 p.745

Further information

Health Protection Agency (HPA) Topics A-Z: *E. coli* enteritis, pertussis, HiB, pseudomonas, chlamydia 🖳 http://www.hpa.org.uk

Bacterial infection: tuberculosis[ND]

Caused by *Mycobacterium tuberculosis*. Worldwide, 1½ billion people have TB. In the UK, 7000 cases are reported each year. Incidence is increasing and 10% cases are antibiotic-resistant.

Primary TB: Initial infection. Transmitted by droplet infection. A lesion forms (usually pulmonary) which drains to local LNs. Immunity develops and the infection becomes quiescent.

- *Symptoms:* May be none. Cough, sputum, haemoptysis, pneumonia, pleural effusion, fever, sweats, lassitude, anorexia, erythema nodosum.
- *Investigations:* CXR, sputum samples for culture (state on the form that you are looking for acid-fast bacilli), +ve Tuberculin test (may be –ve if immunocompromised).
- *Management:* Refer for treatment and contact tracing.

Post-primary TB: Reactivation of a primary infection. *Risk factors:* old age, malignancy, DM, steroids, HIV, poor nutrition, chronic illness. Initial lesions progress and fibrose (usually upper lobe of lung). Other sites may develop disease. Multiple small lesions throughout the body result in miliary TB, common in immunocompromised patients. Symptoms and signs relate to the organs infected. Refer for specialist treatment.

Tuberculin skin test: Useful in diagnosis of TB and must be carried out before BCG immunization, except for infants <3mo. old who have not had any recent contact with TB. Interpretation—Table 14.2. The tuberculin test can be suppressed by:

- Glandular fever infection
- Viral infections
- Live viral vaccines—do not do a tuberculin test within 3wk. of vaccination
- Hodgkin's disease
- Sarcoidosis
- Corticosteroid therapy
- Immunosuppressant treatment or diseases, including HIV.

⚠ If a patient has a +ve tuberculin test—DON'T give BCG vaccination.

Table 14.2 Tuberculin testing and interpretation of results

Heaf test	Mantoux test	Grade
No induration at puncture sites	0mm induration	0—Negative
Discrete induration at ≥4 sites	1–4mm induration	1—Negative
Ring of induration with clear centre	5–14mm induration	2—Positive*
Disc of induration 5–10mm wide	≥15mm induration	3—Refer to chest clinic
Solid induration >10mm wide ± vesiculation or ulceration.		4—Refer to chest clinic

* In school children, a grade 2 response requires no further action. In other circumstances, refer to a chest clinic.

Treatment[G]

Preventing infected individuals developing clinical disease
Asymptomatic people with +ve tuberculin skin test (Mantoux >10mm)
but normal CXR are treated with isoniazid for 6mo. or isoniazid + rifampicin for 3mo.

Treatment of symptomatic patients: Combination of 3–4 antibiotics for the 1st 2mo. then 2 antibiotics for a further 4mo. Antibiotics used
are rifampicin, isoniazid, pyrazinamide, and ethambutol. All have potentially
serious side-effects and require blood monitoring. Compliance is imperative
to prevent antibiotic resistance. Those found to be non-compliant are best
treated with directly observed therapy (DOT) in which drugs are dispensed
by and taken in the presence of a health professional.

Screening: TB is a notifiable disease and this initiates contact tracing—
usually through chest clinics. All contacts are screened for TB. New
immigrants (and refugees) and school children are also routinely
screened for TB.

Prevention: BCG vaccination—live attenuated strain of bacteria
derived from *M. bovis*. Provides immunity lasting ≥15y. to 70–80% of
recipients. Given by intradermal injection into the left upper arm to:
• All non-immune school children at 13y.
• Health workers
• Staff who may have contact with animal sources of TB
• Staff working in prisons, old peoples homes, refugee hostels, and
  hostels for the homeless
• Contacts of TB cases
• Immigrants from countries with a high incidence of TB and their
  newborn infants
• Those going to Asia, Africa, South or Central America for >1mo.

⚠ Do not give other immunizations into the same arm for 3mo.

Further information

British Thoracic Society 🖳 http://www.brit-thoracic.org.uk
• Chemotherapy and management of tuberculosis in the UK. *Thorax* (1998) **53**: 7: 536–48
• Control and prevention of tuberculosis in the UK: Code of Practice. *Thorax* (2000) **55**: 887–901
Health Protection Agency (HPA) Topics A-Z: tuberculosis. 🖳 http://www.hpa.org.uk

Patient information

Health Protection Agency (HPA) TB and BCG 🖳 http://www.hpa.org.uk
British Lung Foundation 🖳 http://www.britishlungfoundation.org

Viral infection

The common cold: Acute, usually afebrile, respiratory tract infection.
- *Causes:* Rhino (30–50%), picorna, echo, and coxsackie viruses. At any one time, only a few viruses are prevalent.
- *Spread:* Contaminated secretions on fingers and droplet infection. Most people are infected 2–3x/y..
- *Management:* Advise patients to take plenty of fluids and paracetamol for symptom relief. Usually symptoms resolve in 4–10d.
- *Complications:* Exacerbation of asthma/COPD; 2° infection (bronchitis, pneumonia, conjunctivitis, OM, sinusitis, tonsillitis).

Influenza: Sporadic respiratory illness during autumn and winter causing ≈600 deaths/y. with epidemics every 2–3y. → 10x ↑ in deaths.
- *Causes:* Influenza viruses A, B, or C. Similar symptoms are also caused by the adeno and parainfluenza viruses.
- *Spread:* Droplet infection, person-to-person contact, or contact with contaminated items.
- *Incubation:* 1–7d.
- *Presentation:* In mild cases, symptoms are like those of a common cold. In more severe cases, fever begins suddenly, accompanied by prostration and generalized aches and pains. Other symptoms follow: headache, sore throat, respiratory tract symptoms (usually cough ± coryza). Acute symptoms resolve in <5d. but weakness, sweating, and fatigue may persist longer. 2° chest infection is common.
- *Risk factors for developing severe disease:* Chronic lung disease, heart disease, DM, pregnancy, immunosuppression, asplenism or hyposplenism, the elderly and the bedridden.

Management[G]
- *Symptomatic:* Rest, fluids, and paracetamol for fever/symptom control.
- *Antivirals:* zanamivir (Relenza™) and Oseltamivir (tamiflu™) are not a 'cure' but may shorten duration of symptoms and ↓ incidence of complications if started <48h. after onset of symptoms. Only use for treatment of patients in high-risk groups (above—except pregnancy) and only when influenza is prevalent in the community[G].
- Oseltamivir is recommended for prophylaxis in high-risk patients >13y. who are not effectively vaccinated or who live in residential care where a staff member has influenza-like symptoms. Use for 7–10d. from diagnosis of latest case in the establishment[G].

Prevention: Influenza vaccine is prepared each year from viruses of the 3 strains thought most likely to cause 'flu' that winter. It is ~70% effective (range 30–90%). Protection lasts 1y.

Indications for influenza vaccination
- ≥65y.
- Chronic renal disease
- DM
- Chronic lung disease e.g. asthma, COPD
- Cardiovascular disease (except ↑BP alone)
- Immunocompromised or asplenic patients
- Patients living in long-stay residential care establishments
- Health professionals expected to be in contact with influenza

Childhood infections

- Chicken pox 📖 p.494
- Measles 📖 p.492
- Mumps 📖 p.492
- Molluscum contagiosum 📖 p.671

- Rubella 📖 p.492
- Poliomyelitis 📖 p.493
- Gladular fever/Epstein–Barr virus (EBV) 📖 p.915

Other common childhood infections: Table 14.3. All are treated supportively with tepid sponging, paracetamol, and fluids, as needed. Mouth lesions in hand, foot, and mouth disease may benefit from teething gels e.g. Calgel.

Table 14.3 Common childhood viral infections

Condition	Duration	Main symptoms
Roseola infantum	4–7d.	Child <2y.
		High fever
		Sore throat and lymphadenopathy
		Mavcular rash appears after 3–4d. when fever ↓
Erythema infectiosum (5th disease) *Parvovirus**	4–7d.	Erythematous maculopapular rash starting on the face ('slapped cheeks')
		Reticular, 'lacy' rash on trunk and limbs
		Mild fever
		Arthralgia (rare)
Hand, foot, and mouth disease *Coxsackie virus*	5–7d.	Oral blisters/ulcers
		Red-edged vesicles on hands and feet
		Mild fever

* Contact in pregnancy—📖 p.791.

Viral skin infections: 📖 p.670.

Further information

NICE (2002) Zanamivir, oseltamivir and amantadine for the treatment and prophylaxis of influenza 🖥 http://www.nice.org.uk
Health Protection Agency (HPA) Topics A-Z: influenza 🖥 http://www.hpa.org.uk

Measles, mumps, rubella, and polio

Measles[ND]

- *Incubation:* 10–14d.
- *Presentation:*
  - Early symptoms—fever, conjunctivitis, cough, coryza, LNs
  - Later symptoms—Koplik's spots (tiny white spots on bright red background found on buccal mucosa of cheeks), rash (florid maculopapular appears after 4d.).
- *Complications:* Bronchopneumonia, otitis media, stomatitis, corneal ulcers, gastroenteritis, appendicitis, encephalitis (1:1000 affected children), subacute sclerosing panencephalitis (rare).
- *Management:* Supportive—paracetamol, fluids, antibiotics for 2° infection. Symptoms usually last ≈10d.

Rubella/German measles[ND]

- *Incubation:* 14–21d.
- *Symptoms:* Mild and may pass unrecognized. Fever, LNs (including suboccipital nodes), pink maculopapular rash which lasts 3d.
- *Complications:* Birth defects if infected in pregnancy (📖 p.791); arthritis (adolescents); thrombocytopoenia (rare); encephalitis (rare).
- *Management:* Supportive—paracetamol, fluids. Symptoms last 10d.

Mumps[ND]

- *Incubation:* 16–21d.
- *Symptoms:* Subclinical infection is common. Fever, malaise, tender enlargement of 1 or both parotids ± submandibular glands.
- *Complications:* Aseptic meningitis; epididymo-orchitis; pancreatitis.
- *Management:* Supportive—paracetamol, fluids.

Prevention of measles, mumps, and rubella

- Measles, mumps, and rubella (MMR) vaccination consists of live attenuated measles, mumps, and rubella viruses.
- Vaccine viruses are not transmitted so there is no risk of infection from people who have just been immunized.
- Routinely administered to all children after their 1st birthday and again pre-school. Re-immunization is needed if given to children of <1y.
- Children with chronic illness (e.g. CF) are at particular risk from measles and should be immunized.
- Malaise, fever, and rash are common ~1wk. after immunizations and usually last 2–3d. Advise on fever prevention.

✒ Suggestions that MMR vaccine may be associated with autism and inflammatory bowel disease are controversial. Scientific opinion is strongly in favour of there being no link but ↓ public confidence in MMR → ↓ uptake, risk of measles outbreaks, and debate over the use of single vaccines (see websites).

Rubella vaccination: Attenuated virus. Use for girls aged 10–14y. who have not received MMR and non-pregnant women who lack immunity to rubella. Check rubella status at any opportunity in women of child-bearing age and vaccinate any women not immune. Advise women to avoid pregnancy for 3mo. after vaccination. If lack of immunity is detected on routine antenatal screening, vaccinate after delivery.

Poliomyelitis[ND]

- *Spread:* droplet or faeco-oral.
- *Incubation:* 7d.
- *Presentation:* 2d. flu-like prodrome then fever, tachycardia, headache, vomiting, neck stiffness, and unilateral tremor ('pre-paralytic stage'). 65% who experience the pre-paralytic stage go on to develop paralysis (myalgia, LMN signs ± respiratory failure).
- *Management:* Supportive—admit to hospital.
- *Prognosis:* <10% of those developing paralysis die. Permanent disability may result. Post-polio syndrome (with worsening of neurological deficit) may occur many years later.

Prevention: Since 2004 in the UK, polio vaccine in the form of inactivated polio vaccine (IPV) has been combined with diphtheria, tetanus, ± whooping cough, ± *Haemophilus influenzae* vaccine to form a single 3, 4 or 5-part vaccine. Live polio vaccine is no longer used in the UK.

- *Primary immunization in babies and children <10y.:* 3 doses of the 5 part vaccine (DTaP/IPV/Hib) protecting against polio, diphtheria, whooping cough, tetanus and haemophilus influenza, each 1mo. apart-usually at 2mo., 3mo., and 4mo.. If the schedule is disrupted resume the course from where it was stopped.
- *Booster doses in children:* 1 dose of 4 part vaccine (DTaP/IPV) protecting against polio, diphtheria, whooping cough, and tetanus >3y. after the 1° course of immunization (usually pre-school) and another dose of 3 part vaccine (Td/IPV) protecting against tetanus, diphtheria and polio, 10y. later between the ages of 13y. and 18y. (usually on leaving school).
- *Primary immunization in children >10y. and adults:* 3 doses of 3 part vaccine (Td/IPV) each 1mo. apart. Booster doses are required 3y. and 10y. after the primary course.
- *Booster doses for travel:* Not required unless at special risk e.g. travelling to endemic/epidemic area. Boosters of Td/IPV are then given every 10y.

Further information

Health Protection Agency (HPA) Topics A-Z: measles, mumps, rubella, polio.
  🖳 http://www.hpa.org.uk

Patient information

Health Protection Agency (HPA) MMR information sheet and weblinks
  🖳 http://www.hpa.org.uk
Immunization 🖳 http://www.immunisation.org.uk
NHS 🖳 http://www.mmrthefacts.nhs.uk

Herpes virus infection

Herpes zoster: Infections caused by *Varicella zoster* (VZ).

Chickenpox: Very common, especially in spring. Most common in <10y.. 90% adults are immune.

- *Incubation:* 10–21d.
- *Presentation:* Rash ± fever. Spots appear in crops on skin and mucus membranes and progress from macule → papule → vesicle. Crops appear for 5–7d. Vesicles dry out and scab over (usually in <14d.). Infectious for 1–2d. before rash develops and for 5d. after. Exclusion from school until 'all lesions crusted over' is not necessary—see HPA guidance for schools. Scabs fall off usually without scarring.
- *Complications:* Eczema herpeticum (📖 p.636); encephalitis (cerebellar symptoms are most common); pneumonia; birth defects (📖 p.790); neonatal infection (📖 p.790).
- *Management:* Supportive—paracetamol, fluids, topical calamine lotion to lesions. Admit if complications are suspected.

⚠ Non-immune immunosuppressed patients, pregnant women or neonates (📖 p.790) with significant exposure to chickenpox or shingles, should receive zoster immunoglobulin (ZIG) as soon as possible (<3d. after contact). Check antibody levels if immune status is unknown.

Shingles: Reactivation of latent chickenpox virus. Contacts may develop chickenpox but there is no evidence that shingles can be acquired by exposure to chickenpox. Infectious until all lesions have scabbed.

- *Incidence:* 1:25 population. More common in elderly and immunocompromised patients but can occur any age.
- *Presentation:* Unilateral pain precedes a vesicular rash by 2–3d. Crops of vesicles appear over 3–5d., following the cutaneous distribution of ≥1 adjacent dermatomes. The affected area is usually hyperesthetic, and pain may be severe. Lesions scab over and fall off in <14d.
- *Management:* Symptomatic—analgesia, calamine lotion. Oral acyclovir (or similar) is only effective if initiated <48h. after onset—controversial as expensive and of limited benefit in immunocompetent patients.
- *Complications:*
  - Postherpetic neuralgia—may persist for months/years after infection. Can be sharp and intermittent or constant, and may be debilitating. If simple analgesia is ineffective, try neuropathic painkillers e.g. amitriptyline or carbamazepine (📖 p.173). If pain is relentless, refer to a pain clinic.
  - Dissemination to other regions of the skin ± visceral organs (immunosuppressed patients) admit for iv acyclovir.
  - Eye involvement—refer urgently to ophthalmology (📖 p.937).
  - Ramsay Hunt syndrome—📖 p.923.

Chickenpox (Varicella) Immunization: 2 doses 4–8wk. apart. Now recommended for non-immune healthcare workers who have direct patient contact. Those with a definite history of varicella infection can be considered immune—antibody test the others. Vaccination is contraindicated if pregnant or immunocompromised.

Herpes simplex (HSV) infection: 2 types:
- HSV-1 commonly causes herpes labialis (cold sore), herpetic stomatitis, and keratitis.
- HSV-2 usually causes genital herpes.

Both are transmitted by direct contact with lesions. Lesions may appear anywhere on the skin or mucosa but are most frequent around the mouth, on the lips, conjunctiva, cornea, and genitalia. Diagnosis is usually clinical. Can be confirmed with a viral swab of the ulcer (usually undertaken in GUM clinics).

Primary infection: May be asymptomatic and go unnoticed. After a prodromal period (generally <6h.) of tingling, discomfort, or itching, small tense vesicles appear on an erythematous base. Single clusters vary in size from 0.5–1.5cm, but groups may coalesce. Vesicles persist for a few days, then dry, forming a thin yellowish crust. Healing occurs 8–12d. after onset. Infection may be accompanied by systemic symptoms e.g. fever, malaise, and tender lymph nodes.

Recurrent infection: After initial infection, HSV remains dormant in the nerve ganglia. Recurrent eruptions can occur, precipitated by overexposure to sunlight, febrile illnesses, physical or emotional stress, or immunosuppression. The trigger stimulus is often unknown. Recurrent disease is generally less severe and more localized.

Complications
- Aseptic meningitis
- Encephalitis (📖 p.1044)
- Erythema multiforme (📖 p.654)
- Eczema herpeticum—severe disease in skin regions with eczema (📖 p.636)
- Generalized infection in immunocompromised patients—oesophagitis, colitis, perianal ulcers, pneumonia, and neurological syndromes

Management
- *Severe infections:* e.g. disseminated neonatal disease, HSV encephalitis, severe eczema herpeticum, immunocompromised patients—admit for systemic treatment with acyclovir.
- *Eye involvement:* Refer for urgent ophthalmology assessment. *Treatment:* Topical ± oral acyclovir.
- *Suppression of recurrent eruptions:* Oral acyclovir (and similar drugs).
- *Cold sores:* Topical acyclovir—if started early. Available OTC.
- *2° infections:* Topical or systemic antibiotics.
- See also: Genital infection (📖 p.744); neonatal infection (📖 p.744); infection in pregnancy (📖 p.788).

Herpetic whitlow: Swollen, painful, and erythematous lesion of the distal phalanx, results from inoculation of HSV through a skin break or abrasion and is most common in health workers.

Further information
Health Protection Agency (HPA): Guidance on management of communicable diseases in schools and nurseries. 🖥 *http://www.hpa.org.uk*
DoH: The Green Book 🖥 *http://www.dh.gov.uk*

Viral hepatitis[ND]

Acute and chronic hepatitis: 📖 p.442.

Hepatitis A (HAV): Common.
- *Spread:* Faecal-oral route. Patients are infectious 2wk. before feeling ill.
- *Incubation:* 2–7wk. (average 4wk.).
- *Risk factors:* Travel to high-risk areas, institutional inhabitants/workers, iv drug abuse, high-risk sexual practices.
- *Presentation:* May be asymptomatic (especially young children); fever; ↓ appetite; nausea ± vomiting; pale stools ± diarrhoea; fatigue; jaundice; dark urine; abdominal pain ± tender hepatomegaly.
- *Investigation:* LFTs (hepatic jaundice—📖 p.270), hepatitis serology—IgM antibodies signify recent infection, IgG remains detectable lifelong.
- *Management:* Supportive. Avoid alcohol until LFTs are normal. Most recover in <2mo. There is no carrier state and hepatitis A does not cause chronic liver disease. After infection, immunity is lifelong.

Prevention: Vaccination (Havrix®) is indicated for travellers to high-risk areas, people with chronic liver disease, or those working in high-risk situations. Passive immunization with human immunoglobulin gives protection for ≤3mo. and is used for short-term travel or protecting household contacts of sufferers.

Hepatitis B (HBV): Common. Endemic in much of Asia and the Far East. The virus has 3 major structural antigens: surface antigen (HBsAg), core antigen (HBcAg), and e antigen (HBeAg).
- *Spread:* Infected blood, sexual intercourse, mother → newborn (📖 p.788), human bite.
- *Incubation:* 6–23wk. (average 17wk.).
- *Risk factors:* Travel to high-risk areas; babies of infected mothers; sexual partners of infected patients or patients with high-risk sexual practices; iv drug abusers; healthcare workers.
- *Presentation:* May be asymptomatic or present with fever, malaise, fatigue, arthralgia, urticaria, pale stools, dark urine, and/or jaundice.
- *Investigation:* LFTs (hepatic jaundice—📖 p.270), hepatitis serology.
  - HBsAg is present from 1–6mo. post-exposure. If present >6mo. after the acute episode, defines carrier status.
  - HBeAg suggests high infectivity. Present from 6wk.–3mo. after acute illness.
  - Anti-HBs antibodies appear >10mo. after infection. Imply immunity.

Management: In all cases, advise patients to avoid alcohol. Refer for specialist advice. Treatment is supportive for acute illness. Chronic hepatitis is treated with interferon and lamivudine with varying success.

Prognosis
- ~85% recover fully
- 10% develop carrier status
- 5–10% develop chronic hepatitis—may lead to cirrhosis and/or liver carcinoma
- Fulminant hepatitis and death are rare (<1%)

Prevention

- Advise patients re 'safe sex'
- Immunize high-risk groups
- Passive immunization with human immunoglobulin is used to protect non-immune high-risk contacts of infected patients.

Hepatitis C (HCV): Common. A major cause of post-transfusion hepatitis. Prior to 1989 known as non-A, non-B hepatitis.

- *Spread:* Contact with infected blood; mother → baby. NOT easily spread through sexual contact. In 10%, no source of infection is identified.
- *Incubation:* 2–25wk. (average 8wk.).
- *Patients at high risk of infection:* Recipients of blood transfusions; health-care workers; iv drug abusers; haemodialysis patients; infants born to infected mothers; multiple sexual partners.
- *Presentation:* As for HBV.
- *Investigation:* LFTs (hepatic jaundice—📖 p.270), hepatitis serology— anti-HCV antibody detectable 3–4mo. post-infection.
- *Treatment:* Refer for expert advice. Avoid alcohol.
- *Prognosis:* ½ develop chronic infection; 5% develop cirrhosis and 15% of those, hepatoma.

Hepatitis D (HDV): Incomplete virus which only exists with HBV.

Hepatitis E (HEV)

- *Spread:* Faeco-oral route.
- *Incubation:* 2–9wk. (average 40d.).
- *Risk factors:* Travel to developing countries (especially pregnant women).
- *Presentation and management:* Similar clinical presentation to HAV infection. Diagnosis is made after serological confirmation. Treatment is supportive. There is no chronic state. No vaccine exists. Mortality in pregnancy can be as high as 20%.

EBV: 📖 p.915

Further information

Health Protection Agency (HPA) Topics A-Z: Hepatitis A,B,C 🖥 http://www.hpa.org.uk
DoH: The Green Book 🖥 http://www.dh.gov.uk

Human immunodeficiency virus (HIV)

HIV is a retrovirus infecting T-helper cells bearing the CD4 receptor. Worldwide, the HIV epidemic continues, but prophylaxis and treatment is improving prognosis in developed countries where treatment is available.

Transmission: Sexual (60–70%); heterosexual intercourse—50% cases. *Other causes:* iv drug abuse (3%); infected blood products; mother → child; accidental exposure (e.g. needle stick injuries).

Clinical disease

Primary HIV: Symptoms in ≈ ½ infected patients—glandular-fever like syndrome of diffuse maculopapular rash, fever, fatigue, and lymphadenopathy. Rarely, acute neurological symptoms (aseptic meningitis, transverse myelitis, encephalitis). FBC may show atypical lymphocytes.

Early HIV: Follows seroconversion. Plasma viral load ↓ to a plateau. Level of the plateau is prognostic—'fast progressors' have high and 'slow progressors' have low plateau levels. Most patients are asymptomatic. *Symptoms:* night sweats or generalized lymphadenopathy.

Advanced HIV: Accompanied by immunosuppression or AIDS (if CD4 count <200 cells/mm^3). Patients are at risk from opportunistic infections (e.g. pneumococcal infection, TB, CMV, *Pneumocystis carinii*, toxoplasmosis, and cryptosporidial diarrhoae) and AIDS-associated malignancies (e.g. Kaposi's sarcoma, lymphoma).

Death: Due to multiple causes, including chronic incurable systemic infections, malignancies, neurological disease, wasting and malnutrition, and multisystem failure.

Prevention

* Promotion of safe sex.
* ↓ iv drug abuse and ↓ needle sharing.
* Screening blood donors—seroconversion can take up to 3mo., so still small risk of transmission.
* Prevention of transmission from mother to child—risk can be ↓ to <5% by treatment with zidovudine given to the mother antenatally, during delivery, and to the neonate for 1st 6wk.; elective LSCS; and advising against breast-feeding.
* Trials of HIV vaccines are in advanced stages.

Management of HIV infection^G: Specialist treatment is essential.

Antiviral drugs: 3 groups:
* Nucleoside analogues (e.g. zidovudine)
* Non-nucleoside reverse transcriptase inhibitors (e.g. nevirapine)
* Protease inhibitors (e.g. indinavir).

HAART (highly active antiretroviral therapy) is a combination of ≥3 drugs with ≥1 drug penetrating the blood-brain barrier. Many of the drugs have severe side-effects. Adherence to therapy is essential to avoid resistance. Patients who present with clinical manifestations of HIV, CD4 counts <350cells/mm^3, or viral loads >30,000 copies are considered for HAART.

Treatment failure requires switching or increasing therapy with at least 2 new drugs.

Prophylaxis against opportunistic infection: Patients with low CD4 counts are started on prophylactic antibiotics:
- <200 cells/mm^3—*Pneumocystis carinii* (co-trimoxazole)
- <100 cells/mm^3—toxoplasmosis (co-trimoxazole)
- <50 cells/mm^3—*Mycobacterium avium* (azithromycin)

Psychological support: Perhaps the most important role of the GP and community services. Patients often lack the support offered by the community for most other terminal illness. Many HIV sufferers choose to remain at home for palliative care or be cared for by local hospices. As with any palliative care (📖 p.999–1015), the GP and primary care team form an integral part of this service.

❶ For more detailed and updated information, see British HIV Association Guidelines (below).

Kaposi sarcoma: Purple papules or plaques on skin or mucosa of any organ. Metastasizes to lymph nodes. 2 types:
- *Endemic*—occurs in central Africa. Peripheral lesions. Good response to chemotherapy.
- *Associated with AIDS or transplant patients*—commonly, skin or pulmonary lesions. Lymphatic obstruction predisposes to cellulitis. If suspected, get expert help.

(M.K. Kaposi (1837–1902)—Hungarian dermatologist)

Needle stick injury: Exposure is significant if the source is HIV +ve, the material is blood or another infectious body fluid (semen, amniotic fluid, genital secretions, CSF), and exposure is caused by inoculation (risk transmission 1:300 if HIV +ve source) or by a splash onto a mucous membrane (risk transmission 1:3000).

⚠ **Immediate action:** Irrigate site of exposure with running water. Establish potential risk of HIV—history of HIV infection and (if possible) blood sample from the source and victim. Refer to A&E immediately for instigation of HIV prevention policy.

Essential reading
British HIV Association (2003) HIV treatment guidelines 🖳 http://www.bhiva.org

Further information
Health Protection Agency (HPA) HIV 🖳 http://www.hpa.org.uk
DoH (2004) Winning ways: reducing healthcare associated infection in England 🖳 http://www.dh.gov.uk

Patient information
NAM Aidsmap ☎0207 840 0050 🖳 http://www.aidsmap.com
National AIDS Helpline ☎0800 567 123 (24h. helpline)
Terrence Higgins Trust ☎0845 1221 200 🖳 http://www.tht.org.uk.
Children with AIDS Charity (CWAC) ☎020 7247 9115 🖳 http://www.cwac.org

Creutzfeldt–Jakob disease (CJD) or human spongiform encephalopathy

A degenerative brain disease due to a rogue form of brain protein or 'prion' which is transmitted like an infectious agent, though CJD is not transmissible from person to person by normal contact.

Types:

Sporadic or classical: Most common form in the UK. Incidence: ≈50 cases/y.. Rare <40y. Median duration of symptoms 3–4mo. *Cause:* unknown.

Variant: Only recently recognized. Affects younger people than classical CJD and duration is longer, lasting a median of 14mo. *Cause:* transmitted by ingestion of nervous tissue in beef infected with bovine spongiform encephalitis or 'mad cow disease'. In June 2004, there were 146 cases of vCJD in the UK.

Iatrogenic: Cases associated with treatments using human growth hormone and human dura mater grafts. Rarely associated with corneal grafts or contaminated instruments used in surgery.

Familial prion disease: ~20–30 families in the UK are affected with a version of CJD which is passed from generation to generation in an autosomal dominant pattern. Median duration of symptoms from onset is 2–5y.

Presentation: Long incubation (>25y. in some cases). *Clinical features:* vary according to the areas of brain most affected but are always rapidly progressive. *Common features:* personality change; psychiatric symptoms; cognitive impairment; neurological deficits (sensory and motor deficits, ataxia); myoclonic jerks, chorea or dystonia; difficulty with communication, mobility, swallowing, and continence; coma and death.

Differential diagnosis: Dementia, depression, MS, MND, SOL.

Management: There is no simple diagnostic test and often families feel frustrated by early misdiagnosis. Refer to neurologist if suspected. Genetic testing is possible for patients with familial CJD. Warn families about the likely course of the disease and symptoms/signs they might expect. *Consider:* social services input, advice on benefits (can apply for DLA/AA under special rules—⬚ p.107), referral to other services (e.g. DN, physiotherapy, OT), voluntary sector services (e.g. Crossroads). Reassess needs frequently as patients change rapidly.

Palliative care: ⬚ p.999–1015.

Compensation to victims: The government introduced a compensation scheme for victims and families of vCJD in 2000. Further information is available from 🖳 http://www.vcjdtrust.co.uk

Infection control: Detailed advice has been published by the Department of Health 🖳 http://www.dh.gov.uk
- CJD disease: guidance for healthcare workers (2000)
- Transmissible spongiform encephalopathy agents: safe working and prevention of infection (June 2000)
- Winning ways: reducing healthcare associated infection in England (2004)

Further information

Health Protection Agency (HPA) Infections: topics A-Z— CJD
🖳 http://www.hpa.org.uk
National CJD Surveillance Unit ☎0131 537 2128
🖳 http://www.cjd.ed.ac.uk
The Prion Unit ☎020 7594 3769. Imperial College School of Medicine, St Mary's Campus, Norfolk Place, London W2 1PG.
The Human BSE Foundation ☎0191 389 4157
🖳 http://www.hbsef.org

Patient support
CJD Support Network ☎01630 673 973 🖳 http://www.cjdsupport.net

Other infections

Aspergillosis A spectrum of diseases. *Cause:* Aspergillus fungus present in the soil and decaying vegetation. Its spores can be inhaled any time of the year but reach peak levels in autumn and winter. Inhaled fungal spores colonize bronchial mucosa and nasal sinuses. If suspected, refer to a chest physician.

Presentations

- *Extrinsic asthma:* 📖 p.376.
- *Allergic bronchopulmonary aspergillosis:* Grows in the walls of the bronchi. Presents with episodes of eosinophilic pneumonia (characterized by wheeze, cough, fever, and malaise) throughout the year but worse in late autumn. CXR shows fleeting lung shadows (cleared by expectorating firm, brown plugs of mucus). Untreated → upper lobe fibrosis and 'proximal' bronchiectasis.
- *Invasive aspergillosis:* Only occurs in the immunocompromised. Aspergillus disseminates from the lung → brain, kidneys, and other organs. Carries very poor prognosis.
- *Aspergillus sinusitis:* Nasal congestion, headache, and facial discomfort.
- *Aspergilloma:* Growth within existing lung cavities (e.g. from previous TB or sarcoidosis). A ball of fungus forms. CXR shows a round lesion with air halo above it. Occasionally results in haemoptysis.

Management: Refer for specialist management.

Lyme disease: *Cause: Borrelia burgdorferi.*
- *Spread:* Transmitted by ticks—usually from deer or sheep.
- *Presentation:* Erythema migrans (75%—red macule/papule on upper arm, leg, or trunk 3–32d. after a tick bite which expands to form a ring with central clearing; diameter can be up to 50cm; further smaller lesions then develop elsewhere); flu-like illness; lymphadenopathy ± splenomegaly; arthralgia. Symptoms are typically intermittent and changing.
- *Complications:* Neurological abnormalities, aseptic meningitis, myocarditis, arthritis.
- *Management:* Confirm diagnosis with serology. Treatment is usually with doxycycline or erythromycin—take microbiology advice. Treatment with antibiotics after a tick bite but before symptoms have arisen is controversial.

Removal of ticks: Place a large blob of petroleum jelly (Vaseline™) over the tick. It suffocates over a few hours and can be removed easily with a pair of tweezers.

Cryptosporidium: Protozoan causing diarrhoeal disease. *C. parvum* causes most cases. Infections result from zoonotic spread, direct person-to-person contact, or waterborne transmission. Children, travellers to foreign countries, and immunocompromised patients are at high risk. Responsible for ~5% of all gastroenteritis in both industrialized and developing countries.
- *Incubation:* 2–5d. Clinical illness occurs in 80% infected individuals.

- *Symptoms:* profuse watery diarrhoea, abdominal cramp ± nausea, anorexia, fever, and malaise.
- *Management:* Confirm diagnosis with stool microscopy. Treatment is supportive (fluid replacement—📖 p.255). Usually symptoms last 1–2wk. (rarely >1mo.). Immunocompromised patients develop profuse intractable diarrhoea which is difficult to clear and may continue intermittently for life.

Pneumocystis carinii (PCP): May be classified as a protozoan or fungus. Causes pneumonia in immunocompromised patients.
- *Presentation:* Fever, breathlessness, tachypnoea, dry cough, respiratory failure (± cyanosis).
- *Investigation:* CXR normal or 'ground glass' appearance, sputum culture may be diagnostic.
- *Management:* If suspected, refer for specialist care. Treatment is with septrin or dapsone.
- *Prevention:* Prophylactic antibiotics are given to AIDS patients with low CD4 counts (📖 p.499).

Threadworm: Common in the UK—especially amongst children. *Enterobius vermicularis* causes anal itch as it leaves the bowel to lay eggs on the perineum. Often seen as silvery thread-like worms at the anus of children. *Treatment:* Mebendazole (available OTC). Treat household contacts as well as the index case.

Fungal skin infection: 📖 p.672

Syphilis: 📖 p.742

Trichomonas: 📖 p.745

Gastroenteritis: 📖 p.452

Further information

Health Protection Agency (HPA) Topics A-Z: aspergillus; lyme disease; cryptospordium; pneumocystis carinii 🖥 http://www.hpa.org.uk
The Aspergillus Website 🖥 http://www.aspergillus.man.ac.uk
The Lyme Disease Network 🖥 http://www.lymenet.org

Infections in immunocompromised patients

Infections in patients whose host defense mechanisms are compromised range from minor to fatal. They are often caused by organisms that normally reside on body surfaces.

Opportunistic infections: Infections from endogenous microflora that are non-pathogenic or from ordinarily harmless organisms. Occur if host defence mechanisms have been altered by:

- Age
- Infection
- Burns
- Neoplasms
- Metabolic disorders
- Irradiation
- Foreign bodies
- Corticosteroids
- Immunosuppressive or cytotoxic drugs
- Diagnostic or therapeutic instrumentation

The precise character of the host's altered defences determines which organisms are likely to be involved. These organisms are often resistant to multiple antibiotics.

Organisms commonly involved

- Non-pathogenic streptococci
- E. coli
- Herpes viruses—📖 p.494
- CMV
- Cryptococcal infection
- Toxoplasmosis
- Mycobacteria—📖 p.488
- Pneumocystis—📖 p.503
- Candida—📖 p.672 and 741

Management: Expert care is always required—refer promptly to the consultant responsible for the patient.

Prophylaxis

Antibiotics: Used for prevention of:
- Rheumatic fever and bacterial endocarditis
- TB and meningitis in exposed patients
- Recurrent UTIs and otitis media
- Bacterial infections in granulocytopenic patients
- Pneumocystis in AIDS patients

⚠ Watch for signs of superinfection with resistant organisms.

Active immunization

- *Influenza vaccine:* Give annually—see 📖 p.490 for list of indications.
- *Haemophilus influenzae type b vaccine:* For asplenic/hyposplenic patients—children should complete routine HiB vaccinations. Individuals immunized in infancy who then become asplenic should receive 1 booster dose aged >1y. Unimmunized adults and children >10y. should receive a single dose of HiB.
- *Meningococcal vaccine:* Give to close contacts of patients with type A or C meningococcal meningitis. In some cases, given to patients with immunosuppression—take specialist advice.

- *Pneumococcal vaccine:* Single dose—give to chronically ill, asplenic, and elderly patients and those with sickle cell and HIV disease. Booster doses are not required except for patients with asplenia or nephrotic syndrome, when a booster should be given after 5–10y.
- *Hepatitis B vaccine:* Give to patients who repeatedly receive blood products as well as to medical and nursing personnel and others at risk.

Passive immunization: Can prevent or ameliorate herpes zoster (ZIG), hepatitis A and B, measles, and cytomegalovirus infection in selected immunosuppressed patients. If a patient is in contact with any of these diseases, ask advice from the consultant looking after the patient or a consultant in communicable disease control.

Immunoglobulin administration: Effective for patients with hypo-gammaglobulinemia. Given on a regular basis by iv infusion.

Asplenic patients: All asplenic patients (or functionally asplenic patients e.g. patients with sickle cell disease) are at ↑risk of bacterial infection. Ensure patients have:
- *Vaccinations:* Haemophilus influenzae b, pneumococcal, influenza, and, in some cases, meningococcal vaccine. If possible, vaccinations should be given >2wk. prior to splenectomy.
- *Prophylactic antibiotics:* Oral penicillin continuously until age 16y. or for 2y. post-splenectomy—whichever is longer.
- *Stand-by amoxicillin:* To start if symptoms of infection begin.
- *Patient-held card:* Alerting health professionals to infection risk.

⚠ Warn patients about risk of severe malaria and other tropical infections.

⚠ Admit patients to hospital if infection develops despite prophylactic measures.

Patient cards and information sheets are available from: Department of Health, PO Box 410, Wetherby, LS23 7LL. Patients should also be encouraged to wear a Medic-Alert bracelet or necklace.

HIV: 📖 p.498

Prevention of travel-related illness

Pre-travel assessment: 8 wk. pre-departure where possible. *Check:*
- Age
- General health
- Where and when intending to travel (including areas within a country and stop-overs elsewhere)
- Type of accommodation
- Purpose of travel
- Previous experience (including experience with antimalarials)
- Current vaccination status

Health risks

- *Environmental hazards* (e.g. changes in altitude/climate): Avoid rapid changes of altitude and take time to readjust; avoid sunburn.
- *Accidents:* Avoid potentially dangerous tasks under the influence of alcohol e.g. swimming, driving. Avoid motorbikes—especially without helmets and protective clothing.
- *Illness abroad:* MI causes 61% deaths related to international travel. Don't travel if unwell. Ensure adequate insurance including repatriation costs. Take enough supplies of regular medication when travelling to last the entire trip and take preventive steps to avoid infection.
- *Transport-related problems*
  - Fitness to fly—📖 p.208
  - Motion sickness—take OTC medication if afflicted
  - Jet lag
  - DVT—drink plenty of water on long haul flights; avoid alcohol; regularly get up and walk around; consider prophylactic aspirin ± support stockings
- *Psychological effects of travel*

Vaccination: 4% deaths related to travel are due to infectious disease—ensure fully vaccinated for areas intending to visit. Charts are available in GP and Pulse magazines and via travel information clinics (opposite).

Travellers' diarrhoea: 50% travellers experience some diarrhoea. Most cases last 4–5d.; 1–2% last >1mo.

Prevention

- Take care to eat and drink uncontaminated food and water
- Food should be freshly cooked and hot
- Avoid salads and cold meats/fish
- Eat fruit that can be peeled
- Stick to drinks made with boiling water or bottled drinks and water with intact seal; avoid ice in drinks
- Use water purification tablets if necessary

Action: If diarrhoea occurs when abroad, advise patients to use oral rehydration fluids. Only take anti-diarrhoeals if impossible to get to a toilet. Seek medical advice if blood in stool, fever, or not resolving in 72h. (24h. for the elderly or infants).

⚠ Don't use anti-diarrhoeals if blood in stool, fever, or <10y. old.

Prevention of malaria[ND]

- *Awareness of risk:* High-risk areas are Central and S. America; SE Asia; Pacific islands; Sub-Saharan Africa—however brief the time there. Pregnant and asplenic patients are at particular risk.
- ↓ *mosquito bites:* Mosquitos bite at night.
  - *Accommodation*—sleep in screened accommodation spraying screens with insecticide each evening, and use a prethroid vaporiser. If screens are not available, use permethrin impregnated bed net (kits available).
  - *Person*—in the evenings wear long-sleeved shirts and trousers; protect limbs with diethyl-toluamide-containing repellant.
- *Chemoprophylactic drugs:* Regimes vary with location and time of year. Charts are available in GP and Pulse magazines and via travel information clinics (see below). For all anti-malarials, apart from mefloquine, start 1wk. prior to departure. Start mefloquine 3wk. before leaving to allow change to alternative if adverse side-effects. Continue all antimalarials for 4wk. after return.
- *Awareness of residual risk:* Chemoprophylaxis is not 100% effective. Advise all travellers to malaria regions to seek medical advice if unwell for up to 6mo. after return. Malaria is a great mimic. Have a high level of suspicion.

Prevention of HIV/hepatitis B and C

- Avoid casual sexual contacts. If these occur, use barrier methods of contraception (Femidom, condoms).
- Avoid shared needles (e.g. tattooing/ear piercing/drugs).
- Medical kits—if traveling to a high-risk area, take a clearly labelled medical kit containing sutures, syringes, and needles for use in an emergency.
- Avoid blood transfusion—$^2/_3$ blood donations in the developing world are unscreened. Know your blood group. Have good travel insurance including repatriation costs. In an emergency, the Blood Care Foundation can arrange screened blood to be provided anywhere in the world (☎01293 425 485).
- Vaccination for hepatitis B prior to travelling.

Useful information

Health Protection Agency (HPA) (2003) Guidelines for malaria prevention in travellers from the UK 🖳 http://www.hpa.org.uk

DoH: Health advice for travellers 🖳 http://www.dh.gov.uk

National Travel Health Network and Centre (funded by DoH): Information for travellers and health professionals including Yellow fever vaccination centres. Advice line for health professionals: ☎020 7380 9234 🖳 http://www.nathnac.org

Fit for Travel NHS (Scotland) travel site ☎09068 44 45 46 (Premium rate) 🖳 http://www.fitfortravel.scot.nhs.uk

Medical Advisory Service for Travellers Abroad (MASTA) Travellers advice line: ☎0906 822 4100 (Premium rate). General contact: ☎0113 283 7575 🖳 http://www.masta.org

Illness in travellers returning from abroad

⚠ In all returned travellers who present unwell, consider imported disease in addition to the usual differential diagnosis. Tropical medicine is a specialized field. If unsure, seek expert advice by telephone or admit the patient.

History: *Ask about:*
- Symptoms
- Areas travelled to (including brief stop-overs)
- Duration of travel
- Immunizations received prior to travel
- Malaria prophylaxis
- Health of members of the travel party
- Sexual contacts whilst abroad
- Medical treatment received abroad

Examination: Full examination. Particularly check for fever, jaundice, abdominal tenderness, chest signs, rashes, lymphadenopathy.

Investigations: Depend on symptoms and examination findings. *Consider:* FBC, thick and thin blood films for malaria, LFTs, viral serology, blood culture, stool culture (ensure it is fresh), MSU.

Fever: *Consider:*

Malaria^ND: 2000 cases/y. are notified in the UK. Easy to miss.
- *Symptoms:* Malaria is a great mimic and can present with virtually any symptoms. Usually consists of a prodrome of headache, malaise, myalgia, and anorexia followed by recurring high fevers, rigors, and drenching sweats—lasting 8–12h. at a time.
- *Examination:* May be normal—look for anaemia, jaundice ± hepatosplenomegaly.
- *Investigation:* In all cases of fever in patients who have returned from a malarial endemic area—even if the plane just landed there and they did not get off, send a thick and thin film for malaria.
- *Management:* Admit for further investigation and treatment if:
  - Very unwell
  - Unable to check a thick and thin film (e.g. presentation at a weekend or out of hours)
  - Thick and thin film +ve
  - Persistent fever despite −ve thick and thin film

Falciparum malaria: Caused by *Plasmodium falciparum.* Accounts for ~½ UK cases. It may not present for up to 3mo. after return from a malarial area. Can be fatal in <24h.—especially if it occurs in pregnant women or small children (<3y.). *Complications:* cerebral malaria (80% deaths); hypoglyceamia; renal failure; pulmonary oedema; splenic rupture; disseminated intravascular coagulation; death.

Benign malaria: Caused by *P. vivax, P. ovale,* and *P. malariae.* May cause illness up to 18mo. after return. All have very low mortality. Relapse may occur at intervals after initial infection as parasites lie dormant in the liver (*P. vivax* and *P. ovale*) or blood (*P. malariae*).

TyphoidND and paratyphoidND: Caused by *Salmonella typhi* and *Salmonella paratyphi*. ~200 cases/y. are notified in the UK.
- *Spread:* By the faeco-oral route.
- *Incubation:* 3d.–3wk..
- *Symptoms:* Usually presents with malaise, fever, headache, cough, constipation (or diarrhoea), nose bleeds, bruising, and/or abdominal pain.
- *Examination:* Pyrexia; relative bradycardia; rose-coloured spots on the trunk (40%); splenomegaly; CNS signs (coma, delirium, meningism).
- *Management:* Admit for further investigation and treatment with antibiotics.
- *Prognosis:* 10% die if untreated; <0.1% if treated. 1% become chronic carriers after infection.

Traveller's diarrhoea: In all cases send a fresh stool sample for M,C & S at first presentation, noting on the form areas visited. Consider the usual causes for diarrhoea (📖 p.255) including gastroenteritis (📖 p.452). In addition, consider:

CholeraND: Caused by gram –ve bacterium *Vibrio cholerae*.
- *Spread:* By faeco-oral route
- *Incubation:* Few hours to 5d.
- *Presentation:* Profuse watery stools, fever, vomiting, and rapid dehydration.
- *Management:* Admit. Requires expert treatment with rehydration ± antibiotics

Giardiasis: Common flagellate protozoan. Infection is suggested by an incubation period (≥2wk.); watery stool with flatus ++ (explosive diarrhoea); no fever. Stool microscopy may be –ve. If suspected, treat with metronidazole 2g daily for 3d.. Rapid response is diagnostic.

Amoebic dysenteryND: May begin years after infection. Diarrhoea begins slowly, becoming profuse and bloody ± fever ± malaise. Diagnosis is confirmed by microscopy of fresh stool. Take specialist advice on management.

Sexually transmitted diseases: 📖 p.742–45

HIV: 📖 p.498

TB: 📖 p.488

Viral hepatitis: 📖 p.496

Meningitis: 📖 p.1044

Further information
Health Protection Agency (HPA) Topics A-Z: malaria, giardia, cholera.
  🖳 *http://www.hpa.org.uk*

Breast disease

Presentation of breast disease

Conditions requiring referral to a breast surgeon

- *Lump:* New, discrete lump; new lump in pre-existing nodularity; asymmetrical nodularity that persists after review following menstruation; breast abscess; cyst persistently refilling/recurrent cyst.
- *Pain:* If associated with a lump; intractable pain not responding to reassurance and simple measures; unilateral persistent pain in postmenopausal women.
- *Nipple discharge:* Women <50y. with bilateral discharge sufficient to stain clothes, bloodstained discharge, or persistent single duct discharge; all women aged >50y.
- *Nipple retraction, distortion, or nipple eczema*
- *Change in skin contour*
- *Family history:* Request by any woman with a strong family history.

⚠ **Refer urgently** if a discrete lump and >35y. *or* definite signs of cancer e.g. ulceration, skin nodule, skin distortion.

Breast lump

History: Age (malignancy rare <30y.); how and when noticed; relationship to menstrual cycle; changes in shape or size since noticed; pain; nipple discharge; pregnancy and breastfeeding; family history; current medication (in particular, contraceptive pill or HRT).

Examination: Seat the woman at 45° supported on a couch. Look at contour of the breast, skin changes, arm swelling. Ask the woman to point to or find the lump. Ask her to place the hand on the side being examined behind her head. Palpate each quadrant of the breast with a flat hand. Check the tail of the breast in the axilla. Examine both breasts. If a lump is found, assess shape, size, surface, edge, consistency, mobility, and attachments. Check local LNs in axilla and supraclavicular region and hepatomegaly.

Differential diagnosis

- Breast cancer 📖 p.518
- Fibroadenoma 📖 p.514
- Benign mammary dysplasia 📖 p.514
- Mammary duct ectasia 📖 p.515
- Fat necrosis 📖 p.515
- Lipoma 📖 p.665
- Sebaceous cyst 📖 p.664

Management

- *No lump:* Reassure. Ask the woman to check her own breasts. Consider reviewing in 6wk.
- *Discrete lump:* Refer.
- *Asymmetrical nodularity*
  - If <35y. old with FH of breast cancer or ≥35y.—refer.
  - If <35y. and no family history, review in 6wk.—if the nodularity has gone, reassure, else refer.

Breast pain

History and examination: As for breast lump (📖 p.512). Use a pain chart to distinguish cyclical from non-cyclical pain.

Differential diagnosis
- Benign mammary dysplasia 📖 p.514
- Mammary duct ectasia 📖 p.515
- Breast cancer 📖 p.518
- Breast abscess 📖 p.515
- Referred pain (e.g. cervical root pressure)

Management
- *Cyclical pain ± nodularity:* Common
  - *If mild/moderate:* Reassure. Advise simple analgesia or OTC NSAID prn.
  - *If severe* (~15%—pain >7d./month and interfering with life): Discontinue any oral contraceptives and if pain persists, try either danazol (200–300mg daily for 1mo. then 100mg daily for 5 mo.) or bromocriptine (consult local protocols). Discontinue treatment after 6 mo. Breast pain will recur in 50% but often will be milder and not require treatment. If severe, repeat previously successful treatment.
- *Non-cyclical pain*
  - If mild/moderate—reassure.
  - If severe (~50%)—assess whether localized or diffuse. If localized, then refer. If diffuse, try NSAID or, if ineffective, danazol or bromocriptine. Refer if persistent or refractory to treatment.

Discharge from the nipple

History and examination: As for breast lump (see p.512).

Differential diagnosis
- Physiological (e.g. pregnancy)
- Mammary duct ectasia 📖 p.515
- Breast cancer 📖 p.518
- Mammary dysplasia 📖 p.514
- Intra-duct papilloma

Management
- *If ≥50y. of age:* Refer
- *If <50y. of age*
  - Large-volume, bloodstained, or persistent discharge from a single duct—refer.
  - Bloodstained or serous fluid which tests +ve for blood from multiple ducts—refer.
  - Coloured or clear discharge –ve for blood—check medication to exclude iatrogenic cause. If small volume, then reassure; if large volume or persistent, then refer.

Eczema of the nipple: Always suspect underlying breast cancer. Refer for specialist assessment—📖 p.519 (Paget's disease of the breast).

Essential reading
Cancer Research UK (2003) Guidelines for referral of patients with breast problems. Available from NHS Responseline ☎08701 555 455; e-mail: doh@prolog.uk.com; 🖳 http://www.cancerscreening.nhs.uk

Benign breast disease

Benign mammary dysplasia: Aberration of the normal cyclical changes. Various terms used e.g. epitheliosis, adenosis, fibroadenosis.

Presentation: Women <60y.; most common in teens or age 40–60y. Often history of premenstrual breast pain. Patients may notice a lump or diffuse lumpiness which may be tender/painful. Lumps may change through the cycle, becoming larger prior to menstruation and smaller afterwards.

Examination: Isolated lump or several diffuse areas of thickening scattered throughout both breasts. Characteristically, lumps are diffuse, difficult to define, not fixed, and not associated with skin changes/skin tethering.

Management
- Breast lump; breast pain; asymmetrical nodularity/lumpiness—📖 p.512.
- Diffuse symmetrical lumpiness—review regularly until satisfied that there is no enlarging mass.

Breast cysts: Breast acini coalesce to form cysts. Cysts may be of any size, single or multiple, and occur at any age pre-menopause.

Presentation: Breast lump ± pain ± past history of breast cysts.

Examination: Firm, rounded lump which is not fixed and not associated with skin changes/skin tethering.

Management
- If no past history of breast cysts, refer to a breast surgeon for exclusion of malignancy.
- If past history of breast cysts and lump is accessible, it is reasonable to attempt aspiration. Send aspirated fluid for cytology. Refer if fluid aspirated is bloodstained; lump does not disappear completely; cyst refills >2x; aspiration fails; cytology reveals malignant or suspicious cells.

Galactocoele: Milk-containing cyst which arises during pregnancy. Refer any new lump arising in pregnancy to a breast surgeon. Once diagnosis is confirmed, repeated aspiration may be needed. Resolves spontaneously.

Mastitis: 📖 p.808

Fibroadenoma: 75% all benign breast neoplasms. Common in women <35y. old. Giant fibroadenomas may occur in older women. Presents with painless, hard, extremely mobile lump, often difficult to locate. Typically slips around under examining fingers ('breast mouse'). Refer to a breast surgeon. Usually removed.

Mammary duct ectasia: Occurs around the menopause. Ducts become blocked and secretions behind become 'stagnant'. Ducts can rupture and contents cause *'plasma cell mastitis'*.

Presentation: Perimenopausal woman; discharge from ≥1 duct which may be bloodstained; breast lump; breast pain.

Examination: Nipple discharge ± breast lump ± inflammation of breast.

Management: Breast lump, nipple discharge, breast pain—📖 p.512. Usually no treatment is needed.

Fat necrosis: Usually history of injury ± bruising. As bruising settles, scarring results in palpable lump ± puckering of skin. Most common in women with large breasts. Always refer for biopsy. No treatment is needed.

Breast abscess: Usually occurs in a lactating breast following mastitis; occasionally in a non-lactating breast in association with indrawn nipple or mammary duct ectasia.

Presentation: Gradual onset of pain in 1 breast segment.

Examination: Hot, tender swelling of the affected area.

Management: Refer for surgical drainage.

Mamillary fistula: Rare. Usually as result of a breast abscess. Refer.

Gynaecomastia: Hypertrophy of the male breast. May be unilateral or bilateral. The whole breast is enlarged. No discrete lumps or fixation to the skin or underlying muscle. Check testes for testicular tumours; look for evidence of liver failure or hyperthyroidism.

Differential diagnosis
- Physiological (neonatal, pubertal)
- Idiopathic
- Hormonal
  - Drug induced e.g. cyproterone
  - Hypogonadism
  - Testicular, adrenal, or liver tumour
- Cirrhosis
- Hyperthyroidism
- Other drugs e.g. digoxin, cimetidine, spironolactone

Management: Treat cause.

Breast cancer screening

In the UK, there has been a national screening programme for breast cancer since 1988. The aim of the screening programme is to detect breast cancer at an early stage in order to ↑ survival chances (stage I tumours—5y. survival 84%; stage IV tumours—5y. survival 18%).

Breast awareness: Trials of breast self-examination have not demonstrated ↓ mortality. Instead, less formal 'breast awareness' is advocated. The DoH has produced a leaflet 'Be breast aware' (available at 🖥 *http://cancerscreening.org.uk/breastscreen/breastawareness*). It advises women to: know what is normal for them; look and feel; know what changes to look for; report any changes without delay; and attend for breast screening if aged ≥50y.

Effectiveness of breast cancer screening in the UK: Screening of women aged 50–69y. results in a 25% ↓ in mortality[S].

Screening test: 2-view mammographic screening performed 3 yearly. Screening detects 85% of cancers in women aged >50y. (60% of which are impalpable). ~70–80% screening-detected cancers have good prognosis. Screening more frequently does not ↓ mortality[R].

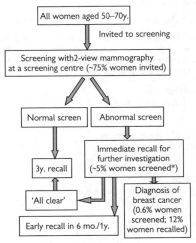

* 8% first-time screens; 4% subsequent screens

Figure 15.1 Organization of breast cancer screening in the UK

Interval cancers: Cancer occurring in the interval between screens. Can occur through failure to detect a cancer at screening or as a result of a new event after screening took place. In the 1st year after screening, 20% breast cancers are interval cancers. This ↑ to ~60% in the 3rd year.

Screening population: Available to women age 50–70y. (older women can request screening 1x/3y.). There is no evidence routine screening of women aged 40–49y. ↓ mortality[S]. A large study is under way investigating effectiveness of annual mammography in screening women <50y. with strong FH of breast cancer. Until results are available, local policies apply—contact local breast surgeon for advice. Genetic screening is also available for women with strong FH.

Acceptability of screening: 81% women find mammography uncomfortable but 90% return for subsequent screens. GPs have an important role—sending personalized invitations for screening to women from their GPs ↑ uptake rates[R].

Anxiety due to screening: False +ve results cause anxiety as well as prompting further invasive investigations. Anxiety levels in women who are recalled and then found to be disease-free are higher during the year after their recall appointment than women who receive –ve results at screening. In some women, the anxiety lasts years.

Patient choice: The breast screening programme has designed a leaflet for women, to facilitate informed choice. Copies can be obtained from the NHS response line ☎08701 555 455 or e-mail: *doh@prolog.uk.com*

Further information

NHS Breast Screening ▣ *http://www.cancerscreening.nhs.uk*
Cancer Research UK (2003) Breast screening—UK. Available from: ▣ *cancerresearchuk.org/cancerstats*

Table 15.1 Pros and cons of breast cancer screening

Benefits	Adverse effects
• Earlier diagnosis	• Discomfort and inconvenience of screening
• Improved prognosis and lower mortality	• Radiation risks of screening (very small)
• Less radical and invasive treatment needed	• Reassurance to those women who have false –ve result
• Reassurance for those with –ve result	• Reassurance to those who develop an interval cancer and possibly later presentation due to false sense of security
	• Anxiety and adverse effects of further investigation for those with false +ves
	• Overdiagnosis of minor abnormalities that would never develop into breast cancer
	• Earlier knowledge of disease and overtreatment for those who, despite early diagnosis, have unchanged prognosis

Breast cancer

Most common cancer in the UK. Accounts for 18% of all female cancers—British women have a 1:9 lifetime risk of developing the disease. Although mortality is falling, breast cancer is the 3rd most common cause of cancer death in the UK accounting for ~13,000 deaths/y.

Risk factors

- *Age:* ↑ with age—80% in women >50y.
- *Socioeconomic status:* Higher incidence in more affluent social classes.
- *Geographic variation:* More common in the developed world—migrants assume the risk of the host country within 2 generations.
- *Reproductive history:* ↑ risk if early menarche or late menopause; late age at 1st birth ↑ risk; ↑ parity → ↓ risk; breastfeeding ↓ risk.
- *Hormones:* Slight ↑ risk in current and recent users of combined oral contraceptives—excess risk disappears >10y. after stopping; risk ↑ by 6 cases/1000 after 5y. combined HRT use and 19 cases/1000 after 10y. use—also ↓ sensitivity of mammography; ↑ risk in postmenopausal women with higher endogenous levels of sex hormones.
- *Lifestyle:* Obesity ↑ risk post menopause; 30% ↓ risk if taking regular physical activity; high-fat diet is probably associated with ↑ risk; alcohol ↑ risk by 7%/unit consumed/d.
- *Physical characteristics:* Taller women have ↑ risk; women with denser breasts have 2–6x ↑ risk.
- *Ionizing radiation:* Exposure ↑ risk.
- *Previous breast disease:* Past history of either benign or malignant breast disease ↑ risk.
- *Family history:* 1 1st degree relative with breast cancer (mother or sister) ↑ risk x 2—but 85% of women with breast cancer have no FH. If several family members with early onset breast cancer, refer for genetic screening—BRCA1 and BRCA2 genes account for 2–5% all breast cancers.

Prevention

- *Lifestyle measures:* ↓ alcohol intake; ↓ weight; avoid exogenous sex hormones (e.g. HRT); breast feed.
- *Chemoprophylaxis:* Tamoxifen ↓ risk of breast cancer by 40% in high-risk women but limited by side-effects (thromboembolism and endometrial carcinoma). Other drug trials in progress.
- *Prophylactic surgery:* ↓ risk by 90% in very high-risk women.

Presentation

- Found at breast screening (p.516)
- Clinical presentation: Breast lump (90%); breast pain (21% present with painful lump; pain alone <1%); nipple skin change (10%—see opposite); family history (6%); skin contour change (5%); nipple discharge (3%). Rarely presents with distant metastases e.g. bone pain. In the elderly, breast cancer may grow slowly and present with extensive local lesions.

Paget's disease of the breast: Intra-epidermal, intraductal cancer. Any red, scaly lesion or eczema around the nipple suggests Paget's disease—refer to a breast surgeon. (*J. Paget (1814–99)—British surgeon*)

Management: Refer for urgent assessment to a breast surgeon. Specialist investigation includes: USS; mammography ± fine needle aspiration; investigations to evaluate spread (e.g. CT, liver USS, bone scan).

Classification: Virtually all breast cancers are adenocarcinomas—85% ductal; 15% lobular.

• *In situ* (non-invasive)
• *Stage I:* ≤2cm diameter; no LNs affected; no spread beyond breast
• *Stage II:* 2–5cm diameter and/or LNs/armpit affected; no evidence of spread beyond armpit
• *Stage III:* >5cm diameter; LNs/armpit affected; no evidence of spread beyond the armpit
• *Stage IV:* Any sized tumour; LNs/armpit affected; spread to other parts of the body

Treatment: Includes surgery (lumpectomy ± axillary clearance, mastectomy), radiotherapy, and/or chemotherapy. Tamoxifen ↑ survival of patients with oestrogen receptor +ve tumours (60% tumours) of any age but rarely causes endometrial carcinoma—warn to report any untoward vaginal bleeding. Continue tamoxifen for ≥5y.—take advice from a specialist prior to stopping. Anastrozole (Arimidex®) is an alternative in postmenopausal women and oophorectomy, radiotherapy, or goserelin can be used to suppress the ovaries in premenopausal women.

Lymphoedema: All patients who have breast surgery are at risk. Injury to the arm on the surgery side may precipitate/worsen lymphoedema. *Do not* take blood from that limb, use it for iv access, or vaccination. *Management* of lymphoedema—📖 p.1013.

Psychological impact of breast cancer: Depression, anxiety, marital and sexual problems are common. Be sensitive. Discuss possibilities of reconstruction surgery or breast prostheses, as appropriate. Refer to breast care nurse for support and advice.

Palliative care: 📖 p.999–1015

Breast cancer in men: <1% breast cancers. *Associations:* pre-existing gynaecomastia; Klinefelter's syndrome. Usually presents as a painless lump ± skin ulceration in a man >60y. Refer to a breast surgeon. Prognosis is poor.

Patient information and support

Breakthrough Breast Cancer: ☎08080 100 200 🖥 *http://www.breakthrough.org.uk*
Breast Cancer Care: ☎0808 800 6000 🖥 *http://www.breastcancercare.org.uk*
Breast Cancer Campaign: 🖥 *http://www.bcc-uk.org*
BACUP (British Association of Cancer United Patients): ☎0808 800 1234 (helpline). 🖥 *http://www.cancerbacup.org.uk*
Against Breast Cancer: 🖥 *http://www.aabc.org.uk*

Other relevant pages

Haematology and immunology

Anaemia (1)

Definition: Anaemia is a lack of sufficient red blood cells and thus haemoglobin ($\male$: Hb <13 g/dL; $\female$: Hb <11 g/dL). It results if there is:

- ↓ *red cell production:* Defective precursor proliferation and/or maturation;
- ↑ *loss or rate of destruction:* Bleeding or haemolysis;
- ↓ *tissue requirement for oxygen:* In practice—hypothyroidism.

Presentation

- Patients who become anaemic slowly may remain asymptomatic for a long time.
- As anaemia progresses, pallor, exertional dyspnoea, tachycardia, palpitations, angina (especially if past history of coronary artery disease), night cramps, and cardiac bruits appear.
- Ultimately, with severe anaemia, high-output cardiac failure may develop.

Investigation: Table 16.1

Table 16.1 Investigation and differential diagnosis of anaemia

MCV	Causes	Further investigations
Low— <76fl	• Iron deficiency • Thalassaemia • Haemoglobinopathy • Anaemia of chronic disorder	• Blood film • Ferritin • Hb electrophoresis (if indicated) • Reticulocyte count • Rectal examination • Faecal occult blood test
Normal	• Acute blood loss • Haemolysis • Anaemia of chronic disorder • Uraemia • Haemoglobinopathy • Marrow failure	• Blood film • Reticulocyte count • Hb electrophoresis (if indicated) • Ferritin • Serum B_{12} (+ intrinsic factor levels if ↓) • Serum and red cell folate • Renal function • Serum bilirubin
High—>96fl	• Folate deficiency • B_{12} deficiency • Alcohol • Liver disease • Thyroid disease • Myelodysplasia	• Blood film • Serum B_{12} (+ intrinsic factor levels if ↓) • Serum and red cell folate • Liver function • Thyroid function tests

Management: Treat the cause. If no cause for anaemia is found, refer for specialist investigation.

Vitamin B$_{12}$ deficiency: Vitamin B$_{12}$ is found in liver, kidney, fish, chicken, meats, and dairy products. Absorption takes place by active and passive mechanisms—the latter being dependent on intrinsic factor, (a protein produced by gastric parietal cells).

Presentation: Deficiency may be an incidental finding or present with anaemia, sore mouth (glossitis, angular cheilosis, and/or mouth ulcers), and/or neurological features (peripheral neuropathy, optic atrophy, subacute combined degeneration of the cord, or, rarely, psychosis).

Causes of deficiency
• *Inadequate dietary intake:* e.g. vegans—give dietary advice and/or dietary supplements.
• *Malabsorption:* After gastrectomy (total or partial) or ileal resection; pernicious anaemia—treat with regular doses of parenteral vitamin B$_{12}$ (hydroxocobalamin im—initially 1mg on alternate days for 1–2wk., then 250mcg weekly until blood count is in the normal range; maintenance dose is 1mg every 2–3mo.)

Pernicious anaemia: Caused by severe lack of intrinsic factor 2° to gastric atrophy. *Risk factors:* FH, other autoimmune disease (e.g. vitiligo), premature greying, blood groups A and HLA3. Long term, patients have ↑ risk of stomach cancer. Intrinsic factor antibodies (either blocking or binding antibodies) are diagnostic. *Treatment:* see B$_{12}$ deficiency.

Folate deficiency: Folate is found in highest concentrations in liver and yeast but is also in spinach, other green vegetables, and nuts.

Presentation: Deficiency may be an incidental finding or presents with symptoms and signs of anaemia ± polyneuropathy or dementia. Always check serum B$_{12}$ as deficiencies may coexist.

Causes of deficiency
• *Inadequate dietary intake:* Common e.g. old age, poor social conditions, malignancy, anorexia, excess alcohol.
• *Malabsorption:* Coeliac disease, Crohn's disease, partial gastrectomy, tropical sprue, lymphoma, diabetic enteropathy.
• *Excess use:* Pregnancy, lactation, prematurity, ↑ cell turnover e.g. malignancy, haemolysis.
• *Drugs:* Anticonvulsants, trimethoprim.

Management: In all cases, treat the cause. Supplement folate with folic acid 5mg od for 4mo. If malabsorption, may need ↑ dose to 15mg od. For prophylaxis in chronic haemolytic states or for renal dialysis, 5mg od long term is used (take advice).

⚠ **Folate supplements in pregnancy:** Advise women to take supplements from planning pregnancy to 12wk. gestation to prevent neural tube defect. *Dose:* to prevent first occurrence—400mcg od; to prevent recurrence or if on anticonvulsants—5mg od

Anaemia (2)

Iron deficiency anaemia^G: The most common form of anaemia.

Presentation: Usually found incidentally, though may present with symptoms and signs of anaemia. *Specific features of iron deficiency:* koilonychia (spoon-shaped nails); glossitis; angular stomatitis.

Causes of deficiency

- *Blood loss:* Major cause in the UK. Women <55y.—consider menstrual loss; take menstrual history; remain alert to the possibility of other causes. Patients >50y.—consider GI neoplasm. Ask about bowel symptoms, stools. Do a DRE. Check FOBs. Consider referral for gastroscopy ± colonoscopy.
- *↑ demand:* Common in pregnancy and lactating mothers; adolescence and infants (especially premature infants). No specific investigations are available.
- *Poor diet:* Common in the elderly, alcoholics, and vegetarians/vegans. It is also common in areas of the world where food is scarce.
- *Malabsorption:* Common post-gastrectomy (□ p.441) and may be the presenting feature of coeliac disease (□ p.454).

⚠ If the cause of the iron deficiency is not apparent, refer for further investigation.

Management: Treat the underlying cause where possible. Give oral iron supplements e.g. ferrous sulphate 200mg tds—iron may cause constipation and turn stools black. Hb should ↑ by 1 g/dL/wk.—confirm response to treatment 2–3wk. after starting. Continue treatment until iron stores are replenished (usually about 3mo.).

Failure to respond to iron supplements: Consider continuing bleeding, non-compliance with iron tablets or that oral iron is not absorbed, diagnosis is incorrect, or anaemia is mixed.

Haemolysis: Normal red cells survive 120d. before being removed from the circulation, mainly by the spleen. In haemolytic anaemia—red cells are destroyed faster than they are produced and anaemia develops.

Presentation: Anaemia often accompanied by jaundice due to bilirubin released when the red cells are destroyed. *FBC:* ↓ Hb; ↑ reticulocytes. Film shows polychromasia ± abnormal shaped cells (e.g. spherocytes) or other clues as to the cause of the haemolysis (e.g. fragmented cells suggest mechanical damage).

Causes: Table 16.2

Management: Refer to haematology for advice on management or if the cause is unclear. Rarely, spleenectomy is needed.

Table 16.2 Causes of haemolytic anaemia

Cause	Examples
Congenital	
Membrane abnormalities	Hereditary spherocytosis or elliptocytosis
Haemoglobin abnormalities	Abnormal Hb e.g. sickle cell anaemia (📖 p.526)
	Defective synthesis e.g. thalassaemia (📖 p.526)
Metabolic abnormalities	Glucose-6-phosphate dehydrogenase (G6PD) or pyruvate kinase deficiency
Acquired	
Immune	Autoimmune (warm or cold); isoimmune (e.g. transfusion reaction; haemolytic disease of the newborn —📖p.794), or drug-induced
Hypersplenism	Malaria, lymphoma, RA, portal hypertension
Red cell fragmentation	Artificial heart valves
Activated complement	Paroxysmal nocturnal haemoglobinuria
Secondary	Renal disease, liver disease
Miscellaneous	Infections (e.g. malaria), burns, chemicals, toxins, drugs

Aplastic anaemia^G: Bone marrow failure. Characterized by pancyto-poenia. Generally caused by damage to the haematopoietic stem cells by drugs (inform Medicines and Healthcare Products Regulatory Agency on yellow card—📖 p.128) or toxins. No cause is found in 50%.

Presentation: Anaemia, thrombocytopenia (📖 p.304), and neutro-poenia (recurrent infection). FBC reveals pancytopoenia and lack of reticulocytes.

Management: Refer urgently to haematology. Treatment is:
- *Supportive*—transfusions and antibiotics *or*
- *Definitive*—Aims to restore a healthy, working bone marrow. Bone marrow transplant is curative. Immunosuppressive therapy is an alternative when transplant is not an option

Further information

British Society of Gastroenterologists (2000) Management of iron deficiency anaemia
📖 http://www.bsg.org.uk
British Committee for Standards in Haematology 📖 http://www.bcshguidelines.com
- Diagnosis and management of acquired aplastic anaemia (2003)
- Diagnosis and management of hereditary spherocytosis (2004)

Patient information and support

Aplastic Anaemia Trust: 📖 http://www.theaat.org.uk

Haemoglobinopathy

Thalassaemia: Common in populations from Africa, the Middle East, Mediterranean, Indian subcontinent, and SE Asia. Results from ↓ production of either the α (α thalassaemia) or β (β thalassaemia) globin chains of haemoglobin. 2 main types of each are recognized:

- $α^{o}$ and $β^{o}$ thalassaemia: no gene product is produced
- $α^{+}$ and $β^{+}$ thalassaemia: α and β chains but produced at ↓ rate

β thalassaemia

- Defective β chain production → excess α chain synthesis.
- The excess α chains are unstable and precipitate in red cell precursors causing their destruction in bone marrow and spleen → proliferation of marrow, bony deformity (mongoloid facies, bossing of skull, thinning of long bones), and progressive splenomegaly.
- Homozygotes develop profound anaemia from 3mo. of age and without repeated transfusions would die in <1y.
- Patients who receive repeated transfusions grow and develop normally but iron accumulates due to the transfusions and death is usual in the 2nd/3rd decade due to iron overload (📖 p.444).
- Prenatal and antenatal diagnosis is possible. Refer all at-risk patients for genetic counselling/screening (📖 p.770 and 773).
- If suspected in an infant, refer urgently to paediatrics or haematology. Specialist on-going care is essential.

β thalassaemia trait (thalasaemia minor): Heterozygous patients. Asymptomatic but red cells are hypochromic and microcytic. May be confused with iron deficiency anaemia but ferritin is normal and does not respond to iron supplements.

α thalassaemia

- Prenatal diagnosis—refer all at-risk patients for genetic counselling/screening (📖 p.770 and 773). Antenatal screening is routinely offered in high-prevalence areas and will be extended to the whole UK by 2006.
- The heterozygous state for $α^{+}$ thalassaemia is haematologically silent.
- Heterozygotes for $α^{o}$ thalassaemia and homozygotes for $α^{+}$ thalassaemia have mild hypochromic anaemia which is normally asymptomatic.
- Haemoglobin H results from inheritance of $α^{o}$ from 1 parent and $α^{+}$ from the other. Patients are moderately anaemic with splenomegaly and have haemoglobin H (4 β chains combined with a haem molecule) in their red cells. Specialist management is needed.
- The homozygous state for $α^{o}$ thalassaemia is associated with foetal death at ~38wk. (Barts hydrops).

The sickling disorders: Most common amongst people originating from areas in which malaria is endemic—Africans (1–2% newborns) and certain Mediterranean, Middle Eastern, and Indian populations. *Varieties:*

- Heterozygous state for haemoglobin S (sickle cell trait—AS);
- Homozygous state (sickle cell anaemia/disease—SS);
- Heterozygous states for haemoglobin S and haemoglobins C, D, E, or other structural variants;
- Combination of haemoglobin S with any form of thalassaemia.

Mechanism: In Haemoglobin S valine replaces glutamic acid at position 6 in the β chain. Haemoglobin S undergoes liquid crystal formation as it becomes deoxygenated causing sickling of affected blood cells. The effect of sickling is to shorten survival of red cells → haemolytic anaemia. Aggregation of the sickled cells leads to:

- Tissue infarction—resulting in pain and/or tissue damage e.g. stroke (10% children with sickle cell anaemia have a stroke; 5% have recurrent strokes) *and/or*
- Sequestration in the liver, spleen, or lungs—producing sudden and profound anaemia.

Prenatal and antenatal screening: 📖 p.770 and 773

Diagnosis: FBC and film—chronic anaemia with sickling on film. Confirm diagnosis with haemoglobin electrophoresis.

Sickle cell trait: Patients with <40% of haemoglobin S have no symptoms unless they are subjected to anoxia e.g. anaesthesia.

Sickle cell anaemia: Low Hb level (typically 8–9g/dL) with high reticulocyte count. Patients compensate well. Illness is due to complications arising as a result of acute exacerbations or 'crises' and by the effects of recurrent tissue damage due to microinfarction over a long period of time. Prognosis is variable. In Africa, children usually die within 1y. In the UK, patients frequently survive into adulthood (average survival 42–48y.). Most common cause of death is infection.

Management:
- There is no medication to prevent sickling.
- Treat as if hyposplenic—give HiB and pneumococcal vaccination, annual influenza vaccination ± prophylactic antibiotics (📖 p.504).
- Advise patients to avoid cold and maintain adequate hydration.
- Warn about the dangers of anaesthetics (Medic Alert bracelet is helpful).
- Treat infection early.
- Give analgesia for painful crises—admit if severe.
- Admit if significant crisis of any sort (e.g. stroke, dyspnoea, acute abdomen, aplastic anaemia).
- Refer for early management of long-term complications (e.g. renal failure, epilepsy).

Patient information and support
UK Thalassaemia Society ☎0800 73 111 09 🖥 http://www.ukts.org
Sickle Cell Society ☎020 8961 7795 🖥 http://www.sicklecellsociety.org

Bleeding and clotting disorders

The purpuras

Vascular purpuras: Result from damage to the vessel wall. *Due to:*
- Infection (e.g. meningococcal septicaemia, EBV)
- Immune dysfunction (e.g. Henoch Schönlein purpura—📖 p.284)
- Vitamin C deficiency
- Part of the ageing process (senile purpura)
- Local stasis or ↑ venous pressure (e.g. varicose veins)
- Drug reaction (e.g. steroid-induced purpura)

Thrombocytopoenic purpuras: Pupura is related to the level of the platelet count. Bleeding is inevitable if platelet count ↓ to <5–10 x 10^9/l.
- *Non-immune thrombocytopoenic purpura:* Results from conditions which damage the bone marrow e.g. aplastic anaemia (📖 p.525), leukaemia (📖 p.532), myeloproliferative disorders (📖 p.530–1), CLL (📖 p.530), multiple myeloma (📖 p.530).
- *Immune thrombocytopoenic purpura:* Usually idiopathic (ITP). May be associated with SLE, transfusions, or drug reactions (e.g. heparin).

Idiopathic thrombocytopoenic purpura (ITP)
- *In children:* Self-limiting disorder often occurring after viral illness. The child is purpuric with a platelet count of <10 x 10^9/l. Despite this, severe bleeding is rare. *Management:* Refer to paediatrics as an emergency. Often no specific treatment is needed.
- *In adults:* Chronic relapsing illness. Insidious onset with haemorrhage and bruising. Platelet count is ↓. Ask about drug history (particularly thiazides, quinine, or digoxin). Look for evidence of SLE or lymphoma. Examine for presence of an enlarged spleen. Refer to haematology.

Impaired platelet function: May occur with any haematological malignancy resulting in bleeding—even if the platelet count is normal.

Clotting factor deficiencies: Genetic deficiencies of every clotting factor have been described but the majority of them are rare. Acquired clotting factor deficiencies are common e.g. vitamin K deficiency in newborns (📖 p.816), anticoagulation (📖 p.366), liver disease.

Haemophilia: 2 common forms—haemophilia A (factor VIII deficiency) and haemophilia B (factor IX deficiency—Christmas disease). Sex-linked recessive disorders. ♂>>♀. *Prevalence:* 90/million population (haemophilia A) and 16/million population (haemophilia B).

Classification: Carrier (♀ heterozygotes—>25% clotting factor activity); mild (5–25% clotting factor activity); moderate (2–5% clotting factor activity); severe (50% haemophiliacs—≤1% clotting factor activity).

Clinical features: Bleeding → joints or muscles is often delayed following trauma. If untreated, results in permanent damage. Pressure effects occur if bleeding takes place into a confined space e.g. intracranial bleed. Severity of bleeding is related to levels of clotting factors.

Management: All haemophiliacs need long-term follow-up via a specialist haemophilia centre. Prenatal and antenatal screening is available—refer to genetics. Treatment can be 'on demand' or 'prophylactic'.
* *On-demand treatment*
  * Transfusion of factor VIII or IX preparation as soon as possible after bleeding has started—most administer it to themselves.
  * Symptomatic treatment of bleeds e.g. rest, analgesia ± physiotherapy for bleeds in muscles/joints.
* *Prophylactic:* Prevents bleeds and their consequences.
  * Tranexamic acid—prevents bleeding after minor surgical procedures for patients with mild haemophilia / carriers with symptoms.
  * Desmopressin—stimulates production of factor VIII (not factor IX). Prevents bleeding in patients with mild/moderate haemophilia A.
  * Factor VIII or IX—factor VIII 3x/wk. or factor IX 2x/wk.

Problems with treatment
* *Inhibitors:* 25% of patients have antibodies to factor VIII or IX products. Treated with iv factor VIIa or, in children, through an 'immune tolerization programme' involving daily administration of factor VIII/IX.
* *Infection from blood products:* ~1500 UK haemophiliacs have been infected with HIV through contaminated blood products—more with hepatitis B and C. Whenever possible, genetically engineered 'recombinant' products are used rather than blood products.

von Willebrand's disease: Autosomal dominant deficiency of a clotting factor (vW factor). ♂ = ♀. Prevalence: 1% population. Most are mildly affected with easy bruising, nose bleeds, and/or menorrhagia. Severe cases may bleed into joints. FBC—normal platelets; clotting screen—↑ bleeding time. Refer to haematology. Mild cases are managed with tranexamic acid, desmopressin, and/or COC pill (for menorrhagia). Severe cases may need treatment with vW factor. No recombinant form available as yet. *(E.A. von Willebrand (1870–1939)—Finnish physician)*

Thrombophilia[G]**:** ↑ tendency to clot. Screen for a clotting tendency (blood test for factor V Leiden) if:
* Venous thromboembolism <45y.
* Arterial thrombosis <40y.
* Recurrent thromboembolism/ thrombophlebitis
* Unexplained prolonged APTT
* Clear FH of venous thrombosis
* FH of thrombophilic abnormality
* Patients with SLE, ITP, or recurrent foetal loss
* Skin necrosis (especially if on warfarin)
* Unexplained neonatal thrombosis

Refer to haematology. Patients may need short-term prophylaxis with anticoagulants at times of risk (e.g. surgery, pregnancy) or, rarely, long-term anticoagulation.

Further information
British Committee for Standards in Haematology (2001) Diagnosis and management of heritable thrombophilia 🖥 http://www.bcshguidelines.com

Patient information and support
Haemophilia Society ☎0800 018 6068 🖥 http://www.haemophilia.org.uk

Haematological malignancy

⚠ **Urgent referral of suspected haematological cancers**
- Blood count/film suggestive of ALL or CML
- Lymphadenopathy (>1cm) persisting for 6wk.
- Hepatosplenomegaly
- Bone pain associated with anaemia and ↑ESR
- Bone X-rays reported as being suggestive of myeloma
- Constellation of ≥3 of the following symptoms: fatigue, night sweats, weight loss, itching, breathlessness, bruising, recurrent infections, bone pain

Acute leukaemia: 📖 p.532

Lymphoma: 📖 p.534

Chronic lymphocytic leukaemia (CLL)^G: Occurs in the elderly, accounting for 40% leukaemias in that age group.

Presentation: Widespread painless lymphadenopathy often noted over a period of months/years. *Examination:* Lymphadenopathy, spleno- ± hepatomegaly.

Investigation: 70–80% all diagnoses follow FBC done for another reason—↑lymphocyte count. Blood film—small lymphocytes, many of which are disrupted to form characteristic 'smear'cells.

Management: Refer to haematology. Treatment is often unnecessary due to the benign nature of the disease. May require chemotherapy and/or radiotherapy.

Multiple myeloma^G: *Age:* Usually >50y. 2500 new cases/y. in the UK. A mutant B lymphoid clone is present. The proliferating cells grow mainly in the bone marrow where they cause infiltration, localized tumours and bone erosion. Main sites of myeloma involvement are: skull, vertebral column, thoracic cage, pelvis, and proximal long bones.

Presentation
- Bone pain ± tenderness—particularly back, pelvis, or femur
- Infection e.g. chest infection
- Anaemia
- Renal failure
- Pathological fractures and/or bleeding
- Hyperviscosity syndrome

Investigation: *FBC:* anaemia; *ESR* ↑↑; *blood film:* rouleaux formation. *U&E:* U and Cr may be ↑; *Ca^{2+}:* frequently ↑; *serum electrophoresis:* para-protein band; *urine electrophoresis:* Bence Jones protein. *X-ray:* erosive lesions in skull, ribs, pelvis. Fractures and vertebral collapse are common.

Management: Refer to haematology. Survival is increasing, with some reports of median survivals >5y.. Treatment is with chemotherapy.

Essential thrombocythaemia: Rare disorder. Patients have ↑ risk of both thrombosis and haemorrhage due to abnormal platelet function. *FBC*—platelet count >1000 x 10^9/l; WCC is normal or ↑; Hb is ↑ or ↓. Refer to haematology.

Chronic myeloid (granulocytic) leukaemia: *Peak age:* 30–60y. Found by chance in 20% patients. Otherwise, presents with non-specific symptoms e.g. weight ↓, lassitude, gout, anaemia. Splenomegaly is common and the spleen may be so enlarged that patients present with abdominal pain, digestive symptoms, or pleuritic pain due to splenic infarction. Rarely, abnormal bleeding occurs due to abnormal platelet function. *FBC:* ↑ WCC (usually >50 x 10⁹/l) ± anaemia. *Blood film:* bone marrow pre-cursors of myeloid cells. Refer to haematology. Median survival is 3–4y. from diagnosis due to transformation to acute leukaemia.

Polycythaemia rubra vera: Haematological malignancy resulting in overproduction of red cells. *Age range:* most >50y.

Presentation: Non-specific symptoms e.g. night sweats, headaches, skin itching (especially after a bath) dizziness, vertigo, and tinnitus. On examination—splenomegaly ± hepatomegaly; red-faced but skin has a dusky, cyanotic hue. Associated with gout, thrombosis and haemorrhage (due to abnormal platelet function and hyperviscosity), and peptic ulceration. *FBC:* ↑ Hb (usually >20g/dL). Differential diagnosis—□ p.304.

Management: Refer to haematology. Patients remain at risk from thrombosis and haemorrhage unless the Hb level is ↓ by regular venesection. Slowly progressive and survival for 10–20y. is not unusual—10–20% eventually transform to acute leukaemia; 1:3 to myelofibrosis.

Myelofibrosis (myelosclerosis): Progressive accumulation of fibrous tissue in the bone marrow cavity replacing normal marrow. Haemopoietic function is taken over by the spleen and liver. Patients are usually elderly and present with symptoms of anaemia, malaise, fever ± gout. The spleen is massively enlarged. *FBC*—↓ Hb; *blood film*—immature erythroid cells (normoblasts) and myeloid cells (metamyelocytes and myelocytes). Red cells are tear-drop shaped. Refer to haematology. Median survival is 2–3y.—but many live much longer. Occasionally transforms to acute leukaemia.

Myelodysplastic syndromes^G: Comprise a group of disorders characterized by ineffective production of ≥1 haemopoietic cell line. Differs from myeloproliferative disorder as there is no invasion of normal marrow by abnormal cells. Affects elderly patients and may be discovered incidentally or present with anaemia and/or bleeding. The spleen may be palpable but is never grossly enlarged. FBC and blood film are diagnostic. Refer to haematology. Treatment is with transfusion and prompt treatment of infection ± chemotherapy. Tends to evolve gradually to acute myeloid leukaemia (¾ in <2y.).

Further information

British Committee for Standards in Haematology ▣ http://www.bcshguidelines.com
● Diagnosis and management of chronic lymphocytic leukaemia (2004)
● Diagnosis and management of multiple myeloma (2001)
● Diagnosis and management of adult myelodysplastic syndromes (2003)

Patient information and support

Leukaemia Research Fund ☎020 7405 0101 ▣ http://www.lrf.org.uk

Acute leukaemias

The acute leukaemias are clonal malignant disorders (derived from a single cell) affecting all age groups.

Acute lymphoblastic leukaemia (ALL): The abnormal proliferation is in the lymphoid progenitor cells. Incidence: 48/million population/y. ♂>♀. Usual age range: 2–10y. with a peak at 3–4y. Accounts for 85% of childhood leukaemia. Incidence then falls with increasing age, apart from a secondary peak at about 40y.

Acute myeloid leukaemia (AML): Derived from abnormal proliferation of a myeloid progenitor cell. There are at least 7 different subtypes. Most common leukaemia of adulthood with ~5000 cases/y.. Incidence ↑ with age. Median age at presentation ≈60y. ♂=♀. Risk factors include previous chemotherapy or radiotherapy and exposure to radiation.

Presentation
Symptoms/signs resulting from bone marrow failure
- Anaemia: pallor, lethargy, dyspnoea
- Neutropoenia: infections of the mouth, throat, skin, or perianal region
- Thrombocytopoenia: spontaneous bruising, menorrhagia, bleeding from wounds, bleeding of gums, or nose bleeds

Symptoms/signs resulting from organ infiltration
- Bone pain (ALL)
- Superficial lymphadenopathy
- Abdominal distension due to hepatosplenomegaly ± abdominal lymphadenopathy
- Testicular enlargement
- Respiratory symptoms due to mediastinal LNs
- Meningitis-like syndrome
- Gum hypertrophy
- Skin infiltration (AML)

Investigation
- *FBC:* normal or ↓ Hb and platelets; WCC <1×10^9/l to >200×10^9/l
- *Blood film:* abnormal with presence of blast cells
- *U&E:* renal impairment if leucocyte count is very high
- *CXR:* shows mediastinal mass and/or lytic bone lesions

Management: Refer for urgent (same day) paediatric/haematology opinion if:
- Abnormal blood count reported as needing urgent investigation
- Petechiae/purpura/spontaneous bleeding
- Fatigue in a previously healthy individual if accompanied by generalized lymphadenopathy and/or hepatosplenomegaly
- Any other suspicious symptoms/signs

Differential diagnosis
- Infections (e.g. EBV)
- Myeloproliferative or lymphoproliferative disorder
- Myelodysplasia
- Aplastic anaemia
- ITP
- Lymphoma
- Metastatic disease
- Juvenile chronic arthritis (📖 p.874)

Treatment: Involves intensive supportive care and systemic chemotherapy. Bone marrow transplantation may be curative. Prognosis—Table 16.3.

Short-term side-effects of treatment
• *Drug side-effects:* Most chemotherapeutic agents have pronounced side-effects e.g. nausea, vomiting, hair loss, neuropathy.
• *Immunosuppression:* Any fever in a neutropoenic child or adult must be taken seriously and referred immediately back to the unit in charge of care. Likewise, any chickenpox contact must be referred immediately for consideration of administration of Zoster Ig (☐ p.494) or, for measles contact, administration of Measles Ig.

Long-term side-effects of treatment
• Heart—cardiomyopathy, arrythmias
• Lung—fibrosis
• Endocrine system—growth delay, hypothyroidism, infertility
• Kidney—↓ GFR
• 2° malignancies—may appear after many years
• Psychological effects

Table 16.3 Prognosis of acute leukaemia

	5y. survival
Childhood ALL	65–75%
Adult ALL	25–30%
AML age <55y.	40–60%
AML age >55y.	20%

Patient information and support
Leukaemia Research Fund ☎020 7405 0101 🖳 http://www.lrf.org.uk
Leukaemia Care ☎0800 169 6680 🖳 http://www.leukaemiacare.org
Cancer and Leukaemia in Childhood (CLIC) ☎0845 301 0031 🖳 http://www.clic.org.uk

Lymphoma

Non-Hodgkin's lymphoma (NHL)^G: Derived from malignant transformation of lymphocytes—B cells in most cases (85%). Usually develops in lymph nodes but can arise in other tissues almost anywhere in the body. *Incidence:* 5000 cases/y. in England and Wales (3% cancers). Incidence is increasing by 4%/y. ♂>♀.

Presentation: May be detected incidentally on CXR (mediastinal mass) or present with painless peripheral lymphadenopathy, abdominal mass (nodal or spleen), weight ↓, night sweats, or unexplained fevers. Other symptoms are dependent on site e.g. neurological symptoms if CNS involvement; pleural effusion; skin lesions.

Investigation: *FBC:* may be normal or show normochromic, normocytic anaemia. *Monospot:* perform in all patients <30y. with persistent lymphaedenopathy to exclude EBV. *ESR:* Normal or ↑. *LFTs:* may be abnormal if liver involvement. LN biopsy is diagnostic.

Management: Refer urgently to haematology. Treatment is based on histology, spread and prognostic indicators and includes radio- and chemotherapy. Histological types—Table 16.4.

Prognosis: Table 16.4. For DLBCL and follicular lymphoma, prognosis is better if age <60y., affected lymph tissue is confined to 1 side of the diaphragm (Ann Arbor stage I/II), serum lactate dehydrogenase (LDH) is not raised, there is no extra-nodal involvement, and the patient is fit.

Lymphoma associated with HIV: Incidence ↑ ×60. Primarily DLBCL and Burkitt's type. Extra-nodal involvement is common. Poor prognosis.

Hodgkin's lymphoma: Characterized by the presence of Reed Sternberg cells. *Incidence:* 1200 cases/y. in England and Wales. *Peak age ranges:* 15–35y. (>50% occur <40y.) and 50–70y.

Presentation: Painless lymphadenopathy (95%), weight ↓, night sweats or unexplained fevers, pruritus. The spleen is involved in 30% → splenomegaly. Investigation is as for NHL.

Management: Refer urgently to haematology. Treatment includes radio- and chemotherapy.

Prognosis: *Early stage disease* (Ann Arbor stage I/II—Affected lymph tissue is confined to 1 side of the diaphragm): 80% 10y. survival: *late stage disease* (Ann Arbor stage III/IV—affected lymph tissue both sides of diaphragm and/or extralymphatic tissue involvement): 60% 5y. survival. (*T. Hodgkin (1798–1866)—English physician/pathologist*)

Further information

British Committee for Standards in Haematology (2002) Diagnosis and management of nodal non-Hodgkin's lymphoma ▣ *http://www.bcshguidelines.com*

Patient information and support

Lymphoma Association ☎0808 808 5555 ▣ *http://www.lymphoma.org.uk*

Table 16.4 Types of NHL—presentation and prognosis

Type of lymphoma Annual incidence	Peak age	Presentation and features	5y. survival
Aggressive NHL			
Diffuse large B cell (DLBCL) *4/100,000*	64y. ♂=♀	Rapidly enlarging lymphadenopathy. Extranodal involvement is common. 10% have bone marrow involvement at presentation. 40–50% cure rate.	
Primary mediastinal DLBCL *0.24/100,000*	40y. ♀>♂ (3:1)	Bulky mediastinal mass ± vena cava obstruction and/or pericardial/pleural effusion.	80%
Anaplastic large cell *0.24/100,000*	34y. ♀>♂ (3:1)	Affects children/young adults. Often localized.	
Peripheral T cell *0.72/100,000*	61y. ♂=♀	Disseminated nodal and extra-nodal disease.	
Burkitt's *<0.2/100,000—more common in Africa*	31y. ♂>♀ (2:1)	Presents with bulky central nodal disease ± extranodal involvement (typically in the abdomen), bone marrow, and/or CNS involvement.	80–90%
Lymphoblastic (precursor B or T cell) *0.24/100,000*	28y. ♂>♀ (2:1)	In adults > 80% are of T cell lineage. Presents with nodal disease and/or mediastinal mass, bone marrow, CNS, or testicular involvement.	50–60%
Mantle cell *0.72/100,000*	63y. ♂>♀ (4:1)	Nodal, bone marrow, peripheral blood, and splenic involvement are common. Median survival 3–4y.	10–20%
Non-aggressive NHL			
Follicular lymphoma *4/100,000*	60y. ♂=♀	50% present with bone marrow involvement. Treatable but recurs with subsequent recurrences becoming more frequent and more difficult to treat. Resistance to treatment or transformation to DCBCL is the usual cause of death.	20–90%*
Small lymphocytic lymphoma/chronic lymphocytic leukaemia *0.72/100,000*	65y. ♂=♀	Blood, BM, and nodal disease. 3% transform to DCBCL.	50%
Marginal zone/gastric MALT *0.62/100,000*	60y. ♂>♀	70% localized disease. Many patients have a history of autoimmune disease or chronic inflammation e.g. Sjögren's disease or *H. pylori* infection (treatment may → regression)	

* Depending on international prognostic index (IPI) classification.

Immunodeficiency syndromes

A group of diverse conditions caused by immune system defects and characterized clinically by of ↑ susceptibility to infections.

History

⚠ Consider an immunodeficiency disorder in anyone with infections that are unusually frequent, severe, resistant, or due to unusual organisms.

Ask about

- Family history—Immune deficiency, early death, similar disease, autoimmune illness, early malignancy;
- Adverse reaction to immunization or viral infection;
- Splenectomy;
- Tonsillectomy or adenoidectomy;
- Radiation therapy to thymus or nasopharynx;
- Prior prophylactic antibiotic or immunoglobulin therapy.

Primary immunodeficiency: Since many 1° immunodeficiencies are hereditary or congenital, they appear initially in infants and children; about 80% of those affected are <20y. old and, owing to X-linked inheritance, ♂>>♀. Genetic screening is available for some conditions. Refer all suspected cases to immunology.

Classification: >70 primary immunodeficiencies have been described. Classified into 4 groups depending on which component of the immune system is deficient:

- B cells
- T cells
- Phagocytic cells
- Complement

Prevalence: Selective IgA deficiency (usually asymptomatic) occurs in 1:400 people. All other primary immune deficiencies are rare. Excluding IgA deficiency, 50% of affected patients have B-cell deficiency; 30%—T-cell deficiency; 18%—phagocytic deficiencies; and, 2%—complement deficiencies (see Table 16.5).

Secondary immunodeficiency: Impairment of the immune system resulting from illness or removal of the spleen in a previously normal person. Often reversible if the underlying condition or illness resolves. 2° immunodeficiencies are common—most prolonged serious illness interferes with the immune system to some degree. Treat the cause.

Infection in immunocompromised: 📖 p.504

Asplenia and splenectomy: 📖 p.505

Table 16.5 Type of infection and likely immune deficiency

Type of infection	Likely deficiency
Gram +ve organisms (e.g. streptococci)	B cell
Viruses, fungi, and other opportunistic infections	T cell
Staphylococcal and gram −ve infections	Phagocytic
Neisseria infections	Complement

B cell deficiency

- *Selective IgA deficiency and IgG subclass deficiencies:* Variable symptoms with most only mildly affected. When more severely affected, early treatment of infection is usually all that is needed.
- *Congenital X-linked hypogammaglobulinaemia and common variable immunodeficiency* (not inherited—cause unknown): ↓ immunoglobulins. Treatment is with iv immunoglobulin replacement. ↑ risk of leukaemia/lymphoma.

T cell deficiency

- *DiGeorge's syndrome:* Defect on chromosome 22 → absent/hypoplastic thymus (and ↓ T cells), absent parathyroid glands ± cardiac and/or facial abnormalities. Mild deficiency (80%) is treated supportively. Severe deficiency requires thymus/bone marrow transplant. *(A.M DiGeorge (b. 1921)—US physician).*
- *HIV:* 📖 p.498

Combined B and T cell deficiency

- *Severe combined immunodeficiency disease:* Autosomal or X-linked recessive. Absence of both Tcell and B cell immunity. Presents <6mo. old with frequent infections. Treatment is with bone marrow transplant. Untreated most die at <1y.
- *Ataxia telangectasia:* Autosomal recessive. Selective IgA deficiency or hypogammaglobulinaemia and Tcell dysfunction. Presents in early childhood with telangectasias, cerebellar ataxia, and recurrent chest infections. Treatment is supportive. ↑ risk of leukaemia/lymphoma.
- *Wiskott-Aldrich syndrome* (partial combined immunodeficiency syndrome): X-linked recessive. ↑IgA and IgE; normal or ↓ IgG; ↓ IgM. Presents with eczema, thrombocytopenia, and recurrent infections. Treatment is with bone marrow transplant—rarely survive beyond teens without. ↑ risk of leukaemia/lymphoma. *(A. Wiskott (1898–1976)—German paediatrician; R. A. Aldrich (1917–99)—US paediatrician)*

Phagocytic deficiency

- *Chronic granulomatous disease:* X-linked (²/₃) or autosomal recessive. Phagocyte dysfunction. Usually present <6mo. of age with fungal pneumonia, lymphadenopathy, hepatosplenomegaly, and/or osteomyelitis. Treatment is supportive with prophylactic antibiotics and early treatment of infections.
- *Agranulocytosis:* Absence of neutrophils. Patient becomes suddenly unwell with fever ± rigors, sore throat, mouth ulcers, headache, and malaise. Most develop septicaemia. Check urgent FBC. Admit as a medical emergency. Usually caused by drugs. Implicated drugs include:

• Co-trimoxazole	• Clozapine	• NSAIDs
• Chloramphenicol	• Thioridazine	• Maloprim
• Cephalosporins	• Gold	• Fansidar
• Propylthiouracil	• Penicillamine	• Captopril
• Carbimazole	• Sulphasalazine	• Carbamazepine
• Chlorpromazine		

Patient information and support

Immune Deficiency Foundation 🖳 *www.primaryimmune.org*

Allergies

'One man's meat is another man's poison'

Allergic diseases result from an exaggerated response of the immune system to external substances. Affects 1:6 of the British population—and is increasing. Allergic problems include:

- Asthma (📖 p.376)
- Occupational asthma (📖 p.399)
- Eczema (📖 p.636)
- Anaphylaxis (📖 p.1034)
- Rhinitis—both seasonal and perennial (📖 p.920)
- Conjunctivitis (📖 p.936)
- Food intolerance (📖 p.151)

Assessment

- Age
- Symptoms—past and present, main problem, frequency and severity, seasonal/perennial, provoking factors
- Impact on lifestyle—time off work/school, sleep
- Occupation/hobbies
- Treatment—past and present
- Home environment—pets, damp, dust, smoking
- Allergies in the past
- Family history of allergic illness.
- Examination will depend on main symptoms (e.g. asthma—📖 p.376)

Investigation

Skin prick testing: Identifies IgE sensitivity to common allergens, allowing diagnosis or exclusion of atopy. An alternative is measurement of serum IgE levels. In most places this is a 2°care procedure, though a pilot study has shown it is feasible in general practice. Patients should avoid using antihistamines before skin prick testing.

Patch testing: Identifies substances causing contact allergy. A battery of allergens on discs are applied to the skin—usually on the back—and stuck in place with tape. The skin response is then monitored. Only done in specialist allergy or dermatology clinics.

Management

Allergen avoidance: For anaphylaxis may be lifesaving:

- *Pets:* Exclude the offending animal.
- *Pollens:* Keep windows shut (including car windows); wear glasses/sunglasses; avoid grassy spaces; fit a pollen filter in the car.
- *Foods/ drugs:* Avoid the food/drug; avoid hidden exposure (check labels carefully); inform any school/ clubs a child attends; take food with you wherever possible; record drug allergies in medical notes.

House dust mite: Evidence that anti-house dust mite measures are effective in the relief of asthma and eczema is not strong. Measures focus on the bedroom. Advise the room should be ventilated regularly; encase mattresses, pillows, and duvets in mite-proof covers (leave in place 6mo.); wash bed clothes at 60°C every 1–2wk.; use a vacuum cleaner with an adequate filter; remove bedroom carpet; ↓ soft toys to a minimum and wash frequently/put in the freezer to kill house dust mites.

Medication: See individual conditions.

Referral to specialist allergy clinic

- For investigation and management of anaphylaxis;
- If the diagnosis of allergy is in doubt;
- Food allergy;
- Occupational allergy;
- Urticaria in which allergic aetiology is suspected;
- For consideration of immunotherapy.

Bee/wasp sting allergy: Accounts for ~4 deaths/y. in the UK. May result in a local or generalized reaction of varying severity. Intensity of reaction is also variable—because someone has had 1 bad reaction—they will not necessarily get another. Treat local or mild generalized reactions with antihistamine. Supply patients with more severe reactions with an epipen and teach them, and close contacts, to use it. Refer to an allergy clinic for consideration of desensitization.

Food allergy: Affects 1.4% of the adult population and 5–7% of children. Types of adverse reaction to foods include:

- Type I food allergy—acute allergy e.g. acute peanut allergy
- Type IV food allergy—delayed e.g. milk causing eczema
- Non-allergic food intolerance
- Pharmacological e.g. tyramine in red wine or cheese may provoke migraine
- Metabolic e.g. lactase deficiency
- Toxic e.g. reaction to preservative rather than food
- Food aversion—symptoms non-specific and unconfirmed by blinded food challenge.

A limited number of foods are responsible for the vast majority of cases of true food allergy—nuts (especially peanuts), wheat, eggs, fish, shellfish, and cows' milk.

Management: Avoid offending food; refer to allergy clinic for confirmation of diagnosis and dietary advice; supply epipen (and teach to use) in the interim if anaphylactic reaction.

Patient information and support

Allergy UK ☎01322 619864 ▣ http://www.allergyuk.org
Anaphylaxis Campaign ☎01252 542029 ▣ http://www.anaphylaxis.org.uk
Medic Alert Foundation (Supply Medic Alert bracelets) ☎0800 581 420
  ▣ http://www.medicalert.co.uk

Other relevant pages

Musculoskeletal problems

Sports medicine

Benefits of exercise: 📖 p.232

Career options for GPs—sports medicine: 📖 p.33

Nutrition: Recommend a normal varied diet (📖 p.226).

- *Special circumstances:* Particular sports have special requirements (e.g. ↑ protein for strength athletes). Increasing muscle glycogen stores before exercise can ↓ fatigue during prolonged heavy exercise e.g. 'carbohydrate (CBH) loading'—3–4d. of ↑ carbohydrate (8–10g/kg body weight) and a carbohydrate meal 3–4h. before competing.
- *Fluids:* Sufficient fluid during exercise is vital to good performance and health especially in hot conditions. Rehydration fluids containing carbohydrate and electrolytes are absorbed faster than plain water.
- *Supplements:* e.g. vitamins, minerals, amino acids, carnitine, creatine. A good diet generally supplies sufficient nutrients.

Principles of managing sporting injuries

- *First aid* (**A**irway, **B**reathing, **C**irculation)—refer severe injuries to A&E.
- *RICE*
  - **R**est: Relative rest of affected part whilst continuing other activities to maintain overall fitness.
  - **I**ce *and analgesia:* Use immediately after injury (wrap ice in a towel and use for maximum 10min. at a time to prevent acute cold injury).
  - **C**ompression: Taping or strapping can be used to treat (↓ swelling) and also to prevent acute sprains and strains.
  - **E**levation: ↓ local swelling and dependent oedema enabling quicker recovery.
- *Confirm the diagnosis*—clinical examination, X-ray.
- *Early treatment*—according to cause. Don't delay.
- *Liaise*—with sports physician, sports physio, and coach (if elite athlete).
- *Rehabilitation*—regaining fitness, strength, and flexibility; examine and correct the cause of the injury (e.g. poor technique, equipment).
- *Graded return to activity*—discuss with coach.
- *Prevention*—suitable preparation and training (e.g. suitable footwear, warm-up exercises, safety equipment) can ↓ likelihood of injuries.

Drugs and sport: 📖 p.138

Muscle injuries

- *Haematoma* within or between muscles can → dramatic whole limb bruising (due to tracking of blood) and stiffness. Treat with RICE regime; encourage movement in pain-free range.
- *Strain* (e.g. hamstring injury). Refer to physiotherapy. A 2° ligament injury is likely if the patient returns to sport too soon.

Ligament injuries (sprains)

- *Grade1*—local tenderness, normal joint movement. Give NSAIDs, support strain, encourage mobilization.

- *Grade2*—slightly abnormal joint movement. More joint protection, NSAIDs, elevate limb, encourage middle of the range movement.
- *Grade 3*—abnormal joint movement. Refer to orthopaedics.

Overuse injuries: Incidence increasing due to ↑ intensive training regimes—even amongst amateurs.
- *Causes:* Load too great for conditions, poor technique or posture, faulty or poor quality equipment.
- *Types of injury:* Stress fractures, joint tenderness or effusion, ligament and tendon strains, muscle stiffness. Overtraining syndrome—📖 p.584.
- *Management:* Rest, NSAIDs, physiotherapy, improved training regime.
- *Prevention:* Recognize and correct poor posture or technique, check equipment is appropriate and fits, warm up and stretching before exercise, gradually ↑ intensity and duration of training.

Environmental factors
- *Heat cramps:* Painful spasm of heavily exercised muscles (calves and feet)—due to salt depletion. *Treatment:* Rest, massage of affected muscle, and fluid and salt replacement (e.g. dioralyte).
- *Heat stroke/exhaustion:* Exercising in excessive heat → salt and water depletion, dehydration, and metabolite accumulation. *Signs:* Headache, nausea, confusion, incoordination, cramps, weakness, dizziness, and malaise. Eventually, thermoregulatory mechanisms fail → seizures and coma. *Signs:* Flushing, sweating, and dehydration. Temperature may be normal (mild cases) or ↑. *Treatment:* Rest, fluid, and salt replacement (e.g. dioralyte). Admission for iv fluids and supportive measures in severe cases.
- *Hypothermia:* Ensure appropriate clothing and limit time in the cold. *Signs:* Behaviour change, incoordination, clouding of consciousness. *Treatment:* Remove from cold environment, wrap in blankets (including the head), and transfer to hospital. Do not use direct heat.
- *Frost bite:* Freezing of the peripheries (usually feet, hands, ears, or nose). Tissues become hard, insensitive, and white. *Treatment:* Gentle re-warming, Refer if significant dead tissue. Debridement is usually delayed to allow natural recovery.
- *Diving:* Decompression illness is due to rapid ascent causing nitrogen dissolved in blood to form gas bubbles. Usually <1–36h. after surfacing. *Presentation:* Deep muscle aches, skin pain, paraesthesia, itching and burning, retrosternal pain, cough and breathlessness, neurological symptoms. Refer suspected cases urgently to A&E.

'Scrumpox' (herpes gladiatorum): Herpes simplex virus is very contagious and outbreaks among sporting teams are common e.g. spread by close contact and facial stubble grazes whilst scrumming. *Treatment:* Aciclovir (cream or tablets) and exclusion of infected players. Impetigo, erysipelas, and tinea barbare can be transmitted in the same way and are also sometimes called 'scrumpox'.

Fitness to undertake sport: 📖 p.209

Further information
British Association of Sport and Exercise Medicine 🖳 http://www.basem.co.uk
ABC of Sports Medicine. (1999) BMJ Publishing.

Common injuries and accidents

Wounds: Most patients with significant lacerations present directly to A&E. If presenting to general practice, perform immediate care (elevate bleeding limb and apply pressure to arrest bleeding). Advise nil by mouth and transfer to A&E.

Minor lacerations: Ensure no foreign body is in the wound—if in doubt, refer for X-ray/surgical exploration (especially important if injury is with glass). Clean away debris and any necrotic material. Check there is no damage to underlying nerves, tendons, bone, or blood supply before dressing or closing a wound. Check tetanus status. In assault cases, take particular care to document all injuries carefully e.g. with photographs, drawings, and measurements of wounds. Consider NAI in children—📖 p.886.

Closing the wound: Aim to oppose the skin edges without tension to allow healing. Do not attempt if you are not confident that you can achieve an adequate result. Always refer cuts through the lip margin to A&E and consider referral for facial wounds and wounds in children.
- *Skin closure strips* (Steristrips): Useful for small cuts in non-hairy skin that are not under tension. They can also be used in addition to sutures for larger wounds.
- *Skin 'glue'* (e.g. Histoacryl): quick (takes 30s. to set) and can be used on hairy skin such as the scalp.
- *Suturing:* Undertake training before attempting suturing. Infiltrate wound edges with 1% lidocaine (max. 2mg/kg). Addition of adrenaline (epinephrine) can help haemostasis but must not be used on digits or extremities as necrosis can occur. Take care to oppose edges accurately—start interrupted sutures in the middle of the wound. Use appropriate suture (e.g. adult face 5–0 monofilament nylon—remove after 5d.; limbs or trunk 3–0 nylon—remove after 1–2wk.).

Pretibial lacerations: 📖 p.563

Subungual haematoma: 📖 p.556

Animal bites: ~200,000 people are bitten by dogs each year in the UK. Animal bites are contaminated and wound infection is common. Clean carefully with soap and water. Check tetanus status. Do not suture unless cosmetically essential and there is minimal tissue damage—refer if in doubt. Give prophylaxis against infection (e.g. with co-amoxiclav or erythromycin).

Human bites: are especially prone to infection. Also consider risk of Hepatitis B and HIV. If HIV prophylaxis is indicated, it needs to be started immediately—refer urgently to A&E for local policy implementation.

Snake bites: The adder is the only poisonous snake in the UK. Bites are only rarely lethal. Attempt to identify the snake species and refer the patient urgently to hospital. Do not apply a tourniquet or try cutting or sucking the wound.

Weaver fish sting: Common on sandy beaches. The fish lurks under the sand so usually trodden on—presents with severe pain in the foot. Immerse the affected area in uncomfortably hot (but not scalding) water. Give analgesia. Pain resolves after 2–3d.

Jelly fish sting: Remove the patient from the sea as soon as possible. Scrape or wash adherent tentacles off. Alcoholic solutions, including suntan lotions, should not be applied because they may cause further discharge of stinging hairs. Ice packs ↓ pain and a slurry of baking soda (sodium bicarbonate), but not vinegar, may be useful for treating stings from UK species.

Insect stings: 📖 p.674

Removal of ticks: 📖 p.502

Air gun pellets: Common. Refer for X-ray. Can be difficult to remove—and may be left in place if not in a harmful position.

Coin and other foreign body ingestion: Most coins will pass through the gut without any problems. If asymptomatic, they can be left to take their course (advise checking stools to ensure passed). If symptomatic, refer for X-ray and consideration for endoscopic removal. If there is any indication of aspiration, refer urgently.

Fish hooks: Infiltrate with lidocaine. Push the hook forwards through the skin until the barb is exposed. Cut the barb off and then ease the hook back through the skin the same way it entered.

Knocked out teeth: Ask the patient to suck tooth clean, reinsert, or store in milk, and send the patient to the dentist.

Removing a tight ring from a swollen finger: Wind cotton tape around the finger, advancing towards the ring. Then thread tape through the ring and pull on this end to unwind the tape (levers ring over PIP joint). If unsuccessful, use a ring cutter.

Head injury[G]

Severe head injury
- Perform basic life support (📖 p.1020)
- Protect the cervical spine (see below and 📖 p.548)
- Transfer to A&E by ambulance.

Less severe head injuries
History: If possible, take the history from a witness as well as the patient. Ask about circumstances of injury, loss of consciousness (LOC), seizures, current symptoms, and behaviour.

Examination: Check scalp, head for injury, neurological examination (including fundi), other injuries—accompanying neck injuries are common.

⚠ Refer to A&E if [G]:
- Glasgow coma scale <15 at any time since injury (📖 p.1032)
- Loss of consciousness
- Focal neurological deficit since injury—problems speaking, understanding, reading, writing, ↓ sensation, loss of balance, weakness, visual changes, abnormal reflexes, problems walking, irritability, or altered behaviour, especially in young children
- Any suspicion of skull fracture; penetrating head injury; blood or CSF in the nose, ear, or wound; serious scalp laceration; or haematoma
- Amnesia for events before or after injury
- Persistent headache
- Vomiting
- Seizure
- Any previous cranial neurosurgical interventions
- High-energy head injury (e.g. pedestrian hit by motor vehicle, fall >1m. or >5 stairs)
- History of bleeding or clotting disorder or on anticoagulant therapy
- Difficulty in assessing the patient (e.g. very young, elderly, intoxicated, or epileptic) or concern about diagnosis
- Suspicion of non-accidental injury
- Inadequate supervision at home

If there is a history of neck pain/neck injury, immobilize the neck and refer to A&E.

If examination is normal
- Warn the patient (+ carer) they may suffer mild headaches, tiredness, dizziness, tinnitus, poor concentration, and poor memory for the next few days.
- Advise rest and paracetamol (but not codeine-based analgesics) for the headache.
- Young children can be difficult to assess—sleepiness is common and not a worrying sign as long as the child is rousable.
- Give written head injury information regarding warning signs to trigger reconsultation—drowsiness, severe headache, persistent vomiting, visual disturbance, and/or unusual behaviour.

Injury to the face: Mostly due to RTAs and violent incidents. Carefully document injuries, as your notes may be required for legal proceedings. Look for other injuries e.g. airway problems, head injury, neck injury. Palpate the face for signs of a fracture—if present, refer to maxillofacial surgeons for assessment. Check tetanus status. Post-traumatic stress disorder (📖 p.963) is common after facial injury.

Specific injuries:

- *Facial lacerations:* Best sutured by an experienced surgeon. Refer to A&E.
- *Fractured mandible:* A blow to the jaw can cause unilateral or bilateral fractures. Presents with pain (worse on moving jaw), bruising ± bleeding inside the mouth ± discontinuity of the teeth (displaced fracture) ± numbness of the lower lip (if the inferior dental nerve has been damaged). Refer for X-ray.
- *Dislocated jaw:* Presents with pain and the mouth is stuck open. Refer for X-ray and reduction.
- *Fractured zygoma/malar complex:* A blow on the cheek may fracture the zygomatic arch in isolation or, more usually, cause a 'tripod' fracture. *Signs:* bony tenderness, flattening of the malar process—best seen from above (may be masked by swelling), epistaxis, subconjunctival haemorrhage extending posteriorly, and infraorbital numbness ± jaw locked. Refer for X-ray. Advise not to blow nose.
- *'Blow out' fracture of orbit:* Uncommon fracture due to blunt trauma to the eye (e.g. squash ball injury). *Signs:* enophthalmos (may be masked by swelling), infraorbital nerve loss, and inability to look upwards due to trapping of inferior rectus muscle. Refer for X-ray and assessment of eye trauma.
- *Middle third facial fractures (Le Fort):* Usually bilateral. *Signs:* epistaxis, CSF rhinorrhea, crepitus on palpation, swelling, open bite, and risk of airway compromise. Refer for X-ray.
- *Nasal fracture:* 📖 p.918
- *Haematoma of the pinna:* 📖 p.923
- *Whiplash:* 📖 p.549
- *Avulsed tooth:* 📖 p.545
- *Dog bite:* 📖 p.544

Post-concussion syndrome: Seen following even quite minor head injury. Due to neuronal damage. Features include all or some of:

- Headache
- Dizziness
- Poor concentration
- Fatigue
- Depression
- Memory problems

Treatment is supportive and symptoms usually resolve with time (though can take months or even years).

Further information

NICE (2003) Triage, assessment investigation and early management of head injury in infants, children and adults 🖳 http://www.nice.org.uk

Neck problems

Neck pain is common (lifetime incidence 50%) and contributes to 2% of GP consultations. Prevalence is highest in middle age. Most neck pain is acute and self-limiting (within days/weeks) but 1:3 patients presenting to the GP with neck pain have symptoms lasting >6mo. or recurring pain. Pain is often poorly localized and neck problems commonly present with shoulder pain and/or headache (cervicogenic headache), so diagnosis may be difficult. Take a careful history and examine thoroughly:

⚠ **Neck trauma:** Any significant cervical trauma requires neck immobilization with a hard collar and referral to A&E for cervical spine X-rays to exclude vertebral fracture or instability that could threaten the spinal cord.

Spasmodic torticollis (wry neck): Common. Sudden onset painful stiff neck due to spasm of trapezius and sternocleidomastoid muscles. Self-limiting. Heat, gentle mobilization, muscle relaxants, and analgesia can speed recovery. A cervical collar may help in short term but can prolong symptoms. Often caused by poor posture e.g. computer /seating position; sleeping without adequate neck support; carrying heavy uneven loads.

Cervical spondylosis: Degenerative disease of the cervical spine can cause pain but minor changes are normal (especially >40y.) and usually asymptomatic. Pain is usually intermittent and related to activity. Examination reveals ↓ neck mobility. Severe degeneration can cause nerve root signs. Treat with analgesia and a cervical collar. X-ray only if conservative measures fail, troublesome pain, nerve root signs, or the patient has psoriasis (?psoriatic arthropathy).

Nerve root irritation or entrapment: 2° to degeneration, vertebral displacement or collapse, disc prolapse, local tumour, or abscess. Causes neck stiffness, pain in arms or fingers, ↓ reflexes, sensory loss, and ↓ power. The level of entrapment can usually be determined clinically (📖 p.590 and 592–3). In order of frequency:
- C5/6—affects thumb sensation and biceps muscle power
- C7/8/T1—affects little finger sensation and flexor carpi ulnaris power
- C6/7—affects middle finger sensation, triceps reflex may be absent— and, latissimus dorsi weak
- C4/5—gives shoulder pain and upper arm weakness

Management: Analgesia ± cervical collar. X-ray cervical spine—lateral or oblique views. Refer for physiotherapy. Refer for further investigations (e.g. MRI) if conservative management fails and there is objective evidence of a root lesion.

⚠ **Refer urgently to neurosurgery** if there are signs of spinal cord compression:
- Root pain and lower motor neurone signs at the level of the lesion *and*
- Spastic weakness, brisk reflexes, up-going plantars, loss of coordination and sensation below the lesion.

Cervical rib: Congenital condition—C_7 vertebra costal process enlargement. Usually asymptomatic but can cause thoracic outlet compression leading to hand or forearm pain, weakness, or numbness and thenar or hypothenar wasting. Radial pulse may be weak. *Investigation:* X-ray of thoracic outlet may show cervical rib—but symptoms are sometimes due to fibrous bands that are not seen on X-ray. Refer to upper limb orthopaedic surgeon for further assessment.

Whiplash injuries: Neck pain due to stretching or tearing of cervical muscles and ligaments due to sudden extension of neck—often caused by RTA. Pain and ↓ neck mobility typically starts several h. or d. after injury. Pain may radiate to shoulders, arms, and head.

Management: Examine carefully to exclude bony tenderness requiring X-ray. Treat with analgesia and early mobilization—collar may help initially but avoid long-term use. Recovery is often slow and 40% patients suffer long-lasting symptoms. Psychological problems and medico-legal issues can affect progress.

Systemic causes of neck pain: Always consider other causes of neck pain and refer as appropriate:
- Shoulder problems (📖 p.552)
- Temporomandibular joint problems (📖 p.912)
- Ankylosing spondylitis and psoriatic spondylitis (📖 p.576)
- Rheumatoid arthritis (📖 p.572)
- Polymyalgia rheumatica (📖 p.580)
- Calcium pyrophosphate dihydrate disease (pseudogout—📖 p.577)
- Diffuse idiopathic skeletal hyperostosis (DISH)
- Fibromyalgia (📖 p.584)
- Myeloma (📖 p.530)
- Metastatic disease
- Infection e.g. Staphylococcal, TB (📖 p.488)
- Osteomalacia (📖 p.566)

Further information for patients and GPs
Arthritis Research Campaign ☎0870 8505000 *http://www.arc.org.uk*

Low back pain^G

- *Acute low back pain:* New episode of low back pain of <6wk. duration. Common—lifetime prevalence 58%.
- *Chronic low back pain:* Back pain lasting >3mo. If present >1y. → poor prognosis.

Table 17.1 Causes of back pain—age suggests the most likely cause

Age (y.)	Causes
15–30	Postural, mechanical, prolapsed disc, trauma, fractures, ankylosing spondyloarthropathies, spondylosithesis, pregnancy
30–50	Postural, degenerative joint disease, prolapsed disc, discitis, spondylo-arthropathies
>50	Postural, degenerative, osteoporotic collapse, Paget's, malignancy (lung, breast, prostate, thyroid, kidney), myeloma
	Other causes: referred pain, spinal stenosis, cauda equina tumours, spinal infection

Prevention of back pain: Regular exercise; optimal weight; advice re-posture, working environment, and lifting techniques; correct uneven leg length of >2–3cm measured from pubis to medial malleolus.

History
- Circumstances of pain—history of injury; duration.
- Nature and severity of pain—pain/stiffness mainly at rest or at night; easing with movement suggests inflammation e.g. discitis, spondyloarthropathy.
- Associated symptoms e.g. numbness, weakness, bowel or bladder symptoms.
- PMH—past illnesses (e.g. carcinoma), previous back problems.
- Exclude pain not coming from the back. (e.g. GI or GU pain).

Examination
- Assess flexion, extension, lateral flexion, and rotation of the back whilst standing.
- Ask to lie down—this gives a good indication of how severe symptoms are.
- In lower limbs, look for muscle wasting and check power, sensory loss, and reflexes (knee jerk and ankle jerk). Assess straight leg raise (SLR)—sciatica is present if SLR elicits back/buttock pain compared to the other side.

⚠ 'Red flag' signs
- <20y. or >55y.
- Non-mechanical pain
- Thoracic pain
- Past history of carcinoma
- HIV
- Taking steroids
- Unwell
- Weight ↓
- Widespread neurology
- Structural deformity

Triage back problems into 1 of 4 groups

- *Simple backache:* Specialist referral not needed. Age 20–55y.; well; mechanical pain (with no symptoms/signs inflammatory disease) in lumbosacral area, buttocks, or thighs.
- *Nerve root pain:* Specialist referral not needed in first 4wk. assuming signs of resolution. Pain radiates to the foot or toes; unilateral leg pain is worse than the low back pain; numbness or paraesthesia present in the same direction; SLR reproduces leg pain; localized neurological signs (e.g. absent ankle jerk).
- *Possible serious pathology* 'red flag' signs: Check FBC, ESR (↑ in metastases, myeloma, discitis, and, often, ankylosing spondylitis), Ca^{2+}, PO_4 and alkaline phosphatase (↑ in Paget's and tumours); arrange lumbar spine and pelvis X-ray; and refer in <4wk.
- *Cauda equina syndrome:* Immediate referral. Sphincter and/or gait disturbance; saddle anaesthesia.

Management of acute pain in the surgery

- *Explain the likely natural history* of the pain and advise to avoid bed rest and try to maintain normal activities (↓ chance of chronic pain).
- *Don't X-ray routinely:* High radiation dose and +ve findings are rare. *Exceptions:* young (<25y.)—X-ray SI joints to exclude ankylosing spondylitis; elderly—to exclude vertebral collapse/malignancy.
- *Prescribe analgesia* e.g. paracetamol ± NSAIDs.
- *Consider referral for physiotherapy, chiropractic, or osteopathy* in the 1st 6wk. for those in pain or failing to return to normal activities. Avoid spinal pathology if possible. Refer patients not returning to normal activities by 6wk. for back exercises, if available locally.

Management of chronic pain: Aim to help patients accept and cope with pain and to lead as full a life as possible. Education, exercise, and psychological approaches may ↓ disability.

- *Exclude spinal pathology and lesions amenable to surgery* e.g. disc protrusion and spondylolisthesis.
- *Consider referral to a pain clinic.*
- *Analgesics* can help sleep disturbance but are of limited benefit if used regularly long term (use for exacerbations).
- *Tricyclic antidepressants* e.g. amitriptyline 25–75mg nocte may be helpful.
- *Other approaches:* Back supports (e.g. corsets or belts); heel raises (to correct uneven leg length), and TENS are sometimes helpful.

Further information

RCGP: Management of acute low back pain ⬚ http://www.rcgp.org.uk

Patient information and support

HMSO The Back Book.
Arthritis Research Campaign ☎0870 8505000 ⬚ http://www.arc.org.uk

Shoulder problems

⚠ Consider pain referred from neck, cardiac ischaemia, or diaphragmatic irritation (gallbladder disease, subphrenic abscess, PE) in all patients presenting with shoulder pain.

Rotator cuff injury: The shoulder is the most mobile joint in the body and relies on the musculo-tendinous rotator cuff to maintain stability. Disorders of the rotator cuff account for most shoulder pain.

- **Acute tendonitis:** Often caused by excessive use or trauma in the young (<40y.). Severe pain in the upper arm. Patients hold the arm immobile and are unable to lie on the affected side. Usually starts to resolve spontaneously after a few days. In middle age, can be caused by inflammation around calcific deposits—requires steroid injection.
- **Rotator cuff tears:** May accompany subacromial impingement pain (below) and is difficult to diagnose clinically unless the tear is large— suspect if subacromial impingement pain is recurrent. Refer to an upper limb orthopaedic surgeon.
- **Subacromial impingement:** Pain occurs in a limited arc of abduction (60–120°—*painful arc syndrome*) or on internal rotation due to acromial or ligament pressure on a damaged rotator cuff tendon.
  - *Patients <40y.*—associated with glenohumeral instability from generalized connective tissue laxity, or labral injury (see recurrent dislocation below).
  - *Older patients*—often due to chronic rotator cuff tendonitis or functional cuff weakness or tear.

Investigations: X-rays may show calcification of the supraspinatus tendon in acute tendonitis and irregularities/cysts at humeral greater tuberosity if chronic cuff tendonitis.

Treatment: Rest followed by mobilization and physiotherapy, NSAIDs, and/or subacromial steroid injection (📖 p.192). If conservative measures fail, refer for imaging, arthroscopy, and consideration for surgery.

Frozen shoulder (adhesive capsulitis): Overdiagnosed in primary care. Affects patients aged 40–60y. Painful, stiff shoulder with global limitation of movement—notably external rotation. Pain is often worse at night. Cause unknown but ↑ in diabetics and those with intra-thoracic pathology (MI, lung disease) or neck disease.

Management: NSAIDs, physiotherapy, and local steroid injection (📖 p.192). May take >1y. to recover and long term outcome is uncertain. If restricted movements are slow to return, consider orthopaedic referral.

Shoulder OA: Often occurs after history of trauma. Less common than knee or hip OA. Often associated with crystal-induced inflammation and 2° causes of OA (e.g. gout, haemachromatosis). Imaging for synovitis (USS/MRI) is important to rule out disease that may benefit from steroid injection. Shoulder replacement may be considered in severe cases.

Rupture of long head of biceps: Discomfort in arm on lifting and a feeling of 'something going'. A lump appears in the body of biceps muscle on elbow flexion. May be associated with other shoulder pathology. *Management:* Reassure. No treatment necessary.

Shoulder dislocation: Usually due to fall on arm or shoulder—anterior dislocation is most common. Shoulder contour is lost (flattening of deltoid) and the head of humerus is seen as an anterior bulge. Axillary nerve may be damaged → absent sensation on a patch below the shoulder. Occasionally, immediate reduction is possible (i.e. on sports field) but beware of concurrent fractures—refer to A&E for X-ray and reduction.

Recurrent dislocation: Usually anterior and follows trauma—but 5% recurrent dislocations are in teenagers with no history of trauma but general joint laxity. Refer for specialist physiotherapy and consideration of surgery.

Acromioclavicular joint problems: Pain on the top of the shoulder or in the suprascapular area suggests a problem with the acromioclavicular joint or neck. AC joint pain is usually due to trauma or OA. Joint tenderness and pain are present on palpation and passive horizontal adduction. *Management:* NSAIDs ± local steroid injection (📖 p.192).

Fractured clavicle: Common injury (5% all fractures). Occurs in neonates as a birth injury. In children/adults usually results from a fall onto an outstretched arm. 80% fractures are in the middle $^1/_3$; 15% the lateral $^1/_3$; and 5% the medial $^1/_3$. Refer to A&E for confirmation of diagnosis and fracture clinic follow-up. Treatment is with sling support and analgesia. Most heal well. Complications include pneumothorax, malunion, and nerve/vessel damage.

Further information for patients and GPs
Arthritis Research Campaign ☎0870 8505000 🖥 *http://www.arc.org.uk*

Elbow, wrist, and hand problems

Tennis elbow and golfers' elbow (epicondylitis)

- *Tennis elbow*—tenderness over the lateral epicondyle and lateral elbow pain on resisted wrist extension.
- *Golfers' elbow*—tenderness over the medial epicondyle and medial elbow pain on resisted wrist pronation.

Common extensor tendon inflammation at the epicondyle. *Cause:* Repeated strain. *Management:* Stop trigger movements if possible. Often settles with time ± NSAIDs. Recovery is speeded by local steroid injection (📖 p.192). Physiotherapy may help, as may an elbow brace.

Pulled elbow: Common in children <5y. Traction injury to elbow causes subluxation of radial head. Often occurs when the child is pulled up suddenly by the hand. Child will not use the arm. No clinical signs. ♂>♀. Left arm > right. X-rays are unhelpful. *Management:* Apply anterior pressure with the thumb on the radial head whilst supinating and extending the forearm. Immediate recovery is seen after reduction.

Olecranon bursitis: Traumatic bursitis due to repeated pressure on the elbow. Pain and swelling over olecranon. Aspirate fluid from bursa—send for microscopy to exclude sepsis and gout (request polarized light microscopy). Fluid may reaccumulate—if sepsis has been excluded, inject hydrocortisone to help it settle. Refer septic bursitis for drainage.

Dislocated elbow: Usually fall on outstretched hand with flexed elbow. Ulna is displaced backwards, elbow is swollen and held in fixed flexion. May have associated fracture. Refer to A&E for reduction.

Ulnar neuritis: Narrowing of the ulnar grove (from OA, RA, or post-fracture) causes pressure on ulnar nerve → ulnar neuropathy. Clumsiness with the hand is often the first symptom, then weakness ± wasting of hand muscles innervated by the ulnar nerve and ↓ sensation in the little finger and medial ½ of the ring finger. Rule out metabolic and autoimmune causes of a mononeuritis and refer for nerve conduction studies and consideration of surgical decompression if entrapment is likely.

Tenosynovitis: Inflammation of the tendon sheath—often due to unaccustomed activity (e.g. gardening). May affect extensor or flexor tendons. Pain is often worse in morning. Presents with swelling and tenderness over the tendon sheath and pain on using the tendon. *Management:* Rest and NSAIDs. If not settling, an injection of steroid into the tendon sheath can help.

De Quervain tenosynovitis: Tenosynovitis of thumb extensor and abductor tendon sheaths causing pain over radial styloid and on forced adduction and flexion of the thumb. *Management:* Thumb splint, local steroid injection, or surgery as a last resort. (F. de Quervain (1868–1940)—Swiss surgeon)

Ganglion: Smooth, firm, painless swelling—usually around the wrist. No treatment is needed unless causing local problems. May resolve spontaneously. Can be drained (large bore needle)/excised, but often recurs.

Work-related upper limb pain (repetitive strain injury)
Work-related pain in the arm ± wrist e.g. related to keyboard use. Over-use syndrome. Controversial—existence of RSI has been challenged. A country's compensation system has a great effect on the reporting of RSI. Diagnosis of exclusion—no physical signs. Exclude other conditions e.g. carpal tunnel syndrome (CTS), tennis elbow.

Management: Reassure—condition is curable. Continue work but avoid the aggravating activity. Liaise with work to ensure evaluation of workstation ergonomics. Gradually reintroduce activity. Physiotherapy may help. Explore psychological and work-related issues. A multidisciplinary approach is needed.

Carpal tunnel syndrome: Pain in the radial 3½ digits of the hand ± numbness, pins and needles, and thenar wasting. Due to compression of the median nerve as it passes under the flexor retinaculum. Worse at night. Symptoms are improved by shaking the wrist. *Associations:* Pregnancy, hypothyroidism, obesity, and carpal arthritis.

Investigations
- Phalen's test—hyperflexion of wrist for 1min. triggers symptoms
- Tinnel's test—tapping over the carpal tunnel causes paraesthesiae
- Nerve conduction studies

Management: Night splints; carpal tunnel steroid injection (🕮 p.192); surgery to divide the flexor retinaculum is curative in mild/moderate disease.

Osteoarthritis in the hand
- Heberden's nodes—swellings of DIP joints. No treatment needed.
- Bouchard's nodes—swellings of PIP joints. No treatment needed.
- First carpometacarpal OA—pain and swelling at the base of the thumb. A splint or steroid injection can be helpful. Thumb becomes stiff. If pain persists, surgery may help.

Dupuytren contracture: Palmar fascia contracts so that the fingers (typically the right 5th finger) cannot extend. *Prevalence:* 10% of men >65y. (more if FH). Less common in women. *Associations:* Smoking; alcohol; heavy manual labour; trauma; DM; phenytoin; Peyronie's disease; AIDS. *Management:* Often simple reassurance suffices. Ultimately surgery to release the contracture may be required.
(*G. Dupuytren (1777–1835)—French surgeon*)

Hand and wrist injuries: 🕮 p.556

Trigger finger: Nodules on the tendon can occur spontaneously and in RA and DM. Most common in ring and middle fingers. The nodule can be palpated, moving with the tendon. Pain and triggering (the finger is in fixed flexion and needs to be flicked straight by the other hand) occur because the nodule jams in the tendon sheath. *Management:* Local steroid injection or surgery.

Further information for patients and GPs
Arthritis Research Campaign ☎0870 850 5000 🖳 *http://www.arc.org.uk*

Hand and wrist injuries

Colles' fracture: Most commonly due to a fall onto an outstretched hand in an elderly lady. Pain and swelling of the wrist ('dinner-fork' deformity). Refer any suspected fracture for X-ray.
(A. Colles (1773–1843)—Irish surgeon)

⚠ Always consider assessment and treatment for osteoporosis in all men and women >50y. who have had a Colles' fracture (📖 p.568).

Scaphoid fracture: Caused by falling onto an outstretched hand. Pain, swelling, and tenderness in the anatomical snuff box. Symptoms may be mild and a fracture is easily missed—refer all suspect cases for scaphoid view X-rays. If X-ray is inconclusive and pain continues, repeat 2wk. later—bone scan can help if still –ve. Non-union and avascular necrosis of the proximal fragment is a potential complication, which can lead to long-term problems of arthritis and pain.

Fractured fingers: Refer all suspected fractures for X-ray ± reduction.
- *Fractured metacarpal* (fractured 5th metacarpal is most common)—normally heals if immobilized in a wool and crepe bandage for 10d.
- *Fracture proximal phalanx*—normally associated with a rotation deformity and may require open surgical reduction and fixation.
- *Fracture middle phalanx*—often can be manipulated into position and splinted by strapping to the next finger.
- *Terminal phalanx*—usually a crush fracture. Protect with a mallet splint.

Nail injuries
- *Avulsed nail:* Protect the nail bed of an avulsed nail with soft paraffin and gauze, check tetanus status, and give antibiotic prophylaxis (e.g. flucloxacillin 250mg qds for 5d.). Partially avulsed nails need removing under ring block to exclude an underlying nail bed injury—the nail is replaced to act as a splint to the nail matrix.
- *Subungal haematoma:* A blow to the finger can cause bleeding under the nail—very painful due to pressure build-up. Relieve by trephining a hole through the nail using a 19 gauge needle (no force required just twist the needle as it rests vertically on the nail) or a heated point (e.g. of a paper clip or cautery instrument). Of benefit up to 2d. after injury.

Nerve injury: Can occur due to trauma or lacerations. Examine sensory and motor function. Always ensure no other structures are damaged before suturing skin wounds. Refer all injuries for specialist assessment and management—microsurgery can improve the outcome considerably in some cases. Intensive hand physiotherapy is important to regain function. Types of nerve injury:
- *Neuropraxia*—temporary loss of nerve conduction. Often caused by pressure causing ischaemia.
- *Axonotmesis*—damage to the nerve fibre but the nerve tube is intact. The chance of successful nerve regrowth and a good recovery is high.
- *Neurotmesis*—divided nerve. Lack of guidance to the regrowing fibrils gives less chance of a good recovery and a neuroma may develop.

Median nerve damage: The median nerve controls grasp. Damage causes inability to lift the thumb out of the plane of the palm (abductor pollicus brevis failure) and loss of sensation over the lateral side of the hand.

Ulnar nerve damage: Injury distal to the wrist causes a claw hand deformity and sensory loss over the little finger and a variable area of the ring finger.

Radial nerve damage: The radial nerve opens the fist. Injury produces wrist-drop and variable sensory loss including the dorsal aspect of the root of the thumb.

Tendon injury: Can occur due to trauma or lacerations. Examine hand function. Always ensure no other structures are damaged before suturing skin wounds. Extensor or flexor tendons can be affected. Refer—primary surgical repair is usually the treatment of choice.

Vascular injury: Can occur due to trauma or lacerations. Check perfusion and temperature of fingers and examine pulses. Always ensure no other structures are damaged before suturing skin wounds. Refer all injuries for specialist assessment and management.

Mallet finger: The finger tip droops due to avulsion of the extensor tendon attachment to the terminal phalanx. Refer for X-ray. *Management:* A plastic splint which holds the terminal phalanx in extension is worn for 6wk. to help union (must not be removed). Arthrodesis may be needed if healing does not occur.

Gamekeeper thumb: Forced thumb abduction causes rupture of the ulnar collateral ligament. Can occur on wringing a pheasant's neck (hence the name) or, more commonly, by catching the thumb in the matting on a dry ski slope. The thumb is very painful and pincer grip weak. Refer—open surgical repair is the most effective treatment.

Hip problems

Hip disease causes pain on walking, ↓ joint movement, limp or a waddling gait, and shortening of the affected leg. This results in ↓ walking distance, difficulty climbing stairs and getting out of low chairs. Referred pain is often felt in the knee. *Causes of hip pain:*

- **Buttock pain**—PMR, sacroilitis, vascular insufficiency, referred from back.
- **Groin pain**—hip joint disease (OA, RA, Paget's, osteomalacia), fracture, osteitis pubis, hernia, psoas abscess.
- **Lateral thigh pain**—trochanteric bursitis, referred pain from back, enthesitis (spondyloarthropathies), gluteus medius tear, meralgia paraesthetica, fascia lata syndrome.

Osteoarthritis of the hip: Major cause of hip pain and disability. Incidence ↑ with age; ♂≈♀. *Predisposing factors:* past hip disease (e.g. Perthes) or trauma; unequal leg length. Pain may be diffuse and felt in hip region, thigh, or knee. Relieved by rest in early stages of disease. *Signs:* ↓ internal rotation and abduction of hip with pain at extremes of movement; antalgic gait; eventually fixed flexion of the hip. X-ray may confirm diagnosis but is often not needed, and there is poor correlation between X-ray changes and pain felt.

Management: Analgesia (e.g. regular paracetamol, NSAIDs), education, weight ↓, exercise, correction of unequal leg length. Walking stick ± shock-absorbing shoe insoles can help. Consider referral for physiotherapy (muscle strengthening exercises may ↓ pain) or to orthopaedics for consideration of hip resurfacing or replacement.

Total hip replacement >90% achieve good result. Most last 10–15y. *Post-op care:* risk of dislocation in the 1st 6wk.—advise to avoid crossing legs; take care with transfers; use a walking stick; no driving for 6wk. Physiotherapy is usually arranged via 2° care.

Malignancy: Hip and pelvis are common sites for 2° malignancy. Pain is severe and unremitting, day and night. Often accompanied by ↓ weight. X-ray may show no abnormalities or reveal lytic or sclerotic deposits. Bone scan is diagnostic but may miss myeloma. Depending on clinical circumstances, either refer for specialist advice (oncologist, radiotherapist) or palliative care. Treat with analgesia meanwhile (📖 p.172 and 1002).

Hip fracture: Common amongst the elderly—carries high morbidity and mortality (≈25%). ♀>♂. Usually occurs through the neck of the femur. *Risk factors:* maternal hip fracture, osteoporosis, unsteadiness, sedative medication, poor eye sight, and polypharmacy. There may be a history of a fall but not always. Suspect in any patient who is elderly or has risk factors for osteoporosis (📖 p.568) who is 'off legs' . Occasionally, patients may still be able to weight bear with difficulty. *Signs:* external rotation, shortening, and adduction of leg. *Management:* refer urgently to A&E for X-ray.

Hip dislocation: Occurs in front seat passengers in car accidents as the knee strikes the dashboard. Reduction under anaesthetic is required.

Greater trochanter pain (trochanteric bursitis): Can mimic ± coexist with hip OA. May be associated with muscle weakness around the hip. *Diagnosis:* point tenderness over the greater trochanter.

Management: Consider local steroid injection if trochanteric bursitis is likely—though most cases are due to referred back pain. Refer to physiotherapy for exercises to strengthen hip musculature to prevent recurrence or for treatment of back problems if causing the pain.

Fascia lata syndrome: Inflammation of the fascia lata causing pain in the lateral thigh. Often due to overuse or weak musculature around the hip. Treatment is rest ± referral to physiotherapy.

Hip infection: Presents with hip pain, ↓ weight, night sweats, and rigors. Be aware of infection in patients with RA, hip prosthesis, or immunocompromise. Refer for investigation. X-rays are often unhelpful—bone scan is non-specific. *Management:* admit for ultrasound-guided drainage, bed rest, and iv antibiotics.

Avascular necrosis: May present with hip pain. Have a high level of suspicion in patients with risk factors—SLE, sickle cell disease, high alcohol consumption, pregnancy, or corticosteroids. X-ray or bone scan may confirm diagnosis but MRI is most sensitive. Specialist management is needed.

Groin pain in athletes: Consider:
• Conjoint tendon pathology (Gilmour's groin)
• Symphysitis (footballers notably)
• Adductor tendonitis
Liaise with a sports medicine physician or physiotherapist early.

Further information for patients and GPs
Arthritis Research Campaign (ARC) ☎0870 8505000
    🖳 http://www.arc.org.uk

Knee problems (1)

Remember, knee pain can be referred from the hip, so examine the hip as well. Ask about trauma, pain, swelling, mobility, locking, clicking, and giving way.

Non-traumatic knee effusion: *Common causes:*
- Gout
- Calcium pyrophosphate dihydrate disease (pseudogout)
- Spondylarthropathies (includes reactive arthritis)
- RA

Investigation
- Blood: FBC, ESR, rheumatoid factor, anti-nuclear antibody, LFTs, bone biochemistry, and thyroid function tests.
- Drain effusion (or refer to rheumatology to drain) and send fluid for polarized light miscroscopy (for crystals) and microbiology (?infection).

Management
- If no infection, inject with long-acting steroid, immobilize, and advise no weight bearing for 48h.
- Refer to rheumatology.

OA knee: Very common. X-ray evidence of OA is even more common. *Treatment:* education; glucosamine; analgesia (paracetamol ± NSAIDs); exercise (refer to physiotherapy ± exercise programme). Suggest using a walking stick. Steroid injection (📖 p.190) can be helpful in some patients. If pain and disability are severe, refer to orthopaedics for consideration of total knee replacement.

Total knee replacement: Very successful procedure → ↓ pain and ↑ mobility. 95% prostheses last 10y.

Infection of the knee joint: Most commonly, infected joint. *Signs:* hot, red, swollen, painful knee. *Differential diagnosis:* Reiter's disease, gout, pseudogout, traumatic effusion, RA. If infection is suspected, refer to rheumatology or orthopaedics for investigation.

Chondromalacia patellae: Common in teenage girls. Pain on walking up or down stairs or on prolonged sitting. *Signs:* pain on stressing the undersurface of the patella. Arthroscopy (indicated only in severe cases) reveals degenerative cartilage on the posterior surface of the patella. *Management:* analgesia + physiotherapy (vastus medialis strengthening relieves pain in 80%). For persistent cases, exclude spondylarthropathy (enthesitis pain—📖 p.576) and refer to orthopaedics for arthroscopy.

Osgood–Schlatter disease: Seen in athletic teenagers. Pain and tenderness ± swelling over the tibial tubercle. X-rays not required. *Management:* avoid aggravating activities. Usually settles over a few months. If not settling, refer to orthopaedics or rheumatology for further assessment. (*R.B. Osgood (1873–1956)—US orthopaedic surgeon; C.B. Schlatter (1864–1934)—Swiss physician*)

Growing pains: A term often used wrongly for diffuse aches and pains in children. The syndrome involves the child waking at night with leg or arm pain. Rubbing the limb → rapid relief. There is no pain or disability in the morning. Examination is normal and pains resolve spontaneously.

Hypermobility: Associated with knee pain, especially if associated patellar subluxation. A FH of hypermobility is common. Pain may be aggravated by exercise. Extremely hypermobile individuals may have a hereditary connective tissue disorder (e.g. Ehlers-Danlos syndrome) and may suffer from premature OA. Refer for specialist rheumatology advice.

Patellar dislocation: Lateral dislocation of the patella and tearing of the medial capsule and quadriceps can occur due to trauma. More common in young people and in joint hypermobility syndrome. Patient is in pain and unable to flex knee. Refer, via A&E or orthopaedics, for reduction. Recurrent dislocation on minimal trauma can be troublesome—refer to rheumatology to exclude a hereditary connective tissue disorder and/or to orthopaedics.

Recurrent subluxation of the patella: Medial knee pain + knee 'gives way' due to lateral subluxation of the patella. Most common in girls with valgus knees. *Associations:* familial, hypermobility, high riding patella. *Signs:* ↑ lateral patella movement and +ve apprehension test (pain and reflex contraction of quadriceps on lateral patella pressure).

Management: Refer to physiotherapy for vastus medialis exercises. If that is unhelpful, refer to rheumatology to exclude a hereditary connective tissue disorder and/or to orthopaedics for consideration of lateral retinacular release.

Bipartite patella: Detected on X-ray. Usually asymptomatic incidental finding but can cause pain due to excessive mobility of a patella fragment. If troublesome, refer for fragment excision.

Patella tendonitis: Small tear in the patella tendon causes pain. Most commonly seen in athletes. Differential diagnosis includes inferior patellar pole enthesitis (spondylarthropathies), fat-pad syndrome, anterior cartilage lesion, and bursitis. Diagnosis is with USS. *Treatment:* rest, NSAIDs ± steroid injection around (not into) the tendon.

Bursitis: Prepatella bursitis (housemaid's knee) is associated with excessive kneeling. Vicar's knee (infrapatella bursitis) is associated with more upright kneeling. *Management:* avoid aggravating activity, aspirate ± steroid injection (↓ recurrence). If clinically infected, refer to orthopaedics for drainage and antibiotics.

Baker's cyst: Popliteal cyst (herniation of joint synovium) can cause swelling and discomfort behind the knee. Rupture may result in pain and swelling in the calf, mimicking DVT. Treat underlying knee synovitis. Surgical cyst removal may be necessary if persistent problems. (*W.M. Baker (1839–96)—English surgeon*).

Further information for patients and GPs
Arthritis Research Campaign (ARC) ☎0870 8505000
  🖳 http://www.arc.org.uk

Knee problems (2)

Iliotibial tract syndrome: Pain due to inflammation of the synovium under the iliotibial tract from rubbing of the tract on the lateral femoral condyle. Seen in runners. *Management:* rest, NSAIDs, specialist physiotherapy ± steroid injection.

Collateral ligament injury: Common in contact sports. Causes knee effusion (if severe) ± tenderness over the injured ligament. Collateral ligaments provide lateral stability to the knee. Normally there is <5° of movement—if >5° the ligament may be ruptured. *Management:* rest, knee support, analgesia. Refer to orthopaedics if rupture suspected.

Cruciate ligament injury: Cruciate ligaments provide anterior/posterior knee stability.

- *Anterior cruciate tears:* occur due to a blow to the back of tibia ± rotation when foot is fixed on the ground. *Signs:* effusion and +ve draw test (with the patient supine with foot fixed and knee at 90°, apply pressure to pull the tibia forward (it should be stable)—test is +ve if the tibia moves forward on the femur).
- *Posterior cruciate tears:* caused e.g. when the knee hits the dashboard in car accidents. Reverse draw test is +ve (with patient supine and knee at 90°, apply pressure to push tibia backwards (it should be stable)—test is +ve if the tibia moves backward on the femur).

Management: Refer to orthopaedics. Assessment can be difficult—refer if unsure. Plaster cast and then physiotherapy helps most (60%) but some require reconstructive surgery. Consider urgent referral if keen sportsmen.

Meniscal lesions: Twisting with the knee flexed can cause medial (bucket handle) meniscal tears and adduction with internal rotation can cause lateral cartilage tears. *Symptoms/signs:*

- Locking of the knee—extension is limited due to cartilage fragment lodging between the condyles.
- Giving way of the knee.
- Tender joint line.
- +ve McMurrays test—rotation of the tibia on the femur with flexed knee, followed by knee extension, causes pain and a click as the trapped cartilage fragment is released. Reliability of this test is debated.

Management: Refer for MRI ± arthroscopy. Treated by removal of the torn meniscal fragment.

Meniscal cysts: Pain + swelling over the joint line due to a meniscal tear. Lateral cysts are more common than medial. The knee may click and give way. Refer for arthroscopy—removal of damaged meniscus relieves pain.

Loose bodies in the knee: May result in locking of the knee joint in any direction of movement and/or effusion. *Causes:* OA, chip fractures, osteochondritis dissecans, synovial chondromatosis. If problematic, refer for removal.

Osteochondritis dissecans: Necrosis of articular cartilage and underlying bone. Can cause loose body formation. Cause unknown. Seen in young adults → pain after exercise and intermittent knee swelling ± locking. X-ray shows cartilage damage. Predisposes to arthritis. Refer for expert management.

Shin splints: Exercise-related shin pain may be due to a stress fracture of the tibia, compartment syndrome, or periostitis. Fractures are not always obvious on X-ray—bone scan is more sensitive and shows periostitis. *Management:* rest and analgesia. Consider referral to sports physiotherapist.

Pretibial lacerations: The shin has poor blood supply, especially in the elderly. Flap wounds are common, may heal poorly ± break down to form ulcers. *Management:* carefully realign the flap, secure with steristrips, without tension and bandage. Advise elevation of the leg. Review regularly to check healing.

Ankle and foot problems

Ottawa rules for ankle and foot X-ray

Ankle injury

Refer for an ankle X-ray if there is pain in the malleolar area AND

- bone tenderness at the posterior tip of the lateral malleolus *or*
- bone tenderness at the posterior tip of the medial malleolus *or*
- patient is unable to weight bear at the time of the injury and when seen.

Foot injury:

Refer for a foot X-ray if there is pain in the midfoot AND

- bone tenderness at the 5th metatarsal base *or*
- bone tenderness at the narvicular *or*
- patient is unable to weight bear at the time of injury and when seen.

Otherwise diagnose a sprain

Foot and heel pain: 📖 p.262

Osteochondritis: 📖 p563

Acute ankle or foot injury: Twisting of the ankle → pain and swelling is a very common injury. Foot injuries are also common. It can be difficult to distinguish between a sprain and a fracture. The Ottawa rules ↓ need for X-ray by ¼ . Treat sprains with rest, ice, compression, elevation, and analgesia (paracetamol ± NSAIDs). If severe (or the patient is an athlete), refer to physiotherapy.

Achilles tendonitis: Inflammation of the Achilles tendon may be related to overuse or a spondylarthropathy. Presents as a painful local swelling of the tendon. *Management:* Rest, NSAIDs, heel padding, physiotherapy. Steroid injection may help (never inject into the tendon). If persistent, refer to rheumatology.

Ruptured Achilles tendon: Presents with a sudden pain in the back of the ankle during activity (felt as a 'kick'). The patient walks with a limp. There is some plantar flexion, but the patient cannot raise the affected heel from the floor when standing on tip toe. A 'gap' can usually be felt in the tendon. *Management:* Refer immediately for consideration of repair. The alternative is immobilization in plaster with the foot plantar flexed.

Plantar fasciitis/bursitis: Common cause of inferior heel pain. Pain is worst when taking the first few steps after getting out of bed. Usually unilateral and generally settles in <6wk.. *Management:* Advise shoes with arch support, soft heels, and heel padding. Achilles tendon stretching exercises can help (see Arthritis Research Council website for leaflet— 📖 p.561). NSAIDs and steroid injection (📖 p.190) are also helpful. In persistent cases, refer to rheumatology.

Tender heel pad: Dull throbbing pain under the heel. Develops over a few months after heel trauma. May be due to plantar fasciitis, bursitis, or tendonitis. *Management:* Rest and heel padding. Refer to physiotherapy—ultrasound treatment can help. Blind steroid injections into the fat pad are not recommended. In persistent cases, refer to rheumatology.

Flat feet (pes planus): Low medial arch. Normal in young children (📖 p.872). Painless flat foot in which the arch is restored on standing on tiptoe needs no treatment. If painful, may be helped by analgesia, exercises, or insoles. For severe pain, hind foot fusion is an option. Refer if the arch does not restore on tiptoeing.

Pes cavus: High foot arches may be idiopathic, due to polio, spina bifida, or other neurological conditions. Toes may claw. *Management:* Padding under metatarsal heads relieves pressure. Operative treatment— soft tissue release or arthrodesis straightens toes. Can lead to tarsal bone OA causing pain—refer for fusion.

Metatarsalgia (forefoot pain): May be due to synovitis, sesamoid fracture, injury, or ↑ pressure on the metatarsal heads due to mechanical dysfunction (e.g. in RA). Treat with insoles and padding under the MT heads. Surgery may be helpful in RA—discuss with rheumatologist.

Morton's metatarsalgia (interdigital neuroma): Pain due to entrapment of the interdigital nerve between the 3rd/4th metatarsal heads. *Symptoms:* Gradual onset of sudden attacks of pain or paraesthesia during walking. *Management:* Steroid injection and advice re footwear may help. Some need surgical excision of the neuroma.
(T.G. Morton (1835–1903)—US surgeon)

Toe fracture: Often due to dropping a heavy weight onto the toe. Does not need treatment—strapping to the adjacent toe may ↓ pain.

Hammer and claw toes
• *Hammer toes:* Extended MTP joint, hyperflexed PIP joint, and extended DIP joint. Most common in 2nd toes.
• *Claw toes:* Extended MTP joint, flexion at PIP and DIP joints. Due to imbalance of extensors and flexors (e.g. after polio).
If causing pain or difficulty with walking/ footwear, refer for surgery.

Hallux valgus (bunion): Lateral deviation of the big toe at MTP joint exacerbated by wearing pointed shoes ± high heels. A bunion develops where the MTP joint rubs on footwear. Arthritis at the MTP joint is common. Bunion pads can help but severe deformity requires surgery.

Hallus rigidus: Arthritis at 1st MTP joint causes a stiff painful big toe. Refer severe cases to podiatrist or orthotist for offloading or custom-made rocker bottom foot orthoses.

Ingrowing toe nail: Most common in the big toe. Ill-fitting shoes and poor nail cutting predispose to the nail growing into the toe skin → pain. The inflamed tissue is prone to infection. *Management:* Advise re cutting nails (cut straight with edges beyond the flesh). Refer to podiatry. Treat infection with antibiotics (e.g. flucloxacillin 250–500mg qds). If recurrent problems, consider surgery (e.g. wedge resection of the nail).

Patient information
British Orthopaedic Foot Surgery Society 🖥 http://www.bofss.org.uk

Bone disorders

Paget's disease of bone: Accelerated, disorganized bone remodelling due to abnormal osteoclast activity. Affects up to 1:10 of the elderly but only a minority are symptomatic. ♂:♀ ≈ 3:1.

Presentation
- Pain—dull ache, aggravated by weight bearing. Often remains at rest.
- Deformity—bowing of weight-bearing bones, especially tibia (sabre), femur, and forearm. Usually asymmetrical.
- Frontal bossing of forehead.

Investigation: X-rays—distinctive changes; ↑ bone specific Alk phos; normal Ca^{2+}, PO_4, PTH, bone scintigraphy.

Management: Refer to rheumatology. Give analgesia. ↓ pain and long-term complications with bisphosphonates (e.g. risedronate 30mg/d. for 2mo.).

Complications: Pathological fractures; OA of adjacent joints; high output CCF (📖 p.334); hydrocephalus and/or cranial nerve compression → neurological symptoms e.g. deafness, spinal stenosis, bone sarcoma (10% of those affected >10y.).
(J. Paget (1814–99)—British surgeon)

Rickets/osteomalacia: Vitamin D deficiency → rickets in children and osteomalacia in adults.

Clinical features of rickets
- Bone pain/tenderness—arms, legs, spine, pelvis
- Skeletal deformity—bow legs, pigeon chest (forward projection of the sternum), rachitic rosary (enlarged ends of ribs), asymmetrical /odd shaped skull due to soft skull bones, spinal deformity (kyphosis, scoliosis), pelvic deformities
- Pathological fracture
- Dental deformities—delayed formation of teeth, holes in enamel, ↑ cavities
- Muscular problems—progressive weakness, ↓ muscle tone, muscle cramps
- Impaired growth → short stature (can be permanent)

Clinical features of osteomalacia
- Bone pain—diffuse; particularly in hips
- Muscle weakness
- Pathological fractures
- Low calcium → perioral numbness, numbness of extremities, hand and feet spasms, and/or arrhythmias

Causes and management
- *Dietary deficiency (<30nmol/l):* Particularly in children with pigmented skin in Northern climes. Give vitamin D and Ca^{2+} supplements.
- *Age-related deficiency (<30nmol/l):* Vitamin D metabolism deteriorates with age and many >80y. are deficient. Consider giving vitamin D (800IU/d) to all elderly >80y.

- *2° rickets/osteomalacia:* Vitamin D deficiency is due to other disease e.g. malabsorption, liver disease, renal tubular disorders, or chronic renal failure. Treat underlying cause/supplement Ca^{2+} and vitamin D.
- *Vitamin D dependent rickets:* Rare autosomal recessive disorder resulting in an enzyme deficit in the metabolism of vitamin D. Refer for specialist care. Treated with vitamin D and Ca^{2+} supplements.
- *Hypophosphataemic rickets* (vitamin D resistant rickets): X-linked dominant trait resulting in ↓ proximal renal tubular resorption of phosphate. Parathyroid hormone and vitamin D levels are normal. Specialist management is needed. Treatment is with phosphate replacement ± calcitriol.

Osteomyelitis: Infection of bone. May spread from boils, abscesses, or follow surgery. Often no primary site is found. More common in those with DM, impaired immunity, and/or poor living standards.

Organisms involved: S. Aureus, Streptococci, E. coli, Proteus and Pseudomonas species, TB. Before antibiotics, 25% died and 25% were crippled.

Signs: Pain, unwillingness to move affected part, warmth, effusions in neighbouring joints, fever, and malaise.

Investigation: Blood cultures +ve in 60%, ↑ESR/CRP, ↑WCC.

Management: Refer suspected cases for same day orthopaedic opinion. Diagnosis is confirmed with imaging e.g. MRI or bone scanning (X-ray changes take a few days to appear). *Treatment:* iv then po antibiotics (≥6wk.) and surgery to drain abscesses.

Complications: Septic arthritis, pathological fracture, deformity of growing bone, chronic infection.

Chronic osteomyelitis: Occurs after delayed or inadequate treatment of acute osteomyelitis. *Signs:* pain, fever, and discharge of pus from sinuses. It follows a relapsing and remitting course over years. Specialist management is needed.

Bone tumours: Bone is a common site for secondaries from other tumours (e.g. breast, lung, thyroid, kidney and prostate). 1° tumours:
- *Malignant:* All rare—Ewing's sarcoma, osteosarcoma, chondrosacroma
- *Mixed:* Giant cell tumour (osteoclastoma) is benign histologically but may behave in a malignant way
- *Benign:* Osteoid osteoma, chondroma, and osteochondroma

Presentation: Aching bone pain, swelling ± pathological fracture.

Management: Refer all bony swellings for X-ray and specialist management—excision, chemotherapy, radiotherapy, and reconstruction.

Patient information and support
Arthritis Research Campaign ☎0870 8505000 🖳 http://www.arc.org.uk
National Association for the Relief of Paget's Disease ☎0161 7994646
🖳 http://www.paget.org.uk

Osteoporosis

Lifetime risk of osteoporotic fracture is 40% in women and 13% in men. ↑ with age. ♀:♂ ≈ 3:1. Main morbidity and financial costs relate to hip fracture where incidence ↑ steeply >70y. Treatment aims to prevent fracture. Osteopoenia cannot be reliably diagnosed on X-ray—though vertebral fractures may be seen. Hip and lumbar spine bone mineral density (BMD) measurement by dual energy X-ray absorptionometry (DEXA) scan can quantify risk of osteoporotic fracture.

Definition: Osteoporosis is defined as BMD >2.5 standard deviations (SD) below the young adult mean (T score of −2.5). There is ↑ relative risk of fracture x2–3 for each SD ↓ in BMD.

BMD measurement: Check BMD if <75y. and previous fragility fracture or on long-term steroids and <65y. Measure BMD if other risk factors (below) or osteopoenia on X–ray—follow local referral guidelines until national guidance is available. Report should contain information on fracture risk, management, and time interval for re-checking BMD.

Glucocorticoid use: Risk factor for osteoporosis. Minimize steroid dose. All patients taking any dose of oral steroids should take calcium/vitamin D^G. In addition, add a bisphosphonate for patients >65y. taking oral or high-dose inhaled steroids for >3mo. Refer patients <65y. for DEXA scan and add a bisphosphonate if T score is ≤−1.5.

Previous fragility fracture: Fracture sustained falling from ≤ standing height—includes vertebral collapse (may not be a fall). Previous fracture is a risk for future fractures. Common fractures:

- *Wrist*—Colles'
- *Hip*—associated with ↑ mortality
- *Spine*—opsteoporotic vertebral collapse causes pain, ↓ height, and kyphosis. Pain can take 3–6mo. to settle and requires strong analgesia. Calcitonin is useful for pain relief for 3mo. after vertebral fracture if other analgesics are ineffective.

Investigations: DEXA scan if <75y. Exclude other causes of pathological fracture (e.g. malignancy, osteomalacia, hyperparathyroidism). Check FBC, ESR, TSH, Cr, bone and liver function tests—all should be normal. Consider checking serum paraproteins/urine Bence Jones protein, bone scan, and FSH/testosterone/LH (if hormonal status is unclear).

Management^N:

- If ≥75y. treat without DEXA once all non-osteoporotic causes of fracture have been ruled out.
- If 65–74y. treat if DEXA confirms osteoporosis.
- If <65y. and very low BMD (T score ≤−3) *or* T score ≤−2.5 and ≥1 additional age-independent risk factor (below).

Other major age-independent risk factors for osteoporosis:

- Low BMI (<19 kg/m^2) or height loss >3cm.
- FH of maternal hip fracture aged <75y.
- Untreated premature menopause (<45y.), prolonged amenorrhoea or ♂ hypogonadism.
- Conditions associated with prolonged immobility.

- Medical disorder independently associated with bone loss e.g. inflammatory bowel or coeliac disease, chronic liver disease, hyperthyroidism, ankylosing spondylitis, chronic renal failure, type 1 DM, RA

Lifestyle advice: Provide to all at-risk patients.
- *Adequate nutrition:* Maintain body weight so BMI <19kg/m². Give Ca^{2+} supplements to postmenopausal women with dietary deficiency[C]. Supplement with Ca^{2+} (0.5–1g/d.) and vitamin D (800 U/d.). If on long-term steroids[C], >80y., housebound, or institutionalized[C].
- *Regular exercise:* Weight-bearing activity >30min/d. ↓ fracture rate[S].
- *Stop smoking* pre-menopause →25% ↓ fracture rate post menopause.
- *↓alcohol consumption to <21u/wk. (♂) or <14u/wk. (♀)*

Treatment options
- *Bisphosphonates:* e.g. alendronate 10mg od. ↓ bone loss and fracture rate[C]. Mainstay of treatment and prevention of osteoporosis.
- *Selective oestrogen receptor modulator (SERM):* e.g. raloxifene 60mg od— if bisphosphonates are contraindicated/not tolerated or unsatisfactory response (further fracture and/or ↓ in BMD after ≥1y. treatment).
- *HRT (♀):* 📖 p.734—Postpones postmenopausal bone loss and ↓ fractures[C]. Optimum duration of use is uncertain (>5–7y.) but benefit disappears within 5y. of stopping. New evidence suggests ↑ risk of breast cancer[R]. CSM guidance (2003):
  - *Premature menopause:* HRT is still recommended for the prevention of osteoporosis until women reach 51y.
  - *>51y.:* HRT should **not** be considered 1st line therapy for long-term prevention of osteoporosis. HRT remains an option where other therapies are contraindicated, cannot be tolerated, or if there is a lack of response. Risks and benefits should be carefully assessed.
- *HRT (♂):* Supplement testosterone if hypogonadism.
- *Calcitonin/teraparatide:* Consider referral for consultant initiation if other treatment options are exhausted.

Referral: To endocrinology or menopause clinic if premature menopause (<40y.); unexplained cause of osteoporosis; osteoporosis in a man; or problems with management.

Prevention of falls: 📖 p.162   **Falls in the elderly:** 📖 p.996

Further information
NICE 🖥 http://www.nice.org.uk
- Osteoporosis—secondary prevention (2005)
- Osteoporosis—assessment of fracture risk and prevention in high risk individuals—due for publication in 2006.

Royal College of Physicians (2003) Osteoporosis: clinical guidelines for prevention and treatment 🖥 http://www.rcplondon.ac.uk
CSM Guidance (2003) further advice on safety of HRT (12/2003) 🖥 http://www.mca.gov.uk
Million Women Study Collaborators (2003) *Lancet* **362**: 419–27
Women's Health Initiative Study 🖥 http://www.whi.org

Patient information and support
Arthritis Research Campaign ☎0870 850 5000 🖥 http://www.arc.org.uk
National Osteoporosis Society ☎0845 450 0230 🖥 http://www.nos.org.uk

Osteoarthritis (OA)

The single most important cause of locomotor disability. OA used to be considered as 'wear and tear' of the bone and cartilage of synovial joints but is now recognized as a metabolically active process involving the whole joint i.e. cartilage, bone, synovium, capsule, and muscle.

The main reason for patients seeking medical help is pain. Levels of pain and disability are greatly influenced by the patient's personality, levels of anxiety, depression, and activity and often don't correlate well with clinical signs.

Risk factors: ↑ age (uncommon <45y.); ♀>♂; ↑ in black and Asian populations; genetic predisposition; obesity; abnormal mechanical loading of joint e.g. instability; poor muscle function; post-meniscectomy; certain occupations e.g. farming.

Symptoms and signs: Joint pain ± stiffness, synovial thickening, deformity, effusion, crepitus, muscle weakness and wasting, and ↓ function. Most commonly affects hip, knee, and base of thumb. Typically, exacerbations occur that may last weeks to months. Nodal OA, with swelling of the distal interphalageal joints (Heberdens' nodes) has a familial tendency.

Investigations: X-rays may show ↓ joint space, cysts, and sclerosis in subchondral bone, and osteophytes. Check FBC and ESR if inflammatory arthritis is suspected (normal or mildly ↑ in OA—ESR >30 suggests RA or psoriatic arthritis).

Aims of treatment

- Educate the patient
- ↓ pain
- Optimize function
- Minimize progression

Management: Exclude other causes of pain e.g. sepsis, bursitis, gout, inflammatory arthritis, and fibromyalgia. OA may be a coincidental finding and not the cause of the patient's pain.

Information and advice: Give information and advice on all relevant aspects of osteoarthritis and its management. The ARC website has a wide range of information leaflets for patients. Use the whole multidisciplinary team e.g. refer to

- Physiotherapist for advice on exercises, strapping, and splints;
- OT for aids;
- Chiropodist for foot care and insoles;
- Social worker for advice on disability benefits and housing;
- Orthopaedic surgeon for assessment for joint replacement if significant disability or night pain (waiting lists are often long).

↓ load on the joint: Weight reduction can ↓ symptoms and may ↓ progression in knee OA. Using a walking stick in the opposite hand to the affected hip and cushioned insoles or shoes (e.g. trainers) can also help.

Exercise and improving muscle strength: ↓ pain and disability e.g. walking (for OA knee), swimming (for OA back and hip but may make neck worse), cycling (for OA knee but may worsen patellofemoral OA). Refer to physiotherapy for advice on exercises, especially isometric exercises for the less mobile.

Pain control: Regular paracetamol is effective for many patients. NSAIDs are overused (📖 p.174) and there is no evidence of additional benefit over simple analgesics (📖 p.174) except in acute exacerbations. Topical NSAIDs have fewer side-effects than oral NSAIDs and may be helpful for superficial joints, as may rubefacients and counter-irritants (e.g. capsaicin cream). Some patients find local heat or cold soothing. Low-dose antidepressants (e.g. amitriptyline) are a useful adjunct, especially for pain causing sleep disturbance.

Glucosamine: 1500mg/d. may improve knee symptoms—consider 3mo. trial of treatment. There is still controversy as to whether glucosamine can modify OA progression.

Aspiration of joint effusions and joint injections: Can help in exacerbations. Some patients respond well to long-acting steroid injections—it may be worth considering a trial of a single treatment. Hyaluronan injections improve pain in the short/mid term[R].

Psychological factors: Have a major impact on the disability from OA. Education about the disease and emphasis that it is not progressive in most people is important. Seek and treat depression and anxiety.

Refer
- To rheumatology to:
  - Confirm diagnosis if coexistent psoriasis (psoriatic arthritis mimics OA and can be missed by radiologists)
  - Rule out 2° causes of OA (e.g. pseudogout, haemochromatosis) if young OA or odd distribution
  - If joint injection is thought worthwhile but you lack expertise or confidence to do it.
- To orthopaedics if symptoms are severe for joint replacement. Refer as an emergency if you suspect joint sepsis.

❶ Arthroscopy of uncomplicated OA joints can worsen the disease.

Further information for patients and GPs
Arthritis Research Campaign (ARC) ☎0870 8505000 🖥 http://www.arc.org.uk

Patient information and support
Arthritis Care ☎0808 800 4050 🖥 http://www.arthritiscare.org.uk
The Disabled Living Foundation ☎0845 130 9177 🖥 http://www.dlf.org.uk

Rheumatoid arthritis

Rheumatoid arthritis (RA) is the most common disorder of connective tissue, affecting ~1% UK population. $♀:♂ ≈ 3:1$. It is an immunological disease triggered by environmental factors in patients with genetic predisposition. Disease course is variable with exacerbations and remissions.

⚠ Refer all suspected cases to rheumatology—early treatment with disease modifying drugs can significantly alter disease progression.

Presentation
- Can present at any age—most common in middle age.
- Variable onset—often gradual but may be acute.
- Usually starts with symmetrical small joint involvement—i.e. pain, stiffness, swelling, and functional loss (especially in the hands)—joint damage and deformity occur later.
- Irreversible damage occurs early if untreated and can → deformity and joint instability.
- Other presentations—monoarthritis; migratory (palindromic) arthritis; PMR-like illness in the elderly; systemic illness of malaise, pain, and stiffness.

Differential diagnosis: Diagnosis may not be easy—consider psoriatic arthritis, nodal OA, SLE (especially in ♀ <50y.), bilateral carpal tunnel syndrome, other connective tissue disorders, and PMR in the elderly.

Investigations
- Check FBC (normochromic normocytic or hypochromic microcytic anaemia), ESR, and/or CRP (↑). May have ↑ platelets, ↓WCC.
- Rheumatoid factor and anti-CCP antibodies are +ve in the majority. A minority have a +ve ANA titre.
- X-rays—normal, periarticular osteporosis or soft tissue swelling in the early stages; later—loss of joint space, erosions, and joint destruction.

Symptoms and signs: Predominantly peripheral joints are affected—symmetrical joint pain, effusions, soft tissue swelling, early morning stiffness. Progression to joint destruction and deformity. Tendons may rupture.

Specific features
Hands: Ulnar deviation of the fingers, 'z' deformity of the thumb, swan neck (hyperextended PIP and flexed DIP joints), and boutonniere (flexed PIP and extended MCP joints, hyperextended DIP joint) deformities of the fingers. ↓ grip strength and ↓ hand function causes disability.

Legs and feet: Subluxation of the metatarsal heads in feet and claw toes result in pain on walking. Baker's cysts (📖 p.561) at the knee may rupture, mimicking DVT (📖 p.364).

Spine: Especially cervical spine—causing neck pain, cervical subluxation, and atlanto-axial instability leading to a risk of cord compression. X-rays are required prior to general anaesthesia.

Non-articular features: Common. Weight ↓, fever, malaise.
- *Rheumatoid nodules* (especially extensor surfaces of forearms).
- *Vasculitis*—digital infarction, skin ulcers, mononeuritis.

- *Eye*—Sjögren's syndrome, episcleritis, scleritits.
- *Lungs*—pleural effusions, fibrosing alveolitis, nodules.
- *Heart*—pericarditis, mitral valve disease, conduction defects.
- *Skin*—palmar erythema, vasculitis, rashes.
- *Neurological*—nerve entrapment e.g. Carpal tunnel, mononeuritis, and peripheral neuropathy.
- *Felty's syndrome*—see below.

Complications of RA: Physical disability, depression, osteoporosis, ↑ infections, lymphoma, cardiovascular disease, amyloidosis (10%), side-effects of treatment.

Management of RA: 📖 p.574

Felty's syndrome: Combination of RA, splenomegaly, and leucopenia. Occurs in patients with longstanding RA. Recurrent infections are common. Hypersplenism → anaemia and thrombocytopenia. Associated with lymphadenopathy, pigmentation, and persistent skin ulcers. Splenectomy may improve the neutropenia. (*A.R. Felty (1895–1964)—US physician*).

Sjögren's syndrome

Primary Sjögren's syndrome: Under-recognized cause of fatigue and dryness of skin/mucous membranes (may present with dyspareunia). Associated with all autoimmune connective tissue diseases and often presents with nodal OA. Long term, associated with lymphoma. Auto-immune profile is characteristic.

Secondary Sjögren's syndrome: Association of any connective tissue disease (50% have RA) with keratoconjunctivitis sicca (↓ lacrimation → dry eyes) or xerostomia (↓ salivation → dry mouth).

Investigations

- Collect saliva generated in 10min.—<0.5ml/min. suggests xerostomia.
- Put a strip of filter paper over the lower lid and measure the distance along the paper that tears are absorbed (Schirmer's test)—<10mm in 5min. suggests ↓ lacrimation.

Management: Refer to rheumatology. Provide information and support. Use artificial tears for dry eyes. Xerostomia may respond to frequent cool drinks, artificial saliva sprays e.g. glandosane, or sugar-free gum. Inform the dentist of the diagnosis. Skin rashes may respond to antimalarials. Long-term monitoring for mucosal lymphomas is important. (*H.S.C. Sjögren (1899–1986)—Swedish ophthalmologist*).

Further information

Primary Care Rheumatology Society ☎01609 774794 🖳 http://www.pcrsociety.org.uk

Patient information and support

Arthritis Research Campaign ☎0870 8505000 🖳 http://www.arc.org.uk
Arthritis Care ☎0808 800 4050 🖳 http://www.arthritiscare.org.uk
The Disabled Living Foundation ☎0845 130 9177. 🖳 http://www.dlf.org.uk
Arthritis Foundation 🖳 http://www.arthritis.org
British Sjögren's Association ☎0121 455 6549 🖳 http://www.bssa.uk.net

Management of rheumatoid arthritis

A multidisciplinary team approach is ideal e.g. GP, medical and surgical teams, physiotherapist, podiatrist, OT, nurse specialist, and social worker.

General support: Provision of information about the disease, treatments and support available (including equipment and help with everyday activities), self-help and carers groups, 'blue' disabled parking badges, financial support (e.g. DLA, AA—📖 p.107).

Physical therapy: Exercises, splints, appliances, and strapping help to keep joints mobile, ↓ pain, and preserve function.

Medication

NSAIDs and simple analgesics: e.g. regular paracetamol. Provide symptomatic relief but do not alter the course of disease. Patients' response to NSAIDs is individual—start with the least gastric toxic (e.g. ibuprofen 200–400mg tds) and alter as necessary (e.g. to diclofenac 50mg tds). A modified-release form at night may help early morning symptoms. If the patient has a history of indigestion or gastric problems, consider adding gastric protection (e.g. misoprostol or a PPI—📖 p.174).

Corticosteroids

- Intra-articular injections of steroids (e.g. Kenalog) can help settle localized flares (e.g. knee or shoulder) and can be used up to 3x/y. in any particular joint.
- Depot im injections or iv infusions (pulses) can help settle an acute flare but offer short-term benefits, with the risk of systemic side-effects.
- Daily low-dose oral steroids help symptoms and there is some evidence they can modify disease progression, but concerns about adverse side-effects have limited their use.

Disease-modifying drugs (DMARDs)

- Methotrexate
- Sulphasalazine
- Penicillamine
- Gold
- Azathioprine
- Leflunomide
- Hydroxychloroquine
- Ciclosporin
- Cyclophosphamide

Use only under consultant supervision. ↓ disease progression by modifying the immune response and inflammation. Used individually or in combination, they are now started very early in the disease (i.e. first 3–6mo.)—hence the need for early referral. DMARDs can take several months to show an effect. Side-effects and monitoring—Table 17.2.

Surgery: Aims to relieve pain and improve function. Consideration of the risks, benefits, and the most appropriate timing of surgery is vital. *Common procedures:* joint fusion, replacement and excision, tendon transfer and repair, and nerve decompression.

Monitoring patients on DMARDs—baseline measurements

- *Bloods:* FBC, U&E, LFTs, urinalysis.
- *CXR:* within 1y. of start of treatment—for im gold and methotrexate.
- *Baseline pulmonary function tests:* for patients with lung disease given methotrexate.

Table 17.2 Specific drugs—side-effects and monitoring*

Drug	Monitoring	Side-effects to monitor
Methotrexate 7.5–30mg weekly; followed the day after by folate 5mg (i.e. weekly as well)	FBC, U&E, Cr, and LFTs before starting treatment; weekly for 6wk; then every 2–3mo. ❶ Advise patients NOT to self-medicate with OTC aspirin or ibuprofen. Avoid alcohol.	Ask patients to report all symptoms/signs of infection—especially sore throat Severe respiratory symptoms in the 1st 6mo.—refer to A&E
Sulfasalazine 1g bd maintenance	FBC, LFTs + U&E, Cr at 2, 4, 6 & 8wk.; then every 4wk. for 3mo. then 3 monthly. Urgent FBC if intercurrent illness during initiation of treatment.	• Rash (1%) • Nausea/diarrhoea—often transient • Bone marrow suppression in 1–2% in the first months
Intramuscular gold (myocristin) 50mg monthly	FBC, urinalysis, ESR—prior to each injection. LFTs, U&E , Cr—3 monthly.	Ask patients to report: • All symptoms/signs of infection—especially sore throat • Bleeding/bruising • Breathlessness/cough • Mouth ulcers/metallic taste in mouth or • Rashes
D Penicillamine 375mg–1g/d. maintenance	FBC, urinalysis 2 weekly for 8wk. & 1wk. after any ↑ dosage, then monthly. LFTs and U&E; Cr annually.	Altered taste—can be ignored; rash
Azathioprine Up to 2.5mg/kg/d. maintenance	FBC weekly for 6wk. then 1x/mo.. U&E and LFTs 1x/mo. for 3mo. then 3 monthly.	GI side-effects, rash, bone marrow suppression
Ciclosporin Up to 3.5mg/kg/d. maintenance	Cr & BP 2 weekly to stable dose then 1x/mo.. FBC, U&E, LFTs 1x/mo. until stable for 3mo. then 3 monthly. Lipids 6 monthly.	Rash, gum soreness, hirsitism, ↑ Cr, ↑BP, renal failure
Hydroxychloroquine 100–200mg/d. maintenance	Baseline eye check and periodically on advice of local ophthalmologist.	Rash, GI effects, ocular side-effects (rare)
Leflunomide 10–20mg/d. maintenance	FBC, LFTs, U&E, BP—2 weekly for 6mo. then monthly.	Rash, GI, ↑ BP, ↑ ALT

* GMS contract: national enhanced service funding is availbale for shared care drug montoring for: penicillamine, auranofin, sulphasalazine, methotrexate, and sodium aurothiomalate (myocristin).

⚠ **Results requiring action**

- Total WBC <4.0
- Neutrophils <2
- Platelets <150
- LFTs (ALT/AST) >2x baseline
- Persistent proteinuria (>1+ x2) or haematuria.

Discuss with rheumatologist ± stop medication.

Spondylarthropathies and crystal-induced arthritis

Spondylarthropathies

Ankylosing spondylitis: Prevalence 1:2000. $\male:\female \approx 2\frac{1}{2}:1$. 95% HLAB27 +ve. Typically, presents with morning back pain/stiffness in a young man. Progressive spinal fusion (ankylosis) occurs → ↓ spinal movement, spinal kyphosis, sacroiliac (SI) joint fusion, neck hyperextension, and neck rotation. *Other features:* ↓ chest expansion, chest pain, hip and knee arthritis, plantar fasciitis and other enthesitides, iritis, Crohn's, UC, carditis, aortic regurgitation, conduction defects, osteoporosis, psoriaform rashes.

Tests: FBC—normochromic or microcytic hypochromic anaemia, ↑ ESR (may be normal), RhF usually –ve. X-ray—initial signs are widening of the SI joints and marginal sclerosis ; later, SI joint fusion and a 'bamboo spine' (vertebral squaring and fusion).

Management: Exercise helps the back pain. NSAIDs (e.g. diclofenac 50mg tds) also help pain. Refer to rheumatologist early for confirmation of diagnosis, education, disease-modifying drugs, and advice on appropriate exercise regimes to maintain mobility.

Reactive arthritis: Often asymmetrical aseptic arthritis in ≥1 joint. Occurs 2–6wk. after bacterial infection elsewhere e.g. gastroenteritis (salmonella, campylobacter), GU infection (chlamydia, gonorrhoea). ↑ in HLA B27 +ve individuals.

Management: NSAIDs, physiotherapy, and steroid joint injections. Recovery usually occurs within months. A minority develop chronic arthritis requiring disease-modifying drugs. Refer to rheumatology.

Reiter's syndrome: Polyarthropathy, urethritis, iritis, and a psoriaform rash. Affects men with HLA B27 genotype. Commonly follows GU or bowel infection. Joint and eye changes are often severe. (*H.C. Reiter (1881—1969) German public health physician*)

Psoriatic arthritis: Inflammatory arthritis associated with psoriasis. RhF –ve. Presentation variable. Refer suspected cases to rheumatology. Disease modifying drugs (e.g. methotrexate) may improve both skin and musculoskeletal symptoms (🕮 p.574).

Enteropathic spondylarthropathy: Oligoarticular or polyarticular arthritis linked to inflammatory bowel disease. Includes sacroiliitis, plantar fasciitis, inflammatory spinal pains, and other enthsitides (insertional ligament/tendon inflammation). Arthritis may evolve and relapse/remit independently of bowel disease. NSAIDs may help joint pain but aggravate bowel disease. Refer to rheumatology for confirmation of diagnosis, advice on management, and disease-modifying drugs.

Crystal-induced arthritis

Gout: Intermittent attacks of acute joint pain due to deposition of uric acid crystals. *Prevalence:* 3–8/1000. ↑ with age; $\male:\female \approx 5:1$. *Predisposing factors:* FH, obesity, excess alcohol intake, high purine diet, diuretics, acute infection, ketosis, surgery, plaque psoriasis, polycythaemia, leukaemia, cytotoxics, and renal failure. *Associations:* Gout may be linked to ↑ risk of hypertension and coronary heart disease—screen patients.

Presentation of acute gout: Painful swollen joint (big toe, feet, and ankles most commonly); red skin which may peel ± fever. Can be polyarticular, especially in elderly ♀. May mimic septic arthritis.

Investigation
- *Blood*—↑ WCC; ↑ ESR; ↑ blood urate (but may be normal).
- *Microscopy of synovial fluid*—not usually required. Reveals sodium monourate crystals on polarized light microscopy.
- *X-rays*—not usually required. Show soft tissue swelling only unless severe disease, when an erosive pattern is seen.
- *Refer to urology*—if kidney stones or recurrent UTI.

Management of acute gout: Resolves in <2wk.—often after 2–7d. if treated. Exclude infection. Rest and elevate joint. Apply ice packs. NSAIDs are helpful (e.g. diclofenac 75mg bd)—caution if GI problems. Alternatively, if NSAIDs are contraindicated, try colchicine 500mcg bd increased slowly to qds until pain is relieved or side-effects e.g. nausea, vomiting, or diarrhoea (max. 6mg—don't repeat in <3d.). Steroid joint injection or depomedrone 80–120mg im are also effective.

Prevention of further attacks: ↓ weight; avoid alcohol and purine-rich foods (e.g. offal, red meat, yeast extracts, pulses, and mussels); avoid thiazide diuretics and aspirin; consider prophylactic medication if recurrent attacks—allopurinol 100–300mg daily; wait until 1mo. after acute attack and co-prescribe colchicine (500mcg bd) or NSAID for first 1–3mo. to try and avoid precipitation of another acute attack. Check serum urate level after 2mo.—aim for low normal range. Alternatively, or in addition, try an uricosuric e.g. probenecid 250–500mcg bd on a named patient basis.

Chronic gout: Recurrent attacks, tophi (urate deposits) in pinna, tendons and joints, and joint damage. Refer to rheumatology.

Calcium pyrophosphate deposition disease (CPPD— pseudogout): Inflammatory arthritis due to deposition of pyrophosphate crystals. Chondrocalcinosis may be seen on X-ray (calcification of articular cartilage). Knee, wrist, and shoulder are most commonly affected. Associated with OA, hyperparathyroidism, and haemochromatosis. Acute attacks can be triggered by intercurrent illness and metabolic disturbance. Attacks are less severe than gout and may be difficult to differentiate from other types of arthritis. Presence of joint crystals confirms diagnosis. Treat acute attacks like acute gout. A chronic form also occurs—frequently erosive. Refer to rheumatology for confirmation of diagnosis, and advice on management and disease-modifying drugs.

Patient information and support

National Ankylosing Spondylitis Society (NASS) ☎01435 873527 🖳 http://www.nass.co.uk
Psoriatic Arthropathy Alliance. (PAA) ☎0870 7703212 🖳 http://www.paalliance.org
Arthritis Research Campaign ☎0870 850 5000 🖳 http://www.arc.org.uk

Connective tissue diseases

Overlapping group of diseases affecting many organ systems. Associated with fever, malaise, chronic (often relapsing/remitting) course and response to steroids. Often difficult to diagnose—refer suspected cases to rheumatology.

Systemic lupus erythematosus (SLE): Rare autoimmune disease. Prevalence: 1 in 3000. ♀:♂ ≈ 9:1. ↑ in Afro Caribbeans and Asians. Onset 15–40y. Presentation is variable—multisystem involvement must be demonstrated to make a diagnosis:
- *Joints* (95%)—arthritis, arthralgia, myalgia, tenosynovitis
- *Skin* (80%)—photosensitivity, facial 'butterfly' rash, vasculitis, hair loss, urticaria, discoid lesions
- *Lungs* (50%)—pleurisy, pneumonitis, effusion, fibrosing alveolitis
- *Kidney* (50%)—proteinuria, ↑ BP, glomerulonephritis, renal failure
- *Heart* (40%)—pericarditis, endocarditis
- *CNS* (15%)—depression, psychosis, infarction, fits, cranial nerve lesions
- *Blood*—anaemia, thrombocytopoenia, splenomegaly

Investigations: Check an autoimmune profile—95% are ANA (anti-nuclear antibody) +ve. Other immunological abnormalities—↑ double strained DNA, RhF +ve (40%), ↓ complement (C3, C4). FBC—↓Hb, ↓WCC, ↑ESR.

Management: Refer to rheumatology for specialist treatment. NSAIDs help control symptoms, sunscreens protect skin (can be prescribed as ACBS). Be aware that sulphonamides and contraceptive steroids may exacerbate SLE. Steroids are the mainstay of treatment of acute flares (always discuss with a rheumatologist). Hydroxychloroquine can improve skin and joint symptoms. Cyclophosphamide, methotrexate, and ciclosporin are also used (📖 p.575).

Discoid lupus erythematosus (LE): ♀:♂ ≈ 2:1. ≥1 round/oval plaques on the face, scalp, or hands. Lesions are well-defined, red, atrophic, and scaly ± keratin plugs in dilated follicles. Scarring leaves alopecia on the scalp and may result in hypopigmentation. Internal involvement is not a feature.

Investigation: autoimmune profile—as for SLE. Diagnosis is confirmed with lesion biopsy.

Management: Treatment is with potent topical steroids and sunscreen. Remission occurs in 40%. 5% develop SLE.

Antiphospholipid syndrome: May occur with SLE or alone. ↑ clotting tendencies. Associated with thrombosis, stroke, migraine, miscarriage, myelitis, myocardial infarction, and multi-infarct dementia. If suspected, start aspirin 150mg od and refer to rheumatology. May need anticoagulation.

Drug-induced lupus: Occurs with minocycline, isoniazid, hydralazine, procainamide, chlorpromazine, sulfasalazine, losartan, and anti-convulsants. Remits slowly when drug is stopped but may need steroid treatment to settle.

Systemic sclerosis: Rare spectrum of disorders causing fibrosis and skin tightening (scleroderma). Raynaud's is usually present ± ↑ BP, lung fibrosis, GI symptoms, telangiectasias, polyarthritis, and myopathy. *Management:* education and support—treat symptoms (e.g. of Raynaud's) with nifedipine, amlodipine, or angiotensin II receptor blockers. *Prognosis:* variable but early management based on assiduous search for internal organ involvement is vital. Refer urgently to rheumatology. CREST syndrome is a variant with better prognosis.

CREST syndrome: Comprises Calcinosis of subcutaneous tissues, Raynaud's, Oesophageal motility problems, Scerodactyly, and Telagiectasia.

Raynaud's syndrome: Intermittent digital ischaemia precipitated by cold or emotion. Fingers ache and change colour: pale → blue → red on rewarming. Usually presents <25y. of age. Idiopathic. *Prevalence:* 3–20%; ♀:♂ > 1:1; often abates at the menopause; 5% develop autoimmune rheumatic disease—mainly scleroderma and SLE.

Differential diagnosis

- Scleroderma ± CREST sydrome
- SLE
- RA
- Drugs e.g. β-blockers
- Trauma
- Smoking
- Arteriosclerosis
- Hand-arm vibration syndrome from using vibrating tools
- Leukaemia
- Polycythaemia rubra vera
- Cold agglutinins
- Thoracic outlet obstruction
- Thrombocytosis
- Monoclonal gammopathies
- Mixed cryoglobulinaemia

Management: Advise patients to keep warm—woolly socks/gloves in cold weather, hand warmers, stay inside in the cold; avoid drugs that make the condition worse; stop smoking. Nifedipine 10–20mg tds or amlodipine 5mg od help some. Fluoxetine may also be helpful. If any associated symptoms or severe symptoms, refer for rheumatology advice (urgently for iv vasodilation if critical ischaemia e.g. ulceration or infarcts on fingers). (*M. Raynaud (1834–1881)—French physician*).

Sjögren's syndrome 📖 p.573

Dermatomyositis/polymyositis 📖 p.623

Patient support and information

Arthritis Research Campaign (ARC) ☎0870 8505000 🖥 http://www.arc.org.uk
Lupus UK ☎01708 731251 🖥 http://www.lupusuk.com
Raynaud's and Scleroderma Association ☎01270 872776 🖥 http://www.raynauds.org.uk

Vasculitis

Characterized by inflammation within or around blood vessels ± necrosis. Severity depends on size and site of vessels affected. Systemic vasculitis can be life-threatening. *Causes:*

- Idiopathic (50%)
- Connective tissue disease (e.g. RA, SLE)
- 2° to infection (e.g. rheumatic fever, infective endocarditis, Lyme's disease)
- Drug reaction (e.g. NSAIDs, antibiotics)
- Neoplasia (e.g. lymphoma, leukaemia)

Presentation: Variable—may be confined to the skin or systemic involving joints, kidneys, lungs, gut, and nervous system.

- *Skin signs*—palpable purpura (often painful); usually on lower legs or buttocks.
- *Systemic effects*—fever, night sweats, malaise, weight ↓, myalgia, and arthralgia may occur in all types of vasculitis.

Polymyalgia rheumatica (PMR) and giant cell arteritis (GCA) 2 clinical syndromes which are part of the same spectrum. Both affect the elderly (rare <50y.). 50% of patients with GCA also have PMR; 15% with PMR have GCA. ♀:♂ ≈ 3:1. Both conditions typically respond rapidly and dramatically to corticosteroids. Diagnosis is clinical.

Presentation

- *General symptoms*—both PMR and GCA may present with malaise, anorexia, fever, night sweats, weight loss, depression.
- *PMR—typical symptoms*: proximal symmetrical muscle pain and stiffness worse after rest.
- *GCA—typical symptoms*: unilateral throbbing headache, facial pain, scalp tenderness (e.g. on brushing hair) and/or jaw claudication. Visual symptoms: amaurosis fugax, diplopia, sudden loss of vision.

Investigation

- Blood—↑ESR (usually >30) ± normocytic anaemia.
- Temporal artery biopsy—refer urgently if GCA is suspected. Biopsy may be –ve, even in true cases, due to skip lesions. Don't withhold treatment whilst waiting for biopsy; but if the patient has had steroids ≥2wk., +ve biopsy is less likely.
- Exclude other diagnoses, depending on symptoms e.g. malignancy, RA, myeloma. For PMR, consider acute neck pain syndromes with referred pain, bilateral shoulder lesions, arthritis, spinal stenosis, acute discitis with referred pain and myositis.

Initial management: Corticosteroids prevent vascular complications, particularly blindness, and rapidly relieve symptoms—30–60% with GCA became blind before steroids were used to treat the condition.

- *GCA*—prescribe prednisolone 1mg/kg/d. (maximum 60mg od).; refer urgently to ophthalmology or rheumatology.
- *PMR*—prednisolone 15mg od; review after 2–4d.. Good response does not confirm diagnosis but suggests treatment should be continued.

Ongoing management: In all cases, ↓ dose of prednisolone as symptoms allow e.g. by 2.5mg every 4wk. until taking 10mg prednisolone od; then by 1mg/mo. to 5mg od; then more slowly. Check ESR with dose changes and slow regime and recheck ESR if ↑ symptoms. At the start of treatment, give osteoporosis prophylaxis (📖 p.568). If concerned about steroid side-effects, refer to rheumatology for advice on steroid-sparing drug management.

Prognosis: Most patients require >2y. of treatment. Relapse is common after stopping treatment (50% if stopped after 2y.). If relapse occurs, review the diagnosis.

Polyarteritis nodosa (PAN): Uncommon in UK. ♂:♀ ≈ 4:1. Peak incidence in middle age. Multisystem necrotizing vasculitis → aneurysms of medium-sized arteries. Sometimes associated with Hepatitis B.

Presentation: Tender subcutaneous nodules along the line of arteries, coronary arteritis, ↑BP, mononeuritis multiplex, renal failure, GI involvement.

Management: Refer to rheumatology for angiography to confirm diagnosis and advice on management. Treatment is with control of ↑BP, high-dose steroids, and ciclophosphamide.

Churg–Strauss syndrome: Associated with asthma. Vasculitic disease affecting coronary, pulmonary, cerebral, and sphlanchnic circulations ± skin and mononeuritis. Diagnosis is based on clinical features and biopsy. (*J. Churg (b. 1910) and L. Strauss (1913–1985)—US pathologists*)

Management: Refer for specialist treatment with high-dose prednisolone ± ciclophosphamide. Avoid leukotriene receptor agonist drugs for control of asthma as may worsen vasculitis.

Wegener's granulomatosis: Granulomatous vasculitis. Any organ may be involved and symptoms/signs relate to the organs affected e.g. mouth ulcers; nasal ulceration with epistaxis or rhinitis; otitis media; cranial nerve lesions; lung symptoms and shadows on CXR; ↑BP; eye signs (50%). There is often a long prodrome of 'limited Wegener's granulomatosis' characterized by nasal stuffiness, headaches, hearing difficulties, and nose bleeds. (*F. Wegener (1907–90)—German pathologist*)

Management: Refer to rheumatology/general medicine for investigation. ANCA helps diagnostically and in disease monitoring. Treatment is with high-dose steroids, methotrexate, mofetil, and ciclophosphamide.

Vasculitis conditions covered elsewhere
- Erythema nodosum: 📖 p.654
- Kawasaki's disease: 📖 p.854
- Henoch–Schönlein purpura: 📖 p.284

Patient information and support
Arthritis Research Campaign (ARC) ☎0870 8505000 🖥 http://www.arc.org.uk
Stuart Strange Trust 🖥 http://www.vasculitis-uk.org
European Vasculitis Study Group 🖥 http://www.vasculitis.org

Tired all the time

Fatigue is common. 1:400 sustained episodes of fatigue generate a GP consultation. GPs see 30 patients/y. whose main complaint is tiredness and it may be a 2° symptom in many others. 2% of consultations result in 2° care referral. Almost any disease process can cause tiredness—whether physical or psychological. Physical causes account for ~9% of cases; 75% have symptoms of emotional distress.

History

- *Onset and duration*—short history and abrupt onset suggest post-viral cause or onset of DM; protracted course suggests emotional origin.
- *Pattern of fatigue*—fatigue on exertion which goes away with rest suggests organic cause, whilst fatigue worst in the morning which never goes suggests depression.
- *Associated symptoms*—e.g. breathlessness, weight ↓, or anorexia suggest underlying organic disease. Chronic pain may cause fatigue.
- *Sleep patterns*—early morning wakening and unrefreshing sleep may suggest depression, whilst snoring, pauses of breathing in sleep, and sleepiness in the day time suggest sleep apnoea.
- *Psychiatric history*—ask about symptoms of depression, anxiety, and stress; current medication. Ask what the patient thinks is wrong and their underlying fears.

Examination: Full examination unless history suggests cause. Most examinations will be normal.

Common organic causes of fatigue in general practice

- Anaemia
- Infections (EBV, CMV, hepatitis)
- DM
- Hypo-or hyperthyroidism
- Perimenopausal
- Asthma
- Carcinomatosis
- Sleep apnoea

Investigations: Don't over-investigate—1:3 patients have ≥1 abnormal result in a standard battery of tests. Abnormal results are relevant to symptoms in <1:10 of those patients. Suitable initial investigations are: FBC, ESR, TFTs, blood glucose, U&E, LFTs, Ca^{2+}, monospot test, MSU for M,C&S. Viral titres don't help. Screening questionnaires for depression can be useful. Further investigations (e.g. autoimmune profile) may be necessary depending on initial test results, clinical findings, and course.

Management

- Treat organic causes.
- In most, no physical cause is found—reassure. Explaining the relationship of psychological and emotional factors to fatigue can help patients deal with symptoms.
- If lasts >6–12wk. or symptoms/signs of depression, consider a trial of antidepressants. SSRIs (e.g. sertraline 50mg od), are often helpful.
- Refer those with chronic or disabling fatigue with no identifiable cause, suspected sleep apnoea, suspected chronic fatigue syndrome, or if referral is requested by the patient.

Fibromyalgia and over training syndrome: p.584

Chronic fatigue syndrome (CFS, ME): A debilitating and distressing condition. *Prevalence:* 0.2–2.6%; ♀:♂ ≈ 3:2. *Cause:* Poorly understood—viral infections (≈10% after EBV), immunization, chemical toxins (e.g. organophosphates, chemotherapy drugs) are all implicated.

Clinical features: Unexplained fatigue of new/definite onset, not resulting from ongoing exertion, nor alleviated by rest, which results in ↓ activity, and ≥4 of:

- Impaired memory or concentration
- Tender cervical/axillary lymph nodes
- Post-exertional malaise lasting >24h.; typically delayed—usually starting 1–2d. after a period of ↑ physical/mental activity—and may last weeks
- Headaches of new type pattern or severity
- Multi-joint pain without swelling
- Sore throat
- Unrefreshing sleep
- Muscle pain

> ❶ Additional symptoms must not have pre-dated fatigue

Other common symptoms/associations

- Postural dizziness
- Vertigo
- Altered temperature sensation
- Paraesthesiae
- Sensitivity to light or sound
- Palpitations
- IBS
- Food intolerance
- Fibromyalgia
- Feelings of dyspnoea
- Mood swings
- Panic attacks
- Depression (60% have no prior psychiatric diagnosis)

Intercurrent infection, immunization, drugs, caffeine, alcohol, and stress may → setbacks.

Management

- Support and reassurance—explanation, information ± selfhelp groups
- Avoid factors which worsen symptoms e.g. caffeine, alcohol
- Graded exercise is helpful[C]
- Treat symptoms e.g. TCA (e.g. amitriptyline 10–50mg nocte) to help sleep, relieve headache or neuropathic pain; SSRI for depression
- Referral for specialist care e.g. CBT (↓ 2° distress and optimizes rehabilitation) specialist CFS clinic.

Prognosis: Variable. Children tend to recover, though it may take years. 55% of adults presenting with tiredness have symptoms lasting >6mo. Risk ↑ 3x if there is a history of anxiety or depression. Short duration of fatigue with no anxiety/depression improves prognosis. Only 6% of adults with CFS attending specialist clinics return to pre-morbid functioning.

Further information

Royal Australian College of Physicians: Chronic fatigue syndrome
⌨ http://www.mja.com.au/ public/guides/cfs/cfs1.html
King's College ⌨ http://www.kcl.ac.uk/cfs

Patient information and support

ME Association ☎0871 222 7824 ⌨ http://www.meassociation.org.uk
Action for ME ☎01749 670799 ⌨ http://afme.org.uk

Miscellaneous conditions

Fibromyalgia: Pain and fatiguability with multiple hyperalgesic tender sites (>11/18 typical sites). Common. Peak age 40–50y. 90% female. *Cause:* unknown. Often results in significant disability and handicap with inability to cope with a job or household activities.

Clinical picture
- Pain—usually axial and diffuse but may be felt all over.
- Pain is worsened by stress, cold, and activity and associated with generalized morning stiffness.
- Paraesthesiae or dysaesthesiae of hands and feet are common.
- Analgesics, NSAIDs, and local physical treatments are ineffective and may worsen symptoms.
- Sleep patterns are poor—patients tend to wake exhausted and complain of poor concentration.
- Anxiety and depression scores are high.
- Associated symptoms—unexplained headache, urinary frequency, and abdominal symptoms are common.
- Clinical findings are unremarkable.

Diagnosis: Exclude other causes of pain and fatigue (e.g. hypothyroidism, SLE, Sjögrens, psoriatic arthritis, inflammatory myopathy, hyperparathyroidism, osteomalacia). Check FBC, ESR, TFTs, U&E, Ca^{2+}, CK, PO_4, ANA, Rh.F, and immunoglobulins.

Management: Supportive—reassurance that there is no serious pathology, explanation, and information are vital. Low-dose amitriptyline 25–75mg nocte and graded exercise regimes can help, as can counselling and learning of coping strategies. A multidisciplinary approach is helpful—usually accessed through a rheumatology or pain clinic.

Over-training syndrome: Poor performance, fatigue, heavy muscles and depression due to excessive sports training or competing without sufficient rest. Usually diagnosed from history. Exclude other causes of fatigue (📖 p.583). *Management:* rest, reassurance, and alteration of training programme.

Tietze syndrome: Idiopathic costochondritis. Pain is enhanced by motion, coughing, or sneezing. The 2nd rib is most commonly affected. *Examination:* marked localized tenderness. *Differential diagnosis:* muscular sprain; rarely, inflammatory chest wall enthesitis/osteitis 2° sponylarthopathy.

Management: Explanation and reassurance that nothing serious is happening. Simple OTC analgesia e.g. ibuprofen 400mg tds. If pain persists, local steroid or marcaine injections can be helpful. If not settling, consider referral to rheumatology. (*A. Tietze (1864–1927)—German surgeon*).

Musculoskeletal sarcoid: Arthralgia typically of the ankles, associated with changes of acute sarcoid (🕮 p.396). Chronic sarcoid can be associated with erosive arthritis and osteitis/periostitis pains. Erosive arthritis treated effectively with methotrexate. Refer to rheumatology.

Reflex sympathetic dystrophy: 🕮 p.197

Patient information and support

Arthritis Research Campaign (ARC) ☎0870 850 5000 🖳 http://www.arc.org.uk
Fibromyalgia Association UK ☎0870 220 1232
🖳 http://www.fibromyalgia-associationuk.org
STIFF(UK) ☎01782 562 366 🖳 http://www.stiffuk.org

Other relevant pages

Neurology

Cranial nerve lesions

Cranial nerves may be affected at any point from the nerve nucleus within the brainstem to the point of innervation. Think systematically about the level of the lesion. *Potential sites:*

- Muscle
- Neuromuscular junction
- Along the course of the nerve outside the brainstem
- Within the brainstem.

Any cranial nerve may be affected by DM, MS, tumours, sarcoid, vasculitis, or syphilis, and >1 nerve may be affected by a lesion. Refer according to cause (ENT, ophthalmology, neurology).

Table 18.1 Cranial nerve lesions and their causes

Nerve	Clinical test	Causes
I Olfactory	*Smell*—test each nostril for the ability to differentiate different smells.	Trauma, frontal lobe tumour, meningitis.
II Optic	*Acuity*—Snellen chart. *Visual fields*—compare with your own visual fields by standing directly in front of the patient with your head at the same level as theirs. *Pupils*—size, shape, reaction to light, and accommodation. *Ophthalmoscopy*—darken room, dilate pupil with 1 drop tropicamide 0.5% if needed, view optic disc (?pale, swollen), follow each vessel outwards to view each quadrant, track outwards to check lens and cornea.	*Monocular blindness*—lesion in one eye or optic nerve—e.g. MS, giant cell arteritis. *Bitemporal hemianopia*—optic chiasm compression e.g. pituitary adenoma, craniopharyngioma, internal carotid artery aneurysm. *Homonymous hemianopia*—affects half the visual field on the side opposite the lesion. Lesion beyond the optic chiasm e.g. stroke, abscess, tumour. Visual field defects— 📖 p.295
III	Ptosis, large pupil, eye down and out. ❶ Diplopia from a 3rd nerve lesion may cause nystagmus.	DM, giant cell arteritis, syphilis, posterior communicating artery aneurysm, idiopathic. If pupil normal size, due to DM or other vascular cause.
IV	Diplopia on looking down and in—may compensate by tilting head.	Rare in isolation. May occur due to trauma to the orbit.
V Trigeminal	*Motor*—open mouth. Jaw deviates to the side of the lesion. *Sensory*—corneal reflex lost 1st. Check all 3 divisions.	*Sensory*—trigeminal neuralgia (📖 p.599), herpes zoster, nasopharyngeal carcinoma. *Motor*—bulbar palsy (📖 p.256), acoustic neuroma.
VI	Horizontal diplopia on looking outwards.	MS, pontine CVA, ↑ ICP.

Table 18.1 (cont.)

Nerve	Clinical test	Causes
VII Facial	Causes facial weakness and droop. Ask to raise eyebrows, show teeth, puff out cheeks. *LMN lesion*—all one side of face affected. *UMN lesion*—lower 2/3 face affected only.	*LMN*—Bell's palsy, polio, otitis media, skull fracture, cerebellopontine angle tumours, parotid tumours, herpes zoster (Ramsay Hunt syndrome—□ p.923). *UMN*—stroke, tumour.
VIII Vestibulo-auditory	*Auditory*—ask to repeat a number whispered in 1 ear whilst you block the other. *Vestibular*—ask about balance, check for nystagmus (□ p.276)—ask patient to fix on finger ¾ m away; check gaze—upwards, downwards, lateral (both directions), keeping finger <30° from midline.	Noise, Paget's disease (□ p.566), Ménière's disease (□ p.929), herpes zoster, acoustic neuroma, brainstem CVA, drugs (e.g. furosemide).
IX, X	Gag reflex, palate moves → normal side on saying 'Aah'.	Trauma, brainstem lesions, neck tumours.
XI	*Trapezii*—shrug shoulders against resistance. *Sternomastoid*—turn head to right/left against resistance.	Rare. Polio, syringomyelia, tumours near jugular foramen, stroke, bulbar palsy (□ p.256), polio, trauma, TB.
XII	Tongue deviates to the side of the lesion.	Trauma, brainstem lesions, neck tumours.

Bell's palsy: Facial palsy without other signs. Unknown cause—possibly viral. *Peak age:* 10–40y. ♂ = ♀. *Lifetime incidence:* ~1:65. Affects left and right side of the face equally often.

Presentation: Usually sudden onset; may be preceded by pain around the ear. *Other possible symptoms:* facial numbness; ↓ noise tolerance; disturbed taste on the anterior part of the tongue.

Management: ~70% recover completely; 13% have insignificant sequelae; the remainder have permanent deficit. 85% improve in <3wk.—reassure. There is no evidence prednisolone[C] or acyclovir[C] is helpful—though many neurologists advocate the use of oral prednisolone (1mg/kg/d.—maximum 80mg/d.) and aciclovir (800mg 5x/d. for 5d.) for patients with moderate or severe palsy—ideally starting <72h. (max.7d.) after onset of symptoms. Protect eye with lacrilube ointment for sleeping ± tape eye lid closed/protect with eye pad, and advise glasses in the day ± artificial tears if drying. *Refer*:

• If recovery is not starting after 3 wk.
• For tarsorraphy, if complete or longstanding palsy
• If unacceptable cosmetic result—may benefit from plastic surgery.

Patient support: www.bellspalsy.org.uk
(C. Bell (1774-1842)—Scottish physiologist/surgeon)

Neuropathy

Table 18.2 Quick screening test for muscle power

Joint	Movement	Nerve roots
Shoulder	Abduction	C5
	Adduction	C5-7
Elbow	Flexion	C5-6
	Extension	C7
Wrist	Flexion	C7-8
	Extension	C7
Fingers	Flexion	C7-8
	Extension	C7
	Abduction	T1
Hip	Flexion	L1-2
	Extension	L5-S1
Knee	Flexion	S1
	Extension	L3-4
Ankle	Dorsiflexion	L4
	Plantarflexion	S1-2

Test proximal muscle power by asking the patient to sit from lying, pulling you towards him/herself, or to rise from squatting.

Details of more detailed tests of peripheral nerves are available in the *Oxford Handbook of Clinical Medicine*.

Mononeuropathy: Lesions of individual peripheral (including cranial) nerves. *Causes:* trauma, compression, DM, leprosy.

If >1 peripheral nerve is involved, the term *mononeuritis multiplex* is used. *Causes:* DM, sarcoid, cancer, leprosy, PAN, amyloid.

Common mononeuropathies

- *Median nerve* (C5-T1)—Inability to flex the terminal phalanx of the thumb and loss of sensation over lateral 3½ fingers and palm. Wasting of the thenar eminence. *Common causes:* trauma (especially wrist lacerations), carpal tunnel syndrome (📖 p.555).
- *Ulnar nerve* (C7-T1)—Weakness and wasting of interossei muscles (weakness of abduction of fingers) and claw hand deformity, wasting of hypothenar eminence, sensory loss over medial 1½ fingers and ulnar side of the hand. Flexion of 4th and 5th fingers is weak. *Common causes:* trauma or compression at the elbow, trauma at the wrist.
- *Radial nerve* (C5-T1)—Sensory loss is variable but always includes the dorsal aspect of the root of the thumb. This nerve opens the fist. *Common causes:* compression against the humerus, trauma.

- *Sciatic nerve* (L4-S2)—Weakness of hamstrings and all muscles below the knee (foot drop), loss of sensation below the knee laterally. *Common causes:* back injury, pelvic tumours.
- *Common peroneal nerve* (L4-S2)—Inability to dorsiflex the foot (foot drop), evert the foot, extend the toes. Sensory loss over dorsum of the foot. *Common causes:* trauma.
- *Tibial nerve* (S1-3)—Inability to stand on tiptoe, invert the foot, or flex toes. Sensory loss over sole.

Autonomic neuropathy: Results in postural hypotension (dizziness or syncope on standing, after exercise or a large meal), impotence, inability to sweat, vomiting and dysphagia, diarrhoea or constipation, urinary retention or incontinence, Horner's syndrome (📖 p.282). Check BP lying and standing—a postural drop of ≥30/15mmHg is abnormal.

Causes
- *Primary autonomic failure*—No known cause. Occurs alone or as part of multisystem atrophy. Typically, middle-aged/elderly men. Onset is insidious. Survival—rarely >10y. after diagnosis.
- *Ageing*—25% >74y. have postural hypotension. Review medication. Discourage prolonged bed rest. Often associated with disordered thermoregulation making elderly people prone to hypothermia. Exclude other disorders (e.g. DM, multisystem atrophy, drugs) before putting down to ageing alone.
- *Drugs*—Common culprits are antihypertensives (e.g. thiazides), diuretics (over-diuresis), L-dopa, tricyclic antidepressants, phenothiazines, benzodiazepines.
- *Polyneuropathies*—Autonomic neuropathy may occur as part of more general polyneuropathy e.g. due to DM, Guillain-Barré syndrome, or alcoholic/nutritional neuropathy.
- *Other causes*—Craniopharyngioma, vascular lesions, spinal cord lesions, tabes dorsalis (📖 p.742), Chagas' disease, HIV (📖 p.498), familial dysautonomia.

Management
- Treat any underlying cause.
- Advice:
  - stand slowly
  - raise head of the bed at night
  - eat little and often
  - ↓ carbohydrate and alcohol intake.
- Fludrocortisone (100mcg/d., increasing prn) may help those most severely affected.
- Refer if diagnosis is unclear or simple measures are ineffective.

Polyneuropathy: 📖 p.594

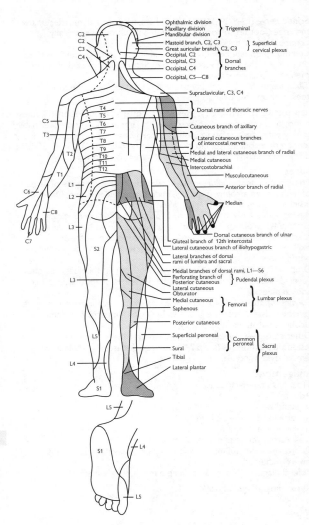

Figure 18.1 Dermatomes and peripheral nerve distribution

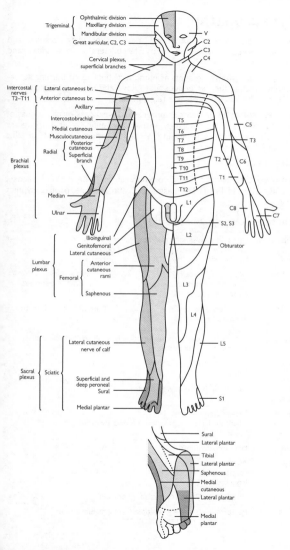

Figure 18.2 Dermatomes and peripheral nerve distribution

Polyneuropathy

Generalized disorder of peripheral nerves, including cranial and autonomic nerves. Distribution is usually bilateral, symmetrical, and widespread.

Sensory neuropathy presents as numbness, tingling, or burning sensation, often affecting the extremities first (glove and stocking distribution), or clumsiness handling fine objects (e.g. needle).

Motor neuropathy presents as progressive weakness or clumsiness of hands, stumbling/falls on walking, respiratory difficulty (can progress rapidly). *Examination:* wasting and weakness most marked distally; reflexes are ↓ or absent.

Causes: Table 18.3

Initial investigations: Exclude common causes—check blood glucose, FBC, ESR, U&E, LFTs, TFTs, plasma B_{12}, autoimmune profile, syphilis serology.

Table 18.3 Causes of polyneuropathy

Inflammatory	Guillain-Barré syndrome (mostly motor) Chronic inflammatory demyelinating polyneuropathy (CDP) Sarcoidosis	
Metabolic	DM (mainly sensory) Renal failure (mainly sensory) Hypothyroidism	Hypoglycaemia Mitochondrial disorders
Vasculitis	Polyarteritis nodosa Rheumatoid arthritis	Wegener's granulomatosis
Malignancy	Paraneoplastic syndromes (especially small cell lung cancer) Polycythaemia rubra vera	
Infection	Leprosy (mainly sensory) Syphilis	Lyme disease HIV
Vitamin deficiency	Lack of B_1, B_6, B_{12} (e.g. alcoholic)	
Inherited	Refsum's syndrome Charcot-Marie-Tooth syndrome (mostly motor) Porphyria	
Toxins	Lead (mostly motor)	Arsenic
Drugs	Alcohol Cisplatin Isoniazid	Vincristine Nitrofurantoin
	Less frequently: metronidazole, phenytoin	
Others	Paraproteinaemias e.g. multiple myeloma, amyloidosis	

Management: Treat cause if possible. Involve physiotherapists and OT. If sensory neuropathy, care of the feet is important to minimize trauma and consequent disability. Refer if a cause is not found.

⚠ If rapid deterioration, admit as acute medical emergency as ventilation may be needed.

Charcot-Marie-Tooth syndrome (peroneal muscular atrophy):
Cause: Unknown.

Presentation: Presents at puberty or in early adult life and begins with foot drop and weak legs. The peroneal muscles are the first to atrophy. The disease spreads to the hands and then arms. Sensation and reflexes are also ↓.

Management: Once diagnosis is confirmed, treatment is supportive.
(*J.M. Charcot (1825–93) and P. Marie (1853–1940)—French neurologists; H.H. Tooth (1856–1925)—English neurologist.*)

Guillain-Barré polyneuritis: Develops within a few weeks of surgery, 'flu vaccination, or infection (URTI, flu, HZ, HSV, CMV, EBV, campylobacter; mycoplasma). In 40%, no precipitating event is found.

Presentation: Ascending motor neuropathy which may advance fast. Proximal muscles are more affected than distal muscles. Trunk, respiratory muscles, and cranial nerves are commonly affected.

Management: If suspected, admit immediately to hospital as an emergency. Ventilation on ITU is frequently required.

Prognosis: 85% make a complete or near complete recovery. 10% are unable to walk alone at 1y. *Mortality:* 10%.
(*C. Guillain (1876–1961) and J.A. Barré (1880–1967)—French neurologists*)

Polio: 📖 p.493

Refsum's syndrome: Rare autosomal recessive disorder which presents in the 2nd decade or later with sensorimotor polyneuropathy, ataxia, visual and/or hearing problems. Treatment involves dietary restriction (avoidance of chlorophyll-containing foods) and plasmapheresis.
(*S. Refsum (1907–91)—Norwegian physician.*)

Headache (1)[G]

Very common presenting complaint in general practice. The skill lies in deciding which headaches are benign, requiring no intervention, and which require action.

History

- *Does the patient have >1 type of headache?* Take a separate history for each.
- *Time*
  - When did the headaches start? New or recently changed headache calls for especially careful assessment
  - How often do they happen?
  - Do they have any pattern (e.g. constant, episodic, daily)?
  - How long do they last?
  - Why is the patient coming to the doctor now?
- *Character*
  - Nature and quality of the pain
  - Site and spread of pain
  - Associated symptoms e.g. nausea/vomiting, visual disturbance, photophobia, neurological symptoms
- *Cause*
  - Predisposing and/or trigger factors
  - Aggravating and/or relieving factors
  - Family history
- *Response*
  - Details of medication used (type, dose, frequency, timing)
  - What does the patient do (e.g. can the patient continue work)?
- *Health between attacks:* Do the headaches go completely or does the patient still feel unwell between attacks?
- *Anxieties and concerns* of the patient

Examination

- In acute, severe headache, examine for purpuric skin rash
- BP
- Brief neurological examination including fundi and visual acuity
- Palpation of the temporal region/sinuses for tenderness
- Examination of the neck
- *In children,* measure head circumference and plot on a centile chart

Investigation: Often not needed. Consider ESR if temporal arteritis is suspected.

Management: Direct treatment at cause.

Differential diagnosis: Table 18.3

❶ ↑BP may cause acute or chronic headache.

Further information

British Association for the Study of Headache (2003) Guidelines for all doctors in the diagnosis and management of migraine and tension type headache, 2nd ed.
⊑ http://www.bash.org.uk

Table 18.4 Differential diagnosis of headache

	Cause	Features	Management
Acute new headache	Meningitis	Fever, photophobia, stiff neck, rash, photophobia	IV or IM penicillin V and immediate admission (📖 p.1044)
	Encephalitis	Fever, confusion, ↓ conscious level	Immediate admission (📖 p.1044)
	Subarachnoid haemorrhage	'Thunder-clap' or very sudden onset headache ± stiff neck	Immediate admission (📖 p.604)
	Head injury	Bruising/injury, ↓ conscious level, periods lucidity, amnesia	Consider admission (📖 p.546)
	Sinusitis	Tender over sinuses ± history of URTI	📖 p.919
	Dental caries	Facial pain ± tenderness	📖 p.912
	Tropical illness	History of travel, fever	📖 p.508
Acute recurrent headache	Migraine	Aura, visual disturbance, nausea/vomiting, triggers	📖 p.600
	Cluster headache	Nightly pain in 1 eye for 2–3mo., then pain free for >1y.	📖 p.599
	Exertional or coital headache	Suggested by history of association	NSAID or propranolol before attacks
	Trigeminal neuralgia	Intense stabbing pain lasting seconds in trigeminal nerve distribution	📖 p.599
	Glaucoma	Red eye, haloes, ↓ visual acuity, pupil abnormality	📖 p.942
Subacute headache	Temporal (giant cell) arteritis	>50y., scalp tenderness, ↑ ESR, rarely ↓ visual acuity	📖 p.580
Chronic headache	Tension type headache	Band around the head, stress, low mood	📖 p.599
	Cervicogenic headache	Unilateral or bilateral, band from neck to forehead, scalp tenderness	📖 p.548
	Medication overuse headache	Rebound headache on stopping analgesics	📖 p.599
	↑ intracranial pressure	Worse on waking/sneezing, neurological signs, ↑BP, ↓ pulse rate	📖 p.602
	Paget's disease	>40y., bowed tibia, ↑ alk phos,	📖 p.566

Headache (2)^G

Asssessment and differential diagnosis of headache: 📖 p.596–7

Chronic daily headache: Prevalence 4%. Defined as any headache that occurs >15d./mo. *Common causes:* tension headache (below), cervicogenic headache (📖 p.548), medication overuse headache (below), migraine, errors of refraction (usually mild, frontal, and in the eyes themselves, and absent on waking). Treat the cause.

Tension type headache: Associated with stress and anxiety and/or functional or structural abnormalities of the head or neck. Prevalence ≈ 2%. ♀:♂≈2:1. Symptoms begin aged <10y. in 15% patients. Prevalence ↓ with age. Family history of similar headaches is common (40%) but twin studies don't suggest a genetic basis. Distinguish between episodic and chronic tension type headache:

- **Episodic:** Defined as headache lasting 30min.–7d. and occurring <180d./y. (<15d./mo.).
- **Chronic:** Headaches on ≥15d./mo. (≥180d./y.) for ≥6mo.

In both cases, pain:
- Is bilateral, pressing, and/or tightening in quality
- Of mild or moderate intensity
- Does not prohibit activities
- Is not aggravated by routine physical activity
- Is not associated with vomiting
- Is associated with ≥1 of: nausea, photophobia, or phonophobia

Management

- Reassure no serious underlying pathology.
- Try measures to alleviate stress—relaxation; massage; yoga; exercise. Cognitive therapy is probably effective but not widely available^{CE}.
- Treat musculoskeletal symptoms with physiotherapy.
- *Drug therapy:* Analgesics are of limited value and might make matters worse (see medication overuse headache).
  - *Headache <2x/wk.:* Simple analgesia e.g. paracetamol, ibuprofen. Avoid codeine-containing preparations.
  - *Chronic headache:* Amitriptyline 25–75mg nocte may help. Stop once improvement maintained for >4–6mo.

Medication overuse (analgesic) headache: Persistent headache may develop in patients with other causes of headache (e.g. tension type headache or migraine) if they overuse the medication used to treat those conditions. Implicated drugs include: ergotamine, triptans, aspirin, paracetamol, and NSAIDs. ♀:♂ ≈ 3:1. Ask any patient complaining of chronic daily headache to give a detailed account of medication use (including OTC)—a diary can be helpful. *Management:* Aim to ↓ consumption of analgesics until taken <15d./mo.

Migraine: 📖 p.600

Cluster headaches (migrainous neuralgia): Clusters of extremely painful headaches focused around 1 eye with associated auto-nomic symptoms (drooping eyelid, red watery eye, runny or blocked nose). May occur at any age but rare <20y. ♂:♀ ≈ 6:1. More common in smokers. Pain lasts up to 1h. and occurs 1–2x/d. every day for 4–12wk. then disappears for 1–2y. Recurrences affect the same side. Onset is often predictable (1–2h. after falling asleep; after alcohol).

Management: Refer for specialist advice. *Drug treatments:*
- *Acute attack*
  - 100% oxygen at a rate of 7–12l/min.
  - 5HT$_1$ agonists e.g. sumatriptan (6mg s/cut)—stops 75% attacks within 15min.
- *Prophylaxis:* Consider if attacks are frequent, last >3wk. or cannot be treated effectively. *Options:*
  - Verapamil (unlicensed)—stops 66% attacks.
  - Lithium (unlicensed)—used as for manic depression (📖 p.973).
  - Ergotamine (unlicensed)—taken ½ h. before the attack is due. Should not be used for prolonged periods.
  - Methysergide—effective but use limited by side-effects. Only used if other drugs are contraindicated, not tolerated, or ineffective.

Trigeminal neuralgia: Paroxysms of intense stabbing, burning, or 'electric shock' type pain lasting seconds to minutes in the trigeminal (V) nerve distribution. 96% unilateral. Mandibular/maxillary > ophthalmic division. Between attacks, there are no symptoms. Frequency of attacks is highly variable ranging from hundreds of attacks/d. to remissions lasting years. Pain is often provoked by movement of the face (talking, eating, laughing) or by touching the skin (shaving, washing). Can occur at any age but more common >50y. ♀ > ♂. *Cause:* Unknown. More common in patients with MS and women with ↑ BP.

Management: Spontaneous remission may occur.
- Carbamazepine 100–400mg tds po ↓ frequency and intensity of attacks
- Refer to neurology if:
  - <50y. old
  - Neurological deficit between attacks
  - Treatment with carbamazepine fails—specialist options include treatment with lamotrigine, phenytoin, or gabapentin, or surgical intervention.

❶ >1 type of headache may coexist—50% migraine sufferers develop tension type headache resulting in background pain between attacks. Consider each separately.

Further information

British Association for the Study of Headache (2003) Guidelines for all doctors in the diagnosis and management of migraine and tension type headache, 2nd ed. 🖥 http://www.bash.org.uk

Migraine[G]

Migraine affects 10% of the UK population. ♂:♀ ≈ 1:2. It is more than just a headache. Attacks can force the patient to abandon everyday activities for several days. Even in symptom-free periods, patients may live in fear of the next attack. 1:3 sufferers will experience significant disability as a result of their migraines at some stage of their lives.

Cause: Disturbance of cerebral blood flow under the influence of 5-HT.

Clinical picture: 3 common types:

- *Aura:* Aura alone with no headache—visual chaos (e.g. zig-zag lines, jumbling of print, dots); hemianopia; hemiparesis; dysphasia; dyspraxia; dysarthria; ataxia (basilar migraine).
- *Classical migraine:* Aura lasting 10–30min. followed by unilateral throbbing headache ± nausea or vomiting ± photophobia.
- *Episodic migraine (common migraine):* Unilateral throbbing headache ± nausea or vomiting ± photophobia but without aura—often premenstrual.

Criteria for diagnosis if no aura: ≥5 headaches lasting 4–72h. + nausea/vomiting or photo-/phonophobia and ≥2 of following:

- Unilateral headache
- Headache interferes with normal functioning
- Pulsating headache
- Aggravated by climbing stairs or other routine activities

History, examination, and differential diagnosis: 📖 p.596–7.

Trigger factors: ½ have a trigger for their migraine. Consider:

- *Psychological factors:* Stress/relief of stress; anxiety/depression; extreme emotions e.g. anger or grief.
- *Food factors:* Lack of food/infrequent meals; foods containing monosodium glutamate, caffeine, and tyramine; specific foods e.g. chocolate, citrus fruits, cheese; alcohol, especially red wine.
- *Sleep:* Overtiredness (physical/ mental); changes in sleep patterns (e.g. late nights, weekend lie-in, shift work, holidays); long-distance travel.
- *Environmental factors:* Loud noise; bright/flickering lights; strong perfume; stuffy atmosphere; VDUs; strong winds; extreme heat/cold.
- *Health factors:* Hormonal changes (e.g. monthly periods, COC pill, HRT, the menopause);↑ BP; toothache or pain in the eyes, sinuses, or neck; unaccustomed physical activity.

Management: Aims to control symptoms and minimize their impact on the patient's life.

Management of an acute attack

- *Advise to rest* in a quiet, dark place and sleep if possible.
- *Analgesia*—dispersible aspirin 900mg, ibuprofen 400mg, or soluble paracetamol 1g at 1st signs of an attack ± antiemetic e.g. domperidone 20mg. If vomiting, consider pr administration e.g. diclofenac 100mg pr.
- *Severe attacks*—in addition, consider 5HT₁ agonists e.g. sumatriptan 50–100mg po, 20mg nasal spray, or 6mg s/cut (not effective if taken before the headache develops; stops 70–85% attacks—start with lowest dose and ↑ as needed; do not give if ergotamine taken <24h. previously).

If called to see a patient with an acute attack
- Administer im diclofenac 75mg ± im chlorpromazine 25–50mg.
- Alternatively, consider 5HT$_1$ agonist (e.g. sumatriptan) unless 2 injections/ tablets/nasal sprays already given in last 24h. (or ergotamine in <24h.).
- Admit if becoming dehydrated.

Treatment of recurrence within the same attack: Repeat symptomatic treatments within their dose limitations—pre-emptively if recurrence is usual/expected. If using triptans, a 2nd dose may be effective, but repeated dosing can cause rebound headache. Naratriptan and eletriptan are associated with relatively low recurrence rates.

Management of chronic migraine
- Reassure about the benign nature of migraine.
- Instruct patients about management of an acute attack.
- Ask the patient to keep a diary to identify possible trigger factors, assess headache frequency, severity, and response to treatment.
- Avoid trigger factors where possible. Give advice on relaxation techniques and stress management to all patients.
- Stop the COC pill if migraine starts or worsens when the pill is started—especially if focal symptoms develop (📖 p.750).
- Consider prophylaxis if frequent or very severe attacks.

Prophylaxis: Consider if ≥4 attacks/mo. or very severe attacks. ↓ attacks by ~50%. Try a drug for 2mo. before deciding it is ineffective. If effective, continue for 4–6mo. then ↓ dose slowly before stopping.
- *β-blockers*: e.g. atenolol 25–100mg bd. Patients who do not respond to one β-blocker may respond to another.
- *Pizotifen*: Start with 1.5mg nocte. If tolerance develops, ↑ dose. Side-effects are common and include sleepiness and ↑ weight.
- *Sodium valproate:* Start at 300mg bd. Unlicensed.
- *Tricyclic antidepressants* e.g. amitriptyline 10–75mg nocte. Unlicensed. Useful if migraine coexists with tension type headache, depression, or sleep disturbance. Start at low dose and ↑ dose every 2–4wk.

Alternative therapies: Feverfew 200mg daily—some evidence of effectiveness after 6wk. use^C. Acupuncture may also be helpful.

Menstrual migraine: Consider:
- *NSAIDs:* e.g. mefenamic acid 500mg tds/qds pc from onset of menstruation to last day of bleeding.
- *Transdermal oestrogen:* e.g. transdermal oestrogen 100mcgm (*avoid if focal migraine*). Apply 3d. before period and continue for 7d.
- *Women on COC pill:* Running 3 packets back to back before pill break and bleed. Alternatively, use an oestrogen-dominant pill e.g. cilest.

Migraine disability assessment score: 📖 p.629

Further information
British Association for the Study of Headache (2003) Guidelines for all doctors in the diagnosis and management of migraine and tension type headache, 2nd ed. 🖥 http://www.bash.org.uk

Patient information and support
Migraine Action Association 🖥 www.migraine.org.uk
The Migraine Trust ☎020 7436 1336 🖥 www.migrainetrust.org

Raised intracranial pressure and intracranial tumours

Raised intracranial pressure (↑ICP): Usually presents with increasing headache associated with drowsiness, listlessness, vomiting, focal neurology, and/or seizures.

Examination
- Drowsiness
- ↓ conscious level
- Irritability
- Focal neurological signs—due to underlying pathology
- VI nerve palsy
- Papilloedema
- Dropping pulse
- Rising BP
- Pupil changes—constriction first, then dilatation

Causes: 1° or 2° tumours, head injury, intracranial haemorrhage, hydrocephalus, meningitis, encephalitis, brain abscess, cerebral oedema (2° to tumour, trauma, infection, ischaemia).

Action: Admit as a medical emergency.

Intracranial tumours
- **2° brain tumours:** 30% brain tumours are 2°—usually from carcinoma of the breast, lung, or melanoma; in 50%, the brain tumours are multiple.
- **1° brain tumours:** 70% brain tumours. Classified according to whether they are benign or malignant and cell type.

Common types of 1° tumour: Glioma is an umbrella term meaning tumour of nervous system origin. Common subtypes:
- Astrocytoma
- Glioblastoma multiforme
- Oligodendroglioma
- Ependymoma

1° tumours of the meninges (meningiomas) and cerebral blood vessels (haemangioblastomas) can also occur.

Presentation of intracranial tumours
- **↑ICP:** Papilloedema 23–50% at presentation; headache 25–35%.
- **Seizures:** 25–30%. Suspect in all adults who have a first seizure—especially if focal or with localizing aura.
- **Evolving focal neurology:** Depends on the site. >50% have focal neurology at presentation. Frontal lobe lesions tend to present late.
- **False localizing signs:** Caused by ↑ICP. VI nerve palsy (causing double vision) is most common due to its long intracranial course.
- **Subtle personality change:** 16–20% at presentation—irritability, lack of application, lack of initiative, socially inappropriate behaviour.
- **Local effects:** Skull base masses, proptosis, epistaxis.

❶ <1% of patients presenting with headache have a brain tumour.

Differential diagnosis
- Other causes of space-occupying lesion:
  - Aneurysm
  - Abscess
  - Chronic subdural haematoma
  - Granuloma
  - Cyst
- Stroke
- MS
- Head injury
- Vasculitis
- Encephalitis
- Todd palsy (📖 p.619)
- Metabolic or electrolyte disturbance.

Action: If suspected, depending on clinical state, admit as an acute medical emergency or refer for urgent neurological assessment.

Prognosis: Gliomas all have <50% 5y. survival. Histological grading determines prognosis; site and grading determine treatment. Depending on site, meningionas and haemangioblastomas tend to have better prognosis.

Benign intracranial hypertension: Presents with symptoms and signs of a space-occupying lesion but none is found. Usually occurs in young, obese women. Cause unknown. Treated with repeat lumbar puncture, ventriculo-peritoneal shunt, diuretics, or dexamethasone. Usually resolves spontaneously, but 10% recur later.

Patient support
The Brain and Spine Foundation ☎0808 808 1000 🖥 http://www.brainandspine.org.uk
Brain Tumour Action (mainly Scotland) ☎0131 315 7299 (evenings and weekends)
🖥 http://www.braintumouraction.org.uk

Intracranial bleeds

Haemorrhagic stroke: 📖 p.606

Subarachnoid haemorrhage (SAH): Spontaneous bleeding into the subarachnoid space. Incidence 15/100,000. ♀ > ♂. Peak age 35–65y. Frequently fatal. *Causes:*

- No cause (15%)
- Rupture of congenital berry aneurysm (70%)
- Arterio-venous malformation (15%)
- Bleeding disorder
- Mycotic aneurysm 2° to endocarditis (rare)

Risk factors: Smoking, alcohol, ↑BP, lack of oestrogen (less common pre-menopause). Berry aneurysms may run in families and are associated with polycystic kidneys, coarctation of the aorta, and Ehlers-Danlos syndrome.

Presentation

- Typically presents as a sudden devastating headache ('thunderclap headache')—often occipital.
- Rarely (6%) preceded by a 'sentinel headache' representing a small leak ahead of a larger bleed.
- Vomiting and collapse with loss of consciousness ± fitting ± focal neurology follow.

Examination: May be nothing to find initially. Neck stiffness takes 6h. to develop. In later stages:

- Papilloedema
- Retinal and other intraocular haemorrhages
- Focal neurology
- ↓ level of consciousness

Action: If suspected, admit immediately as a medical emergency. Only 1:4 admitted with suspected SAH turn out to have one. In most, no cause for the headache is found.

Subdural haemorrhage: Bleeding is from bridging veins between cortex and venous sinuses, resulting in accumulation of blood between dura and arachnoid. *Causes:* trauma (may be trivial); idiopathic.

Risk factors: Age, alcohol, falls, epilepsy, anticoagulant therapy.

Presentation: Often insidious and history may go back several weeks:

- Fluctuation of conscious level (35%)
- Physical and intellectual slowing
- Sleepiness
- Headache
- Personality change
- Unsteadiness on feet
- Slowly evolving stroke (e.g. hemiparesis)
- Sympoms/signs of ↑ICP (📖 p.602)

Differential diagnosis: Stroke, cerebral tumour, dementia.

Action: If suspected, admit as a medical emergency for further investigation. Evacuation of clot is possible even in very elderly patients and normally results in full recovery.

Extradural haemorrhage: Blood accumulated between the dura and bone of the skull. Usually occurs after head injury.

Presentation: Deterioration of level of consciousness after head injury that initially produced no loss of consciousness or after initial post-injury drowsiness has resolved. This 'lucid' interval may last anything from a few hours to a few days. May be accompanied by worsening headache, vomiting, confusion ± focal neurological signs.

Action: If suspected, admit as an emergency for further investigation. Early evacuation of clot carries excellent prognosis. Outlook is less good if coma pre-op.

Acute stroke[G]

Common and devastating condition—most common cause of adult disability in UK. ½ all strokes occur in people >70y.

Definitions
- **Stroke:** A clinical syndrome typified by rapidly developing signs of focal or global disturbance of cerebral functions, lasting >24h. or leading to death, with no apparent causes other than of vascular origin (WHO 1978).
- **Transient ischaemic attack (TIA) or 'mini-stroke':** Neurological symptoms resolve in <24h.

Causes
- **Cerebral infarction** (≈70%): Atherothrombotic occlusion or embolism. *Sources of embolism*: left atrium (AF) or left ventricle (MI or heart failure). Ischaemia causes direct injury from lack of blood supply.
- **Intracerebral or subarachnoid haemorrhage** (≈19%): Haemorrhage causes direct neuronal injury and pressure exerted by the blood results in adjacent ischaemia.
- **Rare causes:** Sudden ↓BP, vasculitis, venous-sinus thrombosis, carotid artery dissection.

Risk factors
- Age
- ↑BP
- DM
- AF
- Previous stroke or TIA
- MI
- Artificial heart valves
- Hyperviscosity syndromes
- Smoking
- Alcohol
- Obesity
- Low physical activity

Presentation
- **History:** Sudden onset of CNS symptoms or stepwise progression of symptoms over hours or days.
- **Examination:** Conscious level may be ↓ or normal; neurological signs (including dysphagia and incontinence); BP; heart rate and rhythm; heart murmurs; carotid bruits; systemic signs of infection or neoplasm.

Differential diagnosis: Decompensation after recovery from previous stroke (e.g. due to infection, metabolic disorder), SOL—1° or 2° cerebral neoplasm, cerebral abscess; trauma—subdural haematoma, traumatic brain injury; epileptic seizure; migraine; MS.

Acute management: All patients who have suffered an acute stroke should be admitted to hospital. Do not give aspirin prior to admission. Treatment of stroke in a stroke unit → ↓ mortality and morbidity[C]. Recent evidence regarding benefits of thrombolysis means acute admission, bypassing the GP altogether, will be the norm in future[C].

Transient ischaemic attack (TIA): History is as for stroke but recovery takes place within 24h. of initial symptoms. Patients with a history of TIA have a 20% risk of stroke in the following month, with highest risk in the first 72h.

Investigations: ECG, CXR, blood—FBC, ESR, U&E, Cr, lipids, glucose. Consider clotting screen ± thrombophilia screeening if FH thrombosis.

Management of TIA

- Once all symptoms have stopped, start aspirin 50–300mg od.
- Start treatment for risk factors e.g. advise to stop smoking, start antihypertensives if ↑ BP.
- Refer for assessment and further investigation to a specialist service e.g. neurovascular clinic. The National stroke guidelines state that all patients with a history of TIA should be seen in a specialist clinic <7d. after the event. Specialist investigations include: CT or MRI scan to confirm diagnosis, carotid dopplers (if carotid artery territory symptoms); echocardiogram (if recent MI, CCF/LVF, or murmur).
- Admit if >1 TIA in 1wk.

Subarachnoid haemorrhage: 📖 p.604

2° prevention of stroke: 📖 p.608

Rehabilitation: 📖 p.176 and 626

After a stroke

- Stroke is a family illness. 40% carers suffer psychological distress 1 year after the stroke. Involve carers and families. Provide information and support.
- Stroke is a devastating illness for the patients. Address psychosocial issues as well as physical disability.
- Monitor and reassess frequently. Continue follow-up even when specialist services have finished. Stroke is a long-term problem. Monitor 2° prevention measures. Refer for more specialist rehabilitation if there is any deterioration in function.
- Remember aids and appliances can help, and patients and carers might be entitled to benefits.
- Concordance with medication—after stroke, most patients will be prescribed ≥1 drugs to ↓ their risk of further stroke, but some have memory loss or problems opening containers. All patients should receive verbal and written information about their medicines and receive help with packaging e.g. non-childproof tops.

Essential reading

Royal College of Physicians (2004) National clinical guidelines for stroke (2nd edition)
📖 http://www.rcplondon.ac.uk

Further information

Cochrane Reviews
Stroke Unit Trialists' Collaboration (2002) Organised inpatient (stroke unit) care for stroke
Wardlaw et al. (2003) Thrombolysis for acute ischaemic stroke

Patient information and support

Stroke Association ☎0845 30 33 100 📖 http://www.stroke.org.uk
Northern Ireland Chest, Heart and Stroke Association ☎0845 76 97 299 📖 http://www.nichsa.com
Chest, Heart, and Stroke Association Scotland ☎0845 077 6000 📖 http://www.chss.org.uk
Different Strokes ☎0845 130 7172 📖 http://www.differentstrokes.co.uk
Speakability ☎0808 808 9572 📖 http://www.speakability.org.uk

Secondary stroke prevention[G]

Patients with a past history of stroke or TIA/amaurosis fugax have a 30–43% risk of recurrent stroke within 5y.. Prevention focuses on ischaemic/embolic events which account for the majority of strokes. Preventive strategies include:

Acute stroke management: 📖 p.606

Lifestyle advice
- Stopping smoking—📖 p.234
- Regular exercise—📖 p.232
- Diet, and achieving a satisfactory weight—📖 p.226
- Reducing salt intake
- Avoiding alcohol excess—alcohol predisposes to both ischaemic and haemorrhagic stroke through effects on BP—📖 p.236

Antiplatelet drugs (usually aspirin): All patients not taking warfarin, who have suffered a non-haemorrhagic stroke (confirmed on CT/MRI) or a TIA should be started on aspirin as soon as possible after the event. Aspirin ↓ long-term risks of cardiovascular events by ¼ . Dose: 50–300mg od for maintenance therapy. Dipyridamole 200mg bd can be used in addition to aspirin (effects are additive). Clopidrel 75mg od is an expensive alternative.

Warfarin
- 1° *prevention:* Patients who have identified potential causes of cardiac thromboemboli should be anticoagulated with warfarin. This includes patients with rheumatic mitral valve disease; a prosthetic heart valve; dilated cardiomyopathy; and AF associated with valvular heart disease or prosthesis. Only anticoagulate patients with non-valvular AF if annual risk of stroke is >3% (Table 18.5). If <3%, start aspirin instead.
- 2° *prevention:* All patients who have suffered a stroke or TIA and have persistent or paroxysmal AF or a major source of cardiac embolism should be anticoagulated with warfarin. Start >14d. after stroke and only if haemorrhagic stroke has been excluded. Target INR 2-3 if no other indication (📖 p.366).

Hypertension management
- Systolic and diastolic BP independently predict stroke. Risk escalates with increasing BP. 5–6mmHg ↓ BP reduces risk by >30%.
- National stroke guidelines recommend treatment with a combination of a thiazide diuretic and ace inhibitor. Aim to keep systolic BP <140mmHg and diastolic BP <85mmHg (<130/80 if diabetic).
- After stroke (but not after TIA), defer treating hypertension until >2wk. after the event as ↑BP may be a physiological response—lowering BP decreases perfusion of the brain and may be harmful.

Cholesterol
- 1° *prevention:* Analysis of data from the coronary prevention trials shows a 22% ↓ in cholesterol using a statin produces a 30% ↓ in stroke

in individuals with no past history of stroke/TIA. Treat if patients meet criteria for coronary prevention (📖 p.322–7).
• 2° **prevention:** There is evidence to suggest all patients with a history of CVD should be treated with a statin regardless of baseline cholesterol. National stroke guidelines suggest treatment with a statin (e.g. simvastatin 40mg od) if total cholesterol is >3.5mmol/l unless contraindicated.

Carotid stenosis and carotid endarterectomy: Carotid endarterectomy ↓ mortality if carotid stenosis is symptomatic. Benefits decrease as the degree of stenosis gets smaller—there is no evidence of benefit if <30% stenosis.
• **Patients with asymptomatic stenosis:** There is a 2% annual risk of stroke, so the place of surgery is controversial—in general, risks outweigh benefits, so start aspirin and ↓ other modifiable risk factors.
• **Patients with a history of stroke /TIA:** Referral for carotid endarterectomy or carotid artery stenting should be considered for any patients who have had stroke/TIA, have >70% carotid artery stenosis, and do NOT have severe disability.

Table 18.5 Non-valvular AF and stroke

Risk group	Annual risk of stroke		
	Untreated	Aspirin	Warfarin*
Very high	12%	10%	5%
Previous ischaemic stroke or TIA			
High	5–8%	4–6%	2–3%
Age >65y. and ≥1 other risk factor (↑BP, DM, heart failure, LV dysfunction)			
Moderate	3–5%	2–4%	1–2%
Age >65y. + no other risk factors Age <65y. + other risk factors			
Low	1.2%	1%	≈0.5%
Age <65y. + no other risk factors.			

* Consider warfarin treatment for all patients in the very high, high, and moderate risk groups. In all cases, weigh the benefit of treatment against potential harms (e.g. bleeding risk in not compliant/unreliable about taking medication) and treatment preference. Target INR 2-3.

Essential reading
Royal College of Physicians (2004) National clinical guidelines for stroke (2nd edition)
🖥 http://www.rcplondon.ac.uk

Patient information and support
Stroke association ☎0845 30 33 100 🖥 http://www.stroke.org.uk
Northern Ireland Chest, Heart, and Stroke Association ☎0845 76 97 299
🖥 http://www.nichsa.com
Chest, Heart, and Stroke Association Scotland ☎0845 077 6000 🖥 http://www.chss.org.uk
Different Strokes ☎0845 130 7172 🖥 http://www.differentstrokes.co.uk
Speakability ☎0808 808 9572 🖥 http://www.speakability.org.uk

Parkinsonism and Parkinson's disease

(J. Parkinson (1755–1824)—English physician)

Parkinsonism: Syndrome of:
- *Tremor:* Coarse tremor, most marked at rest, 'pill-rolling'
- *Rigidity*
  - Limbs resist passive extension throughout movement—'lead-pipe rigidity'
  - Juddering on passive extension of the forearm or pronation/supination—'cogwheel rigidity'
- *Difficulty in initiating movement*
- *Slowness of movement:* 'Mask-like' or expressionless face, ↓ blink rate, ↓ fidgeting, ↓ peristalsis
- *Abnormal gait*
  - Small steps—'marche au petit pas'
  - Flexed posture as if hurrying to keep up with feet—'festinant gait'
- *Micrographia:* Small hand writing

Causes
- Parkinson's disease (PD)
- Other neurodegenerative diseases e.g. Alzheimer's disease, multisystem atrophy
- Following encephalitis
- Drugs e.g. haloperidol, chlorpromazine, metoclopramide
- Toxins e.g. CO poisoning
- Trauma
- Normal pressure hydrocephalus

Treatment of drug-induced parkinsonism: If possible, stop the implicated drug. If on an antipsychotic for schizophrenia, don't stop treatment, add an antimuscarinic (e.g. procyclidine 2.5mg tds), consider switching to an atypical antipsychotic drug, and take specialist advice.

Steel–Richardson–Olszewski syndrome: Parkinsonism accompanied by absent vertical gaze and dementia. Due to progressive supranuclear palsy. *(J.C. Steel, J.C. Richardson, and J.Olszewski—Canadian neurologists.)*

Parkinson's disease (PD): Incurable, progressive, degenerative disease affecting the dopaminergic neurones of the substantia nigra in the brainstem → deficiency of dopamine and relative excess of acetylcholine transmitters. *Cause:* unknown. *Lifetime risk:* ≈1:40. ♂ = ♀. *Peak age at onset:* ≈65y. but 5–10% patients are diagnosed when <40y. old. Prevalence ↑ with age.

❶ ¼ of those diagnosed with PD in life have another cause of their symptoms at autopsy.

Management: Aims to:
- ↓ symptoms and ↑ quality of life
- ↓ rate of disease progression
- Limit side-effects of treatment

Referral: Refer all patients to a specialist with an interest in Parkinson's disease for confirmation of diagnosis, advice on management, and to access a multidisciplinary specialist rehabilitation team.

Rehabilitation: Liaise closely with the specialist rehabilitation team.
● General principles: 📖 p.176 ● Specific issues: 📖 p.627

Drug treatment (*BNF* 4.9): Corrects imbalance of transmitters but not the underlying process. Rarely achieves complete control of symptoms. 5–10% respond poorly to treatment. Treatment for PD should be consultant-initiated and is usually not started until symptoms cause significant disruption of daily activities. Options:

Dopamine receptor agonists: e.g. bromocriptine, pergolide. Often used alone as 1st line treatment. ↑ dose gradually according to response and tolerability. Withdraw gradually. Can also be used in association with L-dopa to ↓ 'off' times and motor impairment (see below).

⚠ Bromocriptine, pergolide, cabergoline, and lisuride have been associated with pulmonary, retroperitoneal, and pericardial fibrosis.
● Check CXR ± spirometry, ESR, and creatinine before starting.
● Monitor for dyspnoea, persistent cough, chest pain, cardiac failure, abdominal pain, or tenderness.

Levodopa (or L-dopa): Precursor of dopamine. ↑ dopamine levels within the substantia nigra. Start with low dose and ↑ in small steps—aim to keep final dose as low as possible and a compromise between ↑ mobility and dose-limiting side-effects (involuntary movements, psychiatric effects). Optimum dose interval varies between individuals.
Only effective for PD. Not effective for patients with parkinsonism due to other degenerative brain disease or drugs. Improves bradykinesia and rigidity > tremor.
Often given with a co-drug (carbidopa or benserazide) which prevents peripheral breakdown of L-dopa to dopamine but does not cross the blood-brain barrier (e.g. sinemet, madopar).
With time, there is ↓ response and troublesome side-effects appear:
● 'On-off' effect—fluctuation between periods of exaggerated involuntary movements and periods of immobility.
● 'End-of-dose' effect—duration of benefit after each dose becomes shorter.
● Abnormal involuntary movements ↑.

Other drugs
Monoamine oxidase B inhibition: e.g selegeline. Used in severe PD in conjunction with L-dopa to ↓ 'end-of-dose' effect (see above). Early use may postpone onset of treatment with L-dopa.
Amantadine: Improves bradykinesia, dyskinesias, tremor, and rigidity. Introduce and withdraw slowly.
Anticholinergic: e.g. benzhexol, orphenadrine. Correct cholinergic excess. Effective for tremor and rigidity (not bradykinesia); ↓ dribbling.
Inhibition of enzymatic breakdown of dopamine: e.g. entacapone. For patients suffering from 'end-of-dose' effect.

Driving: 📖 p.202   **Carers:** 📖 p.178

Patient advice and support
Parkinson's Disease Society ☎0808 800 0303 🖥 *http://www.parkinsons.org.uk*

Multiple sclerosis (MS)

Multiple sclerosis (MS) is a chronic disabling neurological disease due to an autoimmune process of unknown cause. Characterized by formation of patches of demyelination ('plaques') throughout the brain and spinal cord. There is no peripheral nerve involvement.

It is the most common neurological disorder of young adults with a lifetime risk of 1:1000. Peak age of onset is 20–40y. ♀:♂ ≈ 2:1. There is a marked geographical variation—prevalence ↑ with latitude.

Presentation: Depends on the area of CNS affected. Take a careful history—although a patient usually presents with a single symptom, history may reveal other episodes that have gone unheralded. Isolated neurological deficits are never diagnostic. The hallmark of MS is a series of neurological deficits distributed in time and space not attributable to other causes. Predominant areas of demyelination are optic nerve, cervical cord, and periventricular areas.

Common features
- Pain on eye movement (optic neuritis)
- Visual disturbance—↓, blurring or double vision
- ↓ balance
- ↓ coordination
- Sensory disturbance (e.g. numbness, tingling)
- Pain (e.g. trigeminal neuralgia)
- Fatigue
- Depression
- Transverse myelitis (📖 p.616)
- Problems with speech (e.g. slurred or slow)
- Bladder problems (e.g. frequency, urgency, incontinence)
- Constipation
- Sexual dysfunction (e.g. impotence)
- Cognitive changes (e.g. loss of concentration, memory problems)
- Dysphagia

❶ Symptoms may be worsened by heat or exercise.

Prognosis
- **Benign MS** (rare): Few mild attacks and then complete recovery. There is no deterioration over time and no permanent disability.
- **Relapsing-remitting MS (RRMS):** 90% patients. Episodes of sudden ↑ in neurological symptoms or development of new neurological symptoms with virtually complete recovery after 4–6wk. With time, remissions become less complete and residual disability accumulates.
- **Secondary progressive MS (SPMS):** After ~10y. about ½ the patients with relapsing-remitting disease begin a continuous downward progression which may also include acute relapses.
- **Primary progressive MS (PPMS):** 10% patients. Steady progression from the outset, with increasing disability.

Management: If suspected, refer to neurology for confirmation of diagnosis and support from a specialist neurological rehabilitation team.

Disease-modifying drugs: ↓frequency and/or severity of relapses by ~30% and slow course of the disease. Options are β-interferon (for

RRMS and SPMS) and glatiramer (for RRMS only). Prescription must be consultant-led under the NHS risk-sharing scheme—see Table 18.6.

Table 18.6 Indications for β-interferon and glatiramer[N]

	β-interferon	Glatiramer
Age	≥18y.	≥18y.
Contraindications	No contraindications	No contraindications
Walking distance	RRMS: Can walk ≥ 100m without assistance	RRMS: Can walk ≥ 100m without assistance
	SPMS: Can walk ≥ 10m without assistance	
Relapses	RRMS: ≥ 2 clinically significant relapses in the last year	RRMS: ≥2 clinically significant relapses in the last year
	SPMS: Minimal ↑ in disability due to gradual progression and ≥ 2 disabling relapses in the past 2y.	
Stop	• Intolerable side-effects • Pregnant or planning pregnancy • ≥2 disabling relapses within a year • Inability to walk (± help) persisting ≥6mo. • 2° progression with observable ↑ in disability over 6mo.	• Intolerable side-effects • Pregnant or planning pregnancy • ≥2 disabling relapses within a year • Inability to walk (± help) persisting ≥6mo. • 2° progression

Diet: Supplementing the diet with 17–23g a day of linoleic acid (a polyunsaturated fat) may ↓ progression of disability[N]. Rich sources of linoleic acid include sunflower, corn, soya, and safflower oils.

Immunization: Offer influenza vaccination to all MS patients.

Acute relapses: Treat episodes causing distressing symptoms or ↑ limitation with high-dose steroids e.g. prednisolone 500mg–2g od po for 3–5d. Alternatively, refer for high-dose iv steroids. Refer to a specialist neurological rehabilitation team if residual deficit.

Management of symptoms and disability: Liaise closely with the specialist neurological rehabilitation team.
• General principles of rehabilitation: 📖 p.176
• Common neurological rehabilitation problems: 📖 p.626

Essential reading
NICE/RCP (2003) Diagnosis and management of multiple sclerosis in primary and secondary care 🖥 http://www.nice.org.uk
DoH: HSC (2002/004) Cost effective provision of disease modifying therapies for people with MS 🖥 http://www.dh.gov.uk

Patient advice and support
MS Society ☎0808 800 8000 🖥 http://www.mssociety.org.uk

Motor neurone disease (MND)

Motor neurone disease is a degenerative disorder of unknown cause affecting motor neurones in the spinal cord, brainstem, and motor cortex. Prevalence in the UK ~4.5/100,000 population; $\male$:$\female$ ≈ 3:2. Peak age of onset ≈60y. 10% have a FH. There is *never* any sensory loss.

Patterns of disease: There are 3 recognized patterns of MND:
- *Amyotrophic lateral sclerosis (ALS)* (50%)—combined LMN wasting and UMN hyperreflexia.
- *Progressive muscular atrophy* (25%)—anterior horn cell lesions affecting distal before proximal muscles. Better prognosis than ALS.
- *Progressive bulbar palsy* (25%)—loss of function of brainstem motor nuclei (LMN lesions) resulting in weakness of the tongue, muscles of chewing/swallowing, and facial muscles.

Clinical picture: Combination of progressive upper and/or lower motor neurone signs affecting >1 limb or a limb and the bulbar muscles.

Symptoms/signs
- Stumbling (spastic gait, foot-drop)
- Tiredness
- Muscle wasting
- Weak grip
- Weakness of skeletal muscles
- Cramp
- Fasciculation of skeletal muscles
- Fasciculation of the tongue
- Difficulty with speech (particularly slurring, hoarseness, or nasal or quiet speech)
- Difficulty with swallowing
- Aspiration pneumonia.

MND *never* affects external ocular movements (cranial nerves III, IV, VI).

Management: Refer to neurology for exclusion of other causes of the symptoms and confirmation of diagnosis. MND is incurable and progressive. Death usually results from ventilatory failure 3–5y. after diagnosis.
- *Drug therapy*
  - Riluzole (50mg bd) is the only drug treatment licensed in the UK.
  - Evidence suggests it extends life or time to mechanical ventilation for patients with ALS. It may also slow functional decline[N].
  - It should be initiated by a specialist with experience of MND[N].
  - Monitoring of liver function is essential—monthly for the 1st 3mo.; then 3 monthly for 9mo.; then annually thereafter.
- *Support*
  - Involve relevant agencies early e.g. DN, social services, carer groups, self-help groups.
  - Apply for all relevant benefits (p.98–111).
  - Discuss the future and the patient's wishes for the time when they become incapacitated with patient and carer(s).
  - Regular review to help overcome any new problems encountered is helpful for patients and carers.
- *Symptom relief*
  - *Spasticity:* baclofen, tizanidine, botulinum toxin.
  - *Drooling:* propantheline 15–30mg tds po or amitriptyline 25–50mg tds po.

- *Dysphagia:* Blend food; discuss n-g tubes/PEG (📖 p.1004).
- *Depression:* common—reassess support, consider drug treatment and/or counselling.
- *Joint pains:* analgesia.
- *Respiratory failure:* discuss tracheostomy/ventilation—weigh pros and cons of prolongation of life vs. prolongation of discomfort.
- *Palliative care:* 📖 p.999–1015

General principles of rehabilitation: 📖 p.176

Common neurological rehabilitation problems: 📖 p.626

Further information
NICE (2001 and review 2004) Riluzole for motor neurone disease—full guidance.
🖥 http://www.nice.org.uk

Patient support
Motor Neurone Disease Association ☎ helpline: 08457 626262
🖥 http://www.mndassociation.org

Spinal cord conditions

Spinal cord injury tends to affect young people, especially young men. It is devastating and the GP and primary care team are a vital part of the on-going support network. *Causes:* trauma (42% falls; 37% RTAs), herniated disc, transverse myelitis, tumour, abscess.

Transverse myelitis: Inflammation of the spinal cord at a single level. Symptoms develop rapidly over days/weeks and include limb weakness, sensory disturbance, bowel and bladder disturbance, back pain, and radicular pain. Recovery generally begins within 3mo. but is not always complete. *Causes:*

- Idiopathic (thought to be autoimmune mechanism)
- Infection
- Vaccination
- Autoimmune disease e.g. SLE, Sjögren's syndrome, sarcoidosis

- MS
- Malignancy
- Vascular e.g. thrombosis of spinal arteries, vasculitis 2° to heroin abuse, spinal A-V malformation

Management: Depending on severity of symptoms, admit as an acute medical emergency or refer for urgent neurological opinion.

Quadraplegia/tetraplegia: Caused by spinal cord injury above the 1st thoracic vertebra. Usually results in paralysis of all four limbs, weakened breathing, and an inability to cough and clear the chest.

Paraplegia: Occurs when the level of injury is below the 1st thoracic nerve. Disability can vary from the impairment of leg movement, to complete paralysis of the legs and abdomen up to the nipple line. Paraplegics have full use of their arms and hands.

Incomplete spinal cord injuries

- *Anterior cord syndrome:* Damage is towards the front of the spinal cord, leaving the patient with loss of ↓ ability to sense pain, temperature, and touch sensations below the level of injury. Pressure and joint sensation may be preserved.
- *Central cord syndrome:* Damage is in the centre of the spinal cord. Typically results in loss of function in the arms, but some leg movement may be preserved ± some control of bladder/bowel function.
- *Posterior cord syndrome:* Damage is towards the back of the spinal cord. Typically leaves the patient with good muscle power, pain, and temperature sensation, but difficulty coordinating limb movements.
- *Brown-Séquard syndrome:* Damage is limited to 1 side of the spinal cord resulting in loss or ↓ movement on the injured side but preserved pain and temperature sensation, and normal movement on the uninjured side but loss or ↓ in pain and temperature sensation. (*C.E. Brown-Séquard (1817–94)—French neurologist/physiologist.*)

Cauda equina lesion: The spinal cord ends at L1/L2, at which point a bundle of nerves travels downwards through the lumbar and sacral vertebrae. Injury to these nerves causes partial or complete loss of movement and sensation. There may be some recovery of function with time.

Syringomyelia: Tubular cavities (syrinxes) form close to the central canal of the spinal cord. As the syrinx expands, it compresses nerves within the spinal cord. Most common in patients with previous spinal injury—though may be years before. Typically presents with wasting and weakness of hands and arms, and loss of temperature and pain sensation over trunk and arms (cape distribution). *Action:* Refer to neurology.

General principles of rehabilitation: 📖 p.176

Common neurological rehabilitation problems: 📖 p.626

Specific problems associated with spinal cord injury
Autonomic dysreflexia (hyperreflexia): Reflex sympathetic over-activity causing flushing and ↑BP which may be severe. Only occurs in patients with lesions above T5/6. Usually triggered by discomfort below the level of the lesion. Presentation is with pounding headache, sweating, flushing, or mottling above the level of the lesion. *Action:*
• Sit the patient up.
• Remove any obvious cause e.g. pain, bladder distension, constipation.
• Give GTN spray (1–2 puff s/ling) or nifedipine 5–10mg capsule broken sublingually.
• If not settling, admit to hospital.

Loss of temperature control: Most people with complete spinal cord injuries don't sweat below the level of the injury and many quadriplegics can't sweat above the injury either (even though they may sweat due to autonomic dysreflexia). With loss of ability to sweat or vasoconstrict within affected dermatomes, careful control of environmental conditions becomes essential to avoid hypothermia or overheating. In hot weather, advise cooling with wet towels applied to the skin.

Infertility: Many ♂ patients suffer infertility due to:
• Failure of ejaculation
• Retrograde ejaculation
• Thermal damage of the testes (due to sitting in a wheelchair) →
  poor-quality sperm
• Chronic infection of prostate and seminal vesicles (common)

Refer for specialist advice.

Bowel/bladder function: Both bladder and bowel function are reflex actions which we learn to override as children. If the lesion is above the level of this reflex pathway (T12 for bowel and T6 for bladder function), then automatic emptying will still occur when the bladder or bowel is full, though there is no control. If the lesion is below this level—there is no emptying reflex. Bladder/bowel care programmes reflect this. Useful leaflets are available from the Spinal Injuries Association.

Spasticity: 📖 p.627   **UTI:** 📖 p.692

Pressure sores: 📖 p.641   **Depression:** 📖 p.968

Patient support
Spinal Injuries Association ☎0800 980 0501 🖳 http://www.spinal.co.uk

Epilepsy

Epilepsy is a group of disorders in which fits or seizures occur as a result of spontaneous abnormal electrical discharge in any part of the brain. They take many forms but usually take the same pattern on each occasion for a given individual. Prevalence 5–10/1000. 5% of those >21y. old having their 1st fit have cerebral pathology (10% age 45–55y.).

Fits in children: 📖 p.866

Classification of seizures
• *Partial*—simple partial, complex partial, and 2° generalized tonic clonic
• *Generalized*—generalized tonic clonic, absence, myoclonic, tonic, and atonic

Causes
• *Genetic* (20%)
• *Physical*—trauma, SOL, CVA, A-V malformation, sarcoid, vasculitis, ↑BP, following intracranial surgery
• *Metabolic*—drugs (withdrawal of benzodiazepines, TCAs, cocaine, phenothiazines), alcohol/alcohol withdrawal, hypoglycaemia or hyperglycaemia, hypoxia, uraemia, disturbance of electrolytes
• *Infective*—encephalitis or meningitis, cerebral abscess, HIV

Differential diagnosis
• Vasovagal syncope
• Psychogenic non-epileptic attacks (pseudo-seizures)
• Tics
• Panic attack
• Hypoglycaemia
• Normal phenomenom (e.g. déja-vu)
• Cardiac arrythmias
• Other cardiac disorders (e.g. aortic stenosis, HOCM)
• TIA
• Migrainous aura

History
• *Background:* Previous head injury, alcohol/drug abuse, meningitis or encephalitis, stroke, febrile convulsions, FH of epilepsy.
• *Provoking factors:* Sleep deprivation, alcohol withdrawal, flashing lights.
• *Prodrome or aura*
  • *Prodrome*—precedes fit. May be a change in mood or behaviour noticed by the patient or others.
  • *Aura*—part of the seizure that precedes other manifestations—odd sensations e.g. déjà-vu (odd feeling of having experienced that time before), strange smells, rising abdominal sensation, flashing lights.
• *Features of the attack: Eye witness report (*if available)—colour of the patient, movement, length of fit, circumstances, after-effects, etc.; *memories of the patient*—memories of the event and/or 1st memories after the event, frequency of attacks, relationship to sleep, menses, etc.
• *Residual symptoms after the attack:* Bitten tongue, incontinence of urine/faeces (not specific for epilepsy), confusion, headache, aching limbs, temporary weakness of limbs (Todd's palsy after Jacksonian fit).

Examination and investigation
• Neurological examination—any residual deficit, signs of systemic illness.
• First fit—blood for U&E, Cr, LFT, Ca^{2+}, FBC, ESR.

Management of a fitting patient/status epilepticus: 📖 p.1068

Management after first fit: 60% adults who have 1 fit will never have another (90% if EEG normal). Refer *all* patients (unless very frail or elderly) who have fit, who are not known to be epileptic, for neurological assessment to exclude any underlying cause (e.g. tumour) and receive clear guidance on medication, work, and driving.

Ongoing management in general practice: After a new diagnosis of epilepsy, patients are investigated and started on any medication under specialist care, then discharged to their GP. Regular GP review, at least annually, is essential.

Information: Find out how much the patient (and family) understand about epilepsy and what information they have, acknowledge their distress at diagnosis, anger, and fears and answer their questions.
- Heredity—risk for child: no parent with epilepsy (0.5–1%); 1 parent (4%); both parents (15–20%).
- Prognosis—fits are controlled with drugs in 80% patients. Most need drug treatment <5y.
- Driving (📖 p.204)—advise patient to stop driving and notify DVLA and motor insurance company after any seizure. Document your advice. HGV/PSV licenses are withdrawn. Cycling in traffic is unwise.
- Employment—advise patient to inform employer. Patients should not work at heights or with/near dangerous machinery.
- Lifestyle—only swim with lifeguard present.

Drug management: 📖 p.620

Review
- any fits and precipitating causes
- drug compliance (frequency of repeat prescriptions)
- side-effects of drugs
- If fit free >2y., discuss possibility of withdrawing medication (📖 p.620).

Re-refer to a neurologist if:
- control is poor or drugs are causing side-effects
- seizures have continued >5y.
- pointers to a previously unsuspected cause for the fits
- concurrent illness complicates management
- for pre-conceptual advice.

Todd palsy: Focal CNS signs (e.g. hemiplegia) following an epileptic seizure. The patient seems to have had a stroke but recovers in <24h. *(R.B. Todd (1809–60)—Irish anatomist/physician)*

Epilepsy and pregnancy: 📖 p.782

Contraception for epileptic patients: 📖 p.759

Further information
SIGN (2003) *Diagnosis and management of epilepsy in adults* 🖥 http://www.sign.ac.uk

Patient support
Epilepsy Action ☎0808 800 5050 🖥 http://www.epilepsy.org.uk

Epilepsy: drug therapy

BNF 4.8.1

> ❶ **Prescribing tips**
> *Use monotherapy wherever possible:* 2 drugs ↑ toxicity and side-effects. They also frequently interact. Polytherapy offers no advantage over monotherapy for 90% patients.
> *Prescribe by brand name:* Generic prescribing may lead to changing of brand. Changing brand carries 10% risk of worsening of seizure control.

Free prescriptions: Patients on anticonvulsant medication are entitled to free prescriptions (📖 p.119).

Poor fit control
- Check compliance by monitoring the frequency of prescriptions issued. There is no place for routine drug level monitoring in primary care^G. Explore any reasons for poor compliance—it may indicate lack of acceptance of the diagnosis.
- If compliance is acceptable, ↑ dose until fits are controlled, maximum dose is reached, or side-effects occur.
- If fits are still uncontrolled, refer for specialist review.

Withdrawal of drug therapy: Consider if free of fits for 2–3y. The decision to stop medication MUST be the patient's. Balance the problems and inconvenience of drug-taking against the risks of fits returning, with implications for driving, employment, and family.
- *Seizure recurrence is more likely if:*
  - history of generalized tonic-clonic seizures;
  - myoclonic epilepsy or infantile spasms;
  - taking >1 drug to control epilepsy;
  - ≥1 seizure after starting treatment;
  - duration of treatment >10y.
- *Seizure recurrence is less likely if:* seizure free ≥5y.

For adults with grand mal epilepsy, 59% remain fit-free for 2y. after withdrawal of medication compared with 78% on medication.

Drug withdrawal rates: Withdrawal should take >6mo. Withdraw 1 drug at a time. Advise patients not to drive during withdrawal of epileptic medication or for 6mo. afterwards.
- *Decremental doses every 2–4wk.:* carbamazepine (100mg); lamotrigine (50mg); phenytoin (50mg); sodium valproate (200mg); vigabatrin (500mg).
- *Decremental doses every 4–8wk.:* clobazepam (10mg); clonazepam (0.5mg); ethosuximide (250mg); phenobarbitone (30mg); primidone (125mg).

Further information
SIGN (2003) Diagnosis and management of epilepsy in adults 🖳 *http://www.sign.ac.uk*

Table 18.7 Commonly used drugs in epilepsy (Stress the importance of compliance. Start at a low dose and ↑ dose until fits are controlled or side-effects occur.)

		Ethosuximide	Sodium valproate	Carbamazepine	Lamotrigine	Phenytoin
Type of epilepsy	Absence	✓	✓		✓ (unlicensed)	
	Myoclonic		✓			
	Tonic clonic		✓[1]	✓	✓	✓
	Partial ± 2° Generalized		✓	✓	✓	✓
Adult starting dose		500 mg od	300 mg bd	100–200mg od or bd	25 mg od for 2wk[2]	100mg od
Incremental dose		250mg/d. at weekly intervals	200mg/d. at 3-day intervals	100mg/d. at weekly intervals	From starting dose to 50mg od for 2wk, then ↑ by 50mg/d. at weekly intervals	100mg/d. at weekly intervals
Usual daily dose		1–1.5g od	500mg–1g bd	200–1200mg	100–200mg	100–600mg
Common/important side-effects		Blood dyscrasias[3], nausea, sedation, vomiting, dizziness, ataxia	Pancreatitis, liver toxicity[4], blood dyscrasias[3], sedation, tremor, weight ↑, hair thinning, ankle swelling	Blood dyscrasias[3], rash, liver toxicity[4], nausea, sedation, diplopia, dizziness, fluid retention, ↓Na+[5]	Blood dyscrasias[3], rash, fever, influenza-like symptoms, drowsiness, worsening of seizure control	Blood dyscrasias[3], rash, drowsiness, ↓memory, gum hyperplasia, nystagmus, diplopia, tremor, dysarthria, ataxia

1. Drug of choice for primary syndrome of generalized epilepsy.
2. Starting dose is different if used in association with other epileptics—see BNF.
3. Check FBC if bruising, mouth ulcers, or symptoms of infection (sore throat, fevers).
4. Warn about symptoms of liver disease; check soon after starting and at review.
5. Monitor at regular review.

Muscle disorders

Symptoms
- Muscle weakness
- Fatigability
- Pain at rest (suggests inflammation)
- Pain on exercise (due to ischaemia or metabolic myopathy)

Signs
- Myotonia—delayed muscular contraction after relaxation e.g. on shaking hands.
- Local muscular tenderness or firm muscles—may be due to infiltration of muscle with connective tissue or fat.
- Fasciculation—spontaneous, irregular, and brief contractions of part of, a muscle. Suggests LMN disease e.g. MND.
- Lumps—tumours are rare. Lumps may be due to tendon rupture, haematoma, herniation of muscle through fascia.
- Look for associated systemic disease.

Muscular dystrophies: Group of genetic disorders characterized by progressive degeneration and weakness of some muscle groups.

Duchenne's muscular dystrophy: Sex-linked recessive inheritance means almost always confined to boys. 30% of cases are due to spontaneous mutation. Investigation shows markedly ↑ CK (>40x normal). Presents typically at ~4y. with progressively clumsy walking. Few survive to >20y. old. Refer for confirmation of diagnosis and ongoing specialist support. Genetic counselling is important.
(G.B.A. Duchenne (1807–75)—French neurologist)

Patient support
Muscular Dystrophy Campaign ⌨ *http://www.muscular-dystrophy.org*

Myotonic disorders: Characterized by myotonia.

Dystrophia myotonica: Most common of the myotonic disorders. Inherited as an autonomic dominant gene. Typically presents from 20–30y. with weakness of hands, legs, and face and myotonia. Wasting of the face gives a long, haggard appearance. Associated with cataract, frontal baldness in men, atrophy of the testes or ovaries, cardiomyopathy, endocrine abnormaliies (e.g. DM), and mental impairment. Most die in middle age of intercurrent illness. Refer for confirmation of diagnosis and advice on management. Genetic counselling is important.

Toxic myopathies: Certain drugs can cause myopathy including:
- Alcohol
- Labetolol
- Cholesterol-lowering drugs (including the statins)
- Steroids
- Chloroquine
- Zidovudine
- Vincristine
- Ciclosporin
- Cocaine
- Heroin
- PCP

Management: Stop the implicated drug immediately. If symptoms do not resolve, refer for confirmation of diagnosis and advice on further management.

Acquired myopathy of late onset: Often a manifestation of systemic disease e.g. thyroid disease (especially hyperthyroidism), carcinoma,

Cushing's disease. Investigate to find the cause. Treat the cause if found, else refer for further investigation.

Polymyositis: Insidious, symmetrical, proximal muscle weakness due to muscle inflammation. Dysphagia, dysphonia, and/or respiratory muscle weakness may follow. 25% have a purple rash on cheeks, eyelids, and other sun-exposed areas (dermatomyositis) ± nail fold erythema. CK levels are ↑. Associated with malignancy in 10% of patients >40y. Refer for confirmation of diagnosis and advice on management.

Motor neurone disease: 📖 p.614

Poliomyelitis: Acute polio: 📖 p.493

Late effects of polio: 20–30y. after initial infection some patients develop new symptoms, often triggered by a period of immobilization:
- ↑ muscle weakness and fatigue
- Pain in muscles and joints
- Respiratory difficulties (particularly in those who spent some time in an iron lung ventilator)—may present with symptoms relating to sleep

Once other causes are excluded and diagnosis is confirmed, treatment is supportive.

Myaesthenia gravis: Autoimmune disease in which antibodies to the acetylcholine receptor cause a deficit of receptors at the neuromuscular junction → muscle weakness. Antibodies are detectable in 90% of patients. ♀:♂ ≈ 2:1. Associated with thymic tumours and other autoimmune diseases e.g. RA, SLE, hyperthyroidism. Generally follows a relapsing or slowly progressive course. If thymoma present, 5y. survival ≈ 30%.

Presentation: Young adults with easy fatigability of muscles. Commonly affected muscles:
- Orbital muscles causing ptosis and diplopia
- Bulbar muscles causing slurring of speech—ask to count to 50

Weakness is exacerbated by pregnancy, infection, drugs (e.g. β-blockers, opiates, tetracycline, quinine), climate change, emotion, and exercise.

Management: If suspected, refer for confirmation by a neurologist and specialist treatment. Treated with:
- Anticholinesterase e.g. pyridostigmine
- Immunosuppression with prednisolone, methotrexate, or azathioprine
- Thymectomy → remission in 30% and benefit in another 40%
- Plasmapheresis

Patient support

Myaesthenia Gravis Association UK 🖳 http://www.mgauk.org

Lambert–Eaton syndrome (or myaesthenic syndrome): Occurs in association with small cell carcinoma of the lung or, rarely, other auto-immune diseases. Differs from myaesthenia gravis by tendency to hypore-flexia as opposed to hyperreflexia. Autonomic involvement is common. Proximal limb muscles and trunk are most commonly involved. Specialist treatment is essential. (L.M. Eaton (1905–1958) and E.H. Lambert (b.1915)—US neurologists/neurophysiologists)

Other neurological syndromes

Neurofibromatosis
Von Recklinghausen's disease (type 1 neurofibromatosis)
Autosomal dominant trait. Criteria for diagnosis: ≥2 of:
- ≥6 café-au-lait patches (flat, coffee-coloured patches of skin seen in 1st year of life, increasing in number and size with age) >5mm (prepubertal) or >15mm (postpubertal).
- ≥2 neurofibromas
  - Dermal neurofibromas—small violaceous skin nodules which appear after puberty.
  - Nodular neurofibromas—subcutaneous, firm nodules arising from nerve trunks (may cause paraesthesiae if compressed) or a plexiform neurofibroma which appears as a large subcutaneous swelling.
- Freckling in axilla, groin, neck base, and submammary area (women). Present by 10y.
- ≥2 Lisch nodules—nodules of the iris only visible with a slit lamp.
- Distinctive boney abnormality specific to NF1 (e.g. sphenoid dysplasia).
- 1st degree relative with NF1.

Management: Ongoing specialist management is essential.

Complications: affect 1:3 patients:
- Mild learning disability
- Short stature
- Macrocephaly
- Nerve root compression
- GI bleeding or obstruction
- Cystic bone lesion
- Scoliosis
- Pseudoarthrosis
- ↑BP (6%)—due to renal artery stenosis or phaechromocytoma
- Malignancy (5%)—optic glioma or sarcomatous change of neurofibroma
- Epilepsy (slight ↑)

(F.D. von Recklinghausen (1833–1910)—German pathologist.)

Type 2: Much rarer than type 1. Autosomal dominant inheritance.

Diagnosis: 1 of:
- Bilateral vestibular schwannoma (acoustic neuroma—sensorineural hearing loss, vertigo ± tinnitus).
- 1st degree relative with NF2 and *either* a unilateral vestibular schwannoma *or* ≥1 neurofibroma, meningioma, glioma, Schwannoma, or juvenile cataract.

Management: Screen at-risk patients with annual hearing tests. Once diagnosis made, specialist neurosurgical management is needed.

Complications: Schwannomas of other cranial nerves, dorsal nerve roots, or peripheral nerves; meningioma (45%); other gliomas (less common).

Ekbom syndrome (restless legs syndrome): The patient (who is usually in bed) is seized by an irresistible desire to move his legs in a repetitive way, accompanied by an unpleasant sensation deep in the legs. Sleep disturbance is common, as is +ve FH. *Cause:* unknown.

Management
- Exclude drug causes—common culprits: β-blockers, H_2 antagonists, neuroleptics, lithium, TCAs, anticonvulsants.
- Exclude peripheral neuropathy or ischaemic rest pain.
- Iron deficiency (with or without anaemia) is associated in 1:3 sufferers, so check FBC and serum ferritin.
- Codeine (30–60mg tds/qds), carbamazepine (100mg bd), and clonazepam (1–4mg nocte) are helpful. Other drugs which have been used include gabapentin and zopiclone.

Patient support
Restless Leg Syndrome Foundation ⌨ http://www.rls.org
Ekbom Support Group ⌨ http://www.ekbom.org.uk
(K.A. Ekbom (1907–77)—Swedish neurologist).

Wernicke encephalopathy: Thiamine deficiency causing nystagmus, ophthalmoplegia, and ataxia. Other eye signs e.g. ptosis, abnormal pupillary reactions, and altered consciousness or confusion may also occur. Consider in any patient with symptoms and a history of alcoholism.

Management: Refer for confirmation of diagnosis. Meanwhile, start thiamine 200–300mg od po to prevent irreversible Korsakoff's syndrome. In severe cases, admit as a medical emergency.
(K. Wernicke (1848–1904)—German psychiatrist).

Korsakoff syndrome: ↓ ability to acquire new memories. May follow Wernicke encephalopathy and is due to thiamine deficiency. Confabulation to fill gaps in memory is a feature.
(S.S. Korsakoff (1853–1900)—Russian neuropsychiatrist).

Gilles de la Tourette syndrome: 📖 p.891

Huntington's disease (chorea): Autosomal dominant trait. Testing can identify affected individuals before symptoms occur. Pre-conceptual and antenatal testing is available and should be offered to any couple with a FH on either the mother or the father's side. Presents with movement abnormalities (e.g. hemichorea and rigidity) and dementia. Memory is relatively spared compared to cognition.

Management: Refer for expert advice.
(G. Huntington (1851–1916)—US physician.)

Friedreich's ataxia: The most common inherited ataxia (autosomal recessive). Prevalence—1:50,000. Presents in adolescence with progressive gait and limb ataxia, loss of proprioception, pyramidal weakness, and dysarthria. Extra-neurological involvement includes hypertrophic cardiomyopathy (most patients) and DM (10%). Treatment is supportive. Most patients become chairbound within 15y. and die in the 4th or 5th decade from cardiac or pulmonary complications.
(N. Friedreich (1825–82)—German neurologist.)

Common neurological rehabilitation problems

New symptoms or limitations: Consider:

- Is it due to an unrelated disease? e.g. change in bowel habit in someone who has had a stroke might indicate bowel cancer.
- Is it due to an incidental infection? e.g. UTI, chest infection.
- Is it due to a relapse? e.g. acute relapse in MS, TIA or further stroke in a stroke patient.
- Is it due to a side-effect of treatment? e.g. acute confusion, involuntary movements, or the on-off effect in a patient with PD.
- Is it part of a gradual progression? e.g. in MS, MND, brain tumour.

Treat any cause of deterioration identified. If no cause is found, consider re-referring for specialist review and/or referring to the multidisciplinary rehabilitation team involved with the patient.

General principles of rehabilitation: 📖 p.176

Fatigue: Consider and treat factors which might be responsible:

- Depression
- Chronic pain
- Disturbed sleep
- Poor nutrition

Action: Review support, diet, and medication; encourage graded aerobic exercise, consider a trial of amantadine 200mg/d. to improve symptoms[N].

Depression and anxiety: Common. Diagnosis can be difficult. Standardized questionnaires (e.g. hospital anxiety and depression scale—charge payable for usage) may be helpful for screening.

Action: Give opportunities to talk about the impact of the illness on lifestyle. Jointly, identify areas where positive changes could be made e.g. referral to day care to widen social contact. Consider referral for counselling or to a self-help/support group. Consider antidepressant medication and/or referral to psychiatric services.

Emotionalism: If the patient cries (or laughs) with minimal provocation, consider emotionalism—impairment in the control of crying. Reassure.

Sexual and personal relationships: Problems are common. Useful information sheets are available at 🖥 http://www.outsiders.org.uk

Communication problems: Speech therapy assessment is vital. Consider support via dysphasia groups and communication aids e.g. simple pointing board (take advice from speech therapy and OT).

Poor vision: Refer to an optician in the first instance. If corrected vision is still poor, refer for ophthalmology review.

Respiratory infections: Common. Treat with antibiotics unless in terminal stages of disease. Advise pneumococal and influenza vaccination.

Venous thromboembolism: Common but clinically apparent in <5%. Ensure adequate hydration and encourage mobility. Consider use of aspirin 75–150mg od and compression stockings, if immobile. Prophylactic anticoagulation does not improve outcome.

Motor impairment: Aim to maintain physical independence:
- Involve physiotherapy—often only 2 or 3 visits are needed.
- Involve OT—a task-oriented approach is used (e.g. learning how to dress). Can also supply/advise on aids and appliances e.g. velcro fasteners, wheelchairs, adapted cutlery, etc.
- Refer for social services OT assessment if aids, equipment, or adaptations are needed for the home,
- Refer for home care services as necessary.
- Give information about driving (📖 p.202) and/or employment (📖 p.200) where appropriate.

Spasticity ± muscle and joint contractures: Treat with physiotherapy (usually involving exercise ± splinting) ± drugs. Anti-spasticity drugs include dantrolene (25mg od), baclofen (5mg tds or, rarely, through a pump), and tizanidine (2mg od). Botulinum toxin can be directed at specific muscles. Refer via the specialist rehabilitation team.

Pain: Most pain arises from ↓ mobility. *Other causes include:* pre-morbid disease (e.g. osteoarthritis); central pain due to neurological damage; and neuropathic pain.

Action: Chronic pain, especially central pain, may respond to TCAs. Peripheral pain may respond to simple analgesia ± physiotherapy. Other options are TENS and local joint injection. Use of cannibinoids for relief of pain/muscle spasm in MS is currently under assessment. Refer patients with intractable pain to specialist pain clinics.

Bladder problems
- *UTI:* If suspected, check urine dipstick ± send MSU for M,C&S and start antibiotics. If >3 proven UTIs in 1y., refer to specialist incontinence service or urology for further assessment.
- *Incontinence:* 📖 p.694
- *Nocturia:* Desmopressin 100–400mcg po or 10–40mcg intranasally may be helpful.
- *Urgency:* Modify environment (e.g. provide commode); try anticholinergic (e.g. tolterodine 2mg bd or oxybutinin 5mg tds). If not settling, refer for specialist assessment.

Bowel problems
- *Dysphagia:* Common. Fluids are more difficult to swallow than semi-solids. Formal assessment by trained staff is essential. Feeding through N-G tube or percutaneous endoscopic gastrostomy (PEG) may be needed, long or short term. In terminal disease (e.g. MND), weigh provision of nutrition against prolongation of poor-quality life.
- *Constipation:* Difficulty with defaecation or BO <2x/wk.—↑ fluid intake and ↑ fibre in diet. If no improvement, use po laxative ± regular suppositories/enemas.
- *Incontinence:* Exclude overflow due to constipation.

Skin breakdown: *Prevented by:* positioning; mobilization; good skin care; management of incontinence; pressure relieving aids (e.g. special mattresses/cushions). Involve community nursing services.

Neurological assessment scales

Modified Barthel ADL index[*]: Measure of physical disability used widely to assess behaviour relating to activities of daily living for stroke patients or patients with other disabling conditions. It measures what patients do in practice. Assessment is made by anyone who knows the patient well.

Bowels

0 = Incontinent or needs enemas

1 = Occasional accident (1x/wk.)

2 = Continent

Bladder

0 = Incontinent or needs enemas

1 = Occasional accident (1x/wk.)

2 = Continent

Grooming

0 = Needs help with personal care

1 = Independent (including face, hair, teeth, shaving)

Toilet use

0 = Dependent

1 = Needs some help

2 = Independent

Feeding

0 = Unable

1 = Needs help (e.g. cutting)

2 = Independent

Transfer (bed to chair and back)

0 = Unable, no sitting balance

1 = Major help (1 or 2 people); can sit

2 = Minor help (verbal or physical)

3 = Independent

Mobility

0 = Immobile

1 = Wheelchair independent (including corners)

2 = Walks with the help of 1 person (physical or verbal help)

3 = Independent (may use aid)

Dressing

0 = Dependent

1 = Needs help; can do ~½ unaided

2 = Independent (including buttons, zips, laces, etc.)

Stairs

0 = Unable

1 = Needs help (verbal or physical)

2 = Independent

Bathing

0 = Dependent

1 = Independent (bath or shower)

Score

- <15—usually represents moderate disability
- <10—usually represents severe disability

[*] Reproduced with permission from Mahoney FI, Barthel D. (1965) Functional evaluation: the Barthel Index. *Maryland State Medical Journal* **14**: 56–61.

Migraine disability assessment score (MIDAS)[**]: Used to assess the impact of migraine symptoms on lifestyle.

Instructions: Please answer the following questions about ALL the headaches you have had over the last 3mo. If you did not do the activity in the last 3mo., write 0.

1. On how many days in the last 3mo. did you miss work or school because of your headache? □ days

2. How many days in the last 3mo. was your productivity at work or school ↓ by ≥½ because of your headaches? *(Do not include days you counted in question 1 where you missed work or school.)* □ days

3. On how many days in the last 3mo. did you not do house-hold work[*] because of your headache? □ days

4. How many days in the last 3mo., was your productivity in household work ↓ by ≥½ because of your headaches? *(Do not include days you counted in question 3 where you did not do household work.)* □ days

5. On how many days in the last 3mo. did you miss family, social, or leisure activities because of your headaches? □ days

MIDAS score   TOTAL   □ days

A. On how many days in the last 3mo. did you have a head-ache? *(If a headache lasted more than 1 day, count each day.)* □ days

B. On a scale of 0–10, on average how painful were these headaches? *(Where 0 − no pain at all, and 10 − pain as bad as can it be.)* □

Questions A and B measure the frequency of the migraine and the severity of pain. They are not used to reach the MIDAS score, but provide extra information helpful for making treatment decisions.

Table 18.8 Interpreting the MIDAS score

I	Score: 0–5	Minimal/infrequent disability	Tend to have little or no treatment needs. Can often manage with OTC medication. If infrequent, severe attacks may require triptan.
II	Score: 6–10	Mild/infrequent disability	May require medication for acute attacks e.g. NSAID ± antiemetic or triptan.
III	Score: 11–20	Moderate disability	Will need medication for acute attacks. Consider prophylaxis.
IV	Score: ≥21	Severe disability	Consider other causes for headaches e.g. TTH.

[**] Unpaid work such as housework, shopping, and caring for children and others.
Reproduced with permission from BASH headache guidelines 2003.

Dermatology

Skin changes associated with internal conditions

Table 19.1 Systemic conditions associated with skin changes

Condition	Associated skin changes
Addison's disease	Pigmentation, vitiligo.
Cushing's disease	Pigmentation, hirsutism, striae, acne, truncal obesity, moon facies, buffalo hump.
Diabetes mellitus	• *Diabetic dermopathy*—depressed pigmented scars on the shins. • *Necrobiosis lipoidica*—shiny, atrophic yellowish-red plaques on the shins. Affects <1% diabetics but limited to those with DM or who will later develop DM. • *Granuloma annulare*—palpable annular lesions on hands, feet, or face. Only rarely associated with DM. Fades spontaneously in <12mo. Differentiate from ringworm. • Xanthoma (see hypercholesterolaemia below). • Fungal infection (📕 p.672). • Neuropathic ulcers (📕 p.640).
Hyperlipidaemia	• *Xanthoma*— yellowish lipid deposits in the skin; may be eruptive (like a rash), tendinous, plane (palmar creases), tuberous (knees, elbows). • *Xanthelasma*—yellowish plaques on eyelids. Not always associated with hyperlipidaemia.
Inflammatory bowel disease	
Crohn's disease	Perianal abscess, sinus or fistula, erythema nodosum, Sweet's disease (dark red plaques on face, arms, and legs), clubbing.
Ulcerative colitis	Pyoderma gangrenosum, erythema nodosum, Sweet's disease (see Crohn's disease above), clubbing.
Liver disease	Pruritus, spider naevi, erythema, white nails, pigmentation, xanthomas (see hyperlipidaemia above).
Malabsorption	Dry itchy skin, ichthyosis, eczema, oedema.

Table 19.1 (cont.)

Condition	Associated skin changes
Malignancy	• *Acanthosis nigricans*—rare, epidermal thickening and pigmentation in flexures and neck. Associated with GI malignancy. • *Mycosis fungoides*—lymphoma that evolves in the skin. Slowly progressive becoming systemic only in terminal stages. May resemble psoriasis or eczema in early stages. • *Paget's disease of the nipple*—📖 p.519. • *Skin secondaries*—most commonly breast, GI, ovary, lung, or haematological. • *Lymphoedema*—📖 p.1013.

Other conditions occasionally associated with malignancy: flushing, generalized pruritus, hyperpigmentation, ichthyosis, dermatomyositis, erythroderma, hypertrichosis, pyoderma gangrenosum, superficial thrombophlebitis, tylosis.

Condition	Associated skin changes
Malnutrition	• *Iron deficiency*—alopecia, koilonychia, itching. • *Scurvy*—bleeding gums, woody oedema, perifollicular oedema. • *Protein deficiency*—pigmentation, dry skin, oedema, pale brown/orange hair. • *Pellagra*—light-exposed dermatitis, pigmentation.
Neurofibromatosis	📖 p.624
Pregnancy	Pigmentation, spider naevi, abdominal striae, pruritus, pruritic urticarial papules and plaques of pregnancy (PUPP—1:240 pregnancies), pemphigoid gestationis (rare).
Sarcoidosis	Nodules, plaques, erythema nodosum, dactylitis, lupus pernio (dusky-red infiltrated plaques on nose ± fingers).
Thyroid disease	
Hypothyroidism	Alopecia, coarse hair, dry, puffy brownish yellow skin.
Thyrotoxicosis	Pink, soft skin, hyperhydrosis, alopecia, pigmentation, onycholysis, clubbing, pretibial myxoedema (raised erythematous plaques on shins—topical steroids may help).
Tuberous sclerosis	• *Adenoma sebaceum*—red/yellow fibromatous plaques; usually around nose. • *Periungual fibroma*—pink, fibrous projections under nailfolds. • *Ash-leaf macules*—white, oval macules; best seen under Wood's light. • *Shagreen patches*—yellowish naevi with cobblestone surface; found on the back.

Drug eruptions

Common. Any drug can produce any skin change but some patterns are more common with certain drugs. Withdrawal of the offending drug usually results in clearance of the eruption in <2wk.. Simple emollients ± topical steroids may ease symptoms in the interim. Occasionally, patients with severe reactions may require admission for supportive treatment until effects of the drug wear off.

Table 19.2 Common patterns of drug eruption

Type of eruption	Description	Examples of drugs commonly responsible
Toxic erythema	Most common type of drug eruption. May be morbilliform (like measles), urticarial, or like erythema multiforme (📖 p.654). Usually affects trunk > limbs ± fever. *Differential diagnosis:* Scarlet fever, erythematous rash 2° to viral infection.	Antibiotics (e.g. amoxicillin), sulphonamides, thiazides, allopurinol, carbamazepine, gold.
Fixed drug eruption	Round red or purplish plaques that recur in the same site each time the implicated drug is taken. Lesions may blister and heal with pigmentation.	Paracetamol, laxatives (phenolphthalein containing), sulphonamides, tetracycline.
Hypertrichosis	Excess hair (📖 p.659).	Minoxidil, ciclosporin, phenytoin.
Hair loss	Due to either: (a) Abrupt cessation of growth *or* (b) Synchronization of the hair cycle of a large proportion of the hairs so that they are all shed together ~3 mo. later.	(a) Cytotoxics. (b) Anticoagulants, carbimazole, COC pill.
Pigmentation	Either melanin or drug deposition.	Amiodarone, chlorpromazine, minocycline, bleomycin.
Psoriasiform	Some drugs exacerbate psoriasis (a), others provoke a psoriasis-like rash (b).	(a) Lithium, chloroquine. (b) β-blockers, gold, methyl dopa.
Eczematous	Like eczema (📖 p.636–9). Uncommon. Occurs when topical sensitization is followed by ingestion, iv or im use.	Neomycin, penicillin, sulphonamides, local anaesthetics.
Lichenoid	Like lichen planus (📖 p.650).	Thiazides, gold, isoniazid, PAS, quinine, penicillamine.

Table 19.2 (cont.)

Type of eruption	Description	Examples of drugs commonly responsible
Acneiform	Like acne (📖 p.644).	Androgens, lithium, phenobarbitone, steroids, isoniazid.
Urticaria	Like urticaria (📖 p.642).	Penicillin, opiates, salicylates.
Erythema multiforme	📖 p.654	Penicillin, sulphonamides, phenytoin, barbiturates.
Vasculitis	Immune complex reaction.	Thiazides, phenytoin, sulphonamides.
Lupus-like syndrome	Like lupus erythematosis (📖 p.578).	Hydralazine, isoniazid, penicillamine.
Bullous	Fixed drug eruption, phototoxic reaction, drug-induced pemphigus, and barbiturate overdose may all blister.	Barbiturates (overdose), urosemide, nalidixic acid (phototoxic), penicillamine (like pemphigus).
Erythroderma	📖 p.654. Admit immediately.	Allopurinol, gold, phenytoin, sulphonamides, isoniazid, PAS.
Toxic epidermal necrolysis	Serious condition. Skin becomes red, swollen, and separates in sheets. Admit immediately.	Allopurinol, barbiturates, phenytoin, NSAIDs, penicillin, sulphonamides.

Stevens–Johnson syndrome: Systemic illness with fever, arthralgia, myalgia ± pneumonitis and conjunctivitis. Associated with vesicles on the buccal mucosa, GU tract, and/or conjunctivae, and typical target lesions of erythema multiforme (often on the palms) which may blister in the centre.

Causes: Drugs (sulphonamides, penicillin, sedatives); viruses or other infection (e.g. orf, HSV); neoplasia or other systemic disease.

Management: Calamine lotion for the skin. Seek dermatology ± ophthalmology advice.

Prognosis: Illness lasts 10–30d. but usually resolves completely. Occasionally, permanent eye damage may result.
(*A.M. Stevens (1884–1945) and F.C. Johnson (1894–1934)—US paediatricians.*)

Atopic eczema

From the Greek meaning 'to boil over'

Affects 15–20% of schoolchildren and 2–10% of adults—usually starts <6mo. of age and by 1y. 60% of those likely to develop eczema will have done so. Associated with other atopic conditions e.g. asthma, hayfever. Remission occurs by 15y. of age in 90%, though some relapse later.

Differential diagnosis: Scabies; rare syndromes e.g. Wiskott–Aldrich syndrome.

Presentation: Waxing and waning itchy condition:
- *Infants:* Itchy vesicular exudative eczema on face ± hands often with 2° infection. May cause sleep disturbance due to itch. >½ are free of eczema by 18mo..
- *Children >18mo.:* Involves antecubital and popliteal fossae, neck, wrists, and ankles. Lichenification, excoriation, and dry skin are common. Face may be erythematous and have typical infraorbital folds. Loss of self-esteem, behavioural and sleep problems are common.
- *Adults:* The most common manifestation is irritant hand dermatitis in someone with a past history of atopic eczema—see 🕮 p.638. A small number continue to have generalized atopic eczema. May interfere with employment and social activities. Exacerbated by stress.

Diagnosis: Itchy skin PLUS ≥ 3 of:
- Itching in skin creases
- History of asthma or hayfever
- Onset in the first 2y. of life
- Generally dry skin
- Visible flexural eczema

Assessment: Ask about:
- Family (67%) and personal history of atopy and eczema
- Onset and distribution of the disease
- Aggravating factors (e.g. pets, irritants)
- Sleep disturbance due to itching/rubbing
- Impact on quality of life (school work, career, social life)
- Previous treatments (including dietary restrictions), expectations of treatment, and other medications being taken (e.g. steroids for asthma)

Complications
- *Ichthyosis vulgaris:* 🕮 p.649
- *Bacterial infection:* 2° infection (usually with *S. aureus*) commonly causes exacerbations (and may not be seen as obvious infection). Bacterial infection is suggested by presence of crusting or weeping, or sudden deterioration of eczema.
- *Viral infection:* ↑ susceptibility to infection e.g. with viral warts and molluscum contagiosum.
- *Eczema herpeticum:* propensity to develop widespread lesions with HSV and VZ—may require admission and IV aciclovir.
- *Cataracts:* Rarely occur in young adults with very severe eczema.
- *Growth retardation:* Children with severe eczema. Cause unknown. A growth chart should be kept for children with chronic severe eczema.

Management
- Explain the condition and generally good prognosis.
- Advise—loose cotton clothing; avoid wool (exacerbates eczema); avoid excessive heat; keep nails short; gloves in bed.
- If a specific irritant is identified (e.g. house dust mite, pets), then avoid.

Specific treatment
- **Emollients:** e.g. aqueous cream, bath emollients. Use regularly on skin and as soap substitutes. Ideally should be applied 3 or 4 x/d. Best applied to moist skin. Addition of an antipruritic substance e.g. lauromacrogol to the emollient may help break the scratch-itch cycle. Addition of an antiseptic to bath emollient may ↓ bacterial infection.
- **Topical steroids:** Prescribe the least potent strength that is effective. Ointments are preferable on dry, scaly eczema; creams on wet, exudative eczema. Emollients ↓ steroid requirement.
- **Antibiotics:** For infected eczema—can be oral (e.g. flucloxacillin or erythromycin 250mg qds for 2wk.) or topical (alone or in combination with a steroid e.g. fucidin H).
- **Oral steroids:** Rescue therapy while waiting for an urgent consultant opinion. Only use short courses e.g prednisolone 20–30mg od for 5d.
- **Topical immunosuppressants** e.g. tacrolimus—on consultant advice.
- **Antihistamines:** Sedative antihistamines given nocte ↓ desire to itch e.g. promethazine, hydroxyzine.
- **Bandages:** Excoriated or lichenified eczema. Tar bandages (Tarband, Coltapaste) are most effective and messiest; ichthammol (Icthband) or zinc and calamine (Calaband) may be more acceptable. Bandages can be applied at night on top of steroid ointment.
- **Wet wrapping:** Can be used for exudative eczema. Tubigrip bandage or tubular gauze soaked in emollient is applied and covered with a dry bandage. Refer to dermatology.
- **Dietary manipulation:** A few (<10%) benefit. If undertaken at all, advise dietician supervision to avoid malnutrition.

Referral: E = Emergency admission; U = Urgent; S = Soon; R = Routine
- Infection with disseminated HSV (eczema herpeticum)—E
- Severe eczema resistant to treatment. Additional 2° care treatments include phototherapy and immunosuppressive agents—U
- Infection which cannot be cleared in primary care—U
- Severe social/psychological problems due to eczema—S
- Treatment requires excessive amounts of topical steroids—S
- Failure to control symptoms in 1° care—R
- Patient/family might benefit from additional advice on application of treatments (e.g. bandaging techniques)—R
- Patch testing required if contact dermatitis suspected—R
- Dietary factors are suspected (refer direct to dietician)—R

Further information
Barnetson & Rogers (2002) Childhood atopic eczema. *BMJ* **324**:1376–9
NICE: Referral guidelines ⌨ http://www.nice.org.uk

Patient information and support
National Eczema Society ⌨ http://www.eczema.org.uk

Other eczemas

Contact dermatitis[G]: Precipitated by an exogenous agent which is:
- *Irritant* (e.g. water, abrasives, chemicals, detergent) *or*
- *Allergen* (e.g. nickel—10% ♀; 1% ♂; chrome; rubber).

Clinical presentation is often indistinguishable. More common in patients with a past history of atopic eczema. In some patients, contact dermatitis may be an industrial disease (📖 p.114). *Differential diagnosis:* endogenous eczema, psoriasis, fungal infection.

Presentation: Affects any part of the body—site and knowledge of occupation, hobbies, sports, etc. help elucidate cause.
- *Acute:* Itchy erythema and skin oedema ± papules, vesicles, or blisters.
- *Chronic:* Lichenification, scaling, and fissuring.

Management
- *Identification of the allergen or irritant:* Consider referral for patch testing (📖 p.538).
- *Exclusion of the offending allergen or irritant from the environment:* Though may be impossible. There is some evidence that nickel avoidance diets can help patients with nickel sensitivity[G]. Nickel testing kits are available from dermatology departments.
- *Hand care:* Table 19.3.
- *Emollients:* Help skin to recover. Apply frequently.
- *Topical steroids:* Help but are 2° to avoidance measures.

Table 19.3 Hand care

Hand washing	Use warm water and substitute soap with emollient (e.g. aqueous cream); dry with a clean cotton towel—avoid paper towels or drying machines.
Avoidance	Avoid handling hair preparations including shampoos, other detergents, household or industrial cleaning fluids; raw vegetables (e.g. peeling potatoes, tomato juice); fruits (e.g. peeling oranges); raw meat.
Protection	If performing any task where hands would get wet or any of the substances listed above are being handled, wear cotton gloves under PVC gloves. Wear gloves for dusty work or in the cold.
Medication	Use emollients frequently throughout the day (e.g. aqueous cream). If necessary, apply thin layer of steroid ointment twice daily.

Pompholyx
- Sago-like, intensely itchy vesicles on the sides of fingers ± palms/soles.
- No associated atopic eczema or contact dermatitis.
- Young adults. More common in warm weather. Frequently recurrent.
- Treat with emollients and topical steroids (some need potent steroids).
- Treat any infection with oral antibiotics.
- In severe cases, refer to dermatology for wet dressings.

Varicose eczema: 📖 p.640

Discoid (nummular) eczema
- Middle-aged/elderly patients. ♂>♀. Unknown cause
- *Presentation:* Intensely itchy, coin-shaped lesions on limbs. Tend to be symmetrical. May be vesicular or chronic and lichenified.
- *Differential diagnosis:* Tinea corporis; contact dermatitis.
- *Management:* Often clears spontaneously after a few weeks, but tends to recur. If treatment is needed, use a moderate or potent topical steroid. 2° infection is common—treat with topical/systemic antibiotics.

Asteatotic eczema (eczema craquelé)
- *Risk factors:* ↑ age; overwashing; dry climate; hypothyroidism; diuretics.
- *Presentation:* Dry itchy eczema with fine, crazy-paving pattern of fissuring and cracking of the skin of the limbs.
- *Management:* Treat with emollients—occasionally a mild topical steroid is required.

Seborrhoeic dermatitis: Chronic scaly eruption affecting scalp, face, and/or chest. *Differential diagnosis:* psoriasis, rosacea, contact dermatitis, fungal infection. 5 patterns:
- *Scalp and facial involvement:* Most common in young men. Excessive dandruff, itchy scaly erythematous eruption affecting sides of the nose, eyes, ears, hairline. May be associated blepharitis.
- *Petaloid:* Dry, scaly eczema over the pre-sternal area.
- *Pityrosporum folliculitis:* Erythematous follicular eruption with papules/pustules over the back.
- *Flexural:* Most common in the elderly. Axillae, groins, and submammary areas. Moist intertrigo. Associated with 2° candida infection.
- *Infantile:* 📖 p.877.

Treatment
- *Facial, truncal, and flexural involvement:* Imidazole + hydrocortisone (e.g. Canesten HC). Pityrosporum folliculitis may respond to itraconazole 200mg od for 7d. or fluconazole 50mg od for 2 wk.
- *Scalp lesions:* Ketoconazole or coal tar shampoo. In resistant cases, apply 2% sulphur + 2% salicylic acid cream several hours before shampooing.
- Recurrence requiring repeated treatment is common.

Dandruff: Exaggerated physiological exfoliation of fine scales from an otherwise normal scalp. More severe forms merge with seborrhoeic dermatitis and treatment is the same.

Lichen simplex chronicus: Area of lichenified eczema due to repeated rubbing or scratching. May be due to habit or stress. *Treatment:* topical steroids, weak tar paste, and tar impregnated bandages.

Further information
British Association of Dermatologists (2001) Guidelines for the management of contact dermatitis 🖳 http://www.bad.org.uk
Electronic Dermatology Atlas 🖳 http://www.dermis.net/bilddb/index_e.htm

Patient information and support
National Eczema Society 🖳 http://www.eczema.org.uk

Varicose eczema and leg ulcers

Venous (stasis, varicose) eczema
- Middle-aged/elderly patients. ♀ > ♂.
- Associated with underlying venous disease.
- *Early signs:* Capillary veins and haemosiderin deposition around the ankles and over prominent varicose veins.
- *Later signs:* Eczema ± lipodermatosclerosis (fibrosis of the dermis and subcutaneous tissue) ± ulceration.
- *Management:* Treat with emollients ± mild or moderate steroid ointment and compression hosiery. Treat venous disease (🕮 p.362) or ulceration on its own merits.

Leg ulcer: Painful and debilitating condition affecting 1% of the adult population and 3.6% of those >65y.

Cause: >90% due to arterial disease, venous disease, or neuropathy. *Other causes:* trauma, obesity, immobility, vasculitis (rheumatoid arthritis, SLE, PAN), malignancy, osteomyelitis, blood dyscrasias, lymphoedema, self-inflicted.

Common sites
- *Arterial*—shin, toes, over pressure points (under heel, over malleoli);
- *Venous*—above medial or lateral malleoli of the ankle;
- *Neuropathic*—sole of foot, over pressure points.

History: *Ask about:*
- Duration of ulceration
- Pain—painful unless neuropathic, when often painless
- Mobility
- Past history of ulceration, DVT, or varicose vein surgery
- History of trauma to the limb
- Systemic disease, DM, peripheral vascular disease, RA, etc.

Examination
- *Ulcer*
  - Position
  - Evidence of infection
  - Surrounding callus—typical of neuropathic ulcers
  - Evidence of tracking to involve the bones of the foot
- *Leg*
  - Pulses
  - Varicose veins and/or signs of venous hypertension—haemosiderin pigmentation, varicose eczema, atrophie blanche (white lacy scars), lipodermatosclerosis
  - Sensation—↓ when peripheral neuropathy
  - Range of joint movement

Investigation
- Bloods—FBC, ESR, VDRL, blood glucose
- Ankle brachial index (🕮 p.360)
- Swab for M,C&S if any signs of cellulitis/infection
- Diabetic ulcers—if signs infection, X-ray foot to exclude osteomyelitis.

Management
- *Arterial ulcers:* Refer to vascular surgery.
- *Diabetic foot ulcers:* Refer to a specialist diabetic foot team.
- *Venous ulcers:* If ABI >0.8, can be managed in the community with graduated compression bandaging (elastic bandages applied in multiple layers over a non-adherent dressing). Change dressings 1 or 2x/wk. Keep the skin under the bandage moist with simple emollients and treat any surrounding eczema with topical steroids. Give analgesia. Encourage walking, weight ↓ if obese, elevation of leg when resting. 65–70% heal in <6mo.

Referral
- *Non-healing ulcers or ulcers of uncertain cause*—dermatology
- *ABI <0.8*—vascular surgery
- *Varicose veins*—vascular surgery (60% may benefit from vein surgery).

Prevention of recurrence: 5y. recurrence rate 40%—graduated compression hosiery ↓ recurrence. Below knee class 2 stockings are adequate for most and can be, prescribed on NHS prescription but are difficult to apply, especially with arthritic hands. Applicators are available and can be obtained via the OT or bought from specialist disability shops.

Complications
- Infection—treat with systemic antibiotics only if rapidly advancing ulcer edge, cellulites, or systemic symptoms.
- Lymphoedema.
- Contact dermatitis—topical medicaments and dressings. Consider referral for patch testing if suspected.
- Malignant change—squamous cell cancer (rare). Refer for biopsy to confirm diagnosis.

Pyoderma gangrenosum
- *Presentation:* Starts as a pustule/inflamed nodule which beaks down to form an ulcer, which may expand rapidly, with a purplish margin and surrounding erythema. Usually on trunk/lower limbs.
- *Causes:* UC (present in 50% patients with pyoderma gangrenosum); Crohn's disease; RA; Behçet's syndrome; multiple myeloma and mono-clonal gammopathy; leukaemia.
- *Management:* Refer to dermatology.

Bed sores
- Due to pressure necrosis of the skin. Immobile patients are at high risk, especially if frail ± incontinent.
- If at risk, refer to the DN for advice on prevention of bed sores—protective mattresses and cushions, incontinence advice, advice on positioning and movement.
- Warn carers to make contact with the DN if a red patch does not improve 24h. after relieving the pressure on the area. Treat aggressively and admit if not resolving.

Further information
British Vascular Foundation ⌨ http://www.bvf.org.uk
Tissue Viability Society ⌨ http://www.tvs.org.uk

Urticaria (hives) and angio-oedema^G

Urticaria is common. It is characterized by superficial itchy swellings of the skin known as *weals*. Deeper swellings of the skin and alimentary tract are called *angio-oedema*. These may be painful rather than itchy and tend to last longer. Weals and angio-oedema often coexist but either may occur alone. Most urticaria patients do not have systemic reactions but, very rarely, physical urticarias may progress to anaphylaxis. Conversely, urticaria is often a feature of anaphylactic and anaphylactoid reactions.

Clinical classification: It is usually possible to classify urticaria on the basis of clinical presentation.

Ordinary urticaria
- **Acute** (≤6wk. continuous activity)
    - Sudden onset of urticaria ± angio-oedema.
    - May be due to an allergic reaction or childhood viral infection.
    - Typically, individual weals last 2–24h.
    - The offending allergen can often be identified e.g. food (peanuts, shellfish, egg are common culprits); drug (e.g. penicillin); insect sting. Sometimes there is no apparent cause.
    - Treat with antihistamines as needed (e.g. chlorpheniramine 4mg 4–6hrly prn OTC).
    - Oral corticosteroids may shorten the duration of acute urticaria (e.g. prednisolone 50mg/d. for 3d. in adults).
    - Management of anaphylaxis—📖 p.1034–37
    - If recurrent and allergen cannot be identified, refer for allergy testing.
- **Chronic** (≥6wk. continuous activity)
    - Itchy pink weals appear at any site as papules or plaques.
    - Individual weals typically last for <24h. and then disappear without trace.
    - May be associated with angio-oedema affecting tongue ± lips.
    - Usually no cause is found (*chronic idiopathic urticaria*).
    - Treat with antihistamines (e.g. loratadine 10mg od ± sedating antihistamine at night to assist sleep e.g. hydroxyzine 10–50 mg).
    - Drugs (e.g. aspirin, codeine) may act as provoking factors—avoid.
    - Symptoms resolve spontaneously in <6mo. in ~½ of those patients with weals alone. 50% of those with weals *and* angio-oedema still have symptoms 5y. after diagnosis.
    - Consider checking FBC, ESR (to screen for vasculitis—see opposite) ± thyroid function tests (if any symptoms/signs of thyroid dysfunction) and/or dermatology referral if not settling.
- **Episodic** (intermittent): Treat as for acute urticaria.
- **Urticaria of pregnancy:** Often starts in abdominal striae. Treat with chlopheniramine 4mg po 4–6hrly prn for itch.

Contact urticaria: Allergic urticaria or physical urticaria induced by contact with a substance e.g. nettle rash. Usually self-limiting in <2h. if the cause is removed. Manage in the same way as for acute urticaria.

Drug-induced urticarial rash: *Common culprits:* aspirin and other NSAIDs, opiates, ACE inhibitors. Manage as for acute urticaria.

Physical urticaria: Reproducibly induced by the same physical stimulus. Usually short lived (<1h.—except delayed pressure urticaria which takes longer to develop and fade) and self-resolving. Many different stimuli are recognized:

- Dermographism (pressure on skin—5% of the population)
- Delayed pressure urticaria
- Solar urticaria (sunlight)
- Vibratory urticaria
- Aquagenic urticaria (water)
- Cholinergic urticaria (sweat)
- Cold urticaria
- Localized heat urticaria

Anaphylaxis: 📖 p.1034–37

Hereditary angio-oedema
- Due to deficiency of C_1 esterase inhibitor which allows complement activation to go unchecked.
- Autosomal dominant—usually presents in childhood with episodes of angio-oedema without weals. May affect the larynx → respiratory depression, or GI tract → abdominal pain.
- Emergency treatment is with hospital admission for fresh frozen plasma or C_1 inhibitor concentrate infusion.
- Maintenance therapy is only necessary for patients with symptomatic, recurring angio-oedema or related abdominal pain. Anabolic steroids are the treatment of choice for most patients but should only be prescribed under consultant supervision.

Urticarial vasculitis: Indistinguishable from chronic idiopathic urticaria on examination. If individual lesions last >24h., are burning/painful rather than itchy, or leave bruising or scaling, suspect vasculitis. Diagnosis confirmed on skin biopsy. Treatment is as for vasculitis (📖 p.580).

Systemic disease: Lymphoma, thyrotoxicosis, infestation, and infection (especially viral) can all present with urticarial rash.

Differential diagnosis: Pemphigoid, dermatitis herpetiformis, toxic erythema, erythema multiforme, facial erysipelas.

Further information
- **British Association of Dermatologists** (2001) Guidelines for the management of urticaria and angio-oedema. 🖥 http://www.bad.org.uk
- **Electronic Dermatology Atlas** 🖥 http://www.dermis.net

Acne

Chronic inflammatory condition characterized by comedones, papules, pustules, cysts, and scars. Acne vulgaris is common and affects >80% teenagers. Peak age: 18y.; ♂ = ♀.

Cause: Complex. Androgen secretion results in ↑ sebum excretion; pilosebaceous duct blockage (producing comedones); colonization of the duct with *Proprionobacterium acnes* bacteria and release of inflammatory mediators. Inflammatory acne is the result of the host response to the follicular propionibacterium acne.

Rarer causes
- Endocrine—PCOS, Cushings, virilizing tumours
- Squeezing—*acne excoriée*
- Aromatic industrial chemicals—*chloracne*
- Cosmetics
- Drugs—systemic steroids, androgens, topical steroids
- Infantile—faces of male infants; cause unknown
- Physical occlusion e.g. under a violinist's chin

Presentation: Spots on face, neck ± back and chest. Examination reveals blackheads (dilated pores with black plug of keratin = comedones) and whiteheads (small cream-coloured dome-shaped papules); red papules; pustules ± cysts. There may be scarring from old lesions. Burrowing abscesses and sinuses with scarring (*conglobate acne*) are seen in severe cases. Scars may become keloidal.

Differential diagnosis: Rosacea (📖 p.655), bacterial folliculitis (often coexist—📖 p.669).

Classification: Severity of acne is often overestimated by the patient and minimized by the doctor. 4 main types:
- Purely comedonal (non-inflammatory)
- Mild papular
- Scarring papular
- Nodular or scarring acne

Management: *Aims to:* ↓ number of lesions; prevent scarring; ↓ the psychological impact of the condition.
- *Misconceptions:* Explain:
  - Acne is not a disease of poor hygiene. The black tip of a comedone is oxidized sebum, not dirt.
  - Diet is not associated with acne.
- *General measures:* Wash with soap and water twice daily. Apply a moisturizer (e.g. aqueous cream) after washing.
- *Medication:* Table 19.4. Warn patients any treatment takes weeks → months to work fully and usually is continued for months or years. Reassess progress every 2–3mo. and continue treatment until new lesions stop developing.
- *Support:* Acne Support Group ☎0870 870 2263 or 🖥 http://www.stopspots.org

Complications: Acne is not a trivial disease—it can cause scars (both skin and emotional) that last a lifetime. Anxiety, social isolation, and lack of self-confidence are common.

Table 19.4 Treatment of acne (*BNF* 13.6)

	Description	Management
Mild acne	Open and closed come-dones and some papules	Topical treatment applied to the whole area (not just the spots): benzoyl peroxide applied bd—start at lowest strength and build up as needed.
		Topical retinoids (e.g. isotretinoin)—apply low-strength preparation every 2 or 3 nights initially and build up strength and frequency as tolerated. Warn patients they should avoid the sun. Retinoids cause erythema and scaling in most patients which settles with time, and acne may worsen for the first few weeks of treatment.
		Topical antibiotics (e.g. Dalacin T)—resistance is increasing. Use only in combination with benzoyl peroxide or if benzoyl peroxide has failed. Avoid if using oral antibiotics.
Moderate acne	More frequent papules and pustules with mild scarring	Try topical treatment first.
		If not working after 4–8wk. try either long-term oral antibiotics (e.g. tetracycline 500mg bd) for a minimum of 8wk. *or*, for girls, an anti-androgen for >6mo. (e.g. cyproterone acetate in Dianette—also contraceptive).
		Topical preparations may be used simultaneously with systemic therapy.
Severe acne	Nodular abscesses→ more widespread scarring	As for moderate acne.
		If ineffective or relapses rapidly after antibiotics are stopped, refer to a dermatologist for consideration of oral retinoid treatment (e.g. Roaccutane).
		⚠ oral retinoids are teratogenic.

Reasons for dermatology referral
- Acne fulminans: seen in adolescent males, severe acne is associated with fever, arthritis, and vasculitis—U
- Severe acne or painful, deep nodules or cysts that could benefit from oral isotretinoin—S
- Severe social/psychological sequelae—S
- At risk of/developing scarring despite primary care remedies—R
- Poor treatment response—R
- Suspected underlying cause for acne (e.g PCOS—📖 p.712)—R

U = Urgent; S = Soon; R = Routine

Perioral dermatitis: Papules and pustules which appear around the mouth and chin of a woman who has used topical steroids. Treat with oral tetracycline as for acne.

Further information

Webster GF (2002) Acne vulgaris. *BMJ* 325:475–9
NICE: Referral guidelines. Available from 🖥 http://www.nice.org.uk

Psoriasis[G]

Chronic, non-infectious inflammatory skin condition characterized by well-demarcated erythematous plaques topped by silvery scales. Epidermal cell proliferation rate is ↑ x20 and turnover time ↓ from 28d. to 4d. Affects ~2% Caucasian population (less in other races). Presents at any age—mean 28y.; rare <8y. ♂=♀. Presentation—Table 19.5.

Cause: Genetic (polygenic inheritance; 35% have FH; there is a 25% probability that a child with 1 parent with psoriasis will be affected—60% chance with 2). Environmental factors trigger disease.

Precipitating factors
- Trauma (Koebner phenomenon)
- Infection
- Drugs e.g. β-blockers, NSAIDs, lithium, chloroquine
- Alcohol
- Sunlight—aggravates psoriasis in 10%
- Psychological stress

Management >50% experience a lack of self-confidence. Social or psychological problems are common. Be supportive. Explain the condition and treatment options. Advise on self-help groups. *Treatment (BNF 13.5):* Frequent emollients ±
- *Salicylic acid*—2% increasing to 3–6%. ↑ loss of surface scale. When there is significant scaling, use a keratolytic treatment like this first, else other treatments will fail.
- *Coal tar*—anti-inflammatory and anti-scaling properties. The thicker the patch, the stronger the preparation required.
- *Vitamin D analogue* e.g. calcipotriol, tacalcitol—plaque and scalp psoriasis. Effective and no unpleasant smell or staining of clothing.
- *Dithranol*—plaque psoriasis. Apply to lesion only. Stains.
- *Topical retinoids* e.g. tazarotene—mild/moderate plaque psoriasis.
- *Topical steroids*—mild topical steroids can be used for flexural, facial, or scalp psoriasis.

❶ Plaques can become inflamed and/or aggravated on starting topical treatments, after prolonged use of topical steroids, or if steroids are stopped suddenly.

Referral: E = Emergency; U = Urgent; S = Soon; R = Routine
- Generalized pustular or eythrodermic psoriasis—E
- Patient's psoriasis is acutely unstable—U
- Widespread guttate psoriasis (to benefit from early phototherapy)—U
- Severe social or psychological sequelae—S
- Rash is so extensive as to make self-management impractical—S
- Rash is in a sensitive area (e.g. face, hands, feet, genitalia) and the symptoms troublesome—S
- Time off work/school and interfering with employment/education—S
- For management of associated arthropathy—S
- Rash fails to respond to primary care management—R

Additional secondary care treatment options: Phototherapy and PUVA, oral retinoids, cytotoxic and immunosuppressive thearapy, specialist nursing services.

Table 19.5 Patterns of psoriasis

Pattern	Features
Erythroderma	Inflammatory dermatosis affecting >90% skin surface (📖 p.654). Admit.
Generalized pustular	Rare but serious. Unwell with fever and malaise. Sheets of small, sterile, yellowish pustules develop on an erythematous background and spread rapidly. Admit.
Plaque	Most common form. Well-defined, disc-shaped plaques involving the knees, elbows, scalp, hair, margin, or sacrum. Plaques are usually red and covered with waxy white scales which may leave bleeding points if detached. Plaques may be itchy. *Differential diagnosis:* psoriasiform drug eruption; hypertrophic lichen planus.
Scalp psoriasis	Very common. May be confused with dandruff but generally better demarcated and thicker scales.
Guttate	Acute symmetrical raindrop lesions on trunk/limbs. Most common in adolescents/young adults—may follow streptococcal throat infection. *Differential diagnosis:* pityriasis rosea.
Flexural	Affects axillae, sub-mammary areas, and natal cleft. Plaques are smooth and often glazed. Most common in elderly patients. *Differential diagnosis:* flexural candidiasis.
Nail	Nail bed is affected in 50%. Fingernails > toenails. Thimble pitting, onycholysis, and oily patches (oily brownish-yellow discolouration of the nail bed—often adjacent to onycholysis). Associated with arthropathy. Treatment is difficult. *Differential diagnosis:* fungal nail infection.
Palmoplantar pustulosis	Yellow/brown coloured sterile pustules on palms or soles.
Napkin psoriasis	Well-defined eruption in nappy area of infants.

Arthropathy: ~ 40% psoriasis patients. ♂ = ♀.
- *Distal arthritis*—DIP joint swelling of hands/feet ± flexion deformity.
- *Rheumatoid-like*—polyarthropathy similar to rheumatoid arthritis (📖 p.572) but less symmetrical and rheumatoid factor is –ve.
- *Mutilans*—associated with severe psoriasis. Erosions in small bones of hands/feet ± spine. Bones dissolve → progressive deformity.
- *Ankylosing spondylitis/sacroiliitis*—usually HLA B27 +ve (📖 p.576).

Management: Education, physiotherapy, NSAIDs. Refer to rheumatology for confirmation of diagnosis, advice on management, and disease-modifying drugs.

Further information

British Association of Dermatologists (2003) *Recommendations for the initial management of psoriasis* 🖥 http://www.bad.org.uk

Patient information and support

Psoriasis Association ☎0845 676 076 🖥 http://www.psoriasis-association.org.uk
Psoriatic Arthropathy Alliance ☎0870 770 3212 🖥 http://www.paalliance.org

Pityriasis and keratinization disorders

Pityriasis rosea
- Acute self-limiting disorder most commonly affecting teenagers and young adults. *Cause:* unknown.
- Generalized eruption is preceded by the herald patch—a single large, oval lesion 2–5cm diameter.
- Several days later the rash appears, consisting of many smaller lesions, mainly on trunk but also upper arms and thighs.
- Lesions are oval, pink, and have a delicate 'collarette' of scale. May be asymptomatic or cause mild → moderate itch.

Differential diagnosis: Guttate psoriasis; pityriasis versicolor; 2° syphilis.

Management: Treatment does not speed clearance. Topical steroid may relieve itch. Fades spontaneously in 4–8wk.

Pityriasis (tinea) versicolor
- Chronic, often asymptomatic, fungal infection of the skin (*Pityrosporum orbiculare*). Common in humid/tropical conditions.
- In the UK, often affects young adults/teenagers.
- On untanned white skin appears as pinkish-brown, oval or round patches with a fine superficial scale.
- In tanned or darker skin, patchy hypopigmentation occurs. Involves trunk ± proximal limbs.

Differential diagnosis: Vitiligo (🕮 p.657); pityriasis rosea; tinea corporis (🕮 p.673).

Management
- Topical imidazole antifungal (e.g. clotrimazole cream) *or* topical selenium sulphide shampoo to all affected areas at night, washed off the following morning repeated x2 at weekly intervals.
- Resistant cases—systemic antifungal e.g. fluconazole 50mg od for 1wk.
- Recurrences are common.
- Hypopigmentation may take some time to clear.

Pityriasis alba: Finely scaled white patches on face or arms. Affects children/young adults. Associated with atopy.

Management: Usually no treatment is required. Resolves spontaneously over months or years. If severe, refer to dermatology for confirmation of diagnosis. Treatment for severe cases is with topical steroids and/or PUVA.

Callosities: Painless, localized thickenings of the keratin layer—a protective response to friction or pressure. *Management:* keratolytics e.g. 5–10% salicylic acid ointment or 10% urea cream, as needed. Attention to footwear.

Corns: Painful. Develop at areas of high local pressure on the feet e.g. where shoes press against bony protrusions.

Management: Attention to footwear; keratolytics; cushioning (e.g. corn pads); referral to chiropody as needed. Occasionally, surgery may be indicated if deformity of the foot causes recurrent corns.

Ichthyosis: A group of inherited disorders characterized by dry, scaly skin. Vary from mild to severe. Most Common form is *ichthyosis vulgaris*—prevalence 1:300; autosomal dominant; small branny scales on extensor aspects of limbs and back; mild and often undiagnosed.

Management: Topical emollients ± bath additives. Severe cases require expert dermatology advice.

Keratoderma: Hyperkeratosis of palms and soles—may be inherited or acquired. Tylosis is diffuse hyperkeratosis of the palms and soles. It is usually inherited (autosomal dominant) but may rarely be associated with oesophageal cancer. Acquired keratoderma occurs in women around the menopause and patients with lichen planus (🕮 p.650).

Management: Keratolytics e.g. 5–10% salicylic acid ointment or 10% urea cream.

Keratosis pilaris: Common, sometimes inherited condition. Small horny plugs are found on upper thigh, upper arm, and face. Associated with icthyosis vulgaris. Keratolytics (e.g. 5–10% salicylic acid ointment or 10% urea cream) improve symptoms.

Further information
Electronic Dermatology Atlas 🖥 http://www.dermis.net/bilddb/index_e.htm

Patient information and support
Ichthyosis Support Group 🖥 http://www.ichthyosis.co.uk

Lichenoid eruptions

Lichen planus

- Very itchy, polygonal, flat-topped papular lesions 2–5mm diameter, affecting flexor surfaces, palms and soles, mucous membranes (2/3 cases—usually buccal), and genitalia in a symmetrical pattern.
- Koebner phenomenon (lesions occur in the line of damaged skin due to a scratch) exhibited.
- Papules may have a surface network of white lines (Wickham's striae).
- Initially, papules are red but become violaceous. Papules flatten over a few mo. to leave pigmentation or occasionally become hypertrophic.
- 2/3 cases occur in the 30–60y. age group. ♂ = ♀.

Cause: Unknown—possibly autoimmune.

Differential diagnosis

- *Generalized*—lichenoid drug eruption, guttate psoriasis.
- *Genital*—psoriasis, scabies, lichen sclerosus.
- *Hypertrophic*—lichen simplex.

Variants

- *Annular* (10%)—commonly on glans penis.
- *Atrophic*—rare, associated with hypertrophic lesions.
- *Bullous*—blistering is rare.
- *Follicular*—may occur with typical lichen planus or affect the scalp alone (scarring alopecia).
- *Hypertrophic*—plaques may persist for years.
- *Mucous membrane*—may occur alone or with typical lichen planus.

Complications

- *Nail involvement* (10%)—longitudinal pitting and grooving.
- *Scalp*—scarring alopecia.
- *Malignant change*—very rare.

Management: Self-limiting in most patients. Moderate → high-potency topical steroids provide symptomatic relief. Oral lesions can be treated with adcortyl in orabase paste.

Referral: Refer to dermatology if:
- Diagnosis is in doubt
- Extensive involvement
- Potentially scarring nail dystrophy
- Resistant to topical treatment.

Specialist treatment involves oral steroids ± PUVA.

Prognosis: ½ are clear in <9mo.; 15% have continuing symptoms >18mo.; 20% have a further attack.

Lichen planus-like drug eruptions: Recorded after treatment with:

- Thiazide diuretics
- Penicillamine
- Streptamycin
- Quinine
- Tolbutamide
- Isoniazid
- Tetracycline
- Chloroquine
- Phenothiazines
- Gold

Resolution after withdrawal of drug is often slow.

Lichen sclerosus: Itchy genital lesions are characteristic, though trunk, mouth, or limb lesions can occur. Lesions are a few mm in diameter, white, and slightly atrophic. They may aggregate into wrinkled plaques. ♀: ♂ ≈ 10:1. Most common in middle age (though can occur in children).

Differential diagnosis: Lichen simplex chronicus (📖 p.639); Bowen's disease (📖 p.667).

Complications

- *Male*—urethral stricture, recurrent balanitis, phimosis (balanitis xerotica obliterans);
- *Female*—dyspareunia, dysuria;
- *Both* sexes—malignant change (squamous cell carcinoma) is rare.

Management

- *Non-genital lesions*—no treatment;
- *Genital lesions*—mild moderate-potency topical steroid ↓ itch, circumcision/vulvectomy is a last resort;
- *In all cases*—long-term follow-up with biopsy of any suspicious lesions is indicated.

Prognosis: Chronic and usually permanent. May resolve spontaneously in children/young adults.

Further information

Electronic Dermatology Atlas 🖥 http://www.dermis.net/bilddb/index_e.htm

Blistering of the skin

Type of blister depends on level of cleavage of the skin—subcorneal or intraepidermal blisters rupture easily, subepidermal blisters are much tougher. *Causes:*

- *Subcorneal:* Pustular psoriasis (📖 p.646), bullous impetigo (📖 p.668)
- *Intraepidermal:* Eczema (📖 p.636), HSV (📖 p.495), VZ (📖 p.494), pemphigus, friction
- *Subepidermal:* Cold or heat injury (burns—📖 p.1076), pemphigoid, dermatitis herpetiformis, linear IgA disease, dystrophic epidermolysis bullosa
- *Other:* Insect bites (may cause cleavage at any level).

Pemphigus^G: Uncommon, autoimmune disorder affecting skin and mucous membranes. Affects adults (peak incidence 30–70y.). *Cause:* 90% have detectable circulating autoantibodies. Associated with other auto-immune disorders e.g. myaesthenia gravis.

Presentation: 50% present with oral lesions. Suspect in anyone presenting with mucocutaneous erosions/blisters. Flaccid superficial blisters then appear—sometimes months later—over scalp, face, back, chest, and flexures. As blisters are fragile, they burst early and the condition may present as crusted erosions. Untreated, the condition is progressive.

Management: Refer to dermatology. Treatment is with high-dose systemic steroids or other immunosuppressive agents. Treatment is continued long term, though occasional remissions occur. Before treatment with steroids, ¾ patients died in <4y. Now excess morbidity and mortality is due to side-effects of treatment.

Pemphigoid^G: More common than pemphigus. *Cause:* Autoimmune.

Presentation

- *Bullous pemphigoid:* Usually affects the elderly. An urticarial reaction may precede onset of blistering. Large, tense blisters arise on red or normal skin on the limbs, trunk, and flexures. Oral lesions in 20–30%. May be localized to 1 site e.g. lower leg. *Differential diagnosis:* Pemphigus, dermatitis herpetiformis, linear IgA disease.
- *Cicatricial pemphigoid:* Mainly affects mucous membranes in the eyes and mouth. Scarring results and may cause visual loss. Refer to ophthalmologist.
- *Pemphigoid gestationis:* Rare but characteristic bullous eruption associated with pregnancy. Remits after delivery but often recurs in subsequent pregnancies.

Management: Refer to dermatology for skin biopsy and confirmation of diagnosis. Treatment is usually with oral steroids (prednisolone 30–60mg daily initially, reducing as symptoms improve). Other treatments include antibiotics and nicotinamide, azathioprine, or other immunosuppressants.

Prognosis: Self-limiting in 50%. Steroids can often be stopped after ~2y.

Dermatitis herpetiformis: Closely related to coeliac disease (☐ p.454)—2–5% patients with coeliac disease have dermatitis herpetiformis. ♂ > ♀ (2:1). *Peak incidence:* 3rd/4th decade. Consists of itchy vesicular skin rash on elbows (extensor surface), knees, buttocks, and scalp which are often broken by scratching to leave excoriations. Associated with small intestinal enteropathy but symptoms of GI malabsorption are uncommon. *Differential diagnosis:* Scabies, eczema, linear IgA disease.

Management: Refer to dermatology. Responds to withdrawal of gluten—though may take up to 1y.. Controlled in the interim with dapsone or sulfapyridine.

Epidermolysis bullosa: A group of genetically inherited diseases characterized by blistering on minimal trauma. Range from being mild and trivial to being incompatible with life. Most common type is *simple epidermolysis bullosa* (autosomal dominant)—blistering is caused by friction, is mild, and limited to hands and feet. Patients are advised to avoid trauma.

Linear IgA disease: Rare condition of blisters and urticarial lesions on the back and extensor surfaces. Refer to dermatology. Responds to dapsone.

Further information

Electronic Dermatology Atlas ▣ http://www.dermis.net/bilddb/index_e.htm
British Association of Dermatologists ▣ *http://www.bad.org.uk*
● Guidelines for the management of pemphigus vulgaris (2003)
● Guidelines for the management of bullous pemphigoid (2002)

The erythemas

Erythroderma: Inflammatory dermatosis affecting >90% skin surface. Rare, but systemic effects are potentially fatal. σ:φ ≈ 2:1. Typical patient is middle aged or elderly. Patchy erythema becomes universal in <48h. Accompanied by fever, shivering, and malaise. 2–6d. later, scaling appears. The skin is hot, red, itchy, dry, thickened, and feels tight. Hair and nails may be shed.

Cause: Eczema (40%); psoriasis (25%); lymphoma (15%); drug eruption (10%); other skin disease (2%); unknown (8%).

Management: Admit as an acute medical emergency.

Erythema: 📖 p.259

Flushing: 📖 p.261

Erythema multiforme: Immune-mediated disease characterized by target lesions on hands and feet. *Causes:*
- *Idiopathic* (50%)
- *Infective*—streptococcal, HSV, hepatitis B, mycoplasma
- *Drugs*—penicillin, sulphonamide, barbiturate
- *Other*—SLE, pregnancy, malignancy

Presentation: Target lesions (red rings with central pale or purple area) on hands and feet. New lesions appear for 2–3wk. Frequently oral, conjunctival, and genital mucosa is affected. If severe, termed Stevens–Johnson syndrome (📖 p.635).

Differential diagnosis: Toxic erythema (📖 p.634), toxic epidermal necrolysis (📖 p.635), Sweet's disease, urticaria (📖 p.642), pemphigoid (📖 p.652).

Management: Identification and removal of the underlying cause. Mild cases resolve spontaneously and require symptomatic measures only. Admit if extensive involvement.

Erythema nodosum: Tender erythematous nodules (1–5cm diameter) on extensor surfaces of limbs (especially shins) ± ankle and wrist arthritis ± fever. φ:σ≈3:1. Resolves in <8wk. Non-scarring. No treatment needed.

Associations: 20% of cases are idiopathic with no associations.
- Acute sarcoidosis
- Drugs e.g. oral contraceptives, sulphonamides
- Inflammatory bowel disease (UC, Crohn's)
- Malignancy
- TB
- Streptococcal infection

Erythema ab igne: Reticulate pigmented erythema due to heat-induced damage. Common in the elderly—especially from sitting in front of the fire or using hot water bottles to alleviate pain. Explain the cause. Resolves spontaneously.

Palmar erythema: 📖 p.277

Chilblains: Inflamed and painful purple-pink swellings on fingers, toes, or ears. Appear in response to cold. ♀ > ♂. Advise warm housing and clothing, gloves, and woolly socks. In severe cases, oral nifedipine may help.

Livedo reticularis: Marbled, patterned cyanosis of the skin. If not reversible by warming, investigate the cause. Treat the cause. *Causes:* Physiological (e.g. cold); vasulitis (e.g. SLE); hyperviscosity.

Rosacea: Chronic inflammatory facial dermatosis characterized by erythema and pustules. Most common in middle age. ♂ = ♀. *Cause:* Unknown.

Presentation: Earliest symptom is flushing. Erythema, telangiectasia, papules, pustules ± lymphoedema affect cheeks, nose, forehead, and chin. Exacerbated by sunlight and topical steroids.

Complications: Rhinophyma (bulbous appearance of nose); eye involvement—blepharitis and conjunctivitis.

Differential diagnosis: Acne (lacks comedones and older age group); contact dermatitis, SLE, photosensitive eruptions (📖 p.662); seborrhoeic dermatitis.

Management: Repeated treatment is usually needed over many years with prolonged courses of topical or systemic antibiotics (e.g. metronidazole 0.75% gel *or* oral tetracycline 1g daily, decreasing to 250mg od after 3wk. and continuing for 2–3mo.). Refer resistant cases to dermatology.

Erysipelas, cellulitis, scalded skin syndrome: 📖 p.669

Pigmentation disorders

Table 19.6 Causes of hypo- and hyperpigmentation

Hypopigmentation	Hyperpigmentation
Generalized	*Genetic*
Albinism	Racial
PKU (📖 p.846)	Freckles/lentigo
Hypopituarism (📖 p.428)	Neurofibromatosis (📖 p.624)
Patchy	Peutz–Jeghers syndrome (📖 p.465)
Vitiligo	*Drugs*
After inflammation e.g. cryotherapy, eczema, psoriasis, morphoea	Amiodarone—blue-grey pigmentation of sun-exposed areas
Following exposure to chemicals e.g. substituted phenols, hydroquinone	Psoralens
After infection—pityriasis versicolor, leprosy, yaws	Minocycline—blue-black pigmentation in scars and buccal mucosa
Tuberous sclerosis	Chloroquine—blue-grey pigmentation of face and arms
Around a mole	Chlorpromazine—grey pigment in sun-exposed sites
Halo naevus (📖 p.664)	Cytotoxics
	Endocrine
	Addison's disease (📖 p.426)
	Chloasma
	Cushing's syndrome (📖 p.426)
	Nutritional
	Excess ingestion of carrots (carotinaemia)
	Malabsorption (📖 p.451)
	Post-inflammatory
	Eczema (📖 p.636)
	Lichen planus (📖 p.650)
	Systemic sclerosis (📖 p.579)
	Other
	Benign naevi (📖 p.664)
	Malignant melanoma (📖 p.666)
	Chronic renal failure (📖 p.680)
	Acanthosis nigricans (📖 p.633)

Freckles and lentigines
- *Freckles* are small, light brown macules—typically facial—which darken in the sun. They are common particularly in red heads and develop in childhood. Require no treatment.
- *Lentigines* are also brown macules but more scattered and do not darken in the sun. Most common in elderly, sun-exposed skin. Respond to cryotherapy.

Chloasma: Patterned macular symmetrical facial pigmentation, usually involving the forehead, occurring with pregnancy and when taking the COC pill. Reassurance is normally all that is needed. Sunscreens may prevent chloasma becoming more pronounced. Rarely, patients are so worried about their appearance that camouflage cosmetics are warranted (see vitiligo below).

Vitiligo: Affects 1% of the population. ♂ = ♀. *Peak age of onset:* 10–30y. *Cause:* Autoimmune; 30% have a family history. *Associations:* Pernicious anaemia, Addison's, and thyroid disease.

Presentation: May be precipitated by injury or sunburn. Presents as sharply defined white macules which contain no melanocytes. Often symmetrical distribution. *Most common sites:* hands, wrists, knees, neck, face—around eyes and mouth.

Differential diagnosis: Post-inflammatory hypopigmentation, chemical exposure.

Management: Prognosis is variable—some develop a few lesions which remain static, some progress to larger depigmented areas, some even repigment. There is no cure. Advise use of sunscreens for affected areas (ACBS prescription); camouflage cosmetics (refer to Red Cross for advice on application, ACBS prescription). In severe cases, refer for dermatology opinion—high-dose steroids or PUVA may help.

Albinism: *Prevalence:* 1:20,000. Rare genetic syndrome (autosomal recessive inheritance) in which the melanocytes are unable to produce skin, hair, or eye pigment. Patients have white hair, pale skin, pink eyes, poor sight, photophobia, and nystagmus. Several different varieties exist.

Management: Strict sun avoidance, sunglasses, sunscreens, refer any skin lesions for biopsy (↑ risk squamous cell carcinoma).

Morphoea (localized scleroderma): ♀:♂ ≈ 3:1. Localized bands of sclerosis on the skin. Pathologically distinct from lesions of systemic sclerosis. Internal disease is not associated. *Cause:* Unknown—may follow trauma. Presents with round/oval plaques of induration and erythema which become shiny and white, eventually leaving atrophic hairless pigmented patches. Affects trunk/proximal limbs. No established treatment—though topical steroids are often given. Usually spontaneously resolves within a few months.

Hair and sweat gland problems

Hair loss or alopecia: May be diffuse or localized; scarring or non-scarring. Treatment is according to cause. *Differential diagnosis:*

- *Diffuse non-scarring:* Male pattern baldness; hypothyroidism; iron deficiency; malnutrition; hypopituitarism; hypoadrenalism; drug-induced. Male pattern baldness in men and women responds to minoxidil but hair loss returns as soon as the drug is stopped.
- *Localized non-scarring:* Alopecia areata; ringworm; traumatic; hairpulling; traction; SLE; secondary syphilis.
- *Scarring:* Burns; radiation; shingles; teriary syphilis; lupus erythematosus; morphoea; lichen planus.

Alopecia areata^G: Chronic inflammatory disease affecting the hair follicles ± nails (~10%). Presents as patches of hair loss usually on the scalp, but can affect any hair-bearing skin. 20% have a family history.

Management: Investigation is usually unnecessary. Treatment depends on severity of hair loss. Mild cases, reassure and monitor hair loss; more severe cases—refer to dermatology. Treatment options include local injection/systemic steroids and contact immunotherapy. ~40% recover in <1y.; 20% lose all scalp hair—recovery in these cases is unusual (<10%).

Hirsuitism: Affects 10% ♀s. Excess hair in androgenic distribution.

Causes:
- Most cases are idiopathic; there may be a family history
- Drugs—phenytoin; corticosteroids; ciclosporin; androgenic oral contraception; anabolic steroids; minoxidil; diazoxide
- PCOS (📖 p.712)
- Late-onset congenital adrenal hyperplasia (rare)
- Cushing's syndrome (📖 p.426)
- Ovarian tumours (rare)

Assessment
- *History:* Longstanding or recent onset, family history, ethnic origin (more common in Mediterranean countries), menstrual history.
- *Examination:* Distribution of excess hair.
- *Investigation:* Women with longstanding hirsutism (since puberty) and regular periods need no further investigation unless abnormal signs. *Otherwise: Blood*—testosterone (↑ in PCOS, androgen-secreting tumour, late-onset congenital adrenal hyperplasia); LH/FSH ratio (>3:1 suggests PCOS).

Refer to gynaecologist/endocrinologist if: Recent onset, abnormal blood tests, virilism, galactorrhoea, menstrual disturbance, infertility, and/or pelvic mass.

Treatment of idiopathic hirsutism
- Cosmetic—bleaching, shaving, waxing, depilatory creams, electrolysis.
- Weight ↓ in obese individuals.
- Psychological support.
- Drugs—all treatments take ≥6mo. to take effect and none abolish the problem. Relapse follows withdrawal. *Drugs used:* COC pill containing desogestrel or cyproterone (Dianette); spironolactone.

Hypertrichosis: Excess hair in non-androgenic distribution—usually face and trunk. Mostly drug-induced (e.g. phenytoin, ciclosporin A, minoxidil). If not, investigate to find other causes: malnutrition, anorexia nervosa, porphyria cutanea tarda, malignancy. If a cause can't be found, treat symptomatically with electrolysis, bleaching, waxing ± depilatories.

Local hypertrichosis: Can be associated with topical steroid usage, be over a melanocytic naevus, or associated with spina bifida occulta.

Hyperhidrosis: Excess sweating—may be focal or generalized.

Generalized hyperhidrosis: Most likely to occur 2° to other medical conditions. Where possible, treat the cause:
- *Physiological*—after and during exercise; hot, humid conditions; emotional response (e.g. anxiety)
- *Menopause*
- *Infection*—can occur with any bacterial or viral infection; consider malaria if recent history of travel
- *Non-infective*—thyrotoxicosis; phaeochromocytoma; lymphoma; leukaemia
- If no cause can be found a trial of SSRI e.g. fluoxetine 20mg od (unlicensed) may be helpful[R].

Focal hyperhidrosis: Usually a 1° condition, though may occur 2° to other medical conditions. Mainly affects the axillae, palms, soles of the feet, and/or face. 0.6–1% of the population are affected. Onset is typically in the teenage years. May be very distressing and disabling.
- Treat topically with 20% aluminium chloride (e.g. Anhydrol forte) applied to clean skin every night—wash off the following morning.
  ↓ frequency of application as symptoms subside. Treat local irritation with topical steroid e.g. hydrocortisone 1%. Absorbent dusting powder can be helpful for axillary/plantar sweating.
- *Advice for patients:* Avoid clothing made of lycra, nylon, and other man-made fibres and tight clothing; wear colours which don't show the sweat e.g. white, black; use emollient washes and moisturisers rather than soap; try to identify trigger factors for sweating (e.g. alcohol, crowded rooms) and avoid those situations.
- Refer if not responding. 2° care treatment options include: Iontophoresis (immersion of affected areas in warm water with mild electric current—multiple sessions required); Botulinum type A toxin injections; thoracoscopic sympathectomy.

Hidradenitis suppuritiva: Unpleasant chronic inflammatory condition of sweats glands in the axilla, groin, and perineum. Nodules, abscesses, cysts, and sinuses form which result in scarring. Treat with topical antiseptics (e.g. chlorhexidine), systemic antibiotics, and surgical drainage/excision as needed.

Further information
British Association of Dermatologists (2003) Guidelines for the management of alopecia areata
🖳 http://www.bad.org.uk

Patient information and support
Hairline International 🖳 http://www.hairlineinternational.com

Nail changes

May be due to nail disease or indicate other dermatological or systemic disease. *Take a history*—duration, initial changes, evolution of changes, other systemic or local symptoms, FH, drug and alcohol history, occupation, hobbies. *Examine*—colour, shape, extent, and pattern of involvement; consider examination/investigation for other skin or systemic disease (guided by history and appearance of nails).

Table 19.7 Nail changes—description and cause

Change	Description of nail	Differential diagnosis
Colour	Black transverse bands	Cytotoxic drugs
	Blue	Cyanosis, antimalarials, haematoma
	Blue-green	Pseudomonas infection
	Brown	Fungal infection, cigarette staining, chlorpromazine, gold, Addison's disease
	Brown 'oil stain' patches	Psoriasis
	Brown longitudinal streak	Melanocytic naevus, malignant melanoma, Addison's disease
	Red streaks—'splinter haemorrhages'	Infective endocarditis, other vasculitic disease, trauma
	White spots	Trauma to nail matrix
	White transverse bands	Heavy metal poisoning
	White/brown half and half nails	Chronic renal failure
	White (leuconychia)	Hypoalbuminaemia (e.g. associated with cirrhosis)
	Yellow	Psoriasis, fungal infection, jaundice, tetracycline, yellow nail syndrome (defective lymph drainage, nails grow very slowly, may be associated with pleural effusion)
Brittle	Nails break easily—usually at distal end	Effect of water and detergent, iron deficiency, hypothyroidism, digital ischaemia

Table 19.7 (cont.)

Change	Description of nail	Differential diagnosis
Clubbing	Loss of angle between nail fold and plate, bulbous finger tip, nail fold feels bogg.	*Respiratory:* Bronchial carcinoma (not small cell); chronic infection; fibrosing alveolitis; asbestos
		Cardiac: SBE; congenital cyanotic heart disease
		Other: Inflammatory bowel disease (Crohn's > UC); thyrotoxicosis; biliary cirrhosis; congenital; A-V malformation
Koilonychia	Spoon-shaped nails	Iron deficiency anaemia, lichen planus, repeated exposure to detergents
Onycholysis	Separation of the nail from the nail bed	Psoriasis, fungal infection, trauma, thyrotoxicosis, tetracyclines
Pitting	Fine or coarse pits in the nail bed	Psoriasis, eczema, alopecia areata, lichen planus
Beau's lines	Transverse grooves	Any severe illness which affects growth of the nail matrix
Ridging	Transverse	Beau's lines, eczema, psoriasis, tic-dystrophy, chronic paronychia
	Longitudinal	Lichen planus, Darier's disease
Nail fold telangectasia	Dilated capillaries and erythema at the nail fold	Connective tissue disorders (🕮 p.578)
Tumours of the nail fold	Benign	Viral warts, myxoid (mucus) cysts (treat with steroid injection or cryotherapy), periungual fibroma (associated with tuberous sclerosis—appear at puberty)
	Malignant	Melanoma, squamous cell carcinoma

Acute paronychia: Infection of the skin and soft tissue of the proximal and lateral nail fold, most commonly caused by *S. aureus*. Often originates from a break in the skin or cuticle as a result of minor trauma e.g. nail biting. Skin and soft tissue of the proximal and lateral nail fold are red, hot, and tender; nail may appear discoloured/distorted. Treat in the same way as a boil (🕮 p.668).

Sunlight and the skin

Skin cancer: p.666

Sunburn: Susceptibility depends on skin type. Tingling is followed 2–12h. later by erythema. Redness is maximal at 24h. and fades over 2–3d. Desquamation and pigmentation follow. Severe sunburn may cause blistering, pain, and systemic upset. Treatment is symptomatic with calamine lotion prn (some advocate application of vinegar). Rarely dressings are required for blisters or, in severe cases, hospital admission for fluid management. *Complications:* predisposes to skin cancer and photoageing.

Solar keratosis: Single or multiple discrete scaly hyperkeratotic rough-surfaced areas over sun-exposed sites (e.g. dorsum of hands; head and neck). Occasionally occurs on lower lip. More common with fairer skin types. May regress spontaneously or be pre-malignant.

Management: Removal by cryotherapy, currettage, excision biopsy, or application of fluorouracil cream (Efudix) or diclofenac gel (Solaraze). Advise patients to wear sunblock and avoid sun exposure by covering up and wearing a hat with a brim.

Complications: Malignant change; cutaneous horn development (treat with excision or currettage).

Solar elastosis: Sun-exposed skin is yellow, thickened, and wrinkled. No treatment. Advise to avoid sun exposure and wear sunblock.

Skin conditions worsened by sunlight: HSV (cold sores); lupus erythematosis (LE); porphyria; rosacea; vitiligo.

Skin conditions improved by sunlight: Acne; atopic eczema; pityriasis rosea; psoriasis (10% get worse).

Drug-induced photosensitivity: Drugs may produce a light eruption in exposed areas either by dose-dependent or allergic mechanisms. The reaction produced varies according to the drug. *Common examples are:* amiodarone, chlorpropamide, furosemide, griseofulvin, phenothiazines, sulphonamides, tetracyclines, thiazides, nalidixic acid, coal tar, plant—derived psoralens.

Plant-induced photodermatitis: Photocontact dermatitis, similar in appearance to contact dermatitis due to other agents (p.638), results from local sensitization of the skin by contact with psoralens from plants e.g. in carrots, celery, fennel, parsnip, common rue, giant hogweed. Oils used in perfumes derived from plants (e.g. oil of bergamot) may also contain psoralens.

Polymorphic light eruption: Pruritic papules, plaques ± vesicles appear in sun-exposed areas ~24h. after exposure. Most common photodermatosis. ♀:♂ ≈ 2:1. *Cause:* unknown. *Management:* sunscreens and avoidance of sun exposure (sit in the shade, long sleeves, trousers, broad-rimmed hat); a short course of PUVA in spring may help severe cases—refer to dermatology. *Differential diagnosis:* photoallergic contact dermatitis; drug-induced photosensitivity; LE.

Solar urticaria: Rare. Wheals appear within minutes of sun exposure. *Differential diagnosis:* porphyria. *Management:* sunscreens, avoidance. Refer to dermatologist if disabling.

Actinic prurigo: Rare. Starts in childhood. Papules and excoriations on sun-exposed sites. *Management:* sunscreens and avoidance. Refer to dermatology for confirmation of diatgnosis and advice on further management.

Pellagra: Dietary deficiency of nicotinic acid. May give photosensitive dermatitis in association with dementia and diarrhoea. Treatment of underlying deficiency alleviates symptoms.

Porphyria: A group of rare, mostly inherited metabolic disorders. Porphyrins are important in the manufacture of haemoglobin. Deficiency of enzymes in the porphyrin pathway results in build-up of intermediary metabolites which are toxic to skin and nervous system. All require specialist management by either a general physician or dermatologist. The main porphyrias are:

- *Acute intermittent porphyria:* Intermittent attacks precipitated by many drugs. *Presentation:* fever; GI symptoms (vomiting, abdominal pain—can be severe); neuropsychiatric symptoms (hypotonia, paralysis, fits, impaired vision, peripheral neuritis, odd behaviour—even psychosis); *no* skin features. Urine may go deep red on standing.
- *Porphyria cutanea tarda:* Most common porphyria. Typically occurs in male alcoholics with liver damage. Presents with sun-induced sub-epidermal blisters on hands which scar. *Management:* avoidance of alcohol and aggravating drugs (e.g. oestrogens); venesection; chloroquine.
- *Erythropoietic protoporphyria:* Autosomal dominant; starts in child-hood; red blistering eruption leaving scars on hands and nose.
- *Variegate porphyria:* Autosomal dominant. Common in S. Africa. Skin signs are like porphyria cutanea tarda but abdominal pain and neuro-psychiatric symptoms resemble acute intermittent porphyria.

Benign skin tumours

Naevus: Benign proliferation of ≥1 normal constituent of the skin. *Most common type:* melanocytic naevus or 'mole'. Most develop in childhood and adolescence. *Features:*

- **Congenital:** Present at birth in 1% Caucasians (less in darker skinned races). Usually large (>1cm diameter). ≈5% risk of malignancy.
- **Junctional:** Flat, round/oval, brown/black, 2–10mm diameter. Common sites: soles, palms, genitalia.
- **Intradermal:** Dome-shaped papule/nodule commonly on the face or neck. May be pigmented.
- **Compound:** <10mm diameter, smooth surface, variable pigmentation.
- **Blue:** Blue coloured solitary naevus usually found on extremities— especially hands and feet.
- **Halo:** Found in children or adolescents. White halo of depigmentation surrounds the naevus which then disappears. Associated with vitiligo.

Differential diagnosis: Freckle, lentigo, seborrhoeic wart, haemangioma (may be pigmented), dermatofibroma, pigmented BCC, malignant melanoma.

Management: Patients usually present if worried about a mole. Any change merits serious attention. *Reasons for excision biopsy:* concern about malignancy (📖 p.666); ↑ risk of malignant change (e.g. congenital naevi); cosmetic reasons; repeated inflammation; recurrent trauma. Most areas now have specialist 'mole clinics' for assessment and excision of suspicious lesions. Otherwise, refer for urgent dermatology assessment if malignancy is suspected.

Seborrhoeic wart (senile wart, basal cell papilloma): Common >60y. Often multiple—most commonly on trunk. Warty nodules (usually pigmented) 1–6cm diameter with 'stuck on' appearance. Pieces of the wart can be picked off. *Cause:* unknown. *Management:* reassurance. If removal is required, cryotherapy, curettage, shave biopsy and excision biopsy are effective.

Skin tags: Common. Small pedunculated polyps found in axillae, groin, neck, or on the eyelids. *Management:* reassurance. Cosmetic removal can be achieved by snipping across the skin tag with scissors, cryotherapy, or diathermy.

Sebaceous cyst (epidermal cyst): Common. Round or oval, keratin-filled, firm cysts (1–3cm diameter) within the skin. Usually a punctum is seen on the surface. *Management:* reassurance. Treat any complicating bacterial infection with oral antibiotics (e.g. flucloxacillin 250mg qds). Excision is curative.

Milia: Small, white, raised spots (1–2mm diameter) usually on the face (upper cheeks and eyelids). Most common in children, but can occur at any age. *Management:* No treatment required.

Dermatofibroma: Common ($♀ > ♂$; young adult > elderly) and usually asymptomatic. Firm (sometimes pigmented) nodule 5–10mm diameter which may occur following an insect bite or minor trauma. *Most common site:* Lower legs. *Management:* Excision biopsy of symptomatic or diagnostically doubtful lesions.

Lipoma: Common. Benign tumours of fat. Present as soft masses in the subcutaneous tissue. Often multiple; most common on trunk, neck, and upper extremities. Removal by excision is rarely necessary.

Keloid scars: Proliferation of connective tissue presenting as firm smooth nodules/plaques in response to trauma. A scar is termed hypertrophic if changes are limited to the scar but keloid if it extends beyond the limit of the original injury. *Most common sites:* Upper back, chest, ear lobes. More common in negroid races (2nd–4th decades). Refer to dermatologist or plastic surgeon—treated by injection of steroid into the scar, cryotherapy, or topical silicone gel sheeting.

Pyogenic granuloma: Bright red/blood-crusted nodule which bleeds easily. Typically develops at the site of trauma (e.g. small cut) and enlarges rapidly over 2–3wk. *Most common site:* Finger. Usually occurs in children/young adults. *Differential diagnosis:* Malignant melanoma. *Management:* Excision biopsy to exclude malignancy.

Keratoacanthoma: Rapidly growing nodular tumour (<2cm diameter) of sun-exposed skin of face/arms. A central keratin plug may fall out to leave a crater. Heals spontaneously over several months leaving a scar. *Differential diagnosis:* SCC. *Management:* Excision biopsy or curettage and cautery.

Chondrodermatitis nodularis: Small, painful nodule in the upper rim of the pinna. Most common in elderly men. Due to inflammation of the cartilage. Refer for excision.

Campbell-de-Morgan spot (cherry angioma): Small, bright red papules on the trunk in middle-aged/elderly patients. Usually requires no treatment. (*Campbell-de-Morgan (1811–76)—English surgeon*).

Skin cancer

Prevention

⚠ Nearly all skin cancer is caused by the sun and 80% is preventable.

The Sun Safety Code

- Take care not to burn;
- Cover up with loose cool clothing, a hat, and sun glasses;
- Seek shade during the hottest part of the day;
- Apply a high factor sunscreen on any parts of the body exposed to the sun (≥SPF 15);
- Take special care to protect children in the sun.

Malignant melanoma: Incidence: 10/100,000/y. in UK. ♀:♂ ≈ 2:1. It occurs in all races, though particularly common in Caucasians. Frequently metastasizes and may present with metastasis. *Types:*

- *Superficial spreading:* 50% UK cases. ♀ > ♂. Most common site: lower leg (50%). Macular lesion with variable pigmentation.
- *Nodular:* 25% UK cases. ♂ > ♀. Most common on trunk. Pigmented nodule grows rapidly and may ulcerate.
- *Lentigo:* 15% UK cases. A lentigo maligna arises in sun-damaged skin and melanoma develops many years afterwards within it. Most common >60y.—especially if outdoor occupation.
- *Acral lentiginous:* 10% UK cases. Most common form in mongoloid races. Affects palms, soles, and nail beds. Often detected late. Carries poor prognosis.

Causes: Although 30% malignant melanomas arise out of pre-existing moles, risk of change in a benign mole (except dysplastic or congenital naevus) is small; sun exposure is implicated. *Other risk factors:* genetic; multiple benign moles (>50 of >2mm diameter); congenital naevus; previous malignant melanoma; immunosuppression; fair skin type (red hair, blue eyes, and burn easily).

Management: Encourage patients to report early any change in a mole. Changes which warrant further investigation are:

- *Size*—recent ↑
- *Shape*—irregular outline
- *Itch*—common symptom
- *Inflammation*—may be at the edge
- *Crusting*—any oozing or bleeding
- *Colour*—change/variation within the mole

Refer: Any suspected lesions for assessment urgently by a dermatologist ± wide excision. Chemotherapy and radiotherapy are of little benefit in malignant melanoma but immunotherapy treatment looks promising.

Prognosis: Relates to tumour depth at presentation. 5y. survival: <1mm deep—93%; >3.5mm deep—31%.

Basal cell carcinoma (rodent ulcer, BCC): Most common form of skin cancer. Locally invasive but rarely metastasizes. Tends to occur in middle-aged/elderly patients. May be multiple, and appears mainly on light-exposed areas—most commonly the face. 4 main types (all can be pigmented):

* *Nodular* (Most common—starts as small pearly nodule which may necrose centrally leaving a small crusted ulcer with a pearly, rolled edge)
* *Cystic*
* *Multicentric* (plaque-like, large, superficial ± central depression)

Causes: Sun exposure, arsenic ingestion, X-ray irradiation, chronic scarring, genetic predisposition.

Management: Complete excision is ideal. Alternatives are radiotherapy (>60y.), cryotherapy, curettage and cautery. Refer as necessary to radiotherapy or dermatology.

Prognosis: Recurrence rate is 5% at 5y. for all modalities of treatment. Development of new BCC at other sites is common.

Squamous cell carcinoma (SCC): Most common >55y. ♂>♀. May metastasize (10%). Usually develops in light-exposed sites e.g. face, neck, hands. May start within an actinic (solar) keratosis (🔲 p.662) or de novo as a nodule which progresses to ulcerate and form a crust.

Causes: Chronic sun damage, X-ray exposure, chronic ulceration and scarring (aggressive SCC may develop at the edge of chronic ulcers), smoking pipes and cigars (lip lesions), industrial carcinogens (tars, oils), wart virus, immunosuppression, genetic.

Management: Refer to dermatology. Treated with surgical excision ± LN biopsy. Large lesions may require skin grafting. Radiotherapy is an alternative for large lesions in elderly patients.

Bowen's disease: Intraepidermal carcinoma. Common. Typically occurs on the lower leg in elderly women. Lesions are pink/slightly pigmented scaly plaques (<5cm diameter) and may be solitary or multiple. *Risk factor:* exposure to arsenicals. *Management:* biopsy confirms diagnosis. Treatment is with cryotherapy, curettage, or excision. (*J.T. Bowen (1857–1941)—US dermatologist.*)

Further information for GPs and patients

British Association of Dermatologists 🔲 *http://www.bad.org.uk*
* Guidelines for the management of BCC (1999)
* Guidelines for management of Bowen's disease (1999)
* Multiprofessional guidelines for the management of the patient with primary cutaneous squamous cell carcinoma (2002)
* UK guidelines for the management of cutaneous melanoma (2002)

Cancer Research UK Sun Smart Campaign
🔲 *http://www.cancerresearchuk.org/SunSmart*

Meteorological Office UV Index
🔲 *http://www.meto.gov.uk/weather/uv*

Electronic Dermatology Atlas
🔲 *http://www.dermis.net/bilddb/index_e.htm*

Bacterial skin infections

Impetigo

- Superficial skin infection due to S. aureus.
- A thin-walled blister ruptures easily to leave a yellow crusted lesion. May occur anywhere—but most common on face. Lesions spread rapidly and are contagious.
- Avoid spreading to other children—no sharing of towels, face flannels etc.; some schools prohibit attendance until lesions are cleared.
- Localized cases—treat with topical antibiotics (e.g. fucidin cream); widespread infection—treat with oral flucloxacillin or erythromycin.
- *Differential diagnosis:* HSV, fungal infection e.g. ringworm.

Boils and carbuncles

- *Boil (furuncle):* Acute infection of a hair follicle, usually with S. aureus. Starts as a hard, tender, red nodule surrounding a hair follicle becoming larger and fluctuant after several days. Occasionally associated with fever ± malaise. Later may discharge pus and a central 'core' before healing; may leave a scar. *Predisposing factors:* usually absent—DM (evidence conflicting); HIV; obesity; blood dyscrasias; treatment with immunosuppressive drugs.
- *Chronic furunculosis:* Multiple crops of boils that occur over a period of time, either continuously or intermittently.
- *Carbuncle:* Swollen, painful area discharging pus from several points. Occurs when a group of hair follicles become deeply infected, usually with S. aureus. May be associated with fever ± malaise. *Predisposing factors:* malnutrition, cardiac failure, drug addiction, severe generalized dermatosis, prolonged steroid therapy, DM (evidence conflicting).

Differential diagnosis: Cystic acne (📖 p.644); hidradenitis suppurativa (📖 p.659); orf (📖 p.671); anthrax (opposite).

Management

- *For lesions that are non-fluctuant:* apply moist heat to relieve discomfort, help localize the infection, and promote drainage.
- *If there is associated fever/surrounding cellulitis or the lesion is on the face:* treat with oral antibiotics e.g. flucloxacillin 250mg qds for 7d. Erythromycin 250mg qds is an alternative if allergic to penicillin.
- *For lesions that are large but localized, painful, and fluctuant:* Incise and drain; treat with oral antibiotics (as above) until inflammation resolves.
- *Admit:* if not settling with primary care treatment or if boil is in a location where incision and drainage would be difficult in primary care (e.g. genital region).
- *If recurrent or chronic:* take swabs for culture from lesions and carrier sites (nose, axilla, and groin); treat carrier sites with topical antibiotic (e.g. Naseptin qds for 10d.), improved hygiene, and use of antiseptics in bath (e.g. chlorhexidine); consider long-term antibiotics (e.g. erythromycin 250–500mg od).

Acute paronychia: 📖 p.661

Staphylococcal whitlow (felon): Infection involving the bulbous distal pulp of the finger following trauma or extension from an acute paronychia. The finger bulb is red, hot, oedematous, and usually exquisitely tender. Onset of pain is rapid and there is swelling of the entire finger pulp. *Diffferential diagnosis:* herpetic whitlow (📖 p.495). *Management:* admit for drainage and antibiotics.

Folliculitis: Inflammation of the hair follicles caused by infection (usually *S. aureus*), physical injury, or chemical irritation. Classified as superficial or deep by the depth of involvement of the hair follicle. Presents as pustules in hair-bearing areas e.g. legs, beard area. *Risk factors:* obesity, DM (evidence mixed), occlusion from clothing, topical steroid use. *Differential diagnosis:* pityrosporum folliculitis (📖 p.639).

Management: Exclude DM; treat with topical or systemic antibiotics (e.g. Fucidin cream or oral flucloxacillin). *If recurrent or chronic:* see recurrent boils (opposite).

Scalded skin syndrome: Acute toxic illness usually of infants. Characterized by shedding of sheets of skin. May follow impetigo. *Management:* emergency paediatric admission. Requires iv antibiotics.

Erysipelas and cellulitis: Acute infection of the dermis. Preceded by systemic symptoms—fever, 'flu-like' symptoms. Usually affects face or lower leg. May be an obvious entry wound. Appears as a painful, tender reddened area with a well-defined edge. Often the area is swollen and may blister. *Differential diagnosis:* angioedema, allergic contact dermatitis, gout.

Management: Oral penicillin V 250–500mg qds or erythromycin for 7–14d. Severe infections may require hospital admission for iv antibiotics. Recurrent infections (>2 episodes at 1 site) require prophylactic long-term penicillin (e.g. penicillin V 250mg od or bd) and attention to potential entry portals (e.g. tinea pedis).

Complications: Lymphangitis ± permanent damage to lymph drainage; glomerulonephritis (📖 p.682) or guttate psoriasis (📖 p.647).

Necrotising fasciitis: Acute and serious infection. Usually occurs in otherwise healthy individuals after surgery or trauma (may be minor). Ill-defined erythema associated with high fever. Rapidly becomes necrotic. *Management:* emergency admission for iv antibiotics ± surgical debridement.

Anthrax: Rare in UK and only included due to potential use in bioterrorism. Haemorrhagic bulla forms at the site of innoculation. Associated with oedema and fever. Usually from contaminated animal products. Penicillin is curative. Rarely spores are inhaled giving a pneumonia-like picture. Give iv/im penicillin and admit immediately if suspected.

Viral skin infections

Viral warts: Common and benign. Due to infection of epidermal cells with human papilloma virus (HPV)—>50 types identified. Certain types are associated with infection at different sites: common hand warts—type 2; plantar warts—types 1 and 4; genital warts—types 6,11,16, and 18. Genital warts are associated with cervical dysplasia (🕮 p.714). The virus is transmitted by direct contact. Immunosuppressed patients are particularly vulnerable. *Presentation:*

Common warts: dome-shaped papules with papilliferous surface. Usually >1. Most common on hands but may affect other areas. In children, 30–50% disappear spontaneously in <6mo.

Plantar warts (verrucas): on soles of feet. Most common in children/young adults. Pressure makes them grow into the dermis. Often painful. Characterized by dark punctate spots on the surface (may need to pare callus off to see). Warts group together to form mosaics.

Plane warts: smooth, flat-topped papules often slightly brown in colour. Most common on face and backs of hands. Usually >1. Manage as for common/plantar warts. Eventually resolve spontaneously. May show Koebner phenomenon.

Genital warts: 🕮 p.744.

Table 19.8 Treatment of viral warts in general practice

Treatment option	Examples	Notes
Topical salicylic acid	Salactol, duofilm, Bazuka	Avoid use on the face or in patients with atopic eczema. Ensure dead skin is pared off daily before reapplication.
Cryotherapy	Liquid nitrogen	May cause blistering and be painful several days after treatment.
Curettage/cautery		Useful for solitary warts on face. Warts may recur.

⚠ Refer immunosuppressed patients for specialist advice on management.

Further information

British Association of Dermatologists (2001) Guidelines for the management of cutaneous warts 🖥 http://www.bad.org.uk

Molluscum contagiosum: Discrete pearly pink umbilicated papules 1–3mm diameter. If squeezed, papules release a cheesy material. Lesions are multiple and grouped—usually on the trunk, face, and neck. Caused by a DNA pox virus and spread by contact (including towels). Untreated, resolve spontaneously after several months. In the adult or older child, removal by expressing the contents with forceps, curettage, or cryotherapy is possible.

Orf: Solitary, red, rapidly growing papule—often on hand. May reach 1cm diameter. Evolves into a painful purple pustule. Patients usually have had close contact with sheep e.g. vet, farmer. Incubation period ~6d. *Management:* resolves spontaneously in 2–4wk. *Complications:* 2° infection (treat with topical/systemic antibiotics); erythema multiforme; lymphangitis.

HIV infection: 📖 p.498

Cold sore and herpetic whitlow: 📖 p.495

Viral infections: 📖 p.490–95

Fungal infections

There are two major groups of fungal skin infections seen in the UK.

Candidiasis: A virtually uniform commensal of the mouth and GI tract which produces opportunistic infection. *Risk factors:* moist, opposing skin folds; obesity; DM; neonates; pregnancy; poor hygiene; humid environment; wet work occupation; use of broad-spectrum antibiotic. *Presentation*—see Table 19.9.

Dermatophyte infection: Tinea denotes fungal infection. Common. Affects skin, hair, or nails. Skin scrapings or nail clippings may confirm diagnosis. Presentation—see Table 19.10.

General measures for prevention of fungal infections: Keep body folds separated and dry (e.g. with dusting powder) and minimize hot and humid conditions (e.g. advise open footwear).

Management of fungal infections
Topical treatment
- **Genital lesions**—imidazole cream, pessaries.
- **Nail infections**—if confined to 1 or 2 nails, consider using a lacquer or paint e.g. amorolfine lacquer 1–2x/wk. for durations stated in the BNF.
- **Skin lesions**—imidazole cream, spray, powder; terbinafine cream.

Table 19.9 Presentation of candidiasis:

Presentation	Symptoms	Differential diagnosis
Genital infection 'thrush' (📖 p.741)	♀ >> ♂. Itchy, sore vulvovaginitis ± white plaques on mucous membranes, and cheesy discharge. Men develop a similar clinical picture.	Psoriasis; lichen planus; lichen sclerosus; other causes of vaginal discharge.
Intertrigo	Reddened, moist, glazed area in the submammary, inguinal, or axillary folds. In wet workers, may occur between digits. Patients may notice skin changes or present with itch.	Psoriasis; tinea cruris; seborrhoeic dermatitis; bacterial skin infection.
Oral	Sore mouth; poor feeding in infants. Most common in babies, patients with poor oral hygiene, or the elderly with false teeth. White plaques visible on buccal mucosa which can be wiped off ± angular stomatitis.	Lichen planus; epithelial dysplasia.
Nappy candidiasis	Babies; in the nappy area.	📖 p.876
Chronic paronychia	Often seen in wet workers. Presents with chronic nail fold inflammation.	Bacterial infection; chronic eczema.
Systemic candidiasis	Occurs in immunosuppressed individuals (e.g. HIV, malignancy). Red nodules may appear on the skin.	

Table 19.10 Dermatophyte infections

Tinea	Affects	Presentation	Differential diagnosis
Corporis *Ringworm*	Trunk or limbs	Single/multiple plaques with scaling and erythema, especially at the edges. Lesions enlarge slowly and clear centrally (hence 'ringworm').	Discoid eczema; psoriasis; pityriasis rosea.
Cruris *'jock itch'*	Groin ♂ > ♀ Common in athletes	Associated with tinea pedis. Involves upper thigh (+ scrotum rarely). Red plaque with scaling, especially at the edge.	Intertrigo; candidiasis; erythrasma.
Pedis *Athlete's foot*	Feet ♂ > ♀ Young > old	Itchy maceration between toes. *Risk factors*: swimming; occlusive footwear; hot weather.	Contact dermatitis; psoriasis; pompholyx.
Capitis	Hair and scalp	Defined, inflamed scaly areas ± alopecia, with broken hair shafts.	Alopecia areata; psoriasis; seborrhoeic eczema.
Unguium	Nails—prevalence ↑ with age Rare in children Toenails > fingernails	Begins at distal nail edge and progresses proximally to involve the whole nail. Eventually results in thickening, yellowing, and crumbling of the nail plate. Tinea pedis often coexists.	Psoriasis; trauma; candidiasis.

- *Mouth lesions*—remove tongue deposits with a toothbrush by brushing 2x/d.. Oral pastilles, suspensions, or gels (e.g. nystatin, miconazole). If false teeth, advise to place imidazole gel on the teeth before insertion and sterilize overnight with dilute hypochlorite solution (e.g. Milton)

Systemic treatment: Use for recurrent, extensive, systemic, or resistant infection and nail or scalp infection. *Examples:*
- *Oral, mucocutaneous, or systemic candidiasis:* e.g. oral fluconazole 50mg od for 1–2wk. Higher doses/prolonged therapy may be needed if immunosuppressed (seek specialist advice).
- *Genital candidiasis:* single oral dose of 150–200mg fluconazole.
- *Dermatophyte infection:* oral terbinafine (250mg od) or itraconazole (100–200mg od). Warn about possible side-effects.
- *Nail infection:* consider if topical treatment is unsuccessful or >2 nails involved. Confirm diagnosis with nail clipping mycology before treatment. Consider treating with oral terbinafine or pulsed itraconazole— treat at dosage and for durations recommended in the *BNF* (5.2).

Insect bites and infestations

Insect bites: Response depends on the insect involved and the individual's reaction to the bite. Ranges from blisters, through papules, to urticarial wheals. 2° infection is common.

Management

> ⚠ *If anaphylaxis occurs* give s/cut adrenaline, oxygen, and admit via emergency ambulance to A&E (📖 p.1034). *Dose of adrenaline:*
> - **Adult or child >12y.**: 0.5ml epinephrine (adrenaline) 1:1000 solution (500µg) IM. Give half dose if pre-pubertal or adult on tricyclic antidepressants, monoamine oxidase inhibitors, or β blockers.
> - **Child 6–12y.**: ½ adult dose—0.25ml of 1:1000 epinephrine (adrenaline) solution (250µg) IM.
> - **Child 6mo.–6y.**: ¼ adult dose—0.12ml of 1:1000 epinephrine (adrenaline) solution (120µg) IM.
> - **Child <6mo.**: 0.05ml 1:1000 epinephrine (adrenaline) solution (50µg) IM. Absolute accuracy of dose is not necessary.
> *Repeat* after ≥5 min. if improvement is transient, no improvement, or deterioration after initial treatment. May need several doses.

Immediately after the bite—Remove any sting present in the wound. Often no further treatment is needed.
- *If severe local reaction occurs*—Apply an ice pack; give oral antihistamine (e.g. chlorpheniramine 4mg stat); continue antihistamine 4–6 hourly as needed.
- *If 2° bacterial infection occurs*—Treat with oral or topical antibiotics.
- *Remove sources of insects* e.g. remove fleas from carpets with household flea spray (multiple bites on ankles and lower legs).

Scabies: The scabies mite (*Sarcoptes scabei*) is ~½ mm long and spread by direct physical contact. Average infection consists of 12 mites. Symptoms appear 4–6wk. after infection.

Presentation: Intense itching. Examination reveals burrows (irregular, tortuous, and slightly scaly, <1cm long) on sides of fingers, wrists, ankles, and nipples. May form rubbery nodules on genitalia. Itching results in excoriations. Untreated infection becomes chronic.

Differential diagnosis: Lichen planus; dermatitis herpetiformis; papular urticaria; eczema.

Management: Treat with scabicide e.g. malathion lotion. Apply according to manufacturer's instructions. Reapplication may be needed after 1wk. All close contacts need treatment (which may result in all occupants of a residential home being treated). Advise patients to launder all worn clothing and bedding after application. Itching may persist for some time after elimination of infection—use oral antihistamines for symptomatic relief.

Complications: 2° infection (treat with topical or systemic antibiotics).

Headlice: Most common in children age 4–11y. ($\female$ > $\male$) but may occur in anyone. Contrary to popular belief, lice infest clean as often as dirty hair. Adult lice are about the size of a sesame seed, brownish grey in colour, and wiggle their legs. Only adult lice are contagious. *Spread:* only by close head-head contact. Lice don't jump/fly and don't stay viable away from a host.

Symptoms/signs: Normally asymptomatic. Detected by contact tracing of other cases or routine inspection at home or school. Occasionally present as itchy scalp. Presence of 'nits' (egg shells—white dots attached to hair), eggs, or dead lice indicate past infection. A moving louse must be found to confirm active infection.

Detection: After washing hair, apply conditioner and comb with fine-tooth detector comb (available from pharmacy). In at-risk groups (e.g. schoolchildren) repeat weekly. Lice are removed by the comb and seen trapped in its teeth.

Management
- *Prophylactic preparations*—no evidence of effectiveness.
- *Insecticides*—effective. 3 types (no evidence which performs best): Malathion, phenothrin, and permethrin are available OTC but are expensive and NHS prescriptions are often sought. Carbaryl is available on prescription only. Malathion and phenothrin/permethrin are used as 1st and 2nd line; carbaryl reserved for 3rd line. Apply according to manufacturer's instructions asking patients to use 2 applications, 7d. apart. 2–3d. after the final application, check hair with detector comb to ensure lice have cleared. Supply enough for 2 applications. Shampoos are not effective—use lotions, liquids, or cream rinses.
- *Mechanical clearance*—wet-comb conditioned hair with a fine tooth comb until all lice are removed and repeat at 3–4d. intervals for 2wk. Alternative to insecticides, but requires motivation.
- *Other methods of treatment*—electric combs, aromatherapy (tea tree oil), herbal treatments. No evidence supporting their use.
- *Contact tracing*—all cases. Trace those in close contact over the previous month.

Reinfestation/resistance to treatment: If lice have not cleared, there are 3 possible reasons:
- *Reinfestation*—lice found are large adults only. Ask patient to check close contacts again. Re-treat with a different insecticide.
- *Incorrect use of insecticide/mechanical clearance*—lice at mixed stages of development will be seen. Check procedure with the patient and make sure instructions are understood. Repeat treatment with a different insecticide.
- *Resistance to insecticide*—lice are seen at all stages of development. Re-treat with another product.

Crab lice: Similar to head lice. May be sexually transmitted. All hairy areas (including eyelashes, eyebrows, pubic and axillary hair) can be affected. Carbaryl (unlicensed), phenothrin, and malathion are all effective. Apply an aqueous solution to all parts of the body and rinse off after 12h. Repeat after 7d.

Renal medicine and urology

Presentation of renal disease

Table 20.1 Presentation of renal disease

	GN	Interstitial disease			Vascular disease			Outflow tract obstruction
		AIN	ATN	CIN	Small	Large	RVT	
Nephrotic syndrome	++	0	0	0	(+)	0	+*	0
Nephritic syndrome	++	(+)	0	0	(+)	0	+	0
Acute renal failure	+	+	++**	0	+	+	(+)	++
Chronic renal failure	++	(+)	0	++	(+)	+	0	++
Pyelonephritis/UTI	0	0	0	0	0	0	+	+
Hypertension	(+)	(+)	0	(+)	(+)	(+)	0	+

GN: glomerulonephritis (📖 p.682)

AIN: acute interstitial nephritis (📖 p.682)

ATN: acute tubular necrosis

CIN: chronic interstitial nephritis (📖 p.682)

RVT: renal vein thrombosis (📖 p.683)

* RVT is a complication, not a cause, of nephrotic syndrome.
** ATN is the most common cause of acute renal failure.

Acute or chronic renal failure: 📖 p.680

Nephrotic syndrome: Proteinuria >3g/24h. causing hypoalbuminaemia and oedema. Often associated with ↑ cholesterol. *Causes:*

- Minimal change GN (90% children, 30% adults)
- Membranous GN
- Membranoproliferative GN
- Focal segmental glomerulosclerosis
- DM
- Amyloid
- Neoplasia
- Endocarditis
- PAN
- SLE
- Sickle-cell disease
- Malaria
- Drugs (penicillamine, gold)

Presentation: Swelling of eyelids and face; ascites, peripheral oedema; urine froth due to protein. *Nephrotic crisis:* unwell with oedema, anorexia, vomiting, pleural effusions, and muscle wasting.

Investigation: *Urine*—24h. urine collection for protein and creatinine clearance; microscopy for red cells, casts. *Blood*—U&E, creatinine, albumin, cholesterol, FBC, ESR.

Management: Refer all suspected cases of nephrotic syndrome to a renal physician.

Complications
- Thromboembolism
- Hypercholesterolaemia
- Infection—especially pneumococcal. If persistent nephrotic syndrome, offer vaccination
- Hypovolaemia and renal failure
- Loss of specific proteins e.g. transferrin (causes hypochromic anaemia which is iron resistant)

Nephritic syndrome: Central feature is blood in the urine from glomerular bleeding. *Other features:* fluid retention ↑BP, low urine output, rising plasma urea and creatinine. *Causes:* glomerulonephritis, vasculitis.

Acute nephritic syndrome
- Presents 1–3wk. after throat, ear, or skin infection with Gp. A β-haemolytic streptococci.
- *Features:* Oliguria, haematuria and proteinuria, fluid retention, ↑BP, uraemia.
- *Management:* Refer suspected cases immediately to a renal physician.
- *Risks:* Hypertensive encephalopathy, pulmonary oedema, ARF.
- *Prognosis:* Excellent in children; in adults, some proteinuria/urine sediment may persist. CRF is rare.

Nephrocalcinosis: Deposition of Ca^{2+} in the kidneys. X-ray—calcification. May cause symptoms of UTI or renal stones. *Cause:*
- *Medullary* (95%)—hyperparathyroidism, distal renal tubular acidosis, medullary sponge kidney, idiopathic calciuria, papillary necrosis, oxalosis.
- *Cortical*—serious renal disease or chronic GN.

Pyelonephritis/UTI: 📖 p.692

Hypertension: 📖 p.316

Patient support and information
UK National Kidney Federation ☎0845 601 02 09 🖳 http://www.kidney.org.uk

Renal failure

Acute renal failure (ARF): ↓ in renal function over h./d.. No specific symptoms/signs. ↓ in urine output is common. If creatinine and urea are acutely raised, diagnose ARF. Refer all cases immediately to the acute medical team. *Causes:* 80% acute tubular necrosis (renal ischaemia due to acute circulatory compromise); renal tract obstruction (5%); glomerulonephritis.

Chronic renal failure (CRF): Slow ↓ in renal function over mo./y.
Causes:

- Glomerulonephritis
- Chronic pyelonephritis
- DM
- Urinary tract obstruction
- Polycystic kidneys

- ↑BP
- Amyloid
- Myeloma
- SLE
- PAN

- gout
- Ca^{2+}↑
- Interstitial nephritis

Table 20.2 Grading of chronic renal failure

Grade	GFR ml/min	Serum creatinine (approx.) μmol/l
Mild	20–50	150–300
Moderate	10–20	300–700
Severe	<10	>700

❶ Renal function ↓ with age. Many elderly patients have a GFR <50ml/min. which, because of ↓ muscle mass, may not be indicated by a ↑ serum creatinine.

Presentation

- *History:* FH (polycystic kidneys), UTI, drugs (especially analgesics).
- *Symptoms:* Nausea, anorexia, lethargy, itch, nocturia, impotence.
  Later symptoms: Oedema, dyspnoea, chest pain (from pericarditis), vomiting, confusion, fits, hiccups, neuropathy, coma.
- *Signs:* pallor, 'lemon tinge' to skin, pulmonary/peripheral oedema, pericarditis, pleural effusions, metabolic flap, ↑ BP, retinopathy (DM or ↑BP).

Investigation

- *Urine:* M,C&S, 24h. urinary protein and creatinine clearance, RBCs, glucose. Radioisotope clearance is a more accurate way of estimating GFR (usually only available for specialists).
- *Blood:* U&E, creatinine, glucose, Ca^{2+}, PO_4^{2-} urate, protein, FBC, ESR, serum electrophoresis.
- *Radiology:* Renal tract USS.

Management: Refer to a physician with interest in renal medicine. Early referral is essential to find reversible causes, ↓ decline of function, and allow preparation for dialysis. *Treatment:*

- *Treat reversible causes:* If outflow obstruction, refer to urologist; stop nephrotoxic drugs (frusemide, NSAIDs most common).
- *Monitor and treat ↑BP*

- *Seek out* and *treat UTIs*
- *Monitor and treat renal bone disease:* Osteomalacia—📖 p.566–7
- *Dietary advice:* ensure adequate calories, vitamins, and iron; ↓ salt in diet if ↑BP; ↓ protein in diet if proteinuria; ↓ lipids and ↑ carbohydrate. Refer to dietician.

↓ **in renal function:** Generally occurs at a steady rate to end-stage renal failure. Patients are monitored over time. If sudden ↓ in renal function—suspect infection, dehydration, uncontrolled ↑BP, metabolic disturbance (e.g. Ca^{2+}↑), obstruction, nephrotoxins (e.g. drugs). Treatment may delay end-stage renal failure—refer to renal unit.

End-stage renal failure (ESRF): 80 new patients/million population/y.—irreversible. Dialysis starts when GFR is <5% normal. Dialysis is needed lifelong unless a kidney transplant becomes available. In all cases, refer back to the renal unit managing the patient if you have any problems.

Haemodialysis: Blood flows opposite dialysis fluid and substances are cleared along a concentration gradient across a semi-permeable membrane.

Problems: pulmonary oedema; infection (HIV, hepatitis, bacteria); U&E imbalance; BP↓ or ↑; problems with vascular access; dialysis arthropathy (especially shoulders and wrists); aluminium toxicity; expense.

Continuous ambulatory peritoneal dialysis (CAPD): A permanent catheter is inserted into the peritoneum via a subcutaneous tunnel. ~2l dialysis fluid is introduced and kept in the peritoneum. This is changed for fresh fluid up to 5x/d.. This can be done at home and does not tie the patient to a dialysis machine.

Problems: peritonitis; catheter blockage (refer to renal unit as an emergency); weight ↑; poor diabetic control; pleural effusion; leakage.

Anaemia and erythropoietin: $2°$ anaemia due to ↓ kidney erythropoietin production is almost universal amongst people with ESRF. Exclude other causes. Recombinant erythropoietin is given if Hb<8.5g/dL (75% patients).

Renal transplantation: Transplanted kidneys are usually sited in an iliac fossa. Median cadaveric graft survival ≈8y. Closer genetic matches have better survival rates.

Problems
- Rejection
- Persistent ↑BP and ↑ cholesterol
- Atherosclerosis (5x ↑ risk MI death)
- Renal artery stenosis at 3–9mo. post-op
- Obstruction at ureteric anastamosis
- Ciclosporin-induced nephropathy
- Infection due to immunosuppression
- Malignancy from immunosuppressants

Patient support and information
UK National Kidney Federation ☎0845 601 02 09 🖳 http://www.kidney.org.uk
Kidney patient guide 🖳 http://kidneypatientguide.org.uk

Renal disease

Interstitial nephritis: Important cause of ARF and CRF. Associated with inflammatory cell infiltration of the renal interstitium and tubules.
- *Causes*
  - *Acute interstitial nephritis*—Idiosyncratic reaction to drugs (penicillin, NSAIDs, frusemide), infections (Staphylococcal., Streptococcal., Brucella, Leptospira).
  - *Chronic interstitial nephritis*—Idiopathic (most), drugs, sickle-cell disease, analgesic nephropathy.
- *Presentation:* ARF or CRF, raised temperature, arthralgia, eosinophilia.
- *Prognosis:* ARF—good; CRF—gradual deterioration.

Analgesic nephropathy: Caused by prolonged heavy use of analgesics (including NSAIDs). Presents with an interstitial nephritis-like picture. Associated with ↑ incidence UTI. Carcinoma of renal pelvis is a rare complication. Investigate promptly if the patient develops haematuria.

Glomerulonephritis
- *Terminology:* Focal—some glomeruli affected; diffuse—all glomeruli affected; segmental—part of each glomerulus affected; Global—all of each glomerulus is affected.
- *Presentation:* Nephrotic syndrome, renal failure, haematuria, oliguria, hypertension, proteinuria.
- *Investigation:* *Urine*—RBCs, proteinuria; *urine microscopy*—red cells, red cell casts; *blood*—U&E, creatinine, FBC, ESR. Further investigation can only be done in the $2°$ care system and involves renal biopsy ± light microscopy, electron microscopy, and/or immunofluorescence.
- *Management:* Refer all suspected cases urgently to a renal physician.

Table 20.3 Types of glomerulonephritis

Type	Features
Minimal change	Most common in children. Presents with nephrotic syndrome.
Membranous	30% adult nephrotic syndrome. Underlying malignancy in 10% adults. 25% enter remission, 50% progress to CRF in <10y.
Focal segmental glomerulosclerosis	Proteinuria or nephrotic syndrome. Seen with heroin abuse. >50% progress to CRF.
Membrano-proliferative	50% present as nephrotic syndrome. Associations—endocarditis, C3 nephritic factor (autoantibody), measles.
Proliferative	Classically seen 2wk. after Strep. infection. Prognosis is excellent.
IgA disease (Berger's disease)	Causes recurrent haematuria in young men. A similar histological picture is seen in Henoch-Schönlein purpura (📖 p.284). 30% progress to CRF.
Rapidly progressive/ crescentic	Presents with haematuria, oliguria, ↑ BP, acute renal failure. Vigorous treatment can save renal function. Associations—anti-glomerular basement membrane antibodies, Wegener's granulomatosis, Henoch-Schönlein purpura, post-streptococcal infection (rare).

Diabetic nephropathy: 📖 p.416

Adult polycystic kidney disease: Autosomal dominant disease (1:1000). Cysts develop anywhere in the kidney causing gradual ↓ in renal function. Common cause of CRF.

- *Presentation:* Haematuria, UTI, abdominal mass (30% have cysts in liver/pancreas too), lumbar/abdominal pain, ↑ BP.
- *Associated features:* Mitral valve prolapse, SAH/berry aneurysms.
- *Investigation: Blood*—urea, ↓ Hb. *USS*—large kidneys; multiple cysts.
- *Management:* Refer to a renal physician for monitoring of renal function. Treat infections and ↑ BP. Check family members (though cysts may not be seen <30y.).
- *Prognosis:* 45% patients will progress to end-stage renal failure by 60y.

Medullary sponge kidney: Developmental abnormality of the medullary pyramids of the kidney, characterized by dilatation of renal collecting tubules. ♂>♀. There may be a FH.

- *Presentation:* Most are asymptomatic and the condition is an incidental finding (found on 0.5% IVPs). If symptomatic, presents with UTIs, renal stones (found in 12% men and 19% women presenting with Ca^{2+} renal stones without predisposing metabolic abnormalities), haematuria.
- *Management:* Refer if symptomatic.
- *Prognosis:* Usually very good; most require no treatment.

Renal vein thrombosis (RVT)

- *Causes:* Nephrotic syndrome (15–20% develop RVT); membranous GN (30%); acute dehydration.
- *Presentation:* Varied—from no symptoms through to severe pain and loin tenderness. Suspect in at-risk individuals if unexplained loss renal function and RBCs in urine.
- *Management:* Refer to a renal physician for further investigation.

Renal artery stenosis

- *Causes:* Atheroma or fibromuscular hyperplasia (in the young).
- *Presentation:* ↑BP (may be severe or drug resistant); vascular disease elsewhere; abdominal bruit; ↑ urea; proteinuria. If bilateral or extensive—renal failure may be precipitated by dehydration, hypotension, or ACE inhibition (lowers GFR).
- *Management:* Refer for further investigation to a renal physician (if diagnosis is unsure) or vascular surgeon (if diagnosis is known).

Alport's syndrome: X-linked or autosomal recessive disease. Congenital sensorineural deafness with recurrent pyelonephritis, haematuria, and renal failure (from GN). Associated with lens abnormalities, platelet dysfunction, hyperproteinaemia. Causes death in males by 20–30y. without transplantation. Females have normal life expectancy. Renal failure does not recur after transplantation. *(A.C. Alport (1880–1959)—South African physician)*

Patient support and information
UK National Kidney Federation ☎0845 601 02 09 🖥 http://www.kidney.org.uk

Renal stones

Prevalence 0.2%; ♂:♀ ≈4:1; peak age 20–50y. Symptoms are not dependent on size of the stone.

Risk factors

- Dehydration
- Hypercalciuria/hypercalcaemia
- Gout and ↑ plasma urate
- UTI
- Medullary sponge kidney
- Cystinuria
- Renal tubular acidosis
- 1°/2° oxaluria

- Nephrocalcinosis
- Alkali loss from gut e.g. ileostomy—↑ uric acid stones
- Aminoaciduria
- Syndromes (Sjögren's syndrome, Lesch-Nyhan)
- FH (X-linked nephrolithiasis, cystinuria, hyperoxaluria)

Presentation: Usually presents with pain. Location and type of pain gives clues about the site of the stone:

- *Loin pain*—kidney stone
- *Renal colic*—ureteric stone

- *Strangury*—bladder stone
- *Interruption of urine flow*— urethral stone

Renal colic

- *Symptoms:* Severe pain which is always present but has waves of ↑ severity. Usually starts abruptly as flank pain which then radiates around abdomen to groin as stone progresses down ureter. May be referred to testis/tip of penis in man or labia majora in women. Occasionally, frank haematuria. May be past history or FH of renal stones.
- *Signs:* Patient is obviously in pain—usually unable to sit still and keeps shifting position to try to get comfortable (in contrast to peritonitis where patients tend to keep still). May be pale and sweaty. May be mild tenderness on deep abdominal palpation or loin tenderness, though often minimal signs. Occasionally, frank haematuria. If fever, suspect infection.

Other presentations: UTI, haematuria, renal failure.

Differential diagnosis: Acute appendicitis; diverticulitis; salpingitis; ovarian torsion; ruptured AAA; pyelonephritis; pethidine addiction.

Immediate investigations: Dipstick urine if possible for RBCs. If no RBCs, consider alternative diagnosis.

Immediate management: Stones usually pass spontaneously.
- Pain relief (diclofenac 75mg im/100mg pr or pethidine 50–100mg im)
- ↑ fluid intake (though avoid too much fluid)
- Sieve urine to catch stone for analysis
- Consider admission to hospital if: fever, oliguria, uncertain diagnosis, lives alone, analgesia ineffective or short-lived, symptoms continuing >24h.

Further investigation: If not admitted, investigate all patients. Investigations can wait until the next working day.
- *Urine*—M,C&S; RBCs. Consider checking pH of urine (>7.5—infective stones; <5.5—urate stones), checking 'spot' test for urine cystine, and requesting 24h. collection of urine for creatinine clearance, calcium, phosphate, and uric acid secretion.

- **Radiology**—KUB X-ray (90% renal stones are radio-opaque; only urate and xanthine stones are radio-transluscent); IVP.
- **Blood**—U&E, creatinine, Ca^{2+}, PO_4^{3-}, alkaline phosphatase, uric acid, albumin.
- **Recovered stones**—send for biochemical analysis.

Follow-up

- Give general advice on prevention of stones (Table 20.4).
- If investigations show any loss of renal function, renal obstruction, or remaining stones—refer to urology.
- Dependant on composition of stones, give dietary advice/refer to dietician (Table 20.4).

Table 20.4 Prevention of renal stones

Type of stone	Preventive measures
All types	↑ fluid intake (>3l/24h.) especially in hot weather; ↓ milk intake.
Calcium oxalate	Avoid chocolate, tea, rhubarb and spinach, nuts, beans, beetroot; ↓citrus fruits; bendroflumethiazide 2.5mg od may help if hypercalciuria; hyperoxaluria is treated with pyridoxine.
Calcium phosphate	Low Ca^{2+} diet; avoid vitamin D supplements. Bendroflumethiazide 2.5mg od may help if hypercalciuria.
Staghorn/triple phosphate (calcium, magnesium, and ammonium)	Associated with UTI due to Proteus species and urinary stasis. Treat UTI with antibiotics.
Urate	Allopurinol; urinary alkalinization with sodium bicarbonate (pH >6.5).
Cystine	Urinary alkalinization with sodium bicarbonate; d-penicillamine may be used as a chelating agent.

Hyperoxaluria: May be 1°(autosomal recessive condition) or 2° to gut resection/malabsorption. Take specialist advice on management.

- **Type 1 hyperoxaluria**—calcium oxalate stones are widely distributed throughout the body. Presents with renal stones and nephrocalcinosis in children. 80% have CRF in <20y.
- **Type 2 hyperoxaluria**—more benign but less common— Nephrocalcinosis but no CRF.

Cystinuria: Most common aminoaciduria. Usually presents with stones at age 10–30y. *Urine:* cystine ↑, ornithine ↑, arginine ↑, lysine ↑. Take specialist advice on management.

Hypercalcaemia: 📖 p.424

Benign prostatic hypertrophy (BPH)

10–30% of men in their early 70s have symptomatic BPH. There is no clear relation between prostatic volume and symptoms.

Symptoms

- *Obstructive*—↓ and intermittent urinary stream, double micturition, hesitancy, terminal dribbling, feeling of incomplete emptying and straining to void.
- *Irritative* (due to detrusor muscle hypertrophy)—urinary frequency, urgency, urge incontinence, and nocturia.

Complications: 10% at presentation

- Recurrent urinary tract infection (UTI)
- Bladder stones
- Haematuria
- Acute retention of urine—with or without prior obstructive symptoms (📖 p.690)
- Chronic obstruction (📖 p.691)
- Overflow incontinence (📖 p.695)
- Obstructive nephropathy

Assessment: Table 20.5

GP management: Studies suggest that symptoms can improve spontaneously but overall progress very slowly. 1–2%/y. develop urinary retention.

GP options

- *Watchful waiting:* Patients with mild to moderate symptoms at presentation with no complications of BPH and who are not severely troubled by their symptoms. Self-help includes: ↓ evening fluid intake; ↓ caffeine intake; bladder retraining; prevention of constipation.
- *Conventional drug therapy:* Those with mild to moderate symptoms who are troubled by their symptoms. *Consider:*
  - α—adrenoceptor agonists e.g. prazosin, doxazosin—watch for postural hypotension. ↓ symptomatic worsening[R].
  - 5-α-reductase inhibitors e.g. finasteride—best for patients with bulky prostates. Takes up to 6mo. to work. ↓ risk of urinary retention[R].
  - Combination therapy with an α-adrenoceptor agonist and 5-α-reductase inhibitor ↓ progression by 66%—more than either agent alone[R].
- *Alternative therapies:* There is some evidence that Serenoa repens (saw palmetto) is beneficial. Results of a large RCT are awaited.
- *Referral to urologist*
  - Complicated BPH (above)—*E/U*
  - Nodular/firm prostate on DRE—*U*
  - ↑ PSA—*U*
  - Severe symptoms—*S*
  - Failure to respond to drug therapy after 3–12mo. (α-blocker) or 6–12mo. (5-α-reductase inhibitor)—*R*

E = Emergency admission; U = Urgent; S = Soon; R = Routine

Table 20.5 Assessment of BPH

Assessment	Comments
History	<ul><li>General well-being</li><li>Obstructive symptoms</li><li>Irritative symptoms</li></ul> <ul><li>Haematuria</li><li>Pain</li><li>Polyuria and polydipsia</li><li>Neurological symptoms</li><li>Past history of urological instrumentation or STDs</li></ul>
Frequency—volume chart	Assess pattern and type of fluid consumption (e.g. alcohol/caffeine at night ↑ nocturia).
Symptom score (IPSS— 📖 p.704)	Objectively grade symptoms giving measure of severity. IPSS scores: <ul><li>0–7 = mild</li><li>8–19 = moderate</li><li>20–35 = severe</li></ul> A general quality of life measurement can be used to assess impact of symptoms.
Abdominal examination	Look for distended bladder, palpable kidneys. Examine external genitalia.
Digital rectal examination	Anal tone, size, shape, and consistency of prostate (normal prostate—size of a chestnut with smooth, rubbery consistency).
Serum urea and creatinine	Renal function assessment.
MSU	Dipstick for blood and glucose. M,C&S.
Ultrasound measurement of post-micturition residual*	
Maximum voiding flow rate*	<15ml/s. for voided volume >100ml/s is abnormal.
Serum PSA	High values can indicate prostate cancer (📖 p.305).

* May be available through open-access prostate assessment clinics.

Further information

McConnell JD *et al* (2003). The long term effect of doxazosin, finasteride and combination therapy on the clinical progression of benign prostatic hyperplasia *NEJM* **349**: 2387–98

Prostate cancer

Prostate cancer is the 6th most common cancer worldwide and kills 9000men/y. in the UK. 1:6 men have clinical prostate cancer in their lifetimes and the incidence is rising.

Classification

- **Non-metastatic prostate cancer:** Can be divided into:
  - Clinically localized disease—cancer thought after clinical examination, to be confined to the prostate gland.
  - Locally advanced disease—cancer that has spread outside the capsule of the prostate gland but has not yet spread to other organs.
- **Metastatic prostate cancer:** Cancer that has spread outside the prostate gland to local, regional, or systemic LNs, seminal vesicles, or other body organs (e.g. bone, liver, brain).

Risk factors

- **Age:** Uncommon <50y.; 85% of men with prostate cancer are diagnosed aged >65y.
- **Genetic:** ↑ incidence if 1st degree relative affected.
- **Racial:** Incidence varies according to location in the world and ethnic group. Highest rates are in men of black ethnic group in the USA; lowest in Chinese men.
- **Dietary:** Links are proposed between prostate cancer and low intake of fruit (particularly tomatoes) and high intake of fat, meat, and Ca^{2+}.

Screening: 📖 p.160 and p.305

Symptoms and signs

- **Early cancer:** Symptomless. Usually detected following an incidental finding of ↑ PSA. Hard nodule sometimes felt in prostate on DRE.
- **Local disease:** Prostatism, urinary retention, haematuria, lower extremity oedema—prostate is hard, non-tender and sulci lose definition.
- **Metastatic disease:** Weight loss, bone pain, pathological fractures, spinal cord compression, malaise. Ureteric obstruction can cause renal failure. Signs depend on site of metastases.

Investigations: ↑PSA—though in early cancer may be normal and there are other reasons for ↑PSA (📖 p.305).

Management: Refer all suspected cases to urology for histological confirmation and advice on management.

Treatment options

Symptomless local disease: ◆ Controversial. 2 arguments:

As nothing proved beneficial, benefits of treatment are outweighed by risks	*or*	Aggressive treatment before spread is the only way to ensure cure.

The picture is further complicated as >50% men >50 y. of age dying from other causes are found, post-mortem, to have prostate cancer—prostate cancer kills only a small minority of men who have it. The personal and economic cost of treating men whose cancer would never have caused them any problems must be considered.

Options
- *Watchful waiting:* Monitor with PSA /DRE. ↑ in PSA or size of nodule triggers active treatment. At 10y. follow-up <10% with moderately well-differentiated cancer will have died from their cancer. Progression rates are higher in patients with poorly differentiated cancer.
- *Radical prostatectomy:* Has potential for cure but in the age group most affected by prostate cancer mortality is 1.4%. Other common complications: impotence (50%), incontinence (25%).
- *Radiotherapy:* May not be effective—persistent cancer is found in 30% on biopsy.
- *Hormone treatment:* No convincing evidence gives survival benefit in early disease.

Symptomatic disease: 30% 5y. survival. Hormone manipulation is the mainstay of treatment and gives 80% ↓ in bone pain, PSA, or both and a lower incidence of serious complications (e.g. spinal cord compression) if treatment starts at the time of diagnosis. *Options:*
- *Luteinizing hormone releasing hormone (LHRH) analogues:* e.g. goserelin; sc injection every 4–12wk. (depending on the preparation used). Testosterone levels ↓ to levels of castrated men in <2mo. *Side-effects:* impotence, hot flushes, gynaecomastia, local bruising and infection around injection site. When starting LHRH analogues, LH level initially ↑ which can cause increased tumour activity or 'flare'. Counteracted by prescription of anti-androgens (e.g. flutamide) for a few days before administration of the first dose of LHRH and concurrently for 3wk. Response in most patients lasts for 12–18mo.
- *Anti-androgens:* e.g. cyproterone actetate, flutamide, biclutamide. Anti-androgens do not suppress androgen production completely. Used to prevent side-effects due to testosterone flare during initiation of LHRH analogues, as monotherapy in those who find LHRH analogues unsuitable (flutamide 250mg tds—monitor liver function if used long term), and in combination with LHRH analogues to produce maximum androgen blockade.
- *Surgical castration:* ↓ testosterone secretion permanently without the need for medication. Cheap and fewer side-effects than other options.

Bony metastases: In addition to hormone therapy, local radiotherapy and corticosteroids are used for bone pain. Radioactive strontium ↓ the number of new sites of bone pain developed. Mean survival <5y.

Hormone resistant disease: No agreed treatment. There is some evidence that prednisolone 5mg daily or stilboestrol 3mg daily is helpful.

Further information
NICE (2002) Improving outcomes in urological cancers
  ▣ http://www.nice.org.uk

Patient support and information
The Prostate Cancer Charity ☎0845 300 8383 ▣ http://www.prostate-cancer.org.uk
Prostate Cancer Support Association ☎0845 601 0766
  ▣ http://www.prostatecancersupport.co.uk

Urinary tract obstruction

⚠ Consider urinary tract obstruction whenever renal function deteriorates.

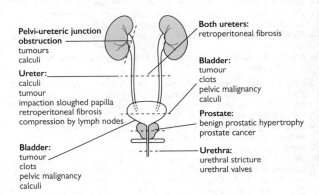

Pelvi-ureteric junction obstruction
tumours
calculi

Ureter:
calculi
tumour
impaction sloughed papilla
retroperitoneal fibrosis
compression by lymph nodes

Bladder:
tumour
clots
pelvic malignancy
calculi

Both ureters:
retroperitoneal fibrosis

Bladder:
tumour
clots
pelvic malignancy
calculi

Prostate:
benign prostatic hypertrophy
prostate cancer

Urethra:
urethral stricture
urethral valves

Figure 20.1 Causes of urinary tract obstruction

Causes of obstruction: Figure 20.1. Obstruction may be:
- unilateral (kidney, pelvi-ureteric junction, or ureter)
- bilateral (bladder, urethra)

❶ Unilateral obstruction may present late if the other kidney remains functioning. Suspect if loin ache worsened by drinking. Confirm with USS. Refer to urology.

Obstructing lesions may be:
- in the lumen e.g. stones
- in the wall e.g. tumours
- impinging from outside e.g. retroperitoneal fibrosis

Acute retention of urine: Sudden inability to pass urine → lower abdominal discomfort with inability to keep still. Differentiate from other causes of anuria. ♂ >> ♀. *Risk factors:* Age >70y., symptoms of prostatism or poor urinary stream.

Causes
- ♂: Prostatic obstruction (82%). Precipitated by constipation, alcohol, drugs (anticholinergics, diuretics), UTI, operation (e.g. day case hernia repair).
- ♀: Gynaecological pathology—ovarian cancer, fibromas, prolapse.
- *Rarer causes:* Urethral stricture, clot retention, spinal cord compression, bladder stone.

Examination
- Abdomen—palpable bladder
- DRE—enlarged ± irregular prostate
- Perineal sensation

Investigation: MSU to exclude infection. U&E, Cr.

Management: Catheterize (record initial volume drained) *or* refer to urology for catheterization—local policies vary. Treat infection. Refer to DN for instruction on management of the catheter. Refer to urology for further assessment and treatment.

Chronic retention of urine: Insidious onset.

Causes: BPH, pelvic malignancy, CNS disease.

Presentation: May present as:
- nocturnal enuresis
- overflow incontinence
- acute or chronic retention
- lower abdominal mass
- UTI
- renal failure

Examination: As for acute retention. Bladder is enlarged (may contain >1.5l) but usually non-tender.

Investigation: MSU to exclude infection, urine dipstick for blood, FBC, U&E, Cr.

Management: Refer to urology for further assessment and treatment. Refer urgently or acutely if pain, UTI, or renal failure (urea >12mmol/l). *Do not* catheterize in the community.

Retroperitoneal fibrosis: Ureters become embedded in dense fibrous plaques in the retroperitoneal space.

Associations: Drugs (methysergide); carcinoma; Crohn's disease; connective tissue disease; Raynaud's syndrome, and fibrotic diseases (e.g. alveolitis).

Presentation: Typically, middle-aged men presenting with fever, malaise, sweating, leg oedema, ↑BP, palpable mass, ARF or CRF.

Management: Refer for specialist care. Options include steroids and nephrostomies.

Horseshoe kidney: Congenital abnormality. Kidneys are fused in the midline to form a horseshoe-shaped mass. The kidney may function normally or may present with obstructive nephropathy or UTIs.

Urinary tract infection (UTI)

UTI is one of the most common conditions seen in general practice accounting for up to 6% consultations ♀>>♂. 20% of women at any time have asymptomatic bacteriuria and 20–40% of women will have a UTI in their lifetime. *Infecting organisms: E. coli* (>70%), Proteus sp., Pseudomonas sp., Streptococci, Staphylococci.

Risk factors
- Prior infection
- DM
- Pregnancy
- Stones
- Dehydration
- GU instrumentation
- Catheterization
- Sexual intercourse
- Diaphragm use
- ↓ oestrogen (menopause)
- Urinary stasis (e.g. obstruction)
- Genito-urinary (GU) malformations
- Delayed micturition (e.g. on long journeys)

Presentations
- *Cystitis:* Frequency, dysuria, urgency, strangury, low abdominal pain, incontinence of urine, acute retention of urine, cloudy or offensive urine, and/or haematuria.
- *Pyelonephritis:* Loin pain, fever, rigors, malaise, vomiting, and/or haematuria.

Initial investigation: If uncomplicated UTI in an otherwise healthy woman, test urine with a leucocyte esterase and nitrate dipstick. If +ve, treat for UTI. *Reasons to send MSU for M,C&S:*

- Unresolved infection after antibiotics
- Recurrent UTI
- Uncatheterized man with UTI
- Catheterized man or woman with symptomatic UTI
- Child—📖 p.852
- Pregnant woman—📖 p.789
- Suspected pyelonephritis
- Haematuria (microscopic or macroscopic) always investigate further—📖 p.265

❶ MSUs should be taken prior to starting antibiotics and sent to the laboratory fresh.

Further investigation: Consider further investigation with blood tests (U&E, Cr, and/or PSA if >40y. and ♂) and/or radiology (renal tract USS, KUB, IVP) if:

- UTI in a man
- UTI in a child (📖 p.852)
- Recurrent UTI in a woman
- Pyelonephritis
- Unclear diagnosis (e.g. persisting symptoms but negative MSU)
- Unusual infecting organism

Management: Catheterized patients—📖 p.697

Pregnant women—📖 p.789

Children—📖 p.852

All other patients:
- ↑fluid intake (>3l/24h.)
- *Alkalinize urine* (e.g. potassium citrate solution) to ease symptoms
- *Oral antibiotics:* Trimethoprim 200mg bd is a good first choice—80% organisms are sensitive. Use a 3d. course for women with uncomplicated UTI. Use a 2wk. course for men, patients with GU malformations

or immunosuppression, relapse (same organism), or recurrent UTI (different organism). Use a 14d. course of a quinolone (e.g. ciprofloxacin 250–500mg bd) for patents with pyelonephritis.

- **Admission to hospital:** Rarely required if dehydrated or extremely systemically unwell.
- **Referral to urology:** If any abnormalities are detected on further investigation or unable to resolve symptoms.

Prevention of recurrent cystitis: Reinfection after successful treatment of infection (90%) or relapse after inadequate treatment.

- **General advice:** Advise patients to urinate frequently; ↑ fluid intake; double void (i.e. go again after 5–10 min.), and void after intercourse. Efficacy of cranberry juice is controversial.
- **Prophylactic antibiotics:** Consider prescribing either post-coitally (e.g. nitrofurantoin 50mg stat) or continuously (trimethoprim 100mg nocte or nitrofurantoin 50mg nocte).
- **Men with BPH:** Finasteride and/or doxazosin ↓ incidence of UTI.
- **HRT:** Topical oestrogen ↓ recurrent UTI in women of all ages[R].
- **Vaccines:** Results of large-scale trials are awaited.

Prostatitis: Consider acute prostatitis in all men presenting with symptoms of UTI. Treat with 4wk. course of oral antibiotic which penetrates prostatic tissue e.g. trimethoprim 200mg bd.

Chronic pyelonephritis: Presents as chronic renal failure or one of its complications. Probably arises from UTIs, vesico-ureteric reflux, and consequent renal scarring in childhood (📖 p.852). Refer for specialist advice on management.

Urethral syndrome: Symptoms of cystitis with –ve MSU. Unknown cause. Associated with cold, stress, nylon underwear, COC pill, and intercourse. Advise patients to drink fluids ++ and wear cotton underwear. Consider changing/stopping COC pill, or trying topical oestrogen if postmenopausal. Tetracyclines (e.g doxycycline 100mg bd for 14d.) or azithromycin (500mg od for 6d.)[R] are helpful in some patients. If not settling, refer to urology. Urethral dilatation/massage may be helpful.

Interstitial cystitis: Predominantly affects middle-aged women. Can cause fibrosis of the bladder wall. Main symptoms—frequency, urgency, and suprapubic pain, especially when the bladder is full. Often misdiagnosed as recurrent UTI. MSU—no bacteriuria. Refer to urologist for confirmation. There is no satisfactory treatment though antispasmodics, amitriptyline, and bladder stretching under anaesthetic may help some patients.

Sterile pyuria: Presence of white cells in the urine in the absence of UTI. *Causes:*

- Inadequately treated UTI
- Appendicitis
- Calculi
- Prostatitis
- Bladder tumour
- Renal TB
- Papillary necrosis
- UTI with failure to culture organism
- Interstitial nephritis or cystitis
- Polycystic kidney
- Chemical cystitis e.g. due to radiotherapy

Management: Initially repeat with clean catch MSU. If finding persists, refer to urology.

Incontinence of urine

Involuntary loss of urine which is objectively demonstrable and a social or hygienic problem. 14% women aged 30–70y. admitted incontinence (♂:♀≈1:2) in a MORI poll. This is probably an underestimate. 1:3 with incontinence consult at outset, 1:3 consult later, 1:3 suffer in silence. Opportunistic questioning can identify sufferers.

Presentation
History
- Frequency of complaint
- Degree of incapacity
- Whether occurs with standing/coughing/sneezing
- Urgency/dysuria/frequency of micturition
- Volume passed
- Past obstetric and medical history
- Medication
- Mobility
- Accessibility of toilets

Examination
- *Abdominal including DRE*—enlarged bladder, masses, loaded colon, faecal impaction, anal tone.
- *Pelvic*—prolapse, atrophy, neurological deficit, retention of urine, and pelvic masses.

Investigation: Intake/output diary—evaluates problem and benchmark for progress (record drinks and passage of urine over a week); urine, glucose, RBCs, MC&S; consider U&E/FBG if renal impairment/DM is suspected.

Drugs that exacerbate/cause incontinence: Diuretics, antihistamines, anxiolytics, α–blockers, sedatives and hypnotics, anticholinergic drugs, TCAs.

GP management: ❶ 30 % have a mixed pattern.
General measures
- Manipulate fluid intake—amount, type (avoid tea, coffee, alcohol), timing
- Alter medication e.g. timing of diuretics
- Treat UTI and chronic respiratory conditions
- Avoid constipation
- Promote weight ↓
- Consider HRT (topical or systemic) for oestrogen deficiency.

Nocturnal enuresis: 📖 p. 894

Stress incontinence
- *Symptoms:* Small losses of urine without warning throughout the day related to coughing/exercise.
- *Causes:* Prostatectomy; childbirth; deterioration of pelvic floor muscles/nerves.
- *Treatment:* Pelvic floor exercises (📖 p.711) continued >3mo. help 60% (taught by physiotherapists/continence advisors; leaflets available)—may be assisted by vaginal cones and/or electrical stimulation. Mechanical devices (e.g. Conveen continence guard®) help 75%.

Urge incontinence: Detrusor instability or hyperreflexia cause the bladder to contract unintentionally.
- *Symptoms:* Frequency, overwhelming desire to void (often precipitated by stressful event), large loss, nocturia.
- *Causes:* Idiopathic, neurological problems (stroke, MS, DM, spinal cord injury, dementia, PD), local irritation (bladder stones, infection), obstruction (BPH), surgery (TURP).
- *Treatment:* Try bladder training programmes—resist the urge to pass urine for increasing periods. Start with an achievable interval based on diary evidence and ↑ slowly. Drugs are helpful e.g. oxybutinin, imipramine (nocturnal symptoms). Spontaneously remits/relapses, so reassess every 3–4mo.

Overflow
- *Symptoms:* Constant dribbling loss day and night.
- *Causes:* BPH, prostate cancer, urethral stricture, faecal impaction, neurological (LMN lesions), side-effect of medication.
- *Treatment:* Aimed at relieving the obstruction (📖 p.690).

Urinary fistula: Communication between bladder and the outside—normally through vagina. Results in constant dribbling loss day and night. Refer to gynaecology/urology. *Causes:* Congenital, malignancy, complication of surgery.

Functional incontinence: No urological problem. Caused by other factors e.g. inaccessible toilets/immobility, behavioural problems, cognitive deficit. Treat the cause.

Table 20.6 Referral for incontinence problems

Specialist continence advisor (or DN)	Urodynamic Studies	Gynaecology/ urology opinion
• Advice on aids or appliances • Advice on primary care management • Patient support	• If type of incontinence is uncertain • Atypical features of incontinence • After unsuccessful surgery • If neurological problem is suspected	• GP management has failed • Severe symptoms • Concomitant gynaecological problems (e.g. prolapse) • Concomitant urological problems (e.g. chronic retention) • Failed incontinence surgery • Vesico-vaginal fistula • Haematuria

Aids and appliances: 📖 p.696

Further information
Association for Continence Advice: Advice for healthcare professionals ☎020 8692 4680
🖥 http://www.aca.uk.com

Patient information and support
The Continence Foundation ☎0845 345 0165 🖥 http://www.continence-foundation.org.uk

Aids and appliances for incontinence

Pads: Many different types. DNs or continence advisors are best aware of those available via the NHS locally. They cannot be prescribed on FP10. Supplied by local NHS Trusts on a 'daily allowance' basis. This varies across the country.

Bed covers: Absorb 1–4l of urine. Good laundry facilities are needed. If left wet can cause skin breakdown. Available via NHS Trusts.

External catheters or sheaths/conveens: Can be prescribed on NHS prescription. Approved appliances are listed in Part IXB of the UK Drug Tariff. Used for men who have intractable incontinence and who are highly physically dependent, don't have urine retention, and don't require an internal catheter. Assessment and fitting is essential by DN or continence advisor. Used in association with drainage bag (opposite).

Types:
- **Self-adhesive** e.g. Bard (Integrity) or attached with adhesive strips e.g. NorthWest Medical (Uridrop and Uristrip). Adhesive sheaths can last several days but daily changing is recommended.
- **Non-adhesive** e.g. Manfred Sauer (Comfort sheath). Replace non-adhesive sheaths 2–3 x/d.. Some are re-usable e.g. Bard (Urosheath).

Problems: Include ↑ susceptibility to UTI, sores on penis, and skin irritation due to the adhesive.

Catheters: Can be prescribed on NHS prescription. Approved appliances are listed in Part IXA of the UK Drug Tariff.

Indwelling catheters: Only use catheters in patients who have:
- Urinary retention or neurogenic bladder dysfunction
- Severe pressure sores
- Inoperable obstructions that prevent the bladder emptying
- Terminal illness
- Housebound without adequate carer support.

Types: Only long-term Foley catheters are suitable for use in primary care. They last 3–12wk.
- Hydrogel coated e.g. Bard (Biocath®)
- Silicone elastomer coated latex e.g. Bard, Rüsch (Sympacath®)
- All silicone e.g. Coloplast, Medasil, Rüsch (Brilliant Aquaflate®)

Catheter size: Unless specified, a 12 or 14Ch catheter is supplied. Use smallest diameter of catheter that drains urine effectively. Catheters >16Ch are more likely to cause bypassing of urine around the catheter and urethral strictures.

Catheter length: Men require longer catheters than women. Specify 'male' or 'female' on the prescription.

Catheter balloon: 10ml balloons are supplied unless specified otherwise. Pre-filled catheters contain sterile water which inflates the retaining balloon with water. They are more expensive but quicker to insert and there are no costs for syringes or sterile water.

Insertion: See Oxford Handbook of Clinical medicine for detailed instructions.

Drainage: Usually attached to a leg bag, though catheter valves are also available allowing the patient to use his/her bladder as a urine reservoir. The valve must be released every 3–4h. to drain out the urine.

Common problems

- *Leakage:* Check no constipation, and catheter not blocked; try smaller gauge catheter.
- *Infection:* 90% develop bacteriuria <4 wk. after insertion. Always confirm suspected UTI with MSU—only treat if symptomatic or *Proteus* species grown. May prove difficult to eliminate. No good evidence bladder instillations help.
- *Encrustation (50%):* Deposition of minerals and other materials from the urine onto the catheter. Worse if there is infection with *Proteus* species. May cause catheter blockage or pain changing catheter. Check pH of urine regularly in patients with problems. Citric acid patency solutions may help if pH >7.4 or a daily dose of vitamin C.
- *Inflammation:* Results from physical presence of a catheter in the urethra. Exacerbated by encrustation and infection. There is no easy solution—try a different brand catheter (e.g. hydrogel catheter rather than silicone).
- *Blockage:* Change catheter. The interval of routine changes should be altered if there is regular blockage towards the end of the life of a catheter.

Intermittent self-catheterization: Patient inserts a catheter into his/her bladder 4–5x/d. to drain urine. ↓ problems of infection and blockage. Useful for neurological bladder dysfunction. *Types:*
- *Reusable silver or stainless steel* e.g. Malvern (Biscath®).
- *Reusable PVC* e.g. Bard (Reliacath®), Rüsch (Riplex®)—can be washed and reused for 1wk. Usually supply 5/mo.
- *Single use* e.g. Astra Tech (Lofric®)—need 125—150 /mo. Expensive. Only use on consultant advice.

Collecting bags: Can be prescribed on NHS prescription. Approved appliances are listed in Part IXB of the UK Drug Tariff.
- *Leg bags:* Drainable bags last 5–7d.. Usually 500/750mls e.g. Bard (Uriplan®). Larger capacity bags are too heavy for mobile patients. A variety of attachment systems are available on prescription. Long tubes are needed to wear a bag on the calf.
- *Night drainage bags:* Connect to night bag attachment of day bags. Single use, disposable, non-draining bags are recommended e.g. Coloplast (Simpla S2®), Bard (Uriplan®). Bag hangers are not available on FP10.

Enuresis alarms: 📖 p.895

Urostomy appliances: 📖 p.470

Further information
PPA Electronic Drug Tariff 🖥 *http://www.ppa.org.uk*

Patient advice and support
The Continence Foundation ☎0845 345 0165 🖥 *http://www.continence-foundation.org.uk*

Penile and testicular conditions

Torsion of the testis: Peak age 15–30y.

Presentation: Sudden onset severe scrotal pain. May be associated with RIF pain, nausea, and vomiting. *Examination:* Tender, hard testis riding higher than contralateral testis.

Action: Admit urgently to surgical/urology team

Epididymo-orchitis: Inflammation of the testis and epididymis due to infection. The most common viral cause is mumps. The most common bacterial infections are gonococci and coliforms. May occur at any age. Chronic infection with TB or syphilis is rare.

Presentation: Acute onset pain in testis; swelling and tenderness of testis/epididymis; fever ± rigors; may be dysuria and ↑ frequency.

Management: May be difficult to distinguish from torsion of the testis. If in doubt, admit for urology/surgical opinion.

Testicular cancer: 📖 p.700

Benign testicular tumours: Rare (<2% tumours). Sertoli cell adenomas; Leydig cell adenomas. Produce sex hormones and cause feminization/masculinization respectively. Refer.

Absent/undescended/retractile testis: 📖 p.248 and p.840

Hydrocoele: Collection of fluid in tunica vaginalis. Occurs at any age.
- 1° *hydrocoele*—no predisposing cause in scrotum.
- 2° *hydrocoele*—reaction to pathology in testis or covering (infection, tumour, torsion). In adults presenting with hydrocoele, always consider impalpable tumour beneath.

Presentation: Swelling in the scrotum. The examiner should be able to get above swelling. Smooth surface, transilluminates, testis is within the swelling and not palpable separately.

Management: Investigation is not required in children; refer adults for USS if testis is not palpable. Further management:
- *Children:* 📖 p.840
- *Adults*
  - Conservative management—reassurance is all that is required for small hydrocoeles.
  - Tapping—may be suitable for large hydrocoeles where surgery is inappropriate—2° infection and recurrence are common.
  - Surgery—refer to urologist.

Hydrocoele of the cord: Arises in part of processus vaginalis in the spermatic cord above the testis. Rounded lump which slips up and down the inguinal canal. No action needed.

Varicocoele: Collection of varicose veins in the pampiniform plexus of cord and scrotum. Can be 2° to obstruction of the testicular veins in the abdomen. L > R. Associated with infertility (thought due to ↑ temperature of testis due to varicocoele).

- *Presentation:* Dull ache in the testis, especially at the end of the day or after exercise.
- *Examination:* Varicocoele is usually visible when standing.
- *Management:* Reassurance. Occasionally surgery may help if symptoms are severe.

Epididymal cysts: Common and often multiple. Found in middle-aged/elderly men. Usually present when the patient finds a lump.
- *Examination:* Smooth-walled cysts in epididymis (palpable above and behind testis), often bilateral.
- *Investigation:* If unsure of diagnosis, refer for USS.
- *Management:* Reassurance. Refer to urology if painful.

Peyronie disease: Hard lumps in the shaft of the penis. Cause un-known. Affects 4% men >40y. 1:3 affected have pain or bending of the penis when erect. Associated with impotence (📖 p.702). 5% have Dupy-trens contracture. (*F. de la Peyronie (1678–1747)—French surgeon*).

Management: Reassurance usually suffices. No proven medical treat-ments, though vitamin E (200mg tds) and para-aminobenzoate in large doses are used. Refer to urology for surgery if pain or severe bending on erection so that intercourse is not possible.

Non-retractile foreskin: Usually noted by parents. May be history of recurrent balanitis. *Examination:* Foreskin adherent.

Management: Age <4y.—do nothing unless recurrent balanitis. If >4y.—refer to paediatric surgery.

Phimosis: Foreskin obstructs urine flow. Common in small children. Time usually obviates need for circumcision. Refer if recurrent balanitis.

Paraphimosis: Foreskin is retracted, then (due to oedema) unable to be replaced. Commonly occurs in catheterized patients when the cathe-ter is changed.

Management: Try to replace foreskin using ice packs (↓ swelling) and lubrication (e.g. KY jelly). If unable to replace the foreskin, admit for surgery.

Balanitis: Acute inflammation of glans and foreskin. Common organ-isms—*staphylococci, streptococci, coliforms, candida.* Can occur at any age. Most common in young boys when associated with non-retractile fore-skin/phimosis. In elderly patients, consider DM.

Management: Oral antibiotics. If recurrent or due to phimosis, consider referral for circumcision.

Balanitis xerotica et obliterans: Chronic fibrosing condition of foreskin thought to be viral in origin. No specific treatment.

Trauma to the foreskin: Torn frenulum—seen after poorly lubri-cated intercourse or if caught in a zip. No treatment required. If recur-rent, consider referral for circumcision.

Priapism: 📖 p.280

Urological malignancy

Bladder cancer: Incidence: 1:5000; $\male : \female \approx 3:1$. Transitional cell carcinoma (TCC) is most common in the UK; squamous cell carcinoma (SCC) worldwide.

Risk factors
- Smoking (½ male and ¼ female cases are attributable to smoking)
- Aromatic amine exposure (textile or rubber industries)
- Schistosomiasis (SCC)
- Stasis of urine
- Chronic UTI

Presentation: Haematuria (painless or painful). Less common—recurrent UTI, frequency, loin pain, pelvic pain, bladder outflow obstruction.

Investigation: MSU—exclude UTI; detection of sterile pyuria and/or microscopic haematuria.

Management: Refer urgently to urology if suspected. Most urology departments have one-stop haematuria clinics offering rapid out-patient assessment of haematuria. Treatment depends on stage at diagnosis:
- *T1:* (80%)   Disease confined to mucosa/submucosa. Transurethral resection of the tumour (TURBT) ± single intravesical chemotherapy treatment. Follow-up is with regular cystoscopy. Very good prognosis—most die from other causes.
- *T2:*   TURBT ± radiotherapy. Follow-up as for T1. 60% survive 5y.
- *T3:*   Radical cystectomy and/or radiotherapy. 40–50% 5y. survival.
- *T4:*   Spread beyond the bladder. TURBT for local symptoms. Palliative radiotherapy ± chemotherapy. Palliative care (📖 p.999–1015). 20–30% 5y. survival; less if para-aortic nodes are involved.

Testicular cancer: Most common malignancy in men age 20–34y.. A devastating disease for sufferers who tend to be young and fit and don't expect to be ill. Screening is not effective. Education to ensure men check their testes for lumps regularly and present early is preferable.

Risk factors
- Undescended testes—bilateral undescended testis → 10x ↑ risk
- Past history testicular cancer—4% risk 2nd cancer

Presentation: Painless lump in testis. Occasionally testicular pain or 2° hydrocoele. May present with metastases—back pain/dyspnoea.

Types of testicular cancer: Table 20.7

Management: Testicular lumps are tumours until proven otherwise. Refer for urgent urological opinion. USS can help diagnosis but *don't* delay referral. Definitive diagnosis is only made at biopsy. Specialist treatment depends on tumour type and extent. Sperm banking is routinely offered in case of ↓ fertility due to treatment. Children conceived of men treated for testicular cancer are not at ↑ risk of congenital abnormality.

Table 20.7 Types and features of testicular cancer

	Seminoma (60%)	**Teratoma**
Typical age	30–40y.	<30y.
Tumour markers	None	β-HCG
		α-FP
		LDH—correlates with volume of metastatic disease
Nature of tumour	Solid	Solid/cystic components
		40% occur within seminomas; mixed tumours are treated like teratomas
Speed of growth	Slow growing	Fast growing—can double in size in days
Stage of presentation	90% stage 1 (tumour confined to testis)	60% stage 1
Treatment	• Treated with inguinal orchidectomy and radiotherapy • Relapses are treated with chemotherapy. • More advanced disease is treated with radio- or chemotherapy.	• Treatment of stage 1 disease is with inguinal orchidectomy and surveillance of tumour markers; 25% relapse in <18 mo. • Treatment of relapses and metastatic disease is with chemotherapy
Survival	98% 5y. survival for stage 1 disease. Overall >85% 5y. survival.	Prognosis depends on stage and degree of differentiation

Hypernephroma: Clear cell adenocarcinoma of renal tubular epithelium. Typical age: 50 y.. ♂:♀ ≈2:1. Spread can be local or haematogenous (bone, liver, lung—causes cannon ball metastases seen on CXR).

Presentation: Haematuria, loin pain, abdominal mass. occasionally night sweats, ↑ PCV (2%), anaemia, hypercalcaemia, left varicocoele.

Investigations: *Urine:* RBCs; *radiology:* USS, CXR.

Management: Refer all suspected cases to urology urgently. Treatment includes nephrectomy ± immunotherapy with interleukin-2. 30–50% 5y. survival.

Wilms nephroblastoma: 📖 p.880

Prostate cancer: 📖 p.688

Carcinoma of the penis: Squamous cell carcinoma (95%) or malignant melanoma. Usually elderly men. Rare in the UK. Refer urgently to urology.

Further information

NICE (2005) Referral guidelines for suspected cancer 🖥 http://www.nice.org.uk

Erectile dysfunction

Persistent inability to obtain or maintain sufficient rigidity of the penis to allow satisfactory sexual performance. 1:10 men suffer to varying degrees but 90% are too embarrassed to seek help from their GP. Incidence ↑ with age.

Causes

- *Organic (80%)*—peripheral vascular disease, DM (>35% of diabetic men are impotent), neurological disorders (e.g. pelvic surgery, spinal injury, multiple sclerosis), side-effects of drugs, smoking, alcohol and drug abuse, Peyronie's disease (🕮 p. 699), testosterone deficiency, or hyperprolactinaemia.
- *Psychogenic*—performance anxiety, depression, stress, relationship failure, fear of intimacy.

Drugs causing impotence: Antihypertensives (especially thiazides), antidepressants (e.g. SSRIs), major tranquillizers, anti-androgens, finasteride and cimetidine.

History: Ensure the presenting problem is erectile dysfunction and not other sexual difficulties; identify risk factors (see above); distinguish psychogenic from organic causes (Table 20.8).

❶ Many whose impotence was originally organic develop a psychogenic component which may perpetuate symptoms.

Table 20.8 Deciding whether impotence is organic or psychogenic

	Psychogenic origin	**Organic origin**
Onset sudden or gradual?	Sudden onset	Gradual onset
Consistent loss of erections?	Inconsistent response	Consistent failure
Does the patient ever wake up with an erection?	Early-morning erections	Loss of early-morning erections
Does the patient want to have intercourse?	Relationship problems	Normal libido
Age?	Usually <60y.	Usually >60y.

Examination and investigation

- Testosterone insufficiency—genitals (small/absent), breasts and beard growth (↓ frequency of shaving); measure serum testosterone ± prolactin if suspected
- Peripheral vascular disease—peripheral pulses
- Psychological distress—mental state
- Check BP and urine for glucose

GP management: Counsel the couple about the problem, its possible causes, and management.

- Advice on lifestyle—↓ smoking and alcohol.
- Discuss pros and cons of available treatment options and select treatment—Table 20.9. All treatments work well for psychogenic and less well for organic causes.

- Review progress—adjust dosage, consider other treatment options or referral to urologist.
- Psychogenic impotence—📖 p.747.

Referral: Options:
- *Urologist:* If the patient has never had an erection, has a severe vascular problem, lack of success in general practice, or severe psychological distress due to impotence.
- *Endocrinologist:* Hormone abnormalities (e.g. ↓ androgen, ↑ prolactin)—treatment does not always restore potency.
- *Psychiatrist/psychosexual counsellor:* Age <40y. and no evidence organic cause; psychosexual problem.

Table 20.9 Treatment of impotence *(BNF 7.4.5)*

Treatment	Notes
Oral drugs	
• Phospho-diesterase type 5 inhibitors e.g. sildenafil[S]	Effective for 70%. Use prn ~1h. before intercourse. Only use 1x/d. Avoid if patient has unstable angina, recent stroke, or MI. **Do not** give a nitrate within 24h. of use.
• Apomorphine	2–3mg prn 20 min. before sexual activity.
• Yohimbine[S]	Available OTC. 10–30mg od is effective. May cause insomnia.
Local drug treatments	
• Intraurethral or intracavernosal alprostadil	Intraurethral preparation is effective for 40% and intracavernosal preparation for 80% patients. Used prn. Requires some manual dexterity. Takes ≈10min. to work. Penile pain is common. Prolonged erection and priapism results in ≈1%. Advise patients to seek medical help if erection >4h.
Mechanical devices	
• Vacuum devices	Effective for 80%. The penis is placed in the device and air withdrawn mechanically sucking blood into the penis. Erection is maintained by placing a constriction band around the base of the penis.
• Penile prosthesis	Last resort. May be inflatable or rigid. Major complication is infection.
Others	
• Androgen supplements	Ineffective unless documented hypogonadism. Only use with specialist advice. Exclude prostatic cancer first and do annual PSA measurement during treatment.
Psychotherapy	Effective for 60%. Time-consuming and expensive but may avert the need for drugs and give permanent resolution.

❶ NHS treatment for impotence is available **only** for men:
- treated for prostate cancer; with kidney failure, spinal cord injury, DM, MS, spina bifida, PD, polio, severe pelvic injury, or who have had radical pelvic surgery or a prostatectomy;
- already receiving drug treatment for impotence on 14.9.98;
- through specialist services, suffering severe distress due to impotence.

Endorse FP10/GP10 with SLS.

International prostate symptom score

	Not at all	Less than 1 time in 5	Less than half the time	About half the time	More than half the time	Almost always	Your score
Over the past month, how often have you had a sensation of not emptying your bladder completely after you finish urinating?	0	1	2	3	4	5	
Over the past month, how often have you had to urinate again in <2h. hours after you finished urinating?	0	1	2	3	4	5	
Over the past month, how often have you stopped and started several times when you urinated?	0	1	2	3	4	5	
Over the past month, how often have you found it difficult to postpone urinating?	0	1	2	3	4	5	
Over the past month, how often have you had a weak urinary stream?	0	1	2	3	4	5	
Over the past month, how often have you had to push or strain to begin urinating?	0	1	2	3	4	5	
Over the past month, typically from the time you went to bed to the time you got up in the morning, how many times did you get up to urinate?	0	1	2	3	4	5+	

Total IPSS

	Delighted	Pleased	Mostly satisfied	Equally satisfied/dissatisfied	Mostly dissatisfied	Unhappy	Terrible
If you were to live the rest of your life with your urinary condition the way it is now, how would you feel about it?	0	1	2	3	4	5	6

0–7 = mildly symptomatic
20–35 = severely symptomatic

8–19=moderately symptomatic

Figure 20.2 International prostate symptom score (IPSS) (Reproduced with permission of the American Urological Association)

Other relevant pages

Gynaecology and genito-urinary medicine

Uterine problems

Congenital abnormalities of the female genital tract

- *Duplication of the cervix and/or uterus; vaginal septum; bicornuate uterus (of varying degrees):* Caused by failure of fusion of the paramesonephric ducts. Usually found incidentally. May cause problems in pregnancy or contraception if pregnancy occurs in uterus without the IUCD. Refer for advice.
- *Imperforate hymen:* May cause cryptmenorrhoea which presents as 1° amenorrhoea (📖 p.728). Refer for surgical release if suspected.
- *Ambiguous genitalia:* 📖 p.882.
- *Cervical incompetence:* 📖 p.715.

Uterine retroversion: 20% women have retroverted retroflexed uterus. May be difficult to palpate bimanually—push on cervix to ante-vert. Rarely it may fail to lift out of pelvis during pregnancy and cause discomfort and urinary retention. Refer. Treated with catheterization.

Fibroids/uterine leiomyoma: Benign tumours of the smooth muscle of the myometrium. Affect ≈20% women (more common in Afro-Caribbeans). Often multiple. Named according to location:
- Pedunculated
- Intramural
- Cervical
- Subserosal (bulge into peritoneum)
- Submucosal (bulge into endometrium)

Risk factors: Low parity; FH. Oestrogen dependent, so more common in premenopausal women and shrink postmenopause.

Symptoms: Usually asymptomatic.
- *Heavy periods*
- *Pelvic pressure or discomfort:* May cause back ache. Can also press on the bladder → ↑ frequency or a feeling of incomplete emptying or difficulty passing urine.
- *Infertility:* 'Natural IUCD' if submucosal; may obstruct fallopian tubes at the cornu.
- *Pain:* Torsion (pedunculated fibroid); degeneration. 'Red degeneration' occurs only in pregnancy (pain, fever, and local tenderness until degeneration is complete).
- *Calcification:* Usually incidental finding on X-ray.

Signs: Bulky uterus ± pelvic mass felt abdominally.

Investigation: Pelvic USS is diagnostic. Blood—FBC (anaemia if menorrhagia; rarely polycythaemia due to fibroids).

Management: Asymptomatic/ mild symptoms—reassure. Else—refer to gynaecology. Options:
- *Medical:* COC pill may ↓ menstrual loss; GnRH analogues (max. use 6mo. due to risk of osteopoenia) cause fibroid shrinkage by up to 50%—used around menopause to avert surgery and pre-surgery to make surgery easier (controversial).
- *Surgical:* Myomectomy—removal of fibroids only; hysteroscopic resection (only suitable for submucosal fibroids); hysterectomy.

Endometrial proliferation: Oestrogen causes endometrial proliferation, progesterone causes endometrial maturation, shedding follows withdrawal of oestrogen and progesterone.

If oestrogen is given alone, the endometrium proliferates unchecked, resulting in irregular, heavy bleeding, polyps, and ↑ incidence of endometrial carcinoma. *Causes:* anovulatory cycles and administration of unopposed oestrogen.

Endometritis: Acute infection of the endometrium ± fallopian tubes and ovaries. Rare except after surgery (including IUCD insertion) or childbirth. Presents with lower abdominal pain, fever, and uterine tenderness. *Investigation:* endocervical swabs for M,C&S (including swab for chlamydia—📖 p.743).

Management: Treat with antibiotics e.g. doxycycline 100mg bd + metronidazole 500mg tds for 1wk. Pyometra is a complication (uterine cavity fills with pus)—suspect if fails to clear. Refer to gynaecology.

Endometrial carcinoma: Peak incidence 55–70y. *Risk factors:* age, obesity, nulliparity, late menopause, DM, drugs (unopposed oestrogen, tamoxifen), granulosa cell ovarian tumour, FH of breast, ovary, or colon cancer.

Presentation: Postmenopausal bleeding (PMB) (>90%). Any woman presenting with PMB has endometrial carcinoma until proven otherwise.

Examination: Usually normal, though the uterus may be bulky. A few cases are detected on routine cervical smear.

Management: Refer any PMB to gynaecology for further investigation. Assessment comprises transvaginal USS to look at endometrial thickness ± endometrial sampling (often performed in outpatients) or D&C. *Treatment:* TAH and BSO ± radiotherapy, progesterone therapy, and/or chemotherapy depending on stage and differentiation of the tumour.

Patient information

Hysterectomy Association 🖥 *http://www.hysterectomy-association.org.uk*
Womens Health: Patient information on fibroids
  🖥 *http://www.womenshealthlondon.org.uk/leaflets/fibroids/fibroids.html*
Cancer Help: Patient information on womb cancer
  🖥 *http://www.cancerhelp.org.uk*

Prolapse

Pelvic organs sag into the vagina due to poor pelvic muscle tone and weakness of pelvic ligaments. *Risk factors:* Childbirth, menopause, coughing, and straining.

Terminology: Named according to organs involved:
• Cystocoele—bladder bulges into the vagina;
• Urethrocoele—urethra bulges into the vagina;
• Rectocoele—rectum bulges into the vagina;
• Enterocoele—loops of intestine bulge into the vagina;
• Uterine—uterus descends into the vagina.

Uterine prolapse is further classified by degree:
• 1st degree—cervix remains in the vagina;
• 2nd degree—cervix protrudes from vagina on coughing/straining;
• 3rd degree (procidentia)—uterus lies outside the vagina and may ulcerate).

Presentation

History: Dragging sensation or feeling of 'something coming down'. Occasionally a 'lump' is felt. Symptoms only present when upright i.e. whilst awake. Often get worse if standing for a long time, coughing, or straining. May be associated with stress incontinence (🕮 p.694), difficulty of defaecation, recurrent cystitis, and/or frequency of micturition (depending on structures involved).

Examination: In left lateral position with Sims speculum. Ask to bear down and watch vaginal walls.

Management: Simple reassurance may be all that is required, depending on the degree of prolapse and severity of symptoms. *Other measures:*
• *Prevention:* Good obstetric practice; low parity; pelvic floor exercises throughout life (opposite).
• *Lifestyle measures:* Weight loss; smoking cessation.
• *General measures:* Treatment of coexisting conditions exacerbating prolapse e.g. COPD, constipation, menopause (🕮 p.732)/atrophic vaginitis (🕮 p.718)
• *Physiotherapy:* Pelvic floor exercises.
• *Ring pessary:* Useful for those too frail for surgery, women who have symptoms but don't want surgery, or as a temporary measure whilst awaiting surgery.
• *Surgery:* Refer to gynaecology if the woman is fit for surgery and:
  • symptoms are of sufficient severity to warrant operation *and/or*
  • incontinence *and/or*
  • recurrent UTI.
  Options: Repair operations, colpo/vaginal suspension, hysterectomy (vaginal or abdominal).

Fitting a ring pessary

- Measure the approximate size required manually (distance between posterior fornix and pubic bone can be measured roughly against the index finger).
- Soften the ring in hot water and lubricate it well.
- Insert the ring into the posterior fornix and tuck above pubic bone.
- Change the pessary every 6mo.

Potential problems

- Discomfort—ring may be too big or atrophic vaginitis.
- Infection—remove, clear infection, then try again.
- Ulceration—remove, allow to heal, consider alternatives or reinsert when fully healed.
- Expulsion—ring may be too small, pelvic musculature inadequate, or retropubic rim unsuitable.

Pelvic floor exercises—basic techniques

- Advise the woman to pull up her pelvic muscles as if stopping herself from passing urine and hold that position for a count of 10.
- Alternatively, or in addition, she could try pulling up her pelvic muscles in the same way but then relaxing them and contracting them rapidly 4 times.
- These exercises should be repeated as many times daily as possible for the rest of her life.

Useful information

Womens Health: Patient information on prolapse
 http://www.womenshealthlondon.org.uk/leaflets/prolapse/prolapse.html

Ovarian disease

Simple cysts: Very common and often incidental finding on USS. May cause pain due to:
- tension within the cyst
- bleeding into the cyst
- cyst rupture or torsion

No need for further investigation if <5cm diameter. Usually resolve spontaneously.

Polycystic ovarian syndrome (PCOS)^G: Common (5–20% premenopausal women). Cause unknown. Hormonal cycling is disrupted and ovaries are enlarged with multiple cysts. Associated with ↑ risk of cardiovascular disease and endometrial cancer. Patients may be asymptomatic or suffer from any or all of the following:
- Acne
- Hirsutism
- Obesity
- Irregular periods
- Infertility
- Insulin resistance

Investigations: Blood—↑testosterone, ↑LH; pelvic USS—polycystic ovaries.

Management: Encourage weight ↓ and exercise.
- If oligomenorrhoeic, consider progestogens to induce a withdrawal bleed every 3–4mo. to ↓ risk of endometrial hyperplasia.
- Metformin (unlicensed) may be helpful for insulin sensitivity, menstrual disturbance, and ovulation.
- Clomifene can be used to induce ovulation—🕮 p.763.
- Hirsutism—🕮 p.658.

Stein-Leventhal syndrome: Polycystic ovarian syndrome with obesity, virilization, acne, and menstrual irregularity. (*I.F. Stein (1887–1976) and M.L. Leventhal (1901–71)—US obstetricians/gynaecologists.*)

Ovarian hyperstimulation: Complication of gonadotrophin or clomifene treatment. *Mild cases:* Lower abdominal discomfort/distension ± nausea. *Severe cases:* Abdominal pain/distension, ascites, pleural effusion, venous thrombosis. Refer.

Tumours: Refer any ovarian mass, except simple cysts <5cm diameter, to gynaecology—a proportion are malignant. *Types:*
- *Serous cystadenoma:* Peak age 30–40y. 30%—bilateral; 30%—malignant.
- *Mucinous cystadenoma:* Large tumours filled with mucinous material. Rupture causes *pseudomyxoma peritonei* (mucin secreting cells are disseminated throughout the peritoneum, continue to secrete mucin, and eventually cause death through intestinal obstruction). Typical age: 30–50y. 5% are malignant.
- *Fibroma:* Small, benign fibrous tissue tumour. Associated with Meigs syndrome ± ascites.
- *Teratoma:* Derives from primitive germ cells. Dermoid cysts (mature teratomas) may contain well-differentiated tissue e.g. teeth. 20%—bilateral. Young > older women. Rarely malignant.

Meigs syndrome: Association of a benign ovarian fibroma with pleural effusion. Mechanism of association is unknown. (*J.V. Meigs (1892–1963)—US obstetrician/gynaecologist*)

Epithelial ovarian cancer (EOC): 90% of ovarian cancers. Responsible for 5% of ♀ deaths.

Risk factors
- Age (peak age 63y.)
- FH (one 1st degree relative ↑ risk from 1.5% → 5%, 2 relatives ↑ risk to 7%)
- Nulliparity
- Infertility (ovarian stimulation e.g. clomifene ↑ risk)

Protective factors
- Pregnancy
- COC pill (↓ risk by ~60%)

Symptoms: Abdominal discomfort and bloating, vaginal bleeding, GI symptoms (constipation, wind), GU symptoms (prolapse, ↑ frequency).

⚠ Refer any postmenopausal bleeding for further investigation (either directly to gynaecology or for USS to assess endometrial thickness).

Signs: Pelvic/adnexal mass, ascites, pleural effusion. Confirm with USS.

Management: Refer urgently to gynaecology. Specialist management is with laparotomy ± adjuvant treatment, dependant on stage of disease. Agents used—chemotherapy (cisplatin); paclitaxel; radiotherapy.

Survival rates
- *Early disease:* 30% of tumours present at early stage. If disease is confined to the ovaries/pelvis, 5y. survival is 50–90% (↑ if well-differentiated). Screening to detect early stage disease—📖 p.160.
- *Advanced disease:* 70–80% respond to initial chemotherapy but the majority relapse. Disease activity is monitored using tumour markers e.g. Ca 125. Relapse <6mo. after treatment or progression during treatment are poor prognostic signs. Further chemotherapy is palliative. Median survival 2–3y.

Sex-cord stromal tumours: Usually present early with symptoms of hormone production e.g. precocious puberty, PMB, or virilism. Granulosa cell tumours are associated with endometrial hyperplasia and carcinoma.

Germ-cell tumours: Peak incidence in early 20s. Present with abdominal pain caused by rupture, torsion, or haemorrhage of the tumour. Most are unilateral. Associated with ↑ AFP and ↑ β-HCG (both are used as tumour markers). Prognosis is good, with the majority being cured.

Further information
RCOG (2003) Long-term consequences of polycystic ovary syndrome
🖥 http://www.rcog.org.uk

Patient information and support
Wellbeing: Information on PCOS 🖥 http://www.wellbeing.org.uk
Verity: PCOS support group 🖥 http://www.verity-pcos.org.uk
Ovacome: Ovarian cancer support group 🖥 http://www.ovacome.org.uk
CancerHelp: Patient information on ovarian cancer
🖥 http://www.cancerhelp.org.uk

Conditions of the cervix

Cervical intraepithelial neoplasia (CIN): Histological diagnosis resulting from biopsy—usually following an abnormal smear.

Classification

- CIN 1   Nuclear atypia confined to basal $1/3$ epithelium (mild dysplasia)
- CIN 2   Nuclear atypia in basal $2/3$ epithelium (moderate dysplasia)
- CIN 3   Nuclear abnormalities through the full thickness of the epithelium (carcinoma in situ/severe dysplasia)

Natural history: Unclear—and unethical to test. CIN 1 may revert to normality. Any stage can progress to cervical cancer.

Treatment: Depends on stage. Ranges from local ablation (diathermy, laser diathermy, cold coagulation) through loop excision of the transformation zone and cone biopsy to hysterectomy.

Cervical cancer: Peak incidence in 6th decade. Squamous cell cancer (80%)—remainder are adenocarcinomas. Incidence is dropping, probably due to the cervical cancer screening programme and changes in sexual practices. *Risk factors:*

- Age
- Social class
- Smoking
- Multiple sexual partners
- HPV infection (types 16, 18, and 33)
- Early age of 1st intercourse and 1st prenancy
- History of dyskaryosis
- Method of contraception (↓ with barrier methods; ↑ with COC use)

Screening: 📖 p.716

Presentation: Routine cervical smear screening, postcoital bleeding, intermenstrual bleeding, offensive vaginal discharge. *Examination:* ulceration or mass on cervix which bleeds easily.

⚠ Refer any woman with postcoital bleeding or intermenstrual bleeding for further investigation

Management: Urgent gynaecology referral. *Treatment:* surgery ± radiotherapy. Most women present with early cervical cancer. Overall 5y. survival rate ≈57%.

Cervical erosion/ectropion: The area of columnar epithelium visible within the vagina when the squamo-columnar junction moves down the cervix at times of high oestrogen exposure (e.g. pregnancy, COC pill, puberty). Physiological. Does not need treatment unless smear is abnormal or causing problems e.g. postcoital or intermenstrual bleeding (refer to gynaecologist for cautery).

Nabothian cysts: Mucus retention cysts on cervix. Usually asymptomatic and need no treatment. If causing troublesome discharge, refer for cautery.

Cervicitis: Presents with vaginal discharge. *Clinically:* speculum examination—mucopurulent discharge, inflamed and friable cervix. *Cause:* Chlamydia (50%); gonococcus; HSV. *Management:* treat cause (📖 p.743–45). Can become chronic.

Cervical polyps: Develop from the endocervix and protrude into the vagina through the external os. Usually asymptomatic, though there may be ↑ vaginal discharge and the lowest part of the polyp may ulcerate and bleed causing intermenstrual, postmenopausal, and/or postcoital bleeding. Vast majority are benign. *Treatment:* avulsion (send for histology). Cauterize base with silver nitrate stick if possible. Frequently recur. If postmenopausal, intermenstrual, or postcoital bleeding, refer to gynaecology.

Cervical incompetence: Diagnosis is usually made on the basis of history of suggestive symptoms in past pregnancies—≥1 late 2nd trimester or early 3rd trimester miscarriage (usually painless leaking of liquor or gradual painless dilatation of the cervix). Refer all women with past history for early obstetric review. *Treatment:* cervical cerclage—a stitch is placed high up around the cervix to keep it closed e.g. Shirodkar suture. The stitch is removed at ~37wk. and labour ensues rapidly if the diagnosis was correct.

Useful information

CancerHelp: Patient information on cervical cancer
💻 http://www.cancerhelp.org.uk

Cervical cancer screening

It is estimated screening prevents 1000–4000 deaths/y. in the UK from squamous cell cancer of the cervix. Adenocarcinoma (20%) is not detected.

Liquid-based cytology: In the UK, the traditional Papanicolou smear (Pap smear) is being replaced by liquid-based cytology. The sample is collected in a similar way to the Pap smear but, rather than smearing the sample from the spatula onto a slide, the head of the spatula, where the cells are lodged, is broken off into a small glass vial containing preservative fluid, or rinsed directly into the preservative fluid. This method should ↓ the number of inadequate smears taken as the new technique enables cervical cells to be examined even if the sample is contaminated with blood, pus, or mucus—which would have obscured the view using the old method.

Taking a smear: Ensure adequate training—poor smear taking misses 20% abnormalities. Courses are available—update skills every 3y. Give all women information about the test, condition being sought, possible results of screening and their implications.

Timing: Avoid menstruation if possible (note on the request form if unavoidable). Ideal time is mid-cycle. Routine bimanual examination is unnecessary—only do a pelvic examination if clinically indicated (e.g. painful/heavy periods).

Screening interval: A smear test is routinely offered to all women age 25–64y. who are sexually active. There is no upper age limit for the 1st smear. Frequency of screening depends on age:
- 25–49y. 3-yearly screening interval
- 50–64y. 5-yearly screening interval
- 65y.+ Only screen those who have not been screened since age 50y. or have had recent abnormal tests

Organization of the cervical screening programme: Cervical screening is an additional service which most practices are expected to provide. Practices undertaking cervical screening must:
- Provide information to eligible women to allow them to make an informed decision about taking part in the programme;
- Perform the cervical screening test (and ensure staff are properly trained and equipped to perform the test);
- Arrange for women to be informed about the results of their tests;
- Ensure that results are followed up appropriately; *and*
- Maintain records of tests carried out, results, and any clinical follow-up requirements.

Payment: As an additional service (unless the practice 'opts out') it is paid for performing cervical screening through the global sum. In addition, quality points and payments are available through the quality and outcomes framework. The practice can obtain maximum points if the service is organized as above, performs smears on >80% eligible women, and regular audit of the process is carried out.

Table 21.1 Interpretation of smear results and action

Result	Action
Inadequate	Repeat smear. If recurrent inadequate smears, refer to gynaecologist.
Normal (94%)	Repeat smear at interval dictated by laboratory.
Metaplasia/squamous metaplasia	Normal finding which should be present. No action needed.
Endocervical cells	Normal cells from the endocervix. No action needed.
Cytolysis	Normal process of cell destruction. No action needed.
Atrophic smear	Common in peri/postmenopausal smears. No action. Similar picture in postnatal smears.
Endometrial cells	May be normal if IUCD in situ or in 1st half of 28d. cycle. Otherwise discuss with laboratory.
Inflammatory changes	Common finding. Significance unclear. Take chlamydial, endocervical, and high vaginal swabs. Treat as necessary.
Actinomyces	Associated with IUCDs. Controversy over best course of action. If asymptomatic, no action. If symptomatic, change IUCD.
Trichomonas, candida, and changes associated with HSV infection	Treat trichomonas. Treat candida if symptomatic. Discuss any new diagnosis of HSV with the patient (📖 p.744).
Borderline changes ± evidence HPV infection	Repeat after 6mo. If recurrent, refer for colposcopy.
Mild dyskaryosis ± HPV change (4%)	Consistent with CIN I. Repeat after 6mo. If recurrent, refer for colposcopy.
Moderate dyskaryosis ± HPV change (<1%)	Consistent with CIN II. Refer for colposcopy.
Severe dyskaryosis ± HPV change (<1%)	Consistent with CIN III. Refer for colposcopy.
Severe dyskaryosis/? invasive carcinoma (<1%)	Consistent with CIN III with features suggesting possible invasive carcinoma. Refer urgently for colposcopy.
Glandular neoplasia	Consistent with carcinoma of the cervix or endometrium. Refer urgently for colposcopy.

Referral for colposcopy is recommended in 2–4% cases.

Further information

DoH 🖳 http://www.cancerscreening.nhs.uk/cervical/index.html

Patient information

Women's Health: Patient information on cervical screening and abnormal smears
🖳 http://www.womenshealthlondon.org.uk/leaflets/cervical/cervical.html

Vaginal and vulval problems

Atrophic vaginitis: Presents with vaginal soreness, dyspareunia, and occasional spotting (❶ refer any postmenopausal bleeding for further assessment—📖 p.713). On examination, the vagina looks pale and dry. Treat with topical oestrogens for up to 3mo. or consider other HRT.

Vaginal cysts: May arise from remnants of the mesonephric ducts (anterolaterally) or occasionally, after healing, following surgery or episiotomy (posterior, lower $^1/_3$). Usually no treatment is needed. If symptomatic or very large, refer for gynaecaology assessment ± removal.

Benign vaginal tumours: Benign leiomyomas or fibro-myomas are common. Refer for surgical removal.

Vaginal intraepithelial neoplasia (VAIN): Multifocal. Occurs in upper $^1/_3$ of vagina. Usually occurs in association with CIN (📖 p.714). May be asymptomatic or present with postcoital staining or abnormal vaginal discharge. Treatment is by local ablation.

Vaginal cancer: Occurs in the 6th or 7th decade. 90% squamous; the rest are clear cell (associated with in utero exposure to stilboestrol), 2° tumours, or sarcomas. Present with postmenopausal bleeding. Most are treated with radiotherapy, though surgery is an option in the early stages. Refer all women with postmenopausal bleeding for gynaecological assessment.

Vaginal discharge: 📖 p.740

Bartholin's gland swellings: Obstruction of the duct leads to cyst formation which presents as painless vulval swelling. If it becomes infected, an abscess results—painful, tender, red vulval lump. Cysts can be left to resolve spontaneously. Abscesses sometimes resolve with antibiotics (if early) or discharge themselves. If they do not resolve, acute admission for surgery (marsupialization) is indicated. The same procedure can be used to remove cysts.

Genital warts: 📖 p.744

Urethral caruncle: Due to prolapse of the posterior urethral wall. Occurs postmenopausally. Seen as a reddened area involving the posterior margin of the urethral opening. Usually asymptomatic, though may bleed or cause dyspareunia. Treatment is with topical oestrogen. Surgical excision is only needed if symptoms do not resolve.

Vulval itching/pruritus vulvae: 📖 p.296

Vulval lumps and bumps: 📖 p.296

Vulval ulceration: 📖 p.264

Vulval dystrophy: Changes in the skin of the vulva which occur in postmenopausal women. Cause unknown. Classified histologically:

- Hyperplastic
- Hypoplastic (lichen scerosus et atrophicus)
- Mixed
- Presence/absence of atypia

Lesions with cell atypia are associated with malignant change.

Presentation: Presents with vulval itching. Vulval skin looks atrophic ± white plaques (leukoplakia). Changes do not extend into the vagina.

Management: Refer to gynaecologist for biopsy. *Treatment:*
- Hyperplastic dystrophy—topical steroids e.g. dermovate bd;
- Hypoplastic dystrophy—topical oestrogen ± testosterone;
- If atypia is present—treated surgically.

Vulval intraepithelial neoplasia (VIN): Previously known as *Bowen's disease* or carcinoma in situ. May be associated with other genital tract neoplasia (e.g. CIN ☐ p.714). *Clinically:* abnormal looking skin of vulva (usually pinky white and altered texture) ± white patches ± itch.

Diagnosis: There is some overlap between vulval dystrophy and VIN. Diagnosis is histological following skin biopsy:
- VIN 1   Epidermis is thickened . Atypia is confined to the basal $1/3$ of the epithelium.
- VIN 2   Nuclear atypia in the lower $1/2$ of the epithelium.
- VIN 3   Carcinoma in situ—nuclear atypia through the full thickness of the epithelium.

Management: Refer all patients with abnormal looking vulval skin (without candidal infection or other obvious cause) to gynaecology for skin biopsy and treatment. *Treatment:* depends on site, histology, and extent. Includes: surgery, cryocautery, laser vaporization, or topical chemotherapy.

Vulval carcinoma[G]: Rare. Mainly affects women in 8th decade. Most are squamous cell carcinoma; others—melanoma, BCC, Bartholins gland carcinoma. The majority occur on the labia and spread to local LNs. Present early with chronic pruritus vulvae ($>2/3$), vulval lump, or ulcer. 3 premalignant changes are identifiable:
- Vulval dystrophy
- Vulval intraepithelial neoplasia (VIN)
- HPV infection (☐ p.744)

Treatment is surgical. 5y. survival rate ≈95%.

Further information
RCOG: Guidelines for management of vulval cancer
   ☐ www.rcog.org.uk

Patient information
CancerHelp: Patient information on vulval cancer
   ☐ http://www.cancerhelp.org.uk

Pelvic pain

Table 21.2 Causes of pelvic pain

Gynaecological		Non-gynaecological	
Acute	**Chronic**	**Acute**	**Chronic**
Ectopic pregnancy	Endometriosis	Appendicitis	Irritable bowel syndrome
Infection	Adhesions	Cystitis	Musculoskeletal
Endometriosis	Fibroids	Neurological	Psychological
Torsion of fibroid	Ovarian cyst	Colitis	Bowel or bladder cancer
Dysmenorrhoea	Venous congestion	Psychological	Neurological
Ovarian cyst (torsion, bleeding, or rupture)	PID		

History: Timing and quality of pain, precipitating and relieving factors, relationship to menstrual cycle (and possibility of pregnancy), dyspareunia, bowel and bladder symptoms, history of ectopic pregnancy, pelvic infection or surgery, psychological problems.

Examination: Abdominal (including DRE), pelvic and vaginal examination (with smear if overdue). Normal pelvic and vaginal examination makes a gynaecological cause unlikely.

Management

- *Acute pelvic pain:* Admit unless cause known and ectopic pregnancy can be excluded.
- *Chronic pelvic pain:* On the basis of history and examination, decide whether the cause is gynaecological or not—patients with gynaecological causes usually have dyspareunia and the pain may be cyclical.
  - If gynaecological, arrange pelvic USS. Most patients are referred for laparoscopy.
  - If GI pain, consider colonoscopy or barium studies.
  - Other investigations: urine—MSU, RBCs ± IVP; spine X-ray.

Mittelschmerz: Mid-cycle pain which occurs around the time of ovulation. Reassure. No action needed.

Psychological causes of pelvic pain: These do occur but be careful not to dismiss organic symptoms as psychological. Psychological pain may be a consequence of and perpetuate physical pain. Diagnosis is one of exclusion.

Pelvic venous congestion: Pelvic veins become dilated and congested. Treatment is with continuous progestogens.

Pelvic inflammatory disease (PID): May be asymptomatic. >10% develop tubal infertility after 1 episode; 50% after 3. Risk ectopic pregnancy ↑ x10 after a single episode.

Acute PID^G: Only 70% of those with clinical acute PID have diagnosis confirmed on laparoscopy. *Causes:* chlamydia (📖 p.743), gonorrhoea (📖 p.745).

History: acute pelvic pain, deep dyspareunia, malaise, dysuria, purulent vaginal discharge, fever >38°C.

Examination: cervical excitation, adnexal tenderness, discharge, pyrexia.

Investigations: endocervical swab for M,C&S and chlamydia screening. FBC—may show leucocytosis. ↑ ESR.

Management: If unwell or ectopic pregnancy cannot be excluded, admit. Otherwise treat with ofloxacin 400mg bd and metronidazole 400mg bd for 2wk. Provide analgesia. Advise rest and sexual abstinence. Arrange contact tracing via GUM clinic. If slow recovery, consider referral for laparoscopy to exclude abscess formation.

Chronic PID: Caused by inadequately treated acute PID.

History: pain and dyspareunia, menorrhagia, dysmenorrhoea.

Examination: generalized lower abdominal/pelvic tenderness, cervical excitation, adnexal mass.

Investigation: screen for chlamydial and gonorrhoeal infection (📖 p.743 and 745). –ve result does not exclude diagnosis.

Management: if suspected or chronic pelvic pain with no obvious cause, refer to gynaecology. Once diagnosis is confirmed, treatment options include long-term antibiotics or surgery.

Further information
RCOG 🖥 *http://www.rcog.org.uk*
● Management of acute PID (May 2003)
● The initial management of chronic pelvic pain (April 2005)

Patient information and support
🖥 *http://www.womenshealthlondon.org.uk/leaflets/pid/pid.html*
Pelvic Inflammatory Disease Support Network. ☎0845 125 5254

Endometriosis^G

Presence of tissue histologically similar to endometrium outside the uterine cavity and myometrium. Most commonly found in the pelvis but can occur anywhere. Affects ~1:5 women. *Risk factors:* age, FH, heavy periods, frequent cycles. Oral contraceptives and pregnancy are protective.

Theories of pathogenesis

- *Reflux and implantation:* Menstrual loss flows backwards through fallopian tubes into the pelvis where it implants into the peritoneum and continues to grow under the influence of oestrogen.
- *Transformation or induction:* Peritoneal tissue transforms into endometrium either under the influence of ovarian steroids or as a result of factors released when menstrual loss refluxes into the peritoneum.
- *Mechanical transplantation:* Endometrium transplanted from one location to another (e.g. during surgery) will grow at that new site.
- *Vascular ± lymphatic spread:* Thought to explain distant deposits e.g. lungs, brain.

Presentation: Pelvic pain (cyclical ± non-cyclical), dyspareunia, dysmenorrhoea, infertility, menorrhagia. *Examination:* pelvic tenderness, pelvic mass, fixation of uterus, occasionally tender nodules can be felt on the utero-sacral ligaments. *Investigation:* refer to gynaecology for laparoscopy/transvaginal USS.

> ❶ Laparoscopic findings of endometriosis are common and extent does not correlate with severity of symptoms. Only treat if symptomatic.

Management

Infertility: Refer for gynaecological opinion.
- If tubal damage—reconstructive surgery or IVF.
- If no tubal damage—laparoscopic ablation may improve fertility.

Pain
- Cyclical—NSAID prn from 1st day of period.
- Constant pain, dyspareunia, or cyclical pain unresponsive to NSAID—progestagen (e.g. norethisterone 10–15mg/d. for 4–6mo.) or continuous COC (4 packets without a break, then 7d. break—effective for 70–80%).
- If symptoms are not controlled, refer. Danazol and GnRH agonists (e.g. goserelin) may be used but side-effects can be troublesome.

Surgical options: Include laparoscopy or laparotomy with ablation of lesions and division of adhesions; tubal surgery; hysterectomy.

> ❶ For all forms of treatment, there is a recurrence rate of 15–20%.
> - If relapse in <6mo., consider treatment has failed and try an alternative.
> - If relapse >6mo. after treatment, consider a relapse and repeat.

Psychological support: Many women will have had pain for years. Often there is delay in diagnosis of the cause—and frequently they have been told it is psychosomatic. Be sympathetic and supportive and use a co-operative strategy for management.

Further information
RCOG (2000) The investigation and management of endometriosis
 www.rcog.org.uk

Patient support
National Endometriosis Society ☎020 7222 2776
 http://www.endo.org.uk

Menorrhagia/heavy periods[G]

Menstrual loss ≥80ml/mo. 10% of women of menstrual age meet this criterion but 1:3 feel their loss is excessive.

Assessment

History: History and pattern of bleeding, presence or absence of pain, contraceptive needs, FH bleeding tendencies, drug history.

Examination: Anaemia; pelvic examination for enlargement, tenderness, or tethering of the uterus (chronic infection or endometriosis) and adnexal tenderness; vaginal examination for endometrial polyps; abdominal examination for pelvic mass/tenderness.

Investigation

- FBC—anaemia;
- Clotting screen—if coagulopathy suspected (e.g. FH);
- TFTs—only if clinical signs/symptoms;
- Cervical smear if needed;
- Endocervical swabs if infection suspected;
- Refer for pelvic USS if pelvic examination is abnormal and/or transvaginal USS to detect endometrial pathology.

Differential diagnosis: Physiological bleeding or dysfunctional uterine bleeding (50%). *Other causes:*

- Fibroids
- Congenital uterine abnormality e.g. bicornuate uterus
- Pelvic infection
- Endometriosis
- Endometrial polyps
- Presence of IUCD
- Endometrial carcinoma
- Bleeding tendency

Dysfunctional uterine bleeding: Excessive menstrual loss in the absence of any detectable abnormality.

Management: Figure 21.1

⚠ *Very heavy bleeding*—stop bleeding with progestogen e.g. norest-histerone 10mg tds. Effective in 24–48h. ↓ dose over 7–10d. and then stop. A lighter bleed will follow. Check FBC and refer for gynaecological assessment.

Reasons for treatment failure: Very high blood loss, low pre-treatment blood loss, unsuspected uterine pathology, lack of compliance.

Referral to gynaecology

- Age >40y.
- Uterus >10/40 size
- Intermenstrual or postcoital bleeding
- Pelvic pain between periods
- Failed medical treatment
- History of tamoxifen/unopposed oestrogens.

Further information

RCOG (1998) The initial management of menorrhagia
🖥 www.rcog.org.uk

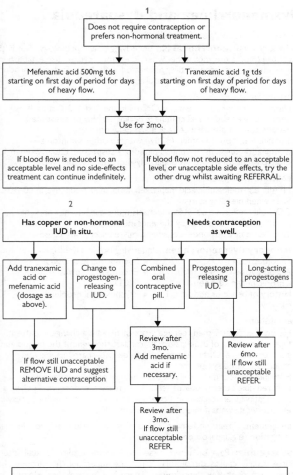

Figure 21.1 Management of menorrhagia in general practice. (Reproduced from *The Initial Management of Menorrhagia* (1998) with permission of the Royal College of Obstetricians and Gynaecologists.)

Dysmenorrhoea and dyspareunia

Dysmennorrhoea/painful periods

Primary dysmenorrhoea: No underlying pelvic pathology. Tends to start 6–12mo. after menarche when ovulatory cycles are established. *Cause:* uterine hypercontractility associated with ↑ prostaglandin production. Ischaemia of the uterine wall during a contraction causes pain.

Presentation
- *History:* Starts when a teenager. Occurs in the first 1–2d. of each period. Lower abdominal cramps ± backache. May be associated gastrointestinal disturbance (e.g. diarrhoea/vomiting).
- *Examination:* Young women (<20y.) with no other symptoms—examination unnecessary unless pathology suspected. Older women or atypical history—see secondary dysmennorhoea (below).

Treatment
- NSAID e.g. mefenamic acid, naproxen, ibuprofen—effective in 80–90%. Start when bleeding starts;
- COC pill—effective 80–90%. Mechanism unclear but may prevent prostaglandin production by the endometrium.
- 10–20% do not respond—consider a missed secondary cause

Secondary dysmenorrhoea: Underlying pelvic pathology:
- Endometriosis
- Adenomyosis
- Chronic pelvic infection
- History of pelvic or abdominal surgery
- Submucous leiomyoma
- Endometrial polyps
- IUCD
- Psychosexual problems

Presentation
- *History:* Starts later than teenage years or may be a change in pattern, type, or intensity of usual pain. Pain can last throughout the period and start just before. Often associated with deep dyspareunia. May be other associated symptoms.
- *Examination:* Abdominal, vaginal, and bimanual pelvic examination—tethered /fixed uterus, uterine tenderness, masses, endocervical polyps.
- *Investigation:* Cervical smear if overdue or clinical abnormality of cervix; endocervical swabs if infection suspected; pelvic USS.

Management: Treat underlying cause if found, else refer for further investigation (e.g. laparoscopy).

Dyspareunia: Pain on intercourse. 10% women admit sexual intercourse usually causes discomfort. It may be *superficial* (felt around the introitus) or *deep* (felt deep inside). There is a psychological element in all cases (a vicious cycle of pain leading to fear of intercourse which exacerbates symptoms). Address both physical and psychological aspects.

Table 21.3 Causes of superficial dyspareunia

Vulval	Vaginal	Urethral
Vulvitis—atrophic, infective (candida, HSV)	Vaginismus	Urethritis
	Lack of lubrication	Urethral caruncle
Dystrophy	Vaginitis—atrophic, infective	Urethral diverticulum
Neoplasm	Congenital—imperforate hymen, atresia	
Lichen sclerosis	Post-surgery e.g. painful episiotomy scar	
	Contracture—atrophy, post-surgery, post-radiotherapy	

Superficial dyspareunia: *Causes:* table 21.3. *Action:* examine if possible (but do not insist); treat cause if possible. If no specific treatment, try lignocaine gel. Most can be treated successfully, especially if the patient has support from a sympathetic partner. *Vaginismus*—🖳 p.746.

Deep dyspareunia: *Causes:* endometriosis, pelvic inflammatory disease, retroverted uterus, rarely ovarian cancer. *Action:* examine, treat any cause found, else refer for further investigation. If no cause is found or cause is untreatable, pain can be ↓ by limiting penetration. Often becomes a chronic problem.

Amenorrhoea

Oligomenorrhoea: Infrequent periods. Manage as for amenorrhoea.

Primary amenorrhoea: No 2° sexual characteristics or menstruation by age 14y. with growth failure *or* no menstruation by age 16y. when growth and sexual development is normal. *Causes:* familial; structural abnormality (e.g. imperforate hymen and haematocolpos); genetic (e.g. Turner's syndrome XO); congenital endocrine abnormality (e.g. testicular feminization); 2° causes of amenorrhoea (see Figure 21.2).

Secondary amenorrhoea: Absence of menses ≥6mo. in a previously menstruating woman. *Causes:* see Figure 21.2.

History: Always consider the possibility of pregnancy.
- *Symptoms:* galactorrhoea (30% prolactinomas), weight change, hirsutism, life crisis or upset (e.g. exams, bereavement), level of exercise (gymnasts are frequently amenorrhoeic), sweats, flushes, cyclical pain;
- Family history of premature menopause or late menarche;
- Drug history (contraceptive particularly);
- Past history of chemo- or radiotherapy or gynaecological surgery.

Examination: Weight and height (common if BMI <19kg/m²); external genitalia (structural abnormality, virilism); vaginal examination (including cervical smear if overdue); pelvic examination (ovarian masses, uterine size); general examination (2° sexual characteristics, hirsutism, ↓ weight, systemic disease).

❶ Replace vaginal and pelvic examination with pelvic USS in young girls.

Investigation: Blood—↑ serum prolactin in 1:3 cases (stress, drugs—phenothiazines, metoclopramide, cimetidine, prolactinoma); TFTs; FSH/LH (↑ FSH menopause, ↑ LH—PCOS); karyotype if phenotypical abnormality; serum testosterone if LH high, hirsutism, or virilism; USS pelvis if structural abnormality or PCOS suspected.

Management: Related to cause:
- *Contraception:* Cessation of COC pill. Normally periods return within 6mo. If not, consider another cause. Progestagen contraception—reassure, no further action.
- *↓Weight:* Investigate and treat reasons (e.g. anorexia). Encourage weight ↑. If no response, refer to gynaecologist.
- *Physical exercise:* Explain reason—many will not cut their level of activity, so consider HRT.
- *Stress:* Reassure, treat any psychiatric problems. Periods should return spontaneously. Set a limit for return (e.g. another 3–4mo.). If periods do not return within that time, consider referral as there may be another cause.
- *Endocrine:* Thyroid dysfunction—📖 p.422; hypothalamic causes—after 6mo. ↑ risk CHD and osteoporosis. Consider use HRT or COC pill. Hyperprolactinaemia—refer to gynaecology or endocrinology.
- *Gynaecological:* Premature menopause—📖 p.733; PCOS—📖 p.712
- *Cause not found:* Refer to gynaecology.

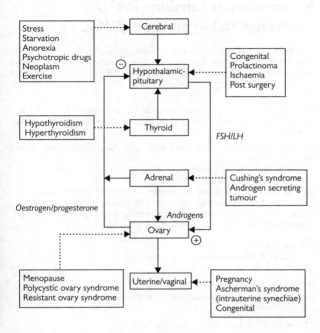

Figure 21.2 Causes of secondary amenorrhoea

Premenstrual tension (PMT)/ premenstrual syndrome (PMS)

A collection of symptoms and bodily changes that occur on a regular basis anything from a few days to several weeks before a woman's period and cease (or ↓ significantly) with its arrival. >95% women have some symptoms—debilitating symptoms occur in 5%. The underlying mechanism is not understood.

Symptoms: >100 symptoms described. Most common are nervous tension, mood swings, irritability, ↑ weight and abdominal bloating, breast tenderness, and headache.

Management: Aims to alleviate symptoms. Usually symptoms return when treatment is stopped.
- Take a history of symptoms and ask patient to keep a diary to establish cyclical nature.
- Be sympathetic and follow-up—the first treatment may not work.
- Treatment is often by trial and error. The range of treatments used (and found effective) reflects the range of symptoms experienced. For most treatments use a 3–6mo. trial

Further information
McRec Bulletin 13(3) Tackling premenstrual syndrome (2003)
🖳 http://www.npc.co.uk/McRec_Bulletins

Patient support
National Association for Premenstrual Syndrome ☎0870 777 2177
🖳 http://www.pms.org.uk

Table 21.4 Treatment of premenstrual tension

Treatment	Effective?	Notes
Hormonal manipulation		
Progesterone/ progestagens[S]	✗	May induce PMT
Oestrogen[R], COC[R], and tibolones[R]	✓	Do not give unopposed oestrogen if the uterus is intact. If progestagen causes PMT, try local application e.g. via IUCD or topical gel.
GNRH analogues[R], danazol[R], bromocriptine[R]	✓	Use limited by side-effects. Bromocriptine helps breast tenderness.
Antidepressants		
SSRIs[C]	✓	↓ physical as well as psychological symptoms.
Lithium[R]	✗	No evidence of effectiveness.
Anxiolytics[CE]	✓	Alprazolam and buspirone are of proven benefit.

Table 21.4 (cont.)

Treatment	Effective?	Notes
Other drugs		
β-blockers[R]	✓/✗	Conflicting evidence.
Diuretics[R]	✓	Spironolactone is effective for bloating/breast tenderness.
NSAIDs[R]	✓	Effective for a range of symptoms.
Surgery		
Hysterectomy ± oophorectomy	✓	Observational studies have found that hysterectomy + bilateral oophorectomy is curative. Hysterectomy alone may also ↓ symptoms.
Complementary therapies		
Oil of evening primrose[S]	✓/✗	Conflicting evidence—may help breast tenderness. May cause fits in patients with epilepsy.
Vitamin B6[S]	✓/✗	Conflicting evidence—high doses (>200mg/d.) may cause reversible peripheral neuropathy.
Magnesium supplements[S]	✓/✗	Conflicting results.
Calcium supplements[S]	✓	↓ symptoms, including breast tenderness and swelling, headaches, and abdominal cramps.
Exercise[R]	✓	High-intensity exercise improves symptoms > low-intensity exercise.
Chiropractic manipulation[S]	✗	No evidence of effectiveness.
Cognitive therapy[R]	✓	Evidence that effective, though size of effect is unclear.
Relaxation[R]	✓/✗	Conflicting evidence—can do no harm.
Reflexology[S]	✓/✗	Insufficient evidence.

Menopause

From the Greek *'men'* (month) and *'pausis'* (halt). Menopause occurs when menstruation stops. It results from loss of ovarian follicular activity through natural mechanisms, surgery, drugs, or radiotherapy. Average age in the UK ≈ 50y. Smoking brings it forwards by ~2y. Impact on a woman's life varies and depends on cultural, health, and social factors.

Diagnosis: >12mo. amenorrhoea with no other cause in women >50y. or >24mo. amenorrhoea in women <50y. The *climacteric* refers to the period of time as the ovaries fail, when production of oestrogen ↓ over a number of years.

What are the symptoms of the menopause?
Periods
- Changes in menstrual pattern are common in the years before the menopause. Typically, cycle shortens after 40y. by up to 7–10d., cycle then lengthens and periods may occur at 2–3mo. intervals until stopping.
- Dysfunctional uterine bleeding (📖 p.724) is common leading up to the menopause but investigate postmenopausal, very heavy, painful, irregular, intermenstrual, or postcoital bleeding.
- Late menstruation (>54y.) requires investigation due to ↑ risk of malignancy.

Flushes and sweats: 80% have flushes—20% seek help. Often associated with palpitations. Most are controlled successfully with oestrogen. *Alternative treatments:* exercise (↓ ≈ 50%), deep breathing exercises, cool ambient temperature. Clonidine and oil of evening primrose are of dubious benefit. Natural progesterone derived from yams has attracted interest—trials are awaited; some evidence may alleviate symptoms but not of +ve benefit on bone or endometrial protection.

Psychological symptoms: Controversial. Some studies report depression and anxiety are more common; others find no association. Depression is multifactorial—consider social, physical, and cultural factors before resorting to HRT as a solution.

Sexual dysfunction: Vaginal dryness and atrophy are common. Manage with systemic or topical oestrogen. Loss of libido post menopause (especially after surgical removal of the ovaries) responds to administration of androgens e.g. testosterone implants in combination with HRT until libido is re-established.

Urinary problems: Common—incontinence, nocturia, and urgency. Stress incontinence does not respond to HRT but topical oestrogen may improve outcome of surgery. Recurrent UTIs in older women ↓ with use of topical vaginal oestrogen.

Ischaemic heart disease: Risk is ↑ x2 after the menopause but there is no evidence to support use of HRT for 1° or 2° prevention of IHD.

Osteoporosis: Consider HRT to prevent osteoporosis in premature menopause (below). In older women, HRT is now *not* recommended as first-line treatment of osteoporosis unless there are other reasons for prescribing the HRT.

Could the symptoms be due to another cause? *Exclude:*
- Physical illness e.g. thyroid disease, anaemia, DM, chronic renal disease
- Side-effects of medication e.g. Ca^{2+} antagonists cause flushing
- Social problems or psychiatric illness—depression screening question-naires can be helpful.

Is the diagnosis in doubt? *Check FSH/LH:*
- Following hysterectomy with conservation of ovaries
- If amenorrhoea age <45y.
- If having regular bleeds due to cyclical HRT/COC pill. ↓FSH/LH in patients taking COC or HRT does not exclude menopause as these preparations can inhibit FSH/LH production—stop medication for 6mo. and await menses (use alternative contraception) or check serum FSH x2 ≥6wk. apart—FSH >20 = menopause.

It is unnecessary to check FSH/LH in other groups.

❶ FSH/LH levels may be normal in the perimenopause.

HRT: 📖 p.734   **Contraception:** 📖 p.758

Premature menopause: Menopause in a woman <45y. old. Associated with ↑ all cause mortality and ↑ risk of osteoporosis and cardiovascular disease. *Causes:*
- Idiopathic
- Radiotherapy and chemotherapy
- Surgery—bilateral oophorectomy → instant menopause; hysterectomy without oophorectomy can also induce premature ovarian failure
- Infection—TB and mumps
- Chromosome abnormalities—particularly the X chromosome
- Autoimmune endocrine disease e.g. DM, hypothyroidism, Addison's
- FSH receptor abnormalities
- Disruption of oestrogen synthesis

Management: Usually HRT is recommended until the average age of menopause i.e. 50y.

Essential reading

RCP (Edinburgh) Consensus conference on hormone replacement therapy: Final consensus statement (October 2003) 🖥 http://www.rcpe.ac.uk/esd/consensus/hrt_03.html

Patient information

British Menopause Society 🖥 http://www.the-bms.org
The Menopause Amarant Trust ☎01293 413000
   🖥 http://www.amarantmenopausetrust.org.uk

Hormone replacement therapy (HRT)

The concept of the menopause as a deficiency state needing replacement therapy with HRT emerged over recent years but recent research has highlighted ↑ breast cancer risks and suggested there is no rationale for using HRT to prevent cardiovascular disease. Thus, long-term use of HRT is not indicated for healthy women without symptoms.

Short-term use of HRT is still recommended for the relief of menopausal symptoms. Carefully balance risks against benefits for each individual*.

Contraindications: Cancer of the breast or endometrium; thromboembolic disease (including AF); kidney or liver disease.

Particular indications

• Early menopause—consider alternatives if prescribing for osteoporosis prevention alone; continue until age 50y.
• Hysterectomy before menopause, even if ovaries are conserved—≈1: 4 have early menopause.
• Relief of symptoms related to oestrogen deficiency peri- and postmenopausally e.g. flushes/sweats.
• 2nd line treatment of osteoporosis for women ≥51y.—🕮 p.568

Things to do before starting HRT

• **Explain pros and cons of HRT:** Support with written information; allow time to consider options.
• **Contraceptive requirement:** HRT does *not* provide contraception. For women of <50y., the COC pill may provide contraception and alleviate menopausal symptoms (🕮 p.732).
• **History:** History of hysterectomy. Ask about bleeding pattern. Investigate any abnormal bleeding prior to starting HRT. Ask about FH of breast cancer. Explore risk factors for osteoporosis and CHD. Check reasons for starting HRT and expectations of treatment. Drug history—HRT ↓ free T_4 and free corticosteroids; anti-epileptics ↑ elimination of oestrogen.
• **Examination:** BP; weight; breasts (check no lumps); check smear is up to date; and consider examining for prolapse /vaginal abnormalities.
• **Health promotion:** Support with general health education about smoking cessation, diet, exercise, alcohol consumption, the breast cancer screening programme, etc.

Choice of preparation: *BNF 6.4.1.1.* Start with low dose and provide a 3mo. supply initially.

• For women without a uterus—give oestrogen alone.
• For women with an intact uterus—progesterone is required for the last 10–13d. of the cycle to prevent endometrial proliferation (🕮 p.709).
• Tablets, patches, gels, and implants are available.
• Consider topical vaginal preparations—these deliver oestrogen locally to vaginal tissues; include pessaries, cream, and rings. No progestogen is needed, though use is limited to 3–6 mo. if the uterus is present.

*See: Consensus conference on hormone replacement therapy: final consensus statement (October 2003) 🕮 http://www.rcpe.ac.uk/esd/consensus/hrt_03.html

Review side-effects after 3mo.: Common side-effects:
- *Oestrogen related*—fluid retention, breast enlargement and tenderness, nausea, headaches
- *Progestogen related*—headache, ↑ weight , bloating and depression (↓ by changing to a preparation with a less androgenic progestogen e.g. dydrogesterone or medroxyprogesterone)

Bleeding may be erratic for the 1st 2–3mo. of cyclical HRT but should appear after progestogen supplement in subsequent months. Continuous combined preparations may cause spotting for up to 12mo. Check BP and weight. ↑ dose if symptoms are not controlled.

Further follow-up: Annually or as needed if any problems. Check BP, weight, breasts, symptoms, and bleeding pattern.

Stopping HRT: Review HRT use every 6–12mo. and reassess risks and benefits. HRT is usually needed for <5y. for vasomotor symptom control. When stopping, withdrawal flushes may be severe and distressing. Stop in cold weather and half the dose for 1mo. first.

Table 21.5 Risks and benefits of HRT

Risks	Short-term benefits	Long-term benefits
↑ Breast cancer (RR 1.35) 2–3x ↑ risk of DVT Gallbladder disease	Alleviation of menopausal symptoms e.g. flushes/ sweats/vaginal dryness ↓ recurrent UTIs	↓ Osteoporosis ↓ Colorectal cancer

RR = relative risk

Essential reading

RCP (Edinburgh) Consensus conference on hormone replacement therapy: final consensus statement (October 2003) ⌨ http://www.rcpe.ac.uk/esd/consensus/hrt_03.html

Patient information

British Menopause Society ⌨ http://www.the-bms.org
The Menopause Amarant Trust ☎01293 413000
⌨ http://www.amarantmenopausetrust.org.uk

Bleeding in early pregnancy

Differential diagnosis

- Spontaneous abortion (miscarriage)
- Bleeding in normal pregnancy
- Ectopic pregnancy (☐ p.738)
- Trophoblastic disease (☐ p.738)
- Non-obstetric conditions e.g. friable cervix, cervical polyp, cervical cancer (☐ p.714)

⚠ Any sexually active woman presenting with abdominal pain and vaginal bleeding after an interval of amenorrhoea has an ectopic pregnancy, until proved otherwise.

Miscarriage[G]: Spontaneous abortion, or miscarriage, is the result of 30% of all pregnancies—8 in 10 miscarriages happen in the 1st 12wk. *Risk factors:* maternal age, smoking, alcohol consumption. *Causes:*
- Foetal abnormalities (50%)
- Uterine (fibroids, incompetent cervix, congenital abnormalities)
- Systemic disease (renal disease, connective tissue disease, DM, systemic infection, SLE)
- Drugs (e.g. cytotoxics, stilboestrol)
- Vascular

History: Date last menstrual period (LMP), result of any pregnancy tests, amount of bleeding, degree of pain, time of onset of pain in relation to bleeding (pain before bleeding—ectopic more likely), whether products passed (though clot/products are difficult to distinguish).

Examination: Cardiovascular status (BP, tachycardia), temperature (? toxic), abdominal examination (guarding/peritonism/unilateral tenderness—suspect ectopic), vaginal examination (exclude other causes of bleeding, sometimes products can be visualized), pelvic exam (size uterus, cervix open—cervix of multiparous woman should only admit a finger tip).

Investigations: Pregnancy test if pregnancy not confirmed. Many areas run rapid access early pregnancy clinics. USS is the definitive test of viability of pregnancy.

Management: Immediate action:
- *Shocked with heavy bleeding*—admit as emergency. Give 0.5mg im ergometrine to ↓ bleeding. Gain iv access if possible.
- *Septic abortion*—admit as acute emergency.
- *Incomplete or inevitable miscarriage*—admit; usually D&C performed.
- *Complete miscarriage*—no action. Follow-up in case of psychological reaction.
- *Threatened miscarriage*—traditionally, bed rest, abstinence from intercourse—though no evidence either makes any difference to outcome.

⚠ **Rhesus –ve women**—if bleeding >12wk. gestation, give anti-D immunoglobulin (250 IU im if gestation <20wk.) within 72h. of bleeding—*whether or not* the pregnancy is lost (☐ p.794).

❶There is no evidence abstinence from pregnancy for time after miscarriage is helpful—fertility may actually ↑ immediately after miscarriage.

Complications:
- *Early*—perforation of uterus during D&C, incomplete evacuation, infection, bleeding;
- *Late*—intrauterine synechiae (Ascherman's syndrome), cervical incompetence, depression and psychological reactions to loss of pregnancy.

Recurrent miscarriage^G: ≥3 miscarriages consecutively. *History:* How many? What gestation? Pain or bleeding? All with 1 partner? Previous cervical dilatation, D&C, or STD; systemic disease; FH of recurrent miscarriage. Refer if pregnancy is wanted—likelihood of pregnancy ~70%.

Psychological effects of early loss of pregnancy: Broach the subject with all women who have suffered a miscarriage or other early loss of pregnancy. Include the woman's partner if possible. Not all women are grieved—adjust your approach accordingly. Legitimize the grief and acknowledge it. Provide information about the condition which caused the loss and reassure, where appropriate, about the future (if <3 miscarriages, risk of further miscarriage is not ↑). Discuss worries and concerns of the woman and her partner. Warn of anniversary phenomenon or sadness they may feel on birth of another's baby. Provide ongoing support as needed.

Essential reading

RCOG ◻ http://www.rcog.org.uk
- **The investigation and treatment of couples with recurrent miscarriage** (2003)
- **The management of early pregnancy loss** (2000)

Patient information and support

Miscarriage Association ☎01924 200799
◻ http://www.miscarriageassociation.org.uk

Ectopic pregnancy and trophoblastic disease

Ectopic pregnancy[G]: A fertilized egg implants outside the uterine cavity—95% in a fallopian tube. Incidence ≈ 1:100 pregnancies and increasing due to ↑ *chlamydia* infections and PID. *Risk factors:* PID (single episode ↑ risk x7), infertility (15%), IUCD (14%), previous ectopic pregnancy (11%), tubal surgery, POP, age, smoking.

History

- *Abdominal pain* (97%): Unilateral or bilateral, usually starts before bleeding, may radiate to shoulder tip, worse on passing urine/opening bowels.
- *Amenorrhoea* (absent in 25%): Peak incidence after 7wk. amenorrhoea.
- *Irregular vaginal bleeding* (79%): Described as 'prune juice' but may be fresh blood, usually not heavy. May pass decidual cast.

Examination: Shock in 15–20%, abdominal tenderness ± rebound or guarding (71%), pelvic examination may reveal enlarged uterus, adnexal mass, cervical excitation.

Management: Admit immediately for further investigation. Resuscitate before admission as needed. Hospital management may be expectant (watch and pregnancy resolves spontaneously), medical (methotrexate), or surgical (laparotomy or laparoscopic surgery). Offer early USS in future pregnancies to confirm pregnancy is intrauterine.

Complications: Death if undetected; infertility (pregnancy rate post ectopic pregnancy is 66% with 10% having a further ectopic pregnancy).

Psychological effects of early loss of pregnancy: 📖 p.737

Trophoblastic disease[G]

Hydatidiform mole: Benign tumour of trophoblast containing 46 chromosomes, all of paternal origin, and no foetal material. Moles may become invasive and penetrate the uterus and/or metastasize to the lungs. 1:30 go on to develop choriocarcinoma.

Presentation

- Bleeding in early pregnancy ± exaggerated symptoms of pregnancy.
- Rarely presents with symptoms of metastatic spread—haemoptysis, pleurisy.
- Uterus is usually large for dates and no foetal heart can be heard. USS has a typical appearance.
- Blood—↑↑↑ Serum β-HCG.

Management: Refer to gynaecology urgently. Patients with confirmed mole are followed up by specialist centres. Incidence in further pregnancies ≈ 1:120. Pregnancy is not advised for 1y. after mole—investigate further pregnancies with early USS and β-HCG estimation. COC pill is contraindicated.

Partial mole: Benign tumour of trophoblast containing 69 chromosomes, 1 set of maternal and 2 of paternal origin, with some foetal tissue. Treat as for mole. No ↑ risk choriocarcinoma.

Choriocarcinoma: Malignant tumour of trophoblast which may follow molar pregnancy (rarely normal pregnancy). Usually presents with vaginal bleeding. May present with metastases (shadows on CXR, dyspnoea, haemoptysis). Can present many years after pregnancy. Treated with chemotherapy—prognosis excellent. Pregnancy is possible after 2y. free from disease.

Further information

RCOG 🖳 http://www.rcog.org.uk
- The management of tubal pregnancy (2004)
- Management of gestational trophoblastic neoplasia (2004)

Patient information and support

Ectopic Pregnancy Trust 🖳 http://www.ectopic.org
Hydatidiform Mole and Choriocarcinoma UK Information and Support Service
  🖳 http://www.hmole-chorio.org.uk

Vaginal discharge

All women have some vaginal discharge. Physiological discharge is white, becoming yellow on contact with air. Amount varies considerably. Discharge is only abnormal when it is different from a woman's normal discharge. The amount is affected by menstrual cycle, sexual activity, use of COC, age, stress, and pregnancy. 95% cases that present in general practice are accounted for by 5 causes:

- Excessive normal secretions
- Bacterial vaginosis
- *Candida albicans*
- Cervicitis (gonococcal, chlamydial, or herpetic)
- *Trichomonas vaginalis*

Rarer causes: Cervical ectropion; chemical vaginitis (avoid perfumed or disinfectant bath additives); foreign body e.g. retained tampon (remove and treat with metronidazole); IUCD; cervical polyp; fistula; necrotic tumour (rare).

History: Pregnancy, DM, recent course of antibiotics, sexual history (recent sexual contact with new partner, multiple partners, presence of symptoms in partner), worries about sexually transmitted disease, vaginal discharge (itchy, offensive, colour), vulval soreness and irritation, lower abdominal pain, dyspareunia, heavy periods, intermenstrual bleeding, fever, vulval pain, attempts at self-medication.

Examination: Abdominal, pelvic, and vaginal examination. Look for lower abdominal tenderness, tenderness on bimanual palpation, cervical erosion or contact bleeding, discharge, warts or ulcers.

Investigation: High vaginal swab for culture and endocervical swabs for gonorrhoea and chlamydia; opportunistic cervical smear. If herpes infection suspected—viral swab (or if unavailable, refer to GUM).

Treatment: Treat cause (📖 p.740–5). If unclear, refer to GUM or gynaecology.

Bacterial vaginosis (BV): Vaginal flora is changed from lactobacillus species to anaerobes. Not sexually transmitted *Prevalence*: 10–40%. ~½ are asymptomatic. Associated with ↑ risk of preterm delivery (and ↓ risk if treated); development of PID and endometritis following abortion or birth; infection post hysterectomy. *History*: Grey-yellow, fishy, offensive discharge; no vulval soreness. *Examination*: Discharge; cervix looks normal. *Investigation*: Endocervical swab—M,C&S.

Management

- 50% remit spontaneously.
- Except in the 1st trimester of pregnancy, treat with metronidazole po (400mg bd for 7d.) or pv (5g bd for 5d).
- In the 1st trimester of pregnancy, treat with clindamycin 2% cream 5g nocte pv for 1wk.
- Cure rates with all methods—85%. No benefit from treating partner.
- Recurrent BV (1:3 recur)—tetracycline 300mg bd for 2wk.

Candidiasis: Fungal infection. ~20% of patients are asymptomatic.
Predisposing factors:

- Cushing's or Addison's disease
- DM
- Pregnancy
- Immunosuppression
- Steroid treatment
- Vaginal trauma
- Broad-spectrum antibiotics
- Radiotherapy/chemotherapy
- Tight-fitting synthetic underwear

History: Well; pruritus vulvae; superficial dyspareunia; thick, creamy, non-offensive discharge.

Examination: Discharge (cottage cheese), sore vulva which may be cracked or fissured.

Investigation: Usually unnecessary. Confirm diagnosis if infection persists or recurs by sending a vaginal swab for M,C&S.

Management: Only treat if symptomatic. Try clotrimazole pessaries (cure rate ≈90%). An alternative is oral fluconazole (contraindicated in pregnancy or lactation—83% cure rate). Sexual transmission is minimal and there is no benefit from treating the partner unless overt infection. Benefits of ingestion or topical application of live yoghurt are not clear, though it is probably not harmful.

Recurrent infection

- If occurs premenstrually, consider prophylaxis with fluconazole 150mg on the 21st day of cycle or 500mg clotrimazole pessary on days 7 and 21.
- If infection at other times, try 2wk. course fluconazole 50mg od po *or* clotrimazole 100mg nocte pv. Advise loose underwear and avoidance of perfumes or disinfectants in bath.

Patient information on thrush

📟 http://www.womenshealthlondon.org.uk/leaflets/thrush/thrush.html

Further information

British Association of Sexual Health and HIV (BASHH)
  📟 http://www.bashh.org
- Management of bacterial vaginosis (2001)
- Management of vulvovaginal candidiasis (2001)

Genito-urinary medicine

GPs are frequently presented with symptoms or signs found incidentally (e.g. when doing a cervical smear) that may indicate sexually transmitted disease. The easiest (and often best) option is to refer suspected cases to GUM clinics. Sometimes the patient is reluctant to go and 40% referrals never attend, so it is still necessary for GPs to know how to prevent, diagnose, and treat STDs themselves.

Contact tracing: Best done by GUM clinics. If a patient refuses to go, then provide the patient with a letter to give to contacts stating the disease they have been in contact with, treatment given, and suggesting contacts visit their local GUM clinic promptly.

Use of GUM clinics: In general, refer patients:
- who require contact tracing;
- if counselling is needed e.g. first attack HSV, HIV
- if diagnosis is still unclear after investigation
- for confirmation of diagnosis e.g. HSV
- if specialist treatment required e.g. treatment of genital warts.

Vaginal discharge 🕮 p.740

Urethritis: Inflammation of the male urethra. Multifactorial condition which is primarily sexually acquired. Mucopurulent cervicitis is the female equivalent. Characterized by discharge and/or dysuria, though may be asymptomatic (found when a swab is taken following contact tracing). Classified by the organisms grown when a swab is taken for M,C&S:
- *Gonococcal urethritis:* N. gonorrhoea is identified on urethral swab.
- *Non-gonococcal urethritis:* 20–30%, no organism is grown. In some cases, associated with bacterial vaginsosis in female partners. Identifiable causes: chlamydia (30–50%); ureaplasmas (10%); mycoplasma genitalium (10%); *Trichomonas vaginalis* (1–17% depending on frequency of TV in the population tested—🕮 p.745); others (<10%—Candida, HSV, bacterial UTI, urethral stricture, foreign body).

Management: Treat cause.

Pelvic inflammatory disease: 🕮 p.721

Behçet disease: Multi-organ disease. *Cause:* unknown—thought to be infective. ♂: ♀ ≈ 2:1. Associated with HLA B5/51 genotype. *Clinical picture (only some features are usually present):* arthritis; ocular symptoms and signs—pain, ↓ vision, floaters, iritis; scarring, painful ulceration of mouth and/or scrotum/labia; colitis; meningoencephalitis.

Management: Refer to GUM clinic, ophthalmologist, or general physician (depending on symptom cluster). Treatment is usually with high dose prednisolone or colchicine. Topical steroids may be useful for ulcers. (*H. Behçet (1889–1948)—Turkish dermatologist*).

Syphilis: Caused by *Treponema pallidum*. Rare in the UK but incidence is increasing. *Incubation:* 9–90d. In all cases refer for specialist care. Contact tracing is essential.

The 4 stages of syphilis:
- *Primary syphilis:* Chancre at the site of contact.
- *Secondary syphilis:* 4–8wk. after chancre. Systemic symptoms: fever, malaise, generalized lymphadenopathy, anal papules (conylomata lata), rash (trunk, palms, soles), buccal snail track ulcers, alopecia.
- *Tertiary syphilis:* 2–20y. after initial infection. Gummas (granulomas) in connective tissue.
- *Quarternary syphilis:* Cardiovascular or neurological complications. *Investigation:* blood for VDRL or TPHA.

Chlamydia Major cause of pelvic pain and infertility in women.

Presentation in women:
- *History:* >50% are asymptomatic.
- *Symptoms:* vaginal discharge (30%); postcoital or intermenstrual bleeding; PID—abdominal pain, fever; urethral syndrome (📖 p.693)
- *Examination:* Mucopurulent cervicitis; hyperaemia and oedema of the cervix ± contact bleeding; tender adnexae; cervical excitation.
- *Investigation:* Send endocervical swab for ELISA ± MSU to confirm diagnosis. Urine samples are used for screening asymptomatic women.

Presentation in men: Usually asymptomatic. May have urethritis (see opposite page). Send urethral swab for ELISA ± MSU to confirm diagnosis.

Presentation in neonates: Conjunctivitis, pneumonia, pharyngitis, otitis media—$^1/_3$ affected mothers have affected babies.

Screening: Chlamydia is a preventable cause of infertility, ectopic pregnancy, and PID. Screening, using first-catch urine testing, ↓ prevalence and incidence of PID[S]. The DoH is implementing a national screening programme, initially aimed at young people aged 16–24y. who access sexual health services, through a phased roll out in England. Similar programmes are being considered in the rest of the UK.

Management
- Doxycycline 100mg bd for 1wk.; azithromycin 1g po as a single dose is an alternative which ensures compliance.
- During pregnancy/breast-feeding use erythromycin 500mg qds 1wk.
- Affected neonates—seek specialist advice.

Further information
DoH (2001) National strategy for sexual health and HIV
 🖳 http://www.dh.gov.uk
British Association of Sexual Health and HIV (BASHH)
 🖳 http://www.bashh.org
- Management of early syphilis (2002)
- Management of late syphilis (2002)
- Management of chlamydia trachomatis genital tract infection (2001)

Patient information and support
Family Planning Association
 🖳 http://www.fpa.org.uk
DoH: Sexual Health Line ☎0800 567 123 (24h.); Sexwise (for under 18s) ☎0800 28 29 30

More sexually transmitted diseases

HIV: 📖 p.498   **Chlamydia:** 📖 p.743   **Syphilis:** 📖 p.742
Lice: 📖 p.675   **Hepatitis B and C:** 📖 p.496 **Scabies:** 📖 p.674

Genital warts: Caused by human papilloma virus (HPV). Usually sexually transmitted and >25% have concomitant STDs. Disease may be clinical (found on examination) or subclinical (changes associated with infection detected on smear). In women, CIN (📖 p.714) is related to infection with HPV infection.

History and examination
- *Women:* Often asymptomatic but may be associated with itching or vaginal discharge. Warts are usually seen on vulva or introitus. Warts enlarge during pregnancy.
- *Men:* Warts are usually found on the penis or perianally.

Management
- *Clinical warts:* Treatment does not eradicate the virus but removes lesions. Usually carried out in GUM clinics. Podophyllin paint 25% is applied weekly, left on 4h, and washed off—cure rates 50–60%. Paint must be applied by doctor or nurse protecting adjacent skin. *Alternative:* surgical treatment e.g. cryotherapy.
- *Subclinical warts:* No treatment. Barrier contraception is needed for at least 3mo. after the warts are gone. Contact tracing is essential.

Genital herpes: May be asymptomatic. *Cause:* HSV 1 and 2. *Differential diagnosis:* 📖 p.264.

History and examination: Diagnostic in 90% cases. Multiple painful genital ulcers <1wk. after sexual contact. Initially redness, then vesicles, ulcers, and finally crusting ± inguinal LNs. Untreated, lasts 3–4wk. *Complications:* Urinary retention, aseptic meningitis.

Management
- Refer to GUM if diagnosis uncertain and for contact tracing.
- Treat with acyclovir (↓ duration, symptoms, and complications), analgesia, ice packs, and salt baths.
- Advice—barrier methods of contraception (risk of transmission in monogamous relationships—10%/y.).
- If pregnant, obtain specialist advice (📖 p.788).

Neonatal infection: Presents at age 5–21d. with vesicular lesions around the presenting part or rarely systemic infection. Usually babies of women with no prior history of genital HSV. Refer as a paediatric emergency.

Recurrent infection: Reactivation of latent virus—HSV2 > HSV1. Less severe than 1° infection. Neonatal transmission rates are low (<3%). Elective LSCS for those with active recurrences at term is controversial. Consider suppressive therapy if >5 attacks/y. e.g. acyclovir 400mg bd. Usually initiated under consultant supervision.

Trichomonas vaginalis (TV)
Presentation in women
- *History:* 5% are asymptomatic. *Symptoms:*
  - Vaginal discharge (25%)—copious, mucopurulent, yellow, smelly discharge. May be frothy.
  - Vaginal soreness.
  - Dysuria.
- *Examination:* Discharge, vaginal inflammation, typical strawberry cervix.
- *Investigation:* Send endocervical swab for M,C&S. May also be detected on cervical smear.

Presentation in men: Almost always asymptomatic. May have dysuria. Take urethral swab for M,C&S.

Management
- Metronidazole po (400mg bd for 7d.) or pv (5g bd for 5d.).
  Clindamycin is a suitable alternative in the 1st trimester of pregnancy.
- Consider referral to GUM clinic for contact tracing.
- Resistant TV—try a combination of po and pr metronidazole (keep total dose <4g/d. due to risk neurotoxicity); for women, treat during menstruation when TV load is at its lowest.

Gonorrhoea
Presentation in women: Infection may cause PID, abscess of Bartholin gland, miscarriage, preterm labour. Babies may have neonatal opthalmia (purulent discharge ± swelling of eyelid <4d. after birth—permanent visual damage can result). Send endocervical swab for M,C&S to confirm diagnosis. Taking rectal and urethral swabs ↑ sensitivity.

Presentation in men: 50% acute infections are asymptomatic. May present with urethritis, prostatitis, urethral stricture, or, more rarely, skin lesions or septic arthritis. Send urethral ± rectal swabs for M,C&S to confirm diagnosis.

Management
- 1 x 500mg ciprofloxacin. Contraindicated in pregnancy or if history of fits—alternative is amoxicillin 3g + probenecid 1g or azithromycin 1g (effective against chlamydia and gonococcus).
- If PID, add co-amoxiclav 250–500mg tds (or erythromycin) for 10d.
- Reculture 3–7d. after treatment. Contact tracing is essential (refer to GUM clinic).
- *Affected neonates:* seek specialist advice.

Further information
British Association of Sexual Health and HIV (BASHH) ⌨ http://www.bashh.org
- Management of trimonas vaginalis infection (2001)
- Management of gonorrhoea in adults (2002)

Patient information and support
Family Planning Association ⌨ http://www.fpa.org.uk
Herpes Association ☎020 7609 9061
  ⌨ http://www.herpes.org.uk

Sexual problems

Sexual problems may have a physical or psychological basis but all develop a psychological aspect in time. Both partners have a problem in ≈30% cases. Be supportive—your response will determine whether the patient receives appropriate help.

History

- What is the problem?
- If new, when did it start?
- Why consult now?
- What outcome does the patient want?
- Is the patient complaining, or his/her partner?
- Past medical and psychiatric history.
- Details of sex education. Attitude towards sex. Sexual history.
- Social history and recent life events.

Consider the following psychological aspects: Poor self-image; anger or resentment (relationship or financial difficulties, children, parents, work stress); ignorance or misunderstanding; shame, embarrassment, or guilt (view that sexuality is 'bad', sexual abuse); anxiety/fear about sex (fear of closeness, vulnerability, letting go, and failure).

Examination: Genitalia for abnormalities and tenderness. Helpful but don't insist—it may scare the patient away.

Lack of sexual interest: Usually needs specialist help. Often underlying psychological difficulties which may relate specifically to sex e.g. previous child abuse, or a general psychological disorder. Women frequently lose interest around the menopause or after operations (especially mastectomy or hysterectomy) or if their partner's performance repeatedly leads to frustration e.g. impotence. Both sexes lose interest if depressed or after traumatic events.

Vaginismus: Usually apparent at vaginal examination—severe spasm of the vaginal muscles and adduction of thighs. Try to find the root cause. *Common causes:* fear of the unknown; past history of rape, abuse, or severe emotional trauma; defence mechanism against growing up. Desensitize simple cases by encouraging the women to examine herself, and also encourage the partner to be confident enough to insert a finger into the vagina. If no success, refer.

Orgasmic problems in women

- *Physical reasons:* Drugs (major tranquillizers, antidepressants), neurological disease, pelvic surgery. Recognized complication of hysterectomy.
- *Psychological reasons:* Women who have never achieved an orgasm may have psychological reasons. Give 'permission' for the woman to investigate her body's own responses further by masturbation or vibrator. When she has learnt how to relax, encourage her to tell her partner and incorporate caressing into their usual lovemaking. Women who have lost the ability to achieve orgasm may need counselling, especially about current relationship or loss of self-image.

Premature ejaculation: Ejaculation sooner than either partner wishes. With practice, men can learn to delay ejaculation. The stop/start technique—when during caressing or intercourse a man feels he is close to climax he should stop being stimulated and relax for 30sec.. Stimulation can then recommence until he is close to climax again, when the relaxation is repeated. If this fails, the woman should squeeze the penis at the base of the glans between finger and thumb during relaxation phases. Consider referral for sex therapy if no improvement.

Delayed ejaculation: Usually a sign of longstanding sexual inhibition. Often the patient can ejaculate by masturbation, but not intravaginally. Explore anxiety and guilt feelings. Use a strategy like that for psychogenic impotence (below). If it fails, refer to a psychosexual counsellor.

Psychogenic impotence: Treatment in general practice is appropriate for couples who do not wish to be referred. See the couple together: Recommend a manual e.g. 'Treat Yourself to Sex'. Forbid sexual intercourse. Explain that stroking should progress slowly from non-genital to genital—if anxiety occurs, go back one step. Progress until erection is achieved. Give permission for intercourse (if not already achieved). If unsuccessful, refer to psychosexual counsellor via Relate or local Family Planning Clinic.

Impotence: 📖 p.702

Dyspareunia: 📖 p.726

Useful information

The British Association for Sexual and Relationship Therapy ☎020 8543 2707
　🖥 http://www.basrt.org.uk
Institute of Psychosexual Medicine 🖥 http://www.ipm.org.uk/
Brown P, Faulder C (1980) *Treat yourself to sex*. Penguin Books. ISBN: 0140463828

Summary of contraceptive methods

'The management of fertility is one of the most important functions of adulthood'

Germaine Greer (1939–)

Emergency contraception

- *<72h. after unprotected intercourse*
  Levonorgestrel 2 tablets of levonorgestrel 750 mcg immediately. Failure rate 2.5% when used day 3–5. ↑ dose by 50% if taking hepatic enzyme-inducing drugs e.g. anticonvulsants. *Side-effects:* nausea and vomiting, PV spotting. *Advice:* contact doctor for more pills if tablets are vomited <2h. after taking them; use barrier method until next period; next period may be early or late.
- *<5d. after unprotected intercourse*
  Insertion of a copper IUCD before implantation. Progestogen-containing IUCDs are not suitable for this purpose. Failure rate <1%.
- *All women*
  Advise to return if abdominal pain, if next period is overdue or abnormally light/heavy, or if need further contraceptive advice.

❶ Discuss transmission of STDs with all women when providing contraceptive service. Advise high-risk groups to use barrier methods in addition to hormonal methods of contraception.

Postponing a period: 2 methods:
- Progesterone e.g. norethisterone 5mg tds starting 3d. before period and stopped when convenient—bleed follows within a few days.
- COC started ≥1mo. before and continued throughout the time when the withdrawal bleed should have occurred (using 2 packs back-to-back). Withdrawal bleed after 2nd pack finished.

Essential reading

Guillebaud J (1993) *Contraception: your questions answered* (2nd Edition) Churchill Livingstone.

Useful information

Family Planning Association (FPA) ☎0845 310 1334
  🖳 http://www.fpa.org.uk
Faculty of Family Planning and Reproductive Health Care
  🖳 http://www.ffprhc.org.uk

Table 21.6 Summary of contraceptive methods

Method of contraception	Failure rate/100 woman y.	Advantages	Disadvantages
Sterilization (♂ or ♀)	<0.05	No contraindications / Once-only procedure / Few side-effects	Difficult to reverse
Progestagen-containing IUCD (e.g. Mirena)	0.1	No need for compliance. Lasts 5y.; ↓ bleeding, dysmenorrhoea, ectopic pregnancy; reversible on removal	Expensive; invasive; may cause erratic bleeding
Injectable progestagen (e.g. depot Provera)	0.1	High compliance; simple; cheap	Breakthrough bleeding/ menstrual irregularity; weight gain; unpredictable return of fertility; no instant reversal. ? ↑ risk osteoporosis
Implanon (single capsule, upper arm)	<0.002	No need for compliance. Lasts 3yrs. Immediately reversible	Needs training to insert and remove. 17% prolonged/heavy bleeding
Combined oral contraceptive (COC)	0.2–0.3	Regular cycle; lighter periods; ↓ dysmen-norhoea; woman has cycle and fertility control	Compliance (missed pill if forget >12h. or failure to absorb patches may ↑ compliance); side-effects common
Progesterone-only pill	0.5–3	Less contraindications than COC pill; woman has fertility control	Compliance (missed pill if forget >3h.); menstrual irregularity
IUCD	0.1–0.4	No need for compliance; lasts 5–8y.	Heavy periods; PID; ectopic pregnancy
Barrier methods— diaphragm; condoms; female sheath	2–15	Woman has fertility control; barrier to transmission of STDs	User-dependant
Natural methods	6–25	No contraindications or side-effects	Requires self-control; high failure rate

Combined oral contraceptive (COC)

Choosing a COC: *BNF 7.3.1.* COCs differ by oestrogen content, type of progestagen and presentation (e.g. patches, ED or phasic preparations). Choose a pill containing ≤35mcg ethinyloestradiol and levonorgestrel or norethisterone for 1st time users. For patients with acne or hirsutism consider a pill containing desogestrel or gestodene.

Women using liver enzyme inducing drugs: 📖 p.759

Before starting the COC:
• Take a history-sexual and reproductive health, medications, and lifesyle. Check BP.
• Risk of taking the COC is > benefit if:
  • Aged >35y. and a smoker
  • BMI >39kg/m² (if >30kg/m² ↑ risk DVT/PE—consider alternatives)
  • BP is consistently >140mmHg systolic and/or 90mmHg diastolic
  • PMH CVD (IHD, stroke or peripheral vascular disease) or DVT/PE or multiple/severe risk factors for either
  • PMH focal migraine
  • Liver disease
  • Female malignancy—breast cancer, genital cancer, mole
  • Hormone related problems in pregnancy (includes pruritus, chorea, pemphigoid gestationis and worsening of otosclerosis)
• Consider a routine thrombophilia screen in FH of DVT/PE in a 1st degree relative aged <45y.—📖 p.529
• Discuss side effects and risks; give directions on administration
• Health education—STDs, cervical smears, smoking

See BNF 7.3.1 for a full list of cautions and contraindications

Starting the COC pill: Contraception begins immediately if started:
• On day 1–3 of the cycle or on day 1 of the cycle and changing from POP (switch to new pill without any break);
• At the end of the 3rd week postpartum;
• <24h. after miscarriage/TOP;
• Changing COC variety and at the end of the previous packet but before the 7d. break (start the new pill omitting the 7d. break).

In all other cases use additional contraception for the first 7d.

> ⚠ **Stop**
> • *Immediately* if sudden severe chest pain, breathlessness, or haemoptysis; calf pain ± swelling; severe stomach pain; unusual severe or prolonged headache; sudden neurological deficit; collapse or first fit; hepatitis, jaundice, or liver enlargement; BP >160/100 (systolic or diastolic); absolute contraindication or >1 relative contraindication.
> • If sustained ↑ BP (2.5% new users); depression.

Taking the pill: 1 pill daily for 21d. then 7d. off (take ED preparations continuously). Use additional contraception (e.g. condom) for 7d. if:
• *Vomiting or severe diarrhoea:* Additional precautions for the period of illness and 7d. afterwards.

- *Missed pill >12h.:* Take missed pill, then the next pill at the normal time; consider emergency contraception if ≥4 pills missed mid-pack or ≥2 pills missed at the start or end of a pack.
- *Antibiotics* (or certain other drugs—*BNF* Appendix 1): Additional contraceptive measures during treatment and for 7d. after (rifampicin—4wk. after). *Long-term antibiotics* : extra precautions for the first 3wk.

If the 7d. of additional contraception runs into the pill-free week (or for ED preparations, inactive pills), omit the pill-free week (or ED tablets) and start a new pack immediately.

Follow-up: 3mo. after starting or changing COC (earlier if complications). Once established, review every 6mo. Assess risk factors and side-effects; give health education e.g. smoking cessation advice; check BP.

Short-term side-effects: Most wear off in the 1st 2 or 3 cycles:
- *Relative oestrogen excess*—nausea; dizziness cyclical weight ↑; bloating; vaginal discharge without infection; breast tenderness. Use a more progestogen-dominated pill.
- *Relative progestogen excess*—dry vagina; sustained weight ↑; depression; PMT; ↓ libido; lassitude; acne; hirsutism. ↑ oestrogen content.
- *Breakthrough bleeding*—exclude cervical causes and problems taking the pill (e.g. vomiting). ↑ progestogen content or change to pill with better cycle control (e.g. containing desogestrel/gestodene or a bi/triphasic pill). If fails, ↑ oestrogen too.

Long-term side-effects:
- ↑ risk CHD (x3 in smokers—except for pills containing desogestrel or gestodene), breast cancer (RR 1.24—returns to normal within 10y. of stopping); and cervical cancer;
- ↓ risk ovarian cancer and endometrial cancer.

Surgery: Stop COC from 4wk. before until 2wk. after major surgery, varicose vein surgery, or any operation followed by immobility.

Travel: If travelling for >5h., ↓ risk DVT with exercise during the journey ± elastic hosiery.

COC patch: Alternative if compliance with daily pill-taking is problematic. Apply patch on day 1 of cycle; change patch on days 8 and 15; remove 3rd patch on day 22 and then apply new patch after a 7d. patch-free interval. If changing from other forms of contraception or starting after pregnancy, miscarriage or TOP, see *BNF* 7.3.1.
- *If patch falls off for <24h. or delayed change of patch for <48h.,* reapply patch immediately and continue cycle.
- *If patch falls off for >24h. (or uncertain of time detached) or delayed change of patch for >48h.* or if application of a new patch at the start of a cycle is delayed, start a new cycle—use additional method of contraception (e.g. condom) for 7d.

Useful information
Family Planning Association (FPA) ☎0845 310 1334 ▤ *http://www.fpa.org.uk*
Faculty of Family Planning and Reproductive Health Care ▤ *http://www.ffprhc.org.uk*

Progestogen-containing contraceptives

BNF 7.3.2.

Progesterone only pill (POP or 'mini-pill'): Alternative to COC pill when oestrogens are contraindicated. Before starting, ensure POP is not contraindicated. *Health education:* side-effects (below); STDs; cervical smears.

Starting the POP

- Day 1 (1st day of the period)—immediate protection. Otherwise, additional contraceptive measures for the 1st 7d.
- Changing from a COC—immediate protection if POP continued directly on from the end of the COC packet (from day 21 pill if ED preparation) i.e. omitting the 7d. break.
- Postpartum—start at 3wk. postpartum. If starting later, use additional precautions for 7d.

Taking the POP: One tablet daily with no pill-free breaks. Patients weighing >70kg are often prescribed 2 pills/d. (unlicensed use); no ↑ dose for cerazette. Not a suitable method for patients concurrently taking enzyme-inducing drugs (e.g. anti-epileptics—🕮 p.620). The POP must be taken at the same time each day (>4h. before usual time for intercourse to give maximum protection).

- *Forgotten pills:* If a pill is missed or delayed >3h. (12h. for Cerazette®), continue taking POP at usual time and use additional precautions for 2d.. If a POP is missed or taken >3h. late and intercourse has occurred before 2 further tablets have been correctly taken, supply emergency contraception.
- *Diarrhoea or vomiting:* Continue taking POP but assume pills 'missed' for duration of attack.
- *Antibiotics:* Do not affect the POP (except enzyme-inducing rifampicin and griseofulvin—treat as missed pills).

Follow-up: Review patients 3mo. after starting POP or changing from COC pill. Earlier if complications. Once established, review 6 monthly. On each occasion ask about side-effects.

Side-effects

- *Menstrual irregularities:* Oligomenorrhoea, menorrhagia, amenorrhoea—examine to exclude a pathological cause (+ pregnancy test if amenorrhoea); consider measuring FSH if oligomenorrhoea/amenorrhoea and age >50y. or menopausal symptoms (🕮 p.732); consider changing progestogen in the pill or giving additional norethisterone or dydrogesterone from d.12 to d.26 for 2–3mo.
- *Ectopic pregnancy:* ↑ risk. If patient presents with abdominal pain, treat as ectopic (🕮 p.738) until proved otherwise.
- *Others:* Nausea and vomiting; headache; dizziness; breast discomfort; depression; skin disorders; disturbance of appetite and weight changes; changes in libido.
- *Long term:* Small ↑ risk breast cancer—risk reverts to normal within 10y. of stopping.

Injectable progestogens: Progestogen in slow-release format.
Preparations:
- Depo-Provera (provides contraception for 12wk.)
- Noristerat (provides contraception for 8wk.—can only be repeated once)

Both are given by deep im injection into the buttock/lateral thigh. Before giving, check the patient knows about possible side-effects (including ↓ in bone density); understands that once given, the injection is not reversible; and that fertility may return after a varying time.

Contraceptive effect is immediate if 1st injection is given:
- within 5d. of onset of menstruation;
- <5d. postpartum if not breast-feeding;
- 6wk. postpartum if breast-feeding;
- 1–5d. after miscarriage or TOP.

Otherwise, advise women to use additional contraception for 7d. after the 1st injection. Repeat injections are effective immediately if given <12wk. + 5d. after previous injection (<8wk. for Noristerat) If not, exclude pregnancy and use additional contraception for 7d.

CSM Advice (2004)
- In adolescents, Depo-Provea should only be used when other methods of contraception are inappropriate.
- In all women balance risks against benefits of use of Depo-Provera for >2y.
- In women with risk factors for osteoporosis (📖 p.568) consider alternative methods of contraception to Depo-Provera.

Progestogen implant: (e.g. Implanon). Side-effects/problems are the same as for injectable progestogens. Insertion and removal requires special training.

Progestogen-releasing IUCD: 📖 p.754

Useful information
Family Planning Association (FPA) ☎0845 310 1334
 🖳 http://www.fpa.org.uk
Faculty of Family Planning and Reproductive Health Care
 🖳 http://www.ffprhc.org.uk

Intra-uterine contraceptive device (IUCD)

Before insertion, ensure no contraindications. *Health education:* possible problems (below); cervical smears.

Insertion and follow-up: Special training is needed. Courses are available and practical experience can be gained via local family planning clinics.

Timing of insertion
- Day 4–14 of a 28d. cycle;
- 4–6wk. postpartum (6–8wk. post Caesarean section);
- Immediately after termination/spontaneous miscarriage at <12wk. gestation.

Follow-up: Review after 1st period, then annually. Ask about periods, pelvic pain, vaginal discharge, and discomfort to partner. Perform pelvic examination to check threads.

Emergency contraception: 📖 p.748

Lifespan of IUCDs
- <40y. of age:
  - Modern copper-containing IUCDs (e.g. Multiload Cu 375) are effective for 8y.
  - Older devices (e.g. Nova T) last 3–5y.
- ≥40y.: most IUCDs are effective until the menopause.

Removal
- *If pregnancy desired:* Remove at any time.
- *If pregnancy not desired:* Remove after establishing a hormonal method or use barrier methods or abstinence ≥7d. prior to removal.
- *Urgent removal* (e.g. for infection): Postcoital contraception needed if intercourse has occurred in the previous 72h.
- *Menopause:* Remove after 1y. amenorrhoea in >50y.; after 2y. amenorrhoea in <50y.. If difficulty removing, try again after a 5d. course of oestrogen (e.g. Premarin 1.25mg od po).

Problems
- *Menorrhagia, intermenstrual bleeding, dysmenorrhoea:* Common for the 1st 3mo. If persistent or any other symptoms, examine for infection (tender uterus or adnexae, vaginal discharge) or malposition (presence of strings, pain). Treat with NSAID (↓ pain and bleeding). If causing anaemia or sustained intermenstrual/postcoital bleeding, remove IUCD.
- *Pelvic infection:* Pelvic pain ± vaginal discharge may indicate infection. Risk greatest for 1st 3wk. after insertion. Examine, take swabs. Treat cause. For most women, if symptoms subside on antibiotics, the IUCD can be left in situ. If nulliparous, remove.

- *Missing threads:* Teach women to feel for IUCD threads after each period. If the threads are not found, advise them to use other contraceptive measures temporarily and visit a GP/family planning clinic. If the threads are not visible/palpable on examination, exclude pregnancy and refer for USS to confirm position of the IUCD. IUCD may have been expelled, be malpositioned, or have perforated the uterus. If in situ and correctly positioned, leave in place until next due to be changed. Else arrange for removal (if known to be in situ, try probing the endocervical canal with a pair of long-handled forceps before referral to gynaecology) ± reinsertion.
- *Actinomyces-like organisms (ALOs) on cervical smear:* 📖 p.717.
- *Pregnancy:* 3–9% of pregnancies occurring with IUCD in situ are ectopic. Consider ectopic pregnancy in any woman presenting with abdominal pain (📖 p.738). If USS confirms intra-uterine pregnancy, removal of the IUCD <12wk. gestation ↓ miscarriage rate (½) and risk of infection, but there is a miscarriage rate associated with removal. If pregnancy >12wk. gestation or no threads are visible, refer to obstetrics.

Table 21.7 Pros and cons of the progestogen-releasing IUCD

Advantages over other IUCDs	Disadvantages
↓ heavy periods	Effective for 5y.
↓ dysmenorrhoea	More difficult to insert than copper IUCD
More reliable	Progesterone side-effects (nausea, breast tenderness)
Protects against ectopic pregnancy	
Suitable for women with history of PID	More expensive
	Associated with irregular bleeding

Useful information
Family Planning Association (FPA) ☎0845 310 1334
🖥 http://www.fpa.org.uk
Faculty of Family Planning and Reproductive Health Care: Run a training scheme leading to the Letter of Competence in Intrauterine Contraception Techniques. ☎020 7724 5669
🖥 http://www.ffprhc.org.uk

Other methods of contraception

Condoms: Give some protection against STDs. Male and female versions. Encourage couples to use a sheath with spermicide, or prescribe separate spermicidal cream/pessaries. Advise about emergency contraception in the event of an accident. Certain lubricants can cause condoms to rupture *(see BNF for list)*.

Vaginal diaphragms or caps: Motivation is crucial. Fitting must be performed by a doctor or nurse trained to fit diaphragms. After fitting, a woman should practise removing and inserting the cap several times under supervision. Then she should practise inserting, wearing, and removing the diaphragm for >1wk. using another form of contraception. Some vegetable/mineral oil-based lubricants can damage caps *(see BNF for list)*.

Advice for women using a diaphragm
- Insert before intercourse and leave in place ≥ 6h. afterwards.
- Place a ribbon of spermicide ≈4cm long on each side of the diaphragm before insertion. If intercourse takes place ≥3h. later, more spermicide is needed (either as cream or pessary).
- After use, wash diaphragm in warm soapy water, dry, and store in its container to maintain shape.

Follow-up: Check fit and comfort after ~1wk. and discuss again the routine for its use, especially the importance of spermicide. See after 3mo. and then annually, but more frequently if there are difficulties or if there is a weight change of >4kg. Prescribe a new diaphragm yearly.

Cervical/vault caps: Attach by suction. Otherwise used in the same way as a diaphragm. Useful for women with poor muscle tone, absent retropubic ledge, or recurrent cystitis when using a diaphragm.

Spermicides to use in combination with caps or condoms
Delfen, Duragel, Gynol II, Ortho-Creme, Orthoforms.

Avoidance of intercourse during times of fertility: 3 methods of estimating time of ovulation are used:
- Urine testing—commercial kit (Persona) is available to buy.
- Temperature—taken orally in the morning before drinking or getting up (thermometer available on FP10). ↑ 0.2–0.4°C indicates progesterone release from the corpus luteum. Unprotected intercourse can take place only from the 3rd day of the ↑ until the next period.
- Mucus texture (Billing's method)—texture of vaginal secretions is felt between finger and thumb daily. Prior to ovulation the mucus becomes profuse and slippery, then abruptly changes to being thicker and more tacky. No unprotected intercourse from the day the mucus becomes more profuse until 3d. after it becomes tacky. Patients with cycles > or <28d. must vary timings.

Coitus interruptus: Penis is withdrawn prior to ejaculation.

Sterilization: There are no contraindications to sterilization of men or women provided they make the request themselves, are of sound mind, and are not acting under external duress. Additional care must be taken when counselling those <25y., without children, pregnant women, those in reaction to a loss of relationship, or who may be at risk of coercion by their partner or others. Prior sanction by a high court judge must be sought in all cases where there is doubt over mental capacity to consent.

Method

- Women—laparoscopic tubal occlusion with clips or rings. Usually done under GA as a day case.
- Men—vasectomy. Usually done under LA as a day case.

Pre-referral counselling

- Alternative long-term contraceptive methods (include sterilization of partner as an alternative);
- Reversibility–sterilization is intended to be permanent, reversal is only 50–60% successful;
- Post-procedure pregnancy rate ('failure rate'—1:200 for women; 1:2000 for men);
- ↑ risk of ectopic pregnancy post tubal occlusion;
- Risk of operative complications;
- Effect on long-term health (no proven long-term risks);
- Need for contraception before and after operation:
  - Women: other contraception until 1st post-procedure period;
  - Men: other contraception until 2 consecutive semen analyses, 2–4wk. apart and ≥8wk. after the procedure show azoospermia.

Useful information

RCOG (2004) Male and female sterilization
  ▣ http://www. rcog.org.uk.
Family Planning Association (FPA) ☎0845 310 1334
  ▣ http://www.fpa.org.uk
Faculty of Family Planning and Reproductive Health Care
  ▣ http://www.ffprhc.org.uk

Contraception for special groups

Under 16y. old: In England and Wales, a doctor is allowed to give advice to a girl aged <16y. if:
- She has sufficient maturity to understand the moral, social, and emotional implications of treatment;
- She has informed her parents, or cannot be persuaded to inform them;
- She is very likely to begin, or continue, sexual intercourse with or without contraception;
- She is likely to suffer if no contraceptive advice or treatment is given; and It is in her best interest that contraceptive advice or treatment is given with or without parental consent.

Don't insist on vaginal examination or taking a smear unless there is a problem that necessitates it. Discuss the merits of delaying sexual intercourse until older. Stress the need for protection against STDs. If prescribing the COC pill for dysmenorrhoea or cycle control in young women, explain its use for contraception too.

Choice of contraceptive method: Low-dose COC pill is the most suitable method. Compliance can be a problem. *Alternatives:* COC patch; progestogen implant/injectables–improved compliance but problems with bleeding and ↑ weight (and see CSM guidance 📖 p.753); IUCD relative contraindication due to ↑ risk PID and ectopic pregnancy. Progestogen-containing IUCD is better but can be difficult to insert in a young woman.

Over 35y. old
- **COC:** Non-smokers without risk factors of IHD and normal BP can use the COC until 50y.. Consider switching to lower dose pills (20μg oestrogen) and lipid-friendly progestogen (e.g. gestodene or desogestrel). Continue until age 50y. then measure FSH at the end of the pill-free week—if normal, continue; if ↑, discontinue and re-check FSH after 6wk. off the COC. If still ↑, use a non-hormonal method until amenorrhoeic for 12mo. HRT is not required until COC is stopped.
- **POP, progestogen injection/implant or progestogen-containing IUCD:** Continue until age 55y. or symptoms suggestive of menopause. Check FSH. If low, continue; if ↑, discontinue or remove IUCD/implant. Re-check FSH after 6wk. (3mo. for injectables). If still ↑, use non-hormonal method until amenorrhoeic 12mo. Avoid progestogen implant if risk factors for osteoporosis
- **Other methods:** Discontinue when complete amenorrhoea for 2y. if age <50y. or 1y. if age ≥ 50y.. (If an IUCD is inserted age >40y., it can be left in situ until the menopause.)
- **HRT before the menopause:** Continue contraception (barrier or IUCD, not POP) until the menopause. Measure FSH at the beginning of the oestrogen-only phase. HRT does not prevent ↑ FSH if menopause has occurred. If ↑ FSH x2, assume menopause has occurred. Continue contraception for a further 1y. then stop.

Contraception after pregnancy: 📖 p.807

Obesity
- *COC pill*—consider a pill containing 20mcg ethinyloestradiol for pa-tients with BMI ≥30kg/m²; avoid in patients >50% over ideal weight or BMI >40. Avoid pills containing desogestrel and gestodene due to ↑ risk venous thrombosis.
- *POP* is less effective if weight >70kg. Prescribe 2 pills/d. (unlicensed).
- *Injectable progestogen* may cause ↑ weight.

DM, ↑BP, IHD, or risk factors for IHD
- *Injectable progestogens*—↓ HDL cholesterol; POP and progestogen-containing IUCD do not significantly alter cholesterol profile.
- *COC pill*—use a preparation that causes minimal disturbance to lipid metabolism e.g. gestodene, desogestrel.
- *For diabetics*—monitor blood sugar more carefully when starting the COC or Progestogen-only methods—if complications of DM, COC is contraindicated.
- *Avoid IUCD* in patients with artificial heart valves or past history of SBE. Use antibiotic prophylaxis for insertion/withdrawal of IUCDs in patients with heart valve lesions who need dental prophylaxis (📖 p.349).

Thrombophilia: COC pill contraindicated.

Epilepsy: COC/POP/progestogen injection may not work in standard dose if on long-term hepatic enzyme-inducing drugs e.g. phenytoin, carbamazepine. Use alternative methods e.g. IUCD or mirena. If none, acceptable use:
- Injectable progestogen—for Noristerat, ↓ interval between injections;
- High-dose COC (aim for >50mcg oestrogen but ≤ 60mcg/d.)
and check d.21 serum progesterone to ensure ovulation is suppressed. Also consider tri-cycling (running 3 packets together) and ↓ pill-free wk to 4d..

Other illness See specialist text. If in doubt, seek consultant advice.

Termination of pregnancy

Legal constraints: The 1967 and 1990 Human Fertilization/Embryology Acts govern termination of pregnancy (ToP) in UK. Termination is allowed at <24wk. gestation if termination:

- ↓ risk to the woman's life.
- ↓ risk to the mother's physical or mental health (90% ToPs are carried out under this clause).
- ↓ risk to the physical or mental health of the mother's existing children.
- The baby is at serious risk of being physically or mentally handicapped.

There is no upper time limit if there is real risk to the mother's life; risk of grave, permanent injury to the mother's physical or mental health; or the baby would be born seriously physically or mentally handicapped. ToPs >24wk. can only be carried out in NHS hospitals. 99% ToPs take place <20wk. Those taking place >20wk. are usually performed when foetal abnormality is found on USS (or amniocentesis) or if pregnancy is concealed in the very young.

The role of the GP

- The earlier in pregnancy an abortion is performed, the lower the risk of complications. General practice is often the 1st stage of the referral procedure—have arrangements which minimize delay.
- Termination of pregnancy, especially for 'social' reasons, is a difficult ethical area for many GPs. We do not sit in moral judgement. Whatever your views, be sympathetic and, if not prepared to refer yourself, arrange for the patient to see someone who will, as soon as possible.
- Confirm pregnancy if unsure. Assess dates by bimanual palpation or arrange dating USS.
- Counselling—unbiased counselling to allow a woman to reach a decision she feels is right for her. This is an important decision she will have to live with for the rest of her life. Why does she want a termination? Has she considered alternatives? Does her partner/parents know? What are their views?
- Ideally, the woman should be given some time, once she has all the information, to make her decision (e.g. follow-up in a few days). Offer a let-out clause—she can always change her mind right up until the time of the procedure and you will support whatever decision she makes.
- Consider signing form HSA1.
- Discuss contraception after ToP (ideally do this before ToP so it can be started immediately after).
- Arrange follow-up after the procedure.

Procedure

- **Medical:** Oral mifepristone, followed by vaginal prostaglandin.
- **Surgical:** Suction termination <15wk.; dilatation and evacuation >15wk.

Follow-up: In many areas, post-procedure follow-up is undertaken by the GP. Worrying symptoms are excessive blood loss, pain, or high temperature. Assess, consider the possibility of infection, and treat if reasonably well. Admit if worried.

❶ Check anti-D has been given if needed (📖 p.794) and chosen method of contraception has been started.

Complications: Haemorrhage, uterine perforation, cervical trauma, failed procedure and on-going pregnancy, infection, pscyhological sequelae. There is no association between ToP and subsequent infertility or miscarriage/pre-term delivery.

Further information
RCOG (2001) The care of women requesting induced abortion
   📖 http://www. rcog.org.uk.

Patient information and support
Marie Stopes International ☎0845 300 8090
   📖 http://www.mariestopes.org.uk
British Pregnancy Advisory Service (BPAS) ☎0845 730 40 30
   📖 http://www.bpas.org.uk
Brook Advisory Centres (patients <25y. only) ☎0800 0185 023
   📖 http://www.brook.org.uk
Antenatal Results and Choices (ARC)—supports parents faced with termination for foetal abnormality ☎0207 631 0285 📖 http://www.arc-uk.org

Infertility^G

Infertility is a cause of considerable psychological distress. It affects ≈1:7 couples. Prevalence is static but the number of couples seeking help is rising. Defined as absence of pregnancy after 2y. of regular unprotected intercourse, though other factors (e.g. woman's age, previous surgery, or irregular menstrual cycles) may justify earlier investigation. Couple-centred management (seeing couples together) is advised.

Management in general practice: See Figures 21.3 and 21.4

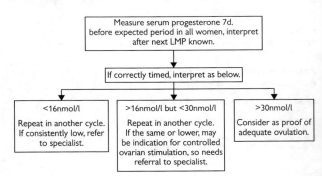

Figure 21.3 Confirmation of ovulation with mid-luteal progesterone level (Reproduced with permission of the Royal College of Obstetricians and Gynaecologists from *The initial investigation and management of the infertile couple* (1999).)

Further information

RCOG (2004) Fertility: assessment and treatment for people with fertility problems
🖳 http://www.rcog.org.uk

Patient information and support

Infertility Network UK (INUK) ☎0870 11 88 088
🖳 http://www.infertilitynetworkuk.com

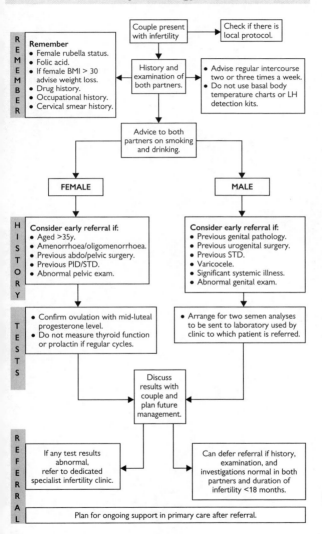

Figure 21.4 Management of infertility in general practice. (Reproduced with permission of the Royal College of Obstetricians and Gynaecologists from *The initial investigation and management of the infertile couple* (1999).)

Obstetrics

Pre-pregnancy counselling

The aim of pre-pregnancy care is to give a woman enough information for her pregnancy to occur under the optimal possible circumstances. Areas to cover are:

Smoking: ↓ ovulation, ↓ sperm count, ↓ sperm motility. Once the woman is pregnant, smoking: ↑ miscarriage rate (x2), ↑ risk of pre-term delivery, and ↓ birth weight (by an average of ≈200g). Smoking is associated with an ↑ rate of cot death, chest infections, and otitis media in children. Explain risks and advise on ways to stop (📖 p.234).

Alcohol: Foetal alcohol syndrome is rare and tends to occur in babies of heavy drinkers—especially those who binge drink. The effects of smaller quantities of alcohol are less clear—20–30y. ago women were advised to drink a Guinness a day and there is no evidence this policy had adverse effects. However, alcohol does cross the placenta and thus may affect the developing brain. Miscarriage rates are ↑ in moderate drinkers. Current advice is to avoid alcohol in pregnancy.

Diet
- Folate-rich foods prior to pregnancy and in the first 12wk.
- Avoid large quantities of vitamin A in vitamin supplements and liver.
- Avoid unpasteurized dairy products, uncooked eggs, pâtés, and pre-prepared salads to prevent infection (e.g. Listeriosis, salmonella) during pregnancy. When preparing food, keep cooked and raw meats separately; wash all soil off fruit and vegetables before eating; wash hands after preparation; only eat well cooked meat.

Folate supplementation: ↓ risk of neural tube defect by 72%.
- *If no previous neural tube defects*—0.4mg od when pregnancy is being planned and for 13wk. after conception.
- *If 1 parent affected, on anti-epileptic medication, or previous child affected*—Advise 5mg od from the time the pregnancy is being planned until 13wk. after conception.
Supplements can be prescribed or are available OTC from chemists and supermarkets.

Contraception: Women contemplating pregnancy are usually still using contraception. Discussion about how to stop/what to expect may be helpful (e.g. injectables, IUCD).

Chronic disease: Review of pre-existing medical conditions with referral for expert advice where necessary.
- Refer women who are diabetic for specialist diabetic review and change women taking sulphonylureas or metformin to insulin.
- Women with epilepsy—review medication (📖 p.782).
- Heart disease—refer for specialist advice if situation not clear.
- GU disease (e.g. HIV, genital warts, bacterial vaginosis)—refer for treatment/advice on mode of delivery if necessary (📖 p.788).
- Discontinue all known possible teratogens prior to conception.

Problems in previous pregnancies
- Recurrent miscarriage—📖 p.737
- Cervical incompetence—📖 p.715
- Congenital abnormalities/inherited disorders—pre-pregnancy counselling and detailed advice on genetic screening for high-risk pregnancies is available via regional genetics services.

Rubella status: If rubella status is unknown, suggest it is checked. Rubella infection in early pregnancy carries a high chance (40–70%) of deafness, blindness, cardiac abnormalities, or multiple foetal abnormalities (📖 p.791). If the woman is not rubella immune, suggest immunization with avoidance of pregnancy for 3mo. afterwards (live vaccine). Re-check rubella status 3mo. after immunization.

Work/ benefits: Discussion of benefits available during pregnancy and employment law is necessary so that women may avoid possible hazards at work, attend for antenatal care, and plan their maternity leave from early in pregnancy.

Discussion of antenatal care and screening available
- Brief discussion of antenatal screening and antenatal care procedures allows women to investigate their choices in pregnancy at their leisure.
- Brief discussion about miscarriage and possibility of infertility allows women to be more confident about asking for help if problems with conception/early pregnancy occur.

Essential reading
NICE (2003) Antenatal care: routine care for the healthy pregnant woman
🖥 http://www.nice.org.uk

Patient information
Family Planning Association: Patient information—planning for pregnancy.
🖥 http://www.fpa.org.uk
Maternity Alliance 🖥 http://www.maternityalliance.org.uk

Obstetric EDD calculator

LMP

Month	January	February	March	April	May	June
Day	*Estimated date of delivery (EDD)*					
1	9-Oct	9-Nov	7-Dec	7-Jan	6-Feb	8-Mar
2	10-Oct	10-Nov	8-Dec	8-Jan	7-Feb	9-Mar
3	11-Oct	11-Nov	9-Dec	9-Jan	8-Feb	10-Mar
4	12-Oct	12-Nov	10-Dec	10-Jan	9-Feb	11-Mar
5	13-Oct	13-Nov	11-Dec	11-Jan	10-Feb	12-Mar
6	14-Oct	14-Nov	12-Dec	12-Jan	11-Feb	13-Mar
7	15-Oct	15-Nov	13-Dec	13-Jan	12-Feb	14-Mar
8	16-Oct	16-Nov	14-Dec	14-Jan	13-Feb	15-Mar
9	17-Oct	17-Nov	15-Dec	15-Jan	14-Feb	16-Mar
10	18-Oct	18-Nov	16-Dec	16-Jan	15-Feb	17-Mar
11	19-Oct	19-Nov	17-Dec	17-Jan	16-Feb	18-Mar
12	20-Oct	20-Nov	18-Dec	18-Jan	17-Feb	19-Mar
13	21-Oct	21-Nov	19-Dec	19-Jan	18-Feb	20-Mar
14	22-Oct	22-Nov	20-Dec	20-Jan	19-Feb	21-Mar
15	23-Oct	23-Nov	21-Dec	21-Jan	20-Feb	22-Mar
16	24-Oct	24-Nov	22-Dec	22-Jan	21-Feb	23-Mar
17	25-Oct	25-Nov	23-Dec	23-Jan	22-Feb	24-Mar
18	26-Oct	26-Nov	24-Dec	24-Jan	23-Feb	25-Mar
19	27-Oct	27-Nov	25-Dec	25-Jan	24-Feb	26-Mar
20	28-Oct	28-Nov	26-Dec	26-Jan	25-Feb	27-Mar
21	29-Oct	29-Nov	27-Dec	27-Jan	26-Feb	28-Mar
22	30-Oct	30-Nov	28-Dec	28-Jan	27-Feb	29-Mar
23	31-Oct	1-Dec	29-Dec	29-Jan	28-Feb	30-Mar
24	1-Nov	2-Dec	30-Dec	30-Jan	1-Mar	31-Mar
25	2-Nov	3-Dec	31-Dec	31-Jan	2-Mar	1-Apr
26	3-Nov	4-Dec	1-Jan	1-Feb	3-Mar	2-Apr
27	4-Nov	5-Dec	2-Jan	2-Feb	4-Mar	3-Apr
28	5-Nov	6-Dec	3-Jan	3-Feb	5-Mar	4-Apr
29	6-Nov	7-Dec	4-Jan	4-Feb	6-Mar	5-Apr
30	7-Nov		5-Jan	5-Feb	7-Mar	6-Apr
31	8-Nov		6-Jan		8-Mar	

LMP

Month	July	August	September	October	November	December
Day			*Estimated date of delivery (EDD)*			
1	7-Apr	8-May	8-Jun	8-Jul	9-Aug	8-Sep
2	8-Apr	9-May	9-Jun	9-Jul	10-Aug	9-Sep
3	9-Apr	10-May	10-Jun	10-Jul	11-Aug	10-Sep
4	10-Apr	11-May	11-Jun	11-Jul	12-Aug	11-Sep
5	11-Apr	12-May	12-Jun	12-Jul	13-Aug	12-Sep
6	12-Apr	13-May	13-Jun	13-Jul	14-Aug	13-Sep
7	13-Apr	14-May	14-Jun	14-Jul	15-Aug	14-Sep
8	14-Apr	15-May	15-Jun	15-Jul	16-Aug	15-Sep
9	15-Apr	16-May	16-Jun	16-Jul	17-Aug	16-Sep
10	16-Apr	17-May	17-Jun	17-Jul	18-Aug	17-Sep
11	17-Apr	18-May	18-Jun	18-Jul	19-Aug	18-Sep
12	18-Apr	19-May	19-Jun	19-Jul	20-Aug	19-Sep
13	19-Apr	20-May	20-Jun	20-Jul	21-Aug	20-Sep
14	20-Apr	21-May	21-Jun	21-Jul	22-Aug	21-Sep
15	21-Apr	22-May	22-Jun	22-Jul	23-Aug	22-Sep
16	22-Apr	23-May	23-Jun	23-Jul	24-Aug	23-Sep
17	23-Apr	24-May	24-Jun	24-Jul	25-Aug	24-Sep
18	24-Apr	25-May	25-Jun	25-Jul	26-Aug	25-Sep
19	25-Apr	26-May	26-Jun	26-Jul	27-Aug	26-Sep
20	26-Apr	27-May	27-Jun	27-Jul	28-Aug	27-Sep
21	27-Apr	28-May	28-Jun	28-Jul	29-Aug	28-Sep
22	28-Apr	29-May	29-Jun	29-Jul	30-Aug	29-Sep
23	29-Apr	30-May	30-Jun	30-Jul	31-Aug	30-Sep
24	30-Apr	31-May	1-Jul	31-Jul	1-Sep	1-Oct
25	1-May	1-Jun	2-Jul	1-Aug	2-Sep	2-Oct
26	2-May	2-Jun	3-Jul	2-Aug	3-Sep	3-Oct
27	3-May	3-Jun	4-Jul	3-Aug	4-Sep	4-Oct
28	4-May	4-Jun	5-Jul	4-Aug	5-Sep	5-Oct
29	5-May	5-Jun	6-Jul	5-Aug	6-Sep	6-Oct
30	6-May	6-Jun	7-Jul	6-Aug	7-Sep	7-Oct
31	7-May	7-Jun		7-Aug		8-Oct

Screening in pregnancy (1)

Most women undergo some form of screening before or during pregnancy. The aim is to identify, prevent, and treat actual or potential problems. Women and their partners must be given unbiased information regarding screening and diagnostic tests, the meaning and consequences of both, what to expect in terms of results, and further options for management. GPs need to be aware of techniques of prenatal diagnosis to:
- identify all women who might benefit from genetic counselling and/or early assessment by the obstetrician;
- counsel patients about the accuracy and risk of prenatal diagnosis;
- make sure that the opportunity for prenatal diagnosis is not overlooked.

Pre-pregnancy genetic screening: There are many inherited diseases and more being discovered all the time. Refer before pregnancy couples who request referral or those with factors which put them at high risk of having a baby with a genetic disorder. Warn patients that most tests give no absolute 'yes' or 'no' but are a risk assessment.

Risk factors that warrant pre-pregnancy genetic screening
- *Personal or family history of genetic abnormality:* e.g. cystic fibrosis; Downs' syndrome; sickle cell; β-thalassaemia; haemophilia; fragile X syndrome; Duchenne and other muscular dystrophies; Huntington's chorea; polycystic kidneys.
- *High-risk ethnic group*
  - *Afro-Caribbean origin*—sickle cell anaemia (📖 p.527 and 773)
  - *Indian subcontinent, Far East, Southern Europe*—thalassaemia (📖 p.526 and 773)
- *Older women:* Risk of Down's syndrome ↑ (📖 p.772).
- *Consanguinous couples:* 1st degree cousins who have a baby together have an ↑ risk of congenital malformations in their offspring.

Tools of antenatal screening
Basic screening tests: Blood and urine tests:

- Hb estimation
- Blood group
- Antibody screening (📖 p.794)
- MSU (📖 p.789)
- Hepatitis B status (📖 p.788)
- Urine dipstick for proteinuria
- Rubella immune status (📖 p.791 and 806)
- HIV status (📖 p.498 and 773)
- Syphilis status (📖 p.742)

❶ Many women are not aware these tests have been done, let alone their purpose or results. Ensure women are given information about the reasons for, significance of, and results of routine tests.

Ultrasound scan: All pregnant women should now be offered early US scan (10–13wk.) for accurate gestational age assessment. High resolution 'anomaly' scan is also routinely offered in most centres at ~18wk.

gestation to detect structural abnormalities e.g. cleft lip and palate; exomphalos; skeletal abnormalities.

α-**fetoprotein (AFP):** Glycoprotein synthesized by the foetal liver which can be measured in the maternal bloodstream and amniotic fluid. AFP alone is a non-specific test requiring those with abnormal values to undergo further investigation. Routinely offered in many centres.

- ↑ *levels are associated with:*
  - Twins
  - Foetal malformation (10%): neural tube defect, exomphalos, posterior urethral valves, nephrosis, GI obstruction, teratomas, or Turner's syndrome
  - Adverse outcome (e.g. abruption , stillbirth) in 30% of those with ↑ levels but no detectable reason
- ↓ *levels are associated with:*
  - Diabetic mothers
  - Chromosomal abnormality (e.g. Down's syndrome—📖 p.772).

Chorionic villus sampling (CVS): At 10–12wk. gestation, the developing placenta is sampled per abdomen or transcervically, with US guidance. Used to detect genetic or metabolic abnormality in high-risk pregnancies.

- *Advantages:* undertaken earlier than amniocentesis to allow termination of affected pregnancies at an earlier stage.
- *Risks:* 4% miscarry; limb defects (rare).

Amniocentesis: Sampling of amniotic fluid via transabdominal needle under US guidance. When undertaken for screening purposes, takes place from 16–19wk. gestation. May be routinely offered to women at high risk of foetal abnormality (e.g. women >35y. of age to exclude Down's syndrome) or to clarify abnormalities found with other screening tests e.g. abnormal AFP or abnormality found on USS associated with genetic syndrome. 1% miscarriage risk.

Fetoscopy: Fibreoptic visualization of the foetus. Carried out from ~18wk. Enables detection of external abnormalities, foetal blood sampling, and organ biopsy. Foetal loss rate ~4%.

Further information

NICE (2003) Antenatal care: routine care for the healthy pregnant woman
  🖥 http://www.nice.org.uk
RCOG (2002) Amniocentesis 🖥 http://www.rcog.org.uk
National Screening Committee: Antenatal and newborn screening programme
  🖥 http://www.nelh.nhs.uk/screening/
The Genetics Interests Group ☎020 7704 3141
  🖥 http://www.gig.org.uk.

Patient information and support

Antenatal Results and Choices (ARC) ☎0207 631 0285
  🖥 www.arc-uk.org

Screening in pregnancy (2)

Spina bifida: USS at 17–19wk. gestation detects 90–95% spina bifida and 100% anencephaly. AFP detects 80% of open defects and 90% of those with anencephaly. Confirmation with USS is required.

Down's syndrome[G]: The most common single cause of mental handicap in children of school age. Incidence: 3/2000 births (📖 p.844). Various screening measures may be used including:

- **Age:** Incidence ↑ with age—1:365 at age 35, rising to 1:110 at age 40 and 1:30 at age 45. Offering amniocentesis to all pregnant women >35y. combined with routine anomaly scanning identifies ≈70% of all cases of Down's syndrome.
- **AFP alone:** Non-specific test. ↓ serum AFP may indicate chromosomal abnormality. Necessitates further evaluation in all cases.
- **Double/triple/quadruple test:** Blood test which measures AFP and hCG ± oestriol (uE₃) ± inhibin A. Blood is taken at 16wk. gestation and a risk value calculated for the individual woman taking into account age, exact gestation, and weight. The result is expressed as a risk assessment (e.g. 1:300) or as a +ve or –ve result. A +ve result usually means the risk of having a Down's syndrome baby is >1:250 and amniocentesis is recommended. A +ve test does not indicate the presence of Down's syndrome—just ↑ risk. Using a cut-off of 1:250 for amniocentesis, ~5% women require amniocentesis which turns out to be normal.
- **Nuchal translucency (NT) test:** USS measurement of the translucency of the nuchal fold in the neck of the foetus at 10–14wk. gestation. Detection rate ≈80%, false +ve rate ≈8%.
- **Integrated test:** Combines blood tests and USS to produce a single estimate of the woman's risk of having a child with Down's syndrome. Uses: woman's age; measurement at 10–13wk. gestation of nuchal translucency and maternal serum level of pregnancy-associated plasma protein A (PAPP-A); measurement 2–4wk. later of maternal serum AFP, unconjugated oestriol, hCG, and inhibin A. Detection rate: 85%. Only 1% of women require unnecessary amniocentesis.

⚠ The UK National Screening Committee has recommended all pregnant women, irrespective of age, should be offered screening for Down's syndrome. Recommended tests:

Gestation	11–14wk.	14–20wk.
Tests	• Nuchal translucency • Combined test (NT, hCG, PAPP-A) • Integrated test (NT, PAPP-A, AFP, hCG, uE3, and inhibin A) • Serum integrated test (PAPP-A, AFP, hCG, uE₃ and inhibin A)—used if NT measurement is not available	• Triple test (AFP, hCG, and uE₃) • Quadruple test (AFP, hCG, uE₃, and inhibin A)

Antenatal HIV testing: HIV testing is now offered as a routine part of antenatal screening in the UK. *Benefits of screening:* Without intervention, ~15% babies born to mothers infected with HIV will become infected with HIV themselves. Administration of zidovudine to HIV infected women during pregnancy and in labour, and to the baby for the first 6wk. of life, together with delivery by LSCS section and avoiding breast-feeding, ↓ risk of transmission to <5%.

Haemoglobinopathies: Antenatal screening, performed as early in pregnancy as possible, is currently offered to all women in areas where the foetal prevalence is >1/10,000. In other areas, haemoglobinopathy screening should be offered to all people in whose racial background the haemoglobinopathies predominately occur. The screening programme is being extended and, by the end of 2005/6, routine screening will be offered to all women.

Women identified as having a trait, or the disorder, should be referred for specialist counselling and their partners offered screening. Follow local guidelines for management in pregnancy and the puerperium.

Table 22.1 High-risk groups for haemoglobinopathy

Haemoglobinopathy	High-risk groups
Sickle cell disease (🕮 p.527)	Blacks of African origin, Saudi Arabians, Indian and Mediterranean populations
Thalassaemia (🕮 p.526)	Mediterranean, Indian, and South East Asian populations

Essential reading

NICE (2003) Antenatal care: routine care for the healthy pregnant woman
  🖳 *http://www.nice.org.uk* or *http://www.rcog.org.uk*
RCOG (2004) Management of HIV in pregnancy
  🖳 *http://www.rcog.org.uk*
National Screening Committee: Information on Down's, HIV, and Haemoglobinopathy screening
  🖳 *http://www.nelh.nhs.uk/screening*

Patient information and support

Antenatal Results and Choices (ARC) ☎0207 631 0285
  🖳 *www.arc-uk.org*

Antenatal care[G]

> ## Objectives of good obstetric care
> - To provide a safe outcome for the mother and baby with the minimum of avoidable complications.
> - To make the birth experience as satisfying as possible for the mother and her family.
> - To make optimal use of available resources.

Pregnancy is a risky business for both mother and baby. Every year women die as a result of pregnancy—the most common causes being eclampsia, haemorrhage, pulmonary embolism, and infection.

Definitions
- *Gravity*—number of pregnancies a woman has had (at any stage).
- *Parity*—number of pregnancies resulting in delivery >28wk. gestation.

Pregnancy tests: Detect β-HCG. +ve from 1st day of missed period until ≈20wk. gestation. Remains positive for ≈5d. after miscarriage/abortion or foetal death.

Antenatal care: Increased emphasis on antenatal screening means the 1st antenatal appointment should now be offered as early into pregnancy as possible. National guidelines suggest further appointments for healthy women should be offered at 16wk., 28wk., 34wk., 36wk., 38wk., and, if not already delivered, at 41wk. Additionally, healthy nulliparous women should be offered appointments at 25wk., 31wk., and 40wk.

First antenatal visit

History
- This pregnancy—LMP, usual cycle, fertility problems, contraception, desirability of pregnancy, any problems so far
- Past pregnancies—outcome and complications of previous pregnancies
- PMH—illness, drugs, varicose veins, abdominal/pelvic surgery
- Family history—↑ BP, DM, congenital/genetic abnormality, twins
- Social history—support at home, housing, financial problems.

Examination
- Check weight and calculate BMI
- Listen to heart and lungs, check BP, and examine abdomen.
- Foetal heart can be heard with a sonic aid per abdomen from 12–14wk. gestation
- Fundus can be felt per abdomen from 12wk.

Investigations
- Arrange routine anomaly scan at 18–20wk. gestation
- Check blood for:
  - Hb, blood group, Rhesus status, and red cell antibodies
  - Syphilis and rubella serology, HBsAg, and HIV with pre-test counselling (📖 p.498)
  - Sickle test and/or Hb electrophoresis (if in high-risk group or area)
- MSU for protein and bacteriuria
- Offer early USS for dating purposes (<16wk.)
- Discuss and offer antenatal screening (📖 p.770) for all women

Health promotion
- Healthy lifestyle—regular exercise and adequate rest
- Intercourse is not harmful if there is no vaginal bleeding
- Diet—avoid liver and vitamin supplements containing vitamin A; avoid soft, unpasteurized cheese, pâtés, pre-prepared salads, uncooked eggs
- Smoking cessation (📖 p.234)
- Alcohol avoidance
- Avoid all unnecessary medication including OTC and complementary medicines
- Wear gloves when gardening and avoid cat faeces in soil and cat litter

Education
- Social security benefits (📖 p.112)
- Employment rights
- Free prescriptions and dental care (📖 p.119)
- Antenatal/parent craft classes
- Local services (e.g. aquanatal classes, yoga for pregnancy)
- Choice of place of delivery and options available (📖 p.776)
- Procedure for antenatal care
- Travel and limitations (e.g. car seatbelt should go above and below bump not across it, airline regulations—📖 p.208); travel to malaria areas is not advisable in pregnancy

Certification: Supply form FW8 which allows application for free prescriptions and dental care. Provide Mat B1 form at 20wk.

Discussion: Worries about pregnancy or social situation.

Follow-up visits: Ask about problems and untoward symptoms.

Routine checks
- BP
- Oedema
- Urine for protein
- Fundal height
- Foetal heart sounds
- Foetal lie and presentation (from 32wk.)

Primiparous women are aware of movements from ≈20wk but multiparous women often feel movements earlier.

Routine laboratory checks: Hb and antibodies at 28wk. (though see 📖 p.794).

Essential reading
NICE (2003) Antenatal care: routine care for healthy pregnant women (and patient information) 🖳 http://www.rcog.org.uk

Patient information and support
National Childbirth Trust (NCT) ☎0870 770 3236 Info line: 0870 444 8707
🖳 http://www.nctpregnancyandbabycare.com

Who should deliver where?

Since the publication of *Changing Childbirth*, all those offering maternity care must give women choices about type of care, place of care and birth, and information that avoids 'personal bias or preference'. Who delivers where ultimately depends on the choice the woman makes. *Options:*

- consultant unit
- midwife or GP/midwife unit integral with/ attached to a consultant unit
- 'isolated unit'—distant from a specialist unit and manned by midwives or midwifes and GPs
- home (≈1% deliveries in UK)

Legal position of GPs: GPs are often fearful of litigation if they accept a woman for delivery outside a specialist unit. Even women with no risk factors can run into problems—rapid intervention to save life is needed in ≈5% deliveries. Due to the low numbers of deliveries most GPs attend, they perceive they lack expertise, which compounds this worry. Changes in the organization of out-of-hours cover and the time commitment to the GP entailed in home deliveries (and inadequate remuneration for that time), mean GP-attended home deliveries are uncommon.

The legal position is that:

- GPs are responsible only for their own acts or omissions.
- Midwives are accountable for their own actions and decisions.
- The GP only becomes responsible for a woman's care in labour when the midwife attending seeks his/her advice. The GP is then bound by terms and conditions of service to offer advice (either over the telephone or by attending), whether or not the woman had been accepted for maternity care.
- If an accident occurs, the GP would be judged against standards of a colleague of similar skills and training, not a specialist obstetrician.

Duties of the GP

- Provision of impartial advice about available services locally.
- Discussion of the available options in a way to enable the woman to make an informed choice.
- To make arrangements for provision of care.

Specialist unit vs. community-based care: Although the perinatal and maternal death rates have ↓ as the proportion of hospital births has ↑ in UK, no evidence exists that hospital is the safest place for women to have normal births. In other countries (e.g. the Netherlands), there is some evidence to the contrary.

△ If a woman decides to deliver away from a specialist unit, she should be informed of what facilities and levels of skill and expertise are and are not available. Record the discussion in her notes.

Table 22.2 Reasons why women choose home or hospital births

Home birth	Hospital birth
To avoid intervention (31%)	Safety (84%)
More in control—in familiar surroundings (25%)	Previous hospital birth (6%)
Previous home birth (11%)	
More relaxed at home (10%)	
Fear of hospitals (10%)	
Continuity of care with midwife (4%)	

Guidelines: Advise to deliver in a consultant unit:

At booking if:

- Pre-existing medical disorders—epilepsy, DM, cardiac, renal, respiratory, hepatitis B, HIV, active genital herpes, iv drug abuse, history of major gynaecological surgery, known uterine abnormality
- Familial disorder with a high risk of transmission
- ↑BP
- Height <150cm and primigravida
- Weight at 1st examination <50kg or >100kg
- Past obstetric history of:
  - Perinatal death
  - Rhesus isoimmunization
  - Pre-eclampsia or eclampsia
  - Antepartum haemorrhage
  - IUGR
  - Caesarean section
  - Postpartum haemorrhage
  - Retained placenta
  - Inverted uterus
  - Shoulder dystocia

If any of the following develop during pregnancy:

- Polyhydramnios
- Malpresentation
- Antepartum haemorrhage
- Prolonged pregnancy (>40wk.+10d.)
- Pre-term labour <37wk.
- Suspected IUGR
- Pregnancy-induced ↑BP
- Multiple pregnancy

Refer women to obstetrics to discuss place of delivery if:

- Primigravida <18y. and >35y. or ≥ para 5
- Excessive maternal weight ↑
- Failure of engagement of the head near term in a primigravida
- Past history of prolonged labour, large baby, subfertility, or cone biopsy.

⚠ Other rarer medical or obstetric conditions may require specialist advice. If in doubt, refer.

Useful information

NICE: Antenatal Care: routine care for healthy pregnant women
 ☐ http://www.rcog.org.uk or http://www.nice.org.uk
RCOG: Home Birth ☐ http://www.rcog.org.uk
National Childbirth Trust (NCT) ☎0870 770 3236 Info line: 0870 444 8707
 ☐ http://www.nctpregnancyandbabycare.com

Usual symptoms of pregnancy[G]

Backache: Due to ↑ joint laxity in lumbar spine and sacro-iliac joints, exaggerated lumbar lordosis, and poor posture. *Management:* encourage light exercise (unless contraindicated e.g. pre-eclampsia)—special classes are run for pregnant women. Treat with simple analgesia. Consider physiotherapy.

Breast soreness: Most common early in pregnancy. Good support bras are essential (can be purchased from specialist clothing stores). Nipples enlarge and darken at ≈12wk.

Constipation: ↑ fluid and fibre intake. If necessary, use laxative—usually bulk forming (e.g. ispaghula husk) or osmotic (e.g. lactulose). Stimulants ↑ uterine activity.

Fatigue: Almost universal symptom in early pregnancy: reaches peak at 12–15wk. *Cause:* unknown. *Treatment:* rest, adjustment of lifestyle and reassurance. *Late pregnancy:* due to ↑ physical effort needed to do everyday tasks and sleep deprivation. Check not anaemic, else reassure.

Haemorrhoids: May be associated bleeding. Treat prolapse with ice packs and replacement. Treat soreness with topical haemorrhoid application.

Headache: Usually tension headache. Check BP and urine for proteinuria to exclude pre-eclampsia (📖 p.786). Treat with rest and analgesia. Migraine may ↑ or ↓ in pregnancy.

Heartburn: Advise bland food, small portions, and frequent meals. Avoid late meals if worse at night and consider raising head of bed (1–2 bricks). Antacid preparations (e.g. magnesium trisilicate) are helpful if lifestyle modifications are ineffective, but may worsen constipation.

Hypotension: Due to ↑ peripheral circulation and venous pooling in lower limbs. Check no bleeding. *Advice:* avoid standing suddenly and hot baths. Sweating and feeling hot are also common.

Insomnia: Due to hormonal change, worries about pregnancy, and physical discomfort. Avoid drug treatment. Reassure. Relaxation techniques and mild physical exercise prior to sleep can help.

Itching
- *Local causes:* usually infective (e.g. scabies, thrush) though stretched abdominal skin may irritate.
- *Generalized itching* (pruritus gravidarum) begins in the 3rd trimester and normally associated with a degree of biliary obstruction.
  - Frank jaundice is rare—refer urgently to obstetrician (📖 p.785).
  - No jaundice—check LFTs, treat with skin lubrication (e.g. aqueous cream). Antihistamines are unhelpful. Disappears after delivery. Recurs in subsequent pregnancies in 50%.

Nausea and vomiting: Most experience nausea from 4–6wk. and ≈½ vomit. Can occur at any time and made worse by odours associated with preparation of food and the sight of food. If severe exclude multiple pregnancy or mole and UTI. Symptoms usually improve by 14–16wk. though may persist in some.

Management: Reassurance. Frequent small meals—avoid greasy/spicy foods, eat foods you can face (varies between women), maintain fluid intake (small amounts frequently), adjust lifestyle (e.g. ask partner to do the shopping). Self-help measures include ginger and P6 acupressure. If severe and disabling, consider use of an antihistamine antiemetic e.g. cyclizine 50mg tds. If dehydrated or >2–5kg weight loss (*hyperemesis gravidarum*), admit for rehydration.

Nose bleeds and bleeding gums: Occur as a result of ↑ peripheral vascularity. Reassure.

Peripheral paraesthesia: Compression of peripheral nerves due to fluid retention. Usually carpal tunnel syndrome (median nerve) but other nerves (e.g. lateral cutaneous nerve of thigh) can be affected. Usually no treatment required. Leg cramp affects 1:3 in late pregnancy. Worse at night. Raising foot of bed by 20cm can help.

Urinary frequency: Check MSU—UTI is common in pregnancy and associated with premature delivery.

Varicose veins and ankle swelling: *Symptoms:* aching legs, fatigue. *Management:* swelling—exclude PET (🕮 p.786). Elevation of legs when sitting, support stockings, encourage walking and discourage standing still. Thrombophlebitis is the most common complication—treat with ice packs, elevation, support stockings, and analgesia. Occasionally, DVT can occur (🕮 p.785). If veins do not settle 2–3mo. after delivery, consider referral for surgery.

Chloasma: 🕮 p.657

Useful information

NICE (2003): Antenatal care: routine care for healthy pregnant women (and patient information) 🖳 http://www.rcog.org.uk

National Childbirth Trust (NCT) ☎0870 770 3236. Info line: 0870 444 8707 🖳 http://www.nctpregnancyandbabycare.com

Medical conditions in pregnancy (A–D)

Anaemia: 📖 p.784

Asthma: Affects ≈5% of pregnant women.
- Generally improves with pregnancy, especially into the 3rd trimester.
- Treat asthma as usual—there is no evidence any of the drugs commonly used cause birth defects, problems in pregnancy or with breastfeeding.
- Women with very badly controlled asthma are more at risk of early labour and IUGR and patients on oral steroids may require iv steroids to cover labour.
- Avoid syntometrine for 3rd stage of labour as it contains ergometrine which can cause a severe attack.
- There is a tendency to worsening of asthma after delivery.

Cardiac disease: Risk of death is greatest in conditions where pulmonary blood flow cannot be ↑ e.g. Eisenmenger's syndrome (maternal mortality 30–50%); primary pulmonary hypertension (mortality 40–50%).

Management: Specialist obstetric care is required for all patients with a pre-existing cardiac condition. Where possible, refer pre-conception to a cardiologist for discussion of risks. Antibiotic prophylaxis is necessary for delivery for women with structural cardiac disease (📖 p.349).

Murmurs in pregnancy: Common. Consider any heart murmurs detected during pregnancy significant and refer for further evaluation—90% will be physiological.

Connective tissue disorders

Antiphospholipid syndrome: Antiphospholipid antibodies (lupus anticoagulant and/or anticardiolipin antibodies) and a history of ≥1 of:
- arterial thrombosis
- venous thrombosis
- recurrent pregnancy loss (typically 2nd trimester).

Can be 1° (occurs alone) or 2° to another connective tissue disease—usually SLE. Associated with ↑ risk of thrombosis and ↑ pregnancy loss (<20% pregnancies result in live birth). Treatment is with aspirin or s/cut heparin throughout pregnancy. Specialist referral is essential.

Rheumatoid arthritis: Symptoms often improve during pregnancy and worsen in the puerperium. Do not use NSAIDs for joint pain >24wk. gestation as can → closure of the foetal ductus arteriosus. Paracetamol or paracetamol + codeine combinations are safe. *2nd line drugs:*
- sulphasalazine—folic acid supplementation is recommended;
- azathioprine—associated with IUGR;
- penicillamine—may weaken foetal collagen;
- methotrexate is contraindicated.

SLE: Exacerbations are common in pregnancy.
- *Effects on foetus:* IUGR; neonatal lupus (from passively acquired maternal antibodies—usually self-limiting skin rash)

- **Effects on mother:** Renal complications may worsen and be associated with ↑BP ± pre-eclampsia; oligohydramnios; premature delivery.

Management: If planning pregnancy, refer for review of drugs. Once pregnant, refer for specialist obstetric care. Pain control—as for RA. *Immunosuppressive drugs:*
- azathioprine—may cause IUGR
- hydroxychloroquine—risk of deposits in foetal eye/ear
- cyclophosphamide and methotrexate are contraindicated

Depression: A significant cause of maternal death. At booking take details of any maternal psychiatric disorder, alcohol and substance abuse, severe social problems (including domestic violence), and previous self-harm. When antidepressants are being used for anything more than mild depression, weigh up the pros and cons of discontinuing treatment during pregnancy. There is no evidence treatment with TCAs or SSRIs is harmful to the foetus. The safety of SSRIs in breastfeeding mothers is unclear—older alternatives (e.g. amitriptyline) are preferable. Postnatally, follow-up women with a history of psychiatric disorder, substance abuse, or self-harm for signs of postnatal recurrence or exacerbation of their problem.

Diabetes: 2–3/1000 pregnancies. 95% have IDDM.
- **Effects on foetus:** Large for dates or IUGR; foetal hyper-insulinaemia; ↑ congenital abnormalities (cardiac, renal and neural tube defects); hypoxia and intrauterine death (especially >36wk.). *Postnatally*—hypoglycaemia during the 1st few hours; transient tachypnoea of the newborn or respiratory distress syndrome; neonatal jaundice.
- **Effects on mother:** Problems are more common if control is poor.
  - *During pregnancy*—1st trimester miscarriage; premature labour; pre-eclampsia; pyelonephritis; polyhydramnios.
  - *During labour*—foetal distress; obstruction (especially shoulder dystocia).

Management
- **Pre-pregnancy**—careful attention to diabetic control (aim BM 4–6mmol/l pre-meals); folate supplementation. ACE inhibitors, sulphonylureas, and biguanides are contraindicated in pregnancy—switch to insulin pre-conception if possible. Suggest pre-pregnancy counselling via diabetic specialist normally involved with care.
- **During pregnancy**—refer to an obstetrician early. Most women continue to use their pre-pregnancy insulin regime but requirements ↑ 2–3x in pregnancy. USS is routinely used to monitor foetal growth and exclude structural abnormalities. Delivery should always take place in a specialist unit with neonatal care facilities.
- **Postnatally**—↓ insulin dose to pre-pregnancy levels (if breastfeeding may need less insulin). Oral hypoglycaemics are contraindicated if breastfeeding.

Gestational diabetes: 📖 p.784

Useful information
Diabetes UK: Professional and patient information on the management of pregnant women with diabetes. 🖥 http://www.diabetes.org.uk

Medical conditions in pregnancy (E–Z)

Epilepsy[G]: 90% have normal pregnancies and deliver healthy babies.

- **Effects on foetus:** 2x ↑ perinatal mortality; ↑ foetal malformation—neural tube defect (↑ risk if taking sodium valproate or carbamazepine); cleft lip and cleft palate (associated with phenytoin and phenobarbitone); non-specific facial abnormalities (5–30% exposed to anticonvulsants). *Postnatally*—haemorrhagic disease of the newborn (associated with carbamazepine, phenytoin, or phenobarbitone); withdrawal symptoms (phenobarbitone—jittery, irritable, fits). Child has ↑ risk of developing epilepsy.
- **Effects on mother:** *During pregnancy*—1st trimester miscarriage; 10% have ↑ fit frequency; status epilepticus is associated with high infant and maternal mortality. *During labour*—1–2% have fit. *During puerperium*—1–2% have fit <48h. post delivery.

Management

- **Pre-pregnancy**—advise folate supplementation (5mg od); suggest referral to consultant neurologist for optimization of drug regime.
- **During pregnancy**—refer for specialist obstetric care. Drug doses may need to ↑ during pregnancy if fit frequency rises; delivery should occur in a specialist centre where any fits can be managed.
- **Postnatally**—breastfeeding is not contraindicated with older anticonvulsants (e.g. phenytoin, sodium valproate, carbamazepine, phenobarbitone). If drug dose has been ↑ in pregnancy, it may need to be ↓ after delivery. All babies should have im vitamin K due to ↑ risk of haemorrhage (📖 p.816).

Further information

SIGN (2003) Diagnosis and management of epilepsy in adults
🖳 http://www.sign.ac.uk

HIV: 📖 p.498

Hypertension: 📖 p.786

Infection: 📖 p.788–91

Jaundice: 📖 p.785

Renal disease: Refer all women for specialist obstetric care. Pre-eclampsia is more common—monitor carefully and refer early. Outcome depends on severity of disease:

Mild renal failure: Cr <125µmol/l and no ↑ BP. 96% have successful pregnancies without adverse effect on underlying disease. Low perinatal mortality.

Moderate (Cr 125–275µmol/l) **and severe** (Cr >275µmol/l) **renal failure:** Maternal complications occur in up to 70% and pregnancy-related loss of renal function in ~½ (10% progress to end-stage renal failure). IUGR in ~40% and pre-term delivery in ~60%.

Women on dialysis: Conception is uncommon. High rate of miscarriage and IUD. ~40–50% live birth rate. Mothers are prone to volume overload, polyhydramnios, and severe exacerbations of ↑BP ± pre-eclampsia. Women need 50% ↑ in duration and frequency of dialysis during pregnancy.

Renal transplant: Risk of 1st trimester miscarriage is ↑, but pregnancies that survive are >90% successful. Immunosuppressant drugs must be continued—they are not harmful to the foetus. Pregnancy does not affect long-term survival of the transplanted kidney. Pelvic position of the transplant does not compromise vaginal delivery.

Thromboembolism: 📖 p.785

Thyroid disease: Refer for specialist obstetric advice.
- *Hyperthyroidism:* Usually Grave's disease. Severity ↓ through pregnancy. May be associated with neonatal goitre, hyperthyroidism, or hypothyroidism. Continue treatment with carbimazole, aiming to keep plasma T_4 at the top of the normal range. Propylthiouracil is preferred postpartum if breastfeeding, as less concentrated in breast milk.
- *Hypothyroidism:* Rare (associated with infertility). If untreated, associated with ↑rate of miscarriage, stillbirth, and foetal abnormality. T_4 needs ↑ in pregnancy and normal maintenance dose is ↑ to accommodate this—the foetus is not affected by maternal thyroxine. Check TFTs at booking and 36wk.

Medical problems arising during pregnancy

Anaemia: Defined as Hb < 11g/dl. Common in pregnancy (20%). Some ↓ in Hb is physiological due to an ↑ in plasma volume. *Risk factors:*
- Starting pregnancy anaemic
- Multiple pregnancy
- Frequent pregnancies
- Poor diet
- Haemoglobinopathy.

Screening: Hb is routinely screened at booking and at 28wk.. In some areas, there is also routine screening for haemoglobinopathy (📖 p.773).

Management
- Routine use of oral iron for all pregnant women is of no proven benefit and may cause harm.
- Women in high-risk groups (e.g. multiple pregnancy) may routinely be given prophylaxis—follow local policies.
- If Hb is <11g/dl at booking or <10.5g/dl at 28wk., start iron (e.g. ferrous sulphate 200mg tds) and folate (5mg od), if indicated. Repeat Hb in 2wk.
- If there is no response to oral iron:
  - exclude occult infection (e.g. UTI)
  - check haematinics
  - consider Hb electrophoresis to exclude haemoglobinopathy regardless of apparent ethnic origin
  - consider referral for parenteral iron

Gestational diabetes: Diabetes mellitus with onset or first recognition during pregnancy. Intensive management can achieve almost normal rates of macrosomia and neonatal hypoglycaemia.

Screening: There is pressure for a screening programme but current screening tests are cumbersome and costly (modified GTT—📖 p.404). Use of a single fasting blood glucose with threshold of 4.8mmol/l is one alternative—only those (30%) with fasting glucose >4.8mmol/l require a GTT. At present, however, only high-risk women (those with past history of gestational DM; past history of a large baby—>4.5kg birth weight; or FH of DM/gestational DM) are screened with a GTT.

Management: As for pre-existing DM in pregnancy (📖 p.781) but insulin is stopped immediately postpartum. Check a 6wk. postpartum GTT. Gestational DM usually recurs in future pregnancies and >30% develop DM in <10y.

Glycosuria in pregnancy: Pregnant women have a ↓ renal threshold for glucose. If glycosuria is detected, repeat the urine test. If still +ve, arrange for a modified GTT (📖 p.404).

Further information
Diabetes UK: Professional and patient information on the management of pregnant women with gestational diabetes 🖳 http://www.diabetes.org.uk

Hypertension and pre-eclampsia: 📖 p.786

Jaundice: Any cause of jaundice may occur in pregnancy. Investigate as usual (📖 p.270) and treat according to cause. Common causes are:
- viral hepatitis (📖 p.496)
- gallstones
- Gilbert's or Dubin–Johnson syndrome.

Jaundice peculiar to pregnancy
- **Cholestatic jaundice of pregnancy:** Pruritus and mild jaundice in the latter half of pregnancy. Associated with ↑ risk of preterm delivery, foetal distress, and perinatal mortality. If suspected, refer for consultant care. Usually this involves monitoring of foetal well-being, with delivery at the 1st signs of foetal compromise. Jaundice clears <4wk. after delivery but often recurs in future pregnancies (40%). Contraindication to taking the COC pill.
- **Acute fatty degeneration of the liver:** Rare. Usually occurs ≥30wk. gestation. *Clinically:* mother develops abdominal pain, jaundice, headache, and vomiting. *Management:* admit for specialist care. Prognosis: ≈15–20% maternal mortality; ≈20% foetal mortality.
- **Pre-eclampsia:** Jaundice is associated with severe pre-eclampsia ± HELLP syndrome (📖 p.787).
- **Hyperemesis:** Jaundice is a complication of severe hyperemesis gravidarum (📖 p.778).

Thromboembolism^G: Pregnancy ↑ risk of thromboembolism ×10. Incidence: ≈1:100 pregnancies (20–50% antenatal). Suspect DVT and/or PE in any woman who is pregnant or in the puerperium who has pain or swelling in the leg, mild unexplained fever, chest pain, and/or breathlessness. *Risk factors:*
- Caesarean section
- Prolonged bed rest
- Previous thromboembolism
- Lupus anticoagulant

Management: 📖 p.364; Warfarin is teratogenic when used in the 1st trimester of pregnancy and can ↑ miscarriage, maternal and foetal haemorrhage, and stillbirth rates. Avoid during pregnancy. Warfarin is safe postpartum and during breastfeeding. Low molecular weight heparin (LMWH) is a safe alternative. Refer for expect advice.

Prevention: Prophylaxis is required if a patient has a thrombophilia (📖 p.529) or past history of pregnancy or pill-associated thromboembolism. LMWH is used antenatally and for up to 6wk postpartum—refer for expert advice.

Useful information
RCOG 🖳 http://www.rcog.org.uk
- Thromboprophylaxis during pregnancy, labour and after vaginal delivery (2004)
- Thromboembolic disease in pregnancy and the puerperium (2001)

Hypertension in pregnancy

Chronic hypertension or essential hypertension: Present before pregnancy. More common in older mothers and there may be a FH. Chronic hypertension may worsen in later pregnancy. Consider changing medication to drugs known to be safe in pregnancy pre-conceptually or as soon as pregnancy is confirmed. Aim to maintain BP <140/90. Risk PET is ↑ x5 (see below).

Pregnancy-induced hypertension (PIH): Like chronic hypertension but appears when the woman is pregnant and resolves after delivery. Treatment is the same. A proportion of women with PIH go on to develop pre-eclampsia and women who have PIH are at greater risk of developing ↑BP later in life.

Pre-eclampsia and eclampsia^G: The most important causes of death resulting from pregnancy in the UK.

Pre-eclampsia or *pregnancy-induced hypertension and proteinuria:* Affects 5–7% of primigravida and 2–3% of all pregnancies. Multisystem disease which develops ≥20wk. gestation and resolves <10d. after delivery. Cause is unclear. It is asymptomatic until its terminal phase, so frequent BP screening is essential. Once present, pre-eclampsia doesn't improve until the baby is delivered. Women who have pre-eclampsia are at greater risk of developing ↑BP later in life.

Eclampsia: Occurs when the woman has a fit as a result of pre-eclampsia. Usually BP is very high and, if the baby is not yet born, it becomes distressed. There is a serious risk of stroke in the mother. Women with pre-eclampsia have a 2% chance of eclamptic seizure. 44% occur after the baby is born—usually <24h. after delivery. Give iv or pr diazepam and admit as emergency.

Risk factors
- Age <20y. or >35y.
- First pregnancy
- Pre-eclampsia in a previous pregnancy
- Past history of ↑BP
- Short stature
- Low maternal weight
- Raynaud's disease
- Renal disease
- Migraine
- SLE
- FH of eclampsia or pre-eclampsia
- Multiple pregnancy
- Gestational trophoblastic disease

Diagnosis: BP >140/90 or >+30/+15 from booking BP; proteinuria >0.3g/24h.

Symptoms: Headaches; vomiting; photophobia; odd visual effects (flashing lights, stripes before the eyes, floaters, or blackouts of vision); epigastric/RUQ pain; general malaise.

Examination
- General appearance (drowsy, confused)
- Anaemia
- Neurological examination: reflexes, fundi, clonus
- Jaundice
- Non-dependant oedema
- Sudden ↑ weight

- *CVS examination:* lung bases
- *Abdominal examination:* RUQ or epigastric tenderness, palpable liver
- *Obstetric examination:* fundal height; liquor volume; presentation; foetal movements; foetal heart sounds and heart rate
- *Urine:* dipstick for proteinuria (as little as 1+ is significant).

△ **Criteria for admission of patients with pre-eclampsia**

- BP has risen by >30/20mmHg over booking BP
- IUGR
- BP ≥140/90 and symptomatic
- BP ≥160/100
- BP ≥140/90 with proteinuria

Prevention: Low-dose aspirin is of benefit in women at risk of severe early pre-eclampsia (i.e. those in whom it has occurred before). Refer for advice.

HELLP syndrome: **H**aemolysis **E**levated **L**iver enzymes **L**ow **P**latelets. Occurs in pregnancy or within 48h. of delivery. Associated with severe pre-eclampsia. *Signs:* hypertension (80%); RUQ pain (90%); nausea and vomiting (50%); oedema. Admit as for pre-eclampsia (opposite).

Renal disease in pregnancy: 📖 p.782

Further information
RCOG (2003) Pre-eclampsia—study group recommendations
🖳 http://www.rcog.org.uk

Patient information and support
Action on Pre-eclampsia (APEC) **UK Group** 🖳 http://www.apec.org.uk
☎020 8863 3271.

Sexually transmitted and GU infection in pregnancy

Bacterial vaginosis: 📖 p.740

Genital herpes^G: Affects ≈ 10% of the UK population (diagnosis made in 1:3). Risk is greatest if the 1° attack occurs at >28wk. gestation 2° attacks are much less of a problem. Risks include: passing the infection to the baby at the time of delivery; early labour; IUGR (1° infection only). Elective Caesarean section is advised at term if a 1° attack occurs during pregnancy at >28wk. gestation or if there is an active 2° attack at the time of labour.

Further information

RCOG (2002) Management of genital herpes in pregnancy
　🖥 http://www.rcog.org.uk

Group B streptococcus^G (GBS): Bacterium carried by 15–20% of pregnant women in the vagina, usually causing no problems. Rarely transmission to the baby during delivery results in septicaemia. Prophylactic treatment is advised in 'high risk' scenarios: early labour (<37wk.); prolonged or early rupture of the membranes; if the woman has a temperature during labour; or if a previous baby has been affected with the condition. Treatment involves iv antibiotics during labour.

Further information

RCOG (2001) Prevention of early onset neonatal group B streptococcal disease
　🖥 http://www.rcog.org.uk

Hepatitis B: Women are routinely offered screening for hepatitis B infection in pregnancy. Transmission to the baby occurs during labour (10–20% of infants of women seropositive for HBsAg and 90% of infants of women seropositive for both HBsAg and HBeAg). Infants infected are at high risk (~90%) of becoming chronic carriers and of developing chronic liver disease ± premature death.

Postnatally: Refer infected women for hepatology assessment. Infected mothers should not donate their milk.

Immunization: Give hepatitis B vaccine as soon as possible after birth to babies born to carrier mothers, with the addition of immunoglobulin (HBIG) if the mother carries the hepatitis B e-antigen or had acute HBV infection during pregnancy. 85–95% effective in preventing neonatal hepatitis B infection. Further doses of vaccine are required at 1 and 2mo. of age, and a booster dose at 1y., at the same time as follow-up testing.

Patient information

DoH: Hepatitis B: how to protect your baby. 🖥 http://www.dh.gov.uk

Hepatitis C: Prevalence 0.1–6%. Except when initial infection of the mother occurs during pregnancy (when transfer rate is much higher), transmission rate to the foetus is 5%. To date, there is no evidence HCV can be transferred to the child by breastfeeding. Infants at risk can be screened for HCV infection at 12mo. (RNA screen) or 18–24mo. (HCV antibody test). The majority of infants who acquire HCV infection via their mothers develop chronic hepatitis. Treatment is with interferon and achieves viral clearance rates of 40%.

HIV: 📖 p.498

Sexually transmitted infection: Both chlamydia (5% pregnancies) and gonorrhoea (<1/1000 pregnancies) can pass to the baby during delivery, causing eye infections. Chlamydia can also cause neonatal chest infections or postpartum womb infection. Both are treatable if detected (📖 p.743 and 745). Follow-up with swabs to confirm eradication.

Thrush: More common in pregnancy. Requires treatment only if causes troublesome itching, soreness, or discharge. *Treatment:* clotrimazole pessaries. Avoid fluconazole.

Urinary tract infections: 1:25 women develop UTI in pregnancy. If suspected, send MSU to confirm diagnosis, and start antibiotics immediately. Routine screening with MSU for UTI is offered at booking. 3–8% of pregnant women have asymptomatic bacteriuria—1:3 will develop symptomatic infection (acute cystitis, pylonephritis) if left untreated. Both untreated bacteriuria and frank UTI are associated with preterm delivery and IUGR. Treat for at least 1wk. with suitable antibiotic. Check MSU following treatment to ensure infection has cleared.

Other infections during pregnancy

Chicken pox^G: Contact with chicken pox in pregnancy is common. If the mother has definitely had chicken pox, there is no risk to herself or the baby. If she doesn't recall having chicken pox, check her immunity with a blood test—80% have antibodies from silent infection.

Risk to the mother: Chicken pox pneumonia is more common (10%)—can be severe.

Risks to the baby
* *<20wk. gestation*—1–2% risk of chicken pox syndrome: eye defects, hypoplasia, microcephaly. If a woman has Varicella-Zoster Ig (VZ-Ig) treatment (see below) after being exposed, risk is even lower.
* *Mother's rash develops <1wk. prior to delivery–1mo. after delivery*—risk of overwhelming infection. Baby may need VZ-Ig treatment.

Management: In cases of 'at risk' exposure, arrange for VZ-Ig to be given to mother and/or baby. This can be lifesaving and significantly ↓ disease severity. It must be given ≤10d. after exposure. If mother develops chicken pox, treat with acyclovir if she presents <24h. after the rash appears and mother is >20wk. gestation.

Further information
RCOG (2001) Chicken pox in pregnancy ◪ http://www.rcog.org.uk

Coughs, colds, and 'flu: Little threat to the pregnancy itself. *Advise* fluids, paracetamol, rest, and TLC. Inhaled decongestants are safe, but avoid cough linctus and OTC composite preparations. Treat any 2° infections as needed. Avoid confusion with other more serious infections of pregnancy.

Cytomegalovirus (CMV): More frequent cause of birth defect than rubella in the UK—5/1000 live births. 10% develop handicap. The foetus is most vulnerable when infection occurs in early pregnancy. Maternal disease may be asymptomatic or a mild flu-like illness. No effective prevention strategy.

Hepatitis B and C: ◫ p.788 and 789   **HIV:** ◫ p.498

Listeriosis: Rare. May occur in epidemics. *Maternal symptoms*—fever, shivering, myalgia, headache, sore throat, cough, vomiting, diarrhoea, vaginitis. *Consequences*: abortion (may be recurrent), stillbirth, premature labour, transmission to the foetus (in 2nd/3rd trimester). Infection of the mother is usually via infected food e.g. pâté, soft cheese, milk. Detection is with blood cultures. Suspect if unexplained fever >48h. and refer for expert advice. Infection in the newborn infant manifests in pneumonia ± meningitis. Prevention—see opposite.

Malaria: Serious complications are more common in pregnancy (cerebral malaria has 50% mortality). Suspect in any pregnant woman who has a fever and has recently visited an infected area. Seek immediate expert advice.

Parvovirus: Presents with febrile illness and often accompanied by acute tenderness of the joints or arthritis affecting hands, wrists, and knees—usually lasts 1–2wk. but 1:10 continue to have symptoms for several months. There may be a fine rash over the trunk and extremeties which comes and goes over a period of several months in response to stress, exercise, sunlight, or bathing.

Parvovirus in pregnancy: Risk of infection in pregnancy ≈1/400. Risk for a non-immune mother with a child who has Fifth disease ≈50–90%. Maternal infection results in 4% ↑ miscarriage (<20wk. gestation). Infection between 9–20wk. may also cause anaemia of the foetus (3% of those infected) resulting in hydrops fetalis developing 2–17wk. afterwards. If known contact, check immune status. If parvovirus infection is suspected (especially if known contact), refer for foetal monitoring. Early transfusion improves chances of the baby's survival. There are no long-term effects from an infection which doesn't cause miscarriage or hydrops.

Rubella: Asymptomatic reinfection of women who have received vaccination can occur, so serology is essential in all pregnant rubella contacts. 50% of mothers who are infected with rubella are asymptomatic. Consequences of infection depend on gestation of the foetus at the time of infection—50–60% are affected if infection occurs in the 1st month; <5% at 16wk. Risk of transmission is much lower with reinfection (<5%). Abnormalities that can occur include: cataract, deafness, cerebral palsy, mental retardation, microcephaly, micropthalmia. If suspected, get expert advice.

Toxoplasmosis: Caused by a parasite found in raw meat and cat faeces. 70% of women have not had toxoplasmosis before pregnancy and ~2/1000 will catch it during pregnancy. 30–40% pass it to their foetus. Infection may result in miscarriage, stillbirth, growth problems, blindness, hydrocephalus, brain damage, epilepsy, or deafness. Risk of transmission to the foetus is related to gestation at the time of infection—3rd trimester ≈70%; 1st trimester ≈15%. If infection is suspected, refer for specialist advice.

Useful information

Toxoplasmosis
  http://www.ridgeway-surgery.demon.co.uk/pregnant/toxoplas.htm

UTI: p.789

Prevention of toxoplasmosis and listeriosis: Advise women to:

- Only eat well cooked meat
- Wash their hands, cooking utensils, and food surfaces after preparing raw meat
- Keep raw meat and cooked foods on separate plates
- Wash all soil from fruit and vegetables before eating
- If possible, get someone else to clean cat litter or use gloves and wash hands afterwards
- Use gloves when gardening and wash hands afterwards

Bleeding in pregnancy

Bleeding in early pregnancy: 📖 p.736

Antepartum haemorrhage (APH): Any bleeding in pregnancy >28wk. gestation (or the point of foetal viability). *Causes:*

Uterine
- Abruption (📖 p.796)
- Placenta praevia (opposite)
- Vasa praevia
- Circumvallate placenta
- Placental sinuses

Lower genital tract
- Cervical
  - Polyp
  - Erosion
  - Carcinoma
  - Cervicitis
- Vaginitis
- Vulval varicosities

> ⚠ **Action**
> - ALWAYS admit to a specialist obstetric unit. If bleeding is severe, admit via an emergency ambulance and whilst awaiting transport raise legs; give O₂ via face mask; if possible, gain iv access, take blood for FBC and cross matching and start iv infusion.
> - NEVER do a vaginal examination—placenta praevia bleeds +++.

Postpartum haemorrhage (PPH)

Primary PPH: Loss of >500ml blood within 24h. of delivery. May occur in the community after home delivery, delivery in a community obstetric unit, or after rapid discharge from a consultant-led unit. *Causes:* uterine atony (90%); genital tract trauma (7%); clotting disorders (3%).

Risk factors
- Past history of PPH
- Retained placenta
- Large placental site
- Low placenta
- Overdistended uterus
- Abruption

- Uterine malformation
- Fibroids
- Prolonged labour
- >5 previous vaginal deliveries
- Trauma to uterus or cervix

> ⚠ **Action**
> - Give ergometrine 0.5mg iv.
> - Call emergency ambulance for transfer to hospital.
> - Give high flow O₂ via face mask as soon as possible.
> - Gain iv access, take blood for FBC and cross matching and start iv infusion if possible.
> - If the placenta has not been delivered, attempt to deliver it by controlled cord traction.
> - Check for trauma and apply pressure to any visible bleeding point/ repair any visible bleeding point. Bimanual pressure on the uterus may decrease immediate loss.
> - Some community units keep carboprost 250mcg (e.g. Haemabate) for emergency use. Use if available (1ml by deep im injection); repeat after 15min.

Secondary PPH: Excessive blood loss pv >24h. after delivery. *Peak incidence:* 5–12d. after delivery. *Causes:* retained placental tissue or clot; postpartum infection.

> ⚠ **Action**
> • Refer for USS.
> • If bleeding is slight and USS normal, then manage conservatively. If any suggestion of infection, start oral antibiotics.
> • If the uterus is tender and the os open, if loss is heavy, or there is any suggestion of retained products on USS, admit to an obstetric unit for further investigation/evacuation of retained products of conception.

Persistent lochia: Lochia/bleeding continuing >6wk. postpartum. Examine uterus per abdomen and with bimanual VE to check involuted. Perform speculum examination. Send vaginal swabs for M,C&S. Causes include infection, retained products of conception, resumption of normal menstrual cycle, side effects of contraception (e.g. if depot given), cervical bleeding due to trauma or other pathology, bleeding from unhealed vaginal or perineal tears and other uterine pathology. If loss is offensive or systemic symptoms or signs of infection, treat blind with antibiotics as for endometritis (📖 p.809). If not settling and no cause is found, refer to gynaecology.

Placenta praevia[G]: Occurs when the placenta lies within the lower uterine segment. *Incidence:* 1:4 routine anomaly scans done at 19wk. gestation show a low lying placenta—5% remain low at 32wk. and <2% at term. *Associations:*

• ↑ with parity
• Age >35y.
• Twins
• Endometrial damage (e.g. history of D&C, TOP)
• Preterm delivery
• Previous LSCS
• Placental pathology (marginal/vellamentous cord insertions, succinturiate lobes, biparite placenta)
• Previous placenta praevia (recurrence rate 4–8%).

Management: If discovered at routine USS at 17–19wk., follow-up USS reveals whether the placenta is moving out of the lower segment. When the placenta remains low, management depends on whether the placenta covers the internal os (major placenta praevia) or not (minor placenta praevia). Major placenta praevia always requires delivery by caesarean section. Normal delivery in a specialist unit may be attempted with minor placenta praevia if the head lies below the lower edge of the placenta.

Complications
• *Maternal*
  • APH—typically painless bleeding with a peak incidence at 34wk.;
  • Malpresentation—35% breech presentation or transverse lie;
  • Abnormal placentation—placenta accreta and percreta especially with a history of previous caesarean section;
  • PPH.
• *Foetal:* IUGR (15%); premature delivery; death.

Useful information
RCOG 🖥 http://www.rcog.org.uk
• Management of postpartum haemorrhage (1998 and update 2003)
• Placenta previa: diagnosis and management (2001)

Haemolytic disease and rhesus isoimmunization

Development of anti-D antibodies results from fetomaternal haemorrhage (FMH) in RhD –ve women carrying a RhD +ve foetus. In later pregnancies, these antibodies cross the placenta causing rhesus haemolytic disease of the foetus which gets successively worse with each pregnancy.

All rhesus –ve mothers are tested for D-antibodies at booking, at 28wk., and 2 weekly thereafter. Testing is not performed once women are given anti-D prophylaxis—see below. Anti-D titres <4IU/ml (<1:16) are unlikely to cause serious disease. If >10u/ml, refer for specialist advice.

Effects on foetus: Hydrops fetalis (oedematous foetus); intra-uterine death.

Effects on neonate: Jaundice; heart failure (oedema, ascites); anaemia; yellow vernix; hepatosplenomegaly; CNS signs.

All neonates with haemolytic disease should be managed by specialist paediatricians. Treatment usually involves UV light for jaundice ± exchange transfusion.

Immunoprophylaxis: Immunoprophylaxis for RhD –ve mothers using anti-D immunoglobulin (anti-D Ig) is given into the deltoid muscle as soon as possible after the sensitizing event—preferably within 72h. (though there is evidence of benefit up to 9d.). Women already sensitized should not be given anti-D Ig.

When should anti-D be administered?
Following spontaneous miscarriage
- ≥20wk.—500IU + test the size of the fetomaternal haemorrhage
- 12–19wk. gestation—250IU
- <12wk.—only give anti-D if there has been an intervention (e.g. D&C) to evacuate the uterus.

Following termination of pregnancy/ ectopic pregnancy: All non-sensitized RhD –ve women.

If threatened miscarriage.
- All non-sensitized RhD –ve women >12wk. gestation.
- If bleeding continues intermittently after 12wk., give anti-D Ig 6-weekly.
- <12wk. gestation—only administer if bleeding is heavy, repeated, or there is associated abdominal pain (particularly if close to 12wk.).

Routine antenatal prophylaxis
- 1–1.5% of RhD –ve women develop anti-D antibodies during pregnancy due to fetomaternal haemorrhage which is usually small and silent—most commonly in the 3rd trimester.
- Routine antenatal prophylaxis can ↓ sensitization to <0.2%. Antenatal prophylaxis should now be routine practice in UK.

- Administration of 500IU anti-D Ig at 28wk. (after blood has been taken for routine antibody screening) and 34wk. gestation ↓ incidence of immunization after birth.
- Women who have been given antenatal prophylaxis may still be sensitized by a large fetomaternal haemorrhage so, following any potentially sensitizing event, additional anti-D Ig should be given and a Kleihauer test (see below) performed.
- Screening for anti-D antibodies after prophylaxis has been given is uninterpretable.

Following sensitizing events before delivery: All non-sensitized RhD –ve women after:

- Invasive prenatal diagnosis (amniocentesis, CVS, foetal blood sampling) or other intrauterine procedures
- APH
- External cephalic version of the foetus
- Closed abdominal injury (e.g. RTA)
- IUD

Dose
- <20wk.—250IU
- >20wk—500IU + test for size of fetomaternal haemorrhage

Postnatal prophylaxis

- 500IU–1500IU is given to every non-sensitized RhD –ve woman <72h. after delivery of a RhD +ve infant.
- >99% women have a fetomaternal haemorrhage of <4mls at delivery—a test to detect fetomaternal haemorrhage >4mls must be done so additional anti-D Ig can be given as needed.
- Risk factors for high fetomaternal haemorrhage include: traumatic delivery, LSCS, manual removal of placenta, stillbirth and IUD, abdominal trauma during the 3rd trimester, twin pregnancy (at delivery), unexplained hydrops fetalis.

Test for the size of fetomaternal haemorrhage: In the UK, blood is taken from the mother (anticoagulated sample) as soon as possible after the sensitizing event (if >20wk. gestation). A Kleihauer acid elution test (which detects foetal haemoglobin (HbF)) identifies women with large fetomaternal haemorrhage who need additional anti-D Ig.

Other causes: Anti-D antibodies are the most common cause of rhesus disease. Other causes: Rh C, E, c, e, Kell, Kidd, Duffy. Anti-Du antibodies are relatively common but usually harmless.

Essential reading

RCOG/NICE (2002) Use of anti-D immunoglobulin for rhesus prophylaxis
🖳 http://www.rcog.org.uk

Abdominal pain in pregnancy

Non-obstetric causes of abdominal pain may be forgotten or signs may be less well localized than in the non-pregnant patient. In all cases consider:

UTI: 📖 p.789

Appendicitis: 1/1000 pregnancies. Mortality is higher in pregnancy and perforation more common (15–20%). Foetal mortality is 5–10% for simple appendicitis but rises to 30% when there is perforation. Due to the pregnancy, the appendix is displaced and pain often felt in the paraumilical region or subcostally. Admit immediately if suspected.

Cholecystitis: 1–6/10,000 pregnancies. Pregnancy encourages gallstone formation. Symptoms include RUQ pain, nausea and vomiting. Diagnosis can be confirmed on USS. Treatment is the same as outside pregnancy, aiming for interval cholecystectomy after birth.

Fibroids: Torsion or red degeneration. Fibroids ↑ in size in pregnancy. They may twist if pedunculated. Red degeneration occurs usually after 20wk. and possibly until the puerperium. It presents as abdominal pain ± localized tenderness ± vomiting and low-grade fever. Treatment is with rest and analgesia. Pain resolves within 1wk.

Ovarian tumours/torsion: 1/1000 pregnancies. Torsion or rupture of a cyst may both cause abdominal pain, as may bleeding into a cyst. USS can confirm the presence of a cyst. Management depends on the nature of the cyst and the severity of the pain. Admit for assessment.

If <20wk. gestation, in addition consider:
- Miscarriage: 📖 p.736
- Ectopic pregnancy: 📖 p.738

If >20wk. gestation, in addition consider:

Labour: 📖 p.802

Abruptio placentae: 1:80–1:200 pregnancies. Part of the placenta becomes detached from the uterus. Consequences depend on the degree of separation and the amount of blood loss. Typically, constant pain (may be felt in the back if posterior placenta); woody hard, tender uterus; shock; foetal heart absent or signs of foetal distress (foetal tachycardia or bradycardia). PV bleeding may occur. If suspected, admit as an acute emergency to the nearest specialist obstetric unit.

Pubic symphysis dehiscence: Painful condition occuring in late pregnancy that may persist after delivery. The pubic symphysis separates resulting in low abdominal pain which may be accompanied by low back pain and radiate down both thighs. Pain is constant and worse on movement. It resolves on rest. Examination reveals a soft abdomen and obstetric examination is normal. Advise simple analgesia (paracetamol 1g qds). Rest in a semi-recumbent position when in pain. Refer for physiotherapy (especially if still a problem in the puerperium). Most resolve spontaneously within several months of delivery. Some persist and need specialist referral.

Haematoma of the rectus abdominis: Rarely bleeding into the rectus sheath and haematoma formation occurs spontaneously or after coughing in late pregnancy. May cause swelling and abdominal tenderness. USS can be helpful. If unsure of diagnosis, admit to exclude acute surgical or obstetric cause of pain.

Uterine rupture: Rare in UK (1:1500 deliveries). Associated with maternal mortality of 5% and foetal mortality of 30%. 70% are due to dehiscence of caesarean section scars. Rupture occurs most commonly during labour but occasionally in the 3rd trimester. Pain and bleeding are variable. Usually associated with profound shock in the mother and foetal distress. Admit as an acute emergency to a specialist obstetric unit.

Intra-uterine growth

Intra-uterine growth retardation^G: Babies may be small because they are premature, small for their gestation, or a combination of the two. Babies small for their gestational age (IUGR—weighing <10th centile weight for their gestational age) have different problems to those of premature babies.

Predisposing factors
- Multiple pregnancy
- Malformation
- Infection
- Maternal smoking
- Maternal DM
- Pre-eclampsia
- Severe maternal anaemia
- Maternal heart or renal disease
- Previous history of small baby

Where the head circumference is relatively spared, suspect placental insufficiency.

Antenatal detection: Difficult to detect—~½ are not detected until after birth. Most GPs will encounter IUGR when they do a routine antenatal check and find the symphysis–fundal height (SFH) is less than would be expected for the gestation. Other suspicious signs are oligohydramnios and poor foetal movements. Confirm suspicions with USS, then seek specialist obstetric advice.

Consequences
- *Labour:* More susceptible to hypoxia in labour so require monitoring in a specialist unit where caesarean section facilities are available and there is paediatric back-up.
- *Postnatal problems:* Susceptible to neonatal hypoglycaemia and jaundice. Babies <2kg may have problems with temperature regulation and require incubator facilities.
- *Long-term effects:* More prone in later life to cardiovascular disease and NIDDM.

Oligohydramnios: Liquor volume <500ml. Rare. Associated with:
- Prolonged pregnancy
- PROM (📖 p.802)
- Placental insufficiency
- Foetal abnormality (renal agenesis, urethral aplasia)

Confirm diagnosis with USS, then refer for specialist obstetric assessment.

Large for dates: Consider:
- Multiple pregnancy
- Large baby (>90th centile)—may have past history of large babies
- Maternal DM
- Foetal abnormality
- Polydramnios

Refer for USS to confirm diagnosis and exclude foetal abnormality or multiple pregnancy. Check maternal fasting blood glucose ± GTT.

Polyhydramnios: Liquor volume >2l. 1:250 pregnancies. *Causes:*
- Foetal abnormality (50%): hydrops fetalis; anencephaly (no swallowing reflex); spina bifida; oesophageal or duodenal atresia; umbilical hernia; ectopia vesicae.
- Maternal (20%): DM, multiple pregnancy.
- No cause found (30%).

Risks: Premature labour; malpresentation; cord prolapse; placental abruption; PPH.

Management: Refer for USS to confirm diagnosis and exclude foetal abnormality or multiple pregnancy. Check maternal fasting blood glucose ± GTT. Refer for specialist obstetric advice.

Useful information
RCOG (2002) The investigation and management of the small-for-gestational-age fetus
 🖳 *http://rcog.org.uk*

Breech babies and multiple pregnancy

Breech babies[G]: 3–4% babies at term.

Risk factors
- Bicornuate uterus
- Fibroids
- Placenta previa
- Oligohydramnios

Management
- Many turn spontaneously—especially if <36wk. gestation.
- If a baby is found to be breech at ≥36wk. gestation, confirm breech position and position of the placenta on USS and refer for specialist obstetric advice. *Options:*
  - Attempt to turn the baby (external cephalic version—ECV)—should only be attempted in specialist unit with facilities for foetal monitoring.
  - Vaginal breech delivery—all breech deliveries should occur in specialist units.
  - Elective caesarean section.
- 10–15% of breech babies are discovered, for the first time, late in labour. If delivering at home or in a community unit, arrange transfer to a specialist unit immediately.

Follow-up: Congenital hip problems are more common in breech babies. Refer all breech babies routinely for hip USS even if examination in the first 24h. is normal.

Further information
RCOG (2001) The management of breech presentation ▣ *http://www.rcog.org.uk*

Multiple pregnancy: *Incidence:*
- Twins—1:105 (1/3 identical)
- Triplets—1:10,000

Predisposing factors
- Previous twins
- FH of non-identical twins
- Race—most common amongst African blacks; least common in Japanese
- ↑ with maternal age
- Infertility treatment—induced ovulation (e.g. clomiphene treatment); IVF

Diagnosis
- Hyperemesis (▢ p.778)
- USS
- Large for dates (▢ p.798)
- Polyhydramnios (▢ p.798)
- Palpation of 2 foetal heads ± multiple limbs
- 2 different foetal heart rates heard (>10bpm different)

Management: Refer for specialist obstetric care.

Complications
- *In pregnancy:* Anaemia; polyhydramnios; pre-eclampsia (x3); APH; placenta praevia; placental abruption.
- *In labour:* Malpresentation; cord prolapse; foetal distress (↑ caesarean section rate); PPH.
- *Foetus:* ↑ perinatal mortality (x5); prematurity; IUGR; malformations (x2–4); twin-twin transfusion may result in 1 twin being plethoric (and jaundiced later) and the other anaemic.

Patient support
Twins and Multiple Births Association (TAMBA) ☎0870 770 3305
🖳 http://www.tamba.org.uk

Labour

Braxton-Hicks contractions: Irregular tightenings of the uterus. Start ≥30wk. gestation (common after 36wk.). May be uncomfortable but not painful. (*J. Braxton-Hicks (1823–97)—English obstetrician*)

Premature rupture of membranes (PROM): Rupture of membranes before labour starts. Usually presents with a history of a gush of clear fluid (± an audible pop) followed by uncontrolled leakage. If chorioamnionitis is present, the woman may have abdominal pain and feel unwell.

Difficult to distinguish clinically from profuse vaginal discharge or incontinence of urine. Check temperature, pulse, and BP and do a routine obstetric examination (including foetal heart). Do not perform a vaginal examination as repeated examinations can introduce infection.

Management
- *Evidence of infection*—admit for specialist obstetric care;
- *<37wk. gestation and suspected PROM*—admit to specialist obstetric unit for further assessment;
- *≥37wk. gestation,* if no signs of spontaneous labour—admit for specialist obstetric assessment within 24h.

Premature labour: Classified as any labour <37wk. gestation. *Prevalence:* 6%. In 1:4 cases, premature delivery is elective due to maternal or foetal problems.

Causes of spontaneous premature labour
- Unknown (40%)
- Cervical incompetence
- Multiple pregnancy
- Uterine abnormality
- Pyelonephritis or other infection
- DM
- Polyhydramnios
- APH

Presentation: Premature rupture of membranes or contractions. If suspected, admit immediately to obstetrics for further assessment.

Normal labour: Occurs ≥37wk. gestation and results in vaginal delivery of a baby in <24h. Often heralded by a 'show' consisting of mucus ± blood and/or spontaneous rupture of membranes ('waters going').
- *1st stage of labour:* Time from the onset of regular contractions until the cervix is fully dilated.
- *2nd stage of labour:* Time from complete cervical dilatation until the baby is born. The mother has a desire to push.
- *3rd stage of labour:* Delivery of the placenta.

Meconium stained liquor: Passage of fresh meconium (dark green, sticky and lumpy) during labour may be a sign of foetal distress. Transfer immediately to a consultant unit for further evaluation.

Management: As the head is born, suck out oropharynx and nose. Aspiration of meconium can cause pneumonitis in the neonate.

Dystocia: Difficulty in labour. May be due to problems relating to the baby, birth passage, or action of the uterus. Neonatal mortality and maternal morbidity both ↑ with duration of labour.

Possible causes

- Pelvic abnormality
- Shoulder dystocia (📖 p.1072)
- Abnormal presentation
- Uterine dysfunction
- Cervical dystocia
- Cephalo-pelvic disproportion

Management: If a patient in labour in the community (at home or in a community unit) fails to progress as expected, admit immediately to a specialist unit for consideration of intervention to speed the labour or caesarean section. Shoulder dystocia is an obstetric emergency (📖 p.1072).

Prolonged pregnancy/post-maturity: The due date is based on pregnancy lasting 40wk. or 280d. from the date of the LMP. It is normal to deliver between 37wk. and 42wk.. At 40wk. gestation, 65% will spontaneously go into labour in the next week. Perinatal mortality rate is ↑ x2 from 42–43wk. and x3 >43wk., so induction of labour is indicated if a pregnancy lasts >42wk.

Pain relief for labour: Most women experience pain in labour.

Strategies for pain relief

- Self-help—keep fit in pregnancy, relaxation techniques, breathing exercises, warm bath;
- TENS—machines are available to hire from most obstetric units;
- Entonox—takes 30–45sec. to have effect; advise women to start inhaling it as soon as the contraction starts;
- Injected opiates (e.g. pethidine);
- Epidural;
- Pudendal block—used for instrumental delivery.

Advise women to discuss options with their midwife.

Epidural: Effective method of analgesia available in most hospital units. Initiated once in established labour (cervix >3cm dilated). Regular BP, pulse, and foetal heart monitoring is required. *Particular indications:*

- OP position
- Breech
- Multiple pregnancy
- Preterm delivery
- Pre-eclampsia
- Forceps delivery

Epidural complications during labour

- Postural hypotension
- ↑ need for instrumental delivery due to pelvic floor muscle paralysis
- Urinary retention

Epidural complications post-delivery: Urinary retention, headache (especially if dural puncture).

Patient information

NCT Information on labour and pain relief (including epidurals)
  📖 http://www.nctpregnancyandbabycare.com

Medical interventions in labour

47% of deliveries are 'normal' i.e. occur without surgical intervention, use of instruments induction, epidural or general anaesthetic. During $^1/_3$ of all deliveries, women have an epidural, general or spinal anaesthetic.

Induction of labour[G]: Carried out when it is felt that the baby is better off out than in (≈20% of deliveries). Only undertaken in units where there are facilities for continuous foetal monitoring and emergency Caesarean section. The procedure involves: assessment of the cervix (+ vaginal prostaglandins if unfavourable); 'sweeping' of the membranes; artificial rupture of the membranes; and/or iv oxytocin to maintain contractions. Reasons for induction of labour include:
• Post-maturity (most common)
• Diseases of pregnancy (e.g. pre-eclampsia)
• Maternal diabetes
• Premature rupture of membranes
• IUGR

Assisted delivery[G]: Forceps and ventouse are used in ≈11% of deliveries in UK (range 4–25% between hospitals). Assisted delivery should only be performed with adequate analgesia (usually epidural or pudendal block) and by experienced practitioners. Forceps and ventouse— Table 22.3.

Caesarian section[G] (CS): Rate in England and Wales is 21.5% (range 10–65% between different hospitals). 10% are elective; the other 11–12% occur after labour has started. Regional anaesthesia for CS is safer for mother and child than a GA.

Reasons for CS: Failure to progress (25%); presumed foetal compromise (28%); breech (14%).

Planned CS is indicated for:
• Breech (where external cephalic version has failed);
• Multiple pregnancies where the first twin is not cephalic;
• Placenta previa (grade 3–4);
• HIV +ve Hepatitis C +ve positive women and those with 1° HSV in 3rd trimester to ↓ virus transmission.

❶ Maternal request is not, on its own, an indication for CS[G] but GPs should discuss risks and benefits if a request is made and, if the patient still requests a CS, refer for a consultant opinion.

Information for women: NICE guidelines highlight the woman's participation in the decision to undertake a CS ('woman-centred care') and suggest information is given antenatally, including:
• Indications (presumed foetal compromise, failure to progress, breech)
• What the procedure involves
• Associated risks and benefits (Appendix 4 of NICE guidelines)
• Implications for future pregnancies and births

Table 22.3 Forceps and ventouse

	Forceps	Ventouse
Indication	Delayed 2nd stage of labour	Delayed 2nd stage of labour
Procedure	'Wrigleys' forceps—for 'lift-out' deliveries	The vacuum extraction cup is applied to the baby's head, suction is applied and traction aids delivery
	'Neville Barnes' forceps—for high deliveries	
	'Keilland's' forceps—if rotation is required	Ventouse allows rotation if the baby is malpositioned
Early complications	Maternal trauma (episiotomy always required)	'Chignon' develops on the baby's head—resolves in 1–2d.
	Foetal facial bruising	Cephalohaematoma
	Facial nerve paralysis	Retinal haemorrhage
		Neonatal jaundice (but no ↑ need for phototherapy)
Longer term complications	Maternal faecal incontinence	
Comparison	Ventouse has an ↑ failure rate compared to forceps but no ↑ CS rate	
	There is ↓ requirement for regional anaesthesia with ventouse deliveries compared to forceps deliveries	
	Forceps deliveries result in more maternal trauma than ventouse deliveries	

Further information

RCOG
● Induction of labour (2001)
● Instrumental vaginal delivery (2000) ▣ http://www.rcog.org.uk
NICE Caesarian Section Guidelines 2004. (Includes a useful table of relative risks of vaginal vs CS for woman and child in Appendix 4) ▣ http://www.nice.org.uk

Patient information

RCOG (2001) About induction of labour—information for pregnant women, their partners and their families ▣ http://www.rcog.org.uk
NCT Information on labour, pain relief (including epidurals) and instrumental deliveries
▣ http://www.nctpregnancyandbabycare.com

Postnatal care

The puerperium is the 6wk. period after delivery. Most women in the UK spend at least 6h. after delivery in hospital. After discharge home, the midwife continues to visit for 2wk. after the birth and then the health visitor takes over. GPs usually see the mother and baby soon after discharge and again routinely for the 6wk. postnatal check. Additional reviews can be arranged as needed.

The mother's 6wk. postnatal check: Discuss any problems in pregnancy or delivery and note for future reference; discuss any problems with the baby. Discuss feeding and contraception.

Examination
- BP
- Abdominal examination—uterus should not be palpable per abdomen
- Vaginal examination—only required if any problems with tears/episiotomy, persistent PV bleeding, or pain
- Consider using depression screening questionnaire e.g. Edinburgh postnatal depression questionnaire

Investigations
- Cervical smear if required
- Check Hb if anaemic postnatally
- Check rubella immunization has been given if not immune antenatally; if not, arrange for vaccination. Check immunity 3mo. after vaccination.

The baby's 6wk. developmental check: 📖 p.818

Breastfeeding: *Advantages:*
- Protection of the baby from infection
- Less chance of atopy in the baby
- Better bonding for mother and baby
- Cheaper than bottle feeding
- More convenient than bottle feeding
- Protects mother against breast and ovarian cancer
- Less postpartum bleeding
- Weight ↓ for the mother

Potential problems
- *Cracked/sore nipples:* 📖 p.808
- *Feeding technique:* Breastfeeding is something some find natural and others find difficult. Teaching a woman and baby to breastfeed takes time and patience. Be supportive and ask a midwife or the local breastfeeding advisor to help if needed.
- *Failing lactation:* Suckling is the strongest stimulus. Advise the mother to devote 2d. to feeding on demand. As a last resort, a short course of metoclopramide may restore prolactin secretion.
- *Working women:* Women who have to go back to work often have problems continuing breastfeeding. Some employers are supportive, but others not. It is possible to breastfeed at home and express enough milk for the next day, but very tiring. An alternative is to express milk from the time the baby is born and store it in the freezer for use when the woman goes back to work.

- *Suppression of lactation:* Takes 4–5d. after breastfeeding has stopped. Breasts become engorged and may be painful. Simple analgesia and a supportive bra are helpful. Stillbirth or neonatal death—📖 p.810

Common postnatal problems: 📖 p.808

Postpartum contraception: Contraceptive needs depend on whether the woman is breastfeeding—see Table 22.4.

Table 22.4 Postpartum contraception

Method	If not breastfeeding*	If breastfeeding**
COC pill	Start ≥3wk. after delivery as ↑ risk of thromboembolism. ❶ Can be started immediately after miscarriage/termination. If PET in pregnancy—start the COC pill only when BP and biochemical abnormalities have returned to normal.	Contraindicated as it may inhibit lactation and enters breast milk in small quantities.
POP	Delay until ≥3wk. postpartum to avoid ↑risk of heavy bleeding. If started >3wk. after delivery, start on 1st day of period for immediate protection or, if cycle not established, use alternative protection for 1st 7d..	↑ quantity of breast milk. Can be started 3wk. after delivery or whenever needed (e.g. if baby weaned or started on supplementary bottle feeds). If started >3wk. after delivery, alternative protection for 1st 7d. is needed.
Injectables/ implants	Delay until ≥3wk. postpartum. If >3wk. postpartum, administer early in period or, if cycle not re-established, check pregnancy test before administration. Delay until ≥3wk. Postpartum.	
IUCD	Delay until >5wk. postpartum—take care with insertion as the uterus may be soft and perforate easily.	
Cap	Refit any time from 5–6wk. postpartum (even after LSCS).	
Condoms	Useful until other methods are established and to prevent transfer of sexually transmitted diseases.	
Sterilization	↑ operative and failure rate at abortion or in postpartum period. Best delayed for a few months.	

* Ovulation can occur within 10d. of abortion and 28d. of delivery.
** If the baby is <6mo. old and the woman is amenorrhoeic and fully breastfeeding, there is no need for additional contraception. If any supplementary bottle feeding, baby is weaned or any vaginal bleeding (except occasional spotting), then assume the mother is fertile.

Patient information
Family Planning Association ☎020 7837 4044 🖳 http://www.fpa.org.uk
National Childbirth Trust 🖳 http://www.nctpregnancyandbabycare.com

Common postnatal problems

Abdominal pain: Cramping, 'period like' for the 1st 1–2wk. after delivery, especially when breastfeeding. These are due to the uterus contracting down or involuting. Suspect infection if offensive lochia, fever, the uterus stops getting smaller day by day, or is still palpable per abdomen 10d. after delivery.

Breast soreness: 3–5d. after birth the breasts become engorged ('the milk comes in') and may be quite painful. Support with a well-fitting maternity bra day and night. Express milk if still painful—a warm bath may help. *Other problems:*
- *Sore/cracked nipples:* Try topical remedies e.g. Kamillosan and/or nipple shields.
- *Skin infection:* Localized soreness, pain around the areola ± nipple or in the breast after a feed—usually due to candida infection. Treat mother and baby with miconazole oral gel.
- *Blocked duct:* Hard, tender lump in the breast. Advise the mother to massage that area of the breast while feeding or expressing milk.
- *Mastitis:* Tender, hot, reddened area of breast ± fever. Treat with flucloxacillin 250mg qds and NSAID e.g. ibuprofen 400mg tds prn. Continue breastfeeding or express the milk to prevent milk stagnation if too painful for feeding.
- *Breast abscess:* Admit for incision and drainage.

Hair loss: Hair becomes thicker in pregnancy and these hairs are all shed at about the same time—~5–6mo. postpartum. Reassure. Hair loss reverts to normal levels within 2–3mo. If severe, persistent, or accompanied by tiredness, consider hypothyroidism (🕮 p.423)—check TFTs.

Haemorrhoids: Common and painful. *Try:*
- Local ice packs (frozen fingers of rubber gloves are the right shape);
- Topical preparations e.g. proctosedyl;
- Resting lying on 1 side;
- Keeping stools soft using a stool softener;
- Advising women to wash the haemorrhoids with cool water after opening bowels and gently push them through the anus (if possible).

Postnatal depression

'Baby blues': Very common—women become tearful and low within the 1st 10d. of delivery. Be supportive. Usually resolves.

Depression: Common (10–15% mothers) reaching a peak ~12wk. after delivery—though symptoms are almost always present at 6wk. Often mothers do not report symptoms as they feel they have failed if they are miserable after the birth of a baby or they just think they are not coping (and may report that to you). Screening questionnaires (e.g. Edinburgh postnatal depression questionnaire) may be useful to detect cases in high-risk women. *Risk factors:*
- Depression during pregnancy
- Social problems (e.g. poor social support, financial problems)
- PMH or FH of depression or postnatal depression
- Alcohol or drug abuse

Management: Talk through problems; give information (e.g. self-help groups); refer to the HV for ongoing support; consider checking TFTs (especially if main presenting symptom is tiredness); consider antidepressant medication (e.g. lofepramine 70mg bd) or counselling. Refer to the mental health team if these measures are not helping.

Puerperal psychosis: Much rarer (1:500 births). Suspect if severe depression; high suicidal drive; mania; psychotic symptoms (📖 p.972). In all cases, seek expert help from a psychiatrist. Consider admission—under a sction if necessary.

Patient information and support
Royal College of Psychiatrists 🖳 http://www.rcpsych.ac.uk

Poor abdominal and pelvic muscle tone: Classes for postnatal exercise to retone the body are available both on dry land and in the swimming pool at most leisure centres. Pelvic floor exercises can be started <1d. after delivery (📖 p.711). Good leaflets explaining these are available from physiotherapists, local maternity units, and the NCT.

Puerperal pyrexia: Temperature >38°C within 14d. of delivery or miscarriage. 90% infections are in the urinary or genital tracts. Ask about:
- Urinary symptoms
- Breast symptoms
- Colour and smell of lochia
- Any other symptoms (e.g. cough, sore throat)
- Abdominal pain

Examine fully including bimanual VE and send MSU and vaginal swabs for M,C&S. *Potential obstetric causes:*
- *Superficial perineal infection:* Complicates tear or episiotomy—treat with flucloxacillin 250–500mg qds.
- *Endometritis:* Presents with offensive lochia, lower abdominal pain, and a tender uterus. Treat with amoxycillin 250–500mg tds and metronidazole 400mg tds. If not settling in <48h. or very unwell, admit for iv antibiotics.
- *Mastitis:* See breast soreness—opposite.
- *DVT or PE:* Can present with pyrexia (📖 p.364).

Persistent lochia: 📖 p.793

Superficial thrombophlebitis: Affects 1% women. Presents with a tender (usually varicose) vein. Exclude DVT. Treat with support (e.g. elasticated stocking); try applying an ice pack to affected area; NSAID prn. Advise not to stand still, and when sitting to elevate the leg above waist level. Recovery usually occurs within a few days.

Tiredness: Very common in the 1st few months after delivery but it may be the presenting feature of postnatal depression, anaemia, or hypothyroidism. Check FBC and TFTs.

Transient autoimmune thyroiditis: Up to 10% women 1–3mo. after delivery. *Presentation:* usually fatigue and lethargy.
- *Hypothyroidism:* Treat with thyroxine for 6mo. then stop for 6wk. and repeat TFTs. Follow-up with annual TFTs—1:5 go on to develop permanent hypothyroidism.
- *Hyperthyroidism:* Refer to an endocrinologist—antithyroid treatment is not normally required but symptom control may be necessary.

Stillbirth and neonatal death

Those babies born dead after 24wk. gestation. Death may occur in utero or during labour. Usually present with a lack of foetal movements and, on examination, no foetal heart can be detected. If suspected, refer as an emergency to the nearest obstetric unit for confirmation of intrauterine death by USS.

Management: In hospital, mothers of babies who have died in utero are usually induced. Samples are routinely taken from mother and baby to try to determine cause of death.

Common causes: Pre-eclampsia; renal disease; DM; infection; malformation; post-maturity; abruption; knots in the cord. No cause is found for 1:5 stillbirths.

After discharge

Lactation suppression: Offer bromocriptine 2.5mg nocte for 2d. then 2.5mg bd for 3wk.

Registration of stillbirth: A certificate of stillbirth is issued by the obstetrician which must be taken to the Registrar of Deaths within 42d. of the stillbirth. Parents are issued with a certificate of burial or cremation and a certificate of registration to keep. The child's name may be entered on the certificate of registration.

Funeral: Parents have the option of a free hospital funeral. Burial is usually in an unmarked multiple occupancy grave. Parents may pay for a single occupancy grave or cremation. Alternatively, parents may pay for a private funeral.

Benefits: In the UK, all maternity benefits are still payable after stillbirth (📖 p.112).

Follow-up: Is routinely arranged by the specialist obstetrician to discuss reasons for the stillbirth and implications for future pregnancies. Primary care follow-up is essential. Stillbirth is a huge burden to come to terms with. Parents do not have the regular contact with medical staff a baby brings. Ensure regular follow-up by a member of the primary care team. Broach the issues brought up by the baby's death directly. Offer an open door. Give information about support organizations e.g. SANDS. Advise waiting 6mo.–1y. before embarking on another pregnancy.

Neonatal death: Death of an infant <28d. old. Rare in the community. If expected, the GP can issue a special death certificate (📖 p.210). If unexpected, refer to the police/coroner. Offer lactation suppression and follow-up as for stillbirth.

Patient support and information

Stillbirth and Neonatal Death Society (SANDS) ☎020 7436 5881 🖳 http://www.uk-sands.org

Other relevant pages

Paediatrics

Paediatric surveillance

> *'Children are one third of our population and all our future'*
> US Select Panel for Promotion of Child Health (1981)

The RCGP has stated that it believes every child should receive 'a comprehensive curative and preventive service, including health surveillance, through general practice'. Recent government publications have emphasized the need to address children's health issues. *Smoking Kills* set a target to ↓ the number of children smoking from 13% to ≤9% by 2010, while in *Towards a Healthier Scotland* the government announced that child health would become a priority health topic.

The care of children forms a significant part of the primary healthcare team's workload. Patients ≤15y. comprise 20% of the average practice list and the under-4s consult their GP more often and have more home visits than any other age group except the elderly.

Diploma in Child Health: A diploma designed to give recognition of competence in the care of children to GP vocational trainees, clinical medical officers, and trainees in specialties allied to paediatrics. Administered, by the Royal College of Paediatrics and Child Health (RCPCH) 🖥 *http://www.rcpch.ac.uk*

Child health surveillance: Includes:
- Developmental screening—🕮 p.816–27
- Immunization—🕮 p.478
- Specific advice on nutrition—🕮 p.836
- Specific advice on safety issues—🕮 p.162 and opposite
- General health education—🕮 p.226–41

GMS practices are expected to perform child health surveillance (excluding neonatal checks) for all children <5y. of age registered with the practice, as an additional service. Opting out → a 0.7% ↓ in the global sum payment.

Developmental screening: The aim of developmental screening is to discover developmental delay or behaviour problems as early as possible so that appropriate management can commence preventing 2° complications. The following pages give a brief guide to developmental screening.

Essential reading
Hall, Hill, Elliman (1994) *The child surveillance handbook.* Radcliffe Medical Press.
  ISBN: 1870905245

Health education for new parents

Reducing the risk of cot death
- Cut smoking in pregnancy
- Do not let anyone smoke in the same room as the baby
- Place the baby on his/her back to sleep
- Do not let the baby get too hot
- Keep baby's head uncovered—place the baby with feet to the foot of the cot, to prevent wriggling down under the covers
- It's safest to sleep the baby in a cot in the parents' bedroom for the first 6mo.
- It's dangerous to share a bed with the baby if either parent:
  - is a smoker—no matter where or when they smoke
  - has been drinking alcohol
  - takes medication or drugs that might make them drowsy
  - feels very tired
- It's very dangerous to sleep together with a baby on a sofa, armchair, or settee
- If the baby is unwell, seek medical advice promptly

Protecting the baby from accidents and infections
- Keep small objects out of the baby's reach
- Stay with the baby when he/she is eating or drinking
- Make sure the baby's cot and mattress are in good condition and that the mattress fits the cot properly
- Install at least one smoke alarm
- Parents should plan a way to escape a fire with the baby
- Never leave the baby alone in a bath or near water
- Immunize the baby
- Make sure the baby can't reach hot drinks or the kettle or iron flex
- Only use toys suitable for the baby's age
- Never shake a baby—ask for help if crying gets too much
- Use a properly fitted baby car seat that is the right size for the baby
- Do not use a baby walker
- Wash hands before feeding the baby and make sure the baby's bottle and teats are properly sterilized

The neonatal check

It is essential that a full neonatal check is carried out <48h. after delivery. Most neonatal checks are carried out by paediatricians in maternity units before discharge. This does not happen if:
- The baby is discharged <24h. after delivery
- The birth occurs at home or in a GP unit
- There is rapid discharge from obstetric unit to a peripheral unit.

Neonatal checks can then be provided by GMS GPs as a national enhanced service or by PMS GPs as part of their negotiated services.

Parental concerns
- Discuss any worries the parent(s) might have about the child
- Review FH, pregnancy, and birth
- Arrange Hepatitis B vaccination if mother is Hepatitis B +ve (📖 p.788) or BCG vaccination if mother is sputum smear +ve (📖 p.489)

History
- *Has the baby passed urine?* If no urine in the 1st 24h. suspect renal abnormality and admit for further investigation.
- *Has the baby passed meconium?* If no meconium in the 1st 24h., suspect meconium ileus and admit for further investigation.

Physical examination: Check the baby systematically—Table 23.1.

Moro reflex: Support head and shoulders about 15cm from the examination couch. Suddenly allow the baby's head to drop back slightly. The response—extension of the arms followed by adduction towards the chest—should be brisk and symmetrical. This reflex disappears by 6mo.

Discuss neonatal screening
- PKU, CF, and thyroid heel prick tests—usually done at 9d.
- Haemoglobinopathy screening (📖 p.774)

Check vitamin K has been given
- Discuss any concerns with the parent(s).
- Deficiency of vitamin K can → *haemorrhagic disease of the newborn* with potentially serious effects including death.
- Vitamin K policies vary widely in the UK. Be aware of local policy.
- Babies at high risk of bleeding (premature, low birth weight, unwell babies, and those who have undergone instrumental deliveries)—routine im administration of vitamin K is the norm.
- Babies given oral vitamin K at birth—1 dose doesn't confer full protection. Formula feeds contain vitamin K supplements but breastfed babies require further doses—ensure they get them.

Check the baby has passed urine and meconium in the 1st 24h.
- Failure to pass meconium may indicate CF or Hirschprung's.
- If the baby fails to urinate, check for low set ears of Potter's syndrome and ensure there is no palpable bladder.

Health education: Discuss:
- Feeding and nutrition
- Sleeping position (📖 p.815)
- Baby care
- Sibling management
- Crying and sleep problems
- Transport in a car

Table 23.1 Checklist for the neonatal examination

General appearance		
Weight • Small for gestation? • Large for gestation? Lanugo or evidence of postmaturity	Syndrome? • Clusters of features e.g. features of Downs syndrome or Turner's syndrome	Pallor, jaundice, or cyanosis Skin • Birth marks • Meconium staining • Purpura

Head and facial features		
Head circumference	Ptosis	Sternomastoid swelling
Cephalhaematoma	Cataract	Hare lip
Fontanelles—size and tension	Red reflex?	Potter's facies
Accessory auricles	Subconjunctival haemorrhage	Pierre Robin jaw (receding jaw with cleft palate)

Mouth		
Cleft palate? (📖 p.839)	Profuse saliva*	Epsteins pearls

Arms and hands		
Proportion of arms/fingers	Number of fingers • Extra digits • Missing digits	Normal movements
Oedema		Erb palsy (📖 p.828)
Palmar creases	Webbing of fingers	

Chest		
Distortion	Respiratory rate**	Air entry
Breast enlargement	Added breath sounds	Recession

Cardiovascular examination		
Pulses (femoral & brachial)	Heart sounds	Murmurs (📖 p.842)

Abdomen		
Umbilical infection	Umbilical hernia	Masses***

Genitalia		
♂: penis—size and shape; position of urethral orifice; testes (normal, undescended or maldescended), hernia, or hydrocoele		
♀: clitoromegaly; vaginal bleeding; posterior vaginal skin tag (common)		

Legs and feet		
Hips (📖 p.824)	Proportion	Club foot (📖 p.869)

Back		
Sacral pit	Spina bifida (📖 p.838)	Scoliosis (📖 p.825)

CNS		
Is the baby behaving normally?	Is the cry normal?	Are all 4 limbs moving equally and is the Moro reflex symmetrical?

* Profuse saliva is associated with oesophageal atresia

** Respiratory rate <60breaths/min is normal

*** Liver is usually palpable as are the lower poles of the kidneys; the spleen is never palpable

The 6-week check

Parental concerns: Ask about any problems in the first 6wk. or any concerns, including worries about vision or hearing.

Physical examination
- Weight and head circumference
- Dysmorphic features
- Murmurs—📖 p.842
- Red reflexes
- Check for congenital dislocation of the hip—📖 p.824
- Testicular descent—📖 p.248

Health education
- Discuss immunizations; feeding; dangers of falls, scalds, and smoking around a baby
- Prevention of cot death—📖 p.815
- Recognition of illness and advice about what to do

Developmental screening
Gross motor development
- *Head control (0–3mo.):* Pull the baby gently from a supine position to a sitting position by the hands/wrists. The baby should hold his/her head upright and steady without wobbling by 6wk.
- *Moro reflex (0–6mo.):* 📖 p.816
- *Ventral suspension (0–10mo.):* Suspend the baby horizontally, face down. The head should be in line with or slightly higher than the body and the hips semi-extended
- *Prone position (from birth):* Place the baby face down on a flat surface. He/she should be able to lift his/her head momentarily from the surface.

Fine motor development and vision
- *Stares (from birth):* Look at baby's face—will usually stare back. If not, ask the mother if the baby looks at her while feeding.
- *Follows horizontally to 90°:* Put baby on his/her back with head turned to 1 side. Move a bright-coloured object 25cm from baby's face from 1 side to the other—should follow the object with eyes ± head across the midline and through ≥90°. If gaze wanders from one side to the other when happy, awake, and >6wk. old, suspect a visual problem.

Hearing and speech
- *Rattle or bell 15cm away at ear level (from birth):* Ensure the baby cannot see the rattle or bell. The baby should quieten to the sound—other satisfactory responses are turning, widening eyes, or change in breathing pattern. If the baby fails to respond, unless the parents are worried about the baby's hearing (when refer immediately), repeat in 2wk. and refer if the baby fails the test a second time.
- *Startle response (from birth):* Clap loudly close to the baby—baby should make some response. If not, ask the parents if he/she reacts to loud noises at home.

Social behaviour
- Smiles (0–10wk.—mean 5wk.)
- Turns to look at observer's face (from birth)

⚠ **Warning signs**
- No visual fixation or following
- Failure to respond to sound
- Asymmetrical neonatal reflexes
- Excessive head lag
- Failure to smile
- Absent red reflex

2,3, and 4 months: Routine immunizations take place at 2,3, and 4mo. Give parents the opportunity to discuss any worries and reinforce health education wherever possible.

The 8- and 18-month checks

Parental concerns: Ask about any concerns—particularly regarding development, behaviour, sleeping problems, or worries about vision or hearing.

Physical examination
- Weight and head circumference (8mo. check) *or* height (18mo. check)
- Dysmorphic features
- Murmurs—📖 p.842
- Congenital dislocation of the hip
    - 8mo. check—📖 p.824
    - 18mo. check—walking gait and thigh creases
- Testicular descent—📖 p.248
- Squint—📖 p.826

Health education
- Accident prevention—falls, drowning, poisoning, scalds, road safety, safety in high chairs and push chairs
- Problems of independent mobility—stair gates, fire guards, cupboard locks, moving dangerous substances to high up cupboards
- Nutrition
- Care of teeth
- Dangers of passive smoking
- Developmental needs—language, play, socialization with other children
- Avoidance and management of behavioural problems

Developmental screening at 8 months
Gross motor development
- Bears weight on legs (3–7mo.)
- Can be pulled to sit (14wk.–6mo.)
- Sits with support (4–6mo.)
- Sits without support (5–8mo.)
- Crawls (6–9mo.)

Fine motor development and vision
- Reaches out to grasp (palmar grasp) (3–6mo.)
- Transfers and mouths (passes an object from 1 hand to the other and puts it in mouth) (18wk.–8mo.)
- Fixes gaze on small objects (5–8mo.)
- Follows fallen toys (18wk.–8mo.)

Hearing and speech
- Vocalizes (4–6mo.)
- Polysyllabic babbling (6–10mo.)
- Laughs (2–5mo.)
- Responds to own name (4–8mo.)
- Distraction hearing test (8–10mo)—usually performed by the health visitor (📖 p.827)

Social behaviour and play
- Puts everything into mouth (4–8mo.)
- Hand and foot regard (4–8mo.)
- Plays peek-a-boo (5½ –10mo.)

> ⚠ **Warning signs**
> - Hand preference
> - Fisting
> - Squint
> - Persistence of primitive reflexes—Moro response, stepping, asymmetrical tonic neck reflex

Developmental screening at 18 months
Gross motor development
- Gets to sitting position (6–11mo.)
- Pulls to standing (6–10mo.)
- Walks holding onto furniture (7–13mo.)
- Walks alone (10–15mo.)—bottom-shufflers later
- Walks backwards (12–22mo.)
- Climbs stairs (14–22mo.)

Fine motor development and vision
- Points with index finger
- Casts (throws) (9–15mo.)
- Delicate pincer grasp (10–18mo.)
- Holds 2 bricks and bangs them together (7–13mo.)
- Scribbles (12–24mo.)
- Builds a tower of 3 or 4 bricks (16–24mo.)

Hearing and speech
- Turns to the sound of name
- Jabbers continually
- Uses 'mama' and 'dada' (11–20mo.—50% by 15mo.)
- Can say ≥3 words other than 'mama' and 'dada' (10–21mo.)
- Points to eyes, nose, and mouth (14–23mo.)
- Obeys simple instructions (15mo.–2½ y.)

Social behaviour and play
- Holds spoon and gets food to mouth (14mo.–2½ y.)
- Explores environment (13–20mo.)
- Takes off shoes and socks (13–20mo.)

> ⚠ **Warning signs**
> - Unable to sit or bear weight
> - Inability to stand without support
> - Persistence of hand regard
> - Absence of babbling or cooing
> - Absence of saving reactions
> - Inability to understand simple commands
> - No pincer grip
> - Casting still present

The 3- and 4-year checks

Parental concerns: Ask about any concerns—particularly regarding development, behaviour, or worries about vision or hearing.

Physical examination
- Height and weight
- Check walking with normal gait
- Murmurs—📖 p.842
- Testicular descent—📖 p.248

Health education
- Accident prevention—falls from heights, fires, drowning, poisoning, road safety
- Nutrition
- Dental care (visiting the dentist)
- Developmental needs—language, play, socialization with other children, preparation for school
- Avoidance and management of behavioural problems

Developmental screening at 3 years

Gross motor development
- Climbs and descends stairs
- Runs (~15mo.)
- Pedals tricycle (21mo.–3y.)
- Jumps in one place (21mo.–3y.)
- Kicks a ball (15–24mo.)
- Stands on 1 foot for 1 second (22mo.–3¼ y.)

Fine motor development and vision
- Picks up 'hundreds and thousands'
- Imitates a vertical line (18mo.–33mo.)
- Copies a circle (2¼ y.–3½ y.)
- Threads beads
- Builds a tower of 8 bricks (21mo.–3½ y.)
- Matches 2 colours

Hearing and speech
- Uses plurals (30mo.–3¼ y.)
- Uses prepositions (3–4½ y.)
- Joins words into sentences (50% by 23mo.; 97% by 3y.)
- Gives own name

Social behaviour and play
- Plays alone
- Eats with spoon and fork
- Puts on clothes (2¼ –3½ y.—with supervision)
- Washes and dries hands
- Separates from mother easily (2–4y.)
- Dry in the day (2–4y.)

⚠ **Warning signs**
- Unable to speak in simple sentences
- Unable to understand speech

Developmental screening at 4 years or pre-school

Gross motor development

- Hops forward on 1 foot for 2min. (3–5y.)
- Stands on 1 foot for 5sec. (2¾ –4½ y.)
- Walks heel-to-toe (3½ –5¼ y.—backwards 4–6y.)
- Bounces and catches a ball (3¼ –5½ y.)

Fine motor development and vision

- Copies a cross (3–4½ y.) and square (4–5½ y.)
- Draws a man with 3 parts (with all features—4½ –6y.)
- Recognizes colours (3y.–4¾ y.)

Hearing and speech

- Speaks grammatically (2½ y.–4¼ y.)
- Counts to 10

Social behaviour and play

- Shares toys
- Brushes teeth
- Dresses without supervision (3¼ –5½ y.)
- Comforts friends in distress (5y.)

⚠ **Warning signs**

Speech difficult to understand due to poor articulation or because of omission or substitution of consonants (confusion of 's', 'f', and 'th' disappears by 6½ y.)

Screening for childhood orthopaedic problems

Congenital dislocation of the hip (CDH): Encompasses varying degrees of instability, subluxation, and dysplasia of the hip joint. Screening should take place at birth, at the 6wk. check, at 6–8mo., and in the second year (15–21mo.). High-risk children (breech babies, FH, foot deformities, sternomastoid tumour) are routinely screened with USS. Screening tests should be taught in vivo by someone experienced in the technique.

Screening a child <3mo.

- In the newborn period, limited abduction is uncommon as a sign of dislocation of the hip and more likely to be due to ↑ tone e.g. spina bifida. At this time, the most important sign is instability of the hip.
- Screening tests should be performed in a warm room with the baby undressed and lying on a firm surface.
- Hips and knees are flexed to 90° with 1 hand, with 1 hand to each leg, thumbs on the inner side of the baby's knee, and ring and little fingers behind the greater trochanters.
- Each hip is tested separately. The examiner's hand on the opposite side from the hip being tested is used to stabilize the pelvis by holding the thumb over the symphysis pubis and fingers under the sacrum.
- Only test once as repeated testing can damage the hips.

Ortolani manoeuvre: Each hip is gently abducted whilst lifting the greater trochanter forward. As a dislocated hip is abducted, a clunk or jumping sensation is felt. It is difficult to tell the difference between a click of a normal hip and clunk, so refer any clicky or clunky hips for further investigation (usually USS or orthopaedic review).
(*M. Ortolani (1904–87)—Italian paediatric orthopaedic surgeon*)

Barlow manoeuvre: This establishes whether the hips are dislocatable. Holding the legs as described above, gently apply pressure along the line of the femur, pushing it backwards out of the acetabulum. The judder of the femoral head slipping in and out of the acetabulum can be felt if the hip is dislocatable. (*J. Barlow (b.1924)—South African physician*)

Screening a child >3mo.

- After 3mo. of age-limited abduction is the most common finding in children with CDH. If the infant lies on his back, with hips flexed at 90°, any hip which cannot abduct >75° should be viewed with suspicion.
- Perform the Ortolani and Barlow tests (see above).
- *Other signs:*
  - Limb shortening on the affected side—compare knee levels.
  - Asymmetry of the thighs—particularly skin creases.
  - Flattening of the buttock—in a prone position, the affected side may look flatter.

Scoliosis: Early treatment of scoliosis prevents progression. Early onset scoliosis (<8y.) is responsible for cosmetic problems, pain, and cardio-pulmonary disturbance. Late onset scoliosis is less severe but also causes pain and significant deformity.

Risk factors
- Congenital malformations of the spine (butterfly vertebra)
- Neuromuscular problems e.g. cerebral palsy
- Connective tissue disorders
- Neurofibromatposis
- Bone dysplasias
- Friedrich's ataxia

Clinical features
- Difference in shoulder height
- Spinal curvature
- Difference in space between trunk and upper limbs

❶ Scoliosis which disappears on bending is postural and of no clinical significance.

Screening tests
- *<1y. old:* Place the child prone on his tummy and feel the shoulder and thoracic cage. There should be no rib hump or shoulder hump.
- *>1y. old:* Ask the child to bend forward whilst standing straight with both feet together and holding both hands straight. Look for a shoulder, thoracic or lumbar hump, difference in shoulder height, obvious spinal curvature, and check the gap between arm and waistline.

⚠ In all cases, if scoliosis is suspected, refer for an orthopaedic opinion.

Vision and hearing screening tests for children

Operational senses are essential for normal development. Conditions which interfere with the normal senses, even if correctable, may lead to permanent impairment if not detected and treated early.

⚠ Warning signs for visual problems
- The child does not fix on the mother's face whilst feeding by 6wk.
- >6wk. old, the child's eye wanders about from one side of the eye socket to the other while awake and happy
- A white spot is seen in the pupil at any age—could be cataract
- The child holds objects close to his face whilst trying to look at them
- A child >6mo. old has a squint in 1 or both eyes

⚠ Warning signs for hearing problems
- There is no startle response to loud noises at 6wk.
- The child does not respond to his name by 8mo.
- Absence of babbling or cooing by 1y.
- Inability to understand simple commands by 18mo.
- Inability to speak in short sentences by 2½ y.

Routine developmental screening: Visual and hearing screening tests are carried out as part of routine child health surveillance at 6wk., 8mo., 18mo., 3y., and pre-school. Refer children for further assessment where there is any parental concern *or* concern about their vision, hearing, or speech as the result of screening.

Tests for squint
- Sit the child on the parent's lap.
- Stand in front of the child and shine a bright light (e.g. pen torch) at arm's length from the child.
- Fix the child's head in the midline and look for the reflection of the light on the child's corneas.
- The reflection should be symmetrical and near the centre of the pupil (usually slightly towards the nose).
- Turn the child's head to 1 side, keeping the eyes fixed on the light. The reflection should remain symmetrical.
- Repeat, turning the head to the other side.
- If reflections are not symmetrical, perform a cover test.

Cover test
- Sit the child comfortably on a parent's lap.
- Shine a bright light or a place a small bright object at arm's length from the child.
- Cover 1 eye with a card.
- Watch for any movement of the uncovered eye to fix on the object.
- Then remove the card and watch the covered eye to see if it moves to fix on the object.
- Repeat with the other eye. If either or both eyes move, a squint is present—refer.

Hearing tests: Young babies have a startle response to loud sounds. There is a routine neonatal hearing screening programme (NHSP) in the UK and by December 2005 all newborn babies in the UK will be offered a routine hearing screen.

Neonatal screening: 2 types of screen are used by the NHSP:
- *Oto-acoustic emission (OAE) screen:* Involves placing a small soft tipped earpiece in the outer part of the baby's ear and playing quiet clicking sounds. In a hearing ear, the cochlea produces sounds in response to the clicks which can be recorded and analysed by the computerized screening system. Screening takes a few minutes and can be done at the bedside when the baby is asleep, but it is not always possible to get clear responses, especially if the baby is <24h. old.
- *Automated auditory brainstem response (AABR) screen:* Involves placing small sensors on the baby's head and neck and then presenting quiet clicking sounds through tiny soft headphones (muffs). A computer analyses the responses to sounds at and around the brain stem.

The distraction hearing test: Can be used from 6mo. of age but is not very reliable. This test requires 2 testers and should be performed in a quiet room. Advise parents not to make any noise during the test.
- The child is placed on the parent's lap facing 1 of the testers.
- This tester attracts attention by moving a soundless toy just out of reach.
- The other tester makes a sound at ear level ~1m. away from the child and slightly behind the child so that any movement cannot be seen.
- Both ears are tested.
- A positive test (implying the child can hear) occurs if the child localizes (searches for and finds) the sound.

Stimuli commonly used:
- Rattle—Manchester rattle (low-frequency sound); Nuffield rattle (high-frequency sounds).
- Cup and spoon—china cup and metal teaspoon. The spoon is run gently around the rim of the cup.
- Voice—high-pitched sound ('ss-ss'); low-pitched sound ('oo-oo'); speech including the child's name.

Pure tone audiometry: From 3y. pure tone audiometry is possible with a co-operative child—📖 p.925.

Further information
NHS Newborn Hearing Screening Programme 🖳 http://www.nhsp.info

Parent and child information and support
LOOK: support for families of blind or visually impaired children
☎0121 428 5038 🖳 http://www.look-uk.org
National Deaf Children's Society ☎0808 800 8880 🖳 http://www.ndcs.org.uk

Birth trauma

Head trauma

- **Caput succedaneum:** Swelling, bruising, and oedema of the presenting portion—usually scalp. Unsightly, but resolves spontaneously.
- **Cephalhaematoma:** Uncommon. Haemorrhage beneath the periosteum. Unilateral and usually parietal. Presents as a lump (the size of an egg) on the baby's head. Treatment is not required, but anaemia or hyperbilirubinemia may follow.
- **Depressed skull fractures:** Rare. Most result from forceps pressure; rarely caused by the head resting on a bony prominence in utero. May be associated with subdural bleeding, subarachnoid hemorrhage, or contusion/laceration of the brain itself. Seen and felt as a depression in the skull. X-ray confirms diagnosis. Neurosurgical elevation may be needed.
- **Intracranial haemorrhage:** Rare. Suggested by lack of responsiveness, fits, respiratory distress ± shock. Admit as an emergency.

Nerve injuries

- **Cranial nerve trauma:** The facial nerve is injured, most often causing facial asymmetry, especially during crying. Usually resolves spontaneously by 2–3mo. of age.
- **Brachial plexus injury:** Follows stretching caused by shoulder dystocia, breech extraction, or hyperabduction of the neck in cephalic presentations. Often associated with other traumatic injuries e.g. fractured clavicle or humerus, subluxations of the shoulder, or cervical spine.
- **Partial injuries of the brachial plexus:** Site and type of nerve root injury determine the prognosis. If a significant deficit persists >3mo., refer to paediatric neurology for further investigation.
  - Injuries of the upper brachial plexus (C5–6) affect muscles around the shoulder and elbow—Erb's palsy (*W.H. Erb (1840–1921)— German neurologist*)
  - Injuries of the lower plexus (C7–8 and T1) affect primarily muscles of the forearm and hand—Klumpke's palsy. (*A.M. Dejerine-Klumpke (1859–1927)—French neurologist*)
- **Injuries of the entire brachial plexus:** No movement of the arm + sensory loss. Refer immediately for neurological opinion. Prognosis for recovery is poor.

Fractures

- **Midclavicular fracture:** Most common fracture during birth. Usually occurs due to shoulder dystocia. Most clavicular fractures are greenstick and heal rapidly and uneventfully. A large callus forms at the fracture site in <1wk. and remodelling is completed in <1mo. Can be associated with brachial plexus injury and/or pneumothorax.
- **Long bone fractures:** The humerus and femur may be fractured during difficult deliveries. Usually long bones heal rapidly without any residual deformity.

Cerebral palsy: The term cerebral palsy identifies children with non-progressive spasticity, ataxia, or involuntary movements. It affects 0.1–0.2% of children (~1% of premature babies/babies small for dates).

Causes
- Prematurity
- In utero disorders
- Neonatal jaundice
- Birth trauma
- Perinatal asphyxia
- CNS trauma
- Severe systemic disease during early childhood (e.g. meningitis, sepsis)

Associated disorders
- Fits (25%)
- Squint and other visual problems
- Deafness
- Learning disability—though intelligence is often normal
- Short attention span
- Hyperactivity

Classification: 3 main categories—but mixed forms are common.

Spastic syndromes: 70%. Upper motor neuron involvement.
- Affects motor function and may → hemiplegia, paraplegia, quadriplegia, or diplegia.
- Affected limbs are underdeveloped and have ↑ tone, weakness, and a tendency toward contractures.
- A scissors gait and toe walking are characteristic.
- In mildly affected children, impairment may occur only during certain activities (e.g. running).
- With quadriplegia, dysarthria is common.

Athetoid and dyskinetic syndromes: 20%. Basal ganglia involvement.
- Characterized by slow, writhing, involuntary movements affecting the extremities (athetoid) or proximal parts of the limbs/trunk (dystonic).
- Abrupt, jerky, distal movements (choreiform) may also occur.
- Movements ↑ with emotional tension and stop during sleep.
- Dysarthria is often severe.

Ataxic syndromes: 10%. Involvement of the cerebellum. Weakness, inco-ordination, and intention tremor produce unsteadiness, wide-based gait, and difficulty with rapid and fine movements.

Diagnosis: Diagnosis is rarely made in infancy with certainty, though often abnormalities in tone, reflexes, and posture are noted during routine developmental screening. Refer for paediatric assessment if suspected. Formal diagnosis is usually made by 2y.

Management: The goal is for children to develop maximal independence within the limits of their handicap. A multidisciplinary, coordinated team approach involving physiotherapists, occupational therapists, speech therapists, social workers, teachers, community paediatricians, and the primary healthcare team, in liaison with the child and his parents, is essential. As with all chronically disabled children, the child and his parents need assistance in understanding the disability, setting realistic goals, and relieving their own feelings.

Information and support
SCOPE (cerebral palsy) ☎0808 800 3333 🖳 http://www.scope.org.uk

Minor problems of neonates and small babies

Table 23.2 Minor problems of neonates and small babies

Condition	Features	Management
Milia	Tiny, pearly white papules on the nose ± palate—blocked sebaceous ducts.	Disappear spontaneously—reassure.
Erythema toxicum (neonatal urticaria)	Red blotches with a central, white vesicle. Each spot lasts ~24h.. Spots are sterile and the baby is well.	If sepsis is suspected—take a swab. Otherwise reassure—resolves spontaneously.
Harlequin colour change	One side of the body flushes red whilst the other stays pale, giving a harlequin effect.	A harmless vasomotor effect—reassure.
Single palmar crease	Common abnormality. Associated with several genetic syndromes e.g. Down's.	Usually of no consequence unless associated with other abnormalities.
Milaria (heat rash)	Itchy red rash which fades as soon as the baby is cooled (e.g. by undressing).	Reassure. Keep the baby cool if the rash appears.
Peeling skin	Common among babies born after their due date.	Apply olive or baby oil, or aqueous cream to prevent the skin cracking.
Petechial or subconjunctival haemorrhage and facial cyanosis	May all occur during delivery.	Resolve spontaneously—reassure. Ensure the baby has had vitamin K supplements.
Swollen breasts	Due to maternal hormones. Occur in both sexes and occasionally lactate (witches' milk).	Breast swelling usually subsides spontaneously. May become infected and require antibiotics.
Sticky eye	Common. Usually due to a blocked tear duct. Swab to exclude ophthalmia neonatorum.	Ophthalmia neonatorum—📖 p.936. Blocked tear duct—bathe with boiled water to clear, when changing nappies. Avoid the use of antibiotics unless overtly infected
Sneezing	Neonates clear amniotic fluid from their noses by sneezing.	Reassure.
Red-stained nappy	Common in the first few days of life. Usually due to urinary urates but may be due to blood from the cord or vagina (oestrogen withdrawal bleed).	Reassure.

Table 23.2 (cont.)

Condition	Features	Management
The umbilicus	After brith, the umbilicus dries, becomes black, and separates at about 1wk. of age.	The umbilical stump can become infected—offensive odour, pus, pre-iumbilical flare, malaise—requiring antibiotics.
		If a granuloma forms at the site of separation, exclude a patent urachus (refer if present) and treat with silver nitrate cautery.
Failure to regain birth weight by 2wk. of age	Usually due to a feeding problem or minor intercurrent illness.	Monitor weight carefully. Refer to paediatrics if no cause is apparent or if, despite treatment of the underlying cause, the baby is not gaining weight.
Possetting	Common.	Only of concern if the baby is otherwise unwell or failing to thrive—see gastro-oesophageal reflux (below).
	The baby effortlessly brings back 5–10mls of each feed during the feed or soon after.	If thriving, advise parents to feed the child propped up and slow down the speed at which feeds are given.
Gastro-oesophageal reflux	Similar to possetting but a greater proportion or all of each feed is brought back.	Advise parents to feed the child propped up.
	Often results in failure to thrive.	Thickening agents (e.g. Carobel, Nestargel) may be helpful as may Gaviscon Infant ± ranitidine.
	More common in babies with cerebral palsy.	Babies usually grow out of the condition after a few months and/or when solids are introduced.
	Rare complications are oesophageal stricture due to acid reflux or aspiration pneumonia.	Refer to paediatrics if failing to thrive despite simple measures, chestiness, or anaemia.
Colic	Very common in newborns up to ~3mo..	Cause is unknown and symptoms resolve spontaneously with time.
	Repeated bouts of intense, unsoothable crying commonly attributed to abdominal pain (though there is no objective evidence).	Advise parents to try colic drops or gripe water.
		There is no evidence that changing from cows' milk to soya-based formula is helpful.
	During an attack, the baby's body becomes tense and rigid, face goes red, and knees draw up.	Refer to paediatrics if diagnosis is in doubt, severe symptoms, other symptoms or signs (e.g. failure to thrive, severe eczema), or fails to resolve by 12wk. of age.
	Usually occurs in early evening.	
	Examination is normal.	
Crying	📖 p.890–891	📖 p.890–891

Neonatal jaundice

In the first few days of life, most babies have ↑ serum bilirubin levels as the liver takes over the excretion of bilirubin from the placenta. Mild jaundice from 2–6d. is therefore physiological.

Very high levels of unconjugated bilirubin are toxic and can cause encephalopathy (*kernicterus*).

Refer to paediatrics if:

Jaundice <24h. after birth: Any jaundice in the first 24h. is assumed to be pathological and needs immediate referral back to hospital to determine cause (usually haemolysis or infection) and for treatment with phototherapy or, in rare, severe cases, exchange transfusion.

Significant jaundice within 1wk. of birth: This may be difficult to assess—particularly in a dark-skinned baby. The opinion of midwives who are dealing with neonates daily can be very valuable. If necessary, arrange bilirubin estimation either by asking the community midwife to take a heel prick sample or by contacting the neonatal SHO. High levels require further investigation and phototherapy. The level at which phototherapy is necessary varies with maturity and age, and may be slightly different in different units. Discuss ↑ levels with the neonatal registrar if worried.

Jaundice persisting >10d.: Although physiological jaundice may persist for some time—particularly in breastfed babies—it is important to rule out pathological causes:
- Hypothyroidism
- Mild haemolysis
- Infection
- Liver disease—results in high levels of conjugated bilirubin.

Early diagnosis is particularly important in congenital biliary atresia so that surgery can be carried out before the liver is irreversibly damaged.

Galactosaemia: Inborn error of metabolism characterized by ↑ plasma galactose. Clinical manifestations depend on the site of enzyme defect.
- *Galactokinase deficiency:* Autosomal recessive inheritance. *Incidence:* 1:40,000. Presents in childhood with cataracts. Treatment involves a galactose-free diet.
- *Classic galactosaemia:* Autosomal recessive inheritance. *Incidence:* 1:44,000. The child appears normal at birth but becomes anorexic and jaundiced within a few days or weeks of consuming breast milk or lactose-containing formula. Vomiting, poor growth, hepatomegaly, and septicemia are common and can be rapidly fatal. Treatment involves eliminating all sources of galactose in the diet. Long-term complications—poor growth, learning difficulty, speech and neurological abnormalities, infertility—are common.

Neonatal hepatitis: Presents with persistent neonatal jaundice.
Always requires specialist investigation and management. Possible causes:

- Congenital infection
- Galactosaemia
- Cystic fibrosis
- Glycogen storage diseases.

Biliary atresia: The end stage of a sclerosing process in an initially patent biliary tree. Cause is unclear. Presents with jaundice in the neonate. Prognosis has improved with laparotomy and porto-enterostomy which can relieve the problem in ~50–70% of babies. The operation must be carried out within 2mo. of birth to stand a chance of success.

Problems of prematurity

Any baby born at <37wk. gestation is considered premature, although most born at 36wk. gestation have few problems, and babies born as early as 32wk. do very well—many needing only tube feeding and warmth. Although some babies of 23–24wk. gestation now survive, survival is rare, and there is a high incidence of disability in these extremely premature babies. Prematurity affects all systems of the body and,—in general, the problems are worse the more premature the baby.

Nutrition: Preterm babies suck and swallow poorly so commonly need naso-gastric tube feeding. They are also at particular risk of hypoglycaemia, so need frequent feeds. Breast milk (sometimes with calorie supplements) or special low birth weight formula is used. Vitamin and iron supplements are routine.

Thermoregulation: Poor in preterm infants, as they have a high surface area:body weight ratio and little subcutaneous fat. A controlled temperature and adequate insulation with clothes and blankets, where appropriate, is important.

Respiration

- *Preterm infants >32wk. gestation:* May have transient tachyopnoea at birth due to inability to express fluid from their lungs. Some need oxygen by headbox.
- *Preterm infants <32wk. gestation:* There may be insufficient surfactant produced causing respiratory distress syndrome and requiring mechanical ventilation. Incidence and severity is ↓ by antenatal corticosteroids.
- *Extremely premature babies:* May develop bronchopulmonary dysplasia (chronic lung disease) and be ventilator and oxygen dependant for many months. These babies are often sent home on oxygen via nasal cannulae. They are at higher risk from respiratory infections particularly RSV—a monoclonal antibody (Palivizumab) is licensed for use monthly during the RSV season to prevent infection in high-risk infants (*BNF* 5.3.5); episodes of bradycardia and apnoea are common. Have a low threshold for readmission.

Jaundice: The immature liver is less able to process bilirubin, so premature babies are at greater risk of developing neonatal jaundice. They are also more likely to develop kernicterus, so have a lower threshold to refer for phototherapy.

Infection: The immune system is poorly developed, so there is greater risk of infection. Furthermore, these babies exhibit few signs, so have a low threshold to refer to paediatrics for a septic screen and antibiotics.

Anaemia: Low iron stores and repeated venepuncture lead to anaemia in premature babies. Some very premature babies may need repeated transfusion, and erythropoeitin is often used to ↓ transfusion requirements. Iron supplements are routinely given to most premature babies.

Neurology: Intraventricular haemorrhages are common. Small ones may have few consequences—more extensive haemorrhages may lead to permanent disability. Hypoxia can also lead to cerebral damage.

Vision: Retinopathy of prematurity, the development of abnormal vascularization at the back of the eye, occurs in very premature babies as a result of high partial pressures of oxygen. This may result in visual impairment—even blindness. Most will have had opthalmological examination whilst in the neonatal unit but may need follow-up and/or laser treatment once home.

Hearing: Premature babies are at greater risk of hearing problems and should have neonatal screening and appropriate follow-up.

Bonding: Separation of mother and premature baby is often necessary. Poor bonding is common, and the problem is added to by fear of losing the baby. Parents may be (quite understandably) very anxious when their babies first come home after a long period in special care and need more support and reassurance than other parents.

Cot death: Premature babies have ↑ risk of cot death.
- Prevention: 📖 p.815
- Management: 📖 p.906

Feeding babies and toddlers

Breastfeeding: Breastfeeding is the preferred way to feed infants from birth until fully weaned, or longer.

Advantages
- ↓ GI and respiratory infections
- ↓ obesity
- Encourages a strong bond between mother and baby
- Cheaper and more convenient than bottle feeding—the milk is ready warmed and does not need sterilized bottles
- Protective effect against breast cancer in the mother

Disadvantages
- Only the mother can feed the baby
- Babies who have had oral vitamin K at birth require additional vitamin K supplements
- Certain diseases can be transferred in breast milk e.g. hepatitis B, HIV
- Drugs or foods taken by the mother can have adverse effects on the baby—📖 p.136
- It is difficult to know how much milk a breastfed baby is taking at each feed
- If a baby is solely breastfed (rare) when >6mo. old, vitamin supplements are needed

Expressing milk for feeding to the baby in a bottle: Mothers who anticipate they will be absent from the baby for a period of time may express milk for someone else to feed to the baby in a bottle whilst they are gone. Advise mothers not to attempt this before breastfeeding is well established as the baby might find the 2 techniques confusing. 2 methods are commonly used:
- Using a commercially available breast pump
- By hand into a sterile bowl

Breast milk can be frozen (special bags are available) and defrosted when required. Bottles should be sterilized and the milk warmed in the same way as for bottle feeding.

Bottle feeding

Cow's milk formula feeds: Prepared from cow's milk altered to simulate the composition of human milk, with added iron and vitamins. Advise parents to choose a formula suitable for their baby and make up the formula exactly as the manufacturer suggests. Feeding bottles and teats should be well washed and, until >6mo. of age, sterilized. Families on low incomes may be entitled to claim free formula milk for their babies.

Unmodified cow's milk: Not recommended until the baby is >1y. old as unmodified cow's milk is less digestible.

Follow-on formula: Not essential unless a child is not taking solids and is >6mo. old. Baby milks suitable from birth can be used until a switch is made to normal cow's milk.

Soya protein based formula: Available, for children with cow's milk allergy, though this group are frequently also intolerant of soya milk. Soya formula is useful for babies who have transient intolerance after gastro-enteritis, but be careful—it contains large amounts of glucose syrup and can damage the teeth of babies fed on it long term. Soya formula is available on NHS prescription.

Special artificial formula: Available for children intolerant to soya and cow's milk formulae. Prescribe on consultant recommendation.

Weaning

- Advise parents to introduce 'solids' at any time from 4–6mo. of age. The baby is ready when he is always hungry, even soon after a feed.
- It is not essential to use ready-made baby meals—often babies like home prepared purées better, and they are cheaper.
- If making purées, advise parents not to add salt or excess sugar.
- Sterilize feeding bowls and cutlery before use until the baby is >6mo. old.
- Start with 1 flavour of finely puréed food e.g. baby rice. It is usual for most of the food to ooze out of the baby's mouth.
- Babies often only take 2–3 teaspoonfuls per meal when they start taking solids.
- It is usual for the baby's stool to change consistency when weaned.
- Add different foods 1 by 1. Avoid eggs and gluten until >6mo. of age.
- Introduce lumpy foods gradually after 6mo. and 'finger foods' the baby can feed itself (e.g. pieces of toast, rusks, biscuits) at 7–9mo.
- Continue giving the baby at least 600ml of milk/d.

Worries about the amount a child is eating: Common worry of most parents. Check the child is gaining weight along his centile line. If so, reassure the parents—often unrealistic expectations of the amount a baby or toddler can eat *or* between meal snacks are the real problem. If not gaining weight along centile line—📖 p.884.

Feeding problems: 📖 p.890. If in doubt, consult the health visitor.

Information and support

Lewis (2003) Practical parenting: weaning and first foods—which foods to introduce and when Hamlyn. ISBN: 0600605647
Parentline ☎0808 800 2222 🖳 http://www.parentlineplus.org.uk

Congenital abnormalities (1)

Major congenital abnormality occurs in ~1:50 babies. Many more have minor abnormalities.

Neural tube defects: Most neural tube defects are detected antenatally by α-fetoprotein screening and routine antenatal USS. Folic acid in the first 12wk. of pregnancy ↓ incidence. Types of defect:

Anencepaly: Absent cerebral cortex and skull vault. Incompatible with life—those infants born alive die within hours of birth.

Cranium defects: Vary in severity from meningocoele (meninges protrude through the defect) to inoperable encephalocoele (brain tissue protrudes through skull).

Spina bifida: The vertebral arch is incomplete.
- *Occulta lesions* are covered with skin and fascia. They are common and usually asymptomatic, though may be associated with mild gait or bladder problems.
- *Cystica lesions* involve herniation of the meninges (meningocoele). They are uncommon but treatable, usually with minor residual defect.
- *Whole cord herniation* (myelomeningocoele) is more common and often results in neurological deficit. It is associated with hydrocephalus, learning and psychological problems.

Primary care management
- Support the child and family
- Ensure receipt of all available benefits
- Liaise with the primary healthcare team and community and specialist services to ensure prompt provision of equipment and services
- Inform carers about local facilities, voluntary organizations, and self-help groups
- Make referrals for new problems promptly
- Liaise with specialist services to provide on-going care
- If the child's mother is planning another pregnancy, advise her to take 5mg folic acid od whilst planning pregnancy and until 13wk. gestation.

Information and support
Association for Spina Bifida and Hydrocephalus (ASBAH)
☎01733 555 988 🖳 http://www.asbah.org.uk

Congenital ENT problems
Branchial and thyroglossal cysts: 📖 p.274

Accessory auricle: *Incidence:* 1.5:100 live births. Small skin lesions consisting of skin or skin + cartilage are present in front of the ear. No treatment is necessary but accessory auricles are often removed for cosmetic reasons.

Bat ears: Common congenital abnormality in which a fold of the pinna is absent. The child is noted to have protruding ears. Runs in families. Referral for surgery is indicated if the condition is causing psychosocial problems.

Congenital deafness: *Causes:*

- Genetic (50%)
- Intrauterine infection e.g. rubella
- Drugs given to the mother in pregnancy e.g. streptomycin
- Birth asphyxia
- Meningitis
- Severe neonatal jaundice

Presentation:

- Neonatal screening will be available for all babies in the UK by 2005/6—📖 p.827.
- Otherwise, diagnosis is made when a parent notices abnormal responses from the child, during routine child health surveillance, or when speech fails to develop.

Management: 📖 p.924

Cleft lip and palate: *Incidence:* 1:600 live births—½ have other abnormalities too (e.g. hypoplastic mandible). Often (though not always) detected at routine antenatal USS. The cleft may be unilateral or bilateral and involve lip and/or palate. Cleft lips are usually repaired in the 1st few days of life; cleft palates at ~3mo., depending on the weight of the baby.

Problems associated with cleft lip and/or palate

- Feeding difficulties with associated poor weight gain
- Aspiration pneumonia
- Hearing problems—particularly glue ear. In some areas children with cleft palate are routinely given grommets at ~18mo. Treat otitis media promptly. Audiology review is important.
- Speech problems—refer for speech therapy.
- Dental problems—universal with cleft palate. Orthodontic treatment is always required.

Information and support

Cleft Lip and Palate Association (CLAPA) ☎020 7833 4883 🖥 http://www.clapa.com

Congenital eye problems

Blocked lacrimal duct: Common—20% babies(📖 p.939).

Congenital cataract: Maybe hereditary or associated with Down's syndrome, galactosaemia, or congenital rubella. Detect by absence of (or dark area in) the red reflex at routine screening checks. In all cases, refer to ophthalmology.

Congenital glaucoma: Usually bilateral. The eyeball becomes enlarged and the pupil large and fixed. Requires early surgical treatment to prevent blindness. Refer urgently to ophthalmology.

Microphthalmios: 1:1000 live births. Small eyes. Associated with Down's syndrome and other genetic abnormalities

Congenital gynaecological abnormalities: 📖 p.708

Congenital orthopaedic abnormalities: 📖 p.868

Congenital abnormalities (2)

Congenital urological abnormalities

Horseshoe kidney, ectopic kidney, double ureter: Common malformations. Usually do not affect kidney function per se but predispose to UTI. Recurrent infections may eventually cause renal damage.

Posterior urethral valves: Folds of mucosa inhibit or block passage of urine causing urethral, bladder, ureter, and renal pelvis dilatation.

Presentation
- Usually detected on antenatal USS.
- Can present in neonates with urinary retention or dribbling urine + distended bladder, UTI, or uraemia.
- Can present later in childhood with recurrent UTI or incontinence.

Investigation and management: MCUG confirms diagnosis. In all cases, refer to urology for surgical disruption of the valves.

Hypospadias: 1:400 male births. The urethral meatus opens on the ventral side of the penis. There is often hooding of the foreskin and ventral flexion of the penis. Refer to urology. Treated with corrective surgery, ideally pre-school.

Undescended testis: Observed in 2–3% of male neonates but most descend during the 1st year. Refer those that don't for surgical descent and fixation to avoid later infertility and ↑ risk of malignancy.

Congenital hydrocoele: Unilateral or bilateral, smooth scrotal swelling which transilluminates. Most congenital hydrocoeles resolve spontaneously in the 1st year of life. Refer to urology if persists >1y.

Congenital gastrointestinal abnormalities

Umbilical hernia: Common. Due to a defect in the umbilical ring when the cord separates. More common in people of black ethnic origin and associated with certain syndromes (e.g. Trisomy 13 and 18). Usually resolves spontaneously. Strangulation is rare. Refer for surgery if an umbilical hernia persists until >2y. of age.

Inguinal hernia

- *Non-acute:* History of intermittent groin ± scrotal swelling—the spermatic cord may be thickened on the affected side. Refer to paediatric surgery for repair (herniotomy).
- *Acute:* Sudden appearance of an irreducible groin or scrotal swelling—necessitates emergency admission for reduction and repair.

Diaphragmatic hernia: *Incidence:* 1:2500 live births. A defect in one hemidiaphragm allows the bowel to herniate into the chest cavity → pulmonary hypoplasia in utero or lung compression postnatally. Detected antenatally on USS or postnatally when the child develops respiratory distress soon after birth. CXR confirms diagnosis. Corrective surgery is associated with high mortality but once successfully repaired, the child usually has no further difficulties.

Exomphalos and gastroschisis

- *Exomphalos:* Complete return of the gut into the abdominal cavity fails to occur during intrauterine life. At birth there is a swelling at the umbilicus consisting of gut covered by a membrane.
- *Gastroschisis:* There is a defect in the abdominal wall through which exposed gut prolapses.

Exomphalos and gastroschisis are usually detected antenatally at routine USS. Delivery then takes place at a specialist centre where surgical repair can be undertaken soon after birth. Once repaired, prognosis is good.

Oesophageal atresia and/or tracheo-oesophageal fistula

1:2500 live births. 5% have oesophageal atresia alone; 5% tracheo-oesophageal fistula (TOF) alone; the remainder have both. Risk factors for sudden infant death syndrome.

Presentation

- *Antenatal:* At routine USS or following investigation of polyhydramnios.
- *Postnatal:* Cough or breathing difficulties in a newborn infant; choking on the first feed; inability to swallow saliva → bubbling of fluid from the mouth developing soon after birth.
- *Later in childhood:* 'H type' fistulas where there is no atresia but just a fistula may present late with recurrent chest infections.

Management: Diagnosis is confirmed with X-ray. Treatment is surgical. Post-operatively, children may have a barking cough (*'TOF cough'*) and/or dysphagia—both settle before 2y.

Duodenal atresia: Usually associated with other abnormalities, particularly Down's syndrome. If not detected on antenatal USS, presents postnatally with bile-stained vomiting. AXR reveals a 'double bubble' with air in stomach and first part of duodenum, but none beyond. Requires surgical correction.

Anorectal atresia (imperforate anus): 1:4000 live births. Usually the baby fails to pass meconium and no anus is visible. There is often a fistula to the urethra (boys) or vagina (girls). Treatment is surgical. In the period after surgery, anal dilation is vital to prevent stricture, and starts 2wk. post-op. It requires use of graded dilators by the baby's parents for several months. Faecal incontinence may be a problem but can usually be managed using a combination of dietary manipulation, enemas, and drug treatment.

Hirschprung's disease: Caused by absence of the ganglion cells of the myenteric plexus in the distal bowel.

Presentation: Presents with delay in passing meconium, abdominal distension, vomiting, and poor feeding in a neonate. If only a short segment is affected, presentation may be much later with chronic constipation. Diagnosis is confirmed with rectal biopsy.

Management: Refer to paediatric surgery. Treatment is surgical removal of the affected area of bowel.
(*H. Hirschprung (1830–1916)—Danish paediatrician*)

Congenital heart disease

Common, affecting ~6:1000 live births—Table 23.3. Neonatal examination only detects 44% of cardiac malformations found in the 1st year. Conversely, only 54% of murmurs heard at neonatal examination are due to underlying cardiac malformation.

Presentation
Murmur on routine examination

- **Ventriculoseptal defect (VSD):** Harsh pansystolic murmur with splitting of the 2nd heart sound.
- **Atrioseptal defect (ASD):** Systolic murmur in the pulmonary area with fixed splitting of the 2nd heart sound. May also present with heart failure or arrhythmia in a young adult.
- **Patent ductus arteriosus (PDA):** Loud, continuous 'machinery' murmur.
- **Aortic stenosis:** Ejection systolic murmur at the apex and left sternal edge with a soft and delayed 2nd heart sound Slow rising pulse, ↓BP. Rarely dizziness, faintness, or loss of consciousness on exertion.
- **Pulmonary stenosis:** Ejection systolic murmur with ejection click.
- **Coarctation of the aorta:** Ejection systolic murmur over the left side and back; absent/delayed femoral pulses and upper limb hypertension.

Innocent murmurs: Murmurs are a common finding in childhood, particularly when examining a febrile child. The majority are not associated with heart disease—so called 'innocent murmurs'. *Features:*
- Asymptomatic
- Soft, systolic murmur—may vary with position and does not radiate
- Normal 2nd heart sound
- No other associated signs of heart disease (normal pulses, no thrill)

Once a murmur has been assessed as being innocent, explain what that means to the parents—otherwise there may be unnecessary ongoing anxiety.

⚠ Unless the child is febrile when the murmur is heard and it disappears once afebrile, refer all children with murmurs for Echo or paediatric evaluation—whether the murmur is detected at routine screening, incidentally when examining the chest for another reason, or when examined because symptomatic.

Heart failure

- Breathlessness, particularly when crying/feeding
- Failure to thrive
- Sweating
- Fast respiratory and pulse rates
- Heart enlargement
- Liver enlargement
- Weight ↑ due to fluid retention

Causes of heart failure in the 1st week of life include:
- Left outflow obstruction
- Severe aortic stenosis
- Coarctation of the aorta
- Hypoplastic left heart

Later causes
- Large VSD
- PDA
- Ostium primum ASD

Table 23.3 Congenital cardiac abnormalities

Condition	Features
ASD	📖 p.356
Coarctation of the aorta	📖 p.356
Fallot tetralogy	Large VSD and pulmonary stenosis.
	In the newborn period, may present with a murmur.
	Progressive cyanosis then develops over the next weeks/years ± ↓ exercise tolerance ± squatting after exercise.
	Treatment is surgical.
Hypoplastic left heart	Left ventricle ± mitral valve, aortic valve, and aortic arch are underdeveloped.
	Presents within the 1st few days of life with heart failure.
	Treatment is surgical.
Patent ductus arteriosus (PDA)	The ductus arteriosus fails to close after birth.
	♀>♂. Associated with prematurity.
	Symptoms depend on the size of the shunt. Presents with murmur ± failure to thrive ± heart failure.
	Treatment is usually surgical closure.
Transposition of the great arteries	The aorta arises from the right ventricle and the pulmonary artery from the left.
	Progressive cyanosis develops within a few hours of birth.
	Treatment is surgical.
Valve disease	📖 p.354
VSD	📖 p.356

Cyanosis
- **<48h. old:** Likely to be due to transposition of the great arteries or severe pulmonary stenosis.
- **Later presentation:** Mostly due to *tetralogy of fallot* (Table 23.3).

Management: In all cases, if new congenital heart disease is detected, refer for specialist paediatric and/or cardiology opinion. Specialist treatment of valve lesions depends on the gradient measured across the valve. Most other congenital cardiac lesions (except VSD and ASD) require surgery—staged for complex lesions.

Prevention of endocarditis: An episode of endocarditis may be the presenting feature of congenital heart disease. There is ↑ risk of developing endocarditis in patients with valve lesions, septal defects (which persists after repair), PDA, and particularly in those with prosthetic valves. All these patients require antibiotic prophylaxis for dental and surgical procedures—📖 p.349.

Information and support
Children's Heart Federation ☎0808 808 5000 🖥 http://www.childrens-heart-fed.org.uk
Personal experiences of parents of children with congenital heart disease 🖥 http://www.dipex.org

Genetic problems (1)

There are 46 chromosomes—22 are matching pairs with matching genes (autosomes); the remaining pair are sex chromosomes which may match (XX—♀) or differ (XY—♂).

General principles: Refer parents of any child affected by a genetic problem for genetic counselling and offer prenatal diagnosis, if available, for any subsequent pregnancies.

Management: Depends on specific problems of each child. Involve the primary healthcare team, specialist healthcare services, social services, community paediatric services, education services, and voluntary organizations, as necessary. Review regularly.

Alteration in number of chromosomes

Down's syndrome: Trisomy 21 (an extra chromosome number 21). Most common chromosomal abnormality affecting 1:600 births. Life expectancy is ↓ but ~½ live to 60y. Incidence ↑ with maternal age at conception but, as most babies are born to mothers <40y. old, the majority are born to younger women. 3 mechanisms:

- *Non-dysjunction:* >90%—when the dividing cell splits, a pair of chromosome 21 goes to 1 cell and none to the other.
- *Translocation:* 6%—chromosome rearrangement (see p.00).
- *Mosaicism:* 2%—some cells have 46 chromosomes, others have 47—the extra being an additional chromosome 21. Due to mitotic non-dysjunction after formation of the zygote.

Clinical features

- Facial abnormalities: flat occiput, oval face (mongoloid facies), low-set eyes with prominent epicanthic folds
- Single palmar crease
- Hypotonia
- Developmental delay
- Congenital heart disease

(J.H.L. Down (1828–96)—English physician)

Edward's syndrome: Trisomy 18. Life expectancy is ~10mo. (♀ > ♂).

Clinical features

- Facial abnormalities: low-set malformed ears, receding chin, protruding eyes, cleft lip or palate
- A short sternum makes the nipples appear too widely separated
- Fingers cannot be extended and the index finger overlaps the 3rd digit
- Developmental delay
- Umbilical or inguinal hernias
- Rocker-bottom feet
- Rigid baby with flexion of the limbs

(J.H. Edwards (b. 1928)—English physician and medical geneticist)

Patau's syndrome: Trisomy 13. 1:7500 births. 50% die in <1mo. Usually fatal in the first year. Multiple abnormalities including:

- Small head and eyes
- Brain malformation
- Heart malformations
- Polycystic kidneys
- Cleft lip/palate
- Skeletal abnormalities e.g. flexion contractures of hands ± polydactyly with narrow fingernails.

(K. Patau (1908–1975)—German-American geneticist)

Structural changes of chromosomes

Translocation: A portion of 1 chromosome is transposed or translocated onto another. If no genetic information is lost, there is no clinical effect (balanced translocation), though offspring of affected individuals often have problems. If an affected infant has a parent with a balanced translocation, the risk of recurrence for subsequent siblings is high. 6% of Down's syndrome is due to translocation.

Deletion: Loss of a portion of a chromosome.

'Cri du chat' syndrome—deletion of the short arm of chromosome 5 is the most common deletion syndrome. Presents with:
- Abnormal cry (cat-like)
- Microcephaly
- Developmental delay
- Marked epicanthic folds
- Moon-shaped face
- Alert expression

Sex chromosome abnormalities

Turner's syndrome: XO—deletion of 1 X chromosome. 1:2500 live births. Mosaicism may occur (XO, XX). Lifespan is normal.

Clinical features
- Female appearance
- Short stature (<130cm)
- Hyperconvex nails
- Wide carrying angle (cubitus valgus)
- Inverted nipples
- Broad chest
- Ptosis
- Nystagmus
- Webbed neck
- Coarctation of the aorta
- Left heart defects
- Lymphoedema of the legs
- Ovaries are rudimentary or absent

Specialist management: Human growth hormone may be considered for short stature.
(H.H. Turner (1892–1970)—US endocrinologist)

Klinefelter's syndrome: XXY or XXYY polysomy—1:1000 live births. Life span is normal.

Clinical features
- Male appearance
- Often undetected until presentation with infertility in adult life
- May present at adolescence with psychopathy, ↓ libido, sparse facial hair, gynaecomastia, and small firm testes

Associations: Hypothyroidism, DM, asthma.

Specialist management: Androgens and plastic surgery may be useful for gynaecomastia.
(H.F. Klinefelter (1912–1990)—US physician)

Advice and support

Genetics Interests Group ☎020 7704 3141 🖥 http://www.gig.org.uk
Down's Syndrome Association ☎0845 230 0372
🖥 http://www.downs-syndrome.org.uk
Turner's Syndrome Support Society ☎01389 380 385
🖥 http://www.tss.org.uk

Genetic problems (2)

Single gene inheritance

Autosomal dominant inheritance: >1000 diseases are known to be inherited in this way. Individually, they are rare, and together account for <1% of all disease. Heterozygotes demonstrate the disease. 1:2 pregnancies of an affected individual will be affected—usually ♂ = ♀. Expression of the gene in a given individual may vary.

Examples: Marfan syndrome (🕮 p.357), myotonic dystrophy (🕮 p.622), neurofibromatosis (🕮 p.624).

Autosomal recessive inheritance: >700 known diseases. Only manifest in the homozygote. Heterozygotes may be asymptomatic or show milder abnormalities. To develop severe disease, the affected gene must be inherited from both parents who must both be heterozygotes. The risk of an affected pregnancy is 1:4—usually ♂ = ♀. Affected individuals have unaffected children unless their partner is a heterozygote.

Glycogen storage diseases: Incidence: ~1:25,000. A group of hereditary disorders caused by lack of ≥1 enzyme involved in glycogen synthesis or breakdown and characterized by deposition of abnormal amounts or types of glycogen in tissues. Inheritance is autosomal recessive for all forms except type VI, which follows an X-linked inheritance. Symptoms and age of onset vary considerably:

- Predominantly liver involvement (types I, III, IV, VI) → hepatomegaly, hypoglycaemia, metabolic acidosis
- Predominantly muscle involvement (types V, VII) → weakness, lethargy, poor feeding, heart failure

Treatment involves frequent small carbohydrate meals; allopurinol (to prevent renal urate stone formation and/or gout) ± limiting anaerobic exercise. A high-protein diet is also helpful for some patients.

Phenylketonuria (PKU): Autosomal recessive trait. *Incidence:* 1:16,000. The enzyme (phenylalanine hydroxylase) needed for excretion of excess phenylalanine is missing. Phenylalanine accumulates in the blood and is excreted unchanged in urine. *Presentation:*

- The baby appears normal at birth but develops severe developmental delay, learning difficulty, and seizures in infancy.
- Prenatal diagnosis is possible if there is a FH.
- In the UK, routine postnatal screening with the Guthrie test (heel prick test) is performed to detect PKU before any permanent damage is done.

Treatment aims to limit the child's phenylalanine intake to prevent accumulation of excess phenylalanine. With treatment, growth and development are normal. Dietary restriction used to be discontinued in adulthood but evidence suggests this may result in a drop in IQ. Dietary restriction should continue lifelong and particularly during pregnancy.

Other examples: Sickle cell disease (🕮 p.526), thalassaemia (🕮 p.526), cystic fibrosis (🕮 p.394).

Sex-linked disorders: ~100 are recognized. Most are recessively inherited from the mother and affect only ♂ offspring.

- A male child of a heterozygote mother has a 1:2 chance of developing the disease.
- A female child of a heterozygote mother has a 1:2 chance of carrying the disease.
- A female child can only be affected by the disease if the father has the disease and mother is a carrier when she has a 1:2 chance of being affected and, if not affected, will be a carrier.

Fragile X syndrome: Affects 1:1250 ♂ births and 1:2500 ♀ births. Genetic abnormality carried on the X chromosome comprising:

- Low IQ (20–70)
- Large testes
- High forehead
- Large jaw
- Facial asymmetry
- Long ears
- Short temper

½ of carrier females have a normal IQ; ½ are affected. Consider fragile X syndrome in any child with developmental delay of unknown cause.

Management: There is some evidence that folic acid supplements ↓ hyperactive and disruptive behaviour tendencies in children with fragile X. Antenatal testing is possible for future pregnancies.

Other examples: Haemophilia (📖 p.528), red-green colour blindness (📖 p.945), Duchenne's muscular dystrophy (📖 p.622).

Polygenic inheritance: Familial trends of disease are commonly seen but there is often no simple inheritance pattern. Usually due to the combination of genes inherited (polygenic inheritance). This field is developing rapidly. Take care with genetic testing as it may unfavourably affect insurance premiums, ability to get a mortgage, etc.

Examples: Neural tube defects, cleft palate, atopy, ischaemic and congenital heart disease, CDH, club foot, type 1 DM, pyloric stenosis, schizophrenia.

Advice and support
Genetics Interests Group ☎020 7704 3141 🖳 http://www.gig.org.uk
Association for Glycogen Storage Disease (UK) 🖳 http://www.agsd.org.uk
National Society for Phenylketonuria (NSPKU) ☎0845 603 9136
🖳 http://www.nspku.org
Sickle Cell Society ☎020 8961 1795 🖳 http://www.sicklecellsociety.org
UK Thalassaemia Society ☎0800 73 111 09 🖳 http://www.ukts.org
Cystic Fibrosis Trust 🖳 http://www.cftrust.org.uk
Fragile X Society ☎01371 875 100 🖳 http://www.fragilex.org.uk
Haemophilia Society ☎0800 018 6068 🖳 http://www.haemophilia.org.uk
Muscular Dystrophy Campaign 🖳 http://www.muscular-dystrophy.org

The sick infant

Infants aged <6mo. can be difficult to assess and may deteriorate rapidly over a short period of time. Physical signs are often absent or deceptive.

General rules

- Always arrange for a sick baby who has not responded to simple measures (e.g. paracetamol and fluids) to be reviewed by a doctor.
- Always trust the mother's instinct.
- Always perform a *full* physical examination. Localizing signs might be absent (e.g. tonsillitis is a frequent cause of vomiting). Petechial rash under the nappy area can be easily missed.
- Remember UTI as a cause of infection.
- If any significant symptoms or signs are present (below), consider acute referral to a paediatrician for further assessment.
- The younger the baby, the lower the threshold for seeking a paediatrician's opinion.

If you are still unsure: Often, despite full assessment, you are left unsure about the nature and severity of a child's disease. If there are no significant symptoms or signs but you are still worried, consider:

- Advising the parents to call you if there is any deterioration or if the child fails to improve within a defined period of time. This is only an option if the parents are able to cope and can be relied upon to call.
- Arranging a review of the child within a few hours of assessment.
- Admitting the child to the paediatricians for observation.

⚠ Significant symptoms

↓ feeding—< ½ usual intake within previous 24h.. With the exception of dehydration, an infant who is feeding well is unlikely to have a serious acute illness.

Persistent vomiting—especially if >½ of the previous 3 feeds has been vomited.

Bile-stained vomiting.

Rapid breathing—particularly if noisy and of sudden onset.

< 4 wet nappies in the previous 24h..

Inappropriate drowsiness or irritability.

Frank blood in the stools.

Persistent unusual cry.

History suggestive of apnoeic episodes.

⚠ Significant signs

↓ muscle tone.

Dehydration—late signs are tachycardia, dry mouth, ↓ skin turgor, sunken fontanelle.

↓ capillary return.

↓ response to stimuli.

Rectal temperature >38.5°C.

Tachypnoea, marked rib recession, or grunting.

Bulging fontanelle—always admit urgently.

Paediatric infection

Table 23.4 A-Z of childhood infection

Infection	Page	Infection	Page
Chicken pox	📖 p.494	Meningitis	📖 p.1044
Conjunctivitis	📖 p.936	Mumps	📖 p.492
Diptheria	📖 p.485	Otitis media	📖 p.922
Epiglottitis	📖 p.917	Pneumonia	📖 p.851
Erythema infectiosum	📖 p.491	Polio	📖 p.493
Gastroenteritis	📖 p.452	Roseola infantum	📖 p.491
Glandular fever	📖 p.915	Rubella	📖 p.492
Hand, foot, and mouth	📖 p.491	Scabies	📖 p.674
Head lice	📖 p.675	Scarlet fever	📖 p.483
Hepatitis A/B	📖 p.496	Sinusitis	📖 p.919
Herpes	📖 p.495	Skin infection	📖 p.668
HIV	📖 p.498	TB	📖 p.488
Impetigo	📖 p.668	Threadworms	📖 p.503
Influenza	📖 p.490	Tonsillitis	📖 p.914
Kawasaki's disease	📖 p.854	URTI	📖 p.850
Malaria	📖 p.508	UTI in childhood	📖 p.852
Measles	📖 p.492	Whooping cough	📖 p.486

In utero infection
- Maternal infection with rubella, CMV, toxoplasmosis, syphilis, and varicella zoster can → congenital malformation (📖 p.790–1).
- Maternal infection with malaria can → poor foetal growth and IUGR.
- Maternal HIV infection: 📖 p.498.

Infections acquired during passage through the birth canal
- Maternal genital herpes can be transferred to the infant during vaginal delivery—📖 p.744 and p.788.
- Maternal gonorrhoea infection may → ophthalmia neonatorum (📖 p.936).
- The presence of β-haemolytic streptococci in the vagina may → neonatal septicaemia or meningitis (📖 p.788).
- HIV (📖 p.498) and hepatitis B infection (📖 p.496) can also be transmitted during birth. Prophylactic treatment is available.

Childhood infections: Very common. Peaks in incidence occur when children start nursery, start and change schools. Due to routine vaccination most of the traditional childhood diseases (with the exception of chicken pox) have been virtually eliminated.

Specific infections: Table 23.4

Viral URTI: Extremely common. Children have >5 URTIs each year. Presents with coryza, runny eyes, and malaise. The child may also have a mild pyrexia and/or a non-specific maculopapular rash.

Management
- Examine to exclude tonsillitis and otitis media.
- If pyrexia but no other symptoms/signs, check urine to exclude UTI.
- Most viral URTIs settle within a few days with paracetamol suspension and fluids.
- Treat complications e.g. tonsillitis, otitis media, or conjunctivitis as necessary.

Bronchiolitis: Occurs in epidemics—usually in the winter months. Due to respiratory syncitial virus (RSV) infection. Usually infects infants <1y. old and presents with coryzal symptoms progressing to irritable cough, rapid breathing ± feeding difficulty.

Examination: Tachypnoea, tachycardia, widespread crepitations over the lung fields ± high pitched wheeze.

Management: Depends on severity of the symptoms.
- *If mild*—paracetamol suspension as required and fluids.
- *If more severe* i.e. if the child or parent is distressed, the child is unable to feed, the child is dehydrated, and/or there is intercostal recession or cyanosis—admit as a paediatric emergency for oxygen ± tube feeding. Rarely ventilation is required.

Croup
- Viral infection occurring in epidemics in autumn and spring.
- Starts with mild fever and runny nose.
- In younger children (<4y.), oedema and secretions in the larynx and trachea → a barking cough and inspiratory stridor.
- The cough typically starts at night and is exacerbated by crying and parental anxiety.
- Some children have recurrent attacks associated with viral URTI.

Management: Steam helps. There is also evidence that nebulized steroids can be helpful[R] but most GPs don't carry them. Admit as a paediatric emergency if there is intercostal recession, cyanosis, or unable to cope.

Acute bronchitis: Occurs when an URTI spreads down the airways. Presents with coughing ± purulent sputum. Chest examination is normal unless asthma is precipitated by the infection. *Management:* advise parents to treat the child with OTC cough linctus, paracetamol, and fluids. Cough may persist for several weeks.

Pneumonia: May be viral, bacterial (pneumococcal, HIB, or staphylococcal) or atypical (e.g. mycoplasma). Presents with fever, malaise, anorexia, cough ± purulent sputum, abdominal pain. *Examination:* localized crepitations ± collapse.

Management: Treat with a broad spectrum antibiotic (e.g. amoxicillin). If dehydrated, distressed, or not responding to simple antibiotics, admit for paediatric assessment.

Urinary tract infection in childhood

8% girls and 2% boys have a urinary tract infection (UTI) in childhood—the majority in the 1st year of life. Amongst neonates, boys have more infections than girls. In all other age groups ♀:♂ ≈ 10:1.

Consequences of UTI in childhood

- 5–15% of children with UTI develop renal scarring within 1–2 y. of the 1st infection.
- There is a higher incidence in children with renal tract abnormalities and vesicoureteric reflux.
- Infections causing renal scarring are associated with adult pyelonephritis, ↑BP, impaired renal function, and renal failure.
- Prognosis is worst for children with recurrent infection, severe reflux, and scarring at 1st presentation.

Causative organisms: Most childhood UTIs are caused by normal bowel flora—*E. coli* (80%), Klebsiella, Pseudomonas, and other gram-negative organisms.

Clinical features of UTI in children

- *Infants and toddlers:* Usually non-specific including vomiting, irritability, fever, abdominal pain, failure to thrive, and prolonged jaundice.
- *Older children:* Dysuria, urinary frequency, abdominal pain, haematuria, enuresis.

Investigation: Suspect diagnosis and check urine in any child with urinary symptoms or any infant with fever >38.5°C with no definite cause. Send urine for M,C & S.

❶ Collecting bag specimens

- Urine collection can be problematical in a young child. A clean catch is best but a bag may be necessary.
- When collecting a bag specimen, the child should be upright and the bag removed as soon as it has been filled to minimize contamination.
- Special pads are also available and are preferred by parents.
- It is important to indicate what method of collection was used for proper interpretation of results.
- Any +ve culture obtained via a bag or pad specimen should be checked with a urine sample taken by clean catch, suprapubic aspirate or catheter specimen (rarely needed).

Management

- The aim of management is to treat infection and prevent long-term complications.
- Treat symptomatic infection without waiting for the result of the urine specimen with trimethoprim for 7–10d.—altering the antibiotic should the responsible organism prove resistant on culture.
- If UTI is confirmed, arrange post-treatment urine sample collection to confirm clearance.
- Prophylactic antibiotics (usually trimethoprim od) should be started after the first infection and continued at least until results of imaging are known.

- Prophylactic antibiotics may be required long term if there is reflux or an underlying abnormality to prevent (further) renal scarring.

Follow-up: Local policies vary—consult local guidelines. Refer all children to a paediatrician after the 1st proven UTI (arrange USS in the meantime if possible). Further imaging will depend on the age of the child and local protocols: infants <1y. generally will need a micturating cystourethrogram (MCUG) to assess for reflux; older children may require IVP or DMSA scans.

Kawasaki's disease

Kawasaki's disease was first reported by Tomisaku Kawasaki, a Japanese paediatrician, in 1967. He observed and described a systemic vasculitic illness predominantly affecting children <5y.

Kawasaki's disease is the most common cause of acquired heart disease in children in developed countries. Epidemiology suggests an infectious aetiology but cause is, as yet, unknown. *Incidence in the UK:* 3.4/100,000 children aged <5y.

Diagnostic criteria for Kawasaki's disease

Presence of ≥5 of the following

- Fever for ≥5d.
- Bilateral (non-purulent) conjunctivitis
- Polymorphous rash
- Changes in lips and mouth:
  - Reddened, dry, or cracked lips
  - Strawberry tongue
  - Diffuse redness of oral or pharyngeal mucosa
- Changes in extremities:
  - Reddening of palms or soles
  - Indurative oedema of hands or feet
  - Desquamation of skin of hands, feet, and groin (in convalescence)
- Cervical lymphadenopathy: >15mm diameter. Usually unilateral, single, non-purulent, and painful

Exclusion of diseases with similar presentation

- Staphylococcal infection (such as scalded skin syndrome, toxic shock syndrome)
- Streptococcal infection (e.g. scarlet fever, toxic shock-like syndrome)
- Rickettsial disease
- Leptospirosis
- Stevens-Johnson syndrome
- Drug reaction
- Measles and other viral exanthems
- Juvenile rheumatoid arthritis

❶ Throat carriage of group A streptococcus does not exclude Kawasaki's disease

Diagnosis

- There is no diagnostic test and many cases are missed.
- Diagnosis is based on clinical criteria—see above.
- Difficulty arises due to the similarity of features of Kawasaki's disease with those of many other childhood infections and the possibility of atypical presentation of Kawasaki's disease.
- Remain alert to the possibility of the diagnosis in any child—particularly if very miserable or with fever for >5d. Poor response to antipyretics heightens suspicion.

Less characteristic features

- Rhinorrhoea
- Cough
- Abdominal pain
- Vomiting
- Diarrhoea
- Pain/swelling of joints
- CNS involvement
- Jaundice
- Sterile pyuria

Complications

- Coronary arteritis with formation of aneurysms (20–30% untreated patients).
- In the acute phase these may cause thrombosis within an aneurysm, MI, or dysrhythmias and even death.
- Long-term morbidity results from scarring of coronary arteries, intimal thickening, and accelerated atherosclerosis.

Management: If suspected, refer for urgent paediatric assessment. Early treatment (<10d. after onset) with iv immunoglobulin and aspirin ↓ incidence and severity of aneurysm formation as well as giving symptom relief. The role of treatment after this time is unclear though iv immunoglobulin is often given >10d. after onset of symptoms if there is evidence of ongoing inflammation.

Support for parents

Kawasaki's Support Group ☎024 7661 2178

Common childhood gastrointestinal complaints

Constipation: Frequent complaint amongst all age groups of children. Differentiate between normal stools a few days apart (which needs no treatment) and infrequent hard stools which suggest constipation.

Infants
- Babies show considerable variation in bowel habit according to their diet (and their mothers' diets if breastfed).
- Babies may change colour alarmingly when opening their bowels and look as if they are straining hard—even to pass a liquid stool.
- Change from breastfeeding to artificial feeds and/or solids can result in a change in stool colour and consistency—with the stool usually becoming harder and more formed.
- Genuine constipation may occur as a result of hunger, poor hydration, or use of overstrength feeds.
- Constipation which causes pain on defaecation results in withholding of stool to avoid pain. This is a vicious cycle which can be hard to break.
- Rare causes include: congenital abnormalities (e.g. spinal cord lesions), imperforate anus (after surgical repair); Hirschsprung's disease; hypothyroidism; cerebral palsy.

Older children
- Acute constipation often accompanies acute febrile illness.
- Once a hard stool causes an anal tear, a cycle of chronic constipation and faecal retention may be started—pain on defaecation results in withholding of stool to avoid pain.
- Symptoms include abdominal pain, anorexia, vomiting, failure to thrive, and a predisposition to UTIs.
- Eventually the child can no longer cope with the mass of faeces and soft stool leaks out around the hard faecal mass causing constant faecal soiling.

Management
- Ensure adequate fluid intake and a high roughage diet.
- Treatment involves regular senna liquid ± a softener (e.g. lactulose) to dislodge the faecal mass and reinstate a regular bowel pattern. The use of laxatives can make faecal soiling worse initially.
- If not controlled with simple laxatives and diet, refer for paediatric assessment.

Rectal bleeding in children: Common. The usual causes are:
- Constipation
- Anal fissure
- Threadworms
- Rectal prolapse
- Meckel's diverticulum

Only refer if profuse or if simple treatment for constipation fails.

Vomiting and/or diarrhoea: Determine:
- Nature and duration of symptoms
- Whether there is blood or mucus in the stool
- Other accompanying symptoms
- Contact with anyone else with similar symptoms
- History of recent foreign travel

Differential diagnosis
- *Physiological*
  - Breastfed babies have loose, often explosive 'mustard grain' stools
  - Babies may posset part of each feed—📖 p.831
  - Toddlers often have intermittent loose stools related to diet
- *Gastrointestinal infection:* The child may have diarrhoea, vomiting, or a combination of the 2. Usually viral in origin—especially rota virus in pre-school children. Consider the possibility of temporary cows' milk intolerance if continuing >2wk.—📖 p.452.
- *Infection elsewhere* e.g. otitis media, UTI, tonsillitis, septicaemia
- *Acute intra-abdominal disease*
  - Intussusception—📖 p.858
  - Appendicitis—📖 p.464
  - Acute obstruction—📖 p.466
  - Pyloric stenosis (vomiting only)—📖 p.858
- *Constipation:* Usually overflow of soft stool with soiling ± vomiting
- *Malabsorption* e.g.coeliac disease (usually only diarrhoea)—📖 p.454
- *Gastro-oesophageal reflux* (usually only vomiting)—📖 p.831
- *Vomiting due to ↑ ICP:* 📖 p.602
- *Ketoacidosis:* 📖 p.1070
- *Anorexia or bulimia:* 📖 p.982
- *Travel/motion sickness*

Examination
- Assess level of hydration: sunken eyes, dry tongue, sunken fontanelle, and ↓ skin turgor are all late signs.
- Look for sources of infection e.g. ENT and chest infection; UTI.
- Examine the abdomen for masses, distention, tenderness, and bowel sounds.

Management
- *Send a stool sample* for M,C&S if diarrhoea + fever, blood in stool, recent return from tropical climate, immunocompromised patient, or lasting >7d.
- *Treat with rehydration:* Encourage clear fluid intake ± rehydration salts. Never give children antidiarrhoeal agents.
- *Food:* Stick to a bland diet avoiding dairy products until diarrhoea has settled. Babies who are breastfed or have not been weaned should continue their normal milk. Some advocate using half-strength milk, though the benefits of this have not been demonstrated.
- *If dehydrated and unable to replace fluids* e.g. concomitant vomiting, child refusing to drink: admit.
- *If no cause found and lasts >3wk. or any atypical features:* Refer for urgent investigation or admit.

Intussusception and pyloric stenosis

Intussusception: The invagination of one part of the bowel into the lumen of the immediately adjoining bowel. It is the most common cause of intestinal obstruction in young children and usually occurs in previously healthy children. *Incidence:* 2:1000 live births. *Peak age:* 5–18mo. ♂:♀ ≈ 2:1.

Associations
- Seasonal variation suggests an underlying viral cause—rota and adeno-viruses have both been implicated
- Intestinal polyps
- Meckel's diverticulum
- Henoch-Schoenlein purpura

Types
- *Ileo-ileal:* Ileum invaginates into adjacent ileum
- *Ileo-colic:* Most common type—an ileo-ileal intussusception extends through the ileo-caecal valve
- *Ileo-caecal:* The apex of the intussusception is the ileo-caecal valve
- *Colo-colic:* Colon invaginates into adjacent colon—may be 2° to bowel tumour

Presentation: Very variable. Always have a high index of suspicion.
- Abdominal colic—paroxysms of pain during which the child draws up his legs. The child often screams with the pain and becomes pale. Episodes usually are 10–15min. apart and last 2–3min. but become more frequent with time.
- Vomiting—early symptom.
- Rectal bleeding—passage of blood ('redcurrent jelly stool') or slime per rectum is a late sign.
- Sausage-shaped mass in the abdomen—usually in the right upper quadrant—though not always present.

⚠ The child rapidly deteriorates if not treated early, becoming toxic and developing an obstructive picture with distended abdomen ± faeculent vomiting.

Differential diagnosis: Other causes of bowel obstruction; gastroenteritis; constipation; haemolytic uraemic syndrome.

Management: Admit as an acute surgical emergency. Untreated intussusception is usually fatal. Treatment is with reduction by barium enema or surgery.

Chronic intussusception: Rare and presents with much milder features than acute intussusception. Can cause failure to thrive.

Pyloric stenosis: Infantile hypertrophic pyloric stenosis usually develops in the first 3–6wk. of life (rare after 12wk.). Failure of the pyloric sphincter to relax → hypertrophy of the adjacent pyloric muscle. Typically affects first-born, male infants. Pyloric stenosis runs in families and is associated with Turner's syndrome, PKU, and oesophageal atresia.

Presentation

- Projectile vomiting—milk; no bile. The child is still hungry after vomiting and immediately feeds again. Rarely there is haematemesis.
- Failure to thrive.
- Dehydration and constipation ('rabbit pellet stools').
- A pyloric mass (feels like an olive) is palpable in the right upper abdomen (95%)—especially if the child has just vomited.
- After a test feed, there is visible peristalsis of the dilated stomach in the epigastrium.

Differential diagnosis

- Posseting/reflux
- Overfeeding
- Gastroenteritis
- Milk allergy
- Other causes of intestinal obstruction
- Infection—especially UTI
- ↑ICP
- Uraemia
- Adrenal insufficiency

Management: Refer to paediatric surgery. After rehydration and investigation to confirm diagnosis, treatment is surgical with a Ramstedt's pyloroplasty. There are usually no long-term consequences.

Diagnosis of asthma in children[G]

Symptoms/signs of a severe asthma attack in children >2y.

- Unable to complete sentences in one breath or too breathless to talk/feed
- Tachycardia:
  - Pulse >120bpm if >5y.
  - Pulse >130bpm if 2–5y.
- Tachypnoea:
  - Respiratory rate >30breaths/min. if >5y.
  - Respiratory rate >50breaths/min. if 2–5y.

Life-threatening signs in children age >2y.

- Central cyanosis
- Silent chest (inaudible wheeze)
- Poor respiratory effort
- Confusion
- Exhaustion
- Hypotension
- Coma

Symptoms/signs of a significant asthma attack if <2y.

- Audible wheezing
- Using accessory muscles
- Cyanosis
- Marked respiratory distress
- Too breathless to feed

Management of an acute asthma attack: 📖 p.1062

Childhood asthma affects ~5% of children in the UK and the prevalence is increasing. Virus-associated wheeze affects up to 20% of children at some point. Peak age of onset is 5y. Despite increased detection and better treatment of asthma in recent years in the UK, 40 children still die every year from the disease.

Risk factors

- Family history of atopy—particularly mother and/or siblings
- Coexistence of atopic disease—this is also a risk factor for persistence of symptoms
- In pre-pubertal children ♂:♀ = 3:2; after puberty ♀ > ♂; boys are more likely to 'grow out' of their symptoms
- Bronchiolitis in infancy
- Parental smoking—particularly the mother
- Prematurity
- Age at first presentation—the earlier the onset, the better the prognosis; the majority of children presenting aged <2y. are free of symptoms by age 6–11y.

Diagnosis: Figure 23.1. Suspect in any child with wheezing.

- *In school children:* Bronchodilator responsiveness, peak flow variability, or bronchial hyper-reactivity tests can all be used to confirm diagnosis as for adults—📖 p.377.
- *In younger children:* It is often not possible to measure airway function in order to confirm the presence of variable airways obstruction.

Differential diagnosis: Table 23.5 (📖 p.865)

Expected PEFR in children: 📖 p.374

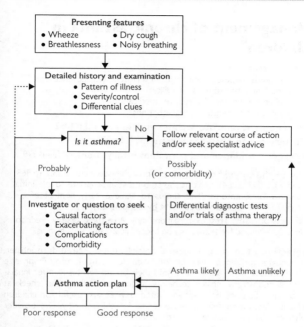

Figure 23.1 Diagnosis of asthma in children. (Reproduced with permission of British Thoracic Society and SIGN.)

❶ In children, asthma tends to be extrinsic. Allergy testing may be useful in making a diagnosis of atopy and in seeking causal factors. Absence of allergy should prompt consideration of alternative diagnoses.

Common precipitating/exacerbating factors

- Exercise
- Emotion
- Weather (fog, cold air, thunder-storms)
- Air pollutants (smoke and dust)
- Household allergens (e.g. house dust mite, animal fur, feathers)
- Infection (commonly viral URTI and chest infections)
- Drugs (NSAIDs)

Essential reading

British Thoracic Society/SIGN (revised 2004) British guidelines on the management of asthma ☐ http://www.sign.ac.uk

Information and support for parents and patients

Asthma UK ☎08457 01 02 03 ☐ http://www.asthma.org.uk

Management of chronic asthma in children[G]

Aims of treatment

- To minimize symptoms and impact on lifestyle (e.g. absence from school; limitations to physical ability)
- To minimize the need for reliever medication
- To prevent severe attacks/exacerbations

Management of acute asthma in children: 📖 p.1062

GP services and self-management: 📖 p.378

Allergen avoidance and complementary therapy: 📖 p.379

> **Drug therapy:** Use a stepwise approach—see Figures 23.2 (p.863) and 23.3 (📖 p.864). Start at the step most appropriate to the initial severity of symptoms. The aim is to achieve early control of the condition and then to ↓ treatment by stepping down.
>
> **Exacerbations:** Treat exacerbations early. A rescue course of prednisolone 30–40mg od for 1–2wk. may be needed at any step and any time.

Selection of inhaler device: If possible, use a metred dose inhaler. Inadequate technique may be mistaken for drug failure. Emphasize patients must inhale slowly and hold their breath for 10sec. after inhalation. Demonstrate inhaler technique before prescribing and check at follow-ups. Spacers or breath-activated devices are useful for children who find activation difficult and essential for children <5y. Dry powder inhalers are an alternative for older children.

Short-acting β_2 agonists: 📖 p.370 (e.g. salbutamol). Work more quickly and/or with fewer side-effects than alternatives. Use prn unless shown to benefit from regular dosing. Using ≥ canister/mo. or >10–12puffs/d. is a marker of poorly controlled asthma.

Inhaled corticosteroids: 📖 p.370. Most effective preventer for achieving overall treatment goals. May be beneficial even for children with mild asthma. Consider if:

- Exacerbations of asthma in the last 2y.
- Using inhaled β_2 agonists >3x/wk.
- Symptomatic ≥3x/wk. or ≥1night/wk.

Oral steroids: 📖 p.370

Add on therapy: Before initiating a new drug, check compliance, inhaler technique, and eliminate trigger factors.

- *Long-acting β_2 agonists:* 📖 p.370—inhaled preparations (e.g. salmeterol) improve lung function/symptoms. Slow-release tablets have similar effect but side-effects greater. Do not use without inhaled steroids. Only continue if of demonstrable benefit.
- *Theophylline:* ↑ lung function/↓ symptoms. Side-effects are common.
- *Leukotriene receptor antagonists:* e.g. montelukast. Provide improvement in symptoms and lung function and ↓ exacerbations.

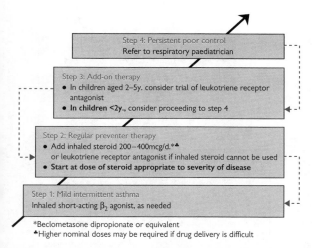

Step 4: Persistent poor control
Refer to respiratory paediatrician

Step 3: Add-on therapy
• In children aged 2–5y. consider trial of leukotriene receptor antagonist
• **In children <2y., consider proceeding to step 4**

Step 2: Regular preventer therapy
• Add inhaled steroid 200–400mcg/d.*♣
  or leukotriene receptor antagonist if inhaled steroid cannot be used
• **Start at dose of steroid appropriate to severity of disease**

Step 1: Mild intermittent asthma
Inhaled short-acting β₂ agonist, as needed

*Beclometasone dipropionate or equivalent
♣Higher nominal doses may be required if drug delivery is difficult

Figure 23.2 Summary of stepwise management in children aged <5y. (Reproduced with permission of British Thoracic Society and SIGN.)

Stepping down: Review and consider stepping down at intervals ≥3mo.. Maintain on the lowest dose of inhaled steroid controlling symptoms. When reducing steroids, cut dose by 25–50% each time.

Referral: Consider referral to a general paediatrician or specialist respiratory paediatrician if:
• Severe exacerbation of asthma—E
• Failure to thrive—U/S
• Unexpected clinical findings e.g. focal signs in the chest, abnormal voice or cry, dysphagia, inspiratory stridor—U/S
• Failure to respond to conventional treatment (particularly inhaled steroid >400mcg/d.)—U/S
• Diagnosis unclear or in doubt—U/S/R
• Excessive vomiting or posseting—S
• Severe upper respiratory tract infections—S
• Symptoms present from birth or perinatal lung problem—S/R
• Persistent wet cough—S/R
• Frequent use of steroid tablets—S/R
• FH of unusual chest disease—R
• Parental anxiety or need for reassurance—R
E = Emergency admission; U = Urgent; S = Soon; R = Routine

❶ This is only a rough guide. Urgency of referral will depend on the clinical state of the child.

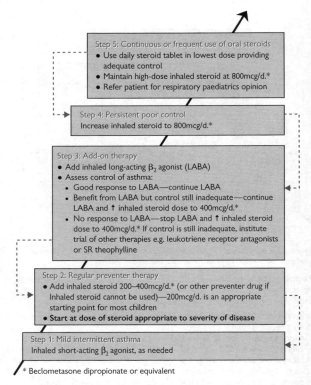

Step 5: Continuous or frequent use of oral steroids
- Use daily steroid tablet in lowest dose providing adequate control
- Maintain high-dose inhaled steroid at 800mcg/d.*
- Refer patient for respiratory paediatrics opinion

Step 4: Persistent poor control
Increase inhaled steroid to 800mcg/d.*

Step 3: Add-on therapy
- Add inhaled long-acting β₂ agonist (LABA)
- Assess control of asthma:
  - Good response to LABA—continue LABA
  - Benefit from LABA but control still inadequate—continue LABA and ↑ inhaled steroid dose to 400mcg/d.*
  - No response to LABA—stop LABA and ↑ inhaled steroid dose to 400mcg/d.* If control is still inadequate, institute trial of other therapies e.g. leukotriene receptor antagonists or SR theophylline

Step 2: Regular preventer therapy
- Add inhaled steroid 200–400mcg/d.* (or other preventer drug if inhaled steroid cannot be used)—200mcg/d. is an appropriate starting point for most children
- **Start at dose of steroid appropriate to severity of disease**

Step 1: Mild intermittent asthma
Inhaled short-acting β₂ agonist, as needed

* Beclometasone dipropionate or equivalent

Figure 23.3 Summary of stepwise management in children aged 5–12y. (Reproduced with permission of British Thoracic Society and SIGN.)

All doses given refer to beclometasone dipropionate (BDP) administered via metred dose inhaler. For other drugs/formulations, adjust dose accordingly (see *BNF* Section 3).

Table 23.5 Differential diagnosis of wheezing in children. (Reproduced with permission of British Thoracic Society and SIGN.)

Clinical clue	Possible diagnosis
Perinatal and family history	
Symptoms present from birth or perinatal lung problem	CF, chronic lung disease, ciliary dyskinesia, developmental anomaly
FH of unusual chest disease	CF, developmental anomaly, neuromuscular disorder
Severe upper respiratory tract disease	Defect of host defence
Symptoms and signs	
Persistent wet cough	CF, recurrent aspiration, host defence disorder
Excessive vomiting or posseting	Reflux ± aspiration
Dysphagia	Swallowing problems ± aspiration
Abnormal voice or cry	Laryngeal problem
Focal signs in the chest	Developmental disease, postviral syndrome, bronchiectasis, TB
Inspiratory stridor as well as wheeze	Central airways or laryngeal disorder
Failure to thrive	CF, host defence defect, gastro-oesophageal reflux
Investigations	
Focal or persistent radiological changes	Developmental disorder, postinfective disorder, recurrent aspiration, inhaled foreign body, bronchiectasis, TB

Essential reading

British Thoracic Society/SIGN (revised 2004) British guidelines on the management of asthma ⌨ http://www.sign.ac.uk

Patient information and support

Asthma UK ☎08457 01 02 03 ⌨ http://www.asthma.org.uk

Childhood epilepsy and febrile convulsions

Childhood epilepsy is a susceptibility to continuing seizures—including febrile convulsions. It occurs in 3–5% of children. Some children continue to have fits into adulthood and 60% of adult epilepsy starts in childhood.

Diagnosis: Seizures, faints, and funny turns can be difficult to distinguish and diagnose. A reliable eye-witness account is the key.

Funny turns in small children: 📖 p.262

Management of the fitting patient: 📖 p.1068

Long-term management: Refer all children where diagnosis is unclear or with suspected epilepsy for specialist assessment, advice on management, and follow-up care.

Education
- Epilepsy is a diagnosis that can cause great alarm and fear. Education is very important.
- Parents need clear information on:
  - What to expect
  - What to do during an attack
  - Avoiding risks e.g. swimming or cycling alone—but not being overprotective
  - Importance of compliance with medication—especially difficult with teenagers
  - When drug withdrawal may be considered, if fit-free.

Drug treatment
- Drug treatment is the mainstay of epilepsy management.
- There is controversy about when to treat—after the 1st, 2nd, or 3rd seizure.
- The drug chosen is matched to the individual patient and type of epilepsy—this is a specialist decision. Often the most suitable drug can only be established by trial and error. Antiepileptic drugs—📖 p.621.

Surgery: Increasingly being used for childhood epilepsy (e.g. lesionectomy). It is useful for intractable partial seizures, hemiepilepsy, and epilepsy with focal EEG and/or radiological features.

Types of epilepsy seen in childhood

Absence seizures (petit mal)
- Absence seizures totally interrupt activities for several seconds. The child stops what he is doing and may stare into middle-space.
- They can occur many times a day.
- Deterioration in school performance may be the first sign.
- Separating them from daydreaming can be difficult.
- ~10% (without other adverse factors) have seizures in adult life.

Management: Refer for specialist investigation and management. There is a typical EEG. Treatment is usually with sodium valproate.

Febrile convulsions

- Epileptic seizures provoked by fever in otherwise normal children.
- *Prevalence:* 3–5% of children aged 6mo.–5y. Often family history.
- Seizures are usually brief (last <5min) and generalized.
- ~10% of children have complex prolonged (>15min) or focal seizures. Intracranial infection (e.g. meningitis) must be excluded.
- The risk of subsequent epilepsy is low—<1% in those with no risk factors and ~10% in those with FH of epilepsy, pre-existing neurological abnormality, or a complex initial seizure.

Management

- Most children are admitted with a first attack.
- Parent reassurance and education are vital. Give practical advice on how to prevent attacks by reducing fevers e.g. early use of paracetamol and tepid sponging.
- Those with recurrent or complex febrile convulsions can be treated with rectal diazepam at the time of attacks—parents need to be taught when and how to administer the diazepam.
- Very rarely prophylaxis with anti-epileptic medication (e.g. sodium valproate) is needed—take specialist advice.

Generalized and partial seizures: 📖 p.618

Rolandic epilepsy

- Clonic, partial sensorimotor attacks affect the face, bulbar muscles (tongue and pharynx), hand and arm and are most common on waking.
- Starts in children aged 2–12y. (peak age 7–10y.). Usually stops by 13y.
- Refer for specialist investigation and management. EEG is characteristic.

Management: Refer for specialist advice. Anti-epileptic medication may be used if attacks are troublesome.

Myoclonic epilepsy

- Sudden involuntary spasm of a muscle or group of muscles (e.g. drop attacks or symmetrical repetitive jerking).
- Consciousness is often maintained.
- Refer for specialist investigation and management
- Lennox-Gastaut syndrome is a severe early onset form—starts age 2–6y. with intractable seizures and a typical EEG. (*W.G. Lennox (1884–1960)— US neurologist; H.J.P. Gastaut (1915–95)—French neurologist*)

Infantile spasms (West's syndrome)

- Starts in the first year of life (peak age: 4mo.).
- Runs of tonic spasms—usually flexion spasms ('salaam' spasms)—occur every 5–10sec.
- Associated with loss of vision and social interaction.
- Refer for specialist investigation and management. There is a typical EEG. Treatment is with steroids and anti-epileptics (usually vigabatrin).
- Poor prognosis: 30–50% have cerebral palsy; 85% have a cognitive disability; 20% death rate.

(*W.J. West (1794–1848)—British physician*)

Information and support for patients and parents

Epilepsy Action ☎0808 800 5050 🖥 http://www.epilepsy.org.uk

Genetic and congenital orthopaedic problems

Genetic problems

Cleido-cranial dysostosis: Autosomal dominant inheritance. Part/all of the clavicle is missing and there is delayed ossification of the skull— sutures remain open. Associated with short stature. No treatment is needed.

Osteogenesis imperfecta: Autosomal dominant inheritance (rarely recessive). Several types but all have an underlying problem with collagen metabolism resulting in fragile bones which fracture easily. Other features include lax joints, thin skin, blue sclerae, hypoplastic teeth, and deafness.

Presentation: Varies according to severity. May be obvious at birth or present early with fractures. Less severe cases present later and may be mistaken for non-accidental injury. Mild cases may not present until adolescence with thin bones on X-ray. Treatment is supportive.

Osteopetrosis (marble bone disease): Autosomal dominant or recessive inheritance.
- Dominant form presents in childhood with fractures, osteomyelitis ± facial paralysis.
- Recessive form is more severe causing bone marrow failure and death. Bone marrow transplantation has been tried but is of limited success.

Congenital malformations

Congenital dislocation of the hip (CDH): 3:2000 live births ($\female:\male \approx 6:1$)—though 10x that number have unstable hips and even more have 'clicks' detected on routine neonatal screening. Often there is a FH of CDH. Associated with breech presentation at term.

Presentation
- Usually detected at routine neonatal screening.
- High-risk infants (e.g. breech babies or those with FH of CDH) are additionally routinely screened with USS at 6wk. of age.
- Despite screening, some cases slip though the net. They present as toddlers with limp/waddling gait; frequent falls; asymmetric thigh creases; or limited hip adduction noted at later developmental checks.
- Rarely some go unnoticed until adulthood when they present with premature osteoarthritis.

Management: Refer to an orthopaedic surgeon specializing in paediatric problems. Treatment depends on when the condition is diagnosed:
- *Young babies:* Splinting—the hips are held in partial abduction using slings under each thigh attached to a body harness (e.g. von Rosen splint). Usually babies wear a splint for ~3mo.
- *Older babies, toddlers and adults:* Surgery is required.

Congenital scoliosis: 📖 p.870

Club foot (talipes): Consists of inversion of the foot, adduction of fore foot relative to hindfoot, and equinus (plantar flexion).
- *Positional talipes:* Moulding deformity seen in neonates. The foot can be passively everted and dorsiflexed to the normal position. Treatment is with physiotherapy. Follow-up to check the deformity is resolving.
- *True talipes:* The foot *cannot* be passively everted and dorsiflexed to the normal position. Refer to orthopaedics. Treatment is with physio-therapy, splints ± surgery.

Polydactyly and syndactyly
- *Polydactyly:* Extra digits can vary from small fleshy tags to complete duplications. They may be an isolated defect or associated with syndromes. Small fleshy tags are removed in the first few months. For extra digits firmly fixed or involving tendons or joints, surgery is delayed until the child is bigger. Refer to orthopaedics or plastic surgery.
- *Syndactyly:* Digits may be joined by a web of skin or more firmly fused. Webbing is usually mild and treatment is for cosmetic reasons, if at all. Where digits are fused, separation and skin grafting is carried out at ~4y.. Refer to plastic surgery.

Hypermobility syndrome: Occurs in children or young adults with lax joints. <½ are symptomatic. Those that have symptoms present with recurrent joint pains—mainly affecting the knees. Other symptoms include joint effusion, dislocation, ligamentous injuries, low back pain, and premature osteoarthritis. The condition is benign, but joints become stiffer with age. Treatment, when needed, is with physiotherapy. Rarely associated with rare congenital disorders e.g. Ehlers-Danlos syndrome.

Information and support

Brittle Bone Society ☎08000 282 459 🖳 *http://www.brittlebone.org*
Osteopetrosis Support Trust 🖳 *http://www.ost.org.uk*
Steps: Support for patients with lower limb conditions and their families ☎0871 717 0044 🖳 *http://steps-charity.org.uk*
Hypermobility Syndrome Association (HMSA) 🖳 *http://www.hypermobility.org*

Musculoskeletal problems in childhood

Children and sports injuries

- Exercise is good for children—it stimulates development of the musculoskeletal and cardiovascular systems.
- It should be fun and not physically or emotionally over-demanding.
- Children are more prone to sports injuries due to continuing growth (bone growth plates are prone to damage) but are more flexible so have ↓ injury rate.
- Children's temperature control is not as good as adults.
- Equipment must be checked regularly to ensure it fits.
- Encourage warm-up and stretching exercises before sport.
- Refer children with suspected overuse or sports injuries which don't recover rapidly with simple analgesia for specialist assessment—especially injuries of growth plates—to ensure correct alignment and continued growth.

Nocturnal musculoskeletal pains (growing pains): Episodic, muscular pains, usually in the legs, lasting ~30min. and waking the child from sleep. Diagnosis can be made on the history, if there are no associated symptoms and examination is normal. If in doubt, check ESR—which should be normal. In most cases, analgesia and reassurance are all that is needed. In resistant cases, physiotherapy may help.

Idiopathic musculoskeletal pain: Pain for which no cause can be found. Pain can become chronic. Exclude other causes by careful history and examination. Investigate further with blood or X-rays only if history or examination suggest a pathological cause. Treatment is with analgesia and reassurance. Advise affected children to return for reassessment ± orthopaedic referral if the pain worsens, continues beyond 6wk., changes in nature, or other symptoms develop.

Scoliosis: Lateral curvature of the spine.

- *Structural (true) scoliosis:* Fixed deformity. Scoliosis is associated with rotation of the vertebrae ± ribs and wedging of the vertebrae.
- *Non-structural (mobile) scoliosis:* Curvature is 2° to another condition outside the spine and disappears when that is corrected—e.g. leg length disparity (disappears on sitting). No rotation of the vertebrae.

Causes of true scoliosis

- *Idiopathic* (opposite).
- *Congenital:* Vertebral malformations produce severe scoliosis which is rapidly progressive. Major causes: hemivertebra; Klippel-Feil syndrome; congenital vertebral bar due to failure of segmentation.
- *Neuromuscular imbalance* e.g. polio, cerebral palsy, muscular dystrophy, neurofibromatosis, syringomyelia.
- *Trauma* resulting in damage to the vertebral growth plate and uneven growth.
- *Neoplasm*
  - 1°: Osteoid osteoma and osteoblastoma cause a painful scoliosis
  - 2°: Lytic metastases
  - *Treatment:* Treatment of tumours (e.g. radiotherapy) may result in scoliosis

- *Metabolic:* Osteoporosis and crush fracture.
- *Infection:* TB of the spine (Potts' disease).

Screening tests: 📖 p.825

Presentation: Usually found incidentally or on screening. Look for:
- Difference in shoulder height
- Spinal curvature
- Difference in space between trunk and upper limbs

❶ Structural scoliosis is often made more obvious by asking the child to bend forwards. Scoliosis which disappears on bending is postural and of no clinical significance.

Management: Refer children with structural scoliosis to orthopaedics.

⚠ If scoliosis is painful (especially at night) in a child or young person, consider spinal tumour and refer for urgent orthopaedic assessment.

Complications: Deformity; pain and limitation of activities; respiratory restriction.

Idiopathic scoliosis: >10° of lateral curvature of the spine—thoracic curves tend to be more severe than lumbar. *Incidence:* 1–3%.
- *Infantile idiopathic scoliosis:* ♂:♀ ≈ 6:4. 90% are left-sided convex scolioses. Associated with ipsilateral plagiocephaly (flattening of the skull). May resolve spontaneously (more likely if ♂ onset at <1y. of age and/or the rib-vertebral angle is <20°) or progress as the child grows. Progressive scoliosis is treated with braces and surgery. As a general rule, the younger the child and the higher the curve, the worse the prognosis.
- *Late onset idiopathic scoliosis:* Affects children aged 10–15y. ♀:♂ ≈ 9:1. The scoliosis is usually right-sided convex. The condition always gets worse without treatment as the child grows. Treatment is with observation (if the scoliosis is mild and the child has nearly completed growth), braces, and/or surgery.

Conditions affecting the lower limbs: 📖 p.872

Septic arthritis: 📖 p.873

Pulled elbow: 📖 p.554

Information and support
Scoliosis Association (UK) ☎020 8964 1166 🖥 http://www.sauk.org.uk
Arthritis Research Campaign (ARC) ☎0870 8505000 🖥 http://www.arc.org.uk

Conditions affecting the lower limbs

- If a child is limping, take it seriously and look for a problem.
- Children find it difficult to localize pain and pain can be referred from the hip to the knee, so examine the whole limb carefully.
- Other causes of referred pain include: spinal pathology, psoas spasm from GI pathology (e.g. appendicitis).
- Limping without pain is uncommon and may be due to undiagnosed congenital hip dislocation—📖 p.868.

Foot problems

Flat feet: All babies and toddlers have flat feet. The arch develops after 2–3y. of walking. Persistent flat feet may be familial or due to joint laxity. If pain free, foot is mobile and the child develops an arch on standing on tiptoe. No action is required. Else refer to orthopaedics.

Kohler's disease: Osteochondritis of the navicular bone. *Peak age:* 3–5y. Presents with pain and tenderness over the dorsum of the mid-foot. X-ray—small navicular bone of ↑ density. The pain usually resolves with simple analgesia and rest. (*A. Kohler (1874–1947)—German radiologist*)

Freiberg's disease: Osteochondritis of the 2nd and 3rd metatarsal heads. Most common in teenagers and young adults. ♀ > ♂. Presents with pain in the foot on walking. The head of the metatarsal is palpable and tender. X-ray shows a wide, flat metatarsal. Treatment is usually conservative with cushioning of shoes and simple analgesia. If severe, refer for orthopaedic assessment. Excision of the metatarsal head may relieve the pain. (*A.H. Freiberg (1868–1940)—US surgeon*)

Sever's disease: Apophysitis of the heel. *Peak age:* 8–13y. Treated with analgesia, raising the heel of the shoe a little, calf-stretching, and avoiding strenuous activities for a few weeks. (*J.W. Sever (1878–1964)—US surgeon*)

In-toe and out-toe gait

- *In-toe:* Originates in the femur (persistent anteversion of the femoral neck), tibia (tibial torsion), or foot (metatarsus varus). Does not cause pain or affect mobility. Usually resolves by age 5–6y.
- *Out-toe:* Common <2y. May be unilateral. Corrects spontaneously.

Knee problems

Bow legs and knock knees

- *Genu varum (bow legs):* Outward curving of the tibia usually associated with internal tibial torsion. Except in severe cases, always resolves spontaneously. Severe cases raise the possibility of rickets or other rare developmental disorders—refer for orthopaedic opinion.
- *Genu valgum (knock knees):* Common amongst 2–4y. olds. Innocent if symmetrical and independent of any other abnormality. Severe, progressive cases suggest rickets—refer for X-ray.

Osgood–Schlatter disease: 📖 p.560

Hip problems

Transient synovitis of the hip (irritable hip): The most common reason for limping in childhood. *Peak age:* 2–10y.. ♂ >> ♀. The child is usually well but complains of pain in the hip or knee and may refuse to weight bear. Cause is unknown. Exclude septic arthritis—refer to orthopaedics. Usually resolves in 7–10d. without treatment.

Perthes' disease: Pain in the hip or knee, limp, and limited hip movement developing over ~1mo. Due to avascular necrosis of the femoral head. Bilateral in 10%. *Peak age:* 4–7y. (range 3–11y.). ♂:♀ ≈ 4:1.

Management: If suspected, refer for X-ray and to orthopaedics. Treatment is with rest, X-ray surveillance, bracing, and/or surgery depending on severity.

Prognosis: Usually the condition heals over 2–3y. Joint damage may lead to early arthritis. Young patients do best. Risk factors for poor outcome include:

- ♀
- Onset >8y.
- Involvement of the whole femoral head
- Pronounced metaphyseal rarefaction
- Lateral displacement of the femoral head

(G.C. Perthes (1869–1927)—German surgeon)

Slipped upper femoral epiphysis: The upper femoral epiphysis slips with respect to the femur, usually in a postero-inferior direction. Bilateral in 20%. Incidence: 1:100,000. *Peak age:* 10–15y. ♂:♀ ≈ 3:1. Typically affects obese, underdeveloped children or tall, thin boys.

Presentation
- Pain at rest in the groin, hip, thigh, or knee—may be mild.
- Limp and/or pain on movement.
- ↓ hip movements—particularly abduction and medial rotation. The affected leg may be externally rotated and shortened.

Management: Conform diagnosis on X-ray (include lateral views)—shows backwards and downwards slippage of the epiphysis. Refer to orthopaedics—surgical pinning or reconstructive surgery is needed. Monitoring of the other hip is essential.

Complications: Avascular necrosis; coxa vara; early arthritis; slipped epiphysis on the contralateral side.

Septic arthritis: Most common in children <5y. old. Tends to affect the hip or knee. The child is usually systemically unwell and holds the affected joint completely still. The joint may be swollen, hot, and tender. This is an emergency—if suspected, admit. Treatment is with iv antibiotics.

Sports injuries: 📖 p.542

Information and support

Steps: Support for patients with lower limb conditions and their families ☎0871 717 0044 🖥 http://steps-charity.org.uk
Arthritis Research Campaign (ARC) ☎0870 8505000 🖥 http://www.arc.org.uk

Arthritis in children

Joint and limb pains are common in children. Arthritis is rare.

Presentation of arthritis in children

- *Older children:* Usually present with well localized joint pains ± hot, tender, swollen joints.
- *Babies and young children:* May present with immobility of a joint or a limp, but the diagnosis can be extremely difficult.

Differential diagnosis of joint pains in children

- Juvenile chronic arthritis (JCA)
- Infections e.g. TB, rubella
- Rheumatic fever
- Henoch-Schönlein purpura
- Traumatic arthritis
- Hypermobility syndrome
- Leukaemia
- Sickle cell disease
- SLE and connective tissue disorders
- Transient synovitis of the hip (irritable hip)
- Septic arthritis
- Perthes disease
- Slipped femoral epiphysis

Septic arthritis: 📖 p.873

Types of childhood arthritis

Still's disease: 10% of JCA. Affects boys and girls equally up to 5y.—then, girls are more commonly affected.

Presentation

- Fever—high, swinging, early-evening temperature
- Rash—pink maculopapular rash
- Musculoskeletal pain—arthralgia, arthritis, myalgia
- Generalized lymphadenopathy
- Hepatosplenomegaly
- Pericarditis ± pleurisy (uncommon)

Differential diagnosis: Malignancy—particularly leukaemia or neuroblastoma); infection.

Investigations: Blood—↑ ESR/CRP; FBC—↑ neutrophils, ↑ platelets. Auto-antibodies are –ve.
(G.F. Still (1868–1941)—English paediatrician)

Oligoarthritis or pauciarticular onset arthritis

- *Persistent:* Most common form of JCA (50–60%) but still rare.
  Peak age: 3y. ♀ >> ♂. Affects ≤ 4 joints—especially wrists, knees, and ankles. Often asymmetrical. Associated with uveitis (often with +ve anti-nuclear antibody) which requires regular screening by slit-lamp examination. Rarely causes blindness. Generally prognosis is good, with remission in 4–5y.
- *Extended:* Chronic arthritis with an oligoarticular onset of the disease, which progresses to involve >4 joints. Joints tend to be stiff rather than hot and swollen.

Polyarticular onset JCA: Develops with or without a preceding systemic illness at any age >1y.. Usually occurs in teenagers, producing widespread joint destruction. There is symmetrical arthritis of hands, wrists, PIPs ± DIPs. Rheumatoid factor is usually –ve (+ve in 3%—often teenage girls).

Juvenile spondyloarthropathy: Affects teenage and younger boys, producing an asymmetrical arthritis of lower limb joints. Associated with HLA-B27 and acute anterior uveitis and represents the childhood equivalent of adult ankylosing spondylitis. ~60% of childhood sufferers develop ankylosing spondylitis later in life.

Psoriatic arthritis: Polyarthritis affecting large and small joints including fingers and toes. The arthritis can be very erosive. Psoriasis may be present in the child or a first-degree relative—📖 p.646.

Management of children with arthritis

- Always refer to a specialist paediatric rheumatology unit to avoid long-term disability. These units have multidisciplinary facilities for rehabilitation, education, and surgical intervention, if necessary, and support both the family and the child.
- NSAIDs and paracetamol help pain and stiffness, but corticosteroids and immunosuppressants (e.g. methotrexate) are often required for systemic disease.
- Ensure families apply for any benefits that might be available to them and support families in any applications made to adapt the home or school environment to their condition.

Information and support
Arthritis Research Campaign (ARC) ☎0870 8505000 🖳 http://www.arc.org.uk

Paediatric dermatology

Birthmarks

Strawberry naevus (capillary haemangioma)
- Not usually present at birth.
- Occurs anywhere on the skin surface.
- Starts as a small, red patch then grows rapidly over a few months into a bright red vascular lump.
- After initial growth, the naevus stays the same size for 6–12mo., then involutes and disappears by 5–7y.
- No treatment is needed but parents may need considerable reassurance.
- If interfering with feeding, breathing, or vision—refer for treatment with intralesional steroids or laser.

Port wine stain (naevus flammeus)
- Present at birth.
- Irregular red/purple macule which often affects 1 side of the face.
- Permanent—may become darker and lumpy in middle age.
- May be associated with other abnormalities e.g. intracranial vascular malformation (Sturge-Weber syndrome).

Salmon patch (stork mark)
- The most common vascular naevus (~50% neonates).
- Small, telangectatic lesion forming a pink macule—most commonly at the nape of the neck or on the upper face.
- Facial lesions resolve spontaneously; those on the neck may persist. No treatment is needed.

Mongolian blue spot
- Bluish discolouration of the skin, usually over buttocks and lower back in dark-skinned babies.
- Of no clinical significance but may occasionally be mistaken for bruising and non-accidental injury.
- Usually disappear by 1y.

Congenital melanocytic naevi: ~1.5% of neonates.
- Noted at birth as raised nodules or plaques of black or brown.
- May be hairy, irregular, and single or multiple.
- Classified by size: <1.5cm—small; 1.5–20cm—medium; >20cm—large.
- There is a risk of malignant change to melanoma. The larger the naevus, the greater the risk.
- Laser therapy can improve cosmetic appearance.

Nappy rash: Most common type of nappy eruption. Usually seen in young infants. Rare >12mo. An irritant dermatitis due to skin contact with urine or faeces.

Presentation: Glazed erythema in the napkin area, sparing skin folds. 2° bacterial or fungal infection is common.

Differential diagnosis
- Seborrhoeic eczema
- Candidiasis
- Napkin psoriasis

Management

- Advise parents to keep the nappy area dry (superabsorbant disposal nappies help).
- Give baby as much time as possible with the nappy off.
- Apply aqueous cream as a moisturiser and soap substitute.
- Apply a barrier cream between nappy changes—though this may interfere with the action of some modern nappies.
- Topical treatment with an antifungal combined with hydrocortisone (e.g. Canesten HC cream) is effective if the nappy rash is not clearing.

Infantile seborrhoeic eczema

- Starts in the first few weeks of life.
- Affects body folds—axilla, groins, behind ears, neck ± face, and scalp ('*cradle cap*').
- Flexural lesions present as moist, shiny, well-demarcated scaly erythema.
- On the scalp, neck, and behind the ears, a yellowish crust is usual.
- Treat flexural lesions with emollients and 1% hydrocortisone ointment or with clotrimazole and hydrocortisone.
- Scalp lesions respond to 2% salicyclic acid in aqueous cream applied od and washed out with baby shampoo.

Candidiasis: Often complicates nappy rash or infantile seborrhoeic eczema. Erythema, scaling, and pustules involve the flexures. There may be associated satellite lesions. Treatment is with a topical antifungal e.g. clotrimazole.

Juvenile plantar dermatosis: Presents with red, dry, fissured and glazed skin, principally over the forefeet. Sometimes involves the whole sole. Usually starts in primary school years and resolves spontaneously in mid-teens. Due to wearing socks and/or shoes made from synthetic materials. Emollients help but topical steroids are ineffective. Advise cotton socks and leather shoes.

Accessory nipples: Commonly seen on the milk line in both male and female infants. Usually small and inconspicuous. No treatment is required.

Psoriasis: 📖 p.646   **Warts:** 📖 p.670

Atopic eczema: 📖 p.636   **Molluscum Contagiosum:** 📖 p.671

Acne: 📖 p.644   **Impetigo:** 📖 p.668

Scalded skin syndrome: 📖 p.669

Further information

Electronic Dermatology Atlas 🖥 *http://www.dermis.net/bilddb/index_e.htm*

Childhood cancer (1)

Prevalence: 12/100,000 children <15y.; *Incidence:* 1200 children aged <15y./y. in England and Wales. Acute leukaemia is the most common form of childhood cancer (1:3 childhood cancers), followed by brain tumours.

Acute leukaemia: Associated with Down's syndrome—though only a very small proportion of children with leukaemia have Down's syndrome. *Peak age range:* 2–4y. 2 major types:
- Acute lymphocytic leukaemia—310 cases/y.
- Acute myeloid leukaemia—60 cases/y.

Presentation: Children usually present with a relatively short history (weeks) of pallor, fatigue, irritability, fever, bone pain, and/or bruising/petechiae. 70% have hepatosplenomegaly and >50% have lymphadenopathy.

Management: If suspected, check FBC and refer for emergency paediatric opinion.

Further information: 📖 p.532

Lymphoma: *Peak age:* 10–14y.
- *Hodgkin's lymphoma:* 50 cases/y.—presents with non-tender cervical/supraclavicular lymphadenopathy. A minority have systemic symptoms. History tends to be long.
- *Non-Hodgkin's lymphoma:* 70 cases/y.—presents with cervical and/or supraclavicular lymphadenopathy and/or disease in the abdomen (hepatosplenomegaly) or mediastinum, pleural effusion, SVC obstruction, or dyspnoea. There tends to be a rapid progression of symptoms.

Differential diagnosis: EBV; other infection; acute leukaemia.

Management: Refer for urgent paediatric opinion if:
- Lymphadenopathy—especially if:
  - No evidence of infection
  - Lymph node(s) is/are >3cm diameter or progressively enlarging
  - Associated with other signs of general ill health (e.g. fever, weight loss)
  - Involves axillary nodes (in the absence of local infection) or supraclavicular nodes
- Mediastinal or hilar mass on CXR
- Symptoms/signs of acute leukemia (see above)

Further information: 📖 p.534

Neuroblastoma: Tumour derived from neural crest tissue. 80 cases/y. in England and Wales—8% of all paediatric tumours. Tends to affect children <4y. old (50% <2y.; 90% <9y.). Sites:
- Adrenal medulla—50%
- Abdominal sympathetic ganglia—25%
- Chest—20%
- Pelvis—5%
- Neck—5%

Presentation: Variable—depends on site of the tumour and extent of metastases. ~½ present with metastatic disease.

- *General effects:* Pallor, fever, anorexia, and weight ↓, irritability, failure to thrive, flushing, ataxia, diarrhoea.
- *Local effects of the tumour:* Abdominal mass, local spread → paraplegia or cauda equine syndrome.
- *Effects of metastases:* Lymphatic spread and haematogenous spread, particularly to liver, lungs, and bone, is common. Associated symptoms include bone pain ± pathological fracture, breathlessness, periorbital bruising (looks like a black eye), proptosis, Horner's syndrome. Skin involvement results in firm nodules ('blueberry muffin appearance').

Management: Refer urgently to paediatrics if suspected. Treated with surgery, radiotherapy, and/or chemotherapy.

Prognosis: Early stage disease has a 95% 5y. survival. Late stage disease has 20% 5y. survival. Children with extra-abdominal tumours, and those who are <1y. at diagnosis have better prognosis.

Brain tumours: 280 cases/y. in England and Wales. Associated with neurofibromatosis and tuberous sclerosis.

Presentation

- Headache (65–70%)
- Vomiting (65–70%)
- Changes in personality/mood (behaviour out of character—45–50%)
- Visual disturbance
- Cranial nerve lesions
- Ataxia
- Seizures
- Deterioration in school performance
- Growth failure
- Rapidly increasing head circumference (infants only)
- Papilloedema (sometimes 1st identified by an optician)

Differential diagnosis: Psychosocial problems; other causes of headache (📖 p.596).

Management

- *Immediate paediatric opinion:* Papilloedema or neurological signs.
- *Urgent paediatric opinion* if headache of recent origin with ≥1 of:
  - Increasing severity or frequency
  - Worse in the mornings/causing waking
  - Associated with vomiting
  - Behavioural change and/or deterioration in school performance.

Further information: 📖 p.602

Information and advice for patients and parents

Leukaemia Research Fund ☎020 7405 0101 🖳 http://www.lrf.org.uk
Cancer and Leukaemia in Childhood (CLIC) ☎0845 301 0031 🖳 http://www.clic.org.uk
Lymphoma Association ☎0808 808 5555 🖳 http://www.lymphoma.org.uk
The Neuroblastoma Society 🖳 http://www.nsoc.co.uk
The Brain and Spine Foundation ☎0808 808 1000 🖳 http://www.brainandspine.org.uk
Brain Tumour Action (mainly Scotland) ☎0131 315 7299 (evenings and weekends) 🖳 http://www.braintumouraction.org.uk

Childhood cancer (2)

Wilms' tumour (nephroblastoma): Type of kidney tumour composed of primitive renal tissue. The left kidney is affected more often than the right and it is bilateral in 10%. 70 cases/y. in England and Wales. Usually affects children <5y. old (peak age: 2–3y.). ♂ > ♀. Rarely associated with Beckwith-Wiedemann syndrome, aniridia, or hemihypertrophy.

Presentation

- *General effects:* Fever, anorexia and weight ↓, anaemia.
- *Local effects of the tumour:* Unilateral abdominal mass ± pain ± haematuria (rare).
- *Effects of metastases:* 20% have metastases to liver, lungs, or bone (rare) at presentation. May present with symptoms/signs of metastases.

Management and prognosis: If suspected, refer for urgent paediatric surgical opinion. Treatment is with surgery ± chemotherapy ± radiotherapy depending on histology and stage at diagnosis. Early stage tumours have 80% 5y. survival; Late stage tumours have 50% 5y. survival. (*M. Wilms (1867–1918)—German surgeon*)

Retinoblastoma: Rare tumour of the eye. 30 cases/y. in England and Wales. Usually affects children <1y. old—most are <5y. old. May be familial (15%—dominant inheritance) when the tumour is usually bilateral. Sporadic tumours are usually unilateral.

Presentation

- Usually detected by a white pupillary reflex found at routine developmental screening.
- Alternatively, may present with squint or inflammation of the eye.

Management: Refer any suspected cases for urgent ophthalmology opinion. Treatment of unilateral tumours is surgical. Bilateral tumours are treated by enucleation of laser ablation of the worst affected eye and radiotherapy to the other eye.

Prognosis: 80% patients with unilateral tumours survive long-term. Bilateral tumours have a poorer prognosis with 40% surviving long-term.

Sarcoma: Affects soft tissue (80 cases/y.) or bone (60 cases/y.).
- *Soft tissue sarcoma:* Presents with a mass at any age. May be at any site. Rarely associated with a FH of early breast cancer.
- *Bone tumour:* Peak age: 10–14y. Osteosarcoma or Ewing's tumour. Present with persistent bony pain—most commonly in a limb. Plain X-ray is helpful.

Management: Refer for urgent specialist opinion if:
- *A mass is found*—especially if it is:
  - growing larger
  - >3cm diameter
  - fixed or deep to the fascia
  - associated with regional lymphadenopathy.
- *A child complains of bone pain*—especially if it is:
  - requiring analgesia
  - limiting activity
  - diffuse or involves the back
  - persistently localized at any site

Treatment is with surgery and chemotherapy. 5y. survival is ~55%.

Gonadal tumours: Usually germ cell tumours (30 cases/y.) of the ovary or testis. Present with:
• Non-transilluminable testicular or paratesticular mass
• Abdominal mass
• Precocious puberty in girls

Management: Refer any suspected case for urgent paediatric surgical or medical opinion as appropriate.

Further information
• Testicular tumours 🔲 p.700   • Ovarian tumours: 🔲 p.712

On-going care: Once the diagnosis is made, most children embark on an intensive regime of treatment which may involve surgery, chemotherapy, and/or radiotherapy. They are usually referred to specialist paediatric oncology units who share care with local hospitals, and have direct access to advice and admission via those units. Outreach nurses provide support in the community (e.g. administration of iv drugs via Hickman lines) with the aim of maintaining as normal a lifestyle as possible.

⚠ Immunosuppression can be a major problem and any febrile episode in a neutropenic child requires immediate referral to a specialist unit. Chicken pox can be very serious—seek specialist advice from the treating unit if the patient is in contact with any other child with chicken pox.

The GP's role: Treatment for childhood cancer is increasingly successful with cure rates of >80% for some forms of cancer. The role of the GP is important at this time, even if it is peripheral:
• Keep in touch with the family and up-to-date with what is going on;
• Provide support to the child and other family members;
• Give advice on any benefits or local services the family might find of assistance;
• Ensure prescriptions requested by specialist services are supplied promptly.

Palliative care: Sadly, despite treatment, some children progress to the terminal stages of their cancers. General principles of palliative care apply (🔲 p.999) but the emotional traumas are often much greater. If possible, engage specialist palliative care services early. Try to maintain continuity of care with as few professionals involved as possible. Provide on-going support to family members after the child has died.

Information and advice for patients and parents
Childhood Eye Cancer Trust (CHECT) 🖳 http://www.rbsociety.org.uk
Sarcoma UK 🖳 http://www.sarcoma-uk.org
Help Adolescents with Cancer (HAWC) ☎0161 688 6244 🖳 http://www.hawc-co-uk.com
Association for Children with Life Threatening or Terminal Conditions and Their Families (ACT) ☎0117 922 1556 🖳 http://www.act.org.uk
Association of Children's Hospices (ACH) 🖳 http://www.childrenshospice.org.uk

Paediatric endocrinology

Congenital adrenal hyperplasia (CAH; adrenogenital syndrome; adrenal virilism): Autosomal recessive trait. There are ↓ levels of circulating cortisol due to absence or deficiency of any of the enzymes needed for synthesis. Each enzyme block causes a characteristic deficiency e.g. 21-hydroxylase deficiency. 2 patterns:
- Androgens accumulate causing virilization of an affected female foetus.
- Androgen synthesis is impaired causing inadequate virilization of an affected male foetus (much rarer).

Presentation: Ambiguity of the external genitalia. Usually detected at the neonatal check but less severe forms may go unnoticed until later in life—even adulthood.

Management: Refer for specialist investigation, management, and follow-up. Treatment is usually with glucocorticoid ± mineralocorticoid replacement.

Male hypogonadism: ↓ function of the testes. 3 types:
- *Primary*—damage to the Leydig cells impairs androgen (testosterone) secretion e.g. Klinefelter's syndrome, anorchia (absent testes).
- *Secondary (hypogonadotropic)*—disorders of the hypothalamus or pituitary impair gonadotropin secretion which may result in impotency and/or infertility e.g. panhypopituitarism (📖 p.428).
- *Resistance to androgen action*—age of onset dictates the clinical presentation:
  - *In utero*—ambiguity of genitalia or female appearance, small penis, incomplete testicular descent
  - *In childhood*—delayed or impaired puberty, impaired development of male 2° sexual characteristics ± gynaecomastia
  - *In adulthood*—↓ libido, impotence, loss of muscle power, testicular atrophy, fine wrinkling of the skin around eyes and lips, sparse body hair, osteopenia, gynaecomastia.

Management: Refer for specialist investigation. Treatment depends on the nature of the deficiency.

Pituitary dwarfism: ↓ function of the anterior pituitary gland causing short stature and failure to thrive. Skeletal maturation, assessed by bone age, is usually >2y. behind chronologic age. *Causes:*
- Idiopathic
- Pituitary tumour e.g. craniopharyngioma
- Midline defect e.g. cleft palate
- Genetic

Management: Close specialist monitoring is critical. Treatment includes:
- Growth hormone—continued until an acceptable height is reached or growth rate falls to <2.5cm/y. Slipped femoral epiphysis is more common among children being treated with growth hormone.
- Cortisol and thyroid hormone replacement if needed.
- Gonadal sex steroids if normal puberty fails.

Diabetes mellitus: 📖 p.404

Congenital goitre: Enlarged thyroid gland present at birth ± hypo- or hyperthyroidism. Hypothyroid babies are treated with thyroxine; if there is tracheal compression or hyperthyroidism, treatment is surgical.

Hypothyroidism

Neonatal (congenital) hypothyroidism: ~1:4000 live births. Usually due to congenital absence of the thyroid gland.

Presentation: Normally detected before clinical signs are evident through routine neonatal screening by heel prick testing (Guthrie test) aged 9d.

Clinical symptoms/signs

- Cyanosis
- Prolonged neonatal jaundice
- Poor feeding
- Hoarse cry
- Umbilical hernia
- Respiratory distress
- Macroglossia
- Large fontanelle
- Delayed skeletal maturation

Management: Refer for specialist advice. Treatment is with thyroxine replacement—requires lifelong therapy. In most treated infants, development is normal.

Juvenile (acquired) hypothyroidism: Usually the result of auto-immune thyroiditis (Hashimoto's thyroiditis).

Presentation

- As for adults (📖 p.423)—↑ weight; constipation; coarse, dry hair; sallow, cool, or mottled coarse skin.
- Signs specific to childhood—growth retardation, delayed skeletal maturation ± delayed puberty.
- TFTs confirm diagnosis.

Management: Refer to paediatrics for specialist advice and follow-up. Treatment is with thyroxine replacement.

Hyperthyroidism

Neonatal hyperthyroidism: Rare but potentially life-threatening. Occurs in infants of mothers with current or prior Graves' disease due to passage of auto-antibodies across the placenta.

Presentation

- Feeding problems
- ↑ BP
- Irritability
- Tachycardia
- Exophthalmos
- Goitre
- Frontal bossing
- Microcephaly
- Failure to thrive
- Vomiting
- Diarrhoea

Management: Refer for specialist management. Affected infants generally recover in <3–4mo. Long-term consequences include premature fusion of the cranial sutures (craniosynostosis) and developmental delay.

Juvenile hyperthyroidism: Usually the result of Graves' disease—characterized by diffuse goitre, thyrotoxicosis, and eye signs (📖 p.422).

Growth disorders

Take every opportunity to weigh and measure a child. Plot height, weight (and head circumference <1y.) on centile charts. Always correct the age of the child for prematurity at birth.

❶ 3% of 'normal' children fall under the 3rd and 3% above the 97th centile.

Calculating expected height: Small parents have small children and tall parents have tall children—always calculate expected height of the child before deciding the child has short stature or excessive height.

> Expected height = (mother's height + father's height) ÷ 2
> *Then:* add 6cm for a boy or subtract 6cm for a girl

Failure to thrive: Common problem. Simply means failure to gain weight in infancy as expected. Defined as:
- Weight consistently <3rd centile for age
- Progressive ↓ in weight to <3rd centile *or*
- ↓ in expected rate of growth based on the child's growth curve.

Usually, head circumference is preserved relative to length and length relative to weight. Failure to thrive is the result of insufficient nutrition to allow weight ↑. Causes are many and varied.

Non-organic causes
- Lack of food due to neglect, lack of education, poverty or famine
- Emotional problems e.g. emotional neglect, unhappy family, or other difficulties at home—most common cause

Organic causes
- Chronic infection
- Gastrointestinal disease e.g. coeliac disease, chronic diarrhoea
- Metabolic disease e.g. DM
- Respiratory disease e.g. cystic fibrosis
- Heart disease
- Physical feeding problems e.g. cleft palate

Presentation: Usually detected by the health visitor when performing routine weighing or developmental checks.

Assessment
- Ask how the child is fed—quantities and times of the day. Check the parent is making up formula feeds correctly.
- Ask about problems feeding the child—specifically about regurgitation of food and vomiting.
- Ask about other physical problems e.g. breathlessness, diarrhoea.
- Examine the child carefully from top to toe looking for any physical abnormalities or signs of developmental delay.
- Watch the way the child interacts with you and the parent. Look for evidence of neglect or maltreatment.
- Look to see how large the parents are—2 small parents will probably have a small child.

Management: Treat any reversible causes. Continue to measure height, length, and head circumference regularly. Try to use the same scales on each occasion.

Refer to paediatrics
- If no cause for failure to thrive is found
- If an abnormality requiring specialist paediatric care is found
- If, despite treatment of a reversible cause, the child continues to lose or fails to gain weight.

Short stature: Defined as height <3rd centile. Occurs mainly in healthy children (80%) but may indicate physical or emotional problems—especially if both parents have heights >3rd centile or serial measurements show growth has fallen below that expected from the centile chart.

Genetic causes
- Familial short stature
- Turner's syndrome
- Familial growth delay (delayed pubertal growth spurt but eventually reach normal height)
- Achondroplastic dwarfism

Physical causes
- Low birth weight conditions
- Endocrine causes e.g. growth hormone deficiency, hypopituitarism, hypothyroidism, DM
- Chronic illness e.g. severe asthma, heart disease, chronic infection

Non-organic causes
- Poor nutrition
- Emotional neglect
- Eating disorders

Management: Manage as for failure to thrive.

Excessive height: Most children with height >97th centile come from tall families and accept their height as normal. Refer if a child is considerably taller than the predicted height. Pathological causes of excess height are rare and include:
- Pituitary adenoma (gigantism)
- Thyrotoxicosis
- Precocious puberty
- Marfan syndrome
- Homocystinuria

Head growth: At birth, head circumference is 32–37cm (term infant). Most head growth occurs in infancy. The anterior fontanelle measures (2.5 x 2.5cm at birth) becoming smaller, until it closes any time from 6mo.–18mo.. Refer children with head circumference <3rd or >97th centile.
- *Microcephaly:* 1:1000 births. Small head out of proportion with the body. Associated with developmental delay. *Causes:* Genetic, intrauterine infection (e.g. rubella, CMV), hypoxia.
- *Macrocephaly:* Large head circumference. *Causes:*
  - *Hydrocephalus*—suspect if the head circumference deviates from the normal curve or if there are signs of ↑ ICP. Refer.
  - *Megalencephaly*—commonly benign and familial. Rarely associated with developmental delay.
- *Asymmetrical skull:* Inequality of growth rates at the sutures. Due to:
  - Postural effects e.g. children who always sleep on 1 side.
  - *Craniosynostosis*—premature fusion of skull sutures. If suspected refer for prompt neurosurgical opinion.

Information and support for patients and parents
Height Matters 🖳 http://www.heightmatters.org.uk

Child abuse and neglect

Estimates suggest that ~2 in every 100 children are abused each year. 1:3 of those children suffer sexual abuse. In retrospective studies 1:10 men and 1:20 women report abuse in their childhood.

Classification: 5 broad categories of abuse are recognized:
- **Physical abuse or non-accidental injury (NAI):** Any physical injury, including poisoning, where there is reasonable suspicion the injury was caused deliberately (or deliberately not prevented) or where the injury is not consistent with the account of its occurrence.
- **Emotional abuse:** Pattern of behaviour impairing a child's emotional development or sense of self-worth e.g. constant criticism, threats, rejection, or withholding love, support, or guidance. Emotional abuse is difficult to prove but often coexists with other forms of abuse.
- **Sexual abuse:** Sexual activities of any sort performed upon a child by an adult or young person able to understand what s/he is doing.
- **Neglect:** Failure to provide for the child's basic needs. Can be:
  - Physical—inadequate food, clothing, shelter, or safe environment
  - Emotional—inattention to a child's emotional needs
  - Educational—persistent absence from school without reason
  - Medical—failure to seek or refusal of required treatment
- **Fabricated or induced illness:** 📖 p.984

❶ In practice, there is often overlap and ≥ 1 type of abuse may co-occur.

Presentation: *Always* have a high index of suspicion. *Suspect abuse if:*
- The child discloses it
- The story is inconsistent with injuries found
- There is late presentation after an injury or lack of concern about the injury by the parent(s)
- Presentation to an unknown doctor
- Accompanying adult is not the parent or guardian
- Sibling has been a victim of abuse
- Reluctance to allow the child to be examined
- Characteristic injuries—look for marks consistent with cigarette burns; scalds (especially if symmetrical or doughnut shaped on buttocks); finger mark or bite mark bruises; perineal bruising or anogenital injury; linear marks consistent with whipping; buckle or belt marks
- Multiple injuries or old injuries coexistent with new
- Unlikely sites for injuries e.g. mouth, ears, genitalia, eyes
- Behaviour of the child is suggestive e.g. withdrawn, 'frozen watchfulness', sexually precocious behaviour, abnormal interaction between child and parents, unwilling to speak about the injury, etc.
- Vaginal discharge, sexually transmitted disease, or recurrent UTI in any child <14y.
- Failure to thrive, developmental delay—and/or behavioural problems, neglect and/or emotional abuse are included in the differential diagnosis of failure to thrive and developmental delay. Any type of abuse may result in behavioural problems.

Risk factors: Child abuse is the result of interaction between the abuser and the child. Several factors are known to be important:

- *Child factors:* age <2y. (1:4 abused/neglected children); prematurity; 'difficult' child (e.g. a demanding child); unrealistic expectations of a child's ability or handicap
- *Parent factors:* parents who have been abused themselves; maternal age <30y.; unwanted pregnancy; substance abuse; psychiatric illness
- *Environmental factors:* social deprivation; inadequate support; family stress or a crisis—especially if no support

Immediate action: Welfare of the child is *paramount*. To not report abuse is to collude with the abuser.

- Wherever possible, arrange for another health professional to be present during the consultation.
- Take a history from any accompanying adult. If possible, also take a history from the child alone too.
- Fully examine the child. Ask for an explanation for any injuries noted.
- Keep thorough notes—recording dates and times, history given, injuries noted, and any explanation of those injuries.

Further action: Depends on nature of the suspected abuse, suspected abuser (e.g. if someone outside the home is suspected, the child is safe to return home), nature of the injuries, and response of the parents. Be familiar with and follow local guidelines and practice policy. *Options are:*

- Hospital admission—protects the child and allows full assessment
- Liaison with the social services child protection team (on-call 24h./d.)
- If admission is refused, contact social services to arrange a Place of Safety Order, or the police to take the child into police protection.

⚠ This guidance appears simple—and *is* when abuse is overt—but often it is *difficult* to decide if a child is being abused. If you have worries but cannot justify them sufficiently to invoke child protection procedures:

- Check, via social services, that the child is not on the 'at risk' register
- Check notes of siblings and other family members to see if there has been any suggestion of abuse in the family before
- Discuss your worries with the health visitor and/or other involved members of the primary healthcare team.

If any of these sources ↑ your suspicion, you may be justified in investigating further or invoking child protection measures at that point.

If you still are not sure what to do, record your worries and the reasons for them in the child's notes and alert all other involved members of the practice team. Review whenever that child is seen again in the practice.

Further information

DoH 🖳 *http://www.dh.gov.uk*
- Working together to safeguard children (1998)
- What to do if you're worried a child is being abused (2003)

RCGP (2003) The role of primary care in the protection of children from abuse and neglect 🖳 *http://www.rcgp.org.uk*

Department for Education and Skills (2004) Every Child matters 🖳 *http://www.everychildmatters.gov.uk*

Behavioural problems

GPs are commonly asked to 'sort out' behaviour problems of children by parents at their wits' end. 2–10% of all children are said to have behaviour problems, depending on how the problems are defined and measured.

Differentiation between normal behaviour and behavioural problems can be difficult—especially if you don't know the child or family well. A significant problem is more likely:
- when the behaviour is frequent and chronic
- when >1 problem behaviour occurs
- if behaviour interferes with social and cognitive functioning.

There is no right or wrong way to deal with these problems and the approach outlined below is just one way to tackle them.

Start by gathering background information: If the child is present, watch interactions between the child and parent/carer. It is useful to interview parents both with and without the child and older children both with and without the parent. Diaries can be helpful. Consider:

The child
- Is the child acutely unwell?
- Does the child have a chronic illness or disability?
- Does the child have a physical deformity?
- Does the child have any learning difficulty?
- What is the child's normal temperament like?

The family
- What were the parents' childhoods like?
- Is there family breakdown or marital stress?
- Does either parent or a sibling have a chronic illness or disability (e.g. depression, schizophrenia, cancer)?
- What were the circumstances of the child being born (IVF, adoption, unwanted pregnancy)?
- Is the child living in care or with short-term foster parents?
- What are the parents' expectations of the child?

The environment
- Social deprivation
- Neighbourhood
- Frequent relocations
- School

Find out about the behavioural problems
- What does the child do?
- When did it start?
- When and where does that behaviour occur?
- How do the parents and other carers/teachers react to the behaviour?

Managing the problem: For simple problems, parental education, reassurance, and a few specific suggestions tailored to the problem are often sufficient. Follow-up is important to ensure that the problem is resolving. If simple measures are not succeeding within 3–4mo., consider referral to other agencies e.g. health visitor, school nurse, child psychiatrist. Specific behavioural techniques include:

Behaviour modification: A learning process that requires caregivers to set consistent rules and limits. Parents should try to minimize anger when enforcing rules and ↑ +ve contact with the child.

Discipline: Ineffective discipline may result in inappropriate behaviour. Scolding or physical punishment may briefly control a child's behaviour if used sparingly but may ↓ the child's sense of security and self-esteem. Threats to leave or send the child away are damaging. *Options:*
• *+ve reinforcement for appropriate behaviour:* This is a powerful tool for controlling a child's behaviour, with no adverse effects.
• *Time-out procedure:* The child must sit alone in a dull place for a brief period. Time-outs are a learning process for the child and are best used for controlling a single inappropriate behaviour or a few at one time.

Breaking vicious circle patterns: The child's behaviour (be it normal for that developmental stage or abnormal) evokes a response in the parent or carer which provokes the child to behave in that manner further—thus generating another response from the parent. Try to identify vicious circle patterns and suggest alternative parental responses which make the behaviour futile.

Common behaviour problems: 📖 p.890

Sleep problems: 📖 p.892

Parent information and support
Green (2002) *Toddler taming: a parents guide to the first four years.* Vermilion. ISBN: 0091875285
Green (2000) *Beyond toddlerdom: every parent's guide to the 5–10s.* Vermilion. ISBN:0091816246
Parentline ☎0808 800 2222 🖥 http://www.parentlineplus.org.uk

Patient information and support
Childline: 24h. confidential counselling service ☎0800 1111 🖥 http://www.childline.org

Common behavioural problems

Excessive crying: Babies vary considerably in the amount they cry and ease with which they are soothed. Likewise, parents vary in their ability to tolerate a crying baby. Babies cry for many reasons—discomfort, hunger, loneliness, separation, boredom, etc. If a baby is crying excessively:

- Take a history from the parent—when does the baby cry? Can s/he be consoled? What do the parents do when the baby cries?
- Examine fully from head to toe to exclude causes of discomfort e.g. nappy rash, otitis media, eczema etc.
- Check the baby is growing along his centile line.
- Consider family stress (including postnatal depression—📖 p.808) as a reason why the parent cannot tolerate the crying.
- Treat any underlying cause found and support the family. Information about behavioural techniques used to manage babies that cry excessively is available from the Cry-sis website 🖳 www.cry-sis.org.uk

Feeding problems: Parents commonly complain their child is not eating enough or eating the wrong foods. Usually the child continues to grow and develop normally. If so, reassure the parents. Advise them to:

- Restrict snacks between meals.
- Show little emotion when putting food in front of the child at meal times and remove the food after 15–20min. without comment about what is or isn't eaten.

⚠ If the child is not growing or developing normally, seek an organic cause—refer to paediatrics.

Rhythmic behaviour: Head rocking or banging, thumb sucking, self-stimulation, baby behaviour, and many other variants all occur during normal development. They usually appear if the child is tired, uncertain, or anxious. Reassure parents. Most resolve spontaneously.

Fears and phobias
Fears

- Fears of the dark, monsters, and spiders are common in 3–4y. olds.
- Fears of injury and death are more common in older children.
- Statements made by the parents in anger or jest may be taken literally by preschool children and can be disturbing.
- Frightening stories, films, or TV programmes may be upsetting and intensify fears.

Phobias: Phobias cause persistent, unrealistic, yet intense anxiety in reaction to external situations or stimuli.

Management: Normal developmental stage-related fears must be differentiated from true phobias. If the phobia is intense and interferes with the child's activity or if the child does not respond to simple reassurance, refer to child psychiatry.

School refusal and truancy

Children <10y.: Younger children may refuse to go to school or recurrently complain of abdominal pain, nausea, or other symptoms that justify staying home. Usually school refusal is a form of separation anxiety, though occasionally it is due to a problem at school e.g. problems interacting with the teacher or friends, or bullying. Advise parents to consult the school—a star chart with a star from the teacher for each morning the child goes to school without a fuss may help. Relapses can occur if the child is absent or after holidays.

Older children: School refusal is a more difficult problem. Speak to parents and child together and separately. Try to ascertain if there is a genuine reason why the child avoids school. Liaise with the school. If not succeeding, refer to child psychiatry.

Conduct disorders: Poor behaviour (e.g. aggression, destructive tendencies, and antisocial behaviour) are common complaints. Tolerance varies from family to family. Try simple strategies such as rewarding good behaviour and ignoring poor behaviour ± 'time-out' strategies (younger children—📖 p.889). If not succeeding, refer to child psychiatry.

Hyperactivity: Not easily defined because claims a child is hyperactive often reflect the tolerance level of the person complaining. More active children with shorter-than-average attention spans create management problems. Hyperactivity may have an underlying cause (e.g. an emotional disorder, CNS dysfunction, a genetic component) or may be an exaggeration of normal temperament. Often it is stage-related—support until that stage has passed. Simple behaviour management techniques (📖 p.888–9) may also help. If persistent and associated with learning difficulty or developmental delay, refer to child psychiatry.

Attention deficit hyperactivity disorder (ADHD): 📖 p.899

Tics: Sudden, repetitive, coordinated movements of no apparent purpose. Commonly involve facial grimacing, head movements, or shoulder movements. Average age of onset ≈2y., Tics are present at some point in ~4% of children. Often a family history is present. The majority are precipitated by stress and disappear spontaneously, though some persist into adulthood.

Gilles de la Tourette syndrome: ♂:♀ ≈ 3:1. Characterized by multiple motor tics and irrepressible verbal outbursts—sometimes obscene. There may also be repetitive blinking, nodding, gesturing, echoing of speech, and/or stuttering. Usually begins in childhood. Associated with obsessive-compulsive disorder and ADHD. Probable genetic aetiology.

Management: Spontaneous remissions do occur. Haloperidol or clonidine may help those severely affected with tics. Treat any associated obsessive-compulsive disorder (📖 p.965) or ADHD (📖 p.899).
(*G. Gilles de la Tourette (1857–1904)—French neurologist*)

Parent information and support
Parentline ☎0808 800 2222 🖳 http://www.parentlineplus.org.uk
Cry-sis: Support for families with crying and sleepless babies ☎020 7404 5011
🖳 http://www.cry-sis.org.uk

Patient information and support
Childline: 24h. confidential counselling service ☎0800 1111 🖳 http://www.childline.org

Sleep problems

Sleeping patterns and habits of children vary considerably and should only be regarded as problems when they are presented as such by the family. First take a careful history. Ask about:

- *Medical problems* e.g. night cough related to asthma, itching from eczema, obstructive sleep apnoea—treat appropriately
- *Physical problems* e.g. hunger or cold
- *Night terrors*
- *The sleep pattern*—usually ≥ 1 of:
  - Difficulty settling
  - Waking during the night
  - Waking early in the morning
- *The amount of daytime sleep*

General advice: In all cases, it is helpful to recommend a regular calming bedtime routine (e.g. bath, story, cuddle, bed) and minimal fuss when a child does wake at night e.g. try to settle back to sleep without taking out of cot, not rewarding waking with games, snacks, etc.

Resistance to going to bed: The baby/child who cries incessantly when put to bed is a common problem, with a peak age of 1–2y. The child cries when left alone or climbs out of bed and seeks the parents.

Causes include:

- Separation anxiety
- Increasing attempts by the child to control his environment
- Long naps late in the afternoon
- Rough, overstimulating play before bedtime
- A disturbed parent-child relationship and/or tension in the home

Management: Letting the child stay up, staying in the room, and comforting or punishing the child are all ineffective. Options include:

- *Leaving the child to cry*—this often does work and the crying diminishes after a few nights, but it is very hard for parents to do and can be impossible if they are in shared accommodation.
- *Controlled crying*—the child is left to cry for a set length of time (e.g. 2–10min) before the parent returns to settle him again, with minimum fuss, and then leaves. Length of time before returning is gradually ↑. Easier for parents than leaving the child to cry and still effective.
- *Staying with the child until he sleeps but gradually withdrawing proximity* e.g. sit on bed with child, after a few nights sit next to bed, then nearer door etc., until child learns to go to sleep alone. This method is gentler than the above but may take longer.

Waking during the night: Occurs in ½ children aged 6–12mo. and is related to separation anxiety. In older children, episodes often follow a stressful event (e.g. moving, illness).

Management: Allowing the child to sleep with the parents, playing, feeding, or punishing the child usually prolong the problem.

- Try the methods used for resistance to going to bed (see above)—but advise parents to always check to see that the child is not ill/needing a clean nappy etc. before being left to cry.

- Scheduled waking where a child is woken 15–60mins. before the time he usually wakes and then resettled has also been shown to improve night waking.
- If a child wakes early, another strategy is to make toys or books accessible. The child may then amuse himself for a period of time without disturbing his parents. Some 2–3y. olds wander around without waking the parents—fitting a stairgate across the child's bedroom door prevents the child coming to any harm doing this.
- Use of sedatives e.g. alimemazine (for children >2y.) is often discouraged but can be useful, particularly when parents feel desperate. Only use as a short-term measure.

Nightmares: Occur during rapid eye movement (REM) sleep. Nightmares can be caused by frightening experiences (e.g. scary stories, television violence), particularly in 3–4y. olds. The child usually becomes fully awake and can vividly recall the details of the nightmare. An occasional nightmare is normal, but persistent or frequent nightmares warrant evaluation by an expert.

Sleepwalking (somnambulism): Involves walking clumsily, usually avoiding objects. The child appears confused but not frightened. 15% of children age 5–12y. have sleepwalked one or more times. It is most common amongst school-aged boys and may be triggered by a stressful event.

- Advise parents/carers not to try to wake the child.
- If the child is in danger, gently steer him away from any harm.
- If the child sleepwalks frequently, consider taking action to prevent the child coming to any harm whilst sleepwalking e.g. stairgate across bedroom door.
- If the sleep walks occur repeatedly at the same time, waking the child ~15mins. before the predicted time can break the cycle.

Night terror: Sudden awakening with inconsolable panic and screaming. Usually occurs in the first 1–3h. of sleep. Episodes last seconds → minutes. *Features:*

- Blank or confused stares
- Incomplete arousal with poor responsiveness to people
- Amnesia for the episode.

Night terrors are most common in children aged 3–8y. and require no treatment apart from simple reassurance. Advise parents not to wake the child as this ↑ the disturbance. If frequent, consider waking the child before episodes occur and keeping the child awake for a few minutes to break the cycle. If the terrors persist beyond 8y., consider a diagnosis of temporal lobe epilepsy.

Parent information and support

Parentline ☎0808 800 2222 🖳 http://www.parentlineplus.org.uk
Cry-sis: Support for families with crying and sleepless babies ☎020 7404 5011
   🖳 http://www.cry-sis.org.uk

Toilet training

Most children can do without nappies by day from 2–3y. and by night from 2–5y.. How to approach toilet training will vary from child to child.

General rules

- *Wait until the child is ready:* This usually means that the child can indicate to the parent that s/he is going to the toilet and has shown an interest in using the potty or toilet. It is helpful to have a potty or child's toilet seat (to put on the normal toilet) for the child to become familiar with before starting toilet training.
- *Pick a good time:* When the child can have a few days at home without nappies in an environment where accidents don't matter. Make sure the child has plenty of spare clothes available.
- *Keep the potty handy or stay within easy reach of the toilet:* When the child says he wishes to go, sit him immediately on the toilet. Reward any result with praise. Don't punish the child for any accidents—advise the parent to ask the child to help clear up any mess and reinforce that it would be better to use the potty/toilet next time.
- *Until the child (and parent) are confident in the child's ability to use the toilet, continue using nappies when out and at night:* Take the child to the toilet at night before bedtime. When dry nappies are consistently noted in the mornings, try the child without nappies at night—a plastic sheet on the mattress is a good idea. Even when a child has been dry day and night for some time, accidents are common if the child is tired, unwell, or unsettled (whether excited or unhappy).

❶ If the child does not succeed within a few days, either try training pants or revert to nappies and try again at a later date.

Nocturnal enuresis: Affects 30% of children aged 4y.; 10% at 6y.; 3% at 12y.; and 1% at 18y.. ♂>♀. Tends to run in families.

Cause

- Enuresis usually represents delay in maturation that resolves with time.
- 1–2% have an underlying physical abnormality—usually UTI. Rare causes (congenital anomalies, sacral nerve disorders, DM, diabetes insipidus, pelvic mass) can be excluded by history, examination, urinalysis for glucose, protein, and M,C & S.
- Enuresis is occasionally caused by emotional distress. The child may have been dry then start wetting the bed at night again. If suspected, ask gently about any problems the child is having and manage those problems before treating the enuresis per se.

Management

- *<6y.*—no need for treatment. Most will resolve spontaneously.
- *≥6y.*—refer to the school nurse who can provide equipment and training to control bedwetting. Techniques used—Table 23.6.

Table 23.6 Methods of enuresis control

Method	Features
Motivational counseling	• The child avoids drinks for 2–3h. before bed; urinates before going to bed; records wet and dry nights; and changes clothing and bedding when wet.
	• Rewards (e.g. star chart) are given for dry nights.
	• The child is reassured throughout that the problem is not his fault and just a developmental problem likely to resolve in time.
Enuresis alarms	• An alarm is triggered when the child starts to pass urine.
	• In the first few weeks, the child wakes after complete emptying of the bladder; in the next few weeks, partial inhibition usually occurs; eventually, the child wakes up in response to bladder contractions before he wets the bed.
	• The alarm should be used for at least 3wk. after the last bed-wetting episode.
	• ~70% effective. Relapse occurs in 10–15%.
Desmopressin	• Synthetic version of antidiuretic hormone.
	• Taken at night as nasal spary or tablet.
	• Adverse effects include headache, nausea, nasal congestion, nosebleed, sore throat, cough, flushing, and mild abdominal cramps.
	• Effective in the short term (for 4–6wk.) e.g. to cover holidays.

Encoparesis: Most children are continent of faeces by 2½ –3y. Faecal soiling after this age usually occurs during the day. If:
• The child has bowel control but passes stool in unacceptable places, the cause is usually emotional. Expert help from child psychiatry is needed—refer.
• A firm stool is passed occasionally in the toilet but usually in the pants, developmental delay (either mental or social) is likely. Try a firm, consistent training programme similar to motivational counselling for enuresis (Table 23.6).
• Soft stool oozes out causing the child to constantly soil himself and smell of faeces, consider overflow incontinence 2° to chronic constipation. Treat underlying constipation. Refer to paediatrics if not settling.

Recurrent pains

Recurrent abdominal pain: Occurs in 1:9 children. $\female:\male \approx$ 4:3. Rare before 4–5y. Peak age of presentation is 8–10y. with another peak in girls during early adolescence.

Presentation: The child complaints of recurrent pain—usually colicky in nature. Site and character is variable, though it is most commonly central. There are 2 types of recurrent abdominal pain:
- Those due to organic disease (such as coeliac disease or constipation)
- Those due to functional illness (~90%).

Differentiating functional and organic pain
- The further away the pain is from the umbilicus, the more likely it is to be organic.
- Investigate all children with loin pain to exclude renal causes.
- Accompanying symptoms (e.g. weight ↓, dysuria or ↑ frequency, regular periodicity) also make an organic cause more likely.
- Other behavioural or psychological problems (e.g. school refusal, irrational fears) make a functional diagnosis more likely.

Examination
- If possible, examine the abdomen both whilst the child is in pain and between painful episodes.
- Check for palpable masses and organomegaly—both require urgent investigation.
- Any guarding or rebound tenderness suggests an organic cause.
- If the pain is functional, examination will be normal.

Investigation
- If examination is normal and there are no symptoms suggesting organic disease, check MSU for M,C & S and consider a FBC and ESR. Record the weight of the child at the first assessment and recheck at subsequent visits.
- If there are any accompanying symptoms or signs, consider abdominal ± renal USS and/or referral to paediatrics.

Management of functional abdominal pain
- Acknowledge the pain is real and the worries of both parents and child. Reassure them that there is no serious underlying cause like appendicitis.
- Suggest a balanced diet with plenty of roughage. Encourage adequate fluid intake.
- Reserve paracetamol for episodes of more severe pain than is usual.
- Stress that if the pain changes or is unusually severe, the child should be reassessed by a doctor.
- Most children recover spontaneously with time, though a proportion develop other recurrent pains and some continue to have pain as adults.

Abdominal migraine or periodic syndrome: Stereotyped attacks in which nausea, vomiting, and headache accompany abdominal pain. Treat as for migraine. Some of these children develop classical migraine later.

Recurrent headache: Differential diagnosis of headache in children is the same as for adults (📖 p.596–7). Recurrent headache with no obvious cause is common in children and a source of much parental anxiety, with parents particularly fearing brain tumours.

Presentation
- Site and character are variable—most commonly frontal.
- Accompanying symptoms (e.g. neurological symptoms, headache worse in the early morning) make an organic cause more likely.
- Increasing severity of headache with time requires investigation.
- Aura preceding the headache may suggest classical migraine (📖 p.600).
- Other behavioural or psychological problems (e.g. school refusal, irrational fears) make a functional diagnosis more likely.
- Nausea and vomiting may accompany any type of headache.

Examination
- Neurological examination—including gait, cranial nerves, fundi for papilloedema, and visual acuity in both eyes (a young child can lose vision in 1 eye without noticing).
- Neck and face—looking for local tenderness e.g. from a tooth abscess or sinusitis.
- If the pain is functional, examination will be normal.

Investigation
- Suggest parents have the child's eyes tested (free <16y.).
- No further investigations are needed if the examination is normal and there are no symptoms suggesting organic disease.
- If there are any symptoms suggesting an intracranial cause, refer to paediatrics—as emergency if neurological signs or papilloedema.

Management of functional headache
- Acknowledge the pain is real and the worries of both parents and child. Reassure them that there is no serious underlying cause like a brain tumour.
- Encourage adequate fluid intake.
- Reserve paracetamol for episodes of more severe pain than usual.
- Stress that if the pain should change or be unusually severe, the child should be reassessed by a doctor.
- Most children recover spontaneously with time.
- If, despite reassurance, there is still significant parental worry, refer to paediatrics.

Poor progress at school

~20% of school-age children require special educational services at some point in their schooling. ♂:♀ ≈ 5:1. Consider:
- Does the child have a physical illness affecting his school work e.g. asthma, eczema?
- Is the child on any drugs that might affect his academic performance (e.g. anticonvulsants)?
- Is the family stable or is there family upset?
- Does another member of the family have a chronic or life-threatening illness?
- Is the child's home environment conducive to doing his school work?
- Is this school refusal?
- Is the child happy at school?
- Is there a problem with vision or hearing?
- Is the child of normal intelligence?
- Does the child interact socially with adults and other children?
- Have developmental milestones been met?
- Does the child have specific difficulty with certain aspects of his school work e.g. mathematics, reading, writing?

Specific learning disorders

Speech and language delay: May be a learning disorder, or due to deafness or neurological problems. Usually detected during routine paediatric developmental screening. Refer for hearing assessment and speech and language assessment promptly.

Dyslexia: Affects 3–5% of the population. ♂ > ♀. There is considerable overlap with other specific learning difficulties such as dyscalculia and dyspraxia. IQ is often normal or high and the child appears bright and alert. There may be a FH. If suspected, liaise with the child's school via the teacher. Formal testing by an educational psychologist can confirm the diagnosis.

Dyscalculia: Rarer than dyslexia but contains many of the same features. The core problem is a difficulty handling numbers and mathematical concepts. Management is the same as for dyslexia.

Dyspraxia: Affects 2% of the population in varying degrees—70% are male. IQ is often normal or high. As with dyslexia, children have varying features. Common features are:
- Clumsiness
- Poor posture
- Awkward gait
- Reading and writing difficulties
- Difficulty holding a pen or pencil properly
- Poor short-term memory
- Poor body awareness
- Confusion about which hand to use
- Difficulties throwing/catching balls
- Poor sense of direction
- Difficulty hopping, skipping, and/or riding a bike
- Slow to learn to dress and feed

Management is as for dyslexia.

Severe learning difficulty: 📖 p.900
Autistic spectrum disorder: 📖 p.900

Attention deficit hyperactivity disorder (ADHD)

- Common neurodevelopmental disorder which interferes with normal social function, learning, and development.
- Aetiology is probably multifactorial with overstimulation, family environment, and genetic factors all contributing.
- Affects 0.5–1% of the school-age population in the UK; rare <7y.; $\male:\female \approx$ 6:1.
- ~50% also have disruptive behaviour/conduct disorders, 20–30% a learning disorder, and 25–40% an anxiety disorder. Emotional problems, low self-esteem, nocturnal enuresis, depression, family and relationship problems are also common.
- Long-term ADHD is associated with low academic achievement, substance misuse, unemployment, and antisocial tendencies.

Diagnosis: ❶ Many of these behaviours are seen in normal children.
- *Inattention:* Poor attention to detail and organization of tasks; appears not to listen; easily distracted; forgetful; lack of concentration on tasks.
- *Impulsivity:* Lack of social awareness; shouts out answers to questions; difficulty waiting (unable to take turns or wait in a queue); excessive talking—interrupts others; lack of social awareness.
- *Hyperactivity:* Fidgets; inappropriate running, climbing or leaving seat.
Diagnosis depends on several symptoms being present for ≥6mo. in >1 setting (e.g. school and home) and exclusion of other diagnoses causing similar behavioural pictures.

Differential diagnosis
- Learning disorder
- Hearing problems
- Epilepsy
- Autistic disorder
- Thyroid disease
- Drug ingestion
- Psychological problems (depression, emotional trauma e.g. divorce)

Management: If suspected, refer to community paediatrics or child psychiatry. Specialist treatment includes behavioural therapy, dietary manipulation (though evidence is slim), and drug therapy (e.g. ritalin—controlled drug, multiple side-effects, growth must be monitored). Self-help and local support groups can be helpful.

Information and support

British Dyslexia Association ☎0118 966 8271 🖳 http://www.bda-dyslexia.org.uk
Dyspraxia Foundation: ☎01462 454 986 🖳 http://www.dyspraxiafoundation.org.uk
Children of High Intelligence 🖳 http://www.chi-charity.org.uk
National Attention Deficit Disorder Information and Support Service (ADDISS)
☎020 8906 9068 🖳 http://www.addiss.co.uk
Independent Panel for Special Education Advice (IPSEA) ☎0800 018 4016
 (Scotland—0131 665 4396; Northern Ireland—0232 705654) 🖳 http://www.ipsea.org.uk

Autism and severe learning difficulty (mental handicap)

Autism: A developmental disorder of unknown cause affecting 2/10,000 children. Though autistic spectrum disorders are much more common (9/1000). ♂:♀ ≈ 4:1. Autism is a severely disabling condition for both child and family which requires a great deal of support from the community services, including the GP.

Diagnosis: Not apparent at birth. Usually detected from 18mo.–3y. when failure of social interaction and lack of speech becomes apparent. GPs play a vital role in detection and diagnosis.

Screening: Consider using a screening tool such as the Checklist for Autism in Toddlers (CHAT) for all toddlers with problems with social interaction or speech and language delay at the 18mo. check (available free from the National Autistic Society website).

Features of autism: Triad of:
• Impaired reciprocal social interaction (A symptoms)
• Impaired imagination associated with abnormal verbal and non-verbal communication (B symptoms)
• Restricted repertoires of activities and interests (C symptoms)

Management: There is no proven treatment. Behaviour therapy is sometimes tried. Be an advocate for the family if they have any problems. Be approachable and willing to listen. Having a child or living with an adult with autism is very hard. Advise families:
• To set unwavering rules for behaviour
• To reward and give more attention to good behaviour
• To contact self-help and support organizations
• To ensure they receive all benefits payable (e.g. Carer's Allowance, Disability Living Allowance).

Prognosis: 70% remain severely handicapped—special schooling is often needed; 50% develop useful speech; 20% develop fits in adolescence; 15% lead an independent life.

Asperger's syndrome (autistic psychopathy): A variety of autism in which a child, from the age of ~2y., shows obsessive preoccupation with routines and stereotyped behaviour with distress if the environment is altered. Social isolation and linguistic difficulties are absent. Better prognosis than autism.
(H. Asperger (1906–80)—Austrian paediatrician)

Severe learning difficulty: Arrested or incomplete development of the mind characterized by subnormality of intelligence. May exist alone or with other disabilities. Often noted by a parent first—take any concerns seriously.

Causes: Varied—many are rare. Divide into:
• *Congenital*
  • Genetic e.g. Down's syndrome

- Metabolic e.g. congenital hypothyroidism
- Others e.g. prenatal rubella
- *Acquired:* e.g. trauma, meningitis, birth injury

Management: Refer to paediatrics/genetics to ensure no treatable cause is missed. *Then:*

- *Communicate with carers:* Explain referrals; test results and their implications; the local system and who is responsible for what. Find out about the condition (as far as possible) and tell the carers where to get more information. Ensure carers receive information about benefits and housing/schooling options available.
- *Refer to other community services* e.g. paediatrician; district handicap team. Ensure follow-up happens and assist with assessment of special needs for schooling, housing, and employment. Continue prescription of medication started by other team members.
- *Manage medical problems not related to disability* e.g. sore throats.
- *Promote compliance* with long-term therapy ± education or rehabilitation programmes.
- *Offer family planning, preconceptual counseling, and/or antenatal diagnosis* for parents of children with severe learning disability and patients with severe learning difficulty reaching reproductive age.

Prognosis

- *IQ 50–70*—80% of people with learning disability. Most lead an independent life and require just special attention to their schooling.
- *IQ 35–49*—special schooling or extra support within mainstream schooling and supervision may be needed.
- *IQ <35* severe learning difficulty. Limited social activity and speech may be impaired. Special schooling and medical services are needed. Support and counselling for families involved is important.

The chronically disabled child: 📖 p.904

Information and support

National Autistic Society of the UK (NAS) ☎0845 070 4004 🖳 http://www.nas.org.uk
MENCAP ☎0808 808 1111 🖳 http://www.mencap.org.uk

Adolescence

Changes of adolescence start gradually—from ~11y. for girls and ~13y. for boys—and are complete by the age of ~17y. Adolescence is characterized by rapid physical development and emotional change. Adjusting to these changes causes problems:

- *Concerns about appearance:* Some become very concerned about their appearance. They need reassurance, especially if not growing or maturing as quickly as their friends.
- *Clothes/style* are important to express solidarity with friends and declare independence.
- *Hormonal changes* result in body shape, voice, hair and skin changes, body hair growth, and menstruation. All can be hard to adjust to.
- *Acne* may need treatment—especially if scarring.
- *Dieting and consumption of junk food* are common. Rarely eating disorders develop.

Emotional problems: In the course of their adolescence, >1:5 children think so little of themselves that life does not seem worth living. Emotional disorders are often not recognized, even by family and friends. Overeating, excessive sleepiness, promiscuity, and a persistent overconcern with appearance may be signs of emotional distress. More obviously, phobias and panic attacks appear.

School problems
- *School refusal:* 📖 p.890.
- *Truancy:* Usually children who are unhappy at home and frustrated at school. They spend their days with others who feel the same.
- *Poor school work:* Emotional problems (e.g. worry about problems at home) often affect school work and make it difficult to concentrate. Pressure to do well/pass exams may be counterproductive. Exams are important, but advise parents not to let them dominate life or cause unhappiness.

Abuse: Physical, emotional, or sexual abuse may occur in adolescence—📖 p.886.

Behavioural problems: It is normal for teenagers and their parents to complain about each other's behaviour and disagree frequently. Parents often feel they have lost control over their child. Adolescents resent parental restrictions on their freedom—but still want parental guidance. Advise parents to lay down sensible ground rules and stick to them. Evidence suggests children are at greater risk of getting into trouble if their parents don't know where they are—advise teenagers to let their parents know where they are going and parents to ask.

Sexual problems: >½ of all children will have had sexual intercourse aged <16y. and so fear and risk of pregnancy are part of adolescent life. Those who start to have intercourse early are at greater risk of early pregnancy and health problems such as sexually transmitted disease and cervical cancer. Worries about sexuality for some can add to the pressure. Sensitive support, clear guidance, and accurate information is helpful.

Contraception: 🕮 p.758

Trouble with the law: ♂ > ♀. Most young people do not break the law—when they do, it usually only happens once. Repeated offending may reflect family culture or may result from unhappiness. Always ask about emotional feelings when an adolescent is repeatedly getting into trouble.

Drugs, solvents, and alcohol: Most teenagers never use drugs or inhale solvents, and of those that do, most never get beyond the experimenting stage. Alcohol is the most common drug causing problems for adolescents, but consider the possibility of any form of drug use when parents notice serious, sudden changes in behaviour.

Psychiatric illness: Rarely, changes in behaviour and mood can mark the beginning of more serious psychiatric disorders. Manic depression and schizophrenia, as well as more common disorders such as anxiety, may emerge during adolescent years. Refer for psychiatric assessment if concerned.

Consent: 🕮 p.60

Confidentiality: 🕮 p.62

Eating disorders: 🕮 p.982

Parent information and support
Parentline ☎ 0808 800 2222 🖥 http://www.parentlineplus.org.uk

Patient information and support
Childline: 24h. confidential counselling service ☎0800 1111 🖥 http://www.childline.org
Brook Advisory Service: Contraceptive advice and counselling for teenagers ☎0800 0185 023
🖥 http://www.brook.org.uk
Sexwise: For under 19s ☎0800 28 29 30

The chronically disabled child

Chronic disability due to a wide variety of causes affects ~10% of children in the UK.

Effects on the child: Vary from child to child, dependent on the nature of the disability, personality of the child, and support the child has at home and in the community. Common problems include:

- Physical discomfort—both due to the disability and to painful or embarrassing treatments.
- Alterations in the normal pattern of growth and development and/or physical differences may lead to social isolation and ↓ motivation.
- Frequent hospitalizations and outpatient visits prevent the child integrating into school or ongoing community activities.
- Dependence—the disability may prevent the child reaching his own goals and achieving his own independence. Many children also realise the additional burden they cause their parents and carers.

Effects on the family: Vary from family to family, depending on financial and/or social support, relationship between parents and other siblings, and many other factors. Stress may cause family break-up, especially when other marital and intra-family problems exist. Common problems:

- Grieving for the loss of the 'ideal child'—conditions that affect the appearance of the child particularly affect attachment between parents and child. The grief might take the form of shock, denial, anger, sadness, depression, guilt, or anxiety and may occur any time in the child's development.
- Neglected siblings.
- Inconsistent discipline—due to demands placed on the family and sympathy for the child—resulting in behaviour problems.
- Marginalization of 1 parent—1 parent tends to take on the bulk of the caring activities. There is a danger the other parent starts to feel inadequate and isolated with respect to the care of the child.
- Major expense and time commitment—frequently 1 parent has to give up work to look after a disabled child resulting not only in loss of income but loss of that parent's independence and opportunities for the future.
- Social isolation.
- Confusion over the health, benefits, and social services available.

Care coordination: Inconsistent policies and funding, inadequate access to facilities (including physical barriers to access), and poor communication and coordination between the healthcare, educational, and community support systems → misery for children with disability and their families. Without coordination of services, care is crisis-oriented.

Care coordination requires knowledge about the child's condition, the family, and the community in which they function. In all cases, *someone* should be designated responsible for coordinating care. The best person to do that will vary according to circumstances and could be the community paediatrician, the GP, the health visitor, a specialist support nurse, or the parents (though the complexities of the health and welfare system in the UK often preclude this). Regardless of who assists in coordination of services, the family and child must be partners in the process

Rehabilitation: The general principles of rehabilitation for adult patients apply to children too (📖 p.176 and 626).

Further information

DoH: Children's NSF. 🖳 http://www.dh.gov.uk
HM Government: Carers and Disabled Children Act (2000)
   🖳 http://www.opsi.gov.uk/acts/acts2000/20000016.htm
Audit Commission: Service for Disabled Children (2003)
   🖳 http://www.audit-commission.gov.uk/disabledchildren

Parent and child information and support

Department of Work and Pensions (DWP) Information on benefits for disabled children and their carers ☎0800 88 22 00 🖳 http://www.dwp.gov.uk
Contact a Family: Support and information for families with disabled children (any disability) ☎0808 808 3555 🖳 http://www.cafamily.org.uk
Whizz-Kidz: Mobility for non-mobile disabled children ☎020 7233 6600
   🖳 http://www.whizz-kidz.org.uk
Holiday Care: Holidays for families with a disabled child ☎0845 124 9971
   🖳 http://www.holidaycare.org.uk
Independent Panel for Special Education Advice (IPSEA) ☎0800 018 4016
   (Scotland—0131 665 4396; Northern Ireland—0232 705654) 🖳 http://www.ipsea.org.uk
National Children's Bureau: Council for disabled children; forum for discussion of policy relating to disabled children 🖳 http://www.ncb.org.uk/cdc

Sudden infant death syndrome (cot death) and child death

Sudden infant death syndrome (cot death): ~1:1500babies/y. are found unexpectedly dead in the 1st year of life in the UK. These deaths are most common in winter months and at night (midnight–9a.m.). An identifiable cause can be found for 1:10 deaths; the rest remain unexplained. Theories include cardiac arrythmia and apnoeic attacks. *Peak age:* 1–4mo. ♂ > ♀.

Risk factors for cot death

- Baby sleeping face down
- Smoking (mother and other family members)
- Overheating
- Minor intercurrent illness
- Twin or multiple pregnancy
- Low birth weight
- Social disadvantage
- Young mother
- Large numbers of siblings

Reducing the risk of cot death: 📖 p.815

Management

If you are the first person contacted

- Check an ambulance is on its way and go immediately to the scene. If in doubt, start resuscitation. Continue until the baby gets to hospital.
- If it is clear the baby is dead and can't be resuscitated, inform the parents sympathetically. Contact the police/coroner. Arrange for the baby to be taken to A&E, not to a mortuary. Contact the paediatrician designated for cot deaths who may wish to see the baby and parents as soon as they get to A&E.
- Take a brief history and record the circumstances of death (e.g. position when found, bedding, vomit) immediately. Your notes might be helpful later. Spend time listening to the parents. Mention the baby by name and don't be afraid to express your sorrow.
- If the baby is a twin, the surviving twin is at ↑ risk of cot death and should be admitted to hospital for observation.

If you learn later that a baby has died: Consider:

- A prompt visit to express sympathy and stress that no-one is to blame. There may be some anger directed towards you as often babies have been seen in general practice within a few days or weeks of the death. Do not be defensive or become angry.
- Explain about formalities—necessary post-mortems and coroner's inquests, arranging a funeral, registering the death, etc.
- Discuss suppression of lactation if breastfeeding (📖 p.810).
- Encourage taking photographs of the baby and other mementoes i.e. lock of hair, hand and foot prints.

Follow-up

- Cancel outstanding appointments for the baby (e.g. developmental screening, immunizations) and inform other involved health/social care professionals.
- Review within a few days. Advise parents about likely grief reactions—guilt, anger, ↓ appetite, sleeplessness, hearing the baby cry. Don't

forget siblings—they can be deeply affected too. Continue regular review as long as it is needed and wanted. Be sensitive to anniversaries. Watch for serious psychiatric illness.
- Ensure parents have received written information about cot death including details of self-help organizations and helplines. Consider referral for counselling—ideal timing for referral varies.
- Ensure you get a copy of the post-mortem findings and try to attend the case discussion which should be held ~1mo. after death.
- Parents should have an opportunity to speak to a consultant paediatrician about the death.
- Refer for specialist obstetric assessment early in the next pregnancy and make sure parents are put in touch with the Care of Next Infant (CONI) scheme. Discuss the use of apnoea alarms.

Death of a child in other circumstances: Death of a child is always difficult. Accidents are the most common cause of death, followed by death from childhood cancer. Principles of management used for cot death can be applied (see above).

Apnoea alarms: Commonly issued to or purchased by parents if they are worried about the risk of cot death. An apnoea alarm cannot be useful unless parents are taught basic life support to a proficient standard. An alarm should not be supplied without this training. There is no evidence that apnoea alarms prevent cot deaths.

Near-miss cot deaths: Parents may rush a child to A&E or the GP after an episode of pallor ± floppiness. Parents may have attempted mouth-to-mouth resuscitation before the baby starts to respond to them or may have simply touched the baby or lifted him up and received a response. Usually there are no residual symptoms or signs.

Management: Difficult. Parents may have misinterpreted normal irregularities in sleep or the child might be unwell and have a physical cause for symptoms e.g. early stages of a viral infection. Usually, parents are very anxious by the time you see the child. Take a careful history and examine the child from top to toe. Treat any cause of symptoms found. Be as reassuring as possible and play down anxieties.

⚠ If the child has any risk factors for cot death, comes from a difficult social background, or parents are unable to cope following the episode—admit the child for observation and further assessment.

Further information and parent support

Foundation for the Study of Infant Deaths (FSID) *Guidelines for general practitioners when a baby dies suddenly and unexpectedly* (2003); information, support, administration of the CONI scheme ▣ *http://www.sids.org.uk/fsid*
Child Bereavement Trust ☎0845 357 1000 ▣ *http://www.childbereavement.org.uk*
Child Death Helpline ☎0800 282 986 ▣ *http://www.childdeathhelpline.org.uk*

Ear, nose, and throat

Useful information

ENT UK: British Association of Otorhinolaryngologists—Head and Neck Surgeons
(BAO-HNS): Professional and patient information ⊑ http://www.entuk.org
British Association of Oral and Maxillofacial Surgeons: Professional and patient
information ⊑ http://www.baoms.org.uk

The mouth

⚠ Refer ALL red or white patches in the mouth (erythroplakia and leucoplakia) and mouth ulcers persisting for >3wk. to an oral surgeon for biopsy to exclude malignancy.

Sore mouth: 📖 p.290   **Oral thrush:** 📖 p.672

Apthous ulcers: Painful white ulcers. Common; affecting ≈20%. Usually idiopathic but may be associated with poor health, stress, Crohn's, coeliac, and Behçet's disease. Most are short-lived. Large ulcers (up to 2cm diameter) can take ~6wk. to heal. *Treatment:* most resolve spontaneously. Topical therapies are effective e.g. adcortyl in orabase paste qds or hydrocortisone lozenges qds (dissolve in contact with the ulcer).

Referral: Any patient with an ulcer that is not significantly improving within 3wk. of presentation to exclude malignancy.

Recurrent ulcers: Check FBC, iron and folate levels. *Refer:* patients whose recurrent ulcers cause them distress.

Primary herpes stomatitis: Causes multiple small painful mouth ulcers. If seen <48h. after onset of symptoms, use oral antivirals e.g. aciclovir. *Symptomatic relief:* analgesic mouth rinses e.g. Difflam. A few become unable to take fluids, dehydrated, and require admission for iv fluids. Recurrent attacks and 'cold sores' can be treated with aciclovir cream 5% 5x/d..

Gingivitis: Gum inflammation. Consider immunodeficiency, vitamin C deficiency, DM, leukaemia, and drug causes e.g. phenytoin, nifedipine, ciclosporin.

Vincent's angina: Pharyngeal infection with ulcerative gingivitis. *Management:* try penicillin V 250mg qds po combined with metronidazole 400mg tds po. *(J.H. Vincent (1862–1950)—French bacteriologist)*

Oral cancer: ↑ incidence in the UK. >2000 new cases are diagnosed each year. ♂ > ♀. Survival is poor (30–40% 5y. survival) mainly due to poor public awareness and late presentation. Usually presents as leucoplakia (white patch), erythroplakia (red patch), or a non-healing ulcer (>3wk.). Refer any suspicious lesions for biopsy. *Main risk factors:* tobacco and alcohol use. *Treatment:* surgery ± radiotherapy and chemotherapy.

Halitosis: 📖 p.266

Tongue problems: 📖 p.294

Salivary glands: Problems with the salivary glands include swelling related to food, lumps, pain, and lack of saliva production. Examine the gland with bimanual palpation. Look for secretions and lymphadenopathy and check the facial nerve.

Mumps: 📖 p.492

Acute parotiditis: Unilateral parotid swelling and pain caused by bacterial infection. *Precipitating factors:* surgery, dehydration, and poor oral hygiene. Treat with antibiotics (e.g. metronidazole 200mg bd for 1wk.) and rehydration. If not settling, there may be abscess formation—refer for drainage.

Salivary stones: Can occur in any of the salivary glands but most common in the submandibular (80%). They cause pain and swelling on eating. The gland may appear normal or may be tender and swollen. Stones predispose to infection in the gland by obstruction of saliva flow. Sometimes stones can be visualized at the salivary duct orifice or felt on bimanual palpation. They usually show up on plain X-rays or on sialography. Some pass spontaneously but most need removal. The whole gland may be removed to prevent recurrent problems.

Salivary gland tumours: Refer all salivary gland swellings that do not resolve in <1mo.. Refer earlier if signs of malignancy—pain, rapid growth, hard fixed mass, weight loss, or facial nerve palsy. 80% of tumours are in the parotid gland. *Investigations:* usually CT or MRI scan followed by excision biopsy. *Treatment:* surgery and radiotherapy.

Behçet's disease: Multi-organ disease. *Cause:* unknown—thought to be infective. ♂:♀ ≈ 2:1. Associated with HLA B5/51 genotype. *Clinical picture (only some features are usually present):* arthritis; ocular symptoms and signs (pain, ↓ vision, floaters, iritis); scarring, painful ulceration of mouth and/or scrotum/labia; colitis; meningoencephalitis.

Management: Refer to GUM clinic, ophthalmologist, or general physician (depending on symptom cluster). Treatment is usually with high-dose prednisolone or colchicine. Topical steroids may be useful for ulcers. (*H. Behçet (1889–1948)—Turkish dermatologist*)

Further information
British Association of Oral and Maxillofacial Surgeons: Professional guidelines and patient information 🖳 http://www.baoms.org.uk
● Salivary gland disorders
● Clinical guidelines for the referral of oral squamous cell carcinoma

Patient information
ENT UK Information on Head and Neck Cancer 🖳 http://www.entuk.org

Dental and maxillofacial problems

Encourage patients to register with a dentist—regular dental care helps prevent dental emergencies and peridontal disease. Patients experiencing difficulty finding an NHS dentist should telephone the local Primary Care Organization for assistance.

Peridontal disease: A disease of the peridontal ligament (not primarily bone) caused by bacterial plaque and exacerbated by smoking and DM. Occurs in the normal population from age 30y. Oral hygiene helps prevent plaque accumulation. Leads to gingivitis, dental abscesses, and tooth loss.

Toothache: Pain and excessive sensitivity to temperature may be a problem with exposed dentine or a pulp infection. Advise the patient to see a dentist.

Dental abscess: Facial swelling and pain related to bacterial infection. Advise the patient to see a dentist. Prescribe analgesia and antibiotics (e.g. metronidazole 400mg bd) if there will be a delay.

Loss of tooth through trauma: ≤24h. after loss, a secondary tooth can be successfully replanted if it is prevented from drying out. The shorter the time since the tooth is lost, the more successful the procedure. If possible, push the tooth back into the socket immediately. If not, then store in milk or in some of the patient's saliva until replantation is possible.

Complications of tooth extraction

- *Haemorrhage*—apply pressure by placing wet gauze over socket and get patient to bite hard for 15min. Refer to dentist if not stopping.
- *Painful socket and bad taste in mouth*—infection. Refer to dentist, give analgesia, and start antibiotics (e.g. metronidazole 400mg bd) if there is likely to be a delay.

Wisdom teeth[G]: Removal of wisdom teeth is one of the most common operations in the UK. NICE guidance is that prophylactic removal of impacted wisdom teeth should be discontinued. They estimate ~½ the 50,000 removals in 1998–9 were prophylactic.

Temporomandibular joint (TMJ) disorders: Common disorders affecting ~70% of the population. Fortunately only 5% seek treatment. Typically presents in early adulthood. ♂:♀ ≈ 1:4. Aetiology is complex—malocclusion and trauma may play a part and psychogenic factors exacerbate the problem.

Presentation: Orofacial pain, joint noises, and restricted jaw function. Non-specific symptoms (e.g. headache, earache, and tinnitus) are common. There are 3 patterns of disease:

- *Myofacial pain and dysfunction:* Due to clenching and teeth grinding. Pain is usually worse in the morning. Stress, anxiety, and depression are key features and poor sleep is common. The patient may have diffuse muscle tenderness.

- *Internal derangement:* The articular disc is in an abnormal position and causes restriction of mandibular movement. Pain is usually continuous and exacerbated by jaw movement.
- *Osteoarthrosis:* Degeneration of the joint seen on older patients. Crepitus and sounds from the joint occur on jaw movement.

Management: Take a careful history, especially noting the nature of the pain. Examine the head and neck including the TMJ and mandibular movement. Exclude other disease. Do not X-ray as this yields little useful information. CT/MRI may be ordered by specialists.

Treatment: Explanation and reassurance of the benign nature of the disorder is important and may be all that is needed. Resting the jaw and avoiding stress may help. Refer those patients who have ongoing problems to the oral surgeons. A bite appliance to wear at night helps 70% patients. Physiotherapy, behavioural therapy, and exercises also help. Drug treatments include NSAIDs, antidepressants, opiates, and muscle relaxants. Surgery is occasionally undertaken if medical treatment fails.

Further information

British Association of Oral and Maxillofacial Surgeons: Temporomandibular joint disorders
  🖳 http://www.baoms.org.uk
NICE (2000) Guidance on the removal of wisdom teeth 🖳 http://www.nice.org.uk

Patient information

British Association of Oral and Maxillofacial Surgeons: Wisdom teeth
  🖳 http://www.baoms.org.uk

Sore throat

Each GP sees ≈120 cases/y., most in children and young adults. 90% patients recover within 1wk.. 70% are viral in origin; the rest bacterial (mostly Group A β-haemolytic streptococcus). Complications are rare. Antibiotic prescription can probably be avoided in most patients. Educating patients of the reasons for not prescribing is vital to maintain a good doctor-patient relationship.

Clinical picture: Pain on swallowing, fever, headache, tonsillar exudate, nausea and vomiting, abdominal pain (especially children, due to abdominal lymphadenopathy). Viral and bacterial infections are indistinguishable clinically but association with coryza and cough may point to a viral aetiology.

Differential diagnosis: Glandular fever, especially in young adults with persistent sore throat.

Investigation: Not usually undertaken. Throat swabs cannot distinguish commensal organisms (40% carry Group A β-haemolytic streptococci) from clinical infection, are expensive, and do not give instant results. Therefore rarely used. Rapid antigen tests give immediate results but have low sensitivity, limiting usefulness.

Treatment

- Analgesia and antipyretics, ↑ fluid intake, and gargle with salt water.
- Antibiotics give a modest benefit in symptom relief (8h. less symptoms) and may confer slight protection against some complications (e.g. quinsy and otitis media). There is no evidence antibiotics protect against rheumatic fever or acute glomerulonephritis. Weigh benefits against:
  - The possibility of side-effects with antibiotic use
  - ↑ in community antibiotic resistance
  - 'Medicalizing' the condition—prescribing ↑ faith in antibiotics and encourages re-attendance with future sore throats.
- If prescribing antibiotics, use penicillin V or erythromycin 250mg qds for 5–10d.. Avoid amoxicillin as this causes a rash in those with sore throat due to glandular fever.
- An alternative prescribing strategy is to issue a 'delayed prescription'— for patients to collect if no better in 2–3d. (70% don't collect).

Complications: All rare:

- ***Quinsy (peritonsillar abscess):*** Usually occurs in adults. *Signs:* unilateral peritonsillar swelling, difficulty swallowing (even saliva), and trismus (difficulty opening jaw). *Refer:* for iv antibiotics ± incision and drainage.
- ***Retropharyngeal abscess:*** Occurs in children. *Signs:* inability to swallow, fever. *Refer:* for iv antibiotics ± incision and drainage.
- ***Rheumatic fever:*** 📖 p.350
- ***Glomerulonephritis:*** 📖 p.682

Indications for referral for tonsillectomy

- *Recurrent acute tonsillitis:* Young children have a lot of throat infections and most will 'grow out' of the problem without the need for surgery. Tonsillectomy is only considered if children miss a lot of school: e.g. >5 attacks causing school absence/y. for 2y.
- *Airway obstruction:* Very large tonsils causing sleep apnoea—📖 p.400.
- *Chronic tonsillitis:* >3mo. + halitosis.
- *Recurrent quinsy*
- *Unilateral tonsillar enlargement:* to exclude malignancy.

Tonsillectomy carries a small risk of severe haemorrhage. Readmit any patient with bleeding post op for observation.

Glandular fever (infectious mononucleosis): Consider in teenagers or young adults with sore throat lasting >1wk. Caused by Epstein-Barr virus (EBV). *Incubation:* 4–14d.. *Signs:* sore throat, malaise, fatigue, LNs, enlarged spleen, palatal petechiae, rash (10–20%). Send blood for FBC (atypical lymphocytes) and glandular fever antibodies (Monospot or Paul-Bunnell).

Complications: 2° infections; rash with amoxicillin; hepatitis; jaundice; pneumonitis; neurological disturbances (rare).

Treatment: Rest; fluids; paracetamol; aspirin gargles (if >14y.); avoid alcohol; consider a short course of prednisolone for severe symptoms; treat 2° infection with antibiotics. DON'T prescribe amoxycillin—causes a severe rash. Counsel re the possibility of prolonged symptoms (up to several months).

Tonsillar tumours: Most often seen in the elderly. *Signs:* unilateral tonsillar swelling, dysphagia, sore throat, earache. Refer for excision biopsy.

Further information

SIGN (1999) Management of sore throat and indications for tonsillectomy 🖳 *http://www.sign.ac.uk*

Patient information

ENT UK: Patient information on sore throat and tonsillectomy 🖳 *http://www.entuk.org*

Hoarseness and stridor

Hoarseness: Change in quality of the voice affecting pitch, volume, or resonance. Occurs when vocal cord function is affected by a change in the cords or a neurological or muscular problem. *Causes:*

- *Local causes:* URTI (most common); laryngitis; trauma—shouting, coughing, vomiting, reflux, instrumentation; carcinoma; hypothyroidism (📖 p.423); acromegaly (📖 p.429)
- *Neurological problems:* Laryngeal nerve palsy; motor neurone disease (📖 p.614); myaesthenia gravis (📖 p.623); MS (📖 p.612)
- *Muscular problems:* Muscular dystrophy (📖 p.622)
- *Functional problems:* (below)

History and examination: Weight ↓; dysphagia or neck lumps add to suspicions of malignancy. Check TFTs in those with weight gain. Indirect laryngoscopy with a mirror can be difficult and give a poor view. ENT departments have thin fibreoptic scopes for direct visualization in outpatients.

⚠ Refer all patients with hoarseness lasting >3wk. for ENT assessment to exclude carcinoma.

Laryngitis: Hoarseness, malaise ± fever and/or pain on using voice. Usually viral and self-limiting (1–2wk.) but occasionally 2° bacterial infection occurs. *Treatment:* Rest voice, analgesia, steam inhalations. Consider antibiotics if bacterial infection suspected e.g. penicillin 250mg qds for 1wk..

Vocal cord nodules: Can cause hoarseness. Usually precipitated by overuse of the voice—typically in singers. They can be visualized at laryngoscopy. Initial treatment is resting the voice, but sometimes nodules need to be removed.

Functional disorders: Hysterical paralysis of the vocal cord adductors due to psychological stress can cause the voice to ↓ to a whisper or be lost completely. More common amongst young women. Refer for laryngoscopy to exclude organic cause. *Treatment:* Speech therapy and psychological support.

Laryngeal carcinoma: ♂ > ♀. Smoking is the main risk factor. First sign is usually hoarseness followed by stridor, dysphagia, and pain. *Investigations:* Laryngoscopy and biopsy. *Treatment:* Surgery ± radiotherapy. Early tumours confined to the vocal cord have 80–90% 5y. survival.

Stridor: Children > adults. Noise created on inspiration due to narrowing of the larynx or trachea. *Signs of severe airway narrowing:* Distress, ↑ respiratory rate, pallor and cyanosis, use of accessory muscles, and tracheal tug. *Causes:* Congenital abnormalities of the larynx, epiglottis, croup (laryngotracheobronchitis), inhaled foreign body, trauma, and laryngeal paralysis.

Croup: 📖 p.851

Acute epiglottitis: Bacterial infection causing a swollen epiglottis. Can potentially obstruct the airway. Much rarer since introduction of HIB immunization (📖 p.487).

Presentation: Look for stridor, drooling, fever, upright leaning forward posture.

⚠ If suspected, DON'T examine the child's throat as this can precipitate complete obstruction.

Management
- *Child:* Refer urgently but try to maintain a calm atmosphere to avoid distressing the child. Examination will be undertaken in hospital with full resuscitation facilities on hand. *Treatment:* iv antibiotics.
- *Adult:* Adult epiglottitis is much less common and less likely to cause complete airway obstruction. Refer for iv antibiotics.

Laryngomalacia (congenital laryngeal stridor): Common—due to floppy aryatic folds and the small size of the airway in young children. Stridor becomes more noticeable during sleep, excitement, crying, and with concurrent URTIs. Normally resolves without treatment but parental concern may necessitate referral.

Inhaled foreign body: Refer to ENT for assessment.

Post-laryngectomy problems: After laryngectomy, patients have a permanent tracheostomy and require practical and psychological support. Problems include excessive secretions and stenosis of the tracheostomy site, recurrent pneumonia, communication difficulties. Ensure referred to speech therapy and maintaining an adequate diet.

Patient information and support
ENT UK: Patient information on hoarseness and laryngitis ▣ http://www.entuk.org
Cancer Research UK: Patient information on laryngeal cancer
▣ http://www.cancerhelp.org.uk

Nasal problems

Nasal polyps: Most common in men age >40y.. Associated with asthma, allergic rhinitis, and chronic sinusitis. Consider cystic fibrosis in children <16y..

Symptoms: Nasal blockage; watery discharge; post nasal drip; change in voice; loss of smell; and taste disturbance.

Signs: Polyps are smooth and pale, usually bilateral, and commonly arise from the middle meatus and middle turbinates. They may completely block the nasal passage. They can be confused with enlarged inferior turbinates but are more mobile and lack sensation.

Management
- Try medical treatment: steroid nasal drops e.g. beclometasone 0.1% bd until polyps shrink (max 1mo.) and then maintenance on steroid nasal sprays.
- Swab and give antibiotics if purulent nasal discharge.
- Refer for assessment and consideration of surgical treatment (polypectomy) if medical treatment fails. ❶ Polyps often recur after surgery.

⚠ Refer unilateral polyps with an unusual or irregular appearance, especially if ulcerating and/or bleeding, for exclusion of malignancy.

Deviated nasal septum: Common in adults—usually 2° to injury. May be associated with external deformity. Nasal blockage is unilateral. Treat mucosal swelling due to rhinitis first as that may be sufficient to control symptoms. If unsuccessful, refer for surgery (submucous resection).

Foreign bodies in the nose: Common in young children. Refer all children with unilateral offensive discharge for exploration under GA. Do not try to remove a foreign body yourself unless the object is very superficial and the child cooperative. You might push the object further in and cause trauma.

Injury to the nose: Injury can be to the nasal skin (lacerations), bone (fracture), or cartilage (septal haematoma and deviation). The upper $1/3$ of the nose has bony support; the lower $1/3$ and septum are cartilaginous. Isolated skin lacerations can be closed with sutures or steri-strips.

⚠ DON'T use local anaesthetic containing adrenaline to anaesthetize the nose.

Fractured nose
- Undisplaced nasal fractures can usually be allowed to heal without intervention. X-rays are unhelpful.
- Give adequate analgesia and advise that bruising may be extensive and the nose will feel blocked for 1–2wk.
- Assessment for permanent deformity can be difficult at the time of the injury due to soft tissue swelling. Reassess 7–10d. after injury and refer any patient with significant deformity, or if the patient is unhappy with the appearance of their nose, to the ENT department for reduction under GA. Ideally, reduction should take place within 1–2wk. (and max. 3wk.) after fracture—so refer promptly.

- Deviation of the nasal septum may not be correctable at the time of manipulation and, if symptomatic, will need a later submucous resection.

⚠ **Neurological assessment** is required if the patient has had a head injury or loss of consciousness (📖 p.546). Always look for associated fractures of the zygoma and maxillary bones ('step' deformity in the orbit, dental malocclusion, difficulty opening the jaw, diplopia) and refer urgently to the maxillofacial surgeons, if present.

Septal haematoma: May occur after injury and causes nasal blockage. Presents as a bilateral soft bulging of the septum. Refer urgently to ENT for evacuation to prevent cartilage destruction.

CSF rhinorrhoea: Clear fluid dripping from the nose after trauma can indicate a fracture of the roof of the ethmoid labyrinth and CSF leak. Fluid tests +ve for glucose. It suggests significant trauma—consider referral for head injury assessment. Spontaneous healing of the CSF leak is the norm but if it persists, refer to neurosurgery for assessment for dural closure.

Septal perforation: Can cause bleeding, crusting, and discomfort. *Causes:* trauma, nose picking, cocaine use, post-operative, malignancy. Refer if suspicion of malignancy, otherwise treat symptomatically (e.g. vaseline or naseptin for crusting). Surgical closure is often not successful.

Sinusitis

Acute sinusitis: Usually follows URTI, though 10% due to tooth infection. *Features:* frontal headache/facial pain (may be difficult to distinguish from toothache)—typically worse on movement/bending ± purulent nasal discharge ± fever. *Management:* steam inhalation; short course decongestants; antibiotics (e.g. amoxicillin 250–500mg tds, erythromycin 250–500mg qds—limited evidence of benefit); steroid nasal spray.

Chronic/recurrent sinusitis: Post-nasal drip (may cause chronic cough—📖 p.254); frontal headache/facial pain; blocked nose. Associated with nasal polyps and vasomotor rhinitis (📖 p.921). Treat as for acute sinusitis. Refer to ENT if symptoms are interfering with life—surgery may help.

Patient information

ENT UK: Information on nasal polyps, nasal injury, sinusitis, nasal obstruction 🖥 http://www.entuk.org

Rhinitis

Allergic rhinitis: Common disorder that may be seasonal or perennial.

Symptoms: Bilateral intermittent nasal blockage; itchy nose, eyes, palate, and throat; sneezing; watery nasal discharge.

Signs: Swollen inferior turbinates; ↓ nasal airway; pale or mauve mucosa; nasal discharge; 'allergic crease' on bridge of nose from persistent rubbing (especially in young sufferers). Ask about potential allergens e.g. pollen, feathers, house dust mite, moulds, and animals.

Investigation: If symptoms are intrusive and difficult to control, refer to allergy clinic for skin prick testing or RAST (radio-allergosorbent) testing. Blood tests for IgE may help identify allergens.

Management

- *↓ allergen exposure:* 📖 p.379
- *Inhalation of steam* ± menthol may give some temporary relief from the discomfort of nasal blockage and can be repeated every 2h.
- *Medication:* Table 24.2
- *Surgical intervention:* e.g. referral for nasal cautery or partial excision of the inferior nasal turbinates. Consider if severe blockage and failure of medical treatment.
- *Desensitization:* Desensitization to allergens by courses of injections has been used in the past and is still used in other countries. 50–70% success rate. Risk of anaphylaxis is high so, in the UK, provision is limited to specialist centres with observation areas and full resuscitation facilities. Refer via an allergy clinic.

Hayfever: Allergic rhinitis and/or allergic conjunctivitis and/or wheeze due to an allergic reaction to pollen. The type of pollen that causes hayfever is connected to where the sufferer lives. In the UK, most hayfever is caused by grass pollen (60%) and silver birch pollen (25%). It occurs at different times in the year depending on which pollen is involved (Table 24.1).

Management

- *When the pollen count is high:* Keep windows shut (including car windows—consider pollen filter for the car); wear glasses/sunglasses; avoid grassy spaces.
- Treat with systemic antihistamine e.g. loratadine 10mg od and/or topical steroid nasal spray e.g. beclometasone 2 puffs bd to each nostril and/or eye drops e.g. nedocromil sodium 1 drop to each eye bd. Start treatment 2–3wk. before the pollen season starts.

Table 24.1 Predominant pollen types in the UK

Jan	Feb	Mar	Apr	May	Jun	Jul	Aug	Sep	Oct	Nov	Dec
Alder Hazel		Elm Willow Ash	Silver birch	Oak	Weed pollen						
					Grass pollen			Fungal spores			

Table 24.2 Drug treatment of allergic rhinitis (BNF 12.2.1 and 12.2.2)

Category	Example	Notes
Intranasal steroid sprays	Beclometasone 2 puffs bd to each nostril	Effective and can be used safely long term. Take >1wk. to show benefit—try for >2mo. before abandoning.
Nasal steroid drops	Beclometasone 0.1% 2 drops tds to each nostril	More systemic absorption than intranasal steroid sprays—only use for a limited period (e.g. 1mo.) and restrict to adults unless prescribed under specialist supervision.
		Method of administration: 'head down' position—kneel with forehead on floor and nostrils pointing skyward; instill drops and maintain this position for 2min.
Topical antihistamines	Azelastine 1 bd to each nostril	Can be used as an alternative to topical steroids.
Topical decongestants	Ephedrine 1 or 2 drops to each nostril tds/qds prn	Short term (e.g. 5–7d.) for nasal blockage. Of dubious value.
		Longer term may cause a vicious circle—**rhinitis medicamentosa:** vasoconstriction → mucosal damage → rebound engorgement and oedema → more decongestant use.
Antimuscarinic nasal spray	Ipratropium 2 sprays to each nostril bd/tds	Helps ↓ watery nasal discharge but has little effect on itch, sneezing, or nasal obstruction.
Other nasal sprays	Sodium cromoglicate 1 puff to each nostril bd/tds or qds	Less effective than topical steroids but can be useful, particularly in children, to give some relief.
Oral antihistamine	Loratidine 10mg od	Can be helpful used alone or in addition to nasal preparations.
Oral or intramuscular steroids	Prednisolone 10mg od or kenalog depot	May be used occasionally for short-term control of severe symptoms e.g. at exam times. A last option.

Vasomotor rhinitis: May be difficult to distinguish from allergic rhinitis as signs and symptoms are similar. Both are common and they may coexist in the same patient. Vasomotor rhinitis tends to have less itch and symptoms may be exacerbated by tobacco, change in air temperature, and perfumes.

Management
- Try measures for allergic rhinitis, as appropriate. Often less successful.
- Ipratropiun bromide helps watery nasal discharge.
- Decongestant tablets (e.g. pseudoephedrine) used short term may help.

Patient information
BBC pollen index ⌨ http://www.bbc.co.uk/weather/pollen

Painful and discharging ears

Earache is a common presenting symptom in general practice. It is often a sign of an ear infection, but if the ears are normal on examination, you should look for a cause of referred pain i.e. from the throat, teeth, sinuses, facial nerve, lymph glands, or wounds in neck.

⚠ Always exclude a perforated drum in discharging ears—beware of cholesteatoma. If you cannot visualize the drum, review the patient.

Otitis media: Infection of the middle ear. Can be bacterial or viral—clinically impossible to distinguish.

Prevention: Parental smoking ↑ children's risk.

Presentation
- *Symptoms:* Painful ear (often unilateral), deafness, systemic illness, and pyrexia. May have purulent and bloody discharge associated with relief of pain if there is a spontaneous perforation.
- *Signs:* Red, bulging drum.

Management
- 80% resolve in ≤3d. without treatment.
- Advise paracetamol and/or NSAIDs for analgesia.
- *Antibiotics:* Symptoms resolve 24h. earlier with antibiotics but they have side-effects and ↑ community antibiotic resistance. Many GPs are now using a 'delayed' approach—prescribing if symptoms are no better in 3d.
- *Perforated ear drum:* Most GPs prescribe antibiotics (e.g. amoxicillin 250–500mg tds for 5–7d.) at presentation if a perforation is present.
- *Refer:* If recurrent attacks or if acute perforation does not heal in <1mo..
- Chronic secretory otitis media: 📖 p.926

Complications: Mastoiditis (rare)—tenderness ± swelling over mastoid, low-grade fever, malaise, hearing loss, persistent discharge, ear may stick out. Suspect if >10d. discharge. Refer to ENT for assessment and iv antibiotics as can lead to labyrinthitis, facial palsy, meningitis, and brain abscess.

Barotrauma: Due to changes in atmospheric pressure (e.g. air travel, diving) in those with poor Eustachian tube function. *Symptoms:* ear pain, vertigo, conductive hearing loss, perforation. *Prognosis:* spontaneous resolution within 2–3wk. *Prevention:* valsalva manoeuvre during flight, decongestants (e.g. pseudoephedrine 120mg 30min. prior to flight). Patients with middle ear effusions should not fly.

Furunculosis: Infection of the hair follicles of the outer $^1/_3$ of the ear canal. *Symptoms:* severe pain—may be exacerbated by moving tragus or opening jaw. *Signs:* boil in the ear canal. *Investigations:* exclude DM. *Treatment:* analgesia, topical antibiotics, and steroid drops e.g. Gentisone HC 3 drops qds for 1wk.; oral antibiotics if cellulitis e.g. flucloxacillin 250–500mg qds for 1wk..

Ramsay Hunt syndrome (Herpes zoster oticus): Severe pain in the ear precedes facial nerve palsy. Zoster vesicles appear around the ear, in the external ear canal, on the soft palate, and in the tonsillar fossa. Often accompanied by deafness ± vertigo which are slow to resolve and may result in permanent deficit. Pain usually abates after 48h. but post-herpetic neuralgia can be a problem. If detected <24h. after the rash appears, treatment with antivirals (e.g. aciclovir 800mg 5x/d. for 1wk.) may be effective. (*J. Ramsay Hunt (1872–1937)—US neurologist*)

Otitis externa: Often occurs in itchy ears—due to scratching or after swimming. *Symptoms:* pain (often severe), discharge (may be offensive), pain on moving pinna. *Signs:* swollen ear canal with discharge and debris, may have swollen lymph glands behind or in front of ear.

Management
* Except in mild cases, need to remove infected material. Gentle syringing may work; if not, needs aural toilet—*refer* to ENT.
* Antibiotic ear drops can be used after removal of debris e.g. gentamicin 0.3%. They are often used in combination with a steroid (e.g. Gentisone HC) to ↓ inflammation and settle eczema.
* Strong analgesia may be needed.
* Severe cases require frequent aural toilet (every few days) and a wick placed in the ear canal.
* Refractory disease may indicate candida or aspergillus infection—swab and treat with clotrimazole solution tds for 14d.

Prevention
* No cleaning ears with cotton buds.
* Avoid getting ears wet in the shower/bath.
* Itchiness (eczema)—intermittent short courses of steroid ear drops (e.g. prednisolone 0.5% ear drops 2–3 drops tds).

Haematoma of the pinna: Usually after trauma (e.g. rugby). Must be evacuated urgently (aspirated via large bore needle or surgically) to prevent necrosis of the cartilage and 'cauliflower' ear. Refer.

Foreign bodies in the ear: Most common in children. Try to remove under direct vision with forceps but avoid pushing objects deeper into the canal and causing damage. Don't poke around with forceps in an uncooperative child. Removal under GA may be needed. Insects can be drowned in oil and syringed out.

Useful information
ENT UK: Patient information on ear infections 🖳 http://www.entuk.org

Deafness

Childhood deafness: Temporary deafness is common due to middle ear infections but permanent deafness is rare (1–2/1000). ↓ hearing is often noticed by parents or teachers—take concerns seriously and refer for assessment. Deafness causes long-term speech, language ± behavioural problems and early intervention makes a difference.

Management: History, examination, assess hearing as appropriate for age. Assess development (including speech and language). Treat or refer according to cause:
- *If no earache consider:* Bilateral glue ear; impacted wax; hereditary cause; history of meningitis, head injury, or birth complications.
- *If earache consider:* Acute otitis media; impacted wax.

Hearing assessment in children: 📖 p.827

Adult deafness: Common and debilitating, leading to isolation and depression. Presentation tends to be late. Patients have many underlying fears and concerns (e.g. ability to work and live independently). *Causes:*
- ***Conductive deafness:*** Wax, debris, or foreign body in the ear canal; perforation of the drum (trauma, infection); middle ear effusion (eustachian tube dysfunction due to infection or postnasal space tumour); otosclerosis (📖 p.927).
- ***Sensorineural deafness:*** Presbyacusis (age related). *Rarer causes:* infections (meningitis, measles); Ménière's (📖 p.929); ototoxic drugs (aminoglycosides); acoustic neuroma (📖 p.927).

Presentation: Usually hearing loss develops insidiously with increasing problems understanding others when there is background noise. Tinnitus may be the presenting problem.

Management: Examine drum; exclude wax; consider postnasal space tumour (especially in those of Chinese ethnic origin). If no self-limiting cause found, refer for a hearing test to quantify hearing loss and assess suitability for hearing aid.

> ⚠ *Refer to ENT if:*
> - Conductive deafness of unknown cause;
> - Sudden deafness if no wax visible;
> - Asymmetrical deafness—to exclude rare dangerous diagnoses e.g. acoustic neuroma, cholesteatoma, nasopharyngeal carcinoma.

Useful screening questions
- Do other people mumble a lot?
- Do you find yourself frequently saying 'pardon'?
- Does the family say the TV is too loud?
- Do you miss hearing the door bell or 'phone'?
- Do you occasionally get the wrong end of the stick in a conversation?

Hearing tests

Whispered voice and conversational voice: Obscure lips to prevent lip reading and mask contralateral ear by rubbing the tragus.

Tuning fork tests (512Hz)
* *Rinne:* Hold vibrating tuning fork close to meatus until patient signals that it can no longer be heard, then apply base to mastoid process. If hearing is normal or there is sensorineural hearing loss, air conduction is better than bone—termed +ve Rinnes test. A –ve test suggests conductive deafness.
* *Weber:* A vibrating tuning fork placed on the forehead is normally heard equally in both ears. In conductive deafness, sound localizes to the affected ear; and in sensorineural deafness, to the contralateral ear.

Audiometry and tympanometry: May be available in the GP surgery, by referral to a community audiometry service or ENT department depending on local arrangements.

Benefits for deaf people: Deaf people can claim benefits in the same way as any other person with a disability (📖 p.97–115). Capability for work—Table 24.3.

Table 24.3 Patients considered incapable of work (and able to claim incapacity benefit)

Hearing	Speech
• They can't hear sounds at all	• They can't speak
• They can't hear well enough to follow a television programme with the volume turned up	• Speech can't be understood by family or friends
• They can't hear well enough to understand someone talking in a loud voice in a quiet room	• Speech can't be understood by strangers

❶ Ability to lip read or get clues from the speaker's gestures should not be taken into account. Those with more hearing or clearer speech may still be eligible if their combined speech and hearing problems render them incapable of work or they suffer from other coexisting disabilities.

Patient information and support

National Deaf Children's Society ☎0808 800 8880 🖥 *http://www.ndcs.org.uk*
Royal National Institute for the Deaf ☎0808 808 0123 *Text phone:* ☎0808 808 9000 🖥 *http://www.rnid.org.uk*
British Deaf Association Helpline ☎0870 770 3300 *Text phone* ☎0800 6522 965 🖥 *http://www.signcommunity.org.uk*
Hearing concern ☎0208 233 2929 🖥 *http://www.hearingconcern.org.uk*
ENT UK: Patient information on deafness and hearing aids 🖥 *http://www.entuk.org*

Causes of deafness

Glue ear (otitis media with effusion): Fluid behind the ear drum due to inadequate drainage via the Eustachian tube. Common after acute otitis media (📖 p.922) or URTI. Associated with Down's Syndrome and cleft lip/palate. *Natural history:* 75% resolve in <3mo..

Presentation: *Symptoms:* deafness ± earache, difficulties with speech and language, and behavioural problems. *Signs:* dull, concave drum with visible peripheral vessels. Behind the drum there may be a fluid level or air bubbles.

Management: Refer to community audiology service or ENT if not resolving, especially if speech or language delay. In children, it is an age-related condition that resolves as the child grows older—any treatment is aimed at ↓ impact of symptoms until natural resolution occurs. Watchful waiting can be used in asymptomatic or mild cases.

- **Medical treatment:** decongestants, oral steroids and nasal drops do not help; long-term antibiotics (e.g. amoxycillin 2–6wk.) and mucolytics may have a short-term benefit as may autoinflation with a nasal balloon.
- **Surgical treatment:** grommets ± adenoidectomy have temporary benefits (6–24mo.). Grommets are air-conducting tubes inserted through the ear drum. Most are extruded spontaneously <9mo. after insertion. They may need reinsertion if deafness recurs. Discharge from the ear occurs in some children with grommets—treat with aural toilet and antibiotic/steroid drops (see otitis externa—📖 p.923). Swimming and bathing are allowed after grommet insertion but avoid diving.

Presbyacusis: Bilateral symmetrical sensorineural deafness in the over 50s is most likely to be due to presbyacusis. Deafness is gradual in onset and due to high-frequency loss. Thus speech discrimination particularly of high-pitched voices is lost first. *Management:* assess with hearing test and refer for hearing aid.

Wax in the ear canal and syringing: Wax can be removed by syringing provided perforation of the drum is not suspected. For hard wax, soften with 5% sodium bicarbonate drops or olive oil tds for 5d. prior to syringing. Do not syringe ears after mastoid operations.

Chronic suppurative otitis media and cholesteatoma: Discharge (may be offensive) and hearing loss but no pain.
- **Central perforation:** 'safe disease'. Treat as for otitis externa to dry discharge and encourage drum healing[C]. Refer if persistent discharge, deafness, vertigo, or earache. Surgery to close the drum may help discharge.
- **Attic or marginal perforation:** 'unsafe disease'. May indicate *cholesteatoma* (stratified squamous epithelium invades the middle ear and can cause local damage leading to deafness, vertigo, facial nerve palsy, cerebral abscesses, and meningitis). Refer to ENT—may need surgery to remove invasive tissue.

Otosclerosis: Bilateral conductive deafness due to adherence of the stapes footplate to the bone around the oval window. Often family history (50%). May deteriorate in pregnancy (if does, then avoid prescribing the oral contraceptive pill). *Treatment:* refer for assessment for surgery to replace stapes with an implant.

Acoustic neuroma: A slow-growing neurofibroma arising from the acoustic nerve. *Symptoms:* unilateral sensorineural deafness, tinnitus ± facial palsy. Refer. *Treatment:* surgery.

⚠ Refer all cases of unilateral or asymmetrical deafness to ENT for MRI to exclude an acoustic neuroma.

Noise-induced deafness: Exposure to noise >85dB can cause hearing damage. Employees should be protected from noise and provided with ear protection if working in noisy environments. They may be eligible for compensation if they have not been protected (📖 p.114–5) or if war veterans (📖 p.100). Refer for audiology if in doubt. Noise exposure can also occur in non-work settings e.g. discos, firearm sports. Immediate indications are ringing in the ears or hearing appearing muffled after exposure.

Tinnitus and vertigo

Tinnitus: Ringing or buzzing heard in the ears or head. Occasional tinnitus is common (15% of population) but 2% are severely affected. Patients with tinnitus that interferes with daily life and sleep are prone to depression. *Cause:* Often unknown. May accompany hearing loss, noise exposure, head injury, Ménières, anaemia, ↑BP, drugs (loop diuretics, tricyclics, aminoglycosides, aspirin, NSAIDs).

Management: Reassurance that there is no sinister cause. Refer to audiology for a hearing aid if there is deafness. Drugs are not usually helpful but look for and treat associated depression. Psychological support is important—consider referral to a hearing therapist and support group (e.g. Tinnitus Association). Masking with background music/radio or an aid that produces white noise (available via ENT) can help. Surgical sectioning of the cochlear nerve is a last resort and causes deafness.

Indications for referral to ENT: Objective tinnitus (noise can be heard by an observer—rare and may be due to vascular malformations or tempormandibular joint problems); unilateral tinnitus (especially if associated with deafness—exclude acoustic neuroma).

Vertigo: An illusion that the surroundings are spinning. Ask about duration and frequency, associated nausea, deafness and tinnitus, and recent viral symptoms. *Causes:*

- *Episodic vertigo lasting a few seconds or minutes:* Commonly due to benign positional vertigo.
- *Episodic vertigo lasting minutes to hours:* Consider Ménières.
- *Prolonged vertigo (>24h.):* Peripheral lesion (e.g. viral labyrinthitis or trauma) or a central lesion (usually associated with other signs—e.g. multiple sclerosis, stroke, tumour).

Examination: Look for neurological signs, especially cerebellar signs, cranial nerves, and Romberg's sign; assess nystagmus, ear drums, and hearing; check BP; Hallpike manoeuvre (move patient quickly from sitting to lying with head turned to one side and extended over the end of the bed, look for nystagmus, and ask about vertigo; repeat with head turned to the other side).

Benign positional vertigo: Sudden onset of vertigo lasting only a few seconds or minutes. Occurs with sudden changes in posture. Common after head injury or viral illness. *Cause:* Possibly otoliths in the labyrinth. *Diagnosis:* From history and +ve Hallpike test (see above). Normal tympanic membrane. *Natural history:* Usually self-limiting (few weeks) although in a few cases, may continue intermittently for years.

Management: Reassure. Labyrinthine sedatives are not helpful. Teach the patient to minimize symptoms by sitting and lying in stages. Habituation may occur by maintaining trigger position until vertigo settles. If not settling, refer to ENT for physiotherapy or for Epleys' manoeuvre[C] (rapid repositioning of head to move otoliths out of the labyrinth).

Viral labyrnthitis: Usually follows a viral URTI. *Symptoms and signs:* Sudden onset of vertigo, prostration, nausea and vomiting, no associated loss of hearing, normal tympanic membrane. *Treatment:* Labyrinthine sedatives e.g. cyclizine or prochlorperazine. *Natural history:* Usually resolves in 2–3wk. If persists >6wk., refer.

Ménières syndrome: Overdiagnosed in patients with recurrent vertigo and deafness. It is a complex of symptoms including clustering of attacks of vertigo and nausea, tinnitus, a sense of fullness in the ear, and sensorineural deafness which may be progressive. *Aetiology:* Idiopathic dilation of endolymphatic spaces. *Refer:* All suspected cases for confirmation of the diagnosis. (*P. Ménière (1799–1862)—French ENT surgeon*)

Management: Acute attacks need labyrinthine sedatives e.g. cyclizine or prochlorperazine. Betahistine may help in some patients as may thiazide diuretics and a low salt diet. There are some indications that stress may precipitate attacks. Labyrinthectomy is a last resort and can help vertigo but results in deafness on that side.

Vertebro-basilar insufficiency: Common in older patients, usually diagnosed on the basis of a history of dizziness on extension and rotation of the neck. Normal tympanic membranes. May have associated cervical spondylosis and neck pain. *Treatment:* Lifestyle advice. Some advocate use of a cervical collar.

Patient information and support

ENT UK: Patient information on tinnitus, dizziness, and vertigo ⌨ *http://www.entuk.org*
British Tinnitus Association ☎0800 018 0527 ⌨ *http://www.tinnitus.org.uk*
Ménières Society ☎0845 120 2975 ⌨ *http://www.menieres.co.uk*

Chapter 25

Ophthalmology

Useful websites

Royal College of Ophthalmologists: Published guidelines available on-line and numerous patient information sheets
🖳 *http://www.rcophth.ac.uk*
Royal National Institute for the Blind: Patient information sheets
🖳 *http://www.rnib.org.uk*
Moorfields Eye Hospital: Patient information sheets
🖳 *http://www.moorfields.org.uk*
Good Hope NHS Hospital Trust: GP information, patient information sheets, and lots of useful weblinks
🖳 *http://www.goodhope.org.uk/Departments/eyedept/index.htm*
Eye Atlas: Excellent photographs of many conditions
🖳 *http://www.eyeatlas.com*

Assessment of the eye in general practice

History: Ask about pain, redness, watering, a change in appearance of the eye, altered vision, and if the problem is unilateral or bilateral. Distinguish between blurred and double vision. Enquire about trauma, previous similar episodes, systemic illness, and eye disease in the family.

Examination: The eyelids should be symmetrical—drooping or elevation of the upper lid may be due to nerve lesions (📖 p.588) or thyroid disease (📖 p.422). Check the skin around the lids, position of eyelashes, and any inflammation, crusting, or swelling of the lid or lid margin. Then examine the eye surface—it should be bright and shiny. Use a fluorescein stain if any indication of corneal damage. Note any redness—if most marked around the lid lining and periphery of the eye, conjunctivitis is likely, where as a duskier redness around the margin of the cornea (ciliary congestion) suggests disease of the cornea, iris, or deeper parts of the eye (uvea).

Examining the ocular media: Takes practice. Darken the room and ensure you have good batteries in the ophthalmoscope. Check the red reflex (opacities within the eye appear as a shadow). Then focus onto the retina. Use a systematic approach to avoid missing anything i.e. start at the optic disc (look for shape, colour, and size of the cup) and then follow each of the 4 main vessels to the periphery. End by examining the macula: ask the patient to look directly at the light. Dilating the pupils with a short-acting mydriatic (e.g. 0.5–1% tropicamide) makes examination much easier—warn patients they may have temporarily blurred vision and should not drive home.

Visual acuity: Test and record the central (macular) vision of each eye separately (with glasses on if worn) for both near and distance. Cover the non-test eye carefully. On a full size Snellen chart, line '6' can be read by the normal eye at 6m (📖 p.935). Near vision can be checked using a newspaper or a near vision testing card (📖 p.934). If patients have forgotten their glasses, use a 'pin hole' to look through (it removes most refractive problems).

Visual fields: Test peripheral vision by sitting in front of the patient and comparing their visual field to your own (one eye at a time). The most basic test is to check the patient can see hand movement in each of the four quadrants. This may reveal hemianopia from damage to visual pathways or field loss due to glaucoma (the patient may be unaware of the loss). Refer for formal tests. Visual field defects 📖 p.295.

Eye movements: If the patient complains of double vision, move an object to the 6 positions of gaze—upper, middle, and lower right; follow the object across to the opposite side and then upper, middle, and lower left ('H' shaped movement)—to check when the double vision occurs.

Pupils: Should be round, central, and of equal size. They should respond equally to light and accommodation (see pupil abnormalities 📖 p.283).

Table 25.1 Eye referrals

Emergency referral (direct to A&E or emergency eye clinic)	Sudden loss of vision
	Acute glaucoma
	Perforating injury; intraocular foreign body
	Chemical burns
	Retinal detachment
	Corneal ulcer
	Sudden onset of diplopia or squint + pain
	Temporal arteritis with visual symptoms (📖 p.580)
Urgent (within 24h.)	Hyphema or vitreous haemorrhage
	Orbital fracture
	Sudden onset of ocular inflammation e.g. iritis or ophthalmic herpes zoster
	Corneal foreign bodies or abrasions
Soon (within 1–2wk.)	Central visual loss
	Sinister 'floaters'
	Flashing lights without a field defect
	Chronic glaucoma with pressure >35mmHg
Routine referral	Gradual loss of vision
	Chronic glaucoma (unless pressure >35mmHg)
	Chronic red eye conditions
	Painless diplopia or squint
	Chalazion/stye/cyst
	Ptosis
	Headaches and migraine*

* Urgent if sinister cause suspected

❶ Community-based optometrists, with their experience, equipment, and training are a valuable resource available to GPs to help differentiate eye conditions and refine referral pathways. Getting an optometrist's opinion can also assist in setting the appropriate priority level for referral or prevent unnecessary referrals.

N.48

She waved

N.36

Faces the sun

N.24

Painting the rainbow

N.18

Life was like a flying dogfish

N.14

Quietly a storm drove purple ducks across the road. The chimney top

N.12

Glowed in the dusk and my sister let her biscuit fall through ashes. September was

N.10

In drizzling mood when hedgehogs threw pinecones in the dark. Squirrels played classical music.

N.8

We won a feather duster by encouraging Jessica to bake an enormous apple pie and pirouette between the tables.

N.6

Queuing had never appealed to the young porcupines but swimming held great drama for the blue and pink ostrich.

N.5

Delight was exceeding the pleasures of everyday ambulation and breaking the pattern of a melancholy existence to see the trees.

(Reproduced with permission from *The Oxford Handbook of Clinical Specialties*, 6th Edition.)

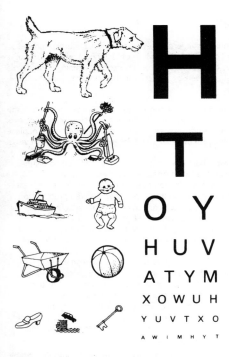

Test types (N. 48–N. 5 opposite) should be read at 30cm.

Reading types are read at 30cm (with reading glasses if used)
Lines on the snellen chart are as follows: (with distance glasses)
6 Able to read to 6m what can normally be read at 6m, ie '6/6'
9 Able to read to 6m what can normally be read at 9m, ie '6/9'
12 Able to read to 6m what can normally be read at 12m, ie '6/12'
18 Able to read to 6m what can normally be read at 18m, ie '6/18'
24 Able to read to 6m what can normally be read at 24m, ie '6/24'
36 Able to read to 6m what can normally be read at 36m, ie '6/36'
60 Able to read to 6m what can normally be read at 60m, ie '6/60'
Counts fingers; counts fingers held 1/2m distance, ie 'CF'
Hand movement; perceives hand moving 1/4m distance, ie 'HM'
Perceives light; can see a torchlight when shone into eye, ie 'PL'
No light perception, abbreviated to 'no PL', ie blind.

Figure 25.1

The red eye

⚠ Signs of a potentially dangerous red eye: ↓ visual acuity, pain deep in the eye (not surface irritation as with conjunctivitis), absent or sluggish pupil response, corneal damage on fluorescein staining, history of trauma. Get the patient seen by a specialist the same day if in doubt—particularly post-op.

Conjunctivitis: Inflammation of the conjunctiva is the most common eye problem seen in general practice. *Symptoms and signs:* red, sore eye; discharge; sticking of eyelids (especially on waking); enlarged papillae under the upper eyelid; pre-auricular LN enlargement; no change in visual acuity.

- *Infective conjunctivitis:* Bacterial or viral—clinically difficult to distinguish. Symptoms usually start in one eye and then affect both. *Investigation:* take a swab if infection does not clear with empiric treatment. *Management:* most self-limiting[C], consider delayed prescription of antibiotic eye drops (e.g. chloramphenicol 2 drops qds for 5d.).

- *Ophthalamia neonatorum:* Caused by N. gonorrhoea (📖 p.745). Presents as a purulent discharge from the eyes of an infant <21d. old. Send swabs for M,C & S. Treat with topical antibiotics. Refer for ophthalmology opinion.

- *Allergic conjunctivitis:* Bilateral symptoms appear seasonally (e.g. hay fever) or on contact with an allergen (e.g. animal fur). Presents with red, watery, itchy eyes ± photophobia ± family or personal history of atopy. *Examination:* follicles in the lower tarsal conjunctiva and 'cobblestones' under the upper lid. Treat with topical or systemic antihistamines (e.g. sodium cromoglycate eye drops, loratidine). Avoid topical steroids due to long-term complications (cataract, glaucoma, fungal infection). Refer if persistent.

Blepharitis: Inflammation of the lid margins causes chronically irritable red eyes. Eyelids have red margins ± scales on the eyelashes. There may be a burning sensation on the lids ± conjunctivitis. Prolonged treatment is often needed:

- *Removal of scales and crusts from the lid margins:* Apply warm compresses and massage lids and then scrub the lid margins with a cotton bud moistened with a few drops of baby shampoo (or sodium bicarbonate) diluted in an egg cup full of warm water. Advise patients to repeat this 2x/d. Sterile impregnated wipes (Lid-Care®) are a more convenient alternative.

- *Exacerbations:* Treat with Fucithalmic ointment rubbed into the lid margins. Topical steroids may occasionally be useful (only use on specialist advice and for ≤2wk.). Refer persistent cases.

Orbital cellulitis: Usually due to spread of infection from the paranasal sinuses. *Signs:* fever, eyelid swelling, proptosis, and inability to move the eye. Refer immediately for iv antibiotics/drainage surgery. *Complications:* meningitis, cavernous sinus thrombosis, blindness.

Subconjunctival haemorrhage: Spontaneous, painless, localized haemorrhage. Common in the elderly. Often recurrent. Looks alarming but clears spontaneously in 1–2wk. *Associations:* ↑BP, clotting disorders, ↑ venous pressure. Consider referral if it follows trauma—especially if the posterior edge of the haemorrhage can't be seen (may be associated with orbital haematoma, penetrating injury, or orbital fracture).

Ophthalmic shingles: Zoster (📖 p.494) in the ophthalmic branch of the trigeminal nerve. Pain, tingling, or numbness around the eye precedes a blistering rash and inflammation. In 50% the eye is affected with conjunctivitis, scleritis, episcleritis, keratitis, iritis, visual loss, and/or oculomotor nerve palsy. Nose tip involvement makes eye involvement likely (nerve supply is the same as the globe). Prescribe oral aciclovir (800mg 5x/d.) and refer immediately.

Scleritis/episcleritis: Presents with diffuse inflammation of the eye with minimal tenderness and no discharge. Try NSAID initially. If pain ↑ then refer—may require treatment with steroids.

Iritis (anterior uveitis): Acute onset pain, photophobia, blurred vision, watering, circumcorneal redness, small or irregular pupil ± hypopyon (anterior chamber pus). Pain ↑ as eyes converge and pupils constrict. Most common in young and middle-aged adults. Associated with ankylosing spondylitis. Refer urgently. Steroid drops ↓ inflammation and mydriatics dilate the pupil and prevent adhesions. Relapses are common.

Other causes of red eye: Acute glaucoma (📖 p.948); foreign body (📖 p.940); dry eye syndrome (📖 p.938); corneal ulceration (📖 p.941); corneal abrasion (📖 p.940); arc eye (📖 p.940).

Useful information

Good Hope NHS Hospital Trust: Patient leaflet on allergic conjunctivitis and blepharitis
📾 http://www.goodhope.org.uk/Departments/eyedept/index.htm
Uveitis Information Group ☎01806 577310
📾 http://www.uveitis.net

The external eye

Entropion: In-turning of the eye lids due to degenerative changes. Most commonly affects the lower lid. ↑ with age (rare <40y.). The eyelashes rub on the cornea and irritate the eye. Taping the lower lid to the cheek can give temporary relief. Refer for rapid surgical correction.

Ectropion: Turning out of the lower eyelid causes eye irritation, watering ± exposure keratitis. Most common in elderly or those with facial nerve palsy. Refer for consideration of surgery.

Ptosis: Drooping of the upper eyelid. *Causes:* congenital, 3rd nerve palsy, Horner's syndrome, mechanical (oedema, xanthelasma, or tumour of upper eyelid), muscular dystrophy, myasthenia gravis. Refer congenital ptosis that obstructs vision for surgical correction (can cause ambylopia). Treat other causes.

Stye: Inflammatory eyelid swelling.
- *Hordeolum externum:* Abscess or infection of a lash follicle or glands of Moll (sweat glands) or Zeis (sebum-producing) causes swelling and inflammation of the eyelid. The abscess points outwards. Treat with a hot compress and antibiotic eye drops e.g. chloramphenicol or fuscithalmic ointment.
- *Marginal cyst of Zeis or Moll:* Non-infected swelling. No treatment needed unless troublesome.
- *Hordeolum internum:* Abscess of meibomian gland. Less common. Points inwards onto the conjunctiva and causes less swelling than hordeolum externum but can persist as a *Chalazion or Meibomian cyst.*, which may eventually resolve or may need surgical incision and curettage.

Pinguecula/pterygium: Common in adults. Creamy coloured, raised, triangular plaque on the conjunctiva on either side of the cornea—more common, nasal side. If grows over the edge of the cornea termed pterygium, else termed pinguecula. Can become inflamed. May respond to steroid eye drops (extreme care if prescribing—exclude corneal ulceration before starting and avoid prolonged use). Otherwise, no need to treat unless encroaching over the pupil → refer for surgical excision. Recurrence is possible.

Dry eye syndrome (keratoconjunctivitis sicca): Dry eyes cause eye irritation and redness often worse in centrally heated buildings. Tear secretion ↓ with age. *Causes:* ↓ tear production (e.g. Sjögrens syndrome), ↑ evaporation of tears (e.g. exposure keratitis), or mucin deficiency in the tears. Schirmers test—place a 5mm wide strip of filter paper under the lower lid for 5min. and then assess length of wetness (>15mm is normal). Treat with artificial tears e.g. hypromellose, lacrilube. If one preparation does not help, try another (may need v. frequent application). Refer for ophthalmology assessment if continuing problems.

Watering eyes (epiphoria): Due to overproduction of tears or outflow obstruction. Caused by emotion, irritation of the cornea (e.g. corneal abrasion, foreign body, conjunctivitis, entropion), iritis, acute glaucoma, ectropion, blocked tear duct.

Lacrimal duct problems

- *Acute dacryocystitis:* Acute inflammation of the tear sac. Can spread to surrounding tissues and cause systemic upset. Treat immediately with antibiotics. Abscess can form—if it does, surgical drainage is required.
- *Infantile dacryocystitis:* Due to delay in canalization or obstruction of the lacrimal duct. Presents with persistently watery or sticky eyes. *Examination:* normal vision and eye appearance. If lower lid conjunctiva is reddened, take a swab to exclude chlamydia infection (□ p.743). *Management:* advise the parents to bathe the lids with cooled boiled water. Avoid antibiotic eye drops unless there is clear infection. Spontaneous resolution is the norm. If fails to clear by 1y. (4%), refer to a paediatric ophthalmologist. Treatment is by probing of the duct to clear it.
- *Chronic dacryocystitis:* Seen in the middle-aged and elderly. There is discharge of mucopus and blockage of the nasolacrimal duct. Refer for syringing of the lacrimal system or surgery.

Useful information

Good Hope NHS Hospital Trust: Patient information on stye, dry eyes, watery eyes and blocked lacrimal duct in children
  ▣ *http://www.goodhope.org.uk/Departments/eyedept/index.htm*

Eye trauma

Measure and record acuity and examine both eyes carefully. If the patient is unable to open the injured eye, try to instill local anaesthetic drops and then examine (if unable to do so, then refer for assessment). Encourage accident prevention i.e. wearing protective goggles.

Corneal abrasions: Can cause severe pain. If so, apply a few drops of local anaesthetic before examining with fluorescein. Ensure no foreign body is left in the eye (evert upper lid). Abrasions normally heal in <48h.. Prescribe antibiotic drops until healing occurs. Eye padding is not needed except to protect the eye after local anaesthetic use.

Superficial foreign bodies: Cause discomfort, a 'foreign body sensation', and watering. They can be difficult to see so examine very carefully, including everting the eyelids. The foreign body sensation may come from an abrasion. If metal or a penetrating injury is suspected, refer for an orbit X-ray. Superficial foreign bodies can be removed (after instilling local anaesthetic) with a corner of clean card. Refer if you are not confident you can remove the foreign body.

Arc eye: Seen in welders, sunbed users, skiers, mountaineers, and sailors who do not use adequate eye protection. Causes severe eye pain, watering, and blepharospasm a few hours after exposure due to corneal epithelial damage from the UV light. Pad the eye and give analgesics and mydriatics. Recovery should occur within 24h.—if not, refer. Advise patients on suitable protective wear for future exposure.

Blunt injury: Caused by fists, squash balls, etc. The result may be anything from a 'black eye' to globe rupture. Globe rupture is usually obvious with a wound and severely ↓ vision. More minor injuries are subconjunctival haemorrhage or corneal abrasion. *Refer if:*
- visual acuity is affected
- double vision
- conjunctiva is lacerated (may be a concealed globe rupture)
- hyphema is present (blood in the anterior chamber)
- unable to see posterior limit of a subconjunctival haemorrhage (may indicate orbital fracture)
- persistent pupil dilation (usually recovers spontaneously but may indicate a torn iris)
- any signs of retinal damage (oedema or detachment)
- if you cannot assess the eye (e.g. if lid swelling prevents examination).

Penetrating wounds: Refer urgently if penetrating injury is a possibility (i.e. history of flying object or working with hammers, lathes, or chisels where a metal fragment may fly off). The wound may be tiny, vision is usually impaired, the eye waters, there is photophobia, and the pupil may be distorted. X-ray can help locate the foreign body. Do not remove large foreign bodies (dart or knife)—support the object with padding whilst transferring the patient, supine, to A&E. Cover the other eye to prevent damage from conjugate movement.

Burns: Chemical burns can cause great damage. Hold lids open, brush out any powder and irrigate with large amounts of clean water immediately. Do not try to neutralize the acid or alkali. Refer urgently.

Corneal ulceration: Presents with pain, photophobia, watering of the eye ± blurred vision. *Examination:* stain with fluorescein. Use a bright light with a blue filter; ulcers show up green.

Non-infective: *Causes:* contact lenses, trauma, previous corneal disease. Remove the cause if possible. Prescribe prophylactic topical antibiotics (e.g. chloramphenicol qds). Refer same day for everything but a simple abrasion. Risk of scarring and visual loss.

Infective

- *Ulcerative keratitis*—may be bacterial, herpetic, fungal, or protozoal. Presents with a very painful eye, blurred vision, photophobia, and profuse watering. On examination, there is circumcorneal injection and conjunctivitis and a creamy white, disc-shaped lesion can often be seen on the central or inferior cornea. Refer the same day—sight threatening.
- *Dendritic ulcer*—corneal ulcer caused by herpes simplex. There is a danger of massive amoeboid ulceration and blindness if steroid eye drops are given. Diagnose by staining with fluorescein. Refer. Treatment is with 3% aciclovir eye ointment 5x/d. continued for 3d. after healing.

Blindness and partial sight

'The eye is the window of the mind'
Richard II, William Shakespeare (1564–1616)

Incidence: 2:1000 in UK. Blindness is defined as inability to perform any work for which eyesight is essential (not the total absence of sight). In practice this means <3/60 vision (may be >3/60 if patient has severe visual field defect e.g. glaucoma). Partial sightedness does not have a standard definition but usually implies vision in the range 3/60–6/60.

Registration of blindness: Voluntary in England. Only ~1:3 of those eligible are registered. Refer patients with low vision for assessment. Application is made by a consultant ophthalmologist to social services. Registration makes a patient eligible for additional benefits that help maintain independent living e.g. ↑ income support/disability living allowance; ↑ tax allowance; assessment of special educational needs; training in Braille; disabled parking badge; ↓TV licence fee; some travel concessions; access to talking books and large print libraries; special visual aids; assessment and retraining for employment. Partial sightedness can also be registered and entitles the patient to some of these additional benefits.

Major causes of blindness in the UK: Macular degeneration, cataract, glaucoma, DM, ophthalmia neonatorum (used to be a major cause—now rare), retrolental fibroplasia (seen in premature infants exposed to high levels of oxygen therapy—now less common).

Driving and impaired vision: 📖 p.202–205

Sudden painful loss of vision in 1 eye

⚠ Always refer urgently to ophthalmology (unless migraine or stroke).

Angle closure glaucoma: Usually preceded by blurred vision or halos around lights. Dilation of the pupils at night can precipitate an attack. Most common in middle or old age and in long-sighted patients. *Cause:* blockage of aqueous drainage from the anterior chamber causes a sudden ↑ in intra-ocular pressure from 15–20 to 60–70mmHg. *Signs:* ↓ vision; hazy cornea (due to oedema); fixed dilated pupil (may be slightly oval); circumcorneal redness; eyeball feels hard (due to ↑ pressure).

Management: Refer as an emergency to ophthalmology. Treatment is with miosis to open drainage channels (e.g. pilocarpine drops) and acetazolamide to reduce aqueous production. Surgery or laser treatment (peripheral iridectomy) to allow free aqueous circulation is undertaken once pressure has been ↓.

Retinal vein occlusion: If central vein occlusion occurs, there is sudden visual loss in one eye, the fundus looks like 'a stormy sunset' (haemorrhages and engorged veins). Branch retinal vein occlusion causes partial visual loss. Incidence ↑ with age. More common than arterial occlusion. *Causes:* glaucoma, arteriosclerosis, ↑BP, polycythaemia, hypercholesterolaemia, ↑ homocystein.

Management: Refer for fluorescin angiography and expert opinion. Laser treatment may prevent neovascular glaucoma ('90-day glaucoma'), retinal neovascularisation, and macular oedema.

Retinal artery occlusion: Usually due to thromboembolism. *Signs:* Sudden visual loss in 1 eye (counting fingers or light perception), afferent pupil defect (💷 p.283). Retina appears white ± cherry red spot at the macular. Exclude temporal arteritis (💷 p.580).

Treatment: If the patient presents <1h. after onset—applying then releasing firm eyeball pressure can sometimes dislodge an embolus into one of the smaller branches and thus preserve some vision. Refer for confirmation of diagnosis. There is no reliable treatment[C]. Optic atrophy and blindness is the usual outcome. Treat any risk factors for atherosclerosis (i.e. ↑BP, hyperlipidaemia, smoking, DM, carotid/cardiac disease).

Vitreous haemorrhage: *Signs:* sudden ↓ in vision, loss of red reflex, difficulty visualizing the retina. *Risk factors:* DM with new vessel formation, bleeding disorders, retinal detachment, central retinal vein occlusion, trauma, head injury.

Management: Refer for confirmation of diagnosis. Treat the cause (e.g. photocoagulation of new vessels). Most bleeds disperse spontaneously in <3mo. Vitrectomy may be required to remove persisting blood.

Optic neuritis: *Presentation:* loss of vision (over hours or days); painful eye movements; ↓ colour discrimination (red desaturation); optic disc swelling (papilloedema). Recovery usually occurs over 2–6wk. but ~50% develop multiple sclerosis (💷 p.612) in <15y. DM can also cause papillitis. Treatment is with high-dose steroids. Refer urgently.

Other causes of sudden loss of vision
- Migraine (💷 p.600)
- Stroke (💷 p.606)
- Amaurosis fugax (💷 p.954)
- Wet AMD (rapid rather than sudden loss of vision—💷 p.944)
- Retinal detachment (💷 p.945)
- Temporal arteritis (💷 p.580)

Patient information and support
DWP: Blindness and partial sight ☎0800 88 22 00 🖳 http://www.dwp.gov.uk
Royal National Institute for the Blind: Information and talking book service
☎0845 766 9999 🖳 http://www.rnib.org.uk
Partially Sighted Society ☎01302 323 132
**Association for Education, Training and Support of Blind and Partially Sighted People
(OPSIS)** ☎0121 428 5037 🖳 http://www.opsis.org.uk
LOOK (for families of blind/visually impaired children) ☎0121 428 5038
Good Hope NHS Hospital Trust: Patient information (glaucoma and retinal vein occlusion)
🖳 http://www.goodhope.org.uk/Departments/eyedept/index.htm

Gradual loss of vision and colour blindness

Macular degeneration: Cause of blindness of 1:2 people registered blind in the UK—2% of >65y. old are blind in 1 or both eyes due to age-related macular degeneration (AMD). Always a bilateral disease but 1 eye is usually more severely affected than the other. *Types:*

• *Dry AMD:* Atrophy of the neuro-retina. Causes gradual loss of vision.
• *Wet (neovascular) AMD:* Subretinal blood vessel formation. Causes rapid blindness.

Risk factors: ↑ age, +ve FH, smoking, ↑BP.

Presentation: Deterioration of central vision (affects reading, face recognition first—worse with changes in lighting); a dark patch that rapidly fades may be noticed on waking (can be interpreted as 'seeing a shadowy figure' and be very frightening—do not confuse with a hallucination). *Examination:* ↓ acuity; normal visual fields; macular exudate (yellow/white spots—drusen); pigment and haemorrhage ± oedema; normal disc.

Treatment: Laser photocoagulation and photodynamic therapy can help some patients with the rapidly progressive neovascular form but for many there is no effective treatment. Treatment of other coexisting conditions (e.g. cataract and glaucoma) can help. Provision of visual aids, registration of blindness, and social support are important.

Refer

• *Urgently*—if there is recent onset distortion or visual loss (<1mo.) but reasonably good vision (6/12). This suggests exudative disease that may respond to laser treatment.
• *Non-urgently*—those with significant loss for confirmation of diagnosis ± registration of partial sight or blindness if visual acuity <6/60.

Prognosis: Varies, depending on the type of AMD, from gradual visual deterioration to rapid progression to blindness.

Optic atrophy: *Signs:* gradual visual loss; pale optic disc. *Causes:* glaucoma, MS, ischaemia (e.g. retinal artery occlusion), retinal damage (choroiditis, retinitis pigmentosa), toxic (tobacco ambylopia, methanol, arsenic, quinine). Refer for confirmation of diagnosis to ophthalmology or neurology.

Chronic glaucoma: 📖 p.948

Diabetic retinopathy: 📖 p.415 and 954

Retinal vein occlusion: 📖 p.942

Cataract: 📖 p.946

Hypertensive retinopathy: 📖 p.954

Retinoblastoma: 📖 p.880

Compressive lesions of the optic pathway: e.g. meningioma, glioma, abscess, A-V malformation can cause visual field defects—type depends on the site of the lesion (📖 p.588 and p.295).

Retinal detachment: Painless loss of vision—'like a curtain' coming across the vision. The rate of detachment can vary (upper retinal detachments tend to occur more quickly, causing loss of lower part of vision). 50% have premonitory symptoms—flashing lights or spots before eyes due to abnormal retinal stimulation prior to the detachment. If the macular is detached (more common in upper detachments), central vision is lost and does not completely recover (even after retinal replacement).

Signs: Grey retina may balloon forward, visual field loss.

Causes: Idiopathic, trauma, DM (fibrous bands in the vitreous), after cataract surgery, myopia. Refer urgently to ophthalmology for treatment to secure the retina. Laser, cryotherapy and silicone implants are used.

Retinitis pigmentosa: Familial disorder resulting in retinal degeneration. *Signs:* night blindness, black pigment flecks in the retina, optic atrophy. Usually first noticed in adolescence. Progresses to blindness.

Colour blindness

- *Congenital colour blindness:* Inherited as a sex-linked characteristic. Much more common in men than women (♂:♀ ≈ 20:1). Patients may request to be tested. This is done using a standard set of cards (Ishihara test). Each card consists of a number in coloured dots against a contrasting background of more coloured dots. Coloured dots are paired to detect different patterns of colour blindness. Lack of red/green discrimination is most common. Colour blindness prohibits certain types of employment (e.g. airline pilot, train driver).

- *Impaired colour recognition:* Occurs later in life. Red is the most common colour affected. May be an early sign of an optic nerve disorder. Patients complain of colour looking 'washed out' (desaturated) in one eye compared to the other. Refer.

Patient information and support

Royal College of Ophthalmologists: Patient information leaflets on age-related macular degeneration, retinitis pigmentosa, and retinal detachment.
🖳 http://www.rcophth.ac.uk

Moorfields Eye Hospital: Patient information sheets on glaucoma, retinal detachment, and macular degeneration 🖳 http://www.moorfields.org.uk/EyeHealth

Royal National Institute for the Blind ☎0845 766 9999 🖳 http://www.rnib.org.uk

The Partially Sighted Society ☎01302 323132

The Macular Disease Society ☎0845 241 2041 🖳 http://www.maculardisease.org

British Retinitis Pigmentosa Society 🖳 http://www.brps.org.uk ☎0845 123 2354

Cataract

Lens opacity is found in 75% >65y. olds. Most do not need treatment.

Risk factors for cataract: Old age, DM, +ve FH, steroids, ↑BP, excessive alcohol, smoking, prolonged steroid treatment, prenatal rubella/toxoplasma (congenital cataract), hypocalcaemia, eye trauma, or radiation exposure.

Presentation: Blurred vision; gradual loss of vision; dazzles and halos around objects (especially in sunlight); frequent spectacle changes due to changing refractive index. Unilateral cataract may not be noticed but loss of binocular vision affects judgement of distance.

In children: Cataracts present with squint, white pupil, nystagmus, amblyopia, or loss of binocular vision.

Signs: A shadow in the red reflex or an absent red reflex, difficulty visualizing the fundus.

Types of cataract
- Nuclear cataracts—central (most common in old age);
- Polar cataracts—localized and usually inherited;
- Subcapsular cataracts—usually linked to steroid use;
- Dot cataracts—common causes DM; trauma.

Management

Childhood cataract: 📖 p.839

Adult cataract: Check blood glucose to exclude DM. Advise patients to have their visual acuity checked regularly. Refer to ophthalmology if symptoms or ↓ sight interferes with social functioning, driving, or independence. Treated with surgery (removal of the natural lens ± posterior chamber lens implantation) as a day case procedure under LA. Healing takes 2–6wk. depending on technique used. 75–95% without other ocular pathology have 6/12 vision or better 3mo. post-op. Patients require testing for new spectacles 6wk. post-op to allow refractive changes to settle.

Complications
- Intraocular infection—rare. Presents with a painful/red/discharging eye ±↓ vision. Refer back to the operating surgeon urgently.
- Posterior capsule rupture.
- Broken or protruding sutures—cause sensation of a foreign body on the cornea or pain. May need to be removed.
- Vitreous haemorrhage.
- Glaucoma.
- Posterior capsule opacification—5–30% <5y. post-op. Symptoms are similar to the original cataract. Treatment is with laser therapy to create a hole in the capsule.

Floaters: Small dark spots in the visual field usually caused by vitreous degeneration which leads to opacities that cast shadows on the retina. Floaters continue to move when the eye comes to rest. *Risk factors:* myopia, cataract operation, trauma. Usually harmless and may settle with time.

⚠ Sudden showers of floaters appearing in 1 eye ± flashing lights can indicate retinal detachment which may be difficult to see on examination. Refer immediately for assessment, especially if there is any visual field loss or ↓ acuity.

Patient information

Moorfields Eye Hospital: Patient leaflets on cataract and floaters
  🖥 http://www.moorfields.org.uk/Eyehealth
Royal College of Ophthalmologists: Patient leaflet on cataract
  🖥 http://www.rcophth.ac.uk
Good Hope NHS Hospital Trust: Patient information on cataract
  🖥 http://www.goodhope.org.uk/Departments/eyedept/cataracts.htm

Chronic simple glaucoma (open angle)

Common. *Incidence:* ~2% of >40y. olds. Accounts for ~1:4 ophthalmology outpatient appointments and 7% of new blindness registrations. *Risk factors:* ↑ IOP >21mmHg—the major risk factor (but 30% of newly diagnosed glaucoma patients have 'normal' pressure), FH (↑ risk ×10), ↑ age, black race, abnormal BP (↑ in elderly), myopia, ↑ plasma viscosity.

Presentation: May be detected during routine optometrist examination or through routine screening for diabetics or patients with FH. Otherwise, patients present late as asymptomatic and visual acuity is preserved until visual fields are severely impaired. *Signs:* optic nerve damage (glaucomatous disc cupping), visual field loss (sausage-shaped blind spots), ↑intraocular pressure (IOP). Distinguishing disc cupping can be difficult. *Look for:* high disc-cup ratio; vertically oval cup; asymmetrical cups; haemorrhage at the disc margin; disc pallor; retinal vein occlusion.

Management: Advise all patients with a FH of glaucoma to have their intraocular pressures (tonometry) and visual fields checked regularly (usually annually) at an optician from 40y. of age. Refer patients with ↑ pressures or in whom you notice (or are doubtful about) disc cupping to ophthalmology for assessment.

Treatment^G: Patients with ↑ intraocular pressure must be followed up life-long. Aim is to ↓ intraocular pressure to slow disease progression (even with 'normal' pressures).

Medical treatment:
- *Topical prostaglandin* (e.g. latanoprost od in the evening)—↑ outflow of aqueous secretion.
- *Topical β-blockers* (e.g. timolol bd)—↓ aqueous secretion.
  Caution in patients with asthma or heart failure. *Side-effects:* allergy and dry eyes.
- *Topical carbonic anhydrase inhibitors* (e.g. dorzolamide tds, or bd if in combination with a β-blocker)—↓ aqueous secretion. *Side-effects:* blurred vision, tiredness, dyspepsia.
- *Topical α-agonists* (e.g. brimonidine bd)—↓ aqueous secretion and ↑ outflow. *Side-effects:* local reactions, headache, dry mouth, tiredness.

Surgery: Trabeculoplasty is considered when the 'target' intraocular pressure is not met with medical treatment (especially in patients <50y.). *Side-effects:* failure, worsening cataract. Argon laser trabeculoplasty can also be used. It is most effective in the elderly (effect is relatively short term).

Further information

European Glaucoma Society (1998) Terminology and guidelines for glaucoma
    🖳 http://www.eugs.org

Patient information and support

Royal College of Ophthalmologists: Patient leaflet on glaucoma
 🖳 *http://www.rcophth.ac.uk*
The International Glaucoma Association, Kings College Hospital, Denmark Hill, London SE5
 9RS ☎020 7737 3265
Good Hope NHS Hospital Trust: Patient information on glaucoma
 🖳 *http://www.goodhope.org.uk/Departments/eyedept/glaucoma.htm*

Refraction errors and squint

Screening for visual abnormalities: 📖 p.826

Amblyopia (lazy eye): ↓ acuity in an eye, after refractive correction, when there is no detectable disorder in the eye or visual pathways. Squint, ptosis, cataract, unequal refractive errors, or astigmatism can cause the image from one eye to be disregarded. This neglect leads to amblyopia. If it persists after 7–8y. old, it is irreversible and the vision is permanently impaired. Thus, referral of children for treatment of these problems is important. Treatment is with glasses ± patching.

Refraction errors

- *Hypermetropia (long sight):* Most common refractive error. Common in infants and lessens with age. Distant objects focus behind the retina so continuous ciliary muscle contraction (to make the lens more convex) is needed to achieve a focused image. This can cause eye tiredness, headache, and a convergent squint in children. Convex lenses are used for correction.
- *Myopia (short sight):* Close objects can be focused on the retina but distant objects focus in front of the retina. There is often a +ve FH. Concave lenses (glasses or contact lenses) are used to correct the defect. Myopia is unusual <6y. old. It tends to worsen until the late teens. Thus, regular eye checks are needed to change lenses (may be every 6mo.). In adults, increasing myopia can indicate developing cataracts. Extreme myopia (6–20 dioptres) predisposes to retinal detachment—recommend these patients have an annual eye examination (more frequent if they have 'floaters'—📖 p.947).
- *Astigmatism:* The degree of curvature across the cornea or lens differs in the vertical and horizontal planes. Thus, objects are distorted longitudinally or vertically. Lenses can be made to correct this defect.
- *Presbyopia:* Age-related long sightedness. The lens becomes larger and stiffer (less easy to deform) between 45–65y. Focusing on close objects is more difficult and glasses may become necessary for near work (e.g. reading).

Refractive procedures: Are increasingly being undertaken as an alternative to spectacles.

Lasik (laser-assisted in situ keratomileusis): Combination of surgery and laser and is now the most common procedure. It can be used for higher degrees of refractive error and astigmatism. Complications are rare but this is still a relatively new procedure, so there is little long-term follow-up data.

Squint: Abnormality of coordinated eye movement. Common, especially in childhood—5% of 5y. olds. May be constant or intermittent, convergent (esotropia) or divergent (exotropia), non-paralytic (full range of eye movement) or paralytic (diplopia in direction of pull of the paralysed muscle).

Predisposing factors: FH of squint, high refractive errors, neurological disease (e.g. cerebral palsy), cataract, Down's syndrome, Turner's syndrome, retinoblastoma, optic atrophy, craniofacial anomalies, retinal disease.

Management: Refer all squints as soon as recognized for ophthalmology assessment. Without treatment, children with squint risk developing amblyopia, failure of binocular vision, and long-term visual problems. Visual maturity occurs at 7–8y. Eye patching, correction of refractive errors (spectacles), and realignment surgery can improve sight up to this age.

Pseudosquint

- **Wide epicanthic folds:** Give the appearance of a squint—corneal reflections are symmetrical.
- **Intermittent deviation of the eyes in neonates:** Common. Check red reflex is present. Normally settles by 3mo.—squint after this time is significant. Refer.

Ocular nerve palsies

3rd (oculomotor) nerve palsy

- **Surgical:** Caused by Berry aneurysm (posterior communicating artery), cavernous sinus lesions, tumour. Presents with ophthalmoplegia (eye looks down and out), proptosis, pain, ptosis, and fixed pupil dilation. Refer for urgent neurosurgical assessment.
- **Medical:** Caused by microvascular disease e.g. DM. Presents with ptosis and ophthalmoplegia but no pain or pupil involvement. Refer to neurology/ophthalmology.

4th (trochlear) nerve palsy: Superior oblique paralysed. Diplopia ± ocular torticollis (holding head tilted), eye cannot look down and in. *Causes:* trauma (30%), DM (30%), tumour, idiopathic.

6th (abducens) nerve palsy: Lateral rectus paralysed. Diplopia, eye turned in and cannot move laterally from the midline. *Causes:* tumour, trauma to base of skull, vascular.

Useful information

Royal College of Ophthalmologists (2000) Patient and GP information: Guidelines for the management of strabismus and amblyopia in childhood.
🖳 www.rcophth.ac.uk
Moorfields Eye Hospital: Patient leaflet on squint
🖳 www.moorfields.org.uk/EyeHealth
Good Hope NHS Hospital Trust: Patient information on refractive surgery
🖳 http://www.goodhope.org.uk/Departments/eyedept/index.htm

Contact lenses and drugs for the eye

Contact lenses: 20% are worn because they are more suitable for the eye condition than spectacles; 80% for cosmetic/convenience reasons. Some are worn just to change eye colour. Contact lenses are used in high myopia or hypermetropia, presbyopia, and after cataract removal (because thick spectacle lenses cause visual field distortion). They are also useful when the cornea has been damaged e.g. after ulceration or trauma and in keratoconus (a rare corneal degenerative disease).

Types of lens: Hard, gas-permeable (larger hard lenses designed to allow air to reach the cornea) and soft lenses are available. Some soft lenses are daily or monthly disposable. Hard and gas-permeable lenses can correct for minor astigmatism, normal soft lenses cannot as the lens is too flexible. A high astigmatism requires spectacles or a special (toric) soft lens (delicate and needs careful cleaning). Patients with poor tear secretion do not tolerate contact lenses well.

Care of lenses: Careful cleaning of the lenses and contact lens container is vital—particular solutions are used for each type of lens and these should not be interchanged. Contact lenses can be stained by fluorescein or rifampicin—ask before prescribing.

Complications: Eye infection, corneal abrasion or ulceration (painful, watering eye after lens removal), sensitization to cleaning agents (redness, stinging, swollen eyelids), losing the lens within the eye, keratitis, acanthamoeba infection.

Drugs and the eye: Many eye complaints can be treated with topical medication. Ointments last longer in the eye than drops (which may need 2hrly application) but can cause blurring of vision. They are particularly useful at night. Antibiotic preparations (e.g. chloramphenicol, fusidic acid) can potentially become contaminated with bacteria so should be discarded after 1mo.

Mydriatics: (e.g. tropicamide, cyclopentolate) dilate the pupil and cause cycloplegia, thus producing blurred vision. They are used to dilate the pupil for examination and to prevent adhesions in iritis. They can precipitate acute closed angle glaucoma in susceptible patients.

Miotics: (e.g. pilocarpine) constrict the pupil and ↑ aqueous drainage. They are used in glaucoma. They can cause systemic side-effects e.g. sweating, ↑ BP, pulmonary oedema.

Local anaesthetic drops: (e.g. amethocaine) can help examination of painful eyes and foreign body removal. Protect the eye with an eye pad until the anaesthetic has worn off to prevent corneal damage (corneal reflex is suppressed).

Steroid eye drops: Used in scleritis, episcleritis, iritis. Prescribe only after slit lamp examination and on the advice of an ophthalmologist. They can cause severe eye damage if used when a dendritic ulcer is present. Long-term may cause glaucoma, thinning of the cornea/sclera, and/or fungal infection.

β-blocking drops: (e.g. timolol, betaxolol) are used in glaucoma. Beware of systemic side-effects (bronchospasm, bradycardia).

α₂ receptor agonists: (e.g. brimonidine) are used in glaucoma. May cause dry mouth, headache, fatigue.

Systemic drugs: Some systemic drugs can have effects on the eye e.g. steroids and TCAs can aggravate glaucoma. Ethambutol and chloroquine can cause retinal problems—e.g. loss of acuity and colour perception problems—refer. Amiodarone can cause corneal microdeposits.

The eye in systemic disease

Diabetes mellitus: 📖 p.414

Table 25.2 Classification of diabetic retinopathy

Group	Classification	Symptoms	Features
I	Background retinopathy	None	Microaneurysms (dots), micro-haemorrhages (small blots), hard exudates not affecting the macula
II	Mild, non-proliferative	Central visual loss	Leakage in macular region ± macular oedema, capillary occlusion, hard exudates within 1 disc space of the macula
III	Severe, non-proliferative	None	Venous abnormalities, large blot haemorrhages, cotton wool spots (small infarcts)
IV	Proliferative retinopathy	None, though complications cause visual loss	New vessel formation either at the disc (NVD) or elsewhere (NVE)
V	Advanced diabetic eye disease	Visual loss or blindness	Extensive fibrovascular proliferation, retinal detachment, vitreous haemorrhage, glaucoma

❶ Refer patients with retinopathy in groups II–V for specialist ophthalmology assessment and treatment

Hypertensive eye disease (📖 p.316): Leads to arteriolar vasoconstriction, arterio-venous 'nipping' (narrowing where vessels cross), flame haemorrhages, hard exudates, retinal infarcts (cotton wool spots), macular oedema, and rarely papilloedema (due to accelerated hypertension). ↑ BP predisposes to retinal vein occlusion.

Arteriosclerosis: Can cause cranial nerve palsies leading to paralytic squint. *Amaurosis fugax* (a form of TIA) is due to emboli passing through the retina and causes brief loss of vision (few mins)—'like a curtain'. Management is: as for TIA (📖 p.606).

Papilloedema: Swollen optic disc with blurred disc margins. Can be due to ↑ ICP (📖 p.602), malignant hypertension (📖 p.317), cavernous sinus thrombosis or optic neuritis (📖 p.943). Refer urgently.

Thyroid eye disease

- *Hyperthyroidism*—proptosis, lid retraction, lid lag (leading to exposure keratitis), double vision, retinal or optic nerve circulatory impairment (sight-threatening), and secondary glaucoma (📖 p.948).
- *Hypothyroidism*—oedema of conjunctiva and periorbital tissues.

Parathyroid disorders

- *Hyperparathyroidism*—gritty red eyes due to Ca^{2+} deposits in conjunctiva, cornea, and sclera.
- *Hypoparathyroidism*—cataract due to ↓ Ca^{2+}.

Blood disorders

- *Anaemia and leukaemia*—vitreous haemorrhage; retinal haemorrhages with white centre (Roth's spots) seen on the fundi. They can also occur in infective endocarditis (📖 p.348).
- *Sickle cell disease*—peripheral retinopathy, arterial occlusion and sclerosis, new vessel formation, vitreous haemorrhage and retinal detachment. Annual retinal examination advised.

Down's syndrome: Epicanthic folds and upward slanting eyelids. Brushfield spots (white dots) in the iris. ↑ prevalence of keratoconus. Cataract, refractive errors and squint are common.

Turner's syndrome: Incidence of squint is ↑ x10.

Collagen disorders: RA, PAN, SLE, Wegener's—dry eyes (📖 p.938), episcleritis and scleritis (📖 p.937).

Ankylosing spondylitis and Reiter's: Intermittent acute red eye and iritis (📖 p. 937 and p.938 respectively).

Psoriatic arthropathy: Associated with uveitis (📖 p.937).

Temporal arteritis: Ischaemic optic neuropathy.

Crohn's and ulcerative colitis: Episcleitis or uveitis occurs in 10% of patients (📖 p. 937).

AIDS: Retinitis due to CMV.

MS: Optic neuritis may be the first sign of MS (📖 p.943).

Other relevant pages

Mental health

Useful information

WHO Guide to Mental and Neurological Health in Primary Care: Includes guidelines, patient resources, and checklist questionnaires ☐ *http://www.mentalneurologicalprimarycare.org*
Centre for Evidence Based Mental Health: Provides information on research, education, workshops, and links to other sites ☐ *http://www.cebmh.com*

Counselling and cognitive behaviour therapy

Counselling: 1:3 problems brought to the GP have a psychosocial component. To cater for these patients most PCOs (81%) have some provision for practice-based counselling and 50% practices have counselling services. Counselling services may also be available via community psychiatric or clinical psychology services.

What is counselling? There are no universally agreed definitions of the term 'counselling' or 'counsellor' and the distinction between counselling and psychotherapy is often unclear. Usually, the key element in counselling is reflective listening to encourage patients to think about and try to resolve their own difficulties. It does not involve giving advice. Most counsellors use brief (time-limited) therapy, offering patients a mean of 7 sessions, each usually lasting ~50 mins.

Who is a counsellor? There is no formal registration requirement in the UK for counsellors or psychotherapists. The GMC advises that GPs should only refer to practitioners who are members of a recognized disciplinary body (Table 26.2) and thus subject to ethical and disciplinary codes.

Does counselling work? Many patients regard antidepressants as harmful or addictive and are increasingly reluctant to take them. They see counselling as an attractive alternative—a view supported by most GPs. Evidence shows counselling subjectively improves the condition the patient has been referred for, and non-directive counselling is more effective than GP care in reducing anxiety and depression in the short term, but not the long term. However, counselling doesn't ↓ drug costs and practices with counsellors make more referrals to 2° care psychiatric services[5]. More research is needed into cost effectiveness.

Who should be referred? Counsellors see a wide range of patients (Table 26.1). ~²/₃ patients referred for counselling have significant levels of anxiety or depression.

Table 26.1 Conditions suitable and unsuitable for referral to a counsellor

Suitable	Unsuitable
• Anxiety	• Psychotic illness
• Depression—especially minor depression (📖 p.968)	• Phobias
• Relationship problems	• Obsessive-compulsive disorder
• Bereavement	• Eating disorder
• After traumatic events	• Personality disorder
	• Substance abuse

Table 26.2 UK recognized professional bodies for counsellors and psychotherapists

Counsellors

- The British Association for Counselling and Psychotherapy (BACP)
- The UK Register of Counsellors
- The Association of Counsellors and Psychotherapists in Primary Care

Psychologists

- The British Psychological Society (chartered and counselling psychologists)

Psychotherapists

- The UK Council for Psychotherapy
- The British Confederation of Psychotherapists

Problem-solving therapy: Another short-term therapy (typically 5–6 x45min. sessions) which involves drawing up a list of problems, and generating and agreeing solutions, broken down into steps, for patients to work on as homework between sessions. Shown to be as effective as antidepressants for moderate depression[R].

Cognitive behavioural therapy (CBT)

- *Behavioural therapies* aim to change behaviour. Usually the therapist uses a system of graded exposure (systematic desensitization) combined with teaching a method of anxiety reduction.
- *Cognitive therapy* focuses on peoples' thoughts and the reasoning behind their assumptions on the basis that incorrect assumptions → abnormal reactions which then reinforce these assumptions further (a vicious cycle).

What is CBT used for? Of proven effectiveness in the treatment of mild depression, anxiety disorders, phobias, panic disorder, eating disorders, and for the treatment of delusions and hallucinations in psychotic illness.

How can patients be referred for CBT? Usually provided by highly trained psychotherapists accessed via psychiatry services. Guided self-help programmes based on CBT are also effective for mild depression and can be delivered:

- Using books e.g. Gilbert (2000) *Overcoming depression* Constable and Robin
- By computer e.g. *Beating the Blues*© (further information available from ▣ http://www.ultrasis.com)
- Via the Internet e.g. ▣ http://www.psychologyonline.co.uk

Essential reading

NICE (2004) Depression ▣ http://www.nice.org.uk

Further information

Bower et al (2003) The clinical effectiveness of counselling in primary care *Psychol Med* **33**: 203–15
DTB (2003) Mild depression in general practice **4(8)**: 60–4

Anxiety disorders (1)

Generalized anxiety disorder (GAD): Long-term condition, fluctuating in severity and nature, often beginning in adolescence. Lifetime prevalence ≈5%.

Clinical features

Psychological
- Fearful anticipation
- Irritability
- Sensitivity to noise
- Restlessness
- Poor concentration
- Worrying thoughts
- Insomnia
- Nightmares
- Depression
- Obsessions
- Depersonalization

Physical
- Dry mouth
- Difficulty swallowing
- Tremor
- Dizziness
- Headache
- Parasthesiae
- Tinnitus
- Epigastric discomfort
- Excessive wind
- Frequent or loose motions
- Chest discomfort/constriction
- Difficulty breathing/hyperventilation
- Palpitations/awareness of missed beats
- Frequency or urgency of micturition
- Erectile dysfunction
- Menstrual problems

Associations
- *Other psychiatric illness:* Panic attacks; depression; and alcohol dependence.
- *Physical illness:* Thyrotoxicosis; hypoglycaemia; chronic fatigue syndrome; stroke; Cushing's disease; phaeochromocytoma.

Management
- *General measures:* Check TFTs. Avoid caffeine; identify potential causes of anxiety, give support and information.
- *Specific measures:*
  - If immediate treatment is necessary try problem solving (📖 p.959) or benzodiazepines e.g. diazepam 2–5mg tds prn ⚠ Don't use >2–4wk.
  - In all cases offer CBT (📖 p.959), treatment with SSRI (e.g. paroxetine 20–40mg od—don't consider treatment unsuccessful unless no improvement after 12 wk.—if effective continue ≥ 6mo.) or self-help with book- or computer based CBT ± exercise. If one treatment doesn't work—try another.
  - Refer for specialist management if significant symptoms despite treatment with 2 interventions (CBT, medication and/or book-based CBT) *or* if considering initiation of venlafaxine.

Phobias: Same symptoms as GAD but limited to certain situations. 2 main features:
- *Avoidance* of the circumstances that provoke anxiety.
- *Anticipatory anxiety* when there is the prospect of encountering these circumstances.

Simple phobia: Inappropriate anxiety in the presence of ≥1 object/ situation e.g. flying, enclosed spaces, spiders. Common in early life. Most adult phobias are a continuation of childhood phobias. *Lifetime prevalence:* 4% ♂; 13% ♀.

Management: Treatment is only needed if symptoms are frequent, intrusive, or prevent necessary activities. Exposure therapy is effective. Obtain either directly (via trained psychotherapist), by referral to psychiatry, or through the private sector (e.g. British Airways fear of flying course).

Social phobia: Intense and persistent fear of being scrutinized or negatively evaluated by others resulting in fear and avoidance of social situations (e.g. meeting people in authority, using a telephone, speaking in front of a group). Must be significantly disabling, not simple shyness. May be generalized (person fears most social situations) or specific (related to certain activities only).

Management
- *Drug therapy:* SSRIs—continue ≥12mo. or long term if symptoms remain unresolved, there is a comorbid condition (e.g. depression, GAD, panic attacks), a history of relapse, or early onset.
- *Psychological therapies:* Cognitive behaviour therapy (cognitive restructuring) ± exposure. Obtain directly or via local psychiatric services, depending on local arrangements.

Agoraphobia: Usually onset is aged 20–40y. and associated with an initial panic attack.

Symptoms: Panic attacks, fear of fainting and/or loss of control are experienced in crowds, away from home, or in situations from which escape is difficult. Avoidance → patients remaining within their home where they know symptoms will not occur. Other symptoms include depression, depersonalization, and obsessional thoughts.

Management: Difficult to manage in general practice. Diagnosis is often delayed, as patients will not come to the surgery. Ongoing management complicated by refusal to be referred to psychiatric services. Prognosis is best when there is good marital/ social support. *Options:*
- *Behavioural therapy* e.g. exposure, training in coping with panic attacks. Available by direct referral or via psychiatric services, according to local arrangements. Home visits may be required, but should be resisted as part of therapy.
- *Drug treatment:* SSRIs (citalopram and paroxetine are licensed); MAOIs; TCAs (imipramine and clomipramine are commonly used). Relapse rate is high. Benzodiazepines can be used if frequent panic attacks, particularly if initiating other treatment, but beware of dependence.

Essential reading:
NICE Management of anxiety (2004) ⬚ http://www.nice.org.uk

Patient information and support
Triumph Over Phobia (TOP) UK: Self-help materials and groups ☎0845 600 9601
⬚ http://www.triumphoverphobia.com
Royal College of Psychiatrists: Patient information sheets ⬚ http://www.rcpsych.ac.uk

Anxiety disorders (2)

Panic disorder: Panic attacks are very common, but panic disorder is uncommon. Lifetime prevalence—1% ♂; 3 % ♀. Intense feeling of apprehension or impending disaster. Anxiety builds up quickly and unexpectedly without a recognizable trigger and patients often present with any combination of:

- Shortness of breath and smothering sensations
- Choking
- Palpitations and accelerated heart rate
- Chest discomfort or pain
- Sweating
- Dizziness, unsteady feelings, or faintness
- Nausea or abdominal pain
- Depersonalization/derealization
- Numbness or tingling sensations
- Flushes or chills
- Trembling or shaking
- Fear of dying
- Fear of doing something crazy or uncontrolled

Examination: Obvious distress; sweating; tachycardia; hyperventilation. ↑ BP is common and usually settles when the episode is over. Otherwise, examination is normal.

Definitions
- *Panic attack:* ≥ 4 symptoms listed above in 1 attack.
- *Panic disorder:* Chronic disorder; initial diagnosis depends on > 4 attacks in 4wk. *or* 1 attack followed by a persistent fear of having another.

Differential diagnosis: Alcohol withdrawal; other psychiatric disorders (e.g. psychosis); hyperthyroidism; temporal lobe epilepsy; cardiac arrhythmia; labyrinthitis; hypoglycaemia; hyperparathyroidism; phaeochromocytoma (very rare).

Associations: Depression (56% patients are depressed); generalized anxiety; agoraphobia; substance abuse; suicide (↑risk). Panic attacks predict future panic disorder and depression.

Acute management of hyperventilation: 📖 p.1056

Management of panic disorder
- *Assess symptoms:* 'Tell me about your first panic attack'. Clarify ideas associated with the attack ('What is the worst thing that could happen to you during a panic attack?'). Ask about other psychiatric symptoms.
- *Drug treatment:* SSRIs—paroxetine and citalopram are licensed in UK. Treatment period ≥6mo., then discontinue slowly over 4–6mo. Start at low dose (10mg citalopram daily). May cause transient worsening of panic in first few weeks. Warn patient to stop if significant anxiety or agitation develops. Other drugs: tricyclics (imipramine, clomipramine). Treat any other associated psychiatric disorders.
- *Psychological treatment:* CBT (📖 p.959) is effective.

⚠ Don't use benzodiazepines for treatment of patients with panic disorder—associated with less good outcome in the long term.

Referral: Refer to psychiatry if treatment with drugs *and* either CBT or book-based CBT is unsuccessful.

Post-traumatic stress disorder (PTSD): Caused by experiencing or witnessing a traumatic event e.g. major accident, fire, assault, military combat. Symptoms can present months or years after the triggering event and may be misdiagnosed as depression or anxiety. 3 main symptom clusters:

- *Intrusive recollections*—thoughts, nightmares, flashbacks;
- *Avoidant behaviour*—numbing of emotions;
- *Hyperarousal*—↑ anxiety and irritability, insomnia, poor concentration, hypervigilence.

Nearly 2/3 experience chronic symptoms and there is a strong association with other psychiatric conditions especially depression, anxiety, and drug/alcohol abuse and dependence.

Management[N]: Treat any other associated psychiatric illness.

- *Watchful waiting:* Appropriate for patients with mild symptoms which have been present for <4 wk. after the trauma: Be supportive and listen. Arrange a follow up contact within 1 mo.
- *Trauma-focused psychological treatment* (trauma focused cognitive behavioural therapy and/or eye movement desensitisation and reprocessing (EMDR): Refer (usually via the community mental health team) all patients with severe symptoms <4wk. after the trauma or if ongoing symptoms beyond 4 wk. which affect every day life.
- *Drug treatment:* Should not be used as a routine first-line treatment in preference to a trauma-focused psychological therapy. Reserve for those with continuing symptoms despite trauma-focused psychological therapy or who have refused trauma-focused psychological therapy. Drug treatments include paroxetine, mirtazapine (unlicensed), amitriptyline (consultant initiation only—unlicensed) and phenelzine (consultant initiation only—unlicensed).

❶ Debriefing immediately after the traumatic event is unhelpful

Essential reading:
NICE ⌂ http://www.nice.org.uk
- Post-traumatic stress disorder (PTSD)(2005)
- Management of anxiety (2004)

Patient information and support:
Anxiety Care Helpline ☎ 020 8478 3400 ⌂ http://anxietycare.org.uk
No more panic ⌂ http://nomorepanic.co.uk
Royal College of Psychiatrists: Patient information sheets ⌂ http://www.rcpsych.ac.uk

Other anxiety-type disorders

Mixed anxiety and depression: Combinations of anxiety and depression are common in general practice—particularly amongst women. Prevalence ~ 10%. When anxiety and depression occur together, symptoms are more severe, there is ↑ functional impairment, the illness is more chronic and persistent, and there is a poorer response to any treatment given. Treat as for anxiety and/or depression depending on the predominating features. Refer for psychiatric assessment if management strategies are not working.

Somatization or hysteria: Physical symptoms in response to emotional distress. Characterized by an excessive preoccupation with bodily sensations combined with a fear of physical illness. Common feature of depression, anxiety, schizophrenia, and substance use.

Somatization disorder: Chronic condition. History of numerous unsubstantiated physical complaints. Starts at <30y. and often persists many years. ♀:♂≈10:1; lifetime prevalence 0.1–0.2%, though mild symptoms are much more common.

Clinical features
- >2y. history of multiple symptoms with no adequate physical explanation.
- Persistent refusal to be reassured that there is no explanation for the symptoms.
- Impaired social/family functioning due to these symptoms and/or associated behaviour.

Management
- Reattribution involves acknowledging and taking the symptoms seriously, offering any necessary examination and investigations, enquiring about psychosocial problems, and explaining the link between symptoms and stress.
- Treat comorbid psychiatric problems (e.g. depression, anxiety, panic).
- Beware of risks of drug interaction—self-medication with multiple OTC (or even prescription) drugs is common.
- Beware of side-effects of medication—these patients do not tolerate prescribed drugs well and have a heightened awareness of side-effects.
- Refer to psychiatry if risk of suicide, marked functional impairment, impulsive or antisocial behaviour.

Heartsink patients: Characterized by:
- Frequent presentation—top 1% attenders at GP surgeries generate 6% GP workload.
- Highly complex and often multiple problems—some real, others not.
- Exasperation generated between patient and doctor.

❶ It is a 2-way process. Some GPs report more heartsink patients than others. The problem relates to the GP's perception of patients as well as the patients themselves.

GP risk factors: Perception of high workload; low job satisfaction; lack of training in counselling or communication; lack of postgraduate skills.

Management strategy
- Do a detailed review of notes ± chart of life.
- Agree patient contacts (e.g. limit to one partner); agree frequency of appointments etc.
- Agree an agenda within consultations e.g. problem list—only 1 problem/visit.
- Employ reattribution techniques as for somatization disorder (opposite)
- Avoid unnecessary investigation and referral.
- Be aware of your own reaction to the patient.
- Acknowledge even heartsink patients can be genuinely ill.
- Consider psychiatric diagnoses—especially chronic anxiety, depression, somatization disorder. Screening questionnaires can be useful.
- Consider referral for CBT.

Obsessive-compulsive disorder (OCD): Lifetime prevalence ≈2%, though minor obsessional symptoms are much more common. ♂:♀ ≈ 2:3. Tends to present in young adults. Patients often have had symptoms for years before seeking help. Relatives may highlight the problem rather than the patient. Often patients are aware that what they are thinking or doing is irrational and are embarrassed to tell anyone.

Features:
- *Obsessional thinking*—recurrent persistent thoughts, impulses, and images causing anxiety or distress.
- *Compulsive behaviour*—repetitive behaviours, rituals, or mental acts done to prevent or ↓ anxiety.
- *Other features*—indecisiveness and inability to take action, anxiety, depression, and depersonalization.

Note: A new NICE guideline is expected in November 2005.

Management: Refer for psychiatric assessment. Treatment involves a combination of patient education, SSRI or clomipramine, and CBT.

Stress: 📖 p.966

Patient information and support
OCD Action ☎020 7226 4000 🖥 *http://www.ocdaction.org.uk*
Royal College of Psychiatrists: Patient information sheets 🖥 *http://www.rcpsych.ac.uk*

Chronic stress

The word stress derives from the Latin 'stringere' meaning to 'draw tight' and was first used during the 17th century to describe hardships or affliction. We all suffer from stress and, most of the time, the pressures of everyday life are a motivating force. A problem only arises when those pressures exceed the individual's ability to cope with them.

Causes of stress: Virtually anything we do can cause stress. The most common causes of stress-related morbidity in the UK are:
- Work problems
- Family problems
- Financial problems
- Legal problems
- Exam stress

The stress epidemic: 105 million working days are lost each year in the UK due to stress (11% of all sickness absence). The Health and Safety Executive estimate that ~$1/_2$ million people in the UK are experiencing work-related stress at a level they believe is making them ill; up to 5 million people feel 'very' or 'extremely' stressed by their work; and work-related stress costs society >£4 billion every year.

Presentation: Most patients don't consult their GP with stress unless they feel it is affecting their health. Common symptoms include:
- Mood swings
- Anxiety
- Depression
- Low self-esteem
- Poor concentration and/or memory
- Fatigue and/or lethargy
- Sleep disturbance
- Other aches and pains for which no cause can be found e.g. muscular pains, chest pains
- Poor or ↑ appetite
- ↑ smoking, alcohol, and/or caffeine consumption
- Headaches
- Loss of libido
- Menstrual abnormalities
- Dry mouth
- Worsening of pre-existing conditions e.g. irritable bowel syndrome, eczema, asthma, psoriasis, migraine

Management: The GP's role is to:
- Identify that stress is the cause of the presenting symptoms
- Educate the patient about stress and the link between their symptoms and stress
- Try to identify the source of the stress
- Provide the patient with self-management strategies (opposite)
- Support the patient
- Treat any medical problems arising out of the stress e.g. depression
- Provide certification if the stress is so great that the patient is unable to work. ❶ If the stress is work-related, consider putting a statement to that effect on the certificate to allow the employer to take steps to alleviate the stress and facilitate return to work.

Post-traumatic stress disorder: 📖 p.963

The stressed GP: 📖 p.94

10 tips for chronic stress relief

- Ensure you get enough sleep and rest—avoid using sleeping tablets to achieve this (see insomnia—📖 p.242)
- Look after yourself and your own health e.g. don't skip meals, sit down to eat, take time out to spend time with family and friends, make time for hobbies and relaxation, do not ignore health worries
- Avoid using nicotine, alcohol, or caffeine as a means of stress relief
- Work off stress with physical exercise—↓ levels of adrenaline released and ↑ release of natural endorphins which → a sense of well-being and enhance sleep
- Try relaxation techniques
- Avoid interpersonal conflicts—try to agree more and be more tolerant
- Learn to accept what you can't change
- Learn to say 'no'
- Manage your time better—prioritize and delegate (see below); create time buffers to deal with unexpected overruns and emergencies
- Try to sort out the cause of the stress e.g. talk to line manager at work, arrange marriage or debt counseling, arrange more childcare

Time management made easy: This technique aims to transform an overwhelming volume of work into a series of manageable tasks.
- Make a list of all the things you need to do
- List them in order of genuine importance
- Note whether you really need to do the task, what you need to do personally, and what can be delegated to others
- Note a time-scale in which each task needs to be done e.g. immediately, within a day, within a week, month, etc.

Further information
Health and Safety Executive (HSE) 🖥 http://www.hse.gov.uk/stress

Patient advice and support
Stress Management Society ☎0870 199 3260 🖥 http://www.stress.org.uk
International Stress Management Association (UK) ☎07000 780 430 🖥 http://www.isma.org.uk

Depression

2.3 million people suffer from depression in UK at any time. 1:5 seeking help in primary care have psychological problems; 1:10 suffer from depression. ♂:♀ ≈ 1:2.

Recognition: ~30–50% cases are not detected, although most of those missed are mild cases, more likely to resolve spontaneously. Diagnosis of mental illness is stigmatizing. Polls show 60% think people with depression would feel too embarrassed to consult their GP. This can lead to 'collusion' between patient and doctor during consultation to avoid any diagnosis of mental health problems—serving interests of doctor and patient, but doing little to tackle the problem.

Causes /comorbidity: Associated with:
- *Psychiatric disorders* e.g. anxiety disorders, alcohol abuse, substance abuse, eating disorders.
- *Physical disorders* e.g. PD, MS, dementia, endocrine disease (thyroid disorders, Addison's disease), hypercalcaemia, rheumatoid arthritis, SLE, cancer, AIDS and other chronic infections, cardio- and cerebrovascular disease, learning disability.
- *Drugs causing symptoms of depression:* β-blockers, anticonvulsants, Ca^{2+} channel blockers, corticosteroids (though prednisolone sometimes used, especially in terminal care, for the artificial 'high' it can give), oral contraceptives, antipsychotic drugs, drugs used for PD (e.g. Levodopa).

Definitions

Major depression: 2 key features: depressed mood and/or ↓ interest or pleasure, which must be disabling to the patient.

Diagnosis: ≥1 key feature and ≥ 5 symptoms from following list present most of the time for ≥2wk.:
- Change in appetite or weight
- Insomnia or hypersomnia
- Fatigue or loss of energy
- Poor concentration
- Poor appetite or overeating
- Low energy or fatigue
- Low self-esteem
- Psychomotor agitation or retardation
- Sense of worthlessness or guilt
- Recurrent thoughts of death or suicide
- Feelings of hopelessness
- Poor concentration or difficulty making decisions

Mild depression: Some of the above symptoms (but not enough to make diagnosis of major depression) associated with some functional impairment (NICE definition—≤4 symptoms).

Dysthymia: A chronic form of minor depression. Depressed mood for *most* of the day, for more days than not, for ≥2y, *and* the presence of ≥2 of the above symptoms.

History
- Onset including precipitating events
- Nature of symptoms, severity, and effect on life
- Past history of similar symptoms/past psychiatric history

- Current life events—stressors at home and at work
- Family history
- Coexistent medical conditions
- Current medication—prescribed and non-prescribed.

❶ Sleep disturbance and fatigue have high predictive value for depression and should prompt enquiry about other symptoms.

Cultural considerations: Some cultures have no terms for depression and may present with physical symptoms (somatization) or use less familiar 'cultural specific' terms to describe depressive symptoms e.g. 'sorrow in my heart'.

Examination
- *General appearance:* self-neglect, smell of alcohol, weight ↓
- *Assessment of mood:* looks depressed and/or tired, speech monotone or monosyllabic, avoids eye contact, tearful, anxious or jumpy/fidgety, feeling of distance, poor concentration, etc.
- *Psychotic symptoms:* hallucinations, delusions, etc.

Assessing severity of depression: Rapid, self-complete pencil and paper questionnaires can help determine severity. Significant depression which is likely to need drug or psychological therapy is suggested by:
- A depression score of ≥11 on the Hospital Anxiety and Depression Scale (HADS) (available from NFER Nelson 🖳 http://www.nfer-nelson.co.uk) or
- A score of ≥14 or more on the Beck Depression Inventory (BDI) (available from Harcourt Assessment 🖳 http://www.harcourt-uk.com)

❶ A fee is payable for the use of both these instruments.

Assessment of suicide risk: Ask about suicidal ideas and plans in a sensitive but probing way. It is a common misconception that asking about suicide can plant the idea into a patient's head and make suicide more likely. Evidence is to the contrary.

Risk factors for suicide
- ♂>♀
- Age 40–60 y.
- Living alone
- Divorced > widowed > single > married
- Unemployment
- Chronic physical illness

- Past psychiatric history
- Recent admission to psychiatric hospital
- History of suicide attempt/ self-harm
- Alcohol/drug misuse

Management of threatened suicide: 📖 p.980

Management of depression: 📖 p.970

Patient information and support
Depression Alliance ☎ 0845 123 2320 🖳 http://www.depressionalliance.org
Royal College of Psychiatrists: Patient information sheets 🖳 http://www.rcpsych.ac.uk
Samaritans: 24h. emotional support via telephone ☎08457 909 090

Management of depression

Table 26.3 Summary of management of depression

Presentation	Action
Major depression and dysthymia	Antidepressant therapy or CBT
Acute milder depression	Education about depression e.g. information leaflets
	Support, self-help groups, and guided self-help
	Simple problem-solving strategies
	Monitor regularly for development of major depression
Persistent milder depression	Trial of antidepressants
Milder depression with history of major depression	Consider antidepressants
	Monitor closely

Antidepressant medication: *BNF 4.3.*

When should antidepressants be started? Don't prescribe at the first visit as symptoms may improve significantly during 1–3wk. watchful waiting (*'Don't just do something, sit there!'*).

What should I tell the patient? Giving patients information ↑ compliance. When starting antidepressant drugs, explain reasons for prescribing; time-scale of action—unlikely to have any effect for 2wk., effects build up to max. effect at 4–6wk.; and likely side-effects.

Which drugs are available? Major groups are:
- **Selective serotonin re-uptake inhibitors (SSRIs)** e.g. fluoxetine 20mg od—usually 1st choice as less likely to be discontinued due to side-effects. Warn of possible anxiety and agitation and advise patients to stop if significant. GI side-effects including dyspepsia are common.
- **Tricyclic antidepressants (TCAs)** e.g. lofepramine 70mg od/bd/tds—titrate dose up from low dose until patient feels the drug is helping *or* until side-effects intrude[S]. Common side-effects include drowsiness, dry mouth, blurred vision, constipation, urinary retention, and sweating.
- **Monoamine oxidase inhibitors (MAOIs)** e.g. phenelzine 15mg tds. MAOIs should not be started until at least 1–2wk. after a tricyclic has been stopped (3wk. in the case of clomipramine or imipramine). Other antidepressants should not be started for 2wk. after treatment with MAOIs has been stopped (3wk. if starting clomipramine or imipramine).

Follow-up: Review patient every 1–2wk. until stable assessing response, compliance, side-effects, and suicidal risk, then monthly. Continue treatment for at least 4mo. after recovery, and at least 6mo. in all. Patients with ≥2 past episodes of major depression should be advised to continue for 2y.[N]

Discontinuation reactions: Occur once a drug has been used ≥8wk.
↓ risk by tapering dose over ≥4wk. Warn about possible reactions:
• Withdrawal of SSRIs—headache, nausea, paraesthesia, dizziness, and anxiety.
• Withdrawal of other antidepressants (especially MAOIs)—nausea, vomiting, anorexia, headache, 'chills', insomnia, anxiety/panic, and restlessness.

Other treatments

Specific psychological therapies: e.g. CBT (📖 p.959), behaviour therapy, interpersonal psychotherapy, problem-solving therapy (📖 p.959). Possible 1st line therapies in mild/moderate depression, though excessive waiting lists are a limiting factor. Simple problem-solving strategies can be tried in the surgery:

1. Identify the main problem
2. Generate solutions
3. Try out the solutions
4. Feedback and modify

Counselling: 📖 p.958

Exercise: Beneficial in mild depression[N].

St John's Wort: May be effective in mild depression but formulations vary widely in potency, and interacts with many drugs including antidepressants (especially SSRIs), warfarin, oral contraceptives, and theophylline.

Referral to psychiatry: U = Urgent; S = Soon; R = Routine
• High suicide risk—U
• Psychotic major depression—U
• History of bipolar disorder—R/S
• Failure or partial response following ≥2 attempts to treat—R

Management of other specific types of depression

Seasonal affective disorder (SAD): 'Winter blues'—recurrent disorder involving 'seasonal' episodes of depression, usually in the winter months. Affects ≈ 2% adults. ♀:♂ ≈ 2:1. Peak incidence: 3rd decade.

Symptoms: Depression + ↑ sleep, ↑ food intake (with carbohydrate craving), and weight gain. 30% experience elatory mood swings in summer.

Management: SSRIs (particularly sertraline); phototherapy (30–90 mi./d. in early morning—effects should be seen within 3wk.). Light boxes can be borrowed from psychiatry departments, hired, or bought (contact SAD Association for more information—🖳 http://www.sada.org.uk).

Recurrent brief depression (RBD): Recurrent depressive episodes of short duration (2–7d.) which meet criteria for major depression (📖 p.969). High prevalence in primary care. Episodes occur as often as monthly. ≈50% also have seasonal variation. At present there is no effective treatment—antidepressants are ineffective.

Essential reading
NICE (2004) Depression 🖳 http://www.nice.org.uk:
DTB (2003) Mild depression in general practice **4(8)**: 60–4

Psychosis

The archetypal layman's 'madness'. Characterized by a loss of the link between reason and the outside world. Psychosis is not a diagnosis but a class of illnesses characterized by 3 key features:

- Hallucinations—📖 p.266
- Delusions—📖 p.255
- Thought disorder—📖 p.292

If ≥ 1 of these features is present, diagnosis is very limited:

- *Affective psychoses*—psychotic depression, mania, and hypomania (below)
- *Delusional psychoses*—schizophrenia and paranoid psychoses (📖 p.974) *or*
- *Organic psychoses*—the dementias (📖 p.978), acute confusional states (📖 p.976).

Mania and hypomania:

Mania is characterized by a persistently high or euphoric mood out of keeping with circumstances. Other signs include:

- ↑ pressure of speech
- ↑ energy and activity
- ↑ appetite
- ↑ sexual desire
- ↑ pain threshold
- ↓ desire or need for sleep
- ↓ insight
- Grandiose delusions
- Hallucinations
- Labile mood— elation to irritability and hostility when thwarted
- Over-assertiveness
- Spending sprees
- Disinhibition
- Self-important ideas
- Poor concentration— easily distracted

Hypomania is a less severe form of mania.

Differential diagnosis: Hypoglycaemia; alcohol or drug abuse; prescribed drug side-effects (e.g. steroids); temporal lobe epilepsy; frontal lobe dysfunction (e.g. due to tumour or stroke); thyrotoxicosis.

Acute management: Treatment in hospital is usually required for the 1st episode or acute relapses. If unwilling to accept voluntary admission, use compulsory admission under the Mental Health Act (📖 p.986). Sedation whilst awaiting admission may be required—use chlorpromazine 50–100mg po or 50mg im (↓ dose for elderly patients and avoid if the patient is epileptic, has been drinking or taking barbiturates).

Chronic management: Requires long-term follow-up:

- *Regular reviews:* Case registers help ensure regular reviews take place. Check a written care plan has been drawn up by the psychiatric service. Assess—symptoms; compliance with medication; efficacy of treatment; medication side-effects; risks of suicide.
- *Educate* the patient and relatives/friends about early signs of relapse and action in case of relapse
- *Reinforce compliance with treatment*
- *Ensure adequate social support:* Self-help groups, day centres, benefits
- *Monitor drugs for toxic side-effects*

- *Advise patients to inform the DVLA:* Driving should cease during the acute illness (all vehicles) and until stable with insight for 3y. (LGV/PCV drivers)—📖 p.205.

Drug treatment: *BNF 4.2.3*
- Lithium is the drug of choice.
- Check levels weekly until the dose is constant for 4wk., then monthly for 6mo., then every 3mo. thereafter, as long as the dose remains constant.
- If levels are slowly rising, suspect nephrotoxicity.
- Check plasma creatinine and TFTs every 6mo..
- Avoid changing proprietary brands as bioavailability varies (📖 p.122).
- *Toxic effects:* blurred vision, D&V, ↓K⁺, drowsiness, ataxia, coarse tremor, dysarthria, hyperextension, fits, psychosis, coma, and shock.
- *Alternative drugs:* sodium valproate; carbamazepine.

Bipolar disorder or manic depression: Consists of episodes when the patient has mania (bipolar I) or hypomania (bipolar II) against a background of depression. Lifetime prevalence ≈ 1%. ♂:♀ ≈ 1:1. Peak incidence is in late teens and early 20s—90% develop the disorder before 30y. *Management:* as for mania (opposite).

Patient information and support
Manic Depression Fellowship ☎0845 634 0540 🖳 http://www.mdf.org.uk
Royal College of Psychiatrists: Patient information sheets 🖳 http://www.rcpsych.ac.uk

Schizophrenia

Frightening and disabling condition in which the sufferer is unable to distinguish his internal from the outside world. Lifetime prevalence ≈1%. Peak age of onset: ♂ (15–25y.); ♀ (25–35y.).

First-rank symptoms: Reliable markers in ~70% of patients. ≥1 symptom is suggestive of schizophrenia:

- Auditory hallucinations in the form of a commentary
- Hearing thoughts spoken aloud
- Hearing voices referring to the patient, made in the 3rd person
- Somatic hallucinations
- Thought broadcasting

- Thought withdrawal, insertion, and interruption
- Delusional perception
- Feelings or actions experienced as made or influenced by external agents (passivity feelings)

Acute schizophrenia: Typically presents in young people with +ve symptoms (delusions, hallucinations, and/or thought disorder). The patient lacks insight, so initial approach may come from a relative or friend.

Assessment: See the patient.
- Try to elicit any history of drug abuse—amphetamines can give a picture identical to schizophrenia.
- Ask about physical and psychological symptoms—in particular, thoughts and perceptions.
- Assess the patient's behaviour and appearance. Look for evidence of self-care, loss of affect, poverty of thought, and social withdrawal.
- Ask friends, neighbours, or relatives present to tell you about the patient's behaviour.

Differential diagnosis: Illicit drugs, temporal lobe epilepsy, acute confusional state, dementia, affective disorders, personality disorder.

Management: BNF 4.2.1
- Seek expert psychiatric help. Is the patient a risk to himself/others?
  - Patients who are a risk need acute admission either voluntarily or under the Mental Health Act.
  - Patients who are no immediate risk may be assessed urgently by the community psychiatric services as an outpatient.
- Start antipsychotic treatment—if necessary before psychiatric assessment. Delay in treatment ↑ patient risks and → poorer prognosis.
- Oral atypical antipsychotic drugs (e.g. amisulpride, olanzapine, risperidone) are 1st line treatment for newly diagnosed schizophrenia.
- Stick to a single drug and start at the lower end of the dose range e.g. risperidone 1mg bd on day 1 and ↑ to 2mg bd on day 2. Don't use loading doses.
- Advise patients to inform the DVLA. Driving should cease during the acute illness (all vehicles) and until stable with insight for 3y. (LGV/PCV drivers)—📖 p.205

Follow-up: Liaise with the community psychiatric services and reinforce the management plan agreed. Following acute episodes, there is ↓ risk of relapse if antipsychotic medication continues 6–24mo. Provide contacts for patient and relative support groups.

Chronic schizophrenia: Characterized by thought disorder and –ve symptoms (poverty of thought, apathy, inactivity, lack of volition, social withdrawal, and loss of affect). Aim to treat the disease, prevent relapse, and improve quality of life.

Long-term health problems
- ↑ death from suicide (1:10 schizophrenics), accidents, cardiovascular disease, and respiratory disease.
- ↑ obesity due to side-effects of antipsychotic drugs, poor diet, sedentary lifestyle, and lack of exercise.
- Substance abuse—¾ smoke; ↑ prevalence of alcohol and drug abuse.
- Rarely patients drink excessive amounts of water → hyponatraemia.

Regular reviews: Case registers ensure regular reviews take place.
- *Check there is a written care plan* from the psychiatric service.
- *Check mental health*—assess symptoms; compliance with medication; efficacy of treatment; medication side-effects; risks of suicide.
- *Check physical health*—watch for weight ↑, DM, and hyperprolactin-aemia, especially on atypical antipsychotics. Check BP and lipids. ECG if palpitations—look for QT prolongation on atypical antipsychotics.
- *Promote lifestyle changes*—↑ exercise; ↓ smoking; improve diet; encourage sensible drinking and avoidance of illicit drugs (e.g. cannabis and amphetamines) which exacerbate symptoms and ↑risk of relapse.
- *Review social support*—areas where assistance may be needed include: finance, housing, employment, structured daily activity, transport, social network. Those who can help include: social services, community mental health team, housing officer, disablement resettlement officer.

Referral to psychiatry: U = Urgent; S = Soon; R = Routine
- ↑ in risk to self or others—U
- Poor response to treatment—U/S/R
- Problems with adherence; consider depot administration—S/R
- Suspected comorbid substance misuse—R
- Patient new to your practice—R
- Patient is on conventional antipsychotics (e.g. sulpiride, thioridazine) and suffering significant side-effects or persistent symptoms. Refer for consideration of change of medication to atypical antipsychotic—R
- For family interventions to ↓ 'expressed emotion' (smothering, hostility and criticism about the patient by the family). Effective in ↓ relapse—R
- For CBT—for persistent symptoms despite antipsychotics and to ↑ insight—R

Patient information and support
National Association for Mental Health (MIND) ☎020 8519 2122 🖳 http://www.mind.org.uk
Rethink (National Schizophrenia Fellowship) ☎020 8974 6814 🖳 http://www.rethink.org

Acute confusional states (delirium)

Common condition seen in general practice—particularly amongst elderly patients. May occur de novo or be superimposed upon chronic confusion of dementia (📖 p.978) → sudden worsening of cognition.

Presentation
- Global cognitive deficit with onset over hours/days
- Fluctuating conscious level—typically worse at night/late afternoon
- Impaired memory—on recovery, amnesia of the events is usual
- Disorientation in time and place
- Odd behaviour—may be underactive, drowsy, and/or withdrawn *or* hyperactive and agitated
- Disordered thinking—often slow and muddled ± delusions (e.g. accuse relatives of taking things)
- Disturbed perceptions—hallucinations (particularly visual) are common
- Mood swings

Examination: Can be difficult. If possible, do a thorough general physical examination to exclude treatable causes.

Possible causes
- *Infection*—particularly UTI, pneumonia. Rarely encephalitis, meningitis.
- *Drugs*—opiates, sedatives, L-dopa, anticonvulsants, recreational drugs.
- *Metabolic*—hypoglycaemia, uraemia, liver failure, hypercalcaemia, other electrolyte imbalance (rarer).
- *Alcohol or drug withdrawal.*
- *Hypoxia*—e.g. severe pneumonia, exacerbation of COPD, cardiac failure.
- *Cardiovascular*—MI, stroke, TIA.
- *Intracranial lesion*—SOL, ↑ ICP, head injury (especially subdural haematoma).
- *Thyroid disease.*
- *Carcinomatosis.*
- *Epilepsy*—temporal lobe epilepsy, post-ictal state.
- *Nutritional deficiency*—B$_{12}$, thiamine or nicotinic acid deficiency.

Differential diagnosis
- *Deafness*—may appear confused.
- *Dementia*—longer history and lack of fluctuations in conscious level. In practice, may be difficult to distinguish, especially if you come across a patient who is alone and can give no history.
- *Primary mental illness* e.g. schizophrenia (📖 p.974); anxiety state (📖 p.960).

Management: Is aimed at treating all remediable causes.

Admit if:
- The patient lives alone
- The patient will be left unsupervised for any duration of time
- Carers (or residential home) are unprepared/unable to continue looking after the patient
- History and examination have indicated a cause requiring acute hospital treatment—admit as an emergency.

Possible investigations to consider in the community

• Urine—dipstick for glucose, ketones, blood, protein, nitrates, and white cells, send for M,C&S
• Check BM to exclude hypoglycaemia
• Blood—FBC, ESR, U&E, LFTs, TFTs
• ECG
• CXR

Management at home

• Acute confusion is frightening for carers—reassure and support them.
• Treat the cause e.g. antibiotics for UTI or chest infection.
• Try to avoid sedation as this can make confusion worse. Where unavoidable, use haloperidol 1–2mg prn or lorazepam 0.5–1mg prn..
• Involve district nursing services e.g. to provide incontinence aids, cot sides, moral support.
• If the cause does not become clear despite investigation or the patient fails to improve with treatment, admit for further investigation and assessment.

Table 26.4 The 6 cognitive impairment test: Kingshill version (2000)*

Question	Response	Score
1. *What year is it?*	Correct: 0; incorrect: 4	....
2. *What month is it?*	Correct: 0; incorrect: 3	....
Remember the following address: e.g. John Brown, 42 West Street, Bedford		
3. *What time is it (to the nearest hour)?*	Correct: 0; incorrect: 3	....
4. *Count backwards from 20 to1*	Correct: 0; 1 error: 2; >1 error: 4	....
5. *Months of the year backwards*	Correct: 0; 1 error: 2; >1 error: 4	....
6. *Repeat the memory phrase*	Correct: 0; 1 error: 2; 2 errors: 4; 3 errors: 6; 4 errors: 8; all incorrect: 10	....
Total		

Instructions on scoring: Ring the appropriate score results for each question; add up the scores to produce a result out of 28.

Total score:

0–7	Not significant
8–9	Probably significant; refer; possible dementia
10–28	Significant; refer; likely dementia

* Reproduced with permission from Dr Patrick Brooke *patrick.brooke@gp-k81017.nhs.uk.*
Further information ⌨ *http://www.kingshill-research.org*

Dementia

Generalized impairment of intellect, memory, and personality, with no impairment of consciousness. Prevalence ↑ with age (rare <60y.; 5% >65y.; 20% >80y.). Common causes: Alzheimer's disease (60%); vascular (multi-infarct) dementia; dementia with Lewy bodies.

Presentation

History: Patients may be aware of 'being a bit forgetful' but usually relatives complain about their behaviour. Early symptoms are loss of short-term memory and inability to perform normally simple tasks. Alternatively, patients present later with failure to cope at home or self-neglect. To diagnose dementia, there must be a clear history of progressive impairment of memory and cognition ± personality change. Always assess level of support in the home, housing, and ability to cope (both patient and carers).

Examination: Check general appearance—look for evidence of self-neglect, malnutrition, abuse; screen for cognitive deficit e.g. with 6CIT (🕮 p.977).

Investigation: Aimed at detecting treatable causes: check FBC, ESR, U&E, LFTs, Ca^{2+}, TFTs, glucose, B$_{12}$, red cell folate, VDRL (syphilis), HIV (if at risk), CXR, MSU.

Differential diagnosis
- Acute confusion—🕮 p.976
- Depression—🕮 p.968
- Communication difficulties—deafness, dysphasia, or language difficulties

Management
- **Refer:** All patients should be referred to a psychogeriatrician for confirmation of diagnosis, exclusion of treatable causes, and ongoing specialist support and assessment. Refer to a social worker and/or CPN for community support.
- **Apply principles of rehabilitation** (🕮 p.176 and 626).
- **Support carers** (🕮 p.178). Advise re benefits (🕮 p.97–111), self-help groups, respite care. Warn that dementia is progressive and prepare carers for a time when the patient does not recognize them.
- **Treat concurrent problems** e.g. UTI, chest infection, anaemia, depression—they make dementia worse.
- **Management of memory loss:** Notebook to record 'tasks must do'; medication dispensers.
- **Management of agitation**
  - Maintain a constant environment if possible
  - Arrange for door catches to prevent wandering
  - Take up loose carpets to prevent falls
  - Consider fire and electrical safety
  - Avoid sedatives wherever possible as may worsen confusion—if needed, use very low dose, review regularly, and consider newer atypical drugs e.g. risperidone.

Alzheimer's disease: Most common form of dementia. Each GP has ~16 patients with Alzheimer's disease at any time. *Cause:* unknown—defective genes found on chromosomes 14, 19, and 21.

Risk factors: FH, Down's syndrome (onset at ~30y.), late onset depression, hypothyroidism, history of head injury.

Presentation: Presents with steady ↓ in memory and cognition. *Onset:* any age—normally >40y. ♀:♂ ≈ 0.7.

Management: Specific treatment with anticholinesterase inhibitors (e.g. donepezil, rivastimine) is now available. There is some evidence these drugs ↓ rate of decline. They are *only* prescribed for patients presenting with mild or moderate dementia and only under specialist supervision—refer.

Prognosis: Mean survival ~7y. from outset.
(*Alois Alzheimer (1864–1915)—German neuropathologist/psychiatrist*)

Lewy body dementia: Fluctuating but persistent cognitive impairment, parkinsonism, and hallucinations. No specific treatment. Avoid antipsychotics as they can be fatal. Use benzodiazepines if tranquilization is necessary. (*Friedrich H. Lewy (1885–1950)—German neurologist*)

Pick's dementia: Dementia characterized by personality change associated with frontal lobe signs such as gross tactlessness. Lack of restraint may lead to stealing, practical jokes, and unusual sexual adventures. Treatment is supportive. (*Arnold Pick (1851–1924)—Czech neurologist/psychiatrist*)

Vascular (multi-infarct) dementia: Multiple lacunar infarcts or larger strokes cause generalized intellectual impairment. Tends to occur in a stepwise progression with each subsequent infarct. The final picture is one of dementia, pseudobulbar palsy, and shuffling gait with small steps. Treatment is as for secondary prevention of TIA/stroke—📖 p.608.

Patient information and support

Alzheimer's Society ☎0845 300 0336 🖥 http://www.alzheimers.org.uk
Dementia Care Trust ☎0870 443 5325 🖥 http://www.dct.org.uk
Benefits enquiry line ☎0800 882 200
Carers UK ☎0808 808 7777 🖥 http://www.carersonline.org.uk

Suicide and deliberate self-harm (DSH)

❶ People who have self-harmed should be treated with the same care, respect, and privacy as any other patient.

Deliberate self-harm (DSH): Deliberate non-fatal act committed in the knowledge that it was potentially harmful and, in the case of drug overdose, that the amount taken was excessive. 90% DSH is due to self-poisoning and it accounts for 20% of admissions to general medical wards—the most frequent reason for admission for young ♀ patients. Paracetamol or aspirin are the most common drugs used. Self-harm is often aimed at changing a situation (e.g. to get a boyfriend back), communication of distress ('cry for help'), a sign of emotional distress, or may be a failed genuine suicide attempt.

Management of DSH and attempted suicide
- *If any self harm:* Assess the situation and admit to A&E as necessary.
- *Ask about present circumstances:* Ask the patient to explain his feelings and reasons for the act of DSH/attempted suicide.
- *Ask about suicidal ideas and plans:* It is a common misconception that asking about suicide can plant the idea into a patient's head and make suicide more likely—evidence is to the contrary. Risk factors—see below. Useful questions:
  - Do you feel you have a future?
  - Do you feel that life's not worth living?
  - Do you ever feel completely hopeless?
  - Do you ever feel you'd be better off dead and away from it all?
  - Have you ever made any plans (if drug overdose—have you handled the tablets)?
  - Have you ever made an attempt to take your own life?
  - What prevents you doing it?
  - Have you made any arrangements for your affairs after your death?
- *Assess psychiatric state:* Depression, agitation, early schizophrenia with retained insight (young patients who see their ambitions restricted), delusions of control, poverty, or guilt. Hopelessness is a good predictor for subsequent and immediate risk of suicide.
- *Refer for psychiatric assessment*
  - *If risk of suicide is high* (direct statement of intent, severe mood change, hopelessness, alcohol or drug dependence, abnormal personality, living alone) admit either via A&E or as a psychiatric emergency: Use the Mental Health Act for compulsory admission if voluntary admission is declined.
  - *If risk of suicide is lower:* Arrange for someone to stay with the patient until follow-up. Remove all potentially harmful drugs. Liaise with the psychiatric services, according to the individual patient, about psychiatric follow-up.

Support of those bereaved through suicide: Those bereaved through suicide face special problems. Give as much support as possible, try to ↓ stigma, suggest self-help groups and/or counselling.

Risk factors for suicide
- ♂>♀
- ↑ with age
- Divorced > widowed > never married > married
- Certain professions: vets, pharmacists, farmers, doctors
- Admission or recent discharge from psychiatric hospital
- Social isolation
- History of deliberate self-harm (100x ↑ risk)
- Depression
- Alcohol or substance abuse
- Personality disorder
- Schizophrenia
- Serious medical illness (e.g. cancer)

Suicide prevention: 'Our Healthier Nation' set a target to ↓ death by suicide by 17% by 2010. GPs play a crucial role in achieving this target. The UK suicide rate is 1:6000 and the average GP will have 10–15 patients who commit suicide during a career in general practice. In ♂ <35y. suicide is now the most common cause of death. The National Suicide Prevention Strategy for England sets out 6 goals and objectives:
- To ↓ risk in key high-risk groups
- To promote mental well-being in the wider population
- To ↓ availability and lethality of suicide methods
- To improve reporting of suicidal behaviour in the community
- To promote research on suicide and suicide prevention
- To improve monitoring of progress towards the 'Saving Lives: Our Healthier Nation' target to ↓ suicide

What can GPs do to prevent suicide? Early recognition, assessment, and treatment of those likely to attempt suicide is the key to the GP role—many visit their GP just weeks before suicide. Restrict access to lethal agents e.g. avoid tricyclic antidepressants and monitor repeat prescriptions of antidepressants carefully. Plan follow-up care for those discharged from psychiatric hospital. Review all suicides in practice significant event meeting.

Essential reading

NICE (2004) Self-harm: the short-term physical and psychological management and secondary prevention of self-harm in primary and secondary care ▣ http://www.nice.org.uk

Further information

DoH (2002) National Suicide Prevention Strategy for England ▣ http://www.dh.gov.uk

Patient/relative information and support

Self Injury and Related Issues (SIARI) ▣ http://www.siari.co.uk
Samaritans: 24h. emotional support via telephone ☎08457 909 090
Survivors of Bereavement by Suicide ☎0870 241 3337 ▣ http://www.uk-sobs.org.uk

Eating disorders[N]

Identification of and screening for eating disorders: Target groups for screening include:
- Young women with low BMI compared with age norms
- Patients consulting with weight concerns who are not overweight
- Women with menstrual disturbances or amenorrhoea
- Patients with GI symptoms
- Patients with symptoms/signs of starvation—sensitivity to cold, constipation, ↓ BP, bradycardia, hypothermia
- Patients with physical signs of repeated vomiting—pitted teeth ± dental caries, general weakness, cardiac arrythmias, renal damage, ↑ risk of UTI, epileptic fits, ↓K^+
- Children with poor growth
- Young people with type 1 DM and poor treatment adherence

Screen target populations with simple screening questions
- Do you worry excessively about your weight?
- Do you think you have an eating problem?

⚠ Patients who are pregnant or have DM are particularly at risk of complications if they have comorbid eating disorders. Refer early for specialist support and ensure everyone involved in care is aware of the eating disorder.

Anorexia nervosa: Prevalence 0.02–0.04%. ♀>>♂. Usually begins in adolescence. Peak prevalence at 16–17y. *Features*:
- Refusal to maintain body weight >85% of that expected (BMI <17.5 kg/m²)
- Intense fear of gaining weight—though underweight
- Disturbed experience of body weight or shape or undue influence of shape on self-image
- Amenorrhoea in women for ≥3 mo. and ↓ sexual interest.

Patients tend to have a set daily calorific intake (e.g. 600–1000 calories) and may employ strategies (e.g. bingeing and vomiting, purging, or excessive exercise) to try to lose weight. Depression and social withdrawal are common as are symptoms 2° to starvation (see above).

Management
- Give ongoing support and information.
- Check electrolytes.
- Refer to a specialist eating disorders clinic (if available) or psychiatry. Treatment involves family therapy for adolescents, psychotherapy, and possible admission for refeeding.

Follow-up: Patients with enduring anorexia nervosa not under 2° care follow-up should be offered an annual physical and mental health check.

⚠ Many patients with anorexia nervosa have compromised cardiac function. Avoid prescribing drugs which adversely affect cardiac function (e.g. antipsychotics, TCAs, macrolide antibiotics, some antihistamines). If prescribing is essential, then follow-up with ECG monitoring.

Bulimia nervosa: Prevalence 1–2%. Mainly ♀ aged 16–40y. *Features:*
- Recurrent episodes of binge eating, far beyond normally accepted amounts of food.
- Inappropriate compensatory behaviour to prevent weight ↑ e.g. vomiting; use of laxatives, diuretics, and/or appetite suppressants. Bulimics can be subdivided into those that purge and those that just use fasting and exercise to control their weight.
- Self-image unduly influenced by body shape (see anorexia above).
- Normal menses and normal weight. If low BMI, classified as anorexia.

Management
- Give ongoing support and information.
- Check electrolytes.
- First-line treatment:
  - Evidence-based self-help programme e.g. 'Overcoming bulimia'—CD-ROM available from Calipso ▣ *http://www.calipso.co.uk*—telephone-based self-help programme run by the Eating Disorders Association; details below; cost ~£200 *and/or*
  - Antidepressant medication—fluoxetine 60mg od is the drug of choice.
- If unsuccessful, refer to a specialist eating disorders clinic (if available) or psychiatry. CBT may help.

Advice for patients purging
- *Vomiting:* Advise patients to avoid brushing their teeth after vomiting, rinse with a non-acid mouthwash after vomiting, and ↓ acid oral environment (e.g. by limiting acid foods).
- *Laxatives:* Where laxative abuse is present, advise patients to gradually ↓ laxative intake. Laxative abuse does not significantly ↓ calorie absorption.

Binge eating disorder: A pattern of consumption of large amounts of food, even when a patient is not hungry. Common. Usually associated with obsessive feelings about food and body image, feelings of guilt/disgust about the amounts consumed, and/or a feeling of lack of control.

Management
- Give ongoing support and information
- Provide an evidence-based self-help programme as a first step and/or antidepressant medication (SSRI is the drug group of choice).
- If unsuccessful, refer for specialist help. CBT might be helpful.
- In all cases, provide concurrent advice and support to tackle any comorbid obesity.

Essential reading
NICE (2004) Core interventions in the treatment and management of anorexia nervosa, bulimia nervosa and related eating disorders ▣ *http://www.nice.org.uk*

Patient support and information
Eating Disorders Association (EDA) ☎0845 634 1414 (Adults) 0845 634 7650 (Youths)
▣ *http://www.edauk.com*

Other psychological conditions

Personality (behavioural) disorder: Patients may prefer the term 'personality difficulties'. Personality changes through life, and personality disorder should not be diagnosed aged <18 y. *Features:*
- Pervasive and maladaptive patterns of behaviour, thinking, and control of emotions.
- These patterns of behaviour, thinking, and control of emotions must be enduring and not limited to episodes of mental illness.
- There must be significant distress/disturbance in social function.

Types of personality disorder: 3 main types:
- Schizoid—paranoid ideas, difficulty mixing
- Histrionic—impulsive, unstable, 'borderline'
- Dependent—anxious, obsessive

Management
- Be clear about professional boundaries and avoid conflict.
- Involve family or friends in the care plan if appropriate.
- Consider referral to psychiatry:
  - For diagnostic clarification
  - If there is a risk of harm to self or others
  - For treatment of comorbid mental illness
  - For specialist treatment of personality disorder.
- SSRIs can help impulsive behaviour.
- Low-dose atypical antipsychotics may help paranoid ideas.
- Mood stabilizers may help emotional instability,

⚠ Risk of overdose is ↑ amongst patients with personality disorder.

Munchausen syndrome (factitious disorder): Intentional production or feigning of physical or psychological symptoms to assume the sick role (± hospital admission). Can be difficult to detect. Differs from *malingering* as there is no external reward (e.g. financial). Associated with personality disorder.

Common presentations
- *Physical:* Dermatitis artefacta, PUO, bruising disorders, brittle DM, diarrhoea of unknown cause, neurological symptoms e.g. psudoparalysis or pseudofits (neurologica diabolica), abdominal pain (laparotomophilia migrans), chest pain (cardiopathia fantastica).
- *Psychological:* Feigned psychosis, fictitious bereavement, fictitious overdose.

Management: Exclude any other basis for presenting pathology. Explain findings to the patient exploring possible causes. Assess psychological and social difficulties. Consider referral to psychiatry.

Munchausen syndrome by proxy: Caregiver—typically a mother with child—seeks repeated medical investigations and needless treatment for the person he/she is caring for. The child or person being cared for may actually be harmed by the carer to achieve these aims.

Common reported symptoms: Neurological, bleeding, rashes.

Management: Often difficult to detect and even harder to prove. A form of abuse that must be taken seriously and handled with care (📖 p.885). Involve all relevant agencies early (e.g. social services, paediatrics). (*Baron H.K.F.F. von Munchausen (1720–1797)—German traveller/soldier.*)

Malingering: Intentional production or feigning of physical or psychological symptoms to assume the sick role for a known external purpose. Malingering is not considered mental illness or psychopathology, although it can occur in the context of other mental illnesses. *Forms:*

• Pure malingering—the individual falsifies all symptoms.
• Partial malingering—the individual has symptoms but exaggerates the impact they have upon daily functioning.
• Simulation—the individual acts out the symptoms of a specific disability.
• False imputation—the individual has valid symptoms but is dishonest as to the source of the problems e.g. attributing neck pain to a RTA to obtain compensation.

Differential diagnosis

• True medical or psychiatric illness yet to be diagnosed
• Factitious disorder/Munchausen syndrome
• Somatization disorder

Common motivating factors

• Avoidance of going to jail or release from jail
• Avoidance of work
• Avoidance of family responsibility
• Desire to obtain narcotics
• Desire to be awarded money in litigation
• Need for attention

Management: Difficult. As doctors we tend to believe our patients.

• Exclude causes for the presenting symptoms through careful history/examination.
• Avoid prescribing drugs for symptoms and unnecessary referrals as these might perpetuate symptoms.
• Avoid certifying the patient as unfit to work or perform activities— if the patient is unhappy about this, suggest a second opinion.
• Tactfully explain your findings and conclusions to the patient and explore the reasons for the behaviour.
• Provide support to find more appropriate ways to solve problems.

Patient/relative information and support

Borderline UK 🖳 http://www.borderlineuk.co.uk
Borderline Personality Disorder (BPD) Central 🖳 http://www.bpdcentral.com
Self Injury and Related Issues (SIARI) 🖳 http://www.siari.co.uk

Compulsory hospitalization under the Mental Health Act 1983 (England & Wales)*

❶Try to obtain voluntary admission—it is better for both you and the patient.

Compulsory admission to hospital under the Mental Health Act may be used if:
- Voluntary admission is impossible *and*
- The patient is suffering from a mental disorder (i.e. mental illness, mental impairment, or psychopathy**) *and either*
  - Needs treatment of that disorder *or*
  - Poses a risk to self or others

Mental illness is not defined by the Act and left to clinical judgement but *does not* include alcohol or drug abuse.

Section 2: Admission for assessment: Most commonly used section in the community.
- Compulsory admission and detention at a hospital for 28d. for assessment. Not renewable after that time. Patients may appeal within 2wk. of detention via the Mental Health Tribunal.
- Can only be used if the patient needs to be detained for their own safety or the safety of others.
- The application must be made by an approved social worker (ASW) (Form 2) or the nearest relative*** (Form 1). Wherever possible, the ASW should be chosen, rather than the nearest relative to avoid affecting family relationships.
- It is a requirement that whoever makes the application must have seen the patient <2wk. ago.
- Recommendation of 2 doctors (not from the same hospital or practice) is needed—one of whom must be 'approved' under the Act and one, if practicable, must have prior knowledge of the patient (Form 3). Ideally, a GP who knows the patient should attend wherever possible. However, GPs are not obliged to visit a patient outside the practice area. The doctors must examine the patient and complete the form within 5d. of each other. GPs should keep a supply of Form 3 for this purpose.
- The application remains valid for 2wk.

In practice, this means calling in the duty social worker and duty psychiatrist. It can be a time consuming and frustrating business. Deputizing GPs should try and contact the patient's own GP.

Section 3: Admission for treatment
- Admission for treatment for ≤6mo..
- The exact mental disorder must be stated.
- Detention is renewable for a further 6mo. and annually thereafter.

- Application must be made by the nearest relative or an approved social worker on the recommendation of 2 doctors—one approved, and the other who has prior knowledge of the patient (see Section 2 above). The doctors must examine the patient and complete the form within 5d. of each other.
- Application remains valid for 14d.

Section 4: Emergency admission for assessment: Used in situations where admission is urgent and compliance with Section 2 would cause undesirable delay.

- Admission to hospital for 72h. only. Not renewable.
- Application must be made by the nearest relative or an approved social worker. It is only valid for 24h.
- Medical recommendation is from *either* an approved doctor *or* a doctor with prior knowledge of the patient.
- GPs should keep a supply of the relevant (pink) forms, as the duty social worker may not be available—Form 5 for use of the nearest relative; Form 7 for the medical recommendation.
- Usually converted to a Section 2 on arrival at hospital.

Section 115/135: Right of entry of an approved social worker (Section 115) or approved police officer (Section 135) who believes a person is being ill-treated or suffering from self-neglect to remove that person to a place of safety. Requires application to a magistrate. In practice, it is quite difficult to apply.

Scotland: The Mental Health Act Care and Treatment (Scotland) 2003 provides for compulsory admission under Part 5 for 72h. The application is made by a fully registered medical practitioner in consultation with a mental health officer, unless this is impracticable. In hospital Part 6 (lasting 28d.) can be applied and then, if necessary, Part 7 (Compulsory Treatment Order) for 6mo.

Further information
🖳 *http://www.scotland.gov.uk*

Essential reading
Hyperguide to the Mental Health Act 🖳 *http://www.hyperguide.co.uk/mha*

---

* In Northern Ireland, similar provisions apply under the Mental Health (Northern Ireland) Order 1986.
** Personality disorder characterized by inability to make loving relationships, antisocial behaviour, and lack of guilt.
*** Nearest relative is defined in the Act as the 1st surviving person out of: spouse (or co-habitee for >6mo.), oldest child (if >18y.), parent, oldest sibling (if >18y.), grandparent, grandchild (>18y.), uncle or aunt (>18y.), nephew or niece (>18y.), non-relative living with patient for ≥5y.

Other relevant pages

Elderly care

> 'Senescence begins,
> And middle age ends,
> The day your descendants
> Outnumber your friends'

Ogden Nash (1902–71)

Older people

Life expectancy is an indicator of the nation's health.
- Over the last century, life expectancy in the UK has risen from an expected lifespan of 45y. for men and 49y. for women in 1901 to 75y. and 80y. respectively in 2000.
- The population aged >65y. has ↑ >2x since the 1930s.
- Currently 1:5 of us is aged >60y.
- The number of individuals aged >90y. is set to double by 2025.
- By 2014 it is estimated that, for the first time, the number of people aged >65y. will exceed the number aged <16y.

Implications of an ageing population: ↑ life expectancy has consequences for the Health Service and those who work in it. Long-standing illness, restricted activity, and accidental injury all ↑ with age.
- In 1998/9, 40% of the NHS budget and nearly 50% of the social services budget was spent on people >65y. of age.
- $2/3$ of general and acute hospital beds are used by people >65y. of age.
- 35% accidental deaths in men and 73% in women occur in people >65y. of age.

Care of the elderly to maintain health and independence is a priority.

Aims of care: Older people are not a uniform group and have a wide range of needs. However, they can be broadly classified into 3 groups:
- ***Entering old age:*** People who have completed their career in paid employment and/or childrearing. These people are active and independent and many remain so for a considerable time. *Aims of care:* promotion of a healthy active life and prevention of disease.
- ***Transitional phase:*** This group is in transition between healthy, active life and frailty. This transition can occur at any age but most commonly takes place between 70–80y. *Aims of care:* identification and effective management of ongoing and emergent problems.
- ***Frail older people:*** These patients are vulnerable as a result of health, social problems, or a combination of both. Often experienced only in late old age. *Aims of care:* maintenance of quality of life.

The role of the GP: A holistic model of care considering interaction of multiple health problems and effects of medication alongside social and family considerations is essential when dealing with older people. The role of the GP is central to that care as:
- Coordinator of services over time
- Provider and monitor of care
- Advocate for patient and family.

Most problems likely to be encountered are not problems specific to old age, though they might be more common in the older age groups. They are covered within their topic sections.

Routine health checks: All patients >75y. are entitled to a health check every year if they have not been seen in the practice for another reason in that time.

Table 27.1 Normal changes of ageing

	18–50y.	50–70y.	>70y.
CVS	>40y. artery walls lose elasticity causing ↑ BP.	Heart muscle becomes less elastic and less able to respond to ↑ effort.	By 85y. the heart is unable to support strenuous activity → tire more easily.
Respiratory	Max. lung function aged 20–30y.; lung function ↓.	By 65y. lung efficiency ↓ by ~40%.	By 80y. lung efficiency is ↓ by ½ → shortness of breath on exertion.
GI	>30y. energy needs ↓ by 5%/y.—unless diet is adjusted → ↑ weight.	Volume of digestive fluids ↓ as does efficiency of the bowel → hard stool ± constipation.	↓ sense of taste; chewing and swallowing may be hampered by tooth loss ± gum disease.
GU	Women: ↓ pelvic muscle tone after childbirth → urinary incontinence; menopause age 45–55y. Men: testosterone levels start to ↓ from ~40–50y.	Women: ↓ oestrogen levels ↓ pelvic muscle tone further and causes vaginal dryness. Men: prostate gland starts to enlarge >50y. and may cause urinary symptoms.	>75–80y. kidney function ↓ → ↓ drug clearance and ↑ toxic effects. Men: ↓ libido and ↓ viable sperm.
Sensory	By 40y. difficulty in focusing on close objects; ↓ hearing starts in the 30s.	Short-term memory and ability to concentrate ↓; reactions slower; >50y. harder to see in low light/moving objects; by 70y. harder to hear faint/high-pitched sounds.	By 90y., 10% brain tissue is lost. Sight and hearing continue to ↓.
Skin, hair, bones, joints	Bones reach max. density in early adulthood; after 25y. muscle bulk and strength start to ↓; ½ people >40y. have grey hair; wrinkles start to appear due to loss of skin elasticity >40y.	Bones weaken (especially postmenopausal women); muscle mass and strength continue to ↓; skin becomes drier; hair thins ± falls out (M>F); teeth may begin to fall out.	Wearing of joints → pain and stiffness; muscle strength at 85y. = ½ strength at 25y.; skin is less able to regulate body temperature → more susceptible to the effects of outside temperature.

National Service Framework for Older People

'Old age is an illness in itself'
Phormio Act IV, Terence (185–159 BC)

Published in March 2001. Sets new national standards of care for all older people in England and Wales, whether they live at home, in residential care, or are being cared for in hospital. It aims to ensure:
• high-quality care and treatment, regardless of age
• older people are treated as individuals, with respect and dignity
• there is fair allocation of resources for conditions which most affect older people
• the financial burden of long-term residential care is eased

National Service Framework standards
• *Rooting out age discrimination*—NHS and social care services will be provided, regardless of age, on the basis of need alone.
• *Person-centred care*—older people will be treated as individuals and enabled to make choices about their own care. This will be achieved through better integration of health and social care services.
• *Intermediate care*—intermediate care services at home or in designated care settings will promote the independence of older people, prevent unnecessary hospital admission, enable early discharge from hospital, and prevent premature or unnecessary admission to long-term residential care.
• *General hospital care*—older people's care in hospital will be delivered through appropriate specialist care and by hospital staff who have the right set of skills to meet their needs.
• *Stroke*—1° and 2° prevention of stroke is a priority (□ p.608).
• *Falls*—prevention of falls is a priority (□ p.162).
• *Mental health in older people*—effective diagnosis, treatment, and support for older people with mental health problems and their carers (□ p.957–88).
• *Promoting an active healthy life in older age*—health and well-being of older people is promoted through a coordinated programme of action led by the NHS with support from councils.

Patient information and support
Age Concern 🖳 *http://www.ageconcern.org.uk*
DOH Older people's services 🖳 *http://www.dh.gov.uk*
European older-people's platform (AGE) 🖳 *http://www.age-platform.org*
Government over 50s website 🖳 *http://www.over50.gov.uk*
Help the Aged 🖳 *http://www.helptheaged.org.uk*
NHSDirect 🖳 *http://www.nhsdirect.nhs.uk*
Pensioners' guide 🖳 *http://www.info4pensioners.gov.uk*
Pension guide 🖳 *http://www.pensionguide.gov.uk*

Further information
National Service Frameworks—📖 p.168
National Service Framework for Older People 🖥 *http://www.dh.gov.uk*

Long-term care

Older people often require a combination of support from medical, nursing, social care, community health, welfare rights, and housing services in order to meet their long-term care needs. The system of long-term care throughout the UK is complex. Whilst some services are provided by the NHS, others are provided through local authorities, and some people opt for private care. Some care is free but other types are means-tested, and there are further anomalies between countries within the UK. Long-term care could include care provided:
- in a residential care home
- by carers—either unpaid (e.g. relatives) or paid (e.g. home helps)
- by meals on wheels and laundry services.

Informal carers: 📖 p.178

Residential care: GPs often become involved when a person decides (or is forced by circumstances) to go into residential care. *Options are:*
- *Sheltered housing*—usually warden-controlled flats, though may be a shared residence.
- *Local authority care home*
- *Independent care home*—often part funded by social services depending on resources.
- *Nursing home*—registered with the Health Authority, with qualified nurses always on hand.
- *Hospital*—suitable where there are medical needs. GP or cottage hospitals often provide respite care.
- *Hospice*—for terminally ill patients. Usually no charge to patients. May be charity funded or run by the NHS.

Care homes: Many people will spend their later years in residential care homes, recently renamed 'care homes'. Care homes provide different levels of care—some provide personal care alone, others provide personal and nursing care. All care homes are required to be registered and regulated by the Local Care Standards Authority. The regulating authorities in the UK are:
- England—Commission for Social Care Inspection
  🖥 *http://www.csci.org.uk*
- Scotland—Scottish Commission for the Regulation of Care (Care Commission) 🖥 *www.carecommission.com*
- Wales—Care Standards Inspectorate for Wales
  🖥 *http://www.csiw.wales.gov.uk*

Choice of establishment: Depends on needs and financial constraints of the individual and characteristics and capabilities of the establishment. Lists of nursing and rest homes in an area can be obtained from social services.

Financial arrangements: Can be confusing. Nursing costs are met by the NHS through the local PCO. Funding depends on the level of care required. Living costs are paid either by the client, the local authority, or a combination of the 2—dependant on means testing. Age Concern produces a detailed factsheet (🖥 *http://www.ageconcern.org.uk*).

Moving into residential care affects entitlement to benefits

- *Attendance allowance/disability living allowance*—stops after 4wk. unless the individual is fully privately funded.
- *Income support/income-based job seeker's allowance*—varies according to the type of care and whether the move is temporary/permanent.
- *Housing benefit/council tax benefit*—for temporary stays continues to be paid. If a permanent move, both benefits cease.
- *War pensioners*—may be entitled to extra help with costs. Contact the Veterans' Agency (📖 p.100).

GP services to care homes: Care home residents typically generate more work than older people who are still living at home. GPs are not obliged to provide any additional services to care homes. Particularly:

- GPs are not obliged to make any notes in nursing home records.
- GPs are not required to make entries on or annotate nursing home prescription (MAR) sheets. GPs are required to issue prescriptions on NHS FP10 forms.
- GPs are not obliged to visit nursing home patients automatically. Visits should be based on clinical need and not convenience.
- GPs are not required to undertake 'routine' reviews of patients.

Hospital admission: Treatment in NHS hospitals is free at the point of delivery to UK residents. Benefits are not usually affected by admission to a private hospital if privately funded. On admission to an NHS hospital, benefits continue for at least 2wk. Exceptions are benefits payable to people admitted from local authority residential care. After that time:

- *>2wk.*—job seeker's allowance stops; individuals can claim income support and incapacity benefit.
- *>4wk.*—attendance allowance and disability living allowance stop; severe disability premium is ↓.
- *>13wk.*—income support, widows' benefits, incapacity benefit all ↓.
- *>1y.*—incapacity benefit ↓; housing benefit ↓ or stops; council tax benefit stops.

2 admissions separated by <28d. are treated as a single admission. Visitors with low incomes may be entitled to help for travel to and from the hospital.

Intermediate care: Period of admission to residential care on a short-term basis for treatment or therapy, following a period in hospital or to avoid hospital admission. Limited to a 6wk. stay and provided free of charge.

Patient information and support

Age Concern 🖳 http://www.ageconcern.org.uk
Department of Work and Pensions 🖳 http://www.dwp.gov.uk
Citizen's Advice Bureau 🖳 http://www.adviceguide.org.uk
Elderly Accommodation Counsel ☎020 7820 1343
🖳 http://www.housingcare.org

Falls amongst the elderly

Falls are a major cause of disability and the leading cause of mortality due to injury in people aged >75y. The government sets out its strategy for tackling falls in the National Service Framework for Older People. The key interventions proposed include: public health strategies to ↓ incidence of falls in the population, and identification, assessment, and prevention measures for those most at risk of falling.

Incidence: ↑ with age—1:3 adults >65y. living in the community and ½ those living in institutions have fallen in the past year.

Consequences of falling

- 20% experience a fall with injury requiring acute medical attention though <1:10 falls → fracture (mainly Colles' and fractured neck of femur).
- Even if uninjured, older people might not be able to get up off the floor without help. The result may be a prolonged period of lying on the floor until help arrives. Apart from the indignity and helplessness this generates, 2° problems (e.g. pneumonia, pressure sores, hypothermia, and dehydration) may follow.
- Any fall may seriously undermine an elderly person's confidence and make him (and his relatives/carers) worry about the possibility of recurrence. As a result, he may restrict activities, becoming less fit and more dependent on others.

Risk factors for falls: Recurrent falls ↑ with number of risk factors:

- ♀:♂ ≈ 2:1 in the over 75s
- ↑ age
- Multiple previous falls
- Disorders of gait or balance
- Visual impairment
- Cognitive impairment
- Low morale/depression
- High level of dependence
- ↓ mobility
- Lower limb weakness or arthritis
- Foot problems
- History of stroke or PD
- Use of psychotropic drugs, sedatives, diuretics, or β-blockers
- Alcohol
- Environmental factors (e.g. loose rugs, poor lighting, ice on the pavement, high winds)

History: deal with the injuries first—ask about pain, loss of function, headache. Ask carers about behaviour.

Examination: Check for bruising, loss of function, confusion, BP, pulse, neurology, and fundi. Consider hypothermia if on the floor any length of time.

Investigate the cause of the fall: *Consider:*

- ***Physical problems:*** neurological problems (e.g. stroke); visual loss; cardiac abnormalities (e.g. arrythmia, postural hypotension); muscular abnormalities (e.g. steroid-induced myopathy); skeletal problems (e.g. osteoarthritis).
- ***Environmental problems:*** climbing ladders to do routine maintenance; loose/holed carpets; slippery floor or bath; chair or bed too low.

Management

- Treat any acute injury. ❶ Subdural haematoma may take several days or weeks to reveal itself.
- Perform a falls assessment (📖 p.163) or refer to a specialist falls service for a falls assessment.
- Undertake measures to ↓ risk of falls/damage from falling—📖 p.163.
- Specialist referral to the care of the elderly team is appropriate if the cause of recurrent falls remains unclear; the patient or carer are worried about the possibility of further falls; or there is doubt about whether the patient can cope in their current social circumstances.

Prevention of falls: 📖 p.162

Osteoporosis and prevention of fracture: 📖 p.568

Further information

Bandolier: Falls in the elderly
  🖥 http://www.jr2.ox.ac.uk/bandolier/band20/b20-5.html
Cochrane (2002) Interventions for preventing falls in elderly people. Gillespie et al.
British Geriatric Society Falls and Bone Health Special Interest Group
  🖥 http://www.falls-and-bone-health.org.uk
SIGN (2002) Prevention and management of hip fracture in older people
  🖥 http://www.sign.ac.uk
NICE (2004) Guidelines for the assessment and prevention of falls
  🖥 http://www.nice.org.uk
Feder et al. (2000) Guidelines for the prevention of falls in people over 65. *BMJ*
  21:1007–1011 🖥 http://www.bmj.com
National Service Framework for Older People
  🖥 http://www.dh.gov.uk

Patient information and support

Disabled Living Foundation
  🖥 http://www.dlf.org.uk
Royal Society for the Prevention of Accidents
  🖥 http://www.rospa.co.uk

Palliative care

Further information

NICE Improving supportive and palliative care for adults with cancer (2004)
🖳 *http://www.nice.org.uk*
Hospice information ☎0870 903 3903 🖳 *http://www.hospiceinformation.info*
Woodruff, Doyle (2004) *The IAHPC Manual of Palliative Care* (2nd Edition) IAHPC Press
🖳 *http://www.hospicecare.com/manual/IAHPCmanual.htm*

Patient advice and support

British Association of Cancer United Patients (BACUP) ☎0800 800 1234
🖳 *http://www.bacup.org.uk*
DIPEX Project: Patient experiences 🖳 *http://www.dipex.org*

Palliative care in general practice

> 'Any man's death diminishes me because I am involved in mankind'
> Devotions Meditation 17, John Donne (1572–1631).

Palliative care starts when the emphasis changes from curing the patient and prolonging life to relieving symptoms and maintaining well-being or 'quality of life'. GPs have 1 or 2 patients with terminal disease at any time, and get more personally involved with them than any others.

The problems arising are a complex mix of physical, psychological, social, cultural, and spiritual factors involving both patients and carers. To respond adequately, good lines of communication and close multidisciplinary teamwork is needed. Local palliative care teams are invaluable sources of advice and support and frequently produce booklets with advice on aspects of palliative care for GPs.

Symptom control must be tailored to the needs of the individual. A few basic rules apply:
- Carefully diagnose the cause of the symptom
- Explain the symptom to the patient
- Discuss treatment options
- Set realistic goals
- Anticipate likely problems
- Review regularly

The Gold Standards Framework: aims to improve quality and of palliative care provided by the primary care team by developing practice-based organization of care of dying patients. The framework focuses on 7 key tasks—optimising continuity of care, teamwork, advanced planning (including out-of-hours), symptom control, and patient, carer and staff support. Evaluation data show the framework ↑, the proportion of patients dying in their preferred place, and improves quality of care as perceived by the practitioners involved.

Further information
Gold Standards Framework ☎ 020 7840 4673
E-mail gsf@macmillan.org.uk
NICE Improving supportive and palliative care for adults with cancer (2004)
🖳 http://www.nice.org.uk
Hospice information ☎0870 903 3903 🖳 http://www.hospiceinformation.info
Woodruff, Doyle (2004) The IAHPC Manual of Palliative Care (2nd Edition) IAHPC Press.
🖳 http://www.hospicecare.com/manual/IAHPCmanual.htm

Patient advice and support
British Association of Cancer United Patients (BACUP) ☎0800 800 1234
🖳 http://www.bacup.org.uk
Macmillan Cancer Relief ☎0808 808 2020 🖳 http://www.macmillan.org.uk

Syringe drivers: Although drugs to control the symptoms of terminal illness can usually be administered by mouth, occasionally that is not possible. Portable syringe drivers give a continuous subcutaneous infusion and can provide good control of symptoms with little discomfort or inconvenience to the patient. *Indications:*
- The patient is unable to take medicines by mouth owing to nausea and vomiting, dysphagia, severe weakness, or coma
- There is bowel obstruction and further surgery is inappropriate
- The patient does not want to take regular medication by mouth

Drugs which can be used in syringe drivers: Table 28.1

Mixing drugs in syringe drivers: Provided there is evidence of compatibility, drugs can be mixed in syringe drivers. Diamorphine can be mixed with:
- Cyclizine
- Hyoscine hydrobromide
- Hyoscine butylbromide
- Midazolam
- Dexamethasone
- Levomepromazine
- Haloperidol
- Metoclopramide

Common problems with syringe drivers
- *If the syringe driver runs too slowly:* Check it is switched on; check the battery; check the cannula is not blocked.
- *If the syringe driver runs too quickly:* Check the rate setting.
- *Injection site reaction:* If there is pain or inflammation, change the injection site.

Table 28.1 Drugs which can be used in syringe drivers

Indication	Drugs
Nausea and vomiting	Haloperidol 2.5–10mg/24h.
	Levomepromazine 5–200mg/24h. (causes sedation in 50%)
	Cyclizine 150mg/24h. (may precipitate if mixed with other drugs)
	Metoclopramide 30–100mg/24h.
	Octreotide 300–600mcg/24h. (consultant supervision)
	Hyoscine hydrobromide 20–60mg/24h.
Respiratory secretions	Hyoscine hydrobromide 0.6–2.4mg/24h.
	Glycopyrronium 0.6–1.2mg/24h.
Restlessness and confusion	Haloperidol 5–15mg/24h.
	Levomepromazine 50–200mg/24h.
	Midazolam 20–100mg/24h. (and fitting)
Pain control	Diamorphine—$1/3$–$1/2$ dose oral morphine/24h.

❶ Subcutaneous infusion solution should be monitored regularly both to check for precipitation (and discolouration) and to ensure the infusion is running at the correct rate.

⚠ Incorrect use of syringe drivers is a common cause of drug errors.

Pain and general debility

Pain control: Pain control is the cornerstone of palliative care. Cancer pain is multifactorial—be aware of physical and psychological factors.

Principles of pain control: 📖 p.172

Pain-relieving drugs: 📖 p.174

Management of specific types of pain: Table 28.2

Terminal restlessness: *Causes:*
- *Pain/discomfort*—urinary retention, constipation, pain which the patient cannot tell you about, excess secretions in throat.
- *Opiate toxicity*—causes myoclonic jerking. The dose of morphine may need to be ↓ if a patient becomes uraemic.
- *Biochemical causes*—↑ Ca^{2+}, uraemia—❶ If it has been decided not to treat abnormalities, DON'T check for them.
- *Psychological/spiritual distress*

Management
- Treat reversible causes e.g. catheterization for retention, hyoscine to dry up secretions.
- If still restless, treat with a sedative. This does NOT shorten life but makes the patient and any relatives in attendance more comfortable. *Suitable drugs:* haloperidol 1–3mg tds po; chlorpromazine 25–50mg tds po; diazepam 2–10mg tds po, midazolam or levomepromazine via syringe driver.

Weakness, fatigue, and drowsiness: Almost a universal symptom.
Reversible causes
- Drugs—opiates, benzodiazepines, steroids (proximal muscle weakness), diuretics (dehydration and biochemical abnormalities), antihypertensives (postural hypotension)
- Emotional problems—depression, anxiety, fear, apathy
- Hyercalcaemia
- Other biochemical abnormalities—DM, electrolyte disturbance, uraemia, liver disease, thyroid dysfunction
- Anaemia
- Poor nutrition
- Infection
- Prolonged bed rest
- Raised intracranial pressure (drowsiness only)

Management
- Treat reversible causes.
- If drowsiness and fatigue persist, consider a trial of dexamethasone 4–6mg/d. or antidepressant. Although steroids make muscle wasting worse, they may improve general fatigue and improve mobility.
- Psychological support of patients and carers—empathy, explanation.
- Physical support—referral to physiotherapist, review of aids and appliances, review of home layout (possibly with referral to OT), review of home care arrangements.
- Advice on modification of lifestyle.

Table 28.2 Management of specific types of pain

Type of pain	Management
Bone pain	<ul><li>Try NSAIDs</li><li>Consider referral for palliative radiotherapy, strontium treatment (prostate cancer), or iv bisphosphonates (↓ pain in myeloma, breast and prostate cancer)</li><li>Refer to orthopaedics if any lytic metastases at risk of fracture, for consideration of pinning</li></ul>
Abdominal pain	<ul><li>Constipation is the most common cause—📖 p.1007</li><li>Colic—try loperamide 2–4mg qds or hyoscine hydrobromide 300mcg tds s/ling. Hyoscine can also be given via syringe driver.</li><li>Liver capsule pain—use dexamethasone 4–8mg /d, titrating dose down to the minimum that controls pain</li><li>Gastric distention—may be helped by an antacid ± an anti-foaming agent (e.g. Asilone). Alternatively, a prokinetic may help e.g. domperidone 10mg tds before meals.</li><li>Upper GI tumour—coeliac plexus block may help. Refer to palliative care team.</li><li>Consider drug causes—NSAIDs are a common iatrogenic cause</li><li>Acute/subacute obstruction—📖 p.1004</li></ul>
Neuropathic pain	<ul><li>Often burning/shooting and may not respond to simple analgesia</li><li>Titrate to the maximum tolerated dose of opioid</li><li>If inadequate, add a nerve pain killer e.g. amitriptyline 10–25mg nocte increasing as needed every 2wk. to 75–150mg. Alternatives include carbamazepine, gabapentin, phenytoin, sodium valproate, and clonazepam.</li><li>If pain is due to nerve compression caused by tumour, dexamethasone 8mg od may help</li><li>*Other options:* TENS; acupuncture; nerve block</li></ul>
Rectal pain	<ul><li>Topical drugs e.g. rectal steroids</li><li>TCAs e.g. amitriptyline 10–75mg nocte</li><li>Anal spasms—glyceryl trinitrate ointment 0.1–0.2% bd</li><li>Referral for local radiotherapy</li></ul>
Muscle pain	<ul><li>Paracetamol and/or NSAIDs</li><li>Muscle relaxants e.g. diazepam 5–10mg od, baclofen 5–10mg tds, dantrolene</li><li>Physiotherapy, aromatherapy, or relaxation</li><li>Heat pads</li></ul>
Bladder spasm	<ul><li>Try oxybutinin 5mg tds or tolterodine 2mg bd</li><li>Amitriptyline 10–75mg nocte is often effective</li><li>If catheterized, try instilling 20mls of intravesical bupivacaine 0.25% for 15min. tds</li></ul>
Acute pain of short duration e.g. dressing changes	<ul><li>Try a short-acting opiate e.g. meptazinol 200mg po given 20min. prior to procedure</li></ul>

Dysphagia, nausea, and vomiting

Nausea and vomiting are common in patients with advanced cancer. Consider cause and mechanism before choosing an antiemetic (Table 28.3). Remember hypercalcaemia as a cause of persistent nausea. Don't forget non-drug measures to ↓ nausea e.g.

- avoidance of food smells and unpleasant odours
- diversion
- relaxation
- acupressure/acupuncture

⚠ For prophylaxis of nausea and vomiting—use po medication; for established nausea or vomiting—consider a parenteral route (e.g. syringe driver) as persistent nausea may ↓ gastric emptying and drug absorption.

Review antiemetic therapy daily.

Obstruction/subacute obstruction of the bowel: Often of complex origin with functional and mechanical elements. Presents with:

- Vomiting—often faeculent with little preceding nausea
- Constipation
- Abdominal distention

Examination reveals an empty rectum.

Treatment options

- If surgery is an option, then refer for a surgical opinion.
- If the patient is otherwise well, consider referral to an oncologist— ovarian and colonic cancers often respond to chemotherapy.
- Otherwise, treatment is symptomatic:
  - Dexamethasone 4–8mg/d.—antiemetic and minimizes obstruction
  - If colic is a problem, stop prokinetics (metoclopramide/domperidone) and start an antispasmodic (e.g. hyoscine 300mcg tds po)
  - For pain, give an opiate—if there is a risk of malabsorption, give by syringe driver
  - Aim to abolish nausea and keep vomiting to a minimum (may be impossible to abolish vomiting) with cyclizine, haloperidol, or levomepromazine
  - If vomiting cannot be controlled, consider referral for venting gastrostomy
  - Keep stool soft
  - Consider referral to palliative care for antisecretory agents (e.g. octreotide).

Dysphagia: May be due to physical obstruction (by tumour bulk) or functional obstruction (neurological deficit).

- Treat the cause if possible e.g. celestin tube for oesophageal tumour
- If the patient is hungry and wishes to be fed, consider referral for a percutaneous endoscopic gastrostomy (PEG)
- If the patient does not wish to have a PEG, ask whether s/he would like subcutaneous fluids and treat symptomatically with mouth care, anxiolytics, analgesia, and sedation.

Table 28.3 Choice of antiemetic

Mechanism of vomiting	Antiemetic
↑ICP	• Dexamethasone 8–16mg/d. • Cyclizine 50mg bd/tds • Levomepromazine 6–25mg/d.
Anxiety, fear, or pain	• Benzodiazepines e.g. diazepam 2–10mg/d. or midazolam sc • Cyclizine 50mg bd/tds • Levomepromazine 6–25mg/d.
Motion/position	• Cyclizine 50mg tds po/sc/im • Hyoscine po (300mcg tds) or transdermally (1mg/72h.) • Prochlorperazine po (5mg qds) or buccal (3–6mg bd)
Endogenous toxins/drugs	• Ondansetron (particularly for chemotherapy induced vomiting) 8mg bd po or 16mg od pr • Haloperidol 1.5–5mg nocte (particularly for opiate induced vomiting, hypercalcaemia, or renal failure). An antiemetic is usually necessary only for the first 4–5d. of opiate therapy. • Alternatives include: metoclopramide; cyclizine; levomepromazine
Gastric stasis*	• Domperidone 10mg tds or metoclopramide 10mg tds (particularly if multifactorial with gastric stasis and a central component)
Gastric irritation	• PPIs e.g. lansoprazole 30mg od or omeprazole 20mg od • Antacids • Misoprostol 200mcg bd—if caused by NSAIDS
Constipation	• Laxatives/suppositories/enemas
Intestinal obstruction	• See opposite
Cough induced	• 📖 p.1011
Unknown cause	• Cyclizine 50mg tsd • Levomepromazine 6–25mg/d. • Dexamethasone 4–8mg daily po/sc • Metoclopramide 10mg tds po

* Vomits of undigested food without nausea soon after eating.

❶ Drugs with antimuscarinic effects antagonize prokinetic drugs and therefore, where possible, should not be used concurrently.

Use of a syringe driver: 📖 p.1001

Other GI problems

Anorexia
- Treat nausea, mouth problems, pain, and other symptoms
- ↓ psychological distress and treat depression
- Advise small, appetising meals, frequently, in comfortable surroundings

Drugs that may be helpful
- Alcohol pre-meals
- Metoclopramide or domperidone 10mg tds pre-meals—to prevent feeling of satiety caused by gastric stasis
- Dexamethasone 2–4mg od or prednisolone 15–30mg od

Mouth problems

General measures
- Review medication making the mouth sore or dry
- Treat oral infections: oral thrush—fluconazole 50mg od for 7d. and soak dentures in Milton fluid for ≥12h. to prevent reinfection
- Mouthwashes—saline, betadine, oraldene, corsodyl, difflam (for pain)
- ¼ –½ ascorbic acid 1g effervescent tablet/d.—place on tongue and allow to dissolve
- Mouth care—refer to DN for advice; use a toothbrush to keep the tongue clean

Specific measures
- Painful mouth—difflam mouthwash ± xylocaine spray
- Ulcers or painful areas—adcortyl in orabase paste topically qds after eating and nocte
- Oral cancer pain—topical NSAIDs e.g. piroxicam melt
- Chemotherapy induced ulcers—sucralfate suspension
- Dry mouth
  - Review medication which might be causing dry mouth e.g. antidepressants, opioids
  - Salivary stimulants—iced water, pineapple chunks, chewing gum, boiled sweets or mints
  - Saliva substitutes e.g. glandosane spray
- Radiotherapy induced dryness—pilocarpine
- Excessive salivation—amitriptyline 10–100mg nocte, hyoscine or glycopyrronium via syringe driver.

Ascites: Depending on clinical state, consider referring for chemotherapy if appropriate *or* treat symptoms:
- Give analgesia for discomfort
- Refer to the general physicians or surgeons for paracentesis if the patient is well and/or peritoneo-venous shunt if recurrent
- Try diuretics—furosemide 20–40mg od or spironolactone 100–200mg od and/or dexamethasone 2–4mg daily
- Try support stockings and/or massage for leg oedema
- 'Squashed stomach syndrome'—try prokinetics e.g. domperidone or metoclopramide 10mg tds.

Hiccup: A distressing symptom. Treatment is often unsatisfactory.
- *General measures:* Rebreathing with a paper bag; pharyngeal stimulation by drinking cold water or taking a teaspoonful of granulated sugar.
- *Peripheral hiccups:* Caused by irritation of the phrenic nerve or diaphragm. Try metoclopramide (10mg tds), antacids containing dimethicone (e.g. gaviscon), dexamethasone (4–12mg/d.), or ranitidine (150mg bd).
- *Central hiccups:* Due to medullary stimulation e.g. ↑ICP, uraemia. Try chlorpromazine (10–25mg tds/qds), dexamethasone (4–12mg/d.), nifedipine (10mg tds), or baclofen (5mg bd).

Constipation: Very common symptom. *Causes:*
- Immobility
- Poor diet
- Poor fluid intake
- Old age
- Drugs—particularly opiates and antidepressants

⚠ Constipation can herald spinal cord compression. If suspected, do a full neurological examination.

Management
- Pre-empt constipation by putting everyone at risk on aperients.
- Treat with regular stool softener (e.g. magnesium hydroxide) ± regular bowel stimulant (e.g. senna) or alternatively use a combination drug (e.g. co-danthrusate).
- If that is ineffective, add glycerine suppositories (hard stool) or bisocodyl suppositories (soft stool).
- If still not cleared, refer to the district nurse for microlet enemas ± high phosphate or arachis oil enemas.
- Once cleared, leave on a regular aperient with instructions to ↑ aperients if constipation recurs.

Diarrhoea: Less common than constipation but can be distressing for the patient and difficult for the carer—especially if incontinence results.

Management
- Screen for infection.
- Ensure no overflow diarrhoea 2° to constipation.
- Ensure no excessive/erratic laxative use.
- Consider giving pancreatic enzyme supplements e.g. creon 25000 tds prior to meals if malabsorption.
- Consider prednisolone enemas/foam (e.g. colifoam) for radiotherapy induced diarrhoea.
- Otherwise, treat symptomatically with codeine phosphate 30–60mg qds or loperamide 2mg tds/qds.

Gut fistulae: Connections from the gut to other organs—commonly skin, bladder, or vagina. Bowel fistulae are characterized by air passing through the fistula channel.

Management
- If well enough for surgery, refer to a surgeon.
- If not fit for surgery, consider referring to palliative care for octreotide.

Neurological and orthopaedic problems

Raised intracranial pressure: Occurs with 1° or 2° brain tumours. Characterized by
- Headache—worse on lying
- Vomiting
- Confusion
- Diplopia
- Convulsions
- Papilloedema

Management
- Unless a terminal event, refer patients urgently to neurosurgery for assessment. Options include insertion of a shunt or cranial radiotherapy.
- If no further active treatment is appropriate, start symptomatic treatment—raise the head of the bed, start dexamethasone 16mg/d. (stop if no response in 1wk.), analgesia.

Spinal cord compression: Affects 5% of cancer patients—70% in thoracic region. Presentation can be subtle. Maintain a *high* level of suspicion in all cancer patients who complain of back pain, especially those with known bony metastases or tumours likely to metastasize to bone.

Presentation
- Often back pain, worse on movement, appears before neurology.
- Neurological symptoms can be non-specific—constipation, weak legs, incontinence of urine.

Management: Prompt treatment (<24–48h. from 1st neurological symptoms) is needed if there is any hope of restoring function. Once paralysed, <5% walk again. Treat with oral dexamethasone 16mg/d. and refer urgently for radiotherapy, unless in final stages of disease.

Bone fractures: Common in advanced cancer due to osteoporosis, trauma as a result of falls, or metastases. Have a low index of suspicion if a new bony pain develops.

⚠ In the elderly, fracture of a long bone can present as acute confusion.

Management
- Analgesia
- Unless in a very terminal state, confirm the fracture on X-ray and refer to orthopaedics or radiotherapy urgently for consideration of fixation (long bones, wrist, neck of femur) and/or radiotherapy (rib fractures, vertebral fractures).

Hypercalcaemia: Most common with:
- Myeloma (>30%)
- Breast cancer (40%)
- Squamous cell cancers.

Presentation: Symptoms are non-specific:
- Thirst
- Polyuria and polydipsia
- Constipation
- Nausea and vomiting
- Abdominal pain
- ↓ appetite
- Depression
- Fatigue
- Confusion

⚠ Always suspect hypercalcaemia if someone is iller than expected for no obvious reason. Untreated hypercalcaemia can be fatal.

Management: Depending on the general state of the patient, make a decision whether to treat the hypercalcaemia or not. If a decision is made *not* to treat, provide symptom control and don't check the serum calcium again. Active treatment depends on the level of symptoms and hypercalcaemia:
- *Asymptomatic patient with corrected calcium <3mmol/l:* Monitor
- *Symptomatic and/or corrected calcium >3mmol/l:*
  - Arrange treatment with pamidronate via oncologist/palliative care team immediately.
  - Check serum calcium 7–10d. post-treatment. 20% do not respond and there is no benefit from retreating them.
  - Effect of pamidronate lasts 20–30d.. Consider maintenance with oral bisphosphonates (e.g. sodium clodronate) started 1wk. after the initial iv pamidronate or regular iv pamidronate. Many initially responsive to bisphosphonates become unresponsive with time.

Further information: 📖 p.424

Respiratory problems

Breathlessness: Usually multifactorial. Affects 70% of terminally ill patients. It is inevitable that breathlessness has a psychological element as being short of breath is frightening.

General management

Non-drug measures
- General reassurance
- Explanation of reasons for breathlessness and adaptations to lifestyle that might help
- Proper positioning—breathlessness is improved by sitting upright and straight
- Try a stream of air over the face e.g. fan, open window
- Breathing exercises can help—refer to physio. Exercises include diaphragmatic breathing and control of breathing rate; relaxation/distraction training.

Drug treatment
- Tenacious secretions—try nebulized saline
- Oral or subcutaneous opioids ↓ subjective sensation of breathlessness—start with oramorph 2.5mg 4 hrly and titrate upwards
- Try benzodiazepines—diazepam 2–5mg od/bd for background control and lorazepam 1–2mg sl prn in between
- Oxygen has a variable effect and is worth a try.

Specific measures
- *Airway compression, bronchoconstriction, or lymphangitis*—try steroids (dexamethasone 4–8mg/d.)
- *Intrinsic or extrinsic compression*—consider referral for radiotherapy, laser therapy, or stenting
- *Pleural effusion*—consider referral for drainage ± pleuradesis
- *Infection*—antibiotics. Most people with terminal disease have a depressed immune system, so have a low threshold to treat with a broad-spectrum antibiotic
- *Pneumothorax on CXR*—consider referral for chest drain
- *Ascites*—consider referral for paracentesis if causing breathlessness
- *Suspected pulmonary emboli*—consider anticoagulation
- *Wheeze*—try inhaled broncholdilators
- *Excessive upper airway secretions*—try hyoscine 0.4–2.4mg/24h. or glycopyrronium 200–600mcg/24h. (consult local palliative care team)
- *Musculoskeletal pain* can cause hypoventilation—treat with analgesia
- *Anaemia (Hb <9g/l)*—consider referral for transfusion
- *Thick secretions*—consider referral for chest physiotherapy
- *Vocal cord palsy*—consider referral to an ENT surgeon for teflon injection.

Stridor: Coarse wheezing sound that results from the obstruction of a major airway e.g. larynx.

Management
- Corticosteroids (e.g. dexamethasone 16mg/d.) can give relief.
- Consider referral for radiotherapy or endoscopic insertion of a stent if appropriate.
- If a terminal event—sedate with high doses of midazolam (10–40mg repeated prn).

Cough: Troublesome symptom.

Management
General measures
- Exclude any treatable cause for cough (e.g. ACE inhibitors)
- Advise upright body position
- Steam inhalations or inhalations with menthol or tinct. Benz. Co (Friars balsam) can help
- Refer for chest physiotherapy, relaxation, and breathing control exercises, if tolerated
- Simple linctus prn can be helpful. If not, consider low-dose opioid linctus e.g. codeine linctus or oramorph 5mg every 4h.

Specific measures
- *Chest infection*—treat with nebulized saline to make secretions less viscous ± antibiotics (if not considered a terminal event)
- *Tumour*—consider referral for radiotherapy
- *Post-nasal drip*—steam inhalations, steroid nasal spray or drops ± antibiotics
- *Laryngeal irritation*—try inhaled steroids
- *Broncospasm*—try bronchodilators ± inhaled or oral steroids
- *Gastric reflux*—try antacids containing dimethicone (gaviscon, asilone)
- ↓ *of salivary secretions*—try hyoscine (see below).

Excessive respiratory secretion: Excessive respiratory secretion (death rattle) can be distressing for patients and relatives in attendance. It may be ↓ using:
- Subcutaneous injection of hyoscine hydrobromide 400–600mcg 4–8 hourly (or 0.6–2.4mg/24h. via syringe driver)—dry mouth is a side-effect and can be distressing.
- Glycopyrronium 200mcg every 4h. sc or im injection (0.6–1.2mg/24h. via syringe driver).

Haematological and vascular problems

Bleeding/haemorrhage: In all patients likely to bleed (e.g. in end-stage leukaemia) pre-warn carers and give them a strategy.

Severe, life-threatening bleed: Make a decision whether the cause of the bleed is treatable or a terminal event. This is best done in advance—but bleeding can't always be predicted.
- *Severe bleed—active treatment:* 📖 p.1040–2
- *Severe bleed—no active treatment:*
  - Stay with the patient
  - Give sedative medication e.g. midazolam 20–40mg sc/iv or diazepam 10–20mg pr and diamorphine 5–10mg sc/iv
  - Support carers, as big bleeds are extremely distressing.

Non-life threatening bleed

First aid measures
- In all cases—reassure; monitor frequently.
- Surface bleeding—pressure on wound; if pressure is not working, try kaltostat or adrenaline (1mg/ml or 1:1000) on a gauze pad
- Nose bleeds—nasal packing or cautery

Follow-up treatment: Follow-up is directed at cause if appropriate:
- Anticoagulants—check INR
- Treat infection that might exacerbate a bleed
- Consider minimizing bleeding tendency with tranexamic acid 500mg qds
- Upper GI bleeding—stop NSAIDs, start PPI in double standard dose and consider referral for gastroscopy
- Lower GI bleeding—consider rectal steroids to ↓ inflammation or rectal tranexamic acid ± referral for colonoscopy
- Radiotherapy—consider referral if haemoptysis, cutaneous bleeding, or haematuria
- Referral for chemotherapy or palliative surgery (e.g. cautery) are also options

Anaemia: Don't check for anaemia if there is no intention to transfuse.
- *If Hb <10g/dl and symptomatic:* Treat any reversible cause (e.g. iron deficiency, GI bleeding 2° to NSAIDs). Consider transfusion.
- *If transfused:* Record whether any benefit is derived (as if not, further transfusions are futile) and the duration of benefit (if <3wk., repeat transfusions are impractical). Monitor for return of symptoms, repeat FBC, and arrange repeat transfusion as needed.

Superior vena cava (SVC) obstruction: Due to infiltration of the vessel wall, clot within the superior vena cava, or extrinsic pressure. 75% are due to 1° lung cancer (3% of patients with lung cancer have SVC obstruction). Lymphoma is the other major cause.

Presentation
- Shortness of breath/stridor
- Headache worse on stooping ± visual disturbances ± dizziness and collapse

- Swelling of the face—particularly around the eyes, neck, hands and arms, and/or injected cornea
- *Examination:* look for non-pulsatile distention of neck veins and dilated collateral veins (seen as small dilated veins over the anterior chest wall below the clavicles) in which blood courses downwards.

Management
- Treat breathlessness—opiates (oramorph 5mg 4 hourly) ± benzodiazepine, depending on the level of anxiety
- Start corticosteroid (dexamethasone 16mg/d.)
- Refer urgently for oncology opinion. Palliative radiotherapy has a response rate of 70%. Stenting ± thrombolysis is also an option.

Lymphoedema: Due to obstruction of lymphatic drainage resulting in oedema with high protein content. Affects ≥1 limbs ± adjacent trunk. If left untreated, lymphoedema becomes increasingly resistant to treatment due to chronic inflammation and subcutaneous fibrosis. Cellulitis causes rapid ↑ in swelling.

Causes
- Axillary, groin, or intrapelvic tumour
- Extensive axillary or groin surgery
- Post-operative infection/radiotherapy

Presentation
- Swollen limb ± pitting
- Impaired limb mobility and function
- Discomfort/pain related to tissue swelling and/or shoulder strain
- Neuralgia pain—especially when axillary nodes are involved
- Psychological distress

Table 28.4 Management of lymphoedema

Avoid injury to limb	In at-risk patients (e.g. patients who have had breast cancer with axillary clearance) or those with lymphoedema, injury to the limb may precipitate or worsen lymphoedema. Do not take blood from the limb or use it for iv access or vaccination.
Skin hygiene	Skin care with moisturisers e.g. aqueous cream, emulsiderm Topical treatment of fungal infection Systemic treatment of bacterial infection
External support	Intensive—with compression bandages Maintenance—with lymphoedema sleeve (contact breast care specialist nurse for more information on obtaining sleeves)
Exercise	Gentle daily exercise of affected limb, gradually increasing range of movement ❶ Must wear a sleeve/bandages when doing exercises
Massage	Very gentle finger tip massage in the line of drainage of lymphatics
Diuretics	If the condition has developed or deteriorated since prescription of corticosteroid or NSAID or if there is venous component, consider trial of diuretics Otherwise, diuretics are of no benefit

Psychiatric problems

Anxiety: All patients with terminal disease are anxious at times. When anxiety starts interfering with quality of life, intervention is justified.

Management

Non-drug measures: Often all that is needed:
- Acknowledgement of the patient's anxiety
- Full explanations of questions, supported with written information as needed
- Support—self-help groups, day care, patients' groups, specialist home nurses (e.g. MacMillan Nurses)
- Relaxation training and training in breathing control
- Physical therapies e.g. aromatherapy, art therapy, exercise.

Drug measures
- *Acute anxiety:* Try lorazepam 1–2mg sl prn or diazepam 2–10mg prn
- *Chronic anxiety:* Try an antidepressant e.g. fluoxetine 20mg od. Alternatives include regular diazepam 5–10mg od/bd, haloperidol 1–3mg bd/tds, or β-blockers (e.g. propranolol 40mg od tds)—watch for postural hypotension

If anxiety is not responding to simple measures, seek specialist help from either the psychiatric or palliative care team.

Depression: A terminal diagnosis makes patients sad on occasions. Many symptoms of terminal disease (e.g. poor appetite) are also symptoms of depression. 10–20% of terminally ill patients develop clinical depression but, in practice, it is often difficult to decide whether a patient is depressed or just appropriately sad about his diagnosis and its implications. If in doubt, a trial of antidepressants can help.

Management

Non-drug measures
- Support e.g. day and/or respite care; carers' group; specialist nurse support (e.g. MacMillan Nurse; CPN); ↑ help in the home
- Relaxation—often ↑ the patient's feeling of control over the situation
- Explanation—of worries/problems/concerns about the future
- Physical activity—exercise; writing

Drug measures
- Consider starting an antidepressant (📖 p.970)
- All antidepressants take ~2wk. to work
- If immediate effect is required, consider using flupentixol 1mg od (beware as can cause psychomotor agitation).

If not responding or suicidal, refer for psychiatric opinion.

Confusion: 📖 p.976

Insomnia: 📖 p.242

Emergencies

Being prepared

This chapter contains information on conditions in which immediate action is essential. For the sake of brevity, it does not contain all acute situations a GP might face—most are dealt with in their appropriate sections within the book.

Before being on-call for emergencies

- Ensure you have a reliable car with a full tank of petrol
- Have a good street map of the area ± an Ordinance Survey map
- Carry a large, strong torch in the car
- Carry a mobile telephone and make sure it is charged
- Check the drug box is fully stocked and all items are in date
- Check all equipment carried is operational and you have spare batteries
- Carry a list of emergency telephone numbers
- Know which chemists have extended opening hours and carry the chemist's rota.

When on-call for emergencies: *In all cases:*

- Record—the time of any calls, full name, date of birth or age, telephone number, address of the patient and current location.
- Give the patient or the person making the call a clear idea of what you will do (e.g. if you will call an ambulance, when you will be visiting) and what you expect them to do.
- If only advice is given, then make full notes to be filed in the patient's notes.
- If visiting, take directions from the person making the request for a visit if the area is unfamiliar to you.
- Keep a full record of the consultation with the patient, any actions taken, and drugs administered (including expiry date, manufacturer, and batch number).
- Don't go alone to suspected violent patients—call the police to accompany you.
- Ensure someone knows where you are and when to expect you back, at all times.

The doctor's bag: 📖 p.54

Useful telephone numbers:	

Managing a resuscitation attempt outside hospital^G

⚠ Ventricular fibrillation complicating acute MI is the most common cause of cardiac arrest that members of the primary healthcare team will encounter. Success is greatest when the event is witnessed and attempted defibrillation is performed with the minimum of delay.

Resuscitation equipment: See Table 29.1
- Resuscitation equipment is used relatively infrequently. Staff must know where to find equipment at the time it is needed and should be trained to use the equipment to the expected level.
- Each practice should have a named individual with responsibility for checking the state of all resuscitation drugs and equipment, on a regular basis—ideally once a week. In common with drugs, disposable items like the adhesive electrodes have a finite shelf-life and will require replacement from time to time, if unused.

Training: Training and practice are necessary to acquire skill in resuscitation techniques. Resuscitation skills decline rapidly and updates and retraining, using manikins, are necessary every 6–12mo. to maintain adequate skill levels. Level of resuscitation skill needed by different members of the primary healthcare team differs according to the individual's role:
- All those in direct contact with patients should be trained in BLS and related resuscitation skills such as the recovery position.
- Doctors, nurses, and other paramedical workers (e.g. physiotherapists) should also be able to use an automatic external defibrillator (AED) effectively. Other personnel (e.g. receptionists) may also be trained to use an AED.

⚠ It is unacceptable for patients who sustain a cardiopulmonary arrest to await the arrival of the ambulance service before basic resuscitation is performed and a defibrillator is available.

Performance management: Accurate records of all resuscitation attempts and electronic data stored by most AEDs during a resuscitation attempt should be kept for audit, training, and medico-legal reasons. The responsibility for this rests with the most senior member of the practice team involved. Process and outcome of all resuscitation attempts should be audited—both at practice and PCO level—to allow deficiencies to be addressed and examples of good practice to be shared.

Ethical issues
- It is essential to identify individuals in whom cardiopulmonary arrest is a terminal event and where resuscitation is inappropriate.
- Overall responsibility for a 'Do not attempt to resuscitate (DNAR)' decision rests with the doctor in charge of the patient's care.
- Seek opinions of other members of the medical and nursing team, the patient, and any relatives in reaching a DNAR decision.
- Record the patient should not be resuscitated in the notes, the reasons for that decision, and what the relatives have been told.

- Ensure all members of the multidisciplinary team involved with the patient's care are aware of the decision and have it recorded in their notes.
- Review the decision not to attempt resuscitation, regularly, in the light of the patient's condition.

Essential reading

Resuscitation Council (UK) (2001) Cardiopulmonary resuscitation guidance for clinical practice and training in primary care 🖳 http://www.resus.org.uk

BMA, RCN, and Resuscitation Council (UK) (2001) Decisions relating to cardiopulmonary resuscitation 🖳 http://www.resus.org.uk

Table 29.1 Resuscitation equipment needed

Equipment	Notes
Defibrillator with electrodes and razor	• An automated external defibrillator should be available wherever and whenever sick patients are seen • Regular maintenance is needed even if the machine has not been used • After the machine is used, the manufacturers instructions should be followed to return it to a state of readiness with the minimum of delay
Pocket mask with 1-way valve	• All personnel should be trained to use one
Oropharyngeal airway	• Suitable for use by those appropriately trained—keep a range of sizes available
Oxygen and mask with reservoir bag	• Should be available wherever possible • Oxygen cylinders need regular maintenance—follow national safety standards
Suction	• Simple, mechanical, portable, hand-held suction devices are recommended
Drugs	Epinephrine/adrenaline—1mg iv Atropine—3mg iv (give once only)—for bradycardia, asystole, and pulseless electrical activity Amiodarone—300mg iv for VF resistant to defibrillation Naloxone—for suspected cases of respiratory arrest due to opiate overdose ⚠There is no evidence for the use of alkalizing agents, buffers, or calcium salts before hospitalization • Drugs should be given by the intravenous route, preferably through a catheter placed in a large vein (e.g. in the antecubital fossa) and flushed in with a bolus of iv fluid • Many drugs may be given via the bronchial route if a tracheal tube is in place; for epinephrine/adrenaline and atropine, the dose is double the iv dose
Other	• Saline flush, gloves, syringes and needles, iv cannulae, iv fluids, sharps box, scissors, tape

Basic life support[G]

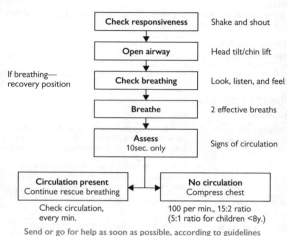

Check responsiveness — Shake and shout

Open airway — Head tilt/chin lift

If breathing— recovery position

Check breathing — Look, listen, and feel

Breathe — 2 effective breaths

Assess 10sec. only — Signs of circulation

Circulation present — Continue rescue breathing ⟷ No circulation — Compress chest

Check circulation, every min.

100 per min., 15:2 ratio (5:1 ratio for children <8y.)

Send or go for help as soon as possible, according to guidelines

Figure 29.1 Basic life support algorithm

Basic life support: Basic life support (BLS) is a holding operation—sustaining life until help arrives. BLS should be started as soon as the arrest is detected—outcome is less good the longer the delay.

1. **D**anger: Ensure safety of rescuer and patient.
2. **R**esponse: Check the patient for any response.
   • Is the patient **A**lert? Yes/No
   • Does he respond to **V**ocal stimuli? Yes/No
   • Does he respond to a **P**ainful stimulus (pinching the lower part of the nasal septum)? Yes/No
   • Is the patient **U**nconscious? Yes/No
3. **If he responds by answering or moving:** Don't move the patient unless in danger. Get help. Reassess regularly.
   If he does not respond: Shout for help; turn the patient on to his back; remove any visible obstructions from the patient's mouth—leave well fitting dentures in place.
4. **A**irway: Open the airway—gently tilt the head back and lift the chin.

   ⚠ Try to avoid head tilt if trauma to the neck is suspected.

5. **B**reathing: With airway open, look, listen, and feel for breathing.
6. **If breathing normally:** Turn the patient into the recovery position (📖 p.1022), get help, and check for continued breathing.
   If not breathing: Or only making occasional gasps/weak attempts at breathing—get help; start rescue breathing.

7. **Give 2 slow, effective rescue breaths**
   - Ensure head tilt and chin lift.
   - Pinch the soft part of the nose closed with your index finger and thumb. Open the mouth a little.
   - Take a deep breath and place your lips around the patient's mouth (or nose/mouth and nose), making sure you have a good seal.
   - Blow steadily into the patient's mouth for ~2 sec. to make the chest rise (1–1.5sec. for a child <8y.). Take your mouth away and watch the chest fall.
   - Repeat the sequence to give 2 effective breaths (max. 5 attempts).
8. **C**irculation: Check the carotid pulse (max. 10 sec.).
9. *If circulation is present:* Continue rescue breathing until the patient starts breathing alone; check signs of circulation every 10 breaths.
   If the patient starts to breath alone but remains unconscious, turn into the recovery position (📖 p.1022) and reassess frequently.
   If there are no signs of a circulation or you are unsure: Start chest compressions:
   - Place the heel of one hand on top of the other over the lower ½ of the sternum (use one hand only in a child <8y. and 2 fingers in an infant <1y.); extend or interlock the fingers of both hands.
   - Position yourself vertically above the patient's chest and, with arms straight, press the sternum down 4–5cm ($1/3$–$1/2$ the depth of the chest in children <8y.). Release the pressure without losing contact between hand and sternum. Compression and release should take an equal amount of time.
   - Repeat at a rate of ~100 compressions/min.
10. **After 15 compressions:** Tilt the head, lift the chin, and give 2 effective breaths. Then without delay, give 15 further compressions, continuing compressions and breaths in a ratio of 15:2 (5:1 if child <8y.).

⚠ Only stop to recheck for signs of a circulation if the patient makes a movement or takes a spontaneous breath; otherwise resuscitation should not be interrupted.

When to go for assistance: It is vital for rescuers to get assistance as quickly as possible.
- **When >1 rescuer is available:** One should start resuscitation while another rescuer goes for assistance.
- **Lone rescuer:** The rescuer must decide whether to start resuscitation or to go for assistance first.
  - If the likely cause of unconsciousness is *trauma; drowning; or if the victim is an infant or a child* the rescuer should perform resuscitation for *1min.* before going for assistance (and may take a young child/infant with him).
  - Otherwise, go for help immediately it has been established the victim is not breathing.

Essential reading

Resuscitation Council (UK) (2000) Resuscitation guidelines 🖳 *http://www.resus.org.uk*

Recovery position[G]

When circulation and breathing have been restored, it is important to:
- Maintain a good airway
- Ensure the tongue does not cause obstruction
- Minimize the risk of inhalation of gastric contents

For this reason, the victim should be placed in the recovery position. This allows the tongue to fall forward, keeping the airway clear.

Action: See Figure 29.2
- Remove the patient's glasses
- Kneel beside the patient and make sure that both legs are straight
- Place the arm nearest to you out at right angles to the body, elbow bent, with the hand palm uppermost
- Bring the far arm across the chest, and hold the back of the hand against the patient's cheek nearest to you
- With your other hand, grasp the far leg just above the knee and pull it up, keeping the foot on the ground
- Keeping the patient's hand pressed against his cheek, pull on the leg to roll the patient towards you, onto his side
- Adjust the upper leg so that both the hip and knee are bent at right angles
- Tilt the head back to make sure the airway remains open
- Adjust the hand under the cheek, if necessary, to keep the head tilted
- Check breathing regularly.

⚠ Monitor the peripheral circulation of the lower arm. If the patient has to be kept in the recovery position for >30min., turn him onto the opposite side.

The unconscious child
- The child should be in as near a true lateral position as possible with his mouth dependant, to allow free drainage of fluid.
- The position should be stable. In an infant, this may require the support of a small pillow or rolled up blanket placed behind the back to maintain the position.

Cervical spine injury
- If spinal cord injury is suspected (e.g. if the victim has sustained a fall, been struck on the head or neck, or has been rescued after diving into shallow water), take particular care during handling and resuscitation to maintain alignment of the head, neck, and chest in the neutral position.
- A spinal board and/or cervical collar should be used if available.

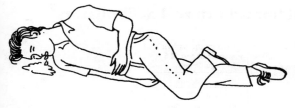

Figure 29.2 Recovery position

Automated external defibrillators[G]

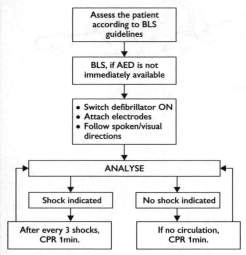

Figure 29.3 Automatic external defibrillator algorithm (Reproduced from *Resuscitation guidelines* (2000) with permission of Resuscitation Council (UK). Full version available from 🖳 http://www.resus.org.uk)

Use of automated external defibrillators (AEDs)

- Modern AEDs have simplified the process of defibrillation considerably.
- ECG interpretation and charging of the machine in preparation to shock are now automated. This has greatly reduced training requirements and extended the range of personnel who can attempt defibrillation.
- The use of such machines should be within the capabilities of all medical and nursing staff working in the community—so ALL practices should have an AED.
- Increasingly, trained lay persons are successfully employing AEDs and it is quite appropriate for reception, administrative, and secretarial staff to be trained in their use.

Cardiac arrest in adults: A high proportion of adults who suffer cardiac arrest in the community will have a VF arrest. Their best chance of survival is to be shocked as soon as possible. If a patient arrests:

- *Perform basic life support* until the defibrillator arrives (🕮 p.1020)
- *Make sure someone has called an ambulance*
- *Prepare the patient* for defibrillation:
  - Expose the chest
  - Shave any chest hair (there should always be a special razor for this purpose stored with the defibrillator)—it is essential there is good contact between the skin and the electrodes
  - Remove any GTN patches visible—if a patch is present and you're not sure what it is, remove it
  - Remove jewellery or move it away from the electrodes
  - Apply the pads—pads should be stored flat, should be unopened, and in date.
- *Pad position:* The pads are marked to show where they should be placed—one on the right side of the chest with the top right corner in the angle between the clavicle and sternum; the other, along the line of the bottom left rib pointing into the axilla
- *Switch the defibrillator on and follow the instructions*
- *Before delivering a shock check:*
  - *Top*—any oxygen has been moved away from the patient and the person looking after the airway is standing clear
  - *Middle*—the person performing cardiac massage and you are standing clear
  - *Bottom*—anyone else in the vicinity is standing clear
- *Announce you are delivering a shock* in a clear, loud voice; check briefly again that everyone is standing clear; and then shock the patient
- *Follow the instructions* from the defibrillator.

Cardiac arrest in children: Ventricular fibrillation is a less common presentation of cardiopulmonary arrest in children, but the same treatment principles apply.

- *Children >8y.:* Modern AEDs designed for use in adults can be used.
- *Children <8y.:* Special infant electrodes are advised—they are available from some manufacturers.

Essential reading

Resuscitation Council (UK) 🖥 http://www.resus.org.uk
- Resuscitation guidelines (2000)—guidelines for the use of automated external defibrillators
- The use of biphasic defibrillators and AEDs in children (revised 2003)

Adult advanced life support^G

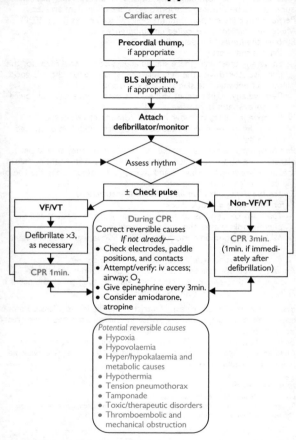

Figure 29.4 Adult advanced life support algorithm (Reproduced from *Resuscitation guidelines* (2000) with permission of Resuscitation Council (UK). Full version available from 🖥 *http://www.resus.org.uk*)

Notes

Precordial thump: Appropriate if arrest is witnessed and defibrillator is not to hand.

Basic life support (BLS) algorithm: 📖 p.1020 or inside back cover. BLS should be started if there is any delay in obtaining a defibrillator, but must not delay shock delivery.

Automated external defibrillator protocol: 📖 p.1024 or inside back cover.

Drugs
- Drugs administered by the iv route must be followed by a flush of ≥20ml of saline to assist delivery.
- Adrenaline (epinephrine)—dose 1mg iv or 2–3mg (diluted in at least 10ml of sterile water) via endotracheal (ET) tube. Give every 3min. during resuscitation but avoid giving within 1min. of defibrillation.

VF/VT arrest
- *Paddle position:* Place 1 paddle under the right clavicle and the other on the left axillary line.
- *Defibrillation:* Up to 3 shocks with energies of 200J, 200J, 360J may be used in any cycle of resuscitation. When all 3 shocks are needed—aim to administer them in <1min. During 1min. after defibrillation, do not administer adrenaline (epinephrine), as it may be harmful. Successful defibrillation is usually followed by at least a few seconds of true asystole.
- *Amiodarone:* Consider, following epinephrine, to treat shock-refractory cardiac arrest due to VF or pulseless VT. Amiodarone 300mg (made up to 20ml with dextrose, or from a prefilled syringe) may be administered into a peripheral vein. A further dose of 150mg may be given for recurrent or refractory VT/VF.

Non-VT/VF arrest
- *Asystole*
  - Check ECG for the presence of P waves or slow ventricular activity—it may respond to cardiac pacing. Repeated precordial blows, lateral to the lower left sternal edge (70/min.), can be used to stimulate the myocardium (percussion pacing).
  - Atropine 3mg iv or 6mg via ET tube (in a volume of 10–20ml of water) may be helpful.
  - If there is any doubt about diagnosis of asystole, treat for VF.
- *Pulseless electrical activity/electromechanical dissociation:* Best chance of survival is prompt identification and treatment of any underlying cause.

Essential reading
Resuscitation Council (UK) (2000) Resuscitation guidelines 🖥 http://www.resus.org.uk

Paediatric advanced life support[G]

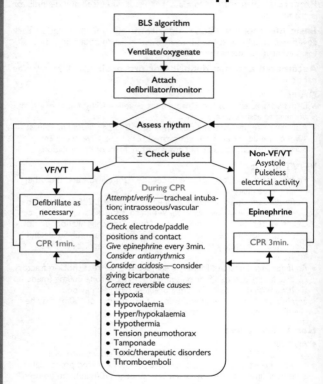

Figure 29.5 Paediatric advanced life support algorithm (Reproduced from Resuscitation guidelines (2000) with permission of Resuscitation Council (UK). Full version available from 🖳 http://www.resus.org.uk)

Basic paediatric life support: Follow the algorithm on 📖 p.1020 or inside the back cover.

Notes
Unable to ventilate? Consider foreign body in the airway and initiate airway obstruction sequence—📖 p.1052.

Checking the pulse
- Child—feel for the carotid pulse in the neck
- Infant—feel for the brachial pulse on the inner aspect of the upper arm.

Adrenaline (epinephrine) dose
- Intravenous or interosseous access—10mcg/kg epinephrine (0.1ml/kg of 1:10,000 solution).
- Via endotracheal (ET) tube—100mcg/kg (1ml/kg of 1 in 10,000 or 0.1ml/kg of 1 in 1000 solution).
- Consider using higher doses (e.g. 100mcg/kg iv or io) if vasodilatation contributed to cardiac arrest (e.g. septicaemia, anaphylaxis).

VF/pulseless VT: Less common in paediatric life support.
- *Defibrillation:* Use up to 3 shocks/resuscitation cycle:
  - 2J/kg, 2J/kg, 4J/kg on the first occasion
  - 4J/kg, 4J/kg, 4J/kg on subsequent occasions.
- *Electrode/paddle position:*
  Child: Place the defibrillator pads or paddles on the chest wall—one just below the right clavicle, the other at the left anterior axillary line.
  Infant: Apply the pads or paddles to the front and back of the infant's chest.
- After each drug, CPR should continue for up to a minute to allow the drug to reach the heart before a further defibrillation attempt.
- For shock resistant VF/pulseless VT, try amiodarone 5mg/kg via rapid iv bolus.

Intravenous fluids: In situations where the cardiac arrest has resulted from circulatory failure, a standard (20ml/kg) bolus of crystalloid fluid should be given if there is no response to the initial dose of epinephrine.

Essential reading
Resuscitation Council (UK) (2000) Resuscitation guidelines 🖥 http://www.resus.org.uk

Resuscitation of the newborn[G]

Follow the algorithm opposite (Figure 29.6).

Rapid assessment of the infant at birth

A healthy baby
- Born blue
- Good tone
- Cries within a few seconds of delivery
- Good heart rate (120–150bpm)
- Rapidly becomes pink during the first 90sec.

A less healthy baby
- Blue at birth
- Less good tone
- ± slow heart rate (<100bpm)
- ± inadequate breathing by 90–120sec.

An ill baby
- Born pale
- Floppy
- Slow/very slow heart rate (<100bpm)
- Not breathing

Notes

Heart rate: Best judged by listening with a stethoscope—in many cases it can also be felt by gently palpating the umbilical cord or by feeling for the apex beat over the anterior chest. Feeling for peripheral pulses is not helpful.

Meconium: Screaming babies have an open airway; floppy babies— have a look.

Airway: Open the airway by placing the head in a neutral position— where the neck is neither extended nor flexed. If the occiput is prominent and the neck tends to flex, place a support under the shoulders. It may be necessary to apply jaw thrust or chin lift if the baby is very floppy.

Breathing: Inflation breaths are breaths with pressures of ~30cms of water for 2–3sec.
- If the heart rate ↑ from its previous rate—you have successfully inflated the chest. If the baby does not then start breathing alone, continue to provide regular breaths at a rate of ~30–40breaths/min. until the baby starts to breathe on its own.
- If the heart rate does not ↑ following inflation breaths, then either you have not inflated the chest or the baby needs more help. By far the most likely is that you have failed to inflate the chest (the chest does not move).

Chest compressions: Only commence after inflation of the lungs. Grip the chest in both hands in such a way that the thumbs of both hands can press on the sternum at a point just below an imaginary line joining the nipples and with the fingers over the spine at the back. Compress the chest quickly, reducing the AP diameter of the chest by ~1/3 with each compression. The ratio of compressions to inflations is 3:1.

Essential reading

Resuscitation Council (UK) (2000) Resuscitation guidelines
🖥 http://www.resus.org.uk

Dry the baby, remove any wet cloth and cover

▼

Initial assessment at birth Start the clock or note the time Assess: COLOUR, TONE, BREATHING, HEART RATE

▼

If not breathing

▼

Control the airway Head in the neutral position

▼

Support the breathing *If not breathing*—5 inflation breaths (each 2–3 sec. duration) Confirm a response—increase in HEART RATE or visible CHEST MOVEMENT

▼

If there is no response Double check head position and apply JAW THRUST 5 inflation breaths Confirm a response—increase in HEART RATE or visible CHEST MOVEMENT

▼

If there is *still* no response Use a 2nd person (if available) to help with airway control and repeat inflation breaths Inspect the oropharynx under direct vision (is suction needed?) and repeat inflation breaths Insert an oropharyngeal (Guedel) airway and repeat inflation breaths *Consider intubation* Confirm a response—increase in HEART RATE or visible CHEST MOVEMENT

▼

When the chest is moving Continue the ventilation breaths if no spontaneous breathing

▼

Check the heart rate If heart rate is not detectable *or* slow (<60bpm) and NOT increasing

▼

Start chest compressions First confirm chest movement—if the chest is not moving, *return to airway* 3 chest compressions to 1 breath for 30sec.

▼

Reassess heart rate If improving—stop chest compressions; continue ventilation if not breathing If heart rate still slow, continue ventilation and chest compressions Consider venous access and drugs at this stage

AT ALL STAGES ASK .... DO YOU NEED HELP?

Figure 29.6 Newborn life support algorithm

Coma

Patients in coma/pre-coma nearly always require emergency admission.

When you receive the call for assistance
- Advise the attendant (unless history of possible spinal injury) to turn the patient onto his/her side
- Call an ambulance to meet you at the scene.

On reaching the patient
- Assess the need for basic life support:
  - **A**irway patent?
  - **B**reathing satisfactory?
  - **C**irculation adequate?
- Turn into the recovery position (□ p.1022) if no contraindications (e.g. spinal injury)
- Call for ambulance support if you have not already done so
- Ensure the patient is warm.
- Record baseline level of responsiveness either using Glasgow Coma Scale (below) or as AVPU Score (□ p.1020). Ensure you note the time the score was recorded.
- Try to establish a diagnosis (see assessment)

As soon as possible
- Insert an airway
- Give oxygen
- Establish iv access
- Transfer to hospital (unless the condition has resolved e.g. hypoglycaemia, fit)

Possible causes
- **Drugs:** Sedatives or hypnotics, opiates, alcohol, solvents, carbon monoxide poisoning
- **Vascular:** Stroke, low cardiac output e.g. post MI, ruptured AAA
- **CNS:** Fit or post-ictal state; hydrocephalus (e.g. blocked shunt); cerebral oedema (e.g. meningitis, SAH, head injury); concussion; extradural or subdural haematoma
- **Metabolic:** Hypo- or hyperglycaemia; hypothermia; hypopituitarism
- **Infection:** Meningitis or septicaemia; pneumonia

Assessment and management: See Figure 29.7

Table 29.2 The Glasgow Coma Scale

Eye opening	Spontaneous	4	To pain	2
	To voice	3	None	1
Best verbal response	Oriented	5	Incomprehensive	2
	Confused	4	None	1
	Inappropriate words	3		
Best motor response	Obeys command	6	Flexion	3
	Localizes pain	5	Extension	2
	Withdraw	4	None	1

Total score = Eye opening + best verbal + best motor response scores

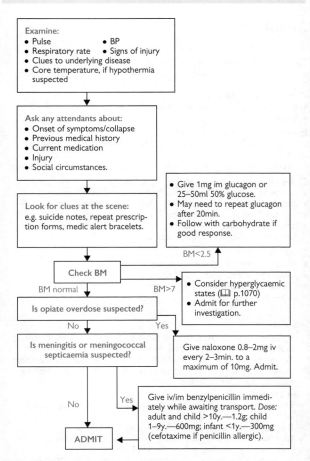

Examine:
- Pulse
- Respiratory rate
- Clues to underlying disease
- Core temperature, if hypothermia suspected
- BP
- Signs of injury

Ask any attendants about:
- Onset of symptoms/collapse
- Previous medical history
- Current medication
- Injury
- Social circumstances.

Look for clues at the scene:
e.g. suicide notes, repeat prescription forms, medic alert bracelets.

Check BM

BM normal

BM<2.5
- Give 1mg im glucagon or 25–50ml 50% glucose.
- May need to repeat glucagon after 20min.
- Follow with carbohydrate if good response.

BM>7
- Consider hyperglycaemic states (☐ p.1070)
- Admit for further investigation.

Is opiate overdose suspected?

No

Yes
Give naloxone 0.8–2mg iv every 2–3min. to a maximum of 10mg. Admit.

Is meningitis or meningococcal septicaemia suspected?

No

Yes
Give iv/im benzylpenicillin immediately while awaiting transport. *Dose:* adult and child >10y.—1.2g; child 1–9y.—600mg; infant <1y.—300mg (cefotaxime if penicillin allergic).

ADMIT

Figure 29.7 Assessment and management of the unconscious patient

Anaphylaxis

Severe systemic allergic reaction.

Common causes
- *Foods:* nuts, fish and shellfish, sesame seeds and oil, milk, eggs, pulses (beans, peas)
- *Insect stings:* wasp or bee
- *Drugs:* antibiotics, aspirin and other NSAIDs, opiates
- *Latex*

Essential features: 1 or both of:
- *Respiratory difficulty* e.g. wheeze, stridor—may be due to laryngeal oedema or asthma
- *Hypotension*—can present as fainting, collapse, or loss of consciousness

Other features: All or some of the following:
- Erythema
- Angio-oedema
- Itching of palate
- Itching of external auditory meatus
- Generalized pruritus
- Rhinitis
- Nausea
- Palpitations
- Urticaria
- Conjunctivitis
- Vomiting
- Sense of impending doom

Examination
- *A*irway—mouth/tongue for oedema
- *B*reathing—chest (wheeze), PEFR
- *C*irculation—pulse, BP
- *Skin*—check for rashes

⚠ Action
- If suspected when the initial call for help comes in, call an emergency ambulance immediately—then visit.
- Ask when the initial call is taken if the patient has had a similar event before. If so, ask if he/she has an Epipen or similar. If yes, advise the caller to use it immediately.

On arrival
- Ensure the patient is comfortable—lie down flat ± leg elevation if ↓BP; sit up if breathing difficulty.
- If available, *give oxygen* at high flow rates (10–15l/min.).
- *Give im adrenaline (epinephrine)* to *all* patients with clinical signs of shock, airway swelling, or breathing difficulty. *Dose:*
  - Adult or child >12y.: 0.5ml epinephrine (adrenaline) 1:1000 solution (500µg) im. Give half dose if: pre-pubertal or adult on tricyclic antidepressants, monoamine oxidase inhibitors, or β blockers.
  - Child 6–12y.: ½ adult dose—0.25ml of 1:1000 epinephrine (adrenaline) solution (250µg) im.
  - Child 6mo.–6y.: ¼ adult dose—0.12ml of 1:1000 epinephrine (adrenaline) solution (120µg) im.
  - Child <6mo.: 0.05ml 1:1000 epinephrine (adrenaline) solution (50µg) im. Absolute accuracy of dose is not necessary.

- *Repeat* after ≥5min. if improvement is transient, no improvement, or deterioration after initial treatment. May need several doses.
- *Give an antihistamine:* Dose of chlorpheniramine:
  - Adults and children >12y.—10–20mg im
  - Children 6–12y.—5–10mg im
  - Children 1–6y.—2.5–5mg im
- *Give hydrocortisone* by im or slow iv injection. *Dose:*
  - Adults and children >12y.—100–500mg
  - Children 6–11y.—100mg
  - Children 1–6y.—50mg
- *Give salbutamol* if bronchospasm
- If severe hypotension does not respond rapidly, start an iv infusion (if available) and *rapidly infuse 1–2l* of saline until BP ↑(children 20ml/kg rapidly, then another similar dose if not responding)
- *Admit the patient to hospital* until ill effects have settled.

❶ The preferred site for im injection is the midpoint of the anterolateral thigh.

Algorithm for management of anaphylaxis in adults: Figure 29.8 (□ p.1036).

Algorithm for management of anaphylaxis in children: Figure 29.9 (□ p.1037).

Follow-up
- Warn patients or parents of the possibility of recurrence.
- Advise sufferers to wear a device (e.g. Medic Alert bracelet) that will inform bystanders or medical staff should a future attack occur.
- Refer all patients after their first anaphylactic attack to a specialist allergy clinic.
- Consider supplying sufferers (or parents) with an Epipen or similar which can be used to administer im epinephrine (adrenaline) immediately should symptoms recur.
- If you supply an Epipen, teach anyone likely to need to use it, how to operate the device. Intramuscular epinephrine is very safe.

Further Information
Resuscitation Council (UK) Emergency Medical treatment of anaphylactic reactions for first medical responders and community nurses (Revised 2005) 🖵 http://www.resus.org.uk

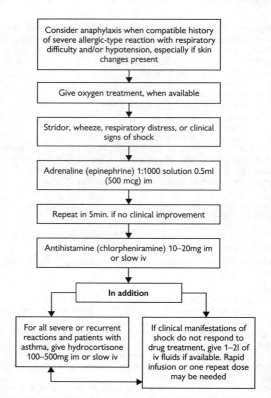

Figure 29.8 Anaphylactic reactions: treatment algorithm for adults (Reproduced with permission of Resuscitation Council UK.)

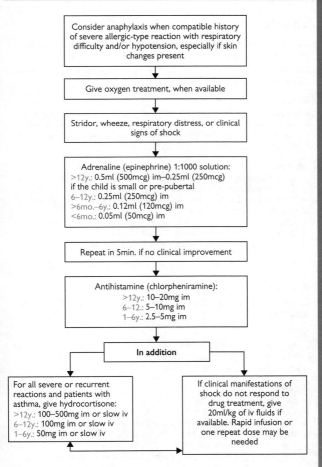

Figure 29.9 Anaphylactic reactions: treatment algorithm for children (Reproduced with permission of Resuscitation Council UK.)

Shock

Due to inadequate blood flow to the peripheral circulation. Usually → ↓ BP (± tachycardia), peripheral cyanosis, and ↓ urinary output.

Hypovolaemic shock: Usually due to haemorrhage e.g. GI bleeding (📖 p.1040), ruptured AAA (📖 p.1042).

Signs
- *Initially*—tachycardia (pulse >100bpm), pallor, sweating ± restlessness.
- *Later*—decompensation—(sudden fall in pulse rate and BP). Young people may decompensate very rapidly. If tachycardic, treat as a medical emergency—speed could be lifesaving.

⚠ Action
- Lie the patient down flat and raise legs above waist height
- Call for ambulance assistance
- Control bleeding by applying pressure, if obvious bleeding point (e.g. nose bleed, laceration)
- Gain iv access and (if possible) take blood for FBC and cross-matching—try to insert 2 large bore cannulae
- If available, start plasma expander/iv fluids; give rapidly over 10–15min.
- If available, give 100% oxygen (unless COPD, when give 24%)

Anaphylactic shock: 📖 p.1034

Cardiogenic shock: Due to heart pump failure e.g. MI, arrythmia, tamponade.

Signs
- Hypotension—systolic BP <80–90mmHg
- Pulse rate may be normal, ↑, or ↓
- Severe breathlessness ± cyanosis

⚠ Action
- Sit the patient up if possible
- Call for ambulance assistance
- Treat any underlying cause found e.g. atropine for bradycardia; diamorphine, frusemide, and GTN spray for acute LVF
- Gain iv access if possible
- If available, give 100% oxygen (unless COPD, when give 24%)

Septic shock: Due to toxins from bacterial infection e.g. meningococcus.

Signs
- Hypotension
- Tachycardia
- Peripheral vasodilation or shut down (peripheral pallor and cyanosis, cool extremities)
- Pyrexia
- Tachypnoea
- ± purpuric rash

⚠ **Action**
- Lie the patient down flat and raise legs above waist height
- Call for ambulance assistance
- Give iv/im benzylpenicillin immediately while awaiting transport.
  Dose:
  - Adult and child ≥10y.—1.2g
  - Child 1–9y.—600mg
  - Infant <1y.—300mg
- If possible, gain iv access whilst awaiting the ambulance and take blood for cultures
- If available, start plasma expander/iv fluids; give rapidly over 10–15min.
- If available, give 100% oxygen (unless COPD, when give 24%)

Other rarer causes of shock: Admit as medical emergencies.
- *Neurogenic*—due to cerebral trauma or haemorrhage e.g. head injury, subarachnoid haemorrhage
- *Poisoning*
- *Liver failure*

Gastrointestinal (GI) bleeding

Causes of GI bleeding

Upper GI bleed
- Peptic ulcer
- Gastritits
- Mallory-Weiss tear
- Oesophagitis
- Oesophageal or gastric cancer
- Oesophageal varices
- Drugs—NSAIDs, steroids, anticoagulants
- Angiodysplasia
- Haemangioma
- Bleeding disorders
- Swallowed blood from nosebleed

Lower GI bleed
- Diverticulitis
- Colitis—infectious or inflammatory
- Large bowel tumour or polyp
- Haemorrhoids
- Anal fissure
- Angiodysplasia (arterio-venous malformations are common)
- Haemangioma
- Bleeding disorders
- Blood from upper GI bleed

Risk factors

Upper GI bleed
- History of alcohol abuse
- History of chronic liver disease
- History of NSAID use
- History of oral steroid use

Lower GI bleed
- Change in bowel habit
- History of diverticulitis
- History of UC

All GI bleeds
- Anticoagulant use
- Serious medical conditions (e.g. cardiovascular, respiratory, or renal disease)
- Recent tiredness (? due to anaemia)

Presentation

Upper GI bleeding: *Typical presentation:*
- Haematemesis—vomiting of blood
- Melaena—passage of black, offensive, tarry stool consisting of digested blood, per rectum (PR)

❶ Iron tablets may cause black stools.

Lower GI bleeding: *Typical presentation:*
- Passage of fresh blood, PR

❶ Very heavy upper GI bleeds can present with fresh red bleeding, PR.

Other features that may be present
- Faintness or dizziness, especially on standing
- Patient feels cold or clammy
- Collapse ± cardiac arrest

Examination
- Pulse—tachycardia
- BP—↓ and/or postural drop
- JVP—↓
- Vomitus

❶ Young people can lose a lot of blood before their BP drops. Be worried if a young person is tachycardic.

⚠ **Action**
- When the call for help is received—arrange immediate emergency transfer of the patient to hospital if a significant acute GI bleed is suspected.
- Attend the patient if diagnosis from history is unclear or (if possible) once the ambulance has been called to assist.
- Regard as an emergency until proved otherwise.

On arrival: Briefly assess the severity of the bleed from history and examination. If a significant GI bleed is suspected:
- Lie the patient flat and lift legs higher than body (e.g. feet on a pillow).
- Insert a large bore iv cannula—the opportunity may be lost by the time the ambulance crew arrive. If possible, take a sample for FBC and X-match on insertion.
- If available, give oxygen.
- If available, start plasma expander/iv fluids.
- Transfer as rapidly as possible to hospital.

Coffee-grounds vomit
- Vomiting of altered blood—looks like coffee granules
- Implies upper GI bleeding—though less severe than fresh red blood
- History and examination as for acute GI bleed
- Always admit to hospital for further assessment

Other bleeds

Bleeding aneurysms

Ruptured abdominal aortic aneurysm (AAA)

- In the community setting, death rate from ruptured AAA ≈ 90% (80% die before reaching hospital and 50% that get to hospital die during surgery).
- Consider a ruptured AAA in any patient with ↓BP and atypical abdominal symptoms (especially if there is a pulsatile abdominal mass).

⚠ In a patient with a known AAA, abdominal pain represents a ruptured AAA unless proven otherwise.

Dissecting thoracic aneurysm

- Consider in any patient with ↓BP and chest pain (especially if the pain radiates through to the back).
- Typically presents with sudden tearing chest pain radiating to the back.
- As the dissection progresses, branches of the aorta are sequentially occluded causing:
  - Hemiplegia—carotid artery
  - Unequal pulses and BP in the two arms—subclavian artery
  - Paraplegia—spinal arteries
  - Acute renal failure—renal arteries
- Proximal extension may cause aortic incompetence and MI (cardiac arteries).

⚠ Action

- Obtain venous access with 2x large bore iv cannulae.
- Admit as 'blue light' emergency, keeping the patient flat in the ambulance.
- Warn relatives of poor prognosis.

Nose bleed/epistaxis: Usually from ruptured blood vessels on the nasal septum (vein behind the comella or Little's area).

Causes

- **Elderly:** Degenerative arterial disease, ↑ BP, nose picking, coryza, allergic rhinitis, blood dyscrasias, teleangiectasia, and tumours. Often no cause is found.
- **Young:** Nose picking, coryza, allergic rhinitis, blood dyscrasias.

⚠ Action

- Check if the patient is on anticoagulants, aspirin, or NSAIDs and enquire about bleeding problems.
- Check BP—often high at time of bleed, so review prior to considering treatment. Watch for signs of shock and airway problems.

Most bleeds can be stopped by:

- Pinching the soft tip of nose for ≥10min.
- If available, applying an ice pack to the bridge of the nose.
- Leaning the patient forward to prevent blood entering the post nasal space.

If the bleeding is not settling and an anterior bleeding point is visualized:
- Try cautery with a silver nitrate stick after application of lignocaine on a piece of cotton wool.
- Prescribe antiseptic cream e.g. naseptin bd for 1wk.

Admit: As an emergency to A&E or ENT if shocked or heavy bleeding cannot be stopped after 30min. Hospital management:
- The anterior nares can be packed to try and stop bleeding using ribbon gauze in paraffin or a nasal tampon. The pack is usually left in place for 24h.
- Posterior nasal packs (e.g. using a foley catheter) are also used.
- Blood transfusion is rarely required.
- Occasionally, surgical exploration is required to find and cauterize the bleeding point or perform arterial ligation.

Referral: Refer recurrent minor bleeds to ENT for non-urgent assessment.

Meningitis and encephalitis

Meningitis: May be preceded with prodrome of fever, vomiting, malaise, poor feeding, and lethargy which is often indistinguishable from a viral infection. Usually rapid onset (<48h.) with signs of:

- **Meningism**
  - Headache
  - Photophobia
  - Stiff neck—can't put chin on chest
  - Kernig's sign +ve—with hips fully flexed, resists passive knee extension
- **↑ICP**
  - Irritability
  - Drowsiness and/or ↓ conscious level
  - Fits
  - Vomiting
  - ↓ pulse rate
  - ↑ BP
  - Bulging fontanelle (baby)
  - Abnormal tone/posturing
- **Septicaemia**
  - Rash—petechiae suggest meningococcus
  - Fever
  - Arthritis
  - Tachycardia
  - Peripheral shut down—cool peripheries, mottled skin, cyanosis
  - Tachypnoea

⚠ Small children, the elderly, or immunocompromised may not present with typical signs. Go on gut feeling.

⚠ Action

- Call an 999 ambulance and get the patient to hospital as soon as possible.
- Give iv/im benzylpenicillin immediately while awaiting transport. *Dose:*
  - Adult and child >10y.—1.2g
  - Child 1–9y.—600mg
  - Infant <1y.—300mg
- Cefotaxime is an alternative for patients allergic to penicillin.
- If possible, gain iv access whilst awaiting the ambulance and take blood for cultures.

Contact tracing/prophylaxis

- Undertaken by the local public health department.
- For a single case, only very close contacts ('kissing contacts' e.g. immediate family members) require prophylactic antibiotics.
- Prophylaxis is with rifampicin 600mg bd for 2d. (child 10mg/kg bd for 2d. unless <1y. when dose is 5mg/kg bd for 2d.) *or* ciprofloxacin 500mg as a single dose (not licensed for this indication and not suitable for children). Rifampicin colours urine red.

Meningitis vaccination
- Group C strains are responsible for 40% of meningococcal disease
- Group B strains are responsible for most of the rest
- Group A strains are common in other parts of the world but rare in the UK.

Meningococcal A&C vaccine: Confers no protection against Group B organisms.

Meningitis C conjugate vaccine
- Confers no protection against group A or group B organisms.
- For infants, doses are given at 2, 3, and 4mo. as part of the routine childhood vaccination programme (📖 p.480).
- For infants >4mo., 2 doses are required; and >1y. of age, only 1 dose is necessary to confer lasting immunity.
- Vaccine may be given to HIV +ve patients.
- A gap of 6mo. is recommended between a dose of the meningococcal A&C vaccine, usually given for travel purposes, and meningitis C conjugate vaccine.
- Do not use meningitis C conjugate vaccine for travel purposes as the greatest risk is from group A infection.
- Immunize individuals travelling abroad to high-risk areas with the meningococcal A&C vaccine, even if they have received the meningitis C conjugate vaccine beforehand.

Helplines for families
Meningitis Research Foundation ☎080 8800 3344 🖥 http://www.meningitis.org.uk
Meningitis Trust ☎0845 6000 800 🖥 http://www.meningitis-trust.org

Encephalitis: Inflammation of brain parenchyma. Usually viral in origin. Typically presents with:
- Fever
- Symptoms and signs of meningitis (see opposite)
- Altered consciousness
- Focal neurological signs/symptoms
- Convulsions
- Psychiatric symptoms

⚠ **Action**
- Admit immediately for further investigation/treatment.
- Treat blind with antibiotics if symptoms/signs of meningitis— see opposite.

Chest pain

On receiving the call for assistance: *Ask:*
- Nature and location of the pain
- Duration of the pain
- Other associated symptoms—sweating, nausea, shortness of breath, palpitations
- Past medical history (particularly heart disease, high cholesterol)
- Family history (particularly heart disease)
- Smoker?

⚠ Action
- Consider differential diagnosis (Table 29.3).
- If MI is suspected, call for ambulance assistance before (or instead of) visiting.
- Otherwise visit, assess, and treat according to cause.
- If a patient is acutely unwell with chest pain, and the cause is not clear, err on the side of caution and admit for further assessment.

Further information: Chest pain (📖 p.251)

Table 29.3 Possible causes of acute chest pain

Diagnosis	Page reference	Features
MI	📖 p.1048	Band-like chest pain around the chest or central chest pressure.
		± radiation to shoulders, arms (L > R), neck, and/or jaw.
		Often associated with nausea, sweating, and/or shortness of breath.
Unstable angina	📖 p.1048	As for MI.
Pericarditis	📖 p.351	Sharp, constant sternal pain relieved by sitting forwards.
		May radiate to left shoulder ± arm or into the abdomen.
		Worse lying on the left side and on inspiration, swallowing, and coughing.
Dissecting thoracic aneurysm	📖 p.1042	Typically presents with sudden tearing chest pain radiating to the back.
		Consider in any patient with chest pain (especially if radiates through to the back) and ↓BP.
PE	📖 p.1054	Acute dyspnoea, sharp chest pain (worse on inspiration), haemoptysis, and/or syncope.
Pleurisy	📖 p.252	Sharp, localized chest pain—worse on inspiration.
		May be associated with symptoms and signs of a chest infection.
Pneumothorax	📖 p.392	Sudden onset of pleuritic chest pain or ↑ breathlessness ± pallor and tachycardia.
Oesophageal spasm, oesophagitis	📖 p.434	Central chest pain. May be associated with acid reflux (though not always).
		May be described as burning but often indistinguishable from cardiac pain.
		May respond to antacids.
Musculoskeletal pain	📖 p.253	Localized pain—worse on movement.
		May be a history of injury.
Shingles	📖 p.494	Intense, often sharp, unilateral pain.
		Responds poorly to analgesia.
		May be present several days before rash appears.
Costochondritis	📖 p.584	Inflammation of the costochondral junctions—tenderness over the costochondral junction and pain in the affected area on springing the chest wall.
Bornholm's disease		Unilateral chest and/or abdominal pain, rhinitis. Coxsackie virus infection. Treat with simple analgesia.
Idiopathic chest pain	📖 p.253	No cause apparent. Common.
		Affects young people > elderly people; ♀ > ♂.

Myocardial infarct (MI) and unstable angina

Myocardial infarct

Typical presentation: Sustained central chest pain not relieved by sublingual GTN.

Other features that may be present
- Collapse ± cardiac arrest
- Breathlessness
- Anxiety/fear of dying
- Nausea ± vomiting
- Sweating
- Pain in 1 or both arms, jaw, back, or upper abdomen.

> ❶ May occasionally be silent, especially in patients with DM.

Examination: Pulse, BP, JVP, heart sounds, chest (? pulmonary oedema).

Investigation: ECG—ST elevation *or* R waves and ST depression in leads V1–V3 (posterior infarction) *or* new LBBB.

⚠ *Action*

When the call for assistance is made

If MI is suspected, arrange immediate transfer to hospital—for thrombolysis to be effective, it must be given as soon as possible after the onset of pain. Seeing the patient before arranging transfer introduces unnecessary delays.

If possible, attend the patient once the ambulance has been called to assist—there is a lot a GP can do that an ambulance crew cannot. If the patient is seen:
- Give aspirin 300mg po (unless contraindicated)
- Insert iv cannula
- Give iv analgesia (diamorphine 2.5–5mg); repeat in 15min. as necessary
- Give iv antiemetic (metoclopramide 10mg)
- Give sublingual GTN to act as a coronary artery vasodilator (if systolic BP >90 and pulse <100bpm)
- If available, give oxygen
- If bradycardia, give atropine 300mcg iv and further doses of 300mcg, if needed, to a maximum of 1.2mg.

Thrombolysis in general practice: May be appropriate in places where transfer to hospital takes >½ h. Special training and equipment is necessary.

Late calls

- If the patient is seen <24h. after an acute episode, admit for specialist assessment.
- If the patient is seen >24h. after an acute episode but still has residual pain or other
  symptoms, admit.
- If the patient is seen >24h. after an acute episode and is well, start regular aspirin, supply with GTN spray, warn what to do if any further episodes of acute chest pain, and follow-up as for MI post-discharge (📖 p.332).

Follow-up care: 📖 p.332

Unstable angina: Defined as rapid acceleration of pre-existing exertional angina or the occurrence of prolonged episodes of ischaemic pain at rest. It is difficult to tell the difference between acute MI and unstable angina in general practice. Treat as for acute MI.

Choking—adult^G

⚠ If blockage of the airway is only partial, the victim will usually be able to dislodge the foreign body by coughing. If obstruction is complete, urgent intervention is required to prevent asphyxia.

Victim is unconscious
- Tilt the victim's head and remove any visible obstruction from the mouth
- Open the airway further by lifting the chin
- Check for breathing by looking, listening, and feeling
- Attempt to give 2 effective rescue breaths (📖 p.1020)

If effective breaths can be achieved in ≤5 attempts
- Check for signs of a circulation
- Start chest compressions and/or rescue breaths as appropriate (📖 p.1020)

If effective breaths *cannot* be achieved in ≤5 attempts
- Start chest compressions immediately, to relieve the obstruction—do not check for signs of a circulation
- After 15 compressions, check the mouth for any obstruction, then attempt further rescue breaths
- Continue to give cycles of 15 compressions, followed by attempts at rescue breaths

If, at any time, effective breaths can be achieved
- Check for signs of a circulation
- Continue chest compressions and/or rescue breaths as appropriate (📖 p.1020)

Victim shows signs of exhaustion or becomes cyanosed but is conscious: Carry out back blows.
- Remove any obvious debris or loose teeth from the mouth
- Stand to the side and slightly behind him
- Support the chest with one hand and lean the victim well forwards
- Give up to 5 sharp blows between the scapulae with the heel of the other hand; each blow should be aimed at relieving the obstruction, so all 5 need not necessarily be given

If the back blows fail, carry out abdominal thrusts
- Stand behind the victim and put both your arms around the upper part of the abdomen
- Ensure the victim is bending well forwards so that the obstructing object comes out of the mouth when dislodged
- Clench your fist and place it between the umbilicus and the xiphisternum. Grasp it with your other hand
- Pull sharply inwards and upwards. Repeat up to 5 times.
  The obstruction should be dislodged.

If the obstruction is still not relieved
- Recheck the mouth for any obstruction that can be reached with a finger
- Continue alternating 5 back blows with 5 abdominal thrusts

Victim is conscious and breathing, despite evidence of obstruction: Encourage him to continue coughing but do nothing else.

Foreign body in the throat: Occurs after eating—fish bone or food bolus are most common. Can cause severe discomfort, distress, and inability to swallow saliva.

Management: Refer immediately to A&E or ENT for investigation (lateral neck X-ray ± laryngoscopy). Most fish bones have passed and the discomfort comes from mucosal trauma. Food boluses often pass spontaneously (especially if the patient is given a smooth muscle relaxant) but occasionally need removal under GA.

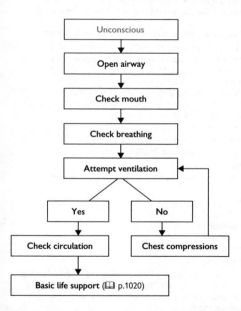

Figure 29.10 Algorithm for the management of choking in adults. (Reproduced with permission of the Resuscitation council (UK) 🖥 http://www.resus.org.uk)

Further information
Resuscitation Council (UK) 🖥 http://www.resus.org.uk

Choking—child^G

⚠ If the child is breathing spontaneously, his own efforts to clear the obstruction should be encouraged. Intervention is necessary only if these attempts are clearly ineffective and breathing is inadequate.

⚠ Do not perform blind finger sweeps of the mouth or upper airway as these may further impact a foreign body or cause soft tissue damage.

Step 1: Perform up to 5 back blows
- Hold the child in a prone position and try to position the head lower than the chest with the airway in an open position
- Deliver up to 5 smart blows to the middle of the back between the shoulder blades
- If this fails to dislodge the foreign body, proceed to chest thrusts

Step 2: Perform up to 5 chest thrusts
- Turn the child into a supine position with the head lower than the chest and the airway in an open position
- Give up to 5 chest thrusts to the sternum
- The technique for chest thrusts is similar to that for chest compressions but chest thrusts should be sharper and more vigorous and carried out at a rate of ~20/min.

Step 3: Check the mouth
- After 5 back blows and 5 chest thrusts, check the mouth
- Carefully remove any visible foreign bodies

Step 4: Open the airway
- Reposition the airway by the head tilt and chin lift (jaw thrust) manoeuvre
- Reassess breathing

Step 5
If the child is breathing:
- Turn the child on his side
- Check for continued breathing

If the child is not breathing
- Attempt up to 5 rescue breaths to achieve 2 effective breaths, each of which makes the chest rise and fall. The child may be apnoeic or the airway partially cleared. In either case, you may be able to achieve effective ventilation at this stage.

If the airway is still obstructed
For a child (>1y.)
- Repeat the cycle (steps 1–5 above) but substitute 5 abdominal thrusts for 5 chest thrusts
- Abdominal thrusts are delivered as 5 sharp thrusts directed upwards towards the diaphragm
- Use the upright position if the child is conscious; kneel behind a small child
- Unconscious children should be laid supine and the heel of one hand placed in the middle of the upper abdomen

- Alternate chest thrusts and abdominal thrusts in subsequent cycles
- Repeat the cycles until the airway is cleared or the child breathes spontaneously

For an infant (<1y.)
- Abdominal thrusts are not recommended in infants because they may rupture the abdominal viscera
- Perform cycles of 5 back blows and 5 chest thrusts only
- Repeat the cycles until the airway is cleared or the infant breathes spontaneously.

Further information

Resuscitation Council (UK) 🖳 *http://www.resus.org.uk*

Acute breathlessness (1)

Attend as soon as possible after receiving the call for help. If there is likely to be any delay, call for emergency ambulance assistance.

On arrival: Be calm and reassuring. Breathlessness is frightening and panic only adds to the sensation of being breathless.

Consider possible causes
- Asthma: 📖 p.1058
- Anaphylaxis: 📖 p.1036
- Acute left ventricular failure: 📖 p.1056
- Arrythmia: 📖 p.342
- Pneumonia: 📖 p.390
- Acute exacerbation of COPD: 📖 p.386
- Hyperventilation: 📖 p.1056
- Pulmonary embolism: See below
- Spontaneous pneumothorax: See opposite and 📖 p.392
- Choking: 📖 p.1050
- Air hunger due to shock: 📖 p.1038

Direct history and examination to finding the cause as quickly as possible. Treat according to the cause. If no cause can be found—don't delay. Admit to hospital as an acute medical emergency.

Pulmonary embolus: Venous thrombi (usually from a DVT) pass into the pulmonary circulation and block blood flow to the lungs. Fatal in ~1:10 cases.

Risk factors
- Immobility—long flight or bus journey, post-op, plaster cast
- Smoking
- COC pill
- Pregnancy or puerperium
- Malignancy
- Past history or FH of DVT or PE

Presentation
- *Symptoms:* Acute dyspnoea, pleuritic pain, haemoptysis, syncope
- *Signs*
  - Hypotension
  - Tachycardia
  - Cyanosis
  - Tachypnoea
  - Pleural rub
  - ↑ JVP
- Look for a source of emboli—though often DVT is not clinically obvious

Differential diagnosis
- Pneumonia and pleurisy
- MI
- Other causes of acute breathlessness (above)
- Acute intra-abdominal emergencies (📖 p.1066)

Action: Give oxygen as soon as possible. Admit as an acute medical emergency.

Further management: After initial anticoagulation in hospital, patients are usually discharged home on oral anticoagulants. Target INR 2.5 (range 2–3). Continue anticoagulation for 3mo. unless on-going risk factors.

Tension pneumothorax
- Complication of traumatic pneumothorax; rare after spontaneous pneumothorax.
- A valvular mechanism develops—air is sucked into the pleural space during inspiration but cannot be expelled during expiration. The pressure within the pleural space ↑, the lung deflates further, the mediastinum shifts to the opposite side of the chest and venous return ↓.
- Can be rapidly fatal.

Clinical features
- Agitated and distressed patient, often with a history of chest trauma
- Tachycardia
- Sweating
- Signs of a large pneumothorax—↓ breath sounds and ↓ chest movement on the affected side
- Mediastinal shift—trachea deviated away from the side of the pneumothorax

⚠ *Action: If suspected:*
- Sit the patient upright if possible;
- Insert a large bore cannula through the 2nd intercostal space of the chest wall in the mid-clavicular line on the side of the pneumothorax to relieve the pressure in the pleural space;
- Transfer as an emergency to hospital.

Acute breathlessness (2)

Acute left ventricular failure (acute LVF): Severe acute breathlessness due to pulmonary oedema. Urgent treatment is needed to save life.

Presenting features
- Sudden acute breathlessness
- Fatigue
- Cough ± haemoptysis (usually pink and frothy)
- Tends to occur at night
- Some relief gained from sitting/standing

Signs
- Dyspnoea
- Tachycardia—gallop rhythm may be present
- Coarse wet sounding crackles at both bases
- Ankle/sacral oedema if right heart failure also present
- ± hypotension

Differential diagnosis: Other causes of acute breathlessness (especially asthma)—🕮 p.1054.

⚠ *Action*
- If severe, call for ambulance support
- Sit the patient up
- Be reassuring—it is frightening to be very short of breath
- Give 100% oxygen if available and no history of COPD (24% if history of COPD)
- Give iv furosemide 40–80mg slowly (or bumetanide 1–2mg)
- Give iv diamorphine 2.5–5mg over 5min.
- Give metoclopramide 10mg iv (can be mixed with diamorphine)
- Give GTN spray 2 puffs sublingually

Admission: Depends on severity and cause of attack, response to treatment, and social support. *Always admit if:*
- Alone at home
- Inadequate social support
- Suspected cause of acute LVF warrants admission (e.g. acute MI)
- Very breathless and no improvement over ½ h. with treatment at home
- Hypotension or arrythmia.

Further information: Heart failure—(🕮 p.334)

Hyperventilation

Features: Fear, terror, and feeling of impending doom accompanied by some or all of the following:
- Palpitations
- Shortness of breath
- Choking sensation
- Dizziness
- Paraesthesiae
- Chest pain/discomfort
- Sweating
- Carpopedal spasm

Differential diagnosis

- Dysrhythmia
- Asthma
- Anaphylaxis
- Thyrotoxicosis
- Temporal lobe epilepsy
- Hypoglycaemia
- Phaeochromocytome (very rare)

⚠ **Action**

Talking down: Explain the nature of the symptoms to the patient.

- Racing of the heart is due to adrenaline produced by the panic.
- Paraesthesiae and feelings of dizziness are due to overbreathing due to panic.

Count breaths in and out, gently slowing breathing rate.

Rebreathing techniques

- Place a paper bag over the patient's mouth and ask him to breath in and out through the mouth. A connected but not switched on O_2 mask or nebuliser mask is an alternative in the surgery.
- This raises the partial pressure of CO_2 in the blood and symptoms due to low CO_2 (e.g. tetany, paraesthesiae, dizziness) resolve. It also demonstrates the link between hyperventilation and the symptoms to the patient.

Propranolol: 10–20mg stat may be helpful—DON'T USE for asthmatics or patients with heart failure or on verapamil.

Recurrent panic attacks: 📖 p.962

Acute asthma in adults

Many deaths from asthma are preventable. Delay can be fatal. Factors leading to poor outcome include:
- Doctors failing to assess severity by objective measurement
- Patients or relatives failing to appreciate severity
- Underuse of corticosteroids

⚠ Regard each emergency asthma consultation as acute severe asthma, until proven otherwise.

Risk factors for developing fatal or near fatal asthma

A combination of severe asthma recognized by ≥ 1 of:
- Previous near fatal asthma definition opposite
- Previous admission for asthma—especially if within 1y.
- Requiring ≥3 classes of asthma medication
- Heavy use of β_2 agonist
- Repeated attendances at A&E for asthma care—especially if within 1y.
- Brittle asthma

And adverse behavioural or psychosocial features recognized by ≥1 of:
- Non-compliance with treatment or monitoring
- Failure to attend appointments
- Self-discharge from hospital
- Psychosis, depression, other psychiatric illness or deliberate self-harm
- Current or recent major tranquillizer use
- Denial
- Alcohol or drug misuse
- Obesity
- Learning difficulties
- Employment problems
- Income problems
- Social isolation
- Childhood abuse
- Severe marital, legal, or domestic stress

Assess and record
- Peak expiratory flow (PEF)
- Symptoms and response to self-treatment
- Heart and respiratory rates
- Oxygen saturation by pulse oximetry (if available)

⚠ Patients with severe or life-threatening attacks may not be distressed and may not have all the characteristic abnormalities of severe asthma. The presence of any should alert the doctor.

Levels of severity of acute asthma exacerbations

Moderate asthma exacerbation
- Increasing symptoms
- PEF >50–75% predicted
- No features of acute severe asthma

Acute severe asthma: Any one of:
- PEF 33–50% best or predicted
- Respiratory rate ≥25 breaths/min.
- Heart rate ≥110/min.
- Inability to complete sentences in 1 breath

Life-threatening asthma: Any 1 of the following with severe asthma:
- PEF <33% best/predicted
- O_2 saturation <92%
- Silent chest
- Cyanosis
- Feeble respiratory effort
- Bradycardia
- Dysrhythmia
- Hypotension
- Exhaustion
- Confusion
- Coma

Near fatal asthma: Respiratory acidosis and/or requiring mechanical ventilation with ↑ inflation pressures.

Brittle asthma
- *Type 1:* Wide PEF variability (>40% diurnal variation for >50% of the time for a period of >150d.) despite intense therapy.
- *Type 2:* Sudden severe attacks on a background of apparently well-controlled asthma.

Management: Figure 29.11—📖 p.1060

Admit to hospital if:
- Life-threatening features
- Features of acute severe asthma present after initial treatment
- Previous near fatal asthma

Lower threshold for admission if:
- Afternoon or evening attack
- Recent nocturnal symptoms or hospital admission
- Previous severe attacks
- Patient unable to assess own condition
- Concern over social circumstances

If admitting the patient to hospital
- Stay with the patient until the ambulance arrives
- Send written assessment and referral details to the hospital
- Give high-dose β_2 bronchodilator via an oxygen-driven nebuliser in the ambulance

Follow-up after treatment or discharge from hospital
- GP review within 48h.
- Monitor symptoms and PEF
- Check inhaler technique
- Written asthma action plan
- Modify treatment according to guidelines for chronic persistent asthma
- Address potentially preventable contributors to admission

Management of chronic asthma: 📖 p.376–81

Essential reading
BTS/SIGN (2004) British guidelines on the management of asthma 🖥 *http://www.sign.ac.uk*

Moderate asthma	Acute severe asthma	Life-threatening asthma
INITIAL ASSESSMENT		
PEF >50% best or predicted	PEF 33–50% best or predicted	PEF <33% best or predicted
FURTHER ASSESSMENT		
Speech normal Respiration <25 breaths/min. Pulse <110 beats/min.	Can't complete sentences Respiration ≥25 breaths/min. Pulse ≥110 beats/min.	Oxygen saturation <92% Silent chest, cyanosis, or feeble respiratory effort Bradycardia, dysrhythmia, or hypotension Exhaustion, confusion, or coma
MANAGEMENT		
Treat at home or in the surgery and ASSESS RESPONSE TO TREATMENT	Consider admission	Arrange immediate admission
TREATMENT		
High-dose β₂ bronchodilator: Ideally via oxygen-driven nebuliser (salbutamol 5mg or terbutaline 10mg) Alternatively, use air driven nebulizer or inhaler via spacer (1 puff 10–20x) *If PEF >50–75: predicted/ best:* Give prednisolone 40–50mg. Continue or step up usual treatment *If good response to first nebulized treatment* (symptoms improved, respiration and pulse setting and PEF >50%) continue or step up usual treatment and continue prednisolone.	*Oxygen 40–60% if available* *High-dose β₂ bronchodilator:* Ideally via oxygen-driven nebulizer (salbutamol 5mg or terbutaline 10mg). Alternatively use air-driven nebulizer or inhaler via spacer (1 puff 10–20x) *Prednisolone 40–50mg or IV hydrocortisone 100mg* *If no response in acute, severe asthma: ADMIT*	*Oxygen 40–60%, if available* *Prednisolone 40–50mg or IV hydrocortisone 100mg immediately* *High-dose β₂ bronchodilator:* Ideally via oxygen-driven nebulizer (salbutomal salbutamol 5mg or terbutaline 10mg). Alternatively use air driven nebulizer or inhaler via spacer (1 puff 10–20x) *ADMIT immediately*

Figure 29.11 Management of acute severe asthma in adults (Reproduced from the *British guideline on the management of asthma* (2004) with permission of SIGN/British Thoracic Society.)

Acute asthma in children

Assess and record
- Pulse rate—increasing heart rate generally reflects ↑ severity
- Respiratory rate and breathlessness
- Use of accessory muscles—best noted by palpation of neck muscles
- Amount of wheezing
- Degree of agitation and conscious level

Levels of severity
Child >5y.: Figure 29.12 (🕮 p.1063)
Child 2–5y.: Figure 29.13 (🕮 p.1064)
Child <2y.: Assessment of children <2y. can be difficult
- Moderate wheezing
  - O₂ saturation ≥92%
  - Audible wheezing
  - Using accessory muscles
  - Still feeding
- Severe wheezing
  - O₂ saturation <92%
  - Cyanosis
  - Marked respiratory distress
  - Too breathless to feed
- Life-threatening
  - Apnoea
  - Bradycardia
  - Poor respiratory effort

⚠ If a patient has signs and symptoms across categories, always treat according to the most severe features.

Management
Child >5y.: Figure 29.12 (🕮 p.1063)
Child 2–5y.: Figure 29.13 (🕮 p.1064)
Child <2y.: Intermittent wheezing attacks are usually in response to viral infection and response to bronchodilators is inconsistent.
- *If mild/moderate wheeze*
  - A trial of bronchodilators can be considered if symptoms are of concern—use a metred dose inhaler and spacer with a face mask.
  - If no response, consider alternative diagnosis (aspiration pneumonitis, pneumonia, bronchiolitis, tracheomalacia, CF, congenital anomaly) and/or admit.
- *If severe wheezing:* Admit to hospital.
- *If any life-threatening features:* Admit immediately as a blue light emergency.

Follow-up after treatment or discharge from hospital
- GP review within 1 week
- Monitor symptoms, PEF, and check inhaler technique
- Written asthma action plan
- Modify treatment according to guidelines for chronic persistent asthma
- Address potentially preventable contributors to admission

Management of chronic asthma
- *Children <12y.:* 📖 p.860–5
- *Children >12y. and adults:* 📖 p.376–81

Essential reading
BTS/SIGN (2004) British guideline on the management of asthma 🖥 *http://www.sign.ac.uk*

ASSESS ASTHMA SEVERITY		
Moderate exacerbation	Severe exacerbation	Life-threatening asthma
Oxygen saturation ≥92% PEF ≥50% best or predicted Able to talk Heart rate ≤120/min. Respiratory rate ≤30/min.	Oxygen saturation <92% PEF <50% best or predicted Too breathless to talk Heart rate >120/min. Respiratory rate >30/min. Use of accessory neck muscles	Oxygen saturation <92% PEF <33% best or predicted Silent chest Poor respiratory effort Agitation Altered consciousness Cyanosis
β₂ agonist 2–4 puffs via spacer Consider soluble prednisolone 30–40mg Increase β₂ agonist dose by 2 puffs every 2min. up to 10 puffs according to response	Oxygen via face mask β₂ agonist 10 puffs via spacer ± face mask or nebulized salbutamol 2.5–5mg (or terbutaline 5–10mg) Soluble prednisolone 30–40mg Assess response to treatment 15min. after β₂ agonist	Oxygen via face mask Nebulize: • salbutamol 5mg or terbutaline 10mg + • Ipratropium 0.25mg soluble predhisolone 30–40mg or iv hydrocortisone 10mg
IF POOR RESPONSE ARRANGE ADMISSION	IF POOR RESPONSE REPEAT β₂ AGONIST AND ARRANGE ADMISSION	REPEAT β₂ AGONIST VIA OXYGEN-DRIVEN NEBULIZER WHILST ARRANGING IMMEDIATE HOSPITAL ADMISSION

GOOD RESPONSE	POOR RESPONSE
Continue up to 10 puffs or nebulised β₂ agonist as needed (max. every 4h.) If symptoms are not controlled repeat β₂ agonist and refer to hospital Continue prednisolone for up to 3d. Arrange follow up clinic visit	Stay with the patient until the ambulance arrives Send written assessment and referral details Repeat β₂ agonist via oxygen driven nebuliser in the ambulance

Figure 29.12 Management of acute asthma in children >5y. (Reproduced from the *British guideline on the management of asthma* (2004) with permission of SIGN/British Thoracic Society.)

⚠ **Lower threshold for admission if**
• Attack in late afternoon or at night
• Recent hospital admission or previous severe attack
• Concern over social circumstances or ability to cope at home

ASSESS ASTHMA SEVERITY		
Moderate exacerbation	Severe exacerbation	Life-threatening asthma
Oxygen saturation ≥92% Able to talk Heart rate 130/min. Respiratory rate 50/min.	Oxygen saturation <92% Too breathless to talk Heart rate >130/min. Respiratory rate >50/min. use of accessory neck muscles	Oxygen saturation <92% Silent chest Poor respiratory effort Agitation Altered consciousness Cyanosis
β_2 agonist 2–4 puffs via spacer Consider soluble prednisolone 20 mg Increase β_2 agonist dose by 2 puffs every 2min. up to 10 puffs, according to response	Oxygen via face mask β_2 agonist 10 puffs via spacer ± face mask or nebulized salbutamol 2.5mg (or terbutaline 5mg) Soluble prednisolone 20mg Assess response to treatment 15min. after β_2 agonist	Oxygen via face mask Nebulize: • salbutamol 5mg or terbutaline 10mg + • Ipratropium 0.25mg soluble predhisolone 20mg or IV hydrocortisone 10mg
IF POOR RESPONSE, ARRANGE ADMISSION	IF POOR RESPONSE, REPEAT β_2 AGONIST AND ARRANGE ADMISSION	REPEAT β_2 AGONIST VIA OXYGEN DRIVEN NEBULIZER WHILST ARRANGING IMMEDIATE HOSPITAL ADMISSION

GOOD RESPONSE	POOR RESPONSE
Continue up to 10 puffs or nebulised β_2 agonist, as needed (max. every 4h.) If symptoms are not controlled, repeat β_2 agonist and refer to hospital Continue prednisolone for up to 3d. Arrange follow-up clinic visit	Stay with the patient until the ambulance arrives Send written assessment and referral details Repeat β_2 agonist via oxygen driven nebulizer in the ambulance

Figure 29.13 Management of acute asthma in children 2–5y. (Reproduced from the British guideline on the management of asthma (2004) with permission of SIGN/British Thoracic Society.).

⚠ **Lower threshold for admission if:**
- Attack in late afternoon or at night
- Recent hospital admission or previous severe attack
- Concern over social circumstances or ability to cope at home

Acute abdominal pain

❶ Signs may be masked in elderly patients or those on corticosteroids. Small children with abdominal pain are difficult to assess.

Consider

GI causes
- Appendicitis (🕮 p.464)
- Gastritis (🕮 p.437)
- Perforated peptic ulcer (🕮 p.438)
- Acute pancreatitis (🕮 p.448)
- Biliary colic (🕮 p.447)
- Acute cholecystitis (🕮 p.447)
- Intestinal obstruction (🕮 p.466)
- Intussusception (🕮 p.858)
- Strangulated hernia (🕮 p.462)
- Ischaemic bowel (🕮 p.466)
- Diverticulitis (🕮 p.467)
- Volvulus (🕮 p.466)
- Impacted faeces (🕮 p.472)
- Inflammatory bowel disease e.g. Crohn's, UC (🕮 p.456)
- Irritable bowel syndrome (🕮 p.460)
- Gastroenteritis (🕮 p.452)

Gynaecological causes
- Ovarian torsion (🕮 p.712)
- Bleed into or rupture of an ovarian cyst (🕮 p.712)
- Ectopic pregnancy (🕮 p.738)
- Dysmenorrhoea (🕮 p.726)
- Pelvic inflammatory disease (🕮 p.720)
- Uterine abruption (🕮 p.796)
- Endometriosis (🕮 p.722)

Other causes
- MI (🕮 p.1048)
- CCF (🕮 p.334)
- Leaking or ruptured AAA (🕮 p.1042)
- Pneumonia (🕮 p.390)
- Sickle cell crisis (🕮 p.527)
- Diabetic ketoacidosis (🕮 p.1068)
- Renal disease (🕮 p.678)
- UTI (🕮 p.692)
- Henoch-Schonlein purpura (🕮 p.284)
- Mesenteric adenitis opposite
- Ruptured spleen below
- Torsion of the testis (🕮 p.698)
- Herpes zoster (🕮 p.494)
- Porphyria (🕮 p.663)

Management: Treat the cause—if unsure, admit as a surgical emergency to hospital. Do not give analgesia prior to surgical assessment as it may mask vital diagnostic signs.

Ruptured spleen: May occur immediately following trauma or present days/weeks later. Diseased spleens (e.g. glandular fever, malaria, leukaemia) rupture more easily.

Presentation
- *History:* of abdominal trauma
- *Signs of blood loss:* tachycardia, ↓ BP ± postural drop, pallor
- *Signs of peritoneal irritation:* guarding, abdominal rigidity, shoulder tip pain
- *Signs of paralytic ileus:* abdominal distention, lack of bowel sounds

⚠ Action: If suspected, admit as a surgical emergency via '999' ambulance.

Mesenteric adenitis: Pain due to mesenteric lymphadenopathy in children. Usually associated with URTI. Treat with simple analgesia and fluids. Review if the pain becomes more severe or changes.

Further information
- Abdominal pain (📖 p.246)
- Epigastric pain (📖 p.259)
- Right upper quadrant pain (📖 p.288)
- Right iliac fossa pain (📖 p.287)
- Left iliac fossa pain (📖 p.273)
- Left upper quadrant pain (📖 p.273)
- Pelvic pain (📖 p.720)

The fitting patient and delirium tremens

When the call for assistance is received: Instruct the attendant:
- to stay with the fitting patient
- to move anything from the vicinity of the patient that might cause injury
- to turn the patient onto his/her side

If the patient is a child, suspect a febrile cause and advise the attendant to cool the child by stripping off layers of clothing and by tepid sponging.

⚠ **Management of a major fit**
- Ensure that the airway is clear
- Turn the patient into the recovery position—🕮 p.1022
- Prevent onlookers from restraining the fitting patient
- Do not give drugs for the 1st 10min.—the fit is likely to stop spontaneously
- After 10min.; treat with diazepam 5–10mg iv or pr (5mg if 2–3y. or elderly; 2.5mg if <2y.)
- If the fit is not controlled, treat as status epilepticus

Admit any patient with a fit if:
- There is suspicion that the fit is 2° to other illness e.g. meningitis, subdural haematoma
- The patient doesn't recover completely after the fit (other than feeling sleepy)
- Status epilepticus

Status epilepticus: If >1 seizure without the patient regaining consciousness *or* fitting continues >20min.
- Give diazepam 5–10mg iv or pr (5mg if 2–3y. or elderly; 2.5mg if <2y.)
- Repeat every 15min. until fits are controlled
- Check BM to exclude low blood sugar
- Arrange immediate admission, even if fits are controlled

Follow-up
- Refer any adult who has a first fit to neurology for assessment
- Refer any child who has a first fit not related to fever to paediatrics for assessment

Delirium tremens (DTs): Major withdrawal symptoms. Usually occur 2–3d. after an alcoholic has stopped drinking. *Features:*
- *General:* Fever, tachycardia, ↑BP, ↑ respiratory rate
- *Psychiatric:* Vivid visual and tactile hallucinations, acute confusional state, apprehension
- *Neurological:* Tremor, fits, fluctuating level of consciousness

⚠ *Action:* DTs have 15% mortality and always warrant emergency hospital admission.

Further information
- Epilepsy: 🕮 p.618–21
- Febrile convulsions: 🕮 p.867
- Alcoholism: 🕮 p.236–9

Endocrine emergencies

Hypoglycaemic coma

History
- Short history
- Known diabetic on oral or insulin therapy
- May or may not have been warning signs/symptoms—sweating, hunger, tremor

Examination: May present with coma, fits or odd/violent behaviour, tachycardia ± ↑ BP.

Investigation: Blood sugar (on blood testing strip) <2.5mmol/l..

⚠ *Action:*
- Give:
  - Glucagon 1mg, sc, im, or iv (0.5mg in children)—takes ≤5min. to act. May have poor effect if the patient is starved or drunk.
    or
  - iv glucose (20–50ml of 20% solution).
- Once the patient has regained consciousness, supplement with oral glucose.
- Monitor frequent blood sugars over the next 4h. (hourly) and 4 hourly for the following 24h. Review reasons for hypoglycaemia— 📖 p.413.
- Maintain a high glucose intake for several hours if the patient has a severe episode of hypoglycaemia due to a sulphonylurea.

Hyperglycaemic ketoacidotic coma: Only occurs in patients with type 1 DM—though may be the way in which it presents (i.e. can occur in young patients not known to be diabetic).

History: 2–3d. deterioration which may have been precipitated by infection.

Examination: Dehydration, hyperventilation, breath smells ketotic, ↓BP + postural drop, tachycardia.

Investigation: Finger prick blood sugar test using reagent strip—usually >20mmol/l. Dipstick of urine is +ve for ketones (if urine available).

⚠ *Action*
Admit immediately to hospital.

Hyperglycaemic hyperosmolar non-ketotic coma: Only occurs in patients with type 2 DM.

History: Up to 1wk. history of deterioration. Often precipitated by other illness e.g. infection, MI. May be a presenting feature of type 2 DM.

Examination: ↓ level of consciousness, dehydration ++, ↓ BP with postural drop.

Investigation: Blood sugar (on blood testing strip) >35mmol/l.

⚠ *Action:*
Admit immediately to hospital.

Myxoedema coma
Presentation
- >65y. old
- History of thyroid surgery/radioactive iodine
- May be precipitated by MI, stroke, infection, or trauma
- Looks hypothyroid
- Hypothermia
- Hyporeflexia
- Heart failure
- Cyanosis
- Bradycardia
- Coma
- Seizures

Investigation: Finger prick blood glucose may be ↓.

⚠ *Action*
- Keep warm
- Treat heart failure with diuretics ± opiates and nitrates—📖 p.1056
- Admit as an emergency to hospital

Hyperthyroid crisis (thyrotoxic storm)
Risk factors
- Recent thyroid surgery/radioactive iodine
- Infection
- Trauma
- MI

Presentation
- Fever
- Agitation and/or confusion
- Coma
- Tachycarida/AF
- D&V
- Acute abdomen
- May have goitre ± thyroid bruit.

⚠ *Action*
Admit as an emergency to hospital.

Obstetric emergencies

Obstetric shock: *Causes:*
- Haemorrhage—remember that in abruption, bleeding may be internal and not seen pv
- Ruptured uterus
- Inverted uterus
- Amniotic fluid embolus
- Pulmonary embolus
- Septicaemia

⚠ **Action**
- Call for help
- Arrange immediate admission to the nearest specialist obstetric unit or failing that, A&E department
- Gain iv access and start iv fluids (if available)
- Treat the cause if apparent

Shoulder dystocia: Affects <1% deliveries but is a life-threatening emergency. Occurs when the anterior shoulder impacts upon the symphysis pubis after the head has delivered, and prevents the rest of the baby following. Most cases of shoulder dystocia are unanticipated. *Clues:*
- Prolonged 1st or 2nd stage of labour
- 'Head bobbing'—the head consistently descends then returns to its original position during a contraction or while pushing in the 2nd stage

If shoulder dystocia occurs in the community, there is usually not time to transfer a woman to a specialist unit.

⚠ **Action:** Call for help. Consider episiotomy. Then try any of these procedures (no particular order):
- Roll the mother onto hands and knees and try delivering posterior shoulder first.
- Flex the mother's legs up to her abdomen (upside down squatting position)—try delivery again.
- Deliver the posterior arm—put a hand in the vagina in front of the baby—ensure the posterior elbow is flexed in front of the body and pull to deliver the forearm. The anterior shoulder usually follows.
- External pressure—ask an assistant to apply suprapubic pressure with the heel of the hand—a rocking movement can help.
- Adduction of the most accessible (preferably anterior) shoulder. Simultaneously put pressure on the posterior clavicle to turn the baby. If unsuccessful, continue rotation through 180 degrees and try again.

Uterine inversion: Rare.

⚠ **Action**
- If noted early, try to replace the uterus. Otherwise, admit by emergency ambulance to the nearest obstetric unit.

The mother may become profoundly shocked so set up an iv infusion before transfer and give O_2 via face mask.

Retained placenta: 3rd stage is complete in <10min. in 97% labours. If the placenta has not delivered within 30min. it will probably not deliver spontaneously. PPH is a risk—📖 p.792.

⚠ *Action*
- Avoid excessive cord traction.
- Check the placenta is not in the vagina—remove if it is.
- Check the uterus—if well contracted, the placenta has probably separated but become trapped in the cervix. Wait for the cervix to relax and remove the placenta.
- If the uterus is bulky, the placenta may have failed to separate. Try:
  - Rubbing up a uterine contraction per abdomen
  - Putting the baby to the breast (stimulates uterine contraction)
  - Giving a further dose of syntometrine
  - If the placenta still will not deliver, transfer as an emergency to a specialist obstetric unit for manual removal

Foetal distress: Signifies hypoxia. *Signs:*
- Passage of meconium during labour
- Foetal tachycardia (>160bpm at term)
- Foetal bradycardia (<100bpm)—seek urgent obstetric assistance

⚠ *Action*
- Give the mother oxygen via a face mask
- Turn the mother on her side
- Transfer immediately to a specialist obstetric unit for further assessment ± delivery

Resuscitation of the newborn: 📖 p.1030

Road traffic accidents (RTAs) and trauma

Road accidents: Doctors are not legally obliged to attend an accident they happen to pass—but most feel morally obliged to do so.

Immediate action
- Assess the scene.
- Ensure police and ambulance have been called.
- Take steps to ensure your own safety and that of others—park your vehicle defensively; turn on hazard lights; use warning triangles.
- Ensure all vehicle ignitions are turned off.
- Triage casualties into priority groups—decide who to attend first.
- Forbid smoking.

Immediate treatment
- Check the need for basic resuscitation:
  - Airway patent?
  - Breathing adequate?
  - Circulation intact?
- Resuscitate as necessary (🕮 p.1020 or inside back cover).
- Control any haemorrhage with elevation and pressure.
- DO NOT attempt to move anyone who potentially could have a back or neck injury until skilled personnel and equipment are available.
- Do not give anything by mouth.
- Use coats and rugs to keep victims warm.
- If available, give analgesia (e.g. opiates—but not if significant head injury or risk of intraperitoneal injury; entonox—from ambulance).
- If shocked, set up iv fluids.
- Take directions from the paramedics—they are almost certainly more experienced than you in these situations.

Medicolegal issues
- Ensure your medic-legal insurance covers emergency treatments.
- Keep full records of events, action taken, drugs administered, origin of drugs, batch numbers, and expiry dates.
- A GP can charge a fee to the victims for any assistance given.

Burns and scalds: 🕮 p.1076

Drowning
Most common in drunk adults and children poorly supervised around water. Children can drown in a few centimetres of water.

⚠ Action
- Call for help
- Start basic life support (Airway, Breathing, Circulation)—🕮 p.1020
- ❶ Attempted resuscitation of a seemingly dead child is worthwhile as cooling ↓ metabolic rate and recovery can occur after prolonged immersion.

Prevention: 🕮 p.162

Fractures

Presentation

- *Symptoms:* Pain at the affected site made worse by movement; loss of function.
- *Signs:* Swelling; bruising; deformity; local tenderness; impaired function; crepitus; abnormal mobility.

⚠ Action
- Immobilize the affected part and give analgesia.
- If available and the patient is shocked, start an iv infusion of plasma expander.
- Refer to A&E for assessment, X-ray and treatment.

Fracture complications
- Often occur after the patient has been discharged from hospital and may present to the GP.
- Patients should not have persistent pain—beware of compartment syndrome (📖 p.197).
- Refer back to the fracture clinic or A&E if:
  - Persistent pain
  - Limb swelling that is not settling
  - Offensive odour or discharge
  - If cast edges are abrading the skin or if the cast has deteriorated in structural strength e.g. from getting wet

Scalds and burns

Assessment

- Cause, size, and thickness of the burn.
- Use the 'rule of nines' to assess extent of burns (see box).
- Partial thickness burns are red, painful, and blistered; full thickness burns are painless and white or grey.
- Always consider non-accidental injury in children—📖 p.886.

Rule of nines: Ignore areas of erythema only.	
Palm	1%
Arm (all over)	9%
Leg (all over)	18% (14% children)
Front	18%
Back	18%
Head (all over)	9% (14% children)
Genitals	1%

⚠ The Rule of Nines is inaccurate for children <10y. For children and for small burns, an alternative method is to estimate the extent of the burn by comparison with the area of the patient's hand. The area of the fingers and palm ≈1% total body surface area burn.

⚠ Action:

- Remove clothing from the affected area and place under cold running water for >10min. or until pain is relieved.
- Do not burst blisters.
- Prescribe/give analgesia.
- Refer all but the smallest (<5%) partial thickness burns for assessment in A&E.
- Refer all electrical burns for assessment in A&E.
- Refer all chemical burns for assessment in A&E unless burn area is minimal and pain-free.
- Consider referral to A&E for smoke inhalation.

If managing the burn in the community:

- Check tetanus immunity and give immunization ± prophylaxis as necessary—📖 p.484.
- Apply silver sulfadiazine cream (flamazine) or vaseline impregnated gauze and non-adherent dressings and review for healing and infection every 1–2d.
- Cover burns on hands in flamazine and place in a plastic bag—elevate the hand in a sling and encourage finger movement.
- Refer if burns are not healed in 10–12d.

Special situations

Chemical burns
- Usually caused by strong acids or alkalis.
- Wear gloves to remove contaminated clothing.
- Irrigate with cold running water for ≥20min.
- Do not attempt to neutralize the chemical—this can exacerbate injury by producing heat.
- Refer all burns to A&E unless the burn area is minimal and pain free.

Electric shock
- Causes thermal tissue injury and direct injury due to the electric current passing through the tissue.
- Skin burns may be seen at the entry and exit site of the current.
- Muscle damage can be severe, with minimal skin injury.
- Cardiac damage may occur and rhabdomyolysis can lead to renal failure.
- Refer all patients for specialist management.

Smoke inhalation
- Refer all patients who have potentially inhaled smoke for assessment— a seemingly well patient can deteriorate later.
- Smoke can cause thermal injury, carbon monoxide poisoning, and cyanide poisoning.
- Airway problems occur due to thermal and chemical damage to the airways, causing oedema—suspect if singed nasal hairs, a sore throat, or a hoarse voice.
- Carbon monoxide poisoning may result in the classic cherry-red mucosa—but this may be absent.
- Cyanide poisoning is commonly due to smouldering plastics and causes dizziness, headaches, and seizures.

Prevention of scalds and burns
- Prevention through public education is important.
- Children often sustain burns by pulling on the flex of boiling kettles or irons, pulling on saucepan handles, or climbing onto hot cookers.
- Refer any children who have sustained accidental burns to the health visitor for follow-up.

Poisoning and overdose

On receiving the call for assistance

- Try to establish what has happened—substances involved, ongoing dangers, state of the patient.
- Advise the caller to stay with the patient until you arrive.
- If the patient is unconscious, arrange for an ambulance to meet you at the scene.
- Arrange for the patient to be removed from any source of danger e.g. contaminated clothing or inhaled gases. DO NOT put yourself or anyone else in danger attempting to do this. If necessary, call the fire brigade, who have protective clothing and equipment, to help remove a patient from a dangerous environment.

Assessment of the unconscious patient
Assess the need for basic life support

- Airway patent?
- Breathing satisfactory?
- Circulation adequate?

Resuscitation (📖 p.1020) takes priority over everything else.

Additionally

- If breathing is depressed and opiate overdose is a possibility, give naloxone 0.8–2mg iv every 2–3min. to a maximum of 10mg..
- Check BM—if low, give 50mls 50% glucose iv.

General examination

- BP
- Pulse
- Temperature
- Level of coma (📖 p.1032)

- Pupil responses
- Evidence of iv drug abuse
- Obvious injury

❶ The coma may not be due to poisoning/overdose

If unconscious, turn into the recovery position: 📖 p.1022.
Check no contraindications first e.g. spinal injury.

Note down any information about the exposure

- *Product name*—as much detail as possible. If unidentified tablets, see if any are left and send them to the hospital in their own container (if there is one), with the patient.
- *Time of the incident*
- *Duration of exposure/amount ingested*
- *Route of exposure*—swallowed, inhaled, injected, etc.
- *Whether intentional or accidental*
- *Take a general history from any attendant*—medical history, current medication, substance abuse, alcohol, social circumstances.

Assessment of the conscious patient
- Note down any information about the exposure, as for the unconscious patient.
- Record symptoms the patient is experiencing as a result of exposure.
- Examine—pulse, BP, temperature (if necessary), level of consciousness or confusion, evidence of iv drug abuse, any injuries.
- If non-accidental exposure, assess suicidal intent (🔲 p.1080).
- Take a general history from the patient and/or any attendant—medical history, current medication, substance abuse, alcohol, social circumstances.

Children: Peak incidence of accidental poisoning is at 2y.—mainly household substances, prescribed or OTC drugs, or plants. Teenagers may take deliberate overdoses—especially of OTC medication e.g. paracetamol.

△ Poisoning can be a form of non-accidental injury (🔲 p.886).

△ **Action**

Consider admission if:
- The patient's clinical condition warrants it: unconsciousness, respiratory depression, etc..
- The exposure warrants admission for treatment or observation:
  - *Symptomatic poisoning:* Admit to hospital.
  - *Agents with delayed action:* Aspirin, iron, paracetamol, tricyclic antidepressants, Lomotil (co-phenotrope), paraquat, and modified-release preparations. Admit to hospital even if the patient seems well.
  - *Other agents:* Consult poisons information.
- You judge there is serious suicidal intent (🔲 p.1080), the poisoning is suspected to be a non-accidental injury to a child, or the patient has another psychiatric condition which warrants acute admission.
- There is a lack of social support.

Poisons information
UK National Poisons Information Service ☎0870 600 6266
TOXBASE—poisons database 🖳 *http://www.spib.axl.co.uk*

Threatened suicide

GPs are frequently called to patients who have deliberately self-harmed themselves, are threatening suicide, or if relatives are worried about risk of suicide.

⚠ Action

If any self-harm: Assess the situation and admit to A&E as needed.

Ask about suicidal ideas and plans: In a sensitive but probing way. It is a common misconception that asking about suicide can plant the idea into a patient's head and make suicide more likely. Evidence is to the contrary. Useful questions:

- Do you feel you have a future?
- Do you feel that life's not worth living?
- Do you ever feel completely hopeless?
- Do you ever feel you'd be better off dead and away from it all?
- Have you ever made any plans to end your life (if drug overdose—have you handled the tablets)?
- Have you ever made an attempt to take your own life—if so, was there a final act e.g. suicide note?
- What prevents you doing it?
- Have you made any arrangements for your affairs after your death?

Ask about present circumstances

- What problems are making the patient feel this way?
- Does s/he still feel like this?
- Would the act of suicide be aimed to hurt someone in particular?

What kind of support does the patient have from friends and relatives and formal services (e.g. CPN)?

Assess suicidal risk: Ask the patient and any relatives/friends present. *Risk factors:*

- ♂ > ♀
- ↑ with age
- Divorced > widowed > never married > married
- Certain professions: vets, pharmacists, farmers, doctors.
- Admission or recent discharge from psychiatric hospital
- Social isolation
- History of deliberate self-harm (100x ↑ risk)
- Depression
- Alcohol or substance abuse
- Personality disorder
- Schizophrenia
- Serious medical illness (e.g. cancer)

Assess psychiatric state: Features associated with ↑ suicide risk are:

- Presence of suicidal ideation (see above)
- Hopelessness—good predictor of subsequent and immediate risk
- Depression
- Agitation
- Early schizophrenia with retained insight—especially young patients who see their ambitions restricted
- Presence of delusions of control, poverty, and/or guilt.

Refer for psychiatric evaluation

High risk of suicide
- Direct statement of intent
- Severe mood change
- Hopelessness
- Alcohol or drug dependence
- Abnormal personality
- Living alone

Admit as a psychiatric emergency, using the Mental Health Act for compulsory admission (📖 p.986) if voluntary admission is declined.

Lower risk of suicide: Arrange for someone to stay with the patient until follow-up. Remove all potentially harmful drugs. Liaise with the psychiatric services, according to the individual patient, about psychiatric follow-up.

⚠ **Mothers of young children:** ↑ risk of child abuse. Assess risks, offer support, arrange for health visitor or social services to visit.

Compulsory admission under the Mental Health Act: 📖 p.986

Disturbed behaviour

When a patient becomes very agitated or violent or starts to behave oddly, the GP is usually called—by the patient, relatives or friends, or police attending the disturbance. After assessing the problem, decide if hospitalization is required and whether this can be done on a voluntary or involuntary basis.

⚠ **Look after your own safety**
- If the patient is known to be violent, get back-up from the police before entering the situation.
- Tell someone you are going in and when to expect an 'exit' call. Advise them to call for help if that call is not made.
- Do not put yourself in a vulnerable situation—sit where there is a clear, unimpeded exit route.
- Do not make the patient feel trapped.
- Do not try to restrain the patient.

Causes of acutely disturbed behaviour
- *Physical illness*—infection (e.g. UTI, chest infection); hypoglycaemia; hypoxia; head injury; epilepsy.
- *Drugs*—alcohol (or alcohol withdrawal); prescribed drugs (e.g. steroid psychosis); illicit drugs (e.g. amphetamines).
- *Psychiatric illness*—schizophrenia; mania; anxiety/depression; dementia; personality disorder (e.g. attention-seeking; uncontrolled anger).

⚠ **Action:**
- Before seeing the patient, gather as much information as possible from notes, relatives, and even neighbours.
- Ask the patient and family for any history of drugs or alcohol excess.
- Listen to the patient and talk calmly—choose your words carefully.
- Try to look for organic causes—this can be difficult in the heat of the moment. Physical examination, except from a distance, may be impossible. Don't put yourself at risk.
- Suspect an organic cause where there are visual hallucinations.
- Discuss and explain your suggested management with the patient and any attendants.
- If the patient is an immediate danger to himself or others, admission is warranted.
- If the cause of the behaviour is unclear, admission for investigation is needed.
- Instigate management of treatable causes identified e.g. admit if MI suspected; treat UTI.
- Consider sedation to cover the period before admission or to alleviate symptoms if admission is inappropriate.

Acute confusion: 📖 p.976

Compulsory admission under the Mental health Act: 📖 p.986

Suitable drugs to use for sedation
- *Oral:* diazepam 5–10mg po or lorazepam 1mg po/s/ling; chlorpromazine 50–100mg po.
- *Intramuscular:* chlorpromazine 50mg; haloperidol 1–3mg.

❶ *Avoid sedating* patients with COPD, epilepsy, or if the patient has been taking illicit drugs, barbiturates, or alcohol.

⚠ **Acute dystonia** can occur soon after giving phenothiazines or butyophenones. *Signs:*
- torticollis
- grimacing
- tongue protrusion
- opisthotonus

Dystonia can be relieved with procyclidine 5–10mg im (repeated prn after 20min. to a maximum dose of 20mg).

Miscellaneous emergencies

Acute limb ischaemia
Causes
- Acute thrombotic occlusion of pre-existing stenotic segment (60%)
- Embolus (30%)
- Trauma e.g. compartment syndrome or traumatic vessel damage

Presentation
- Pain
- Pallor
- Paraesthesia
- Pulselessness
- Paralysis
- Perishing cold

Action
Admit acutely under the care of a vascular surgeon. Treatment can be surgical (e.g. embolectomy) or medical (e.g. thrombolysis).

Hypothermia: Defined as a core temperature of <35°C.
Causes
- Not feeling the cold e.g. neuropathy, confusion, dementia
- Inadequate heat in the home e.g. poor housing, poverty and fear of high fuel bill
- Immobility
- Hypothyroidism
- DM
- ↑ heat loss e.g. psoriasis, erythroderma
- Inadequate protection from the cold e.g. unsuitable clothing whilst doing outdoor sports
- Alcohol
- Drugs—antipsychotics, antidepressants, barbiturates, tranquilizers may lower the level of consciousness and ↓ ability to shiver
- Falls—if unable to rise from the floor may remain still and cold until discovered
- Unconsciousness e.g. overdose, stroke

Presentation
- Skin pale and cold to touch
- Puffy face
- Listlessness, drowsiness, and/or confusion

When severe
- ↓ breathing—slow and shallow
- ↓ pulse volume—faint and irregular
- Stiff muscles
- Loss of consciousness

Investigation
- Rectal temperature on low-reading thermometer <35°C
- ECG—'J' wave on the end of the QRS complex

⚠ *Action*
- Remove from the cold environment
- Wrap in blankets—including head
- *Do not* use direct heat (e.g. hot water bottles) as this can cause rapid fluid shifts and potentially fatal pulmonary oedema.
- Transfer to hospital.
- Consider the cause of the incident and liaise with the hospital, primary healthcare team, and social services to prevent recurrence in the future.

Index

Adult advanced life support algorithm

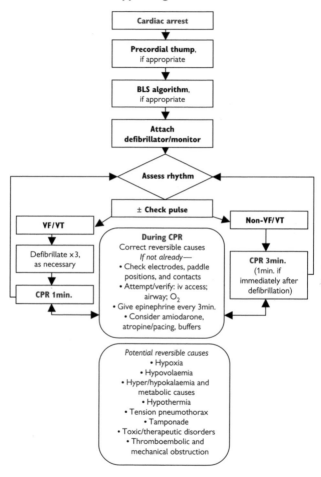

Cardiac arrest

↓

Precordial thump,
if appropriate

↓

BLS algorithm,
if appropriate

↓

**Attach
defibrillator/monitor**

↓

Assess rhythm

± Check pulse

VF/VT

↓

Defibrillate ×3,
as necessary

↓

CPR 1min.

During CPR
Correct reversible causes
If not already—
• Check electrodes, paddle
positions, and contacts
• Attempt/verify: iv access;
airway; O₂
• Give epinephrine every 3min.
• Consider amiodarone,
atropine/pacing, buffers

Non-VF/VT

CPR 3min.
(1min. if
immediately after
defibrillation)

Potential reversible causes
• Hypoxia
• Hypovolaemia
• Hyper/hypokalaemia and
metabolic causes
• Hypothermia
• Tension pneumothorax
• Tamponade
• Toxic/therapeutic disorders
• Thromboembolic and
mechanical obstruction

Paediatric advanced life support algorithm: 📖 p.1028
Newborn advanced life support algorithm: 📖 p.1031

Figures reproduced with permission of Resuscitation Council (UK)

Follicle stimulating hormone (FSH)	P/S	0.8–11.5u/L
		>30u/L post menopause
Prolactin	P	♂ <450u/L
		♀ <600u/L
Prostate specific antigen (PSA)	P	<50y. 0–2.5µg/L (📖 p.305)
		50–59y. 0–3.5µg/L
		60–69y. 0–4.5µg/L
		>70y. 0–6.5µg/L
Thyroxine (free T$_4$)	P	8–22pmol/L
TSH	P	0.35–5.5mIU/L

P = plasma (e.g. heparin bottle); S = serum (clotted—no anticoagulant)

Haematology

	Reference interval
Haemoglobin	♂ 13.0–17.0g/L
	♀ 12.0–15.0g/L
Red cell count (RCC)	♂ 4.5–5.5 × 10^{12}/L
Erythrocytes	♀ 3.8–4.8 × 10^{12}/L
Packed cell volume (PCV) or haematocrit	♂ 0.40–0.50L/L
	♀ 0.36–0.46L/L
Mean cell volume (MCV)	80–100fL
Mean cell haemoglobin (MCHC)	32.0–36.0g/dl
White cell count (WCC)	4.0–11.0 × 10^9/L
Neutrophils	2.0–7.5 × 10^9/L; 40–75% WCC
Lymphocytes	1.5–4.0 × 10^9/L; 20–45% WCC
Eosinophils	0.04–0.50 × 10^9/L; 1–6% WCC
Basophils	0.02–0.10 × 10^9/L; 0–1% WCC
Monocytes	0.2–1.0 × 10^9/L; 2–10% WCC
Platelet count	150–400 × 10^9/L
Reticulocyte count	♂ 25–135 × 0^9/L
	♀ 20–120 × 0^9/L
	0.5–2.5%[*]
Erythrocyte sedimentation rate (ESR)	(📖 p.303)
	<50y. ♂ 10mm, ♀ 19mm
	51–60y. ♂ 12mm, ♀ 19mm
	61–70y. ♂ 4mm, ♀ 20mm
	>70y. ♂ 30mm, ♀ 35mm
International normalized ratio (INR)	Therapeutic ranges (📖 p.366)

[*] Only use % if red cell count is normal. Otherwise use absolute value.